⊘ TABLE B

Age and Race-Specific Reference Ranges for Leukocyte Count and Differential (Compiled from multiple sources. Values may vary among sources and laboratories.)

	Birth	6 Months	4 Years	Adult	Adult of African Descent
Total leukocyte count ($\times 10^9$/L)	9.0–30.0	6.0–18.0	4.5–13.5	4.0–11.0	3.0–9.0
Segmented neutrophil: percent (%)	50–60	25–35	35–45	40–80	45–55
Absolute ($\times 10^9$/L)	4.5–18.0	1.5–6.3	1.5–8.5	2.0–6.8	1.5–5.0
Band neutrophil percent (%)	5–14	0–5	0–5	0–5	0–5
Absolute ($\times 10^9$/L)	0.5–4.2	0–1.0	0–0.7	0–0.5	0–0.5
Lymphocyte percent (%)	25–35	55–65	50–65	25–35	35–45
Absolute ($\times 10^9$/L)	2.0–11.0	4.0–13.5	2.0–8.8	1.0–4.0	1.0–4.0
Monocyte percent (%)	2–10	2–10	2–10	2–10	2–10
Absolute ($\times 10^9$/L)	0.2–3.0	0.1–2.0	0.1–1.4	0.2–1.0	0.2–1.0
Eosinophil percent (%)	0–5	0–5	0–5	0–5	0–5
Absolute ($\times 10^9$/L)	0–1.5	0–0.9	0–0.7	0–0.5	0–0.5
Basophil percent (%)	0–2	0–2	0–2	0–2	0–2
Absolute ($\times 10^9$/L)	0–0.6	0–0.4	0–0.3	0–0.2	0–0.2

⊘ TABLE C

Other Hematology Reference Values

Analyte	Reference Value
Immature reticulocyte fraction (IRF)	0.09–0.31
RDW	12–14.6
Platelet count	150–440 $\times 10^9$/L
MPV	6.8–10.2 fL
Sedimentation rate	
Male	0–10 mm/hr
Female	0–20 mm/hr
Zeta sedimentation rate	
Male	40–52
Female	40–52

CLINICAL LABORATORY
HEMATOLOGY

Shirlyn B. McKenzie, PhD

Department of Clinical Laboratory Sciences
University of Texas Health Science Center at San Antonio

PEARSON
Prentice
Hall

Upper Saddle River, New Jersey 07458

Library of Congress Cataloging-in-Publication Data

McKenzie, Shirlyn B.

   Clinical laboratory hematology / Shirlyn B. McKenzie.

      p. ; cm.

Includes bibliographical references and index.

   ISBN 0-13-019996-6

1.   Blood—Examination. 2.   Hematology. 3.   Blood—Diseases—Diagnosis.

[DNLM: 1.   Clinical Laboratory Techniques. 2.   Hematology—methods.

3.   Hematologic Diseases—diagnosis. 4.   Hematopoietic

System—physiology.   WH 25 M478c 2003] 1. Title.

   RB45 .M385 2003

    616.15—dc21

                                  2003002105

Publisher: Julie Levin Alexander
CLS Series Editor: Elizabeth A. Zeibig
Assistant to Publisher: Regina Bruno
Senior Acquisitions Editor: Mark Cohen
Assistant Editor: Melissa Kerian
Editorial Assistant: Mary Ellen Ruitenberg
Senior Marketing Manager: Nicole Benson
Marketing Assistant: Janet Ryerson
Product Information Manager: Rachele Strober
Director of Manufacturing and Production: Bruce Johnson
Production Managing Editor: Patrick Walsh
Production Liaison: Alex Ivchenko
Production Editor: Karen Fortgang, *bookworks*
Managing Manager: Ilene Sanford
Manufacturing Buyer: Pat Brown
Design Director: Cheryl Asherman
Senior Design Coordinator: Maria Guglielmo Walsh
Cover Design: Joseph DePinho
Manager of Media Production: Amy Peltier
New Media Project Manager: Lisa Rinaldi
Composition: Pine Tree Composition
Printing & Binding: Von Hoffmann Press
Cover Printer: Phoenix Color

Pearson Education, Ltd.
Pearson Education Australia Pty., Limited
Pearson Education Singapore, Pte. Ltd.
Pearson Education North Asia Ltd.
Pearson Education Canada Ltd.
Pearson Educación de Mexico, S.A. de C.V.
Pearson Education — Japan
Pearson Education Malaysia, Pte. Ltd.

10 9 8 7 6 5 4 3 2 1

ISBN 0-13-019996-6

DEDICATION

Dedicated to my family, Gary, Scott, Shawn, Belynda and Dora; my precious granddaughters Lauren and Kristen; my parents George and Helen; and my special friend and sister, Kathy.

CONTENTS

FOREWORD

The author of and contributors to *Clinical Laboratory Hematology* present highly detailed technical information and real-life case studies that will help learners envision themselves as members of the health care team, providing the laboratory services specific to hematology that assist in patient care. The mixture of theoretical and practical information relating to hematology provided in this text allows learners to analyze and synthesize this information and, ultimately, to answer questions and solve problems and cases.

Clinical Laboratory Hematology is part of Prentice Hall's Clinical Laboratory Science series of textbooks, which is designed to balance theory and practical applications in a way that is engaging and useful to students. Furthermore, the books in this series are designed to foster various kinds of learning, and some of the titles, including *Clinical Laboratory Hematology,* will be accompanied by computer applications.

We hope that this book, as well as the entire series, proves to be a valuable educational resource.

Elizabeth A. Zeibig
CLS Series Editor
Prentice Hall Health

PREFACE

Clinical Laboratory Hematology is a comprehensive, yet easy-to-read text of hematology and hemostasis written for students at all levels in clinical laboratory science programs, including clinical laboratory technicians, CLT (medical laboratory technicians, MLT), and clinical laboratory scientists, CLS (medical technologists, MT). Other health professional students and practitioners may also benefit from this book, including pathology residents, physician assistants, and nurse practitioners. This text replaces *Textbook of Hematology* published by Lea & Febiger in 1988 and by Williams & Wilkins in 1996. However this text should be considered as a brand new publication because of its wide variety of changes and enhancements. Included among these changes are the following: we have assembled an extensive team of authoritative contributing authors to write chapters on specialized subjects within their respective fields of expertise; we have developed a striking design that will be conducive to today's visually oriented student; we have developed an exciting set of learning features that will help readers grasp the content more easily; we have developed a book-specific online study guide (*www.prenhall.com/mckenzie*); and finally, we have packaged the text with a free student version of the Chronolab CD-ROM photomicrograph atlas.

ORGANIZATION OF THE BOOK

Understanding hematologic/hemostatic diseases is dependent on a thorough knowledge and understanding of normal processes. Thus, the book begins with a section on normal hematopoiesis and progresses through anemias, nonmalignant and malignant leukocyte disorders. Hemostasis adheres to a similar format with normal hemostasis functions discussed first, followed by abnormalities in hemostasis.

The text is divided into sections and may be studied by section or chapter sequence. This gives the instructor flexibility to fit the book to their specific course design. The first two sections cover an introduction to hematology and normal hematopoiesis. This includes a discussion of the cell morphology, cell cycle, and its regulation. The section includes a discussion on oncogenes emphasizing the concept that neoplasms are the result of mutations in normal genes that control cell proliferation and development. This concept is further discussed in the introduction to hematopoietic neoplasms. The third section, includes procedures that are routine and performed in most laboratories. These are included at the beginning of the book so the students will have basic laboratory test information as they proceed through the subsequent chapters on hematopoietic disorders which focus on laboratory diagnostic protocols.

The next sections cover the hematopoietic disorders and special laboratory procedures. The fourth section includes the anemias and begins with an introduction to anemia chapter. The fifth section is nonmalignant disorders of the leukocytes. The sixth section includes a discussion of special laboratory procedures that are useful in diagnosis and classification of hematopoietic neoplasms: flow cytometry, cytogenetics, and molecular diagnostics. This section may be studied before or after the seventh section on neoplastic hematopoietic disorders, depending on the reader's knowledge level of the neoplasms. If this is the reader's first exposure to the neoplasms, it may be better to cover section 7 before section 6. Alternatively, sections 6 and 7 can be integrated and studied together.

Section 8 is a study of body fluids. Body fluid analysis is often a function of the hematology laboratory, since analysis includes cell counts and review of cell morphology. As much of the analysis includes identification of cells and differentiation of malignant cells from reactive or normal cells, this section has many microphotographs.

Section 9 is a study of hemostasis. It begins with a study of normal hemostasis processes and proceeds to abnormalities that are associated with bleeding and thrombosis. Due to the high frequency of thrombotic disorders and the rapid discovery of mechanisms responsible for thrombosis, the laboratory's role in diagnosis of thrombotic disorders is expanding. Thus, an entire chapter is devoted to hypercoagulability (thrombophilia). This section also includes laboratory testing procedures for evaluation of hemostasis.

The last section includes special hematology procedures and quality assurance and safety in the laboratory. Automation in hematology and hemostasis will be supplemented on the Web page with extensive use of graphics to illustrate abnormal results and teach evaluation and interpretation of data.

The book incorporates ethical issues and management issues of test utilization and value, as well as critical testing pathways. This is the soft side of science but alerts the students to issues they will be facing in their work and communities. In many cases the laboratorian is the one who has the breadth of information needed to help make critical decisions involving the laboratory and its effective, efficient, ethical use.

SUITS ALL LEVELS OF LEARNING

This book has been designed for **both** CLT/MLT and CLS/MT students. Using only one textbook is beneficial and economical in laboratory science programs offering both levels. Use of the book is also helpful to programs that design articulated curricula. The CLS/MT program can be confident of the CLT's/MLT's knowledge level in hematology without doing an extensive CLT/MLT course analysis.

CLT/MLT instructors will need to communicate to their students what is expected of them. They may want their students to find the information in the text that allows them to satisfy the checklist, or they may assign particular sections to read. If not assigned specific sections, the CLT/MLT student may read more than expected which is certainly not a bad thing! The students and instructors should use the checklists to determine the material to be read.

The case study questions and checkpoints are not delineated by level. CLT/MLT students should try to answer as many of these as possible. CLT/MLT instructors should select appropriate chapters for their students. Some chapters, such as molecular techniques, cytogenetics, and flow cytometry may not be included in a CLT/MLT curriculum. Each program will need to assess what fits its particular curriculum.

CLS/MT students should be able to meet both Level I and Level II checklists in most cases, but of course there may be differences among expectations of programs. Therefore, instructors are encouraged to review the checklists to ensure their appropriateness for the course. Although all chapters are appropriate for the CLS/MT student, if the program has two levels of hematology courses, Level I and Level II, instructors may choose to use the book as for a CLT/MLT program in the first course and the remainder of the book in the second course.

In all cases the instructor should begin the course with sections 1 through 3. The remaining sections can be rearranged and used as the instructor desires. The "Background Basics" feature will help the instructor determine which concepts the student should have mastered before beginning a unit of study. This concept should help instructors customize their courses.

UNIQUE PEDAGOGICAL FEATURES

This text has a number of unique pedagogical features that will help the student assimilate, organize, and understand the information. Each chapter begins with a group of components intended to set the stage for the content to follow.

- **Background Basics** alert students to material that should be learned or reviewed before starting the chapter. In most cases it refers readers to previous chapters to help them find the material if they want to review it.
- **Objectives** are comprised of two levels of checklists: Level I for basic or essential information and Level II for more advanced information. These checklists were reviewed by clinical (medical) laboratory technician (CLT/MLT) educators who made recommendations that aimed the Level I checklists to their students. Clinical laboratory science/medical technologist (CLS/MT) educators may expect their students to meet both Level I and Level II checklists requirements.
- **Overview** gives the reader an idea of the chapter content and organization.

Each chapter offers students a variety of opportunities to assess their knowledge and ability to apply it.

- **Case Study** is a running case feature that first appears at the beginning of each chapter and focuses the student's attention on the subject matter that the chapter will cover. Throughout the chapter at appropriate places, additional information on the case may be given such as laboratory test results, and then questions are asked. The questions relate to the material presented in preceding sections. There is a case summary and answers to the questions in the appendix.
- **Checkpoints!** are integrated throughout the chapter. These are questions that require the student to pause along the way to recall or apply information covered in preceding sections. The answers are in the appendix.
- **Summary** concludes the text portion of each chapter in order to help the student bring all the material together.
- **Review Questions** appear at the end of each chapter. There are two sets of questions, Level I and Level II, that are referenced to the Level I and Level II objectives checklists. Answers are in the appendix.

The page design features a number of enhancements intended to aid the learning process.

- **Bold symbols** ✪ ■ are used within the chapter text to help the student quickly cross-reference from the tables and figures to the text.
- **A ∞ symbol** is also used when referring the student to another chapter.
- **Figures and tables** are used liberally to help the student organize and conceptualize information. This is especially important to visual learners.
- **Algorithms** (critical pathways, reflex testing pathways) are used when appropriate to help illustrate effective, cost-efficient use of laboratory tests in diagnosis.
- **The microphotographs** displayed in the book are typical of those found in a particular disease or disorder. Students should be aware that cell variations occur and that blood and bone marrow findings will not always mimic those found in textbooks.

A COMPLETE TEACHING AND LEARNING PACKAGE

The book is complemented by a variety of ancillary materials designed to help instructors be more effective and students more successful.

- **Instructor's Guide** – Prepared by a CLT/MLT educator together with a CLS/MT educator, this guide is designed to equip faculty with necessary teaching resources regardless of the level of instruction. Features include: suggested learning activities for each chapter, test item writing guide, introduction to Bloom's taxonomy, crossword puzzles, transparency masters for selected figures and tables, sample syllabi, and a transition grid to assist instructors in correlating the content of other texts to this text.

- **Companion Web site** – This free online study guide is completely unique to the market. In addition to providing an array of assessment quizzes corresponding to each chapter of the book, the Web site presents up-to-date content in the form of "On the Horizon" features. These short essays present cutting-edge material on new research and technological advancements in the field that can be updated more frequently than the book itself. The quizzes have been developed within an automatic grading system that provides users with instant scoring once users submit their answers. Each student's quiz results can be emailed directly to the educator if desired—as part of a homework assignment. The Web site also will offer instructors the ability to put their syllabus online. Additional figures, tables, and other information are also located on the Web site.

- **CD-ROM** – The book includes a free copy of the student version of *Chronolab's Laboratory Hematology,* a powerful database of hematological images that is useful in the educational setting and beyond. Users may purchase the full version of this database separately through Prentice Hall. More information about obtaining the full version of the Chronolab database can be found on the attached insert that appears on the last page of the book.

ACKNOWLEDGMENTS

I am grateful to the many contributors who gave of their expertise to make this book a comprehensive source of current knowledge in hematology and hemostasis for clinical laboratory science. I am honored to work with so many intelligent people. Thank you for hanging in there until the last edit was done.

Before the writing began, we had a great panel of clinical laboratory educators help us determine the appropriate content for basic and advanced levels. These educators reviewed every chapter's checklists and outline. Their opinions were invaluable in helping assure that this book met the needs of both clinical laboratory technicians (medical laboratory technicians) and clinical laboratory scientists (medical technologists). These individuals include: Linda L. Breiwick, B.S., CLS (NCA), MT (ASCP), MLT Program Director, Medical Laboratory Technology Program, Shoreline Community College, Seattle, Washington; Linda F. Comeaux, CLS (NCA), Program Director, Medical Laboratory Technology Program, Arapahoe Community College, Littleton, Colorado; and Mona Gleysteen, MS, CLS (NCA), CLT/MLT Program Director, Clinical Laboratory Technology Program, Lake Area Technical Institute, Watertown, South Dakota.

Those who assisted in other tasks are invaluable members of the book's team. Thank you to Melissa Nedry, a CLS student at the University of Texas Health Science Center at San Antonio, who edited the glossary. This is a bigger task than anyone can anticipate and she did an outstanding job. Thank you, Linda Comeaux and Dorothy Fike, for composing the accompanying instructor's manual to this book. Thank you to Wayne Lawson for his review of Chapter 5 on hemoglobin.

A very special thanks is not enough for the work that Lynn Williams did for me at a time of great need. Lynn offered to assist with any task that would help me out. Subsequently, I gave her the momentous task of editing the hemostasis chapters as well as coauthoring one of those chapters. Lynn not only edited these chapters but responded expeditiously to any additional requests for information or content. Through this endeavor, I found that Lynn is a beautiful person and she has become a precious, reliable friend. Thank you Lynn, for your help. I am convinced we could not have done this without you.

I am fortunate to have family members who directly or indirectly support all that I take on. A special thanks to my devoted husband who spent many days and nights at the computer making editorial changes, proofreading, and performing various other time-consuming tasks on the book. During this endeavor, he also took on many of my home duties to free me up. His support through this was the reason I was able to finish the task. Thank you also to the rest of my family who are always there for me and help me appreciate what is really important in life: my sons, Scott and Shawn; their wives, Belynda and Dora; my parents, George and Helen Olson; my precious granddaughters, Lauren and Kristen; and my siblings, Kathleen, Skip, Larry, and Gerald.

Thank you also to Beth Zeibig, Mark Cohen, and Melissa Kerian for their assistance in putting this book together. Mark provided many of the new ideas on the book's design as well as encouragement along the way that it could be done. Beth spent many hours reviewing each chapter and giving helpful suggestions for improvement. Melissa provided the gentle prodding and follow through to get the job done. You are a great team. And finally, a special thanks to Prentice Hall for publishing this creation.

REVIEWERS

Nancy L. McQueen, Ph.D.
Professor
Department of Biology and Microbiology
California State University, Los Angeles
Los Angeles, California

Rena E. Goode, MT(ASCP)
Medical Laboratory Technician Program
Ivy Tech State College
Terre Haute, Indiana

Yasmen Simonian, Ph.D., CLS(NCA), MT(ASCP)
Chair and Professor
Department of Clinical Laboratory Science
Weber State University

Ogden, Utah
Larry J. Smith, Ph.D., SH(ASCP)
Director, Coagulation Lab
Memorial Sloan-Kettering Cancer Center
New York, New York

Peggy Simpson, MS, MT(ASCP)
Program Director
Medical Laboratory Technician Program
Alamance Community College
Graham, North Carolina

Dan Southern, MS, CLS (NCA), MT(ASCP)
Program Director
Clinical Laboratory Sciences

Western Carolina University
Cullowhee, North Carolina

Larry Birnbaum, Ph.D., CLS (NCA), MT (ASCP)
Department Chair
Clinical Laboratory Sciences
The College of St. Scholastica
Duluth, Minnesota

Cynthia C. Cowall, M.Ed., MT(ASCP)
Assistant Professor

Medical Technology
Salisbury State University
Salisbury, Maryland
Dorothy J. Fike, MS, MT (ASCP)
Associate Professor
Clinical Laboratory Sciences Department
Marshall University
Huntington, West Virginia

CONTENT LEVEL REVIEW PANEL

Linda L. Breiwick, B.S., CLS (NCA), MT (ASCP)
MLT Program Director
Medical Laboratory Technology Program
Shoreline Community College
Seattle, Washington

Linda Comeaux, B.S., CLS (NCA)
Program Director
Medical Laboratory Technology Program
Arapahoe Community College
Littleton, Colorado

Mona Gleysteen, MS, CLS (NCA)
CLT/MLT Program Director
Clinical Laboratory Technology Program
Lake Area Technical Institute
Watertown, South Dakota

CONTRIBUTORS

Shirlyn B. McKenzie, Ph.D., CLS (NCA)
Professor and Chair
Department of Clinical Laboratory Sciences
University of Texas Health Science Center at San Antonio
San Antonio, Texas

J. Lynn Williams, Ph.D., CLS (NCA)
Visiting Scientist, University of Michigan
Professor, Medical Laboratory Sciences
Oakland University, Michigan

Annette Schlueter, M.D., Ph.D.
Assistant Professor
Department of Pathology
University of Iowa
Iowa City, Iowa

Joel D. Hubbard, Ph.D., MT (ASCP)
Associate Professor
Department of Diagnostic and Primary Care
School of Allied Health
Texas Tech University Health Sciences Center
Lubbock, Texas

Mary Coleman, M.S., CLS (NCA)
Instructor
Department of Pathology
University of North Dakota
Grand Forks, North Dakota

Cheryl Burns, M.S., CLS (NCA)
Associate Professor
Department of Clinical Laboratory Sciences
University of Texas Health Science Center at San Antonio
San Antonio, Texas

Aamir Ehsan, M.D.
Assistant Professor
Department of Pathology
University of Texas Health Science Center at San Antonio
San Antonio, Texas

Carolina Echeverri, M.D.
Hematopathology Fellow
Department of Pathology
University of Texas Health Sciences Center at San Antonio
San Antonio, Texas

Rebecca Laudicina, Ph.D., CLS (NCA)
Associate Professor, Clinical Laboratory Science
University of North Carolina at Chapel Hill
Chapel Hill, North Carolina

Tim R. Randolph, M.S., MT (ASCP)
Assistant Professor
Department of Clinical Laboratory Science
St. Louis University
St. Louis, Missouri

Diana L. Cochran-Black, Dr. P.H., MT (ASCP) SH
Assistant Professor
Department of Medical Technology
College of Health Professions
Wichita State University
Wichita, Kansas

Daniel Bessmer, Major USAF, Biomedical Sciences Corps,
M.S., MT (ASCP) SH
Associate Chief, Core Laboratory
Wilford Hall Medical Center
Lackland AFB, Texas

Linda Smith, Ph.D., CLS (NCA)
Professor
Department of Clinical Laboratory Sciences
University of Texas Health Science Center at San Antonio
San Antonio, Texas

Kathleen M. Mugan, M.Ed., MT (ASCP) SH
Assistant Professor
Department of Medical Technology
University of Arkansas for Medical Sciences
Little Rock, Arkansas

Sue Beglinger, M.S., MT (ASCP)
Education Coordinator/Senior Lecturer
Clinical Laboratory Science Program
Department of Pathology and Laboratory Medicine
University of Wisconsin at Madison
Madison, Wisconsin

Fiona E. Craig, M.D.
Associate Professor of Pathology
University of Pittsburgh School of Medicine
Director Flow Cytometry Laboratory
Division of Hematopathology
UPMC-Presbyterian Hospital
Pittsburgh, Pennsylvania

Nanette Clare, M.D.
Senior Associate Dean
Associate Dean for Academic Affairs
Professor of Pathology
Office of the Dean, School of Medicine
The University of Texas Health Science Center
San Antonio, Texas

Margaret Gulley, M.D.
Associate Professor
Department of Pathology
University of North Carolina
Chapel Hill, North Carolina

Jean Sparks, Ph.D., MT (ASCP)
Senior Scientist
Lexicon Genetics, Inc.
The Woodlands, Texas

Louann Lawrence, Dr. P.H., CLS (NCA)
Professor and Department Head
Department of Clinical Laboratory Sciences
Louisiana State University Health Sciences Center
New Orleans, Louisiana

Susan Leclair, Ph.D., CLS (NCA)
Professor
Department of Medical Laboratory Science
University of Massachusetts Dartmouth
North Dartmouth, Massachusetts

Linda Larson, M.S., MT (ASCP)
Assistant Professor
Department of Pathology
University of North Dakota
Grand Forks, North Dakota

Maryann Weller, Ph.D., MT (ASCP)
Assistant Professor and Program Director
Medical Laboratory Science
Oakland University
Rochester, Michigan

Cheryl Swinehart, M.S., CLS (NCA)
Assistant Professor
Medical Technology Program
University of Minnesota
Department of Laboratory Medicine and Pathology
Minneapolis, Minnesota

Lucia E. More, Major USAF, Biomedical Sciences Corps, M.S. MT (ASCP)
Clinical Laboratory Element Chief
Offutt AFB, Nebraska

Kathryn Hansen, M.S., CLSp(CG)
Supervisor, Cytogenic Laboratory
Department of Pathology
University of Texas Health Science Center at San Antonio
San Antonio, Texas

ABBREVIATIONS

ADCC – Antibody dependent cell-mediated cytotoxicity
AHG – Antihuman globulin
AIDS – Acquired immune deficiency syndrome
AIHA – Autoimmune hemolytic anemia
AL – Acute leukemia
ALL – Acute lymphocytic (lymphoblastic) leukemia
AML – Acute myelocytic (myeloblastic) leukemia
ANLL – Acute nonlymphocytic leukemia
APTT – Activated partial thromboplastin time
ARC – AIDS related complex
Band – Nonsegmented neutrophil
BT – Bleeding time
CBC – Complete blood count
CD – Cluster of differentiation
cDNA – Complementary DNA
CFU – Colony forming unit
CGL– Chronic granulocytic leukemia
CLL – Chronic lymphocytic leukemia
CML – Chronic myelogenous leukemia
CMML – Chronic myelomonocytic leukemia
CMV – Cytomegalovirus
DAF – Decay accelerating factor
DAT – Direct antiglobulin test
DIC – Disseminated intravascular coagulation
dL – Deciliter
DNA – Deoxyribonucleic acid
DVT – Deep vein thrombosis
EBV – Epstein-Barr virus
EPO – Erythropoietin
FA – Fanconi's anemia
FAB – French-American-British
FFP – Fresh frozen plasma
G6PD – Glucose-6-phosphate dehydrogenase
Hb or Hgb – Hemoglobin
Hct – Hematocrit
HDN – Hemolytic disease of the newborn
HPFH – Hereditary persistance of fetal hemoglobin
HUS – Hemolytic uremic syndrome
IAT – Indirect antiglobulin test
Ig – Immunoglobulin
INR – International normalized ratio
IRF – Immature reticulocyte fraction
ISC – Irreversibly sickled cells
ISI – International sensitivity index
ITP – Idiopathic thrombocytopenic purpura

L – Liter
LAP – Leukocyte alkaline phosphatase
LCAT – Lecithin:cholesterol acyl transferase
LD – Lactic dehydrogenase
Lymph – Lymphocyte
MAHA – Microangiopathic hemolytic anemia
MCH – Mean corpuscular hemoglobin
MCHC – Mean corpuscular hemoglobin concentration
MCV – Mean corpuscular volume
MDS – Myelodysplastic syndrome
MHC – Major histocompatibility complex
mL – Milliliter
Mono – Monocyte
MPD – Myeloproliferative disorders
MW – Molecular weight
NRBC – Nucleated red blood cell
PAS – Periodic-acid-Schiff
PCH – Paroxysmal cold hemoglobinuria
PCR – Polymerase chain reaction
PDW – Platelet distribution width
PIVKA – Protein-induced by vitamin-K absence
   (or antagonist)
PK – Pyruvate kinase
PMN – Polymorphonuclear neutrophil
PNH – Paroxsymal nocturnal hemoglobinuria
PT – Prothrombin time
RA – Refractory anemia
RAEB – Refractory anemia with excess blasts
RARS – Refractory anemia with ringed sideroblasts
RBC – Red blood cell
RDW – Red cell distribution width
RER – Rough endoplasmic reticulum
RNA – Ribonucleic acid
RPI – Reticulocyte production index
SCIDS – Severe combined immunodeficiency syndrome
Seg – Segmented neutrophil
SER – Smooth endoplasmic reticulum
SLL – Small lymphocytic lymphoma
TCR – T cell receptor
TIBC – Total iron binding capacity
TRAP – Tartrate resistant acid phosphatase
TTP – Thrombotic thrombocytopenic purpura
vWf – von Willebrand factor
WBC – White blood cell
WHO – World Health Organization

SECTION ONE • INTRODUCTION TO HEMATOLOGY

1

Introduction

Shirlyn B. McKenzie, Ph.D.

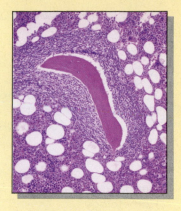

■ CHECKLIST – LEVELS I AND II

At the end of this unit of study the student should be able to:

1. Compare the reference ranges for hemoglobin, hematocrit, erythrocytes, and leukocytes in infants, children, and adults.
2. Identify the function of erythrocytes, leukocytes, and platelets.
3. Describe the composition of blood.
4. Explain the causes of change in the steady state of blood components.
5. Describe clinical pathway, critical pathway, and disease management and identify the laboratory's role in developing these models.
6. Compare capitated payment, prospective payment, and fee-for-service and describe the impact of capitation on the laboratory.

CHAPTER OUTLINE

KEY TERMS

Activated partial thromboplastin time (APTT)
Capitated payment
Complete blood count (CBC)
Diapedese
Erythrocytes
Fee-for-service
Hematocrit
Hematology
Hemoglobin
Hemostasis
Leukocytes
Platelets
Prothrombin time (PT)
RBC indices
Reflex testing
Thrombocytes

BACKGROUND BASICS

Students should complete courses in biology and physiology before beginning this study of hematology.

CASE STUDY

We will address this case study throughout the chapter.
Aaron, a two-year-old male, was seen by his pediatrician because he had a fever of 102–104°F over the past 24 hours. Aaron was lethargic. Prior to this he had been in good health except for two episodes of otitis. Consider why the pediatrician may order laboratory tests and how this child's condition might affect the composition of his blood.

▶ OVERVIEW

The hematology laboratory is one of the busiest areas of the clinical laboratory. Even in small, limited service laboratories, hematology tests are usually offered. This chapter is an introduction to the composition of blood and the testing performed to identify the presence of disease. Also included is a discussion on the laboratory's role in assuring cost-effective and diagnostically efficient testing. The last section gives an overview of the organization of this book and the pedagogical features designed to help students learn hematology and continually assess their progress.

▶ INTRODUCTION

Blood has been considered the essence of life for centuries. One of the Hippocratic writings from about 400 B.C. describes the body as being a composite of four humors: black bile,

blood, phlegm, and yellow bile. Fahraeus, a twentieth-century Swedish physician, suggested that the theory of the four humors came from the observation of four distinct layers in clotted blood. In the process of clotting, blood separates into a dark-red, almost black, jelly-like clot (black bile); a thin layer of oxygenated red cells (blood); a layer of white cells and platelets (phlegm); and a layer of yellowish serum (yellow bile).[1] Health and disease were thought to occur as a result of an upset in the equilibrium of these humors. This may help explain why bloodletting to purge the body of its contaminated fluids was practiced from the time of Hippocrates until the nineteenth century.

The cellular composition of blood was not recognized until the invention of the microscope. With the help of a crude magnifying device that consisted of a biconvex lens, Leeuwenhoek (1632–1723) accurately described and measured the red cells (erythrocytes). The discovery of white blood cells (leukocytes) and platelets (thrombocytes) followed after microscope lenses were improved.

As a supplement to these categorical observations of blood cells, Karl Vierordt in 1852 published the first quantitative results of blood cell analysis.[2] His procedures for quantification were tedious and time consuming. After several years, attempts were made to correlate blood cell counts with various disease states.

Improved methods of blood examination in the 1920s and the growth of knowledge of blood physiology and blood-forming organs in the 1930s, allowed anemias and other blood disorders to be studied on a rational basis. In some cases, the pathophysiology of hematopoietic disorders was realized only after the patient responded to experimental therapy.

Contrary to early hematologists, modern hematologists recognize that alterations in the components of blood are the result of disease, not a primary cause of the disease. Under normal conditions, the production of blood cells in the bone marrow, their release to the peripheral blood, and their survival are highly regulated to maintain a steady state of morphologically normal cells. Quantitative and qualitative hematologic abnormalities may result when an imbalance occurs in this steady state.

▶ COMPOSITION OF BLOOD

Blood is composed of a liquid called plasma and of cellular elements, including **leukocytes**, **platelets**, and **erythrocytes**. The normal adult has about six liters of this vital fluid, which composes from 7% to 8% of the total body weight. Plasma makes up about 55% of the blood volume, whereas about 45% of the volume is composed of erythrocytes and 1% of the volume is composed of leukocytes and platelets (**thrombocytes**). Variations in the quantity of these blood elements are often the first sign of disease occurring in body tissue. Changes in diseased tissue often can be detected by laboratory tests that measure deviations from normal in blood constituents. **Hematology** is primarily the study of the formed cellular blood elements.

The principal component of plasma is water, which contains dissolved ions, proteins, carbohydrates, fats, hormones, vitamins, and enzymes. The principal ions necessary for normal cell function include calcium, sodium, potassium, chloride, magnesium, and hydrogen. The main protein constituent of plasma is albumin, which is the most important component in maintaining osmotic pressure. Albumin also acts as a carrier molecule, transporting compounds such as bilirubin and heme. Other blood proteins carry vitamins, minerals, and lipids. Immunoglobulins and complement are specialized blood proteins involved in immune defense. The coagulation proteins responsible for **hemostasis** (arrest of bleeding) circulate in the blood as inactive enzymes until they are needed for the coagulation process. An upset in the balance of these dissolved plasma constituents may indicate a disease in other body tissues.

Blood plasma also acts as a transport medium for cell nutrients and metabolites; for example, hormones manufactured in one tissue are transported by the blood to target tissue in other parts of the body. Bilirubin, the main catabolic residue of hemoglobin, is transported by albumin from the spleen to the liver for excretion. Blood urea nitrogen, a nitrogenous waste product, is carried to the kidney for filtration and excretion. Increased concentration of these normal catabolites may indicate either increased cellular metabolism or a defect in the organ responsible for their excretion. For example, in liver disease, the bilirubin level in blood increases, indicating the end organ disease. In hemolytic anemia, however, the bilirubin concentration may rise not because of liver disease but because of the increased metabolism of hemoglobin.

When body cells die, they release their cellular constituents into surrounding tissue. Eventually some of these constituents reach the blood. Many of the constituents of body cells are specific for the cell's particular function; thus, increased concentration of these constituents in the blood, especially enzymes, may indicate abnormal cell destruction in a specific organ.

Each of the three cellular constituents of blood has specific functions. Erythrocytes contain the vital protein **hemoglobin,** which is responsible for transport of oxygen and carbon dioxide between the lungs and body tissues. There are five types of leukocytes: neutrophils, eosinophils, basophils, lymphocytes, and monocytes. They are responsible for defending the body against foreign antigens such as bacteria and viruses. Platelets are necessary for maintaining hemostasis. Blood cells circulate through blood vessels, which are distributed throughout every body tissue. Erythrocytes and platelets carry out their functions without leaving the vessels, but leukocytes **diapedese** (pass through vessel walls) to tissues where they defend against invading foreign antigens.

CASE STUDY *(continued from page 2)*

1. If Aaron was diagnosed with otitis media, what cellular component(s) in his blood would be playing a central role in fighting this infection?

▶ REFERENCE RANGES FOR BLOOD CELL CONCENTRATION

Physiologic differences in the concentration of cellular elements may occur according to race, age, sex, and geographic location; pathologic changes in specific blood cell concentrations may occur as the result of disease or injury. Whites have slightly higher cell counts than blacks: their leukocyte counts are higher by 0.5×10^9/L, hemoglobin levels by 0.7 g/dL, **hematocrit** by 0.17 L/L, and erythrocyte counts by 0.05×10^{12}/L.[3]

The greatest differences in reference ranges occur between newborns and adults. Generally, newborns have a higher erythrocyte concentration than any other age group. The erythrocytes are also larger than those of adults. For six months after birth, erythrocytes decrease, and then they slowly increase. In children between the ages of 5 and 17, the hemoglobin and erythrocyte counts increase with age.[3] The leukocyte concentration is also increased at birth but decreases after the first year of life. A common finding in young children is an absolute and relative lymphocytosis. After 12 years of age, males have higher hemoglobin, hematocrit, and erythrocyte levels than females. Tables A through K on the inside covers of this text give hematologic reference ranges for various age groups.

Reference ranges of hematologic values must be determined by each individual laboratory in order to account for the physiologic differences of a population in a specific geographic area. Reference values are determined by calculating the mean for a group of healthy individuals and reporting the reference range as the mean ±2 standard deviations. This range represents the normal value for 95% of normal individuals. A value just below or just above this range is not necessarily abnormal; normal and abnormal overlap. Statistical probability indicates that about 5% of normal individuals will fall outside the ±2 standard deviation range. The farther a value falls from the reference range, however, the more likely the value is to be abnormal.

CASE STUDY *(continued from page 3)*

2. Aaron's physician ordered a complete blood count (CBC). The results are Hb 115 g/L; Hct 0.34 L/L; RBC 4.0×10^{12}/L; WBC 18×10^9/L. What parameters, if any, are outside the reference range? Why do you have to take Aaron's age into account when evaluating these results?

► HEMOSTASIS

Hemostasis is the process of forming a barrier (blood clot) to blood loss when the vessel is traumatized and limiting the barrier to the site of injury. Hemostasis occurs in stages called primary and secondary hemostasis and fibrinolysis. These stages are the result of interaction of platelets, blood vessels, and proteins circulating in the blood. An upset in any of the stages can result in bleeding or abnormal blood clotting (thrombosis). Laboratory testing for abnormalities in hemostasis is usually performed in the hematology section of the laboratory. Alternatively, hemostasis testing may be performed in a separate section of the laboratory.

 Checkpoint! #1

What cellular component of blood may be involved in disorders of hemostasis?

► THE LABORATORY'S ROLE IN DISEASE MANAGEMENT

In the United States, health care spending accounts for about 15% of the gross domestic product.[4] In 1999, there were 5.7 billion laboratory tests performed at a cost of about $35 billion.[5] Yet this is only 3.5% of the amount spent on personal health care.

The rising cost of health care associated with diagnosis and treatment of disease has caused increased scrutiny of the health care system. In an attempt to gain an understanding of these costs and to identify whether there is an inappropriate use of medical resources, researchers studied medical practice patterns. Results revealed overutilization of services and significant variations in diagnosis and treatment of common disorders.[6–8] Concerns over these rising costs and variations in practice resulted in the implementation of cost containment strategies by insurers and health care organizations. Many insurers went from a **fee-for-service** reimbursement to a **capitated payment** system. Under fee-for-service plans consumers choose their own health care providers and the provider determines the fees. Under capitated payment plans, the insurer contracts with certain health care providers who agree to provide services for a defined population on a per-member fee schedule. The insurer determines who the providers will be. Under Medicare (the Federal health care program for older Americans) payment for inpatient services is based on the prospective payment system (PPS). In this payment system, the hospital is reimbursed a fixed amount for services provided to a patient based on medical diagnosis (cost per case). In the capitated payment plan and the PPS plan, every test or service performed is a cost to the provider as they will only be reimbursed a fixed amount regardless of the amount of service provided. These managed cost plans are an attempt by third-party payers (insurers) to ensure that services provided are necessary and reasonably priced. The new reimbursement systems place the provider at risk to provide necessary services while controlling overall costs. Thus, laboratory services must be considered a resource to be managed rather than a source of revenue.

The health care system is now not only interested in managing costs but also in managing care. The goal of managed care is to provide quality care while maximizing efficiency and effectiveness. Disease management (DM) models are an attempt to meet this goal. Under these programs, a protocol is designed to identify patients with a specific disease, and a therapy is developed that is designed to maximize clinical outcomes at an acceptable cost. The DM model for a particular disease is based on evidence in the literature and other sources.[9] Thus, DM is a population-level approach to improving health status rather than a patient-focused approach, as has dominated our health care system. It is designed to improve the value of health care delivery from the perspectives of providers, patients, and insurers. This value concept is broad based and includes maximization of clinical, economic, quality-of-life, and satisfaction outcomes for the lowest expenditure of time and resources.[4]

Many organizations are creating and adopting new strategies to provide cost-effective and diagnostically efficient health care. These strategies include clinical pathways, also known as practice guidelines, and critical pathways (care plans). Sometimes clinical pathways and critical pathways are considered the same and the terms are used interchangeably. Here clinical pathways are defined as plans and procedures developed by physicians, using a foundation of scientific outcomes, for diagnosing and treating a particular disease.[4,8] The guidelines give indications for tests, procedures, and treatments. Critical pathways are the care and services provided by an interdisciplinary health care team after treatment decisions are made. These pathways are developed by teams of practitioners who have the knowledge and perspectives to view the total care process.[10] Clinical and critical pathways are usually designed for common and/or high cost diagnoses. They are not appropriate in complicated cases.

These evolving health care practices require a partnership among the physicians, nurses, allied health practitioners, the patient, and health care administrators. As the complexity of laboratory testing increases, communication between the physician and clinical laboratory provider must increase. The laboratory provider must be able to correlate laboratory test results with clinical disease states, pathophysiology, and treatment, effectively communicate these results to the physician, and suggest cost-effective, follow-up testing when appropriate.[11] The focus should be changing structure and processes to improve patient outcomes. The goal is optimal utilization of laboratory testing, not necessarily less testing.

The laboratory can take proactive approaches to control test utilization. These include:

- Assist in development of critical pathways
- Manage the test ordering system
- Institute sequential testing protocols
- Eliminate incorrect use of tests
- Design wellness panels

As more outcome studies are done to determine which processes and treatments are most effective and as information on the value of laboratory testing is documented, the role of laboratory tests in clinical and critical pathways will become more important. Physicians will want to order the appropriate tests under the guidelines.

LABORATORY TESTING IN THE INVESTIGATION OF A HEMATOLOGIC PROBLEM

The investigation of a hematologic problem by a physician includes taking a medical history and performing a physical examination. Clues provided by this preliminary investigation will help guide the physician's choice of laboratory tests to help confirm the diagnosis. The challenge is to select appropriate tests that contribute to a cost-efficient and effective diagnosis. Laboratory testing usually begins with screening tests, and based on results of these tests, other, more specific tests, are ordered. Repeat tests may be ordered to track disease progression, evaluate treatment, identify side effects and complications, or assist in prognosis.[5]

Hematology screening tests include the **complete blood count** (CBC), which quantifies the white blood cells (WBC), red blood cells (RBC), hemoglobin, hematocrit, and platelets and calculates the **RBC indices.** The indices are calculated from the results of the hemoglobin, RBC count, and hematocrit to define the size and hemoglobin content of RBCs. The indices are important parameters in differentiating causes of anemia and help direct further testing. The CBC may also include a WBC differential. In this procedure the five types of WBCs are enumerated and reported as a percentage of the total WBC count. A differential is especially helpful if the WBC count is abnormal. In these cases the differential will identify which cell type is abnormally increased or decreased and determine if immature and/or abnormal forms are present, thus, providing a clue to diagnosis. The morphology of RBCs and platelets is also studied as a routine part of the differential. If a hemostasis problem is suspected, the screening tests include the platelet count, **prothrombin time (PT),** and **activated partial thromboplastin time (APTT).** These tests will provide clues that guide the choice of follow-up tests to help identify the problem. Follow-up tests may include not only hematologic tests but also chemical, immunologic, and/or molecular analysis.

Follow-up testing that is done based on results of screening tests is referred to as **reflex testing.** As scientists learn more about the pathophysiology and treatment of hematopoietic disease, the number of tests designed to assist in diagnosis expands. To help the physician select the most appropriate tests, the laboratory will collaborate with physicians to design reflex testing protocols for common diseases. These protocols are sometimes referred to as algorithms.

Throughout this text, readers are urged to use the reflex testing concept in their thought processes when studying the laboratory investigation of a disease. Each hematopoietic disorder is discussed in the following order: pathophysiology, clinical findings, laboratory findings, and treatment. The reader should consider which laboratory tests provide the information necessary to identify the cause of the disorder based on the suspected disorder's pathophysiology. Although it is unusual for the physician to provide a patient history or diagnosis to the laboratory when ordering tests, this information is often crucial to direct investigation and assist in interpretation of the test results. Perhaps with the medical necessity guidelines enforced by Medicare, the laboratory will be provided this information in the future. Medical necessity refers to the need for a test to be done, given the diagnosis of the patient. Medicare carriers make the determination of medical necessity and require that the diagnostic code accompany the request for reimbursement of tests done by the laboratory. In any case, if laboratory professionals need more patient information in order to perform testing appropriately, they should obtain the patient's chart or call the physician.

 Checkpoint! #2

A 13-year-old female was seen by her physician for complaints of a sore throat, lethargy, and swollen lymph nodes. A CBC was performed with the following results: Hb 90 g/L; Hct 0.30 L/L; RBC 3.8×10^{12}/L; WBC 15×10^{9}/L. Is reflex testing suggested by these results?

ORGANIZATION OF THE BOOK

This book is organized into ten sections to help the student and instructor design an effective learning experience. The first three sections should be studied in sequence, as they provide the basic background information on which the remainder of the book is based. The fourth section is anemias. The first chapter in this section provides a basis for studying the remaining chapters in the section. Anemias are grouped by a combination of morphology and pathophysiology. Section 5 includes chapters on nonmalignant disorders of leukocytes, both acquired and hereditary. Section 6 is a study of the special laboratory procedures that are used in diagnosis of and in evaluating patient response to treatment for neoplastic hematopoietic disorders. This section may be studied before or after Section 7, Neoplastic Hematopoietic Disorders. Section 8, Body Fluids, is a morphologic study of cells found in body fluids. It uses an atlas approach. The hematology laboratory plays an important role in analyzing cells in body fluids and differentiating benign from malignant. This examination also may reveal other diagnostic findings such as bacteria, crystals, and fungi. Section 9 is a study of hemostasis. The last section, Section 10, includes chapters on special hematology procedures, automation, quality assurance, and safety.

▶ HOW TO USE THIS BOOK

Each chapter begins with a chapter outline, chapter checklists, key terms, background basics, and an overview. These features are designed to help focus the readers' attention on the content and to assure they have the appropriate background knowledge to proceed.

The reader is encouraged to take advantage of the numerous pedagogical features in each chapter to help assimilate and apply the material. Each chapter on hematologic disorders and other selected chapters begin with a case study. The patient's clinical findings are briefly described and the reader's attention is focused on consideration of helpful laboratory tests or a possible diagnosis. Throughout the chapter the case builds periodically by giving more information and asking questions. The case is summarized and answers to questions are given in Appendix B.

Checkpoints are interspersed throughout the chapter. These are questions designed as a self-assessment tool to evaluate understanding of important knowledge or concepts. Answers are provided in Appendix A. Also at the end of the chapter are two sets of review questions, one to assess accomplishment of Level I checklist items and the other Level II checklist items.

▶ SUPPLEMENTAL WEB SITE

A Web site supplements this book. The Web site includes additional teaching and assessment information. For each chapter there is a section called On the Horizon. This section includes information on new developments in the field. It is updated periodically. Additional Level I and Level II questions are included, as well as questions designed to test your ability to apply, or problem solve, based on chapter content. These questions supplement the reader's study of the material. Some chapter Web pages include additional advanced or detailed information on chapter topics as well as tables and figures. The Web site will evolve as users of the book suggest.

SUMMARY

Hematology is the study of the cellular components of blood: erythrocytes, leukocytes, and platelets. Changes in the concentrations of these cells occur from infancy until adulthood. Diseases can upset the steady state concentration of these parameters. A CBC is usually performed as a screening test to determine if there are quantitative abnormalities in blood cells. Reflex tests may be ordered by the physician if one or more of the parameters are outside the reference range.

Changes in the health care system are focused on containing costs while maintaining quality of care. The laboratory's role in this new system is to work with physicians to optimize utilization of laboratory testing.

REVIEW QUESTIONS

LEVELS I AND II

1. In which group of individuals would you expect to find the highest reference ranges for hemoglobin, hematocrit, and erythrocyte count? (Checklist #1)
   a. newborns
   b. males older than 12 years of age
   c. females older than 17 years of age
   d. children between 1 and 5 years of age

2. These cells are important in the transport of oxygen and carbon dioxide between the lungs and body tissues: (Checklist #2)
   a. platelets
   b. leukocytes
   c. thrombocytes
   d. erythrocytes

REVIEW QUESTIONS (continued)

LEVELS I AND II

3. Forty-five percent of the volume of blood is composed of: (Checklist #3)
   a. erythrocytes
   b. leukocytes
   c. platelets
   d. plasma

4. Alterations in the concentration of blood cells generally are the result of: (Checklist #4)
   a. bone marrow abnormalities
   b. an inadequate diet
   c. disease
   d. dehydration

5. Leukocytes are necessary for: (Checklist #2)
   a. hemostasis
   b. defense against foreign antigens
   c. oxygen transport
   d. excretions of cellular metabolites

6. This type of testing can be used by laboratories to help direct the physician's selection of appropriate testing after screening tests are performed: (Checklist #5)
   a. reflexive based on results of screening tests
   b. manual repeat of abnormal results
   c. a second test by a different instrument
   d. standing orders for all inpatients

7. This type of payment system is used by managed care plans to help contain costs of medical care: (Checklist #6)
   a. fee-for-service
   b. cost-per-case
   c. capitation
   d. disease containment

8. A model used to help diagnose and manage the care of the diabetic patient in a cost effective and diagnostically efficient manner while providing quality care is an example of: (Checklist #5)
   a. reflex testing
   b. disease management
   c. capitated payment
   d. critical pathway

9. The Medicare system uses this payment system to contain costs: (Checklist #6)
   a. capitated payment
   b. disease management
   c. fee-for-service
   d. PPS

10. Under the capitation payment system, the laboratory is viewed as a: (Checklist #6)
   a. revenue center
   b. profit center
   c. loss center
   d. cost center

www.prenhall.com/mckenzie

Use the above address to access the free, interactive Companion Web site created for this textbook. Get hints, instant feedback, and textbook references to chapter-related multiple choice questions.

REFERENCES

1. Wintrobe MM. Blood, *Pure and Eloquent.* New York: McGraw-Hill; 1980.

2. Vierordt K. Zahlungen der Blutkorperchen des Menschen. *Arch Physiol Heilk,* 1852; 11:327.

3. Bao W, Dalferes ER, Srinivasan BR, Webber LS, and Berenson GS. Normative distribution of complete blood count from early childhood through adolescence: The Bogulusa Heart Study. *Prev Med.* 1993;22:825–37.

4. Weingarten S, Graber G. Outcome-validated clinical practice guidelines: A scientific foundation for disease management. In: Couch JB, ed. *The physician's guide to disease management.* Gaithersburg, Maryland: Aspen Publishers, Inc; 1997:57–82.

5. Wolman DM, Kalfoglou AL, LeRoy L. *Medicare laboratory payment policy.* Washington DC: National Academy Press. 2000:18–28.

6. Wennberg JE. Variations in medical practice and hospital costs. *Conn Med.* 1985;49:444–53.

7. Wennberg JE, Gittelsohn A. Variations in medical care among small areas. *Sci Am.* 1982;246:120–34.

8. Wennberg JE, Gittelsohn A. Small area variations in health care delivery. *Science.* 1973;12:1102–8.

9. Couch JB. Disease management: An overview. In: Couch JB, ed. *The physician's guide to disease management.* Gaithersburg, Maryland: Aspen Publishers, Inc; 1997:1–27.

10. Keiser JF, Howard BJ. Critical pathways: Design, implementation, and evaluation. *Clin Lab Manage Rev.* 1998; 12:317–32.

11. Fritsma GA, Ens GE. Reflexive protocols and laboratory-clinician communication. *Clin Hem Rev.* April 1997:2–3.

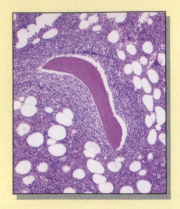

2

Cellular Homeostasis and Hematopoiesis

J. Lynne Williams, Ph.D.

■ CHECKLIST - LEVEL I

At the end of this unit of study the student should be able to:

1. Describe the location, morphology, and function of subcellular organelles of a cell.
2. Differentiate the parts of the mammalian cell cycle.
3. Define *cyclins* and *Cdks* and discuss their role in cell cycle regulation.
4. Define *apoptosis* and explain its role in normal human physiology.
5. Classify and give examples of the major categories of initiators and inhibitors of apoptosis.
6. List the major events regulated by apoptosis in hematopoiesis.
7. Describe the basic concepts of cell differentiation and maturation.
8. Compare and contrast the categories of hematopoietic precursor cells: hematopoietic stem cells, hematopoietic progenitor cells, and maturing cells.
9. Describe the hierarchy of hematopoietic precursor cells and the relationships of the various blood cell lineages to each other (including the concept of colony-forming units/CFUs).
10. Discuss the general characteristics of growth factors and identify the major examples of early acting (multilineage), later acting (lineage restricted), and indirect acting growth factors.
11. List examples of negative regulators of hematopoiesis.
12. Define *hematopoietic microenvironment*.
13. Compare/contrast oncogenes and tumor-suppressor genes (anti-oncogenes).

■ CHECKLIST - LEVEL II

At the end of this unit of study the student should be able to:

1. Describe the periodicity, associated Cdk partners, and function of cyclins D, E, A, and B.
2. Define CAK (Cdk activating kinase) and the two major classes of CKIs (Cyclin dependent kinase inhibitors) and describe their function.
3. Compare the function of cell-cycle checkpoints in cell-cycle regulation.
4. Describe/illustrate the roles of p53 and pRb in cell cycle regulation.
5. Propose how perturbations of cell cycle regulatory mechanisms can lead to malignancy.

■ CHECKLIST—LEVEL II *(continued)*

6. Differentiate, using morphologic observations, the processes of necrotic cell death and apoptotic cell death.

7. Define *caspases* and explain their role in apoptosis.

8. Define and contrast the roles of proapoptotic and antiapoptotic members of the Bcl-2 family of proteins.

9. Explain the function of death receptors in the apoptotic process.

10. Describe apoptotic regulatory mechanisms.

11. Identify the role of apoptosis in hematopoiesis.

12. Give examples of diseases associated with increased apoptosis and inhibited (decreased) apoptosis.

13. Identify the key cytokines required for lineage-specific regulation.

14. Describe the structure and role of growth factor receptors.

15. Outline current clinical uses of cytokines.

16. Describe the cellular and extracellular components of the hematopoietic microenvironment.

17. Discuss the proposed mechanisms used to regulate hematopoietic stem/progenitor cell proliferation/differentiation.

18. Generalize how molecules involved in proliferation, differentiation, cell cycle regulation, and apoptosis can function as oncogenes or tumor suppressor genes.

KEY TERMS

Anti-oncogene/tumor suppressor gene
Apoptosis
Caspase
Cell cycle
Cell cycle checkpoints
Commitment
Cyclins/Cdks
Cytokine
Differentiation
Extracellular matrix
Genome
Hematopoiesis
Hematopoietic microenvironment
Hematopoietic progenitor cells
Hematopoietic stem cells
Homeostasis
Necrosis
Oncogene
Proto-oncogene
Quiescence (G_0)
Restriction point (R)
Stromal cells
Tissue homeostasis

BACKGROUND BASICS

Level I and Level II
Students should have a solid foundation in basic cell biology principles, including the component parts of a cell and the structure and function of cytoplasmic organelles. They should have an understanding of the segments comprising a cell cycle (interphase and mitosis) and the processes that take place during each stage.

► OVERVIEW

This chapter is divided into two parts. The first, Control of Cell Growth and Differentiation, includes a brief review of cell morphology. Cellular processes that maintain tissue homeostasis—cell proliferation and cell death—are discussed. The second part, Hematopoiesis, describes hematopoietic cell differentiation and the role of cytokines and the hematopoietic microenvironment in controlling and directing this process. The chapter concludes with a discussion of what happens when genes controlling cell differentiation and proliferation are mutated.

▶ INTRODUCTION

The maintenance of an adequate number of cells to carry out the functions of the organism is referred to as **tissue homeostasis.** Tissue homeostasis depends on the careful regulation of several cellular processes, including cellular proliferation, cellular differentiation, and cell death (apoptosis). The hematopoietic system presents a challenge when considering the homeostasis of the circulating blood, as the majority of circulating cells are postmitotic cells that are relatively short-lived. Thus, circulating blood cells are intrinsically incapable of providing their replacements when they reach the end of their life spans. **Hematopoiesis** is the process responsible for the replacement of circulating blood cells and depends on the proliferation of precursor cells that still retain mitotic capability. This process is governed by a multitude of cytokines (both stimulating and inhibitory growth factors) and takes place in a specialized microenvironment uniquely suited for regulation of the process. A thorough understanding of cell structural components, as well as the processes of cell division and cell death, allows us to understand not only the normal (physiologic) regulation of hematopoiesis, but also disease processes in which these events become dysregulated (e.g., cancer).

PART I

CONTROL OF CELL GROWTH AND DIFFERENTIATION

▶ CELL MORPHOLOGY REVIEW

A basic understanding of cell morphology is essential to the study of hematology because many hematologic disorders are accompanied by abnormalities or changes in morphology of cellular or subcellular components as well as by changes in cell concentrations.

A cell is an intricate, complex structure consisting of a membrane-bound aqueous solution of proteins, carbohydrates, fats, inorganic materials, and nucleic acids. The nucleus, bound by a double layer of membrane, controls and directs the development, function, and division of the cell. The cytoplasm, where most of the cell's metabolic reactions take place, surrounds the nucleus and is bound by the cell membrane. The cytoplasm contains highly ordered organelles, which are membrane-bound compartments with specific cellular functions (Figure 2-1a ■). The different kinds of organelles and the quantity of each are dependent on the function of the cell and the state of maturation.

CELL MEMBRANE

The outer boundary of the cell, the plasma (cell) membrane is often considered a barrier between the cell and its environment. In fact, it functions to allow the regulated passage of ions, nutrients, and information between the cytoplasm and its extracellular milieu and thus determines the interrelationships of the cell with its surroundings.

The plasma membrane consists of a complex, ordered array of lipids and proteins that serves as the interface between the cell and its environment (Figure 2-1b ■). The plasma membrane is in the form of a phospholipid bilayer punctuated by proteins. The polar (hydrophilic) head groups of the lipids are directed toward the outside and inside of the cell, and the long-chain (hydrophobic) hydrocarbon tails are directed inward. While the plasma membrane has traditionally been described as a "fluid mosaic" structure,[1] it is in fact highly ordered, with asymmetric distribution of both membrane lipids and proteins. The lipid and protein compositions of the outside and inside of the membrane differ from one another in ways that reflect the different functions performed at the two surfaces of the membrane. However, the membrane lipids can freely diffuse laterally throughout their own half of the bilayer, or they may flip-flop from one side of the bilayer to the other in response to certain stimuli. Membrane lipids, including phospholipids, cholesterol, lipoproteins, and lipopolysaccharides, contribute to the basic framework of cell membranes and account for the cell's high permeability to lipid-soluble substances. Different mixtures of lipids are found in the membranes of different types of cells.

Although lipids are responsible for the basic structure of the plasma membrane, most of the specific functions of the membrane are carried out by proteins. The proteins of the membrane provide selective permeability and transport of specific substances, structural stability, enzymatic catalysis, and cell-to-cell recognition functions. The membrane proteins are divided into two general groups: integral (transmembrane) proteins and attached (peripheral) proteins that are located primarily on the cytoplasmic surface of the lipid bilayer. Some of the integral proteins span the entire lipid bilayer, while other integral proteins only partially penetrate the membrane. In some cells, such as erythrocytes (∞ Chapter 4), peripheral proteins on the cytoplasmic side of the membrane form a lattice network that functions as a cellular cytoskeleton, imparting order on the membrane.

Carbohydrates linked to membrane lipids (glycolipids) or proteins (glycoproteins) may extend from the outer surface of the membrane. Functions of the carbohydrate moieties include specific binding, cell-to-cell recognition, and cell adhesion. The sugar groups are added to the lipid or protein molecules in the lumen of the Golgi apparatus after synthesis by the endoplasmic reticulum. Many of the glycoprotein transmembrane proteins serve as receptors for extracellular molecules such as growth factors. Binding of the specific

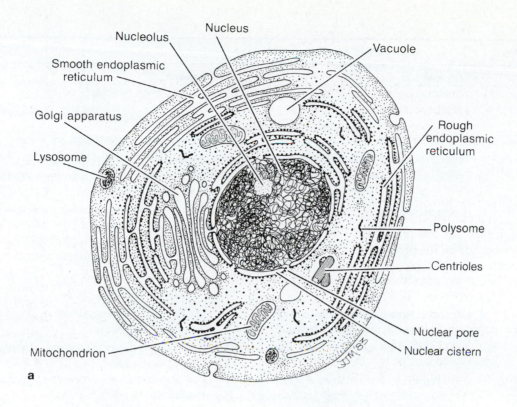

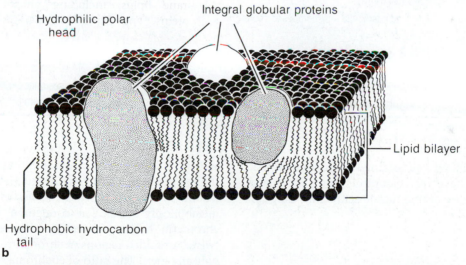

■ **FIGURE 2-1a** Drawing of a cell depicting the various organelles. **b.** The fluid mosaic membrane model proposed by Singer and Nicholson.

CYTOPLASM

The cytoplasm, or cytosol, is where the metabolic activities of the cell take place, including protein synthesis, growth, motility, and phagocytosis. The structural components, called organelles, include the mitochondria, lysosomes, endoplasmic reticulum (ER), Golgi apparatus, ribosomes, granules, microtubules, and microfilaments (Table 2-1 ✪). Organelles and other cellular inclusions lie within the cytoplasmic matrix. The composition of the cytoplasm depends on cellular lineage and degree of cellular maturity. The appearance of cytoplasm in fixed, stained cells is important in evaluating the morphology, classifying the cell, and determining the stage of differentiation. Immature or

ligand to a receptor may result in transduction of a signal to the cell's interior without passage of the extracellular molecule through the membrane.

✪ TABLE 2-1

Cellular Organelles

Structure	Composition	Function
Ribosomes	RNA + proteins	Assemble amino acids into protein
"Free"	Scattered in the cytoplasm Linked by mRNA forming polyribosomes	Synthesis of protein destined to remain in cytosol
"Fixed"	Ribosomes bound to outer surface of RER	Synthesis of protein destined for export from the cell
Endoplasmic reticulum (ER)	Interconnecting membrane-bound tubules and vesicles	Synthesis and transport of lipid and protein
Rough ER (RER)	Studded on outer surface with ribosomes	Abundant in cells synthesizing secretory protein; protein transported to Golgi
Smooth ER (SER)	Lacks attached ribosomes	Important in lipid synthesis, detoxification, synthesis of steroid hormones
Golgi apparatus	Stacks of flattened membranes located in juxtanuclear region	Protein from RER is sorted, modified (e.g., glycosylated) and packaged; forms lysosomes
Lysosomes	Membrane-bound sacs containing hydrolytic enzymes	Destruction of carbohydrates, lipids and proteins (phagocytosed material or metabolites)
Mitochondria	Double-membrane organelle; inner folds (cristae) house enzymes of aerobic metabolism	Oxidative phosphorylation (ATP production) abundant in metabolically active cells
Cytoskeleton	Microfilaments, intermediate filaments and microtubules	Gives the cell shape, provides strength, and enables movement of cellular structures
Microfilaments	Fine filaments (5–9 nm); polymers of actin	Control shape and surface movement of most cells
Intermediate filaments	Ropelike fibers (~10 nm); composed of number of fibrous proteins	Provide cells with mechanical strength
Microtubules	Hollow cylinders (~25 nm); composed of protein tubulin	Important in maintaining cell shape; form spindle apparatus during mitosis
Centrosome	"Cell center"; includes centrioles	Microtubule-organizing center; forms poles of mitotic spindle during anaphase
Centrioles	Two cylindrical structures arranged at right angles to each other; consist of 9 groups of three microtubules	Enable movement of chromosomes during cell division; self-replicate prior to cell division

synthetically active blood cells stained with Romanowsky stains (∞ Chapter 7) have very basophilic (blue) cytoplasm, due to the large quantity of ribonucleic acid (RNA) they contain.

NUCLEUS

The nucleus contains the genetic material, deoxyribonucleic acid (DNA), responsible for the regulation of all cellular functions. The nuclear material, chromatin, consists of DNA and associated structural proteins (histones) packaged into chromosomes. The total genetic information stored in the chromosomes of an organism constitutes its **genome.** The fundamental subunit of chromatin is the nucleosome, a beadlike segment of chromosome composed of about 180 base pairs of DNA wrapped around a histone protein. The linear array of successive nucleosomes gives chromatin a "beads-on-a-string" appearance in electron micrographs. The appearance of chromatin varies, presumably depending on

activity. It is generally considered that the dispersed, lightly stained portions of chromatin (euchromatin) represent unwound or loosely twisted regions of chromatin that are metabolically active. The condensed, more deeply staining chromatin (heterochromatin) is believed to represent tightly twisted or folded regions of chromatin strands that are metabolically inert. The ratio of euchromatin to heterochromatin is dependent on the activity of the cell, with the younger or more active cells having more euchromatin and a finer chromatin structure. The nuclei of most active cells contain from one to four pale staining nucleoli. The nucleolus (singular) consists of RNA and proteins and is believed to be important in RNA synthesis. The nucleolus of very young blood cells is easily seen with brightfield microscopy on stained smears.

The nuclear contents are surrounded by a double membrane, the nuclear envelope. The outer membrane (cytoplasmic side) is continuous with the ER and has a polypeptide composition distinct from that of the inner membrane. The gap between the two membranes (~50 nm) is called the perinuclear space. The nuclear envelope is interrupted at irregular intervals by openings consisting of nuclear pore complexes (NPCs), which provide a means of communication between nucleus and cytoplasm. They constitute envelope-piercing channels that function as selective gates allowing bidirectional movement of molecules. The nucleus exports newly assembled ribosomal subunits, while importing proteins such as transcription factors and DNA repair enzymes.

► TISSUE HOMEOSTASIS: PROLIFERATION, DIFFERENTIATION, AND APOPTOSIS

Tissue homeostasis refers to the maintenance of an adequate number of cells to carry out the functions of the organism. In the human body, somatic cells (including blood cells) generally undergo one of three possible fates: they (1) proliferate by mitotic cell division, (2) differentiate and acquire specialized functions, or (3) die and are eliminated from the body. Cell proliferation is required for the replacement of cells lost to terminal differentiation, cell death, or cell loss. Differentiation provides us with a variety of cells, each of which is capable of executing specific and specialized functions. Recently, it has become apparent that cell death is also an active process (**apoptosis**) that can be initiated by the cell itself. Apoptosis is physiologically as important as cell proliferation and differentiation in controlling the overall homeostasis of various tissues. When the regulation of any of these three cellular processes malfunctions and the processes become unbalanced, the consequence may be tissue atrophy, functional insufficiency, or neoplasia.

THE CELL CYCLE

Cell division is a fundamental process that is required throughout the life of all eukaryotes. Although it has been known for many years that cells have the ability to grow and replicate, the actual mechanisms involved were discovered relatively recently.[2] The biochemical and morphological stages that a cell passes through when stimulated to divide are referred to as the **cell cycle,** which is conveniently divided into several phases: G_1 (Gap-1), S (DNA synthesis), G_2 (Gap-2) and M (mitosis) (Figure 2-2a ■).

Stages of the Cell Cycle

The physical process of cell division is preceded by a series of morphologically recognizable stages referred to as *mitosis (M phase)* (Figure 2-2b ■). During mitosis, cells condense their chromosomes (*prophase*), align them on a microtubular spindle (*metaphase*), and segregate sister chromatids to opposite poles of the cell (*anaphase* and *telophase*). Morphologically, little can be seen during the interval between succeeding mitoses (known as *interphase*) except that cells grow in volume. With the discovery of DNA and the recognition that DNA

carries the information stored in chromosomes, it became clear that during interphase the cell synthesizes molecules and duplicates its components in preparation for mitosis. *S phase* is the phase in which DNA synthesis takes place. However, DNA synthesis occurs during only a narrow window of time during interphase. S phase (DNA synthesis) is separated from M phase (mitosis) by two gap periods: G_1 the time between the end of mitosis and the onset of the next round of DNA replication, and G_2 the time between the completion of S and the onset of mitosis.

Not all of the cells in the body are actively dividing (i.e., are actively engaged in the cell cycle). Cells may exit the cell cycle at G_1 and enter a nonproliferative phase called G_0, or **quiescence.** To proliferate, a cell must enter the cell cycle; in response to specific mitogenic stimuli, quiescent cells exit G_0 and reenter the cell cycle at the level of early G_1. In unicellular organisms such as bacteria, cell division is dependent only on an adequate supply of nutrients. In mammalian cells, all cell division cycles are initiated by specific growth factors, or mitogens, that drive the cell from G_0 to G_1 ($G_0 \rightarrow G_1$).

G_1 is characterized by a period of cell growth and synthesis of components necessary for replication. Cells transit through the G_1 phase of the cell cycle, where in late G_1, they pass through what has been called the **restriction point (R).** R defines a point in the cell cycle after which the cell is no longer responsive to extracellular signals but is committed to completing that cell cycle *independent* of mitogenic stimuli (i.e., cell cycle completion becomes autonomous).[3] Cells then transit across the G_1/S boundary into the S phase of the cycle where DNA synthesis occurs, followed by the G_2 phase and finally mitosis (where nuclear division [*karyokinesis*] and cytoplasmic separation [*cytokinesis*] occur).

Molecular Regulation of Cell Cycle Progression

The fundamental task of the cell cycle is to faithfully replicate DNA once during S phase and to distribute identical chromosomal copies equally to both daughter cells during M phase. Organized progression through the cell cycle normally ensures that this takes place, so that most cells never embark on mitosis before DNA duplication is completed, never attempt to segregate sister chromatids until all pairs are aligned on the mitotic spindle at metaphase, and never reduplicate their chromosomes (reinitiate S phase) before sister chromatids have been separated at the previous mitosis. Cells must ensure that chromosome duplication and segregation occur in the correct order (i.e., $S \rightarrow M \rightarrow S \rightarrow M$). They must also see that the next event in the cycle *only* begins when the previous events have been successfully completed (i.e., chromosome duplication is complete before the chromosomes are segregated into the two daughter cells). Entry into and exit from each phase of the cell cycle are tightly regulated. Research over the past

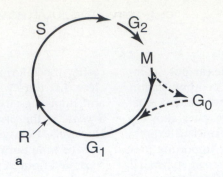

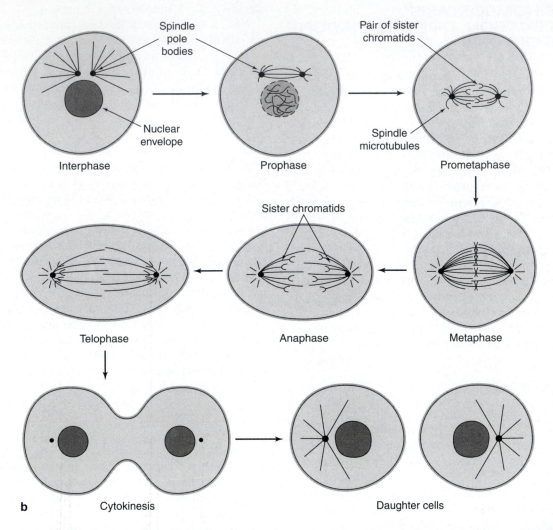

■ **FIGURE 2-2 a** The four phases of the cell cycle: G_1, S, G_2 and M. G_0 represents the state of quiescence, when a cell is withdrawn from the cell cycle. R represents the restriction point—the point in the cell cycle after which the cell is no longer dependent on extracellular signals, but can complete the cycle in the absence of mitogenic stimuli. **b.** The stages of mitosis. During G_1, S, and G_2, the nucleus is in interphase. During interphase, the spindle pole bodies duplicate and nucleate cytoplasmic microtubules. At prophase the chromatin condenses into visible chromosome fibers; the nuclear membrane starts to break down. By prometaphase, the nuclear envelope has disappeared, and each pole body is organizing a set of microtubules. The two sets of microtubules constitute the spindle. At this stage, each condensed chromosome consists of two duplicate DNA molecules called sister chromatids. Each chromatid has a centromere and an associated structure called a kinetchore at which microtubules attach. At metaphase, all the chromosomes are balanced halfway between the poles in a plane called the metaphase plate. After all the chromosomes are aligned, the sister chromatids separate (the beginning of anaphase). The chromosomes (now single chromatids) move along the microtubule bundles to the poles. At telophase, the chromosomes have moved to the poles, and the poles are separated by their maximum distance. The nuclear envelope reforms. At cytokinesis, the cytoplasm pinches to give two separate cells. (Reprinted, with permission, from: *Recombinant DNA,* 2nd ed. New York: W.H. Freeman, 1992.)

20 years has begun to reveal how cells guarantee the orderliness of this process.[2]

Cyclins and Cyclin-Dependent Kinases

Transition between the various phases of the cell cycle is regulated by enzymatic activities of specific and unique kinases. These kinase proteins (**Cdks** or cyclin-dependent kinases) phosphorylate target molecules important for cell cycle control. To be active, the kinase (Cdk) must be complexed with a regulatory subunit named **cyclin** (hence the name, **c**yclin-**d**ependent **k**inase). Numerous cyclins and Cdks exist in the cell. Different kinase complexes with differing cyclin and Cdk components drive the cell from one stage of the cell cycle to the next. The sequential activation of successive cyclin/kinase complexes, each of which in turn phosphorylates key substrates, facilitates or regulates the movement of the cell through the cycle (Figure 2-3a ■). Cdk inhibitors also exist that function to inhibit the active kinase activity by binding to the Cdks or the Cdk/cyclin complexes.

At least 14 cyclins and at least 9 different Cdks have been discovered so far. Not all of them have been shown to play a universal role in regulating the cell cycle. The concentration of the different cyclin proteins rises and falls at specific times during the cell cycle (hence they are *cycling* proteins). Different cyclin/Cdk complexes are functional at different phases of the cell cycle, as summarized in Table 2-2 ✪.

A mammalian cell must receive external signals (growth factors and/or hormones) that trigger the cell to initiate cell cycle progression.[4] These external signals result in an in-

✪ TABLE 2-2

Cell Cycle Regulatory Proteins

Cell cycle phase	Cyclin	Partner Cdk
G_1	D1, D2, D3	Cdk4, Cdk6
G_1/S	E	Cdk2
S	A	Cdk2
M	A	Cdk1 (Cdc2)
	B	Cdk1 (Cdc2)

crease of one (or more) of the D cyclins (of which there are three: D1, D2, and D3). Cyclin D complexes with Cdk4 or Cdk6 and phosphorylates target molecules required for $G_1 \rightarrow$ S progression. The D cyclins are unique in that they are synthesized in response to growth factor stimulation, and will remain active in the cell as long as the mitotic stimulus is present. Toward mid- to late-G_1, levels of cyclin E increase and bind with Cdk2. The cyclin E/Cdk2 complex is required for the G_1 to S transition. Once the cell enters S phase, cyclin E is degraded rapidly, and the activation of Cdk2 is taken over by cyclin A. Cyclin A/Cdk2 is required for the onset of DNA synthesis, progression through S phase, and entry into mitosis. Toward the end of S phase, cyclin A starts to activate another kinase, Cdk1 (previously called cdc2), which signals the completion of S phase and the onset of G_2. Cyclin B takes over from cyclin A as the activating partner of Cdk1, and Cyclin B/Cdk1 controls the onset, sequence of events, and the completion of mitosis. Cyclin B must be destroyed for the cell to exit mitosis and for cytokinesis to take place.

Regulation of Cell-Cycle Kinase Activity

Control of enzyme activity is somewhat unique, in that protein levels of the kinase subunit remain constant throughout the cell cycle and do not require activation from a proenzyme precursor form (unlike the activation of the serine proteases of the blood coagulation cascade; ∞ Chapter 35). Regulation is achieved through varying availability of the regulatory cofactor (the cyclins), through periodic (and cell cycle phase-specific) synthesis, and degradation, of the appropriate cyclin partners (Figure 2-3b ■).[5] It is the periodic accumulation of different cyclins that determines the sequential oscillation of kinase activities, which in turn determines the ordering of events of the cell cycle.

Cell-cycle kinase activity is regulated by multiple mechanisms. In addition to the requirement for the appropriate cyclin partner (controlled by cell-cycle specific cyclin synthesis

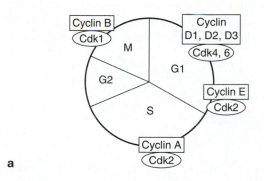

a

Cell Cycle Cyclin Patterns

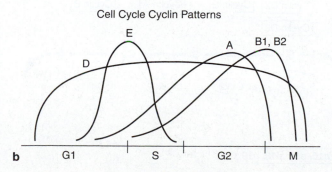

b

■ **FIGURE 2-3a** The phases of the cell cycle with the major regulatory cyclin/Cdk complexes depicted for each. **b.** The levels of the various cyclin proteins during the cell cycle. The cyclins rise and fall in a periodic fashion, thus controlling the cyclin-dependent kinases and their activities.

and degradation), the kinase subunit (Cdk) must be phosphorylated and/or dephosphorylated at specific amino acid residues.[6] Full kinase activity requires the phosphorylation of threonine (Thr) 161 (using the amino acid numbering of Cdk1). The kinase responsible for this activating phosphorylation is called CAK (**C**dk-**a**ctivating **k**inase) and is itself a Cdk (Cdk7, complexed with cyclin H). CAK is responsible for the activating phorphorylation of *all* the kinases important for mammalian cell cycle control, including Cdks 1, 2, 4, and 6. On the other hand, phosphorylation of Thr 14 and tyrosine (Tyr) 15 suppresses kinase activity, and these phosphates must be removed by the phosphatase called CDC25 in order to have a fully active cyclin/Cdk complex.

The final level of regulation involves two groups of proteins that function as inhibitors of Cdks and cyclin/Cdk complexes (Figure 2-4 ■).[7] The first Cdk inhibitor identified was p21; other Cdk inhibitors with structural and functional similarities to p21 include p27 and p57. (This nomenclature indicates they are **p**roteins of the indicated molecular mass in kilodaltons, e.g., p21 is a protein of molecular weight of 21,000.) These three inhibitors bind multiple cyclin/Cdk complexes of both the G_1 and S phases of the cell cycle (cyclin D/Cdk4/6, cyclin E/Cdk2 and cyclin A/Cdk2). The second group of inhibitors is a family of structurally related proteins that include p15, p16, p18, and p19. These inhibitors are more restricted in their inhibitory activity, and inhibit only Cdk4 and Cdk6.

Cell-Cycle Checkpoints

Cell proliferation and differentiation depends on the accurate duplication and transfer of genetic information, which requires the precise ordering of cell-cycle events. Cells achieve this coordination by using **cell-cycle checkpoints** to monitor events at critical points in the cycle and, if necessary, halt progression of the cycle.[8,9,10] The main functions of checkpoints are to detect malfunctions within the system and to assess whether certain events are properly completed before the cell is allowed to proceed through the cycle.

Several major cell-cycle checkpoints have been described. The *G_1 checkpoint* checks for DNA damage, and will prevent progression into S-phase if the integrity of the genome is compromised. The *G_2-M checkpoint* monitors the accuracy of DNA replication during S-phase. It checks for damaged or unreplicated DNA, and can block mitosis if any is found. The *metaphase checkpoint* (also called the *mitotic-spindle checkpoint*) functions to ensure that all chromosomes are properly aligned on the spindle apparatus prior to initiating

chromosomal separation and segregation at anaphase. If defects are detected at any of these checkpoints, the cell-cycle clock is stopped. Activation of repair pathways may be initiated, or if the damage is severe, apoptosis may be triggered (see below).

Two proteins critical for effective function of the G_1 checkpoint are *p53* and *Rb*. Rb is the protein product of the retinoblastoma susceptibility gene, which predisposes individuals to retinoblastomas and other tumors when only one functional copy is present. Rb is present throughout the cell cycle and is an important regulator of cell-cycle progression (Figure 2-5 ■).[11,12] In its *hypo*phosphorylated (active) state, Rb has antiproliferative effects, inhibiting cell cycling. It does so by binding transcription factors (the *E2F* proteins) required for the transcription of genes needed for cell cycling, rendering them transcriptionally inactive. When growth factors induce activation of cyclin D/Cdk4/6, the Rb protein is one of the targets of this kinase activity. As cells progress through G_1, *hyper*phosphorylation of Rb by cyclin D/Cdk4/6 kinase results in inactivation of Rb and release of active E2F, resulting in the activation and expression of genes required for cell-cycle progression. *Rb* functions as a tumor suppressor gene, in that cells lacking functional Rb protein show deregulated expression of cell-cycle regulatory genes and cell proliferation, sometimes resulting in malignancy.

P53 is not required for normal cell function (i.e., it is not required for cell-cycle progression) but serves an important function as a molecular policeman, monitoring the integrity of the genome.[13] It is induced in response to DNA damage and puts the brakes on cell growth and division, allowing time for DNA repair, or triggering apoptosis if repair is not possible. P53 is thus an important component of the G_1 checkpoint, although it is also involved in the G_2/M checkpoint as well. Like Rb, p53 functions as a tumor suppressor

■ **FIGURE 2-4** Cdk inhibitors. There are two families of Cyclin-dependent kinase inhibitors. The first group, including p15, p16, p18, and p19, inhibit only D-type cyclin/Cdk4 or Cdk6 complexes. The second group of inhibitors, including p21, p27, and p57, possess a greater spectrum of inhibitory activity, inhibiting the G_1 as well as S-phase cyclin/Cdk complexes (Cyclin D/Cdk4/6, Cyclin E/Cdk2 and Cyclin A/Cdk2). ⊥ indicates inhibition of the pathway.

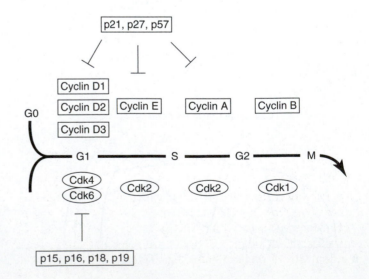

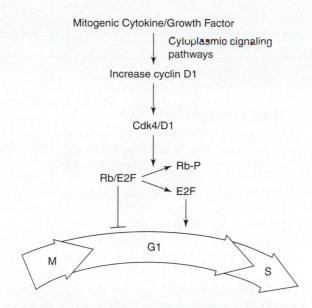

■ FIGURE 2-5 Role of the retinoblastoma susceptibility gene product (Rb) in regulation of the cell cycle. Stimulation of a cell with mitogens or growth factors induces synthesis of the D-type cyclins. Activation of G_1 phase kinase activity (Cyclin D/Cdk4/6) phosphorylates a number of intracellular substrates, including the Rb protein. In the hypophosphorylated (active) state, Rb binds and sequesters transcription factors known as E2F, rendering them inactive. When Cyclin D/Cdk4 or Cdk6 phorphorylates Rb, it releases the E2F transcription factors, which then move to the nucleus, and initiate transcription of genes required for cell-cycle progression (including the genes for Cyclin E and Cyclin A). ↓ indicates stimulation of the pathway; ⊥ indicates inhibition of the pathway.

gene, and is the most commonly mutated gene in human tumors.

 Checkpoint! #1

A cell undergoing mitosis fails to attach one of its duplicated chromosomes to the microtubules of the spindle apparatus during metaphase. The cell's metaphase checkpoint malfunctions and does not detect the error. What is the effect (if any) on the daughter cells produced?

APOPTOSIS

Cells stimulated to enter the cell cycle may experience outcomes other than proliferation (Figure 2-6 ■). Cells can undergo senescence, in which they are permanently growtharrested and no longer respond to mitogenic stimuli. Cells entering the cell cycle can also become terminally differenti-

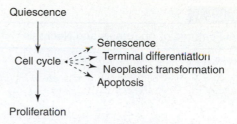

■ FIGURE 2-6 Alternative fates for a cell induced to enter the cell cycle.

ated (committed) into specialized cell types. Uncontrolled transit through the cell cycle is a characteristic feature of neoplastic transformation. Finally, cells can exit at any phase of the cell cycle by undergoing programmed cell death (apoptosis).

Cells can die by either of two major mechanisms: **necrosis** or apoptosis. The criteria for determining whether a cell is undergoing apoptosis or necrosis originally relied on distinct morphologic changes in the appearance of the cell (Table 2-3 ✪).[14] Necrotic death is induced by lethal chemical, biological, or physical events (extracellular assault). Such a death is analogous to "cell murder." In contrast, apoptosis, or "programmed cell death," requires the coordination of gene-directed internal processes, and is analogous to "cell suicide," as death is the consequence of molecular signals contained within individual cells.

Apoptosis is now recognized to play an essential role in the development and homeostasis of all multicellular organisms.[15] Apoptosis is a dominant force in sculpting the developing organism (embryogenesis/organogenesis): it is responsible for the morphogenesis of the hands and feet, the formation of hollow tubes in the body (including the blood vessels, gastrointestinal tract, and heart), and in the development of the immune system, for the selection of appropriate T and B cell clones. In adults, apoptosis is important in tissue homeostasis; it is responsible for the elimination of excess cells (such as expanded clones of T or B cells following immune stimulation, or excess PMNs following cessation of a bacterial challenge). As a defense mechanism, apoptosis is used to remove unwanted and potentially dangerous cells such as self-reactive lymphocytes, cells infected by viruses, or tumor cells. Individual cells that have sustained genotoxic injury (if they are unable to repair the damage to their DNA) will initiate a "self-suicide" program to prevent the cell with an impaired DNA sequence from proliferating. In addition to the beneficial effects of programmed cell death, the inappropriate activation of apoptosis may cause or contribute to a variety of diseases (Table 2-4 ✪).[16,17]

Apoptosis is initiated by three major types of stimuli (see Table 2-5 ✪):

1. Deprivation of survival factors (growth factor withdrawal or loss of attachment to extracellular matrix)

⭐ **TABLE 2-3**

Cardinal Features of Apoptosis and Necrosis

Feature	Necrosis	Apoptosis
Stimuli	Toxins, severe hypoxia, massive insult, conditions of ATP depletion	Physiologic and pathologic conditions without ATP depletion
Energy requirement	None	ATP-dependent
Histology	Cellular swelling; disruption of organelles, death of patches of tissue	Cellular shrinkage; chromatin condensation, apoptotic bodies, death of single isolated cells
DNA breakdown pattern	Randomly sized fragments	Ladder of fragments in internucleosomal multiples of 185 base pairs
Plasma membrane	Lysed	Intact, blebbed, with molecular alterations
Phagocytosis of dead cells	Immigrant phagocytes	Neighboring cells
Tissue reaction	Inflammation	No inflammation

2. Signals by "death" cytokines through apoptotic "death" receptors (tumor necrosis factor-TNF, Fas Ligand)

3. Cell damaging stress

Conversely, apoptosis is inhibited by growth-promoting cytokines and interaction with appropriate extracellular environmental stimuli. The disruption of cell physiology as a result of viral infections can cause an infected cell to undergo apoptosis. The suicide of an infected cell may be viewed as a cellular defense mechanism to prevent viral propagation. To circumvent these host defenses, a number of viruses have developed mechanisms to disrupt the normal regulation of apoptosis within the infected cell. Finally, a number of oncogenes and tumor suppressor genes have been described (see Part II) that may either stimulate or inhibit apoptosis.

Necrosis vs Apoptosis

When a cell is damaged, the plasma membrane loses its ability to regulate cation fluxes, resulting in the accumulation of Na^+, Ca^{++}, and water (Table 2-3 ⭐, and Figure 2-7 ■). Consequently, the necrotic cell exhibits a swollen morphology. The organelles also accumulate cations and water, swell, and ultimately lyse. The rupture of the cytoplasmic membrane and organelles releases cytoplasmic components (including proteases and lysozymes) into the surrounding tissue, triggering an inflammatory response. In contrast, apoptosis is characterized by cellular shrinking rather than swelling, with condensation of both the cytoplasm and the nucleus. Apoptotic cells do not lyse, but portions of the cell bud off in

⭐ **TABLE 2-4**

Diseases Associated with Increased and Decreased Apoptosis

Increased apoptosis	Decreased apoptosis
AIDS	Cancer
Neurodegenerative disorders	Follicular lymphomas
Alzheimer's disease	Other leukemias/lymphomas
Parkinson's disease	Carcinomas with p53 mutations
Amyotrophic lateral sclerosis	Hormone-dependent tumors
Retinitis pigmentosa	breast, prostate, ovarian
Myelodysplastic syndromes	Autoimmune disorders
Aplastic anemia	Systemic lupus erythematosus
Ischemic injury	Other autoimmune diseases
Myocardial infarction	Viral infections
Stroke	Herpes viruses
Reperfusion injury	Poxviruses
Toxin-induced liver disease	Adenoviruses

⭐ **TABLE 2-5**

Inhibitors and Initiators/Inducers of Apoptosis

Inhibitors	Initiators/Inducers
Presence of survival factors	Deprivation of survival factors
Growth factors	Growth factor withdrawal
Extracellular matrix	Loss of matrix attachment
Interleukins	Death cytokines
Estrogens, androgens	TNF
Viral products that block apoptosis	Fas ligand
Cowpox virus CrmA	Cell damaging stress
Epstein Barr virus BHRF-1	Bacterial toxins
Pharmacologic inhibitors	Viral infections
Oncogene and tumor suppressor gene products	Oxidants
(Bcl-2, Bcl-x_L, Mcl-1, Rb, c-Abl)	Glucocorticoids
	Cytotoxic drugs
	Radiation therapy
	Oncogene and tumor suppressor gene products (c-myc, p53, Bax, Bad, Bcl-x_S, c-Fos, c-Jun)

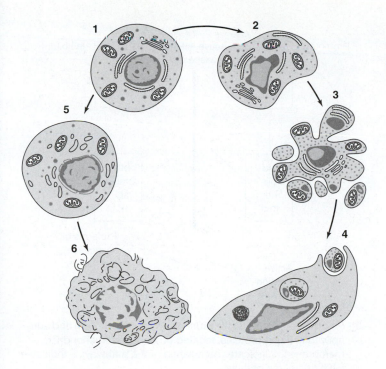

■ **FIGURE 2-7** Diagram illustrating the sequential ultrastructural changes in apoptosis (clockwise arrows) and necrosis (counterclockwise arrows). A normal cell is shown at (1). The onset of apoptosis (2) is heralded by compaction and segregation of chromatin into sharply delineated masses that lie against the nuclear envelope, condensation of the cytoplasm, and mild convolution of the nuclear and cellular outlines. Rapid progression of the process over the next few minutes (3) is associated with nuclear fragmentation and marked convolution of the cellular surface with the development of protuberances. The latter then separate to produce membrane-bound apoptotic bodies, which are phagocytosed and digested by adjacent cells (4). Signs of early necrosis in an irreversibly injured cell (5) include clumping of chromatin into ill-defined masses, gross swelling of organelles, and the appearance of flocculent densities in the matrix of mitochondria. At a later stage (6), membranes break down and the cell disintegrates. (With permission from, Definition and incidence of apoptosis: An historical perspective. In *Apoptosis: the Molecular Basis of Cell Death.* Eds: Kerr, JRF, Harmon, BV. New York: Cold Spring Harbor Laboratory Press, 1991.)

apoptotic bodies that are phagocytosed by neighboring cells or macrophages. Thus, apoptosis is a very efficient process by which the body can remove a population of cells at a given time or in response to a given stimulus *without* the activation of an inflammatory response. Necrosis is a passive event dictated by the external injurious agent and generally leads to the destruction of a large group of cells in the same area. In contrast, apoptosis is an energy-dependent process, orchestrated by the cell itself, and generally affects only single, individual cells. In addition, apoptosis is characterized by a particular type of DNA fragmentation. DNA in an apoptotic cell is enzymatically cleaved by a specific endonuclease into oligonucleotides whose sizes are multiples of ~185 base pairs (corresponding to nucleosomal fragments). When run out electrophoretically on agarose gel, these oligonucleotides make a discrete "ladder pattern" that is considered the hallmark of apoptosis. This is in contrast to the smudge pattern seen in cells undergoing necrosis that indicates the presence of randomly and fully degraded DNA.

Caspases and the Regulation of Apoptosis

The cellular events responsible for apoptotic cell death are directed by a group of proteins called **caspases**.[18,19] Caspases are a family of **c**ysteine proteases that cleave after **asp**artic acid amino acids in a peptide substrate and are responsible for the orderly dismantling of the cell undergoing apoptosis. Apoptosis is a closely regulated physiologic process, with the Bcl-2 family of proteins being particularly important. The Bcl-2 family of proteins includes both proapoptotic and antiapoptotic members and constitutes a critical intracellular checkpoint of apoptosis, determining whether early activation of *initiator* caspases will proceed to full activation of *exe-*

cution caspases and cell death.[20,21] In addition, a number of proteins that modulate cell death by interfering with caspase activity have been described, the so-called **i**nhibitors of **a**poptosis **p**roteins (IAPs).[18,19]

At least 14 caspase enzymes (caspase 1–14) have been identified in humans, although not all play a significant role in apoptosis. Those that are involved in apoptosis form the effector arm of the apoptotic machinery that, once activated, carries out the proteolysis necessary for apoptosis to occur. There is a hierarchical relationship described among the various apoptotic caspases, perhaps analogous to that described for the blood coagulation proteins (∞ Chapter 35). Early acting (initiator) caspases (caspase-2, -8, -9, -10) are recruited in response to apoptotic stimuli and are activated. They then initiate the cascade by activating (downstream) executioner caspases (caspase-3, -6, -7), which activate proapoptotic factors, cleave key proteins required for maintenance of intracellular homeostasis, and orchestrate the ordered dismantling of the cell (Figure 2-8 ■).[19,22] Activation of caspases in apoptosis does not lead to indiscriminate proteolytic degradation but rather to specific cleavage of key substrates including proteins involved in cell structure, proteins involved in cell cycle regulation, DNA repair proteins, proteins involved in RNA splicing, and the activation of a key endonuclease responsible for the characteristic DNA fragmentation.

Bcl-2 was a protein originally cloned from B-cell lymphomas with the characteristic t(14;18) chromosomal translocation (∞ Chapter 31). Since that initial discovery, several additional related proteins have been identified, some of which are proapoptotic while others are antiapoptotic. At present, there are at least eight known apoptosis-

Death Receptor/Death Cytokine
Apoptotic Pathway

Binding of death cytokine to cell receptor

↓

Caspase recruitment

↓

Bcl-2
family   Activation of initiator caspases
⊥

↓

Bcl-2
family   Activation of effector caspases

↓

Cleavage of crucial cellular proteins

↓

Cell death

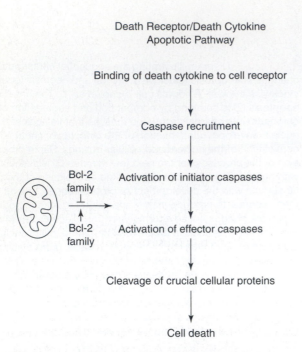

■ **FIGURE 2-8** The apoptotic pathway triggered by death cytokine binding to death receptors. Activation of a death receptor by binding of death cytokine results in the recruitment of specific adapter proteins and activation of initiator caspases. Activated initiator caspases can then proceed to activate downstream effector caspases that mediate the cleavage of various cellular proteins during apoptosis. The contribution of the Bcl-2 family of proapoptotic and antiapoptotic proteins, in determining whether activation of initiator caspases will proceed through to activation of effector caspases, is depicted. ↓ indicates stimulation of the pathway; ⊥ indicates inhibition of the pathway.

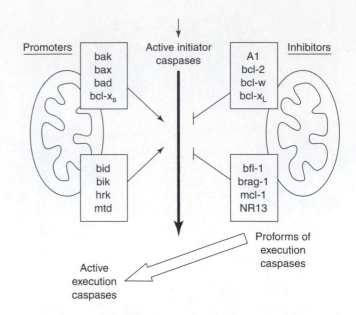

■ **FIGURE 2-9** Bcl-2 family proteins: Proapoptotic (left) and antiapoptotic (right) proteins, located on or near mitochondrial membranes. ↓ indicates stimulation of the pathway; ⊥ indicates inhibition of the pathway.

inhibitory proteins, including the originally described Bcl-2, and at least eight proapoptotic family members (Figure 2-9 ■). The Bcl-2 family of proteins are localized at the mitochondrial membranes and constitute a critical intracellular checkpoint of apoptosis, determining whether early activation of initiator caspases will proceed to full activation of execution caspases (Figure 2-8 ■).[23,24]

It has been suggested that these proteins function at least in part through protein-protein interactions. They all share similar structural regions that allow them to form dimers (either homodimers or heterodimers). Thus Bax (the first proapoptotic member discovered) can heterodimerize with Bcl-2 (an antiapoptotic protein) or homodimerize with itself (Figure 2-10 ■). Bax:Bax homodimers promote apoptosis; with elevated levels of Bcl-2, Bax:Bcl-2 heterodimers are formed, that repress apoptosis. Actually, it is the overall ratio of death agonists (Bax and related proteins) to death antagonists (Bcl-2 and related proteins) and their interactions with each other that determine the susceptibility to a death stimulus. Thus, *death signals* from a variety of sources are received and processed by the cell. They converge on this *rheostat* that de-

termines whether the cell will go on to activate effector caspases, and subsequently whether there will be cleavage of the *death substrates* necessary for the dismantling of the cell in apoptosis.[21]

Although there are multiple initiators of apoptosis, two major pathways of activation have been identified. One pathway involves so-called death receptors at the cell surface, while the second is mediated by other signals such as stress or exposure to cytotoxic agents or radiation. Five death receptors have been described in mammalian cells to date.[25,26] Binding of the specific ligand, or *death cytokine*, to the receptor leads to the recruitment of a number of molecules (adapter molecules) at the cytoplasmic side of the receptor, resulting in activation of initiator caspases (Figure 2-8 ■). The two best-known death cytokines and death receptors are: tumor necrosis factor (TNF) and the TNF receptor, and Fas Ligand and CD95 (Fas receptor). The sequence of events that triggers apoptosis via the second pathway is less well-understood.

Apoptosis and the Lympho-Hematopoietic System

Apoptosis is important in the hematopoietic system (Table 2-6 ✪). The default cellular status of hematopoietic precursor cells is thought to be *cell death* (see below). Cytokines and components of the extracellular matrix function to suppress the apoptotic program, allowing survival of hematopoietic cells when appropriate cytokines are present. As mentioned earlier, apoptosis plays an essential role in the selection of appropriate recognition repertoires of T and

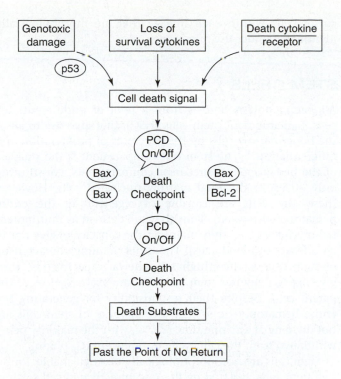

■ **FIGURE 2-10** Model of cell death checkpoints. Following delivery of a cell death signal (genotoxic damage, loss of survival cytokines, or presence of death cytokines), the ratio of proapoptotic components (Bax and related molecules) vs antiapoptotic components (Bcl-2 and related molecules) determines whether or not the death program will continue to completion. A preponderance of Bax:Bax homodimers promotes continuation of the process, while Bax–Bcl-2 heterodimers will shut it down. PCD = programmed cell death (apoptosis). (Adapted, with permission, from: Chao DT, Korsmeyer SJ: Bcl-2 family: Regulators of cell death. *Ann Rev Immunol* 16:395, 1998.)

⊛ **TABLE 2-6**

The Role of Apoptosis in the Hematopoietic and Lymphoid Systems

  I. Default cellular status for hematopoietic stem cells and progenitor cells
     Apoptosis regulated by cytokines and extracellular matrix
 II. Lymphoid Homeostasis:
     Selection of recognition repertoires of T and B cells
     Elimination of autoreactive lymphocytes
     Down regulation of immune response following antigen stimulation
     Cytotoxic killing by CTL and NK cells
III. Elimination of eosinophils, monocytes and neutrophils following infection/inflammatory response

B cells, eliminating those with nonfunctional or autoreactive antigen receptors. Apoptosis helps regulate numbers of mature cells by inducing cell death/elimination of excess cells when expanded numbers of mature cells are no longer needed (i.e., expanded T and B cell clones, following elimination of foreign antigen; elimination of PMNs, eosinophils, and monocytes following an infection/inflammatory response). Finally, apoptosis is the mechanism employed in cytotoxic killing by cytotoxic T lymphocytes and natural killer (NK) cells.

Dysregulation of apoptosis also contributes to hematologic disorders. Apoptosis is increased in the myelodysplastic syndromes, and tends to be decreased in the acute leukemias, perhaps partly explaining the pancytopenias and leukocytosis, respectively, seen in those disorders (∞ Chapters 28–30).

✓ **Checkpoint! #2**

What would be the effect on the hematopoietic system homeostasis if the expanded clone of antigen-activated B lymphocytes failed to undergo apoptosis after the antigenic challenge was removed?

PART II

HEMATOPOIESIS

Whereas cell proliferation and programmed cell death (apoptosis) work together to provide the organism with an adequate number of cells, **differentiation** is the process responsible for generating the diverse cell populations that provide the specialized functions needed by the organism. Differentiation has been defined as the appearance of different properties in cells that were initially equivalent. Since all cells of an organism have the same genetic information, differentiation (or the appearance of specific characteristics) occurs by the progressive restriction of other potentialities of the genome.[27] **Commitment** is the term used to define the instance when two cells derived from the same precursor take a separate route of development.[27] Commitment "assigns the program," and the maturation process executes it (*maturation* encompassing the totality of phenomena that begins with commitment and ends when the cell has all its characteristics).[27]

Hematopoiesis (the development of all the different cell lineages of the blood) has two striking characteristics: the variety of distinct blood cell types produced and the relatively brief lifespan of the individual cells. The cells circulating in the peripheral blood are mature blood cells and, with the exception of lymphocytes, are incapable of replicating (i.e., incapable of mitosis). Also they have a limited lifespan, from days for granulocytes and platelets to ~4 months for erythrocytes. As a result, they are described as *terminally differentiated*. This constant death of mature, functional blood cells means that new cells must be produced to replace those that are removed, either as a consequence of performing their biologic functions (e.g., platelets, granulocytes) or through cellular senescence, or "old age" (erythrocytes). The replacement of circulating, terminally differentiated cells depends on the function of less differentiated hematopoietic cells that still retain significant proliferative capabilities. These hematopoietic precursor cells, located primarily in the bone marrow in adults, consist of a hierarchy of cells with enormous proliferation potential. They maintain a daily production of approximately 10^{11} red blood cells (RBC) and 10^{11} white blood cells (WBC) for the lifetime of the individual. In addition, acute stress (blood loss or infection) can result in a rapid, efficient, and specific increase in production over baseline of the particular cell lineage needed. For example, acute blood loss results in a specific increased production of erythrocytes, while a bacterial infection results in an increased production of phagocytic cells (granulocytes and monocytes).

▶ HEMATOPOIETIC PRECURSOR CELLS

Hematopoietic precursor cells can be divided into three cellular compartments, defined by relative maturity: **hematopoietic stem cells, progenitor cells,** and **maturing cells** (Table 2-7 ✿). There has been a lack of uniformity in the nomenclature used to define these various compartments over the past 20 years. Although there is now general agreement on the designations *stem cells* and *progenitor cells,* the third category has been called by various authors *precursor cells,*[28] maturing cells,[29] or simply morphologically recognizable precursor cells.[30] In this textbook, we use the term *precursor* to include all cells antecedent to the mature cells in each lineage and the term *maturing cells* to include those pre-

cursor cells within each lineage that are morphologically identifiable under the microscope.

STEM CELLS

All hematopoiesis derives from a pool of undifferentiated cells, hematopoietic stem cells (HSC), that give rise to all of the bone marrow cells by the processes of proliferation and differentiation.[31] The stem cell compartment is the smallest of the hematopoietic precursor compartments, constituting only ~0.5% of the total marrow nucleated cells. However, these rare cells are capable of regenerating the entire hematopoietic system. Thus they are defined as multipotential precursors (i.e., they maintain the capacity to give rise to *all* lineages of blood cells). The other defining characteristic of stem cells is their high self-renewal capacity (i.e., they give rise to daughter stem cells that are exact replicas of the parent cell). Despite their responsibility for generating the entire hematopoietic system, the majority of stem cells are not dividing at any one time (<5%), with the majority being withdrawn from the cell cycle, or quiescent (G_0 phase).

Stem cells are not morphologically distinguishable. Primitive stem cells, isolated by fluorescent-activated cell sorting, show a morphology very similar to that of the small lymphocyte. Since stem cells are not morphologically identifiable, they have been defined functionally by the ability to reconstitute both lymphoid and myeloid hematopoiesis when transplanted into a recipient. In mice, the existence of the true HSC has been unequivocally proven by occasional successful transplants with single purified stem cells, thus providing direct proof that single cells capable of sustaining life-long hematopoiesis do exist.[32] There are no practical and quantitative assays for human HSC. Despite the difficulties (both practical and ethical) surrounding an effective assay for human stem cells, a number of characteristics have been used to define their phenotype, and these can be used in cell-separation protocols resulting in a high degree of purity. The currently proposed phenotype of a human HSC is:

$$CD34^+CD38^-Lin^-HLA\text{-}DR^-Rh123^{Dull}$$

✿ TABLE 2-7

Hematopoietic Precursor Cells

Stem Cells	Progenitor Cells	Maturing Cells
• ~0.5% of total hematopoietic precursor cells	• 3 percent of total hematopoietic precursor cells	• >95% of total hematopoietic precursor cells
• Multilineage differentiation potential	• Restricted developmental potential multipotential → unipotential	• Transit population, numerically amplified by proliferation
• Population maintained by self-renewal		
• Quiescent cell population	• Transit population with restricted self-renewal	• Proliferative sequence complete before full maturation
• Stable population/size	• Population amplified by proliferation	
• Not morphologically recognizable	• Not morphologically recognizable	• Morphologically recognizable
• Measured by functional clonal assays in vivo and in vitro	• Measured by clonal assays in vitro	

CD34 is a 110 kDa glycoprotein expressed by human hematopoietic stem cells and progenitor cells.[33] Expression of CD34 is lost as cells mature beyond the progenitor cell compartment. CD38 is a 45 kDa glycoprotein considered to be an early myeloid differentiation antigen. *Lin⁻* refers to the absence of known differentiation markers or antigens present on more lineage-restricted progenitors (e.g., glycophorin A protein, on erythrocytes; glycoprotein IIb/IIIa or CD41 on megakaryocytes and platelets; CD7 on T cells; and CD10 or CD19 on B cells). The HLA-DR antigens are a component of the human major histocompatibility complex antigens. Rhodamine[123] is a supravital dye that is taken up by the mitochondria. Rh^{Bright} cells, with more mitochondria, are thought to be a mitotically active population of cells, while Rh^{Dull} cells are thought to be quiescent. Thus, the long-term reconstituting multipotential stem cells are found in the population of cells that contain no lineage-specific antigens, CD38, or HLA-DR antigens but express CD34 and are largely quiescent, as defined by Rhodamine[123] uptake.

The process of self-renewal, which is a nondifferentiating cell division, assures that the stem cell population is sustained throughout the lifespan of the individual. This small group of cells is able to maintain tremendous hematopoietic cell supplies through the division of only a tiny fraction of its members, keeping the remainder of the stem cells in reserve. The size of the stem cell compartment is relatively stable under homeostatic conditions. In a stem cell compartment that remains stable in size but supplies differentiating cells, a cell must be added to the compartment by proliferation within the compartment (self-renewal) for each cell that leaves by the process of differentiation. Thus the stem cell pool must carefully balance the simultaneous processes of expansion (self-renewal) and differentiation. For an individual stem cell, these two processes are mutually exclusive.

PROGENITOR CELLS

To meet the cell demands imposed upon the hematopoietic system, some stem cells ultimately undergo differentiation. Upon commitment to development, the stem cell enters another compartment, the progenitor cell (PC) compartment. Initially, the daughter cells arising from undifferentiated stem cells retain the potential to generate cells of all hematopoietic lineages (multipotential progenitor cells). After additional divisions, however, the progeny of daughter cells lose their ability to generate cells of progressively more lineages, gradually becoming restricted in differentiation potential to a single cell line (unilineage or committed progenitor cells). The progenitor cell compartment includes precursor cells developmentally located between stem cells and the morphologically recognizable precursor cells.

The PC compartment is larger than the HSC compartment, constituting ~3% of the total nucleated hematopoietic cells. PCs possess limited self-renewal ability; in general their process of cell division is obligatorily linked to differentiation. They are, in essence, transit cells said to be on a suicide maturation pathway (since full maturation and differentiation results in a *terminally differentiated* cell with a finite life span). Like the HSC, PCs are not morphologically identifiable but are functionally defined based on the mature progeny that they produce. Both multipotential and unipotential PCs can be assayed by their ability to form colonies of cells in semisolid media in vitro and are described as *colony-forming units* (CFU) with the appropriate lineage(s) appended. Thus, a CFU-GEMM would be a progenitor cell capable of giving rise to a mixture of all myeloid lineages: **g**ranulocytic, **e**rythrocytic, **m**onocytic, and **m**egakaryocytic, while a CFU-GM would be a bipotential PC with both granulocytic and monocytic differentiation potential, and a CFU-Mk would be a unilineage progenitor giving rise exclusively to cells of the megakaryocytic series. PCs are mitotically more active than stem cells and are capable of expanding the size of the PC compartment by proliferation in response to increased needs of the body. Thus the PC compartment has a potentially *amplifying* population of cells, as opposed to the stable size of the stem cell compartment.

Lineage commitment is a fundamental but poorly understood step in normal hematopoiesis. The factors that regulate this process remain unknown. It is clear, however, that differentiation is accompanied by the increased expression of certain lineage-specific genes. The survival and differentiation of hematopoietic precursor cells is influenced by a number of growth-regulatory glycoproteins, or cytokines (see cytokine section).

MATURING CELLS

After a series of amplifying cell divisions, the committed precursor undergoes a further change when the cell takes on the morphological characteristics of its cell line. Maturing cells constitute by far the majority of hematopoietic precursor cells; proliferation and amplification boosts these cells to over 95% of the total hematopoietic cells. In general, the capacity to proliferate is lost before full maturation of these cells is complete. They exhibit recognizable nuclear and cytoplasmic morphologic characteristics that can be used to classify their lineage. Since these cells can be morphologically categorized, different nomenclature is used. Generally, the earliest morphologically recognizable cell of each lineage is identified by the suffix *-blast,* with the lineage indicated (i.e., lymphoblast [lymphocytes], myeloblast [granulocytes], or megakaryoblast [megakaryocytes/platelets]). In some lineages, additional differentiation stages are indicated by prefixes or qualifying adjectives (i.e., proerythroblast, basophilic erythroblast, etc.). A complete discussion of the stages of maturing cells of each lineage can be found in the appropriate chapters (∞ Chapter 4, erythrocytic; Chapter 6, granulocytic and lymphocytic).

HEMATOPOIETIC PRECURSOR CELL MODEL

The head of this hierarchy of hematopoietic cells is the *pluripotent hematopoietic stem cell (HSC)*. This is the population of cells that has full self-renewal abilities and that gives rise to all the other hematopoietic elements (Figure 2-11 ■).

The earliest differentiating daughters of the HSC are slightly more restricted in differentiation potential. One group of daughter cells are thought to be precursor cells ca-

pable of giving rise to cells of the lymphoid system (the *common lymphoid progenitor cell [CLP]*). (The existence of a common lymphoid progenitor cell common to B and T [and presumably natural killer, NK] lineages has never been established experimentally.) The other group of daughter cells are restricted to producing cells of the myeloid system (the cell lineages of the bone marrow), the *common myeloid progenitor cell (CMP)*. These cells, although multipotential, have restricted self-renewal ability and are ultimately destined to differentiate. Until recently, these early progenitor cells were

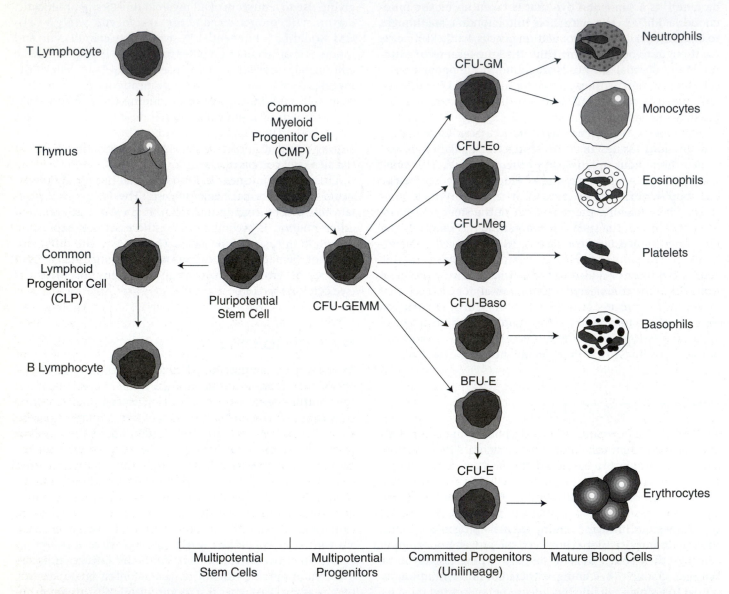

■ **FIGURE 2-11** The differentiation of blood cells from a pluripotential stem cell. The pluripotential stem cell and the colony forming unit-granulocyte, erythrocyte, macrophage, megakaryocyte (CFU-GEMM) have the potential to differentiate into one of several cell lines and are therefore multilineage precursor cells. The committed progenitors—(colony-forming unit) CFU-GM (granulocyte, monocyte), CFU-Eo (eosinophil), CFU-Mk (megakaryocyte), CFU-Baso (basophil), and (burst-forming unit) BFU-E and CFU-E (erythrocyte)—differentiate into only one cell line (unilineage) except for the CFU-GM, which is bipotential. The BFU-E is more immature than the CFU-E. The mature blood cells are those found in the peripheral blood. The common lymphoid progenitor cell (CLP) may differentiate into either T- or B-lymphocytes.

identified as myeloid stem cells (or MSC) and lymphoid stem cells (LSC). However, these cells are not true stem cells, and should not carry labels suggesting they are. They lack the essential defining stem cell characteristics of pluripotential differentiation capabilities and self-renewal.

Following additional differentiation steps, the CLP gives rise to T and B lymphocytes and NK cells, while the CMP gives rise to at least six different lines of cellular differentiation, ultimately producing mature neutrophils, monocytes, eosinophils, basophils, erythrocytes, and megakaryocytes/platelets. One of the first precursor cells defined as arising from the CMP was the CFU-GEMM, a cell capable of producing colonies in culture consisting of granulocytic, eosinophilic, erythrocytic, and megakaryocytic elements. However, it soon was shown that there are layers of functionally defined cells between the true CMP and the CFU-GEMM. Various authors have assigned names to these intermediate cells, including CFU-Blast,[34] HPP-CFC[35] (high proliferative potential, colony-forming cell), CFU-D12[36] (colony-forming unit, day 12), LT-CIC[37] (long-term culture initiating cell). Whether these represent distinct subpopulations of early progenitor cells or overlapping subpopulations is unclear at the present time. In general, they require 2–7 growth factors for optimal growth, are characterized by their capacity to produce large colonies of cells (>50,000 cells per colony) after prolonged growth periods in culture, and represent cell populations more primitive than the CFU-GEMM.[38]

The sequence of events during the differentiation of a myeloid multipotential progenitor cell (CFU-GEMM) to a unilineage, committed progenitor cell is unclear. There is no set program governing the progressive restriction of differentiation potential beyond the CMP/CLP split. Thus, in vitro assays reveal various combinations of bi-, tri-, quatra-, penta-, and hexa-potential progenitors that may be generated by this pathway. Neutrophils and monocytes are derived from a common committed bipotential progenitor cell, the CFU-GM, which ultimately gives rise to lineage restricted and morphologically recognizable precursor cells (myeloblasts and monoblasts). Each of the unilineage or committed progenitor cells is named for the cell line to which it is committed (e.g., CFU-Mk for megakaryocytes, CFU-E for erythrocytes, CFU-M for monocytes, CFU-G for neutrophils, CFU-Eo, for eosinophils, and CFU-B for basophils). Within some lineages, there are designated subpopulations of committed progenitor cells. Thus, committed erythroid progenitors are designated as erythroid burst-forming units (BFU-E) and erythroid colony forming units (CFU-E), with the BFU-E being the more primitive precursor cell, antecedent to the CFU-E. A similar BFU-Mk/CFU-Mk hierarchy has been described for the megakaryocyte lineage.[39] Each committed progenitor cell differentiates into morphologically identifiable precursors of their respective lineage (e.g., CFU-E → Proerythroblast; CFU-G → myeloblast, etc.).

Under normal steady-state physiological conditions, the majority of hematopoietic precursor cells (SC and PC) are retained in the bone marrow. A small population of SC and PC can, however, be found circulating in the peripheral blood. The number of circulating SC/PC can be further increased by the infusion of various cytokines, allowing for the possibility of obtaining "mobilized" peripheral blood SC/PC for transplantation purposes rather than from a direct bone marrow harvest.

✓ **Checkpoint! #3**

Hematopoietic stem cells that have initiated a differentiation program are sometimes described as undergoing death by differentiation. Explain.

► ## CYTOKINES AND THE CONTROL OF HEMATOPOIESIS

The regulation of hematopoietic stem/progenitor cell differentiation and expansion is critical because it determines the concentration of various cell lines in the marrow and eventually in the peripheral blood. Hematopoietic precursor cell survival, self-renewal, proliferation, and differentiation are governed by specific glycoproteins called hematopoietic growth factors, or **cytokines** (Figure 2-12). Growth factor control of hematopoiesis is an extraordinarily complex and highly efficient intercellular molecular communication system that allows the coordinated increases in the production and functional activity of appropriate hematopoietic cell types without expansion of the irrelevant ones. These growth factors were originally described as *colony-stimulating factors* (CSFs) because they sustained the growth of hematopoietic colonies in in vitro cultures, although subsequently the system of nomenclature has changed to that of *interleukins*. Currently, when a new cytokine is discovered, the initial description is based on its biologic properties, and once the amino acid sequence is defined, an interleukin number is assigned. The system has some exceptions and inconsistencies, however. For historic reasons, some cytokines retain their original names (e.g., GM-CSF, G-CSF, M-CSF, EPO, and TPO). For other cytokines, the initial research into their biologic activities focused on activities outside of hematopoietic regulation, and their original names have been retained (e.g., kit-ligand/SCF, Flt ligand).

The growth of hematopoietic precursor cells requires the continuous presence of growth factors (GFs). If the relevant GFs are withdrawn, the cells die within hours, with death occurring by the active process of self-destruction or apoptosis. Thus, the first effect of GFs is to promote cell survival by suppressing apoptosis (programmed cell death). Secondly, GFs promote proliferation. Hematopoietic cells are intrinsically incapable of unstimulated cell division. All cell division or proliferation is dependent on the continuous stimulation by

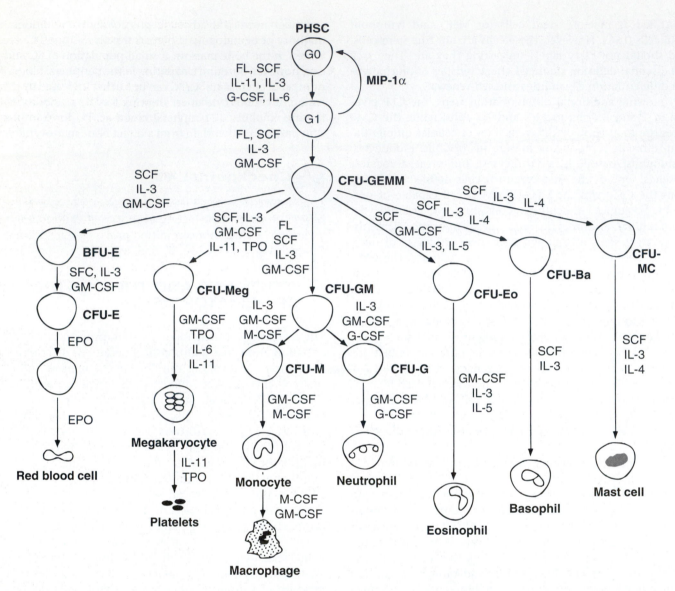

■ **FIGURE 2-12** The pluripotential hematopoietic stem cell (PHSC) gives rise to erythrocytes, platelets, monocytes, macrophages, and granulocytes. This cell can also differentiate into lymphoid cells. Under specific stimulation from growth factors Flt3 ligand (FL); stem cell factor (SCF); and interleukins (IL-3, 6, 11), the PHSC in quiescence (G0) enters the cell cycle (G1) and differentiates to the common myeloid progenitor cell (CMP) and, subsequently, to the colony-forming unit-granulocyte, erythroid, macrophage, megakaryocyte (CFU-GEMM). The CFU-GEMM then differentiates into granulocytes, erythrocytes, monocytes, and megakaryocytes under the influence of specific growth factors, erythropoietin (EPO), thrombopoietin (TPO), granulocyte-monocyte colony-stimulating factor (GM-CSF), granulocyte colony stimulating factor (G-CSF), macrophage colony-stimulating factor (M-CSF), and interleukin-5 (IL-5).

appropriate regulatory cytokines. Finally, GFs control and regulate the processes of differentiation, which ultimately produce the mature functional cells from their multipotential progenitor cell precursors (Figure 2-12 ■).

CHARACTERISTICS OF GROWTH FACTORS

Although many different cytokines have been identified as hematopoietic growth factors, there are a number of characteristics which many of them share (Table 2-8 ✪). Growth factors are produced by a number of different cells, including

monocytes, macrophages, activated T lymphocytes, fibroblasts, and endothelial cells. With the notable exception of erythropoietin (EPO), most GFs are produced by stromal cells in the hematopoietic microenvironment (see below). EPO production is atypical of the lymphohematopoietic GFs in that it is produced mainly in the kidney, released into the peripheral blood, and is carried to the bone marrow where it regulates red blood cell production. As such, it is the only true hormone, as the majority of the other cytokines exert their effects on cells in the local environment where they are produced. Often, a single stromal cell source may produce multiple cytokines.

✪ TABLE 2-8

Characteristics of Hematopoietic Growth Factors

- GFs are produced by stromal cells in the hematopoietic microenvironment.
- GFs have multiple biologic activities.
- Individual GFs, by themselves, are poor stimulators of colony growth; control of hematopoiesis generally involves the interplay of at least several GFs.
- GFs interact with membrane receptors, restricted to cells of appropriate lineage.
- GF requirements change during the differentiation process.
- GFs can affect hematopoiesis directly or indirectly.
- Regulatory cytokines are organized in a complex, interdependent network and exhibit many signal amplification circuits.
- GFs commonly act synergistically with other cytokines.
- GFs that induce proliferation of precursor cells sometimes have the capacity to enhance the functional activity of the terminally differentiated progeny of these precursor cells.

The majority of GFs are not lineage specific; each GF has multiple functions, and most of the GFs act on more than one cell type (i.e., they are *pleiotrophic*) (Table 2-9 ✪). Cytokines must be bound to surface receptors on their target cells to express their activity. They interact with membrane receptors restricted to cells of the appropriate lineage. Since many precursor cells respond to more than one GF, they obviously express receptors for multiple GFs. Some GFs influence hematopoiesis directly by binding to receptors on precursor cells and inducing the appropriate response (survival, proliferation, differentiation). Other GFs influence the process indirectly by binding to receptors on accessory cells, which in turn respond by releasing other cytokines. Some GFs trigger cell division, while others support survival without inducing proliferation.

Hematopoietic regulatory cytokines interact in a highly ordered, interdependent network, creating a complex cell-to-cell communication system. Individual GFs, by themselves, are poor stimulators of colony growth; the control of hematopoiesis generally involves the interplay of at least several GFs. Some GFs act synergistically with other cytokines (synergism is when the net effect of two or more events is greater than the sum of the individual events). The cytokine network often exhibits signal amplification circuits, including autocrine, paracrine, and juxtacrine mechanisms of stimulation/amplification.

GF requirements change during the differentiation process, so that the cytokines/GFs needed by the HSC and early multipotential PC differ from the GF requirements of the later, lineage restricted progenitors and the maturing precursor cells. These are described as early-acting (multilineage) GFs and later-acting (lineage-restricted GFs), respectively. Some GFs that induce the proliferation of precursor cells also have the capacity to enhance the functional activity of the terminally differentiated progeny of those precursor cells. GFs and their receptors share a number of structural features, perhaps explaining some of observed functional redundancies. Most of the GFs have been cloned and characterized, and recombinant proteins are available; certain of these GFs have been shown to have important clinical applications.

Early-Acting (Multilineage) Growth Factors

Several GFs have direct effects on multipotential precursor cells and thus are capable of inducing cell production within several lineages. Early acting cytokines affect primarily proliferation of these noncommitted progenitor cells. These include SCF, FL, IL-3, GM-CSF, IL-6, and IL-11. Although these factors can initiate proliferation in several cell lines, in many instances additional factors are necessary for the production of mature cells in these lineages (Figure 2-12 ■).

Stem Cell Factor and Flt3 Ligand. Stem cell factor (SCF), [also known as steel factor (SF), kit ligand (KL), or mast cell growth factor (MCGF)] promotes the proliferation and differentiation of primitive multilineage progenitor cells as well as committed progenitor cells (CFU-GEMM, CFU-GM, CFU-Mk, BFU-E). SCF also promotes the survival, proliferation, and differentiation of mast cell precursors and has functional activity outside of the hematopoietic system, playing a role in normal melanocyte development and gametogenesis. Flt3 Ligand-responsive (FL-responsive) hematopoietic cells appear to be more primitive than SCF-responsive cells. FL increases recruitment of primitive HPC into the cell cycle and inhibits apoptosis.[40] In contrast to SCF, FL has little effect on unilineage BFU-E/CFU-E, CFU-mast cell, or CFU-Eo but is a potent stimulator of granulomonocytic, B cell, and dendritic cell proliferation and differentiation. FL and SCF have similar protein structures, and share some common characteristics. Both cytokines may be found as either membrane-bound or soluble forms, although the membrane-bound form may be more important physiologically.[41] Neither cytokine has independent in vitro colony stimulating activity, but both act synergistically with IL-3, GM-CSF, G-CSF, and other cytokines to promote early progenitor cell proliferation.

Interleukin 3 and GM-CSF. Interleukin 3 (IL-3) was one of the earliest recognized multipotential growth factors, affecting multilineage progenitor cells and early committed progenitors like BFU-E. IL-3 also has indirect actions and can induce the expression of other cytokines. GM-CSF is also a multipotential GF, stimulating clonal growth of CFU-GEMM, BFU-E, CFU-Mk, CFU-GM, and CFU-Eo. Thus it is a major promoter of granulocyte and monocyte differentiation but lacks a significant effect on basophil production. GM-CSF also activates the functional activity of most mature phagocytes, including neutrophils, macrophages, and eosinophils.

⭐ TABLE 2-9

Hematopoietic Growth Factors (GFs)

GF	Mol. Wt.	Chromosome	Source	Major Target Cells
EPO	34–39,000	7	Kidney (liver)	Erythroid
GM-CSF	18–30,000	5	T cells; E.C.; Fibroblasts; Mast cells	Granulocytes, monos, eos, erythroid, megs, progenitor cells
IL-3	14–28,000	5	Activ T cells, mast cells	Granulocytes, monos, eos, erythroid, megs basos, progenitor cells
G-CSF	18,888	17	Monos, macros, fibroblasts, E.C.	Granulocytes; early progenitor cells
M-CSF	70–90,000	1	Monos, macros, fibroblasts, E.C.	Monos, macros, osteoclasts
IL-1	17,000	2	Monos, lymphs, E.C., fibroblasts	Monos, E.C., fibroblasts, lymphs, PMN, early progenitor cells
IL-2	23,000	4	Activ T cells	Prolif and activ of T, B and NK cells
IL-4	18,000	5	Activ T cells	Stim T_H2, suppress T_H1; B cells, mast cells basos, fibroblasts
IL-5	50–60,000	5	Activ T cells	Eos, B cells, cytotoxic T cells
IL-6	21–26,000	7	Fibroblasts, E.C., macros, T cells	Early progenitor cells; B & T cells; megs; myeloid; myeloma cells
IL-7	17,000	8	Stromal cells	Pre-T, pre-B cells; T_S differentiation
IL-8	8,000	4	Monos, macros, E.C., fibroblasts	Activ of granulocytes (chemokine)
IL-9	40,000	5	Activ T cells	T cells; early erythroid; mast cells
IL-10	18,000	1	T cells, monos, macros, Activ B cells	B cells; mast cells; T_H2 cells; inhib T_H1 cells
IL-11	24,000	19	Stromal cells, fibroblasts	B cells; megs; early progenitor cells
IL-12	75,000	?	B cells; monos; macros	T cells; NK cells
IL-13	18,000	5	T cells; basos	Isotype switching of B cells; inhib cytotoxic & inflamm functions of monos and macros
IL-14	53–65,000	?	T cells	Activ B cells
IL-15	14–18,000	4	Monos, macros, E.C., fibroblasts	T cells (CTL), NK cells (LAK); co-stim for B cells
IL-16	16–18,000	?	T cells, Eos, mast cells	Chemotactic for CD4$^+$ T cells, monos, eos
IL-17	22,000	?	Activ T cells	Induces cytokine production by stromal cells
IL-18	18,000	?	Macros, keratinocytes	Induces IFN production by lymphocytes
SCF/KL	28–36,000	12	Fibroblasts, E.C., stromal cells	Stem cells, progenitor cells; mast cells
FL	18,000	19	Stromal cells, monos, macros, T cells	Stem cells, progenitor cells; B cells; dendritic cells
TPO	65–85,000	3	Stromal cells; hepatocytes	Megs; early progenitor cells

Abbreviations used. T cell, B cell = T or B lymphocytes; NK = natural killer cells; E.C. = endothelial cells; monos = monocytes; macros = macrophages; basos = basophils; eos = eosinophils; megs = megakaryocytes; PMN = neutrophils; activ = activates; inhib = inhibits; activ T cells = T lymphocytes activated by antigens, mitogens, or cytokines; CTL = cytotoxic T lymphocytes; LAK = lymphokine activated killer cells.

Interleukin 6 and Interleukin 11. Interleukin 6 (IL-6) and Interleukin 11 (IL-11) are pleiotropic cytokines with overlapping growth stimulatory effects on myeloid and lymphoid cells as well as on primitive multilineage cells.[42,43] Each cytokine rarely acts alone but functions synergistically with IL-3, SCF, and other cytokines in supporting hematopoiesis. Both cytokines have significant effects on megakaryocytopoiesis and platelet production. Both also mediate the acute phase response of hepatocytes and are major pyrogens in vivo. IL-11 shortens the duration of G_0 of primitive hematopoietic progenitor cells and hastens hematopoietic recovery after treatment with cytotoxic agents or bone marrow transplantation.[44]

Later Acting (Lineage-Restricted) Growth Factors

The growth factors included here tend to have a narrower spectrum of influence and function primarily to induce maturation along a specific cell line. However, most are not lineage-specific, but rather demonstrate a predominant effect on the committed progenitor cell of a single lineage, inducing differentiation of these more mature cells. These include granulocyte colony stimulating factor/G-CSF (granulocytes), monocyte colony stimulating factor/M-CSF (monocytes), erythropoietin/EPO (erythrocytes), thrombopoietin/TPO (megakaryocytes and platelets), interleukin-5/IL-5 (eosinophils), and the other interleukins important in lymphopoiesis (ILs-2, -4, -7, -10, -12, -13, -14, -15).

EPO is the only cytokine to function as a true hormone, as it is produced at a distant site and must travel to the bone marrow to influence erythrocyte production. It is expressed largely by cells in the liver in embryonic life and by cells of the kidney (and to a lesser extent, liver) in adult life. Its release is regulated by the oxygen needs of the body, being induced by hypoxia. EPO stimulates growth, survival, and differentiation of erythroid progenitor cells (with its major effect on CFU-E) and stimulates proliferation and RNA synthesis in more well-differentiated maturing cells. Reticulocytes and mature erythrocytes do not have receptors for EPO and thus are not influenced by this growth factor.

G-CSF, M-CSF, and IL-5 stimulate the proliferation of granulocyte, monocyte/macrophage, and eosinophil progenitor cells, respectively. All three also influence the function of mature cells of their respective lineages, increasing migration, phagocytosis, and metabolic activities and augmenting prolongation of their lifespans. M-CSF also regulates the genesis of osteoclasts, while IL-5 stimulates lymphocyte development.

TPO, also known as mpl-ligand or megakaryocyte growth and development factor (MGDF), is the major physiologic regulator of megakaryocyte proliferation and platelet production. In vitro, TPO primes mature platelets to respond to aggregation-inducing stimuli and increases the platelet release reaction.[45] TPO also synergizes with a variety of other GFs (SCF, IL-3, FL) to stimulate the growth of primitive progenitor cells.

Indirect-Acting Growth Factors

Some cytokines that regulate hematopoiesis do so indirectly, by inciting accessory cells to release direct-acting factors. An example is IL-1, which has no colony-stimulating activity itself. However, when administered in vivo, it induces neutrophilic leukocytosis, resulting from the release of other direct-acting cytokines by accessory cells.

LINEAGE-SPECIFIC CYTOKINE REGULATION

Erythropoiesis

In the erythroid system, progenitor cells give rise to two distinct types of erythroid colonies in culture. A primitive progenitor cell, the BFU-E, is relatively insensitive to EPO and forms large colonies after 14 days in the form of bursts. Production of BFU-E colonies was originally described as being supported by *burst-promoting activity,* or BPA, now known to be due to IL-3 or GM-CSF. CFU-E colonies grow to maximal size in 7 to 8 days and depend primarily on EPO. The CFU-E are the descendants of BFU-E and subsequently give rise to the first recognizable erythrocyte precursor, the pronormoblast. Other cytokines reported to influence production of red cells include IL-9, IL-11, and SCF. However, EPO is the pivotal humoral factor that functions to prevent programmed cell death

of the most committed erythroid progenitor cells and their progeny.

Granulopoiesis and Monopoiesis

Granulocytes and monocytes are derived from a common bipotential progenitor cell, the colony-forming unit-granulocyte, monocyte (CFU-GM) a progeny of the CFU-GEMM. Specific GFs for granulocytes and monocytes, acting synergistically with GM-CSF or IL-3, support the differentiation pathway of each lineage. M-CSF supports monocyte differentiation, while G-CSF induces neutrophilic granulocyte differentiation. Eosinophils and basophils also are derived from the CFU-GEMM under the influence of growth factors.

Megakaryocytopoiesis/Thrombopoiesis

Platelets are derived from megakaryocytes, which are progeny of the CFU-GEMM. CFU-Mk are induced to proliferate and differentiate into megakaryocytes by several cytokines. However, the cytokines that induce the greatest increase in platelet production are IL-11 and TPO.

Lymphopoiesis

The growth and development of lymphoid cells from the common lymphoid progenitor cell occurs in multiple anatomic locations, including the bone marrow, thymus, and lymph nodes and spleen. Multiple GFs play a role in T and B lymphocyte growth and development, most of which act synergistically.

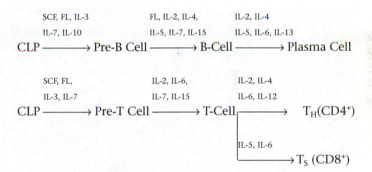

(CLP—common lymphoid progenitor)

> ✔ **Checkpoint! #4**
>
> *Cytokine control of hematopoiesis is said to be characterized by redundancy and pleiotrophy. What does this mean?*

NEGATIVE REGULATORS OF HEMATOPOIESIS

In addition to the well-studied positive GFs that function as positive regulators of hematopoiesis, there exists a second group of polypeptides that inhibit cellular proliferation. The proliferation of hematopoietic precursor cells can be limited by either decreasing production of stimulating factors or increasing factors that inhibit cell growth. There appears to be a homeostatic network of counteracting growth inhibitors secreted in response to GFs, which normally limit cell proliferation after growth stimuli. These negative regulators of hematopoiesis may be responsible for the quiescent state, with respect to DNA synthesis, of stem cells and early progenitor cells. Alternatively, they may oppose the actions of positive regulators that act on these same cells. Whether or not precursor cells synthesize DNA and proliferate depends on a balance between these opposing influences.

Negative regulators of hematopoiesis include:

- Interferons
- TGF-β
- TNF
- PGEs
- Acidic isoferritins
- Lactoferrin
- Di-OH vitamin D_3
- T_s and NK cells
- SCI (MIP-1α)

The interferons and transforming growth factor-β (TGF-β) suppress hematopoietic progenitor cells, largely by inhibiting proliferation or inducing programmed cell death. Tumor necrosis factor (TNF) directly suppresses colony growth of CFU-GEMM, CFU-GM, and BFU-E, while prostaglandins of the E series (PGEs) suppress granulopoiesis and monopoiesis by inhibiting CFU-GM, CFU-G, and CFU-M. Acidic ferritins and lactoferrin are products of mature neutrophils that inhibit hematopoiesis via feedback regulation. Di-hydroxyvitamin D_3 (Di-OH Vitamin D3), classically associated with the stimulation of bone formation, also functions to inhibit myelopoiesis. Additionally, there are cellular components of the immune system, including T-suppressor (Ts) cells and NK cells, that function as negative regulators of hematopoiesis.

Stem cell inhibitor (SCI), also known as macrophage inflammatory protein-1α (MIP-1α), is believed to be a primary negative regulator of stem cell proliferation.[46] It is believed to be a locally acting regulatory element, present in the stromal microenvironment, that controls the steady-state quiescence of stem cells. It functions via juxtacrine interactions between stromal cells and stem cells (see below) to maintain stem cells in the G_0 phase of the cell cycle.

HEMATOPOIETIC GROWTH FACTOR RECEPTORS

Cytokines require surface receptors on their target cells to express their activity. They interact with membrane receptors restricted to cells of the appropriate lineage. Binding of a cytokine (ligand) to its specific receptor transduces an intracellular signal through which the particular survival, prolif-

eration, or differentiation responses are initiated. The intracellular portion of the receptor binds to associated intracellular molecules that activate signaling pathways. These signaling molecules translocate to the nucleus and activate gene transcription. Ultimately, changes in protein synthesis lead to alterations in cell proliferation or other modifications of cellular response induced by the cytokine involved. Many of these receptors have been characterized, and they can be grouped according to certain structural characteristics.

Receptors with Cytoplasmic Tyrosine Kinase Domains

These are all transmembrane proteins with cytoplasmic domains that contain a tyrosine kinase catalytic site. When GF binds to the receptor, the receptor chains dimerize, which enhances the catalytic activity of the kinase domain and activates intracellular signaling pathways. Included in this group are the receptors for M-CSF, SCF, and FL.

Hematopoietic Growth Factor Receptor Superfamily

The receptors for the majority of hematopoietic GFs do not possess intrinsic kinase activity but lead to phosphorylation of cellular substrates by serving as docking sites for adaptor molecules that do have kinase activity. All are multichain integral membrane proteins that demonstrate enhanced binding and/or signal transduction (phosphorylation of cellular proteins) when expressed as a heterodimer or homodimer. The receptors for many of the GF receptors in this large group share peptide subunits with other receptors. There are three major subgroups:

1. IL-3, IL-5, and GM-CSF receptors have unique ligand-specific α chains but share a common β chain. Association of the two chains, induced by ligand binding, results in the formation of a specific high-affinity receptor capable of effective signaling.

2. IL-6 and IL-11 similarly have ligand-specific α chains and share a common β chain called GP 130. The GP 130 β chain is also shared by three other cytokines, leukemia inhibitory factor (LIF), oncostatin M, and ciliary neurotrophic factor (CNTF).

3. The receptor complexes for many of the factors that influence lymphopoiesis are shared as well, including the receptors for IL-2, IL-4, IL-7, IL-9, IL-13, and IL-15. All six receptors have unique, ligand-specific α chains, and share a common γ chain. IL-2 and IL-15 are trimeric structures and share a common β subunit as well.

It has been suggested that the functional *redundancy* seen in the cytokine regulation of hematopoiesis (i.e., the fact that often multiple GFs have overlapping activities) may be at least partly explained by the sharing of common receptor subunits. For example, IL-3 and GM-CSF have very similar spectra of biologic activities and share a common β subunit. Likewise, IL-6 and IL-11 both have megakaryocytic activity and both stimulate the hepatic acute phase response; similarly, they share a common β subunit, GP 130.

A recent finding in receptor biology is the fact that most receptors have discrete functional domains in the cytoplasmic region of one or more of the receptor chains. Thus, mutations disrupting a discrete domain of the receptor may disrupt part, but not all, of the functions of that receptor. Kostmann's syndrome (congenital agranulocytosis) is a rare disorder characterized by a profound absolute neutropenia with a maturation arrest of precursor cells at the promyelocyte/myelocyte stage. Erythropoiesis and thrombopoiesis are normal. In some patients exhibiting this syndrome, molecular studies have revealed a mutation of the G-CSF receptor that disrupts a terminal *maturation-inducing* domain but leaves intact a subterminal *proliferation-inducing* domain.[47] Thus these patients sustain proliferation of neutrophilic progenitor and early maturing cells but fail to complete final maturation of cells in this lineage. Similarly, some individuals with previously unexplained erythrocytosis (i.e., *not* secondary to smoking, high altitude, or increased EPO levels) have been shown to have a mutation affecting their EPO-receptors.[48] The EPO-R has been shown to have two separate domains in the cytoplasmic region of the receptor—one domain closest to the membrane, which constitutes a positive control domain promoting proliferation, and a terminal, negative control domain, which slows down the intracellular signaling from the receptor. In some patients with familial erythrocytosis, studies have revealed a mutation resulting in the generation of a truncated protein receptor that lacks the terminal negative control domain. The loss of this negative control region results in enhanced responsiveness of target cells (BFU-E and CFU-E) to the growth stimulatory effects of EPO, resulting in a (benign) erythrocytosis.

✔ ### Checkpoint! #5

Individuals with congenital defects of the γ chain of the IL-2 receptor suffer from profound defects of lymphopoiesis, far greater than individuals with congenital defects of the α chain of the IL-2 receptor. Why?

Clinical Use of Hematopoietic Growth Factors

The cloning and characterization of genes encoding the hematopoietic GFs have allowed scientists to produce these cytokines in large quantity using recombinant DNA technology. This has provided the opportunity for using GFs in therapeutic regimens for hematopoietic disorders (Table 2-10 ✪).

✪ TABLE 2-10

Clinical Applications of Hematopoietic Growth Factors

- Stimulation of erythropoiesis in renal disease (EPO)
- Recovery from treatment-induced myelosuppression (G-CSF and GM-CSF)
- Therapy of myelodysplastic syndromes (IL-3, GM-CSF, EPO)
- Enhanced killing of malignant cells (IL-2, etc.)
- Priming of bone marrow for donation (IL-3, G-CSF, GM-CSF, FL)
- Stimulation of malignant cells to differentiate (various)
- Enhancement of the acute phase response (IL-1, IL-6)
- Enhancement of the immune system (IL-2, IL-15, etc.)
- Stimulation of marrow recovery in BM transplantation (G-CSF, GM-CSF, EPO, IL-11)
- Treatment in bone marrow failure (IL-3, G-CSF, GM-CSF)

Those cytokines that have been approved by the Food and Drug Administration (FDA) for clinical use include G-CSF and GM-CSF (used primarily to accelerate recovery from granulocytopenia); EPO (for treatment of anemia of various etiologies); IL-11 (for treatment of thrombocytopenia); the interferons (IFNα, IFNβ and IFNγ, used to treat a number of malignant and nonmalignant disorders); and IL-2 (for treatment of metastatic renal cell cancer and melanoma). In vitro studies clearly show that cytokines, used in combination, often show synergy in terms of their biologic effects. Consequently, the use of combinations of growth factors is being evaluated clinically as well, often with dramatic results. For a more thorough discussion of the biologic therapies currently in clinical use or undergoing clinical evaluations, see Gordon and Sosman.[49]

HEMATOPOIETIC MICROENVIRONMENT

It has long been known that hematopoiesis is normally confined to certain organs and tissues (∞ Chapter 3). The proliferation and maturation of hematopoietic precursor cells takes place within the context of a microenvironment that provides the appropriate milieu for these events.[50] Patients undergoing bone marrow transplants receive the donor cells by intravenous infusion; the cells "home in" and initiate significant hematopoiesis only in the recipient's bone marrow. No biologically significant hematopoietic activity occurs in nonhematopoietic organs. For successful engraftment, the HSC require an appropriate microenvironment, which presumably has specific properties that make it a unique site for stem cell renewal, growth, and differentiation.

The term **hematopoietic microenvironment** (HM) is used to refer to this localized environment in the stroma of hematopoietic organs crucial for the development of hematopoietic cells. It consists of a complex network of cells

⊕ TABLE 2-11

Hematopoietic Microenvironment

Cellular (Stroma)		Extracellular	
Components	Function	Components	Function
Adipocytes, endothelial cells, fibroblasts, T-cells, macrophages	• Expression of homing receptors • Production of soluble growth and differentiation factors • Production of integral membrane proteins that function as juxtacrine regulators (SCF, FL) • Production of ECM components	Soluble factors (cytokines and growth factors) Extracellular matrix (ECM) • Collagen, • Glycosaminoglycans (heparan, chondroitin, dermatan-sulfate) • Cytoadhesion molecules	• Regulation of hematopoietic stem/progenitor cell differentiation and expansion. • Structural support • Cell-to-cell interactions; localization of growth factors • Adhesion of hematopoietic precursors to ECM proteins

and extracellular matrix components (Table 2-11 ⊕) that maintains the hematopoietic system throughout the lifetime of the individual. The HM is still relatively poorly understood but is being actively investigated. It includes cellular elements and extracellular components including matrix proteins and regulatory cytokines. The HM provides homing and adhesive interactions important for the colocalization of stem cells, progenitor cells, and growth regulatory proteins within the marrow cavity.

Stromal Cells

The cellular elements of the HM are sometimes referred to as hematopoietic **stromal cells.** They include adipocytes (fat cells), endothelial cells, fibroblasts (referred to by some authors as reticular cells), T lymphocytes, and macrophages. Although the last two cell types are actually hematopoietic cells, they are included in the discussion of stromal cells because they are important sources of cytokine production. The stromal cells' capacity to support hematopoiesis derives from a number of characteristics: they are thought to express homing receptors, although the exact mechanisms involved in mediating homing of hematopoietic cells is unclear; they produce and secrete a number of soluble growth and differentiation factors, as well as a number of membrane-bound cytokines that function as juxtacrine regulators of hematopoiesis (such as SCF and FL); and finally, they produce the various components constituting the extracellular matrix of the HM.

Extracellular Matrix

The **extracellular matrix** (ECM), produced and secreted by the stromal cells, provides the adhesive interactions important for the colocalization of stem cells (SC), progenitor cells (PC), and the growth regulatory proteins. The ECM is composed of collagens, glycoproteins, and glycosaminoglycans. Variations in the type and relative amounts of these components produce the characteristic properties of ECMs in different tissues. Collagen provides the structural support for the other components. Glycosaminoglycans (heparan-sulfate, chondroitin-sulfate, dermatan-sulfate) play a role in cell-cell interactions, helping to mediate progenitor-cell binding to the stroma. They also serve to bind and localize cytokines in the vicinity of the hematopoietic cells.

Within the hematopoietic bone marrow, precursor cells of different lineages and at different stages of differentiation can be found in distinct areas throughout the marrow space. Precursor cells at different stages of differentiation can interact with certain but not all ECM components and can be induced to proliferate or differentiate by some but not all cytokines. It has been proposed that at specific stages of differentiation specialized stromal cells produce extracellular matrix components and hematopoietic supportive cytokines that are conducive for the commitment and/or differentiation of precursor cells of a specific hematopoietic lineage. These interactions could then explain the observed tight regulation precursor cell differentiation and proliferation.[51]

One of the important molecular determinants of the geographic localization of hematopoiesis appears to be the presence of membrane receptors on hematopoietic precursors for ECM proteins. Fibronectin (FN) is a large, adhesive glycoprotein that can bind cells, growth factors, and ECM components. SC/PC and developing erythroblasts have an FN receptor on their surface membrane. As developing erythroblasts mature to the reticulocyte stage, they lose that FN receptor; loss of attachment via FN facilitates the egress of reticulocytes and erythrocytes from the erythroblastic islands in the bone marrow. Likewise, hemonectin (HN) is an adhesive glycoprotein on SC, PC, and granulocytes that is important for the attachment of these cells to the marrow. Loss of HN receptors by developing granulo-

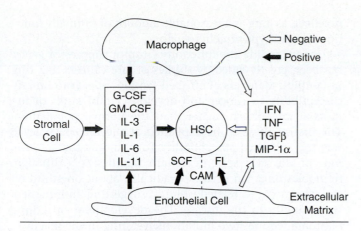

FIGURE 2-13 A model for regulation of hematopoietic precursor cells in the bone marrow microenvironment. The hematopoietic stem cell (HSC) attaches to bone marrow stromal cells via specific receptors and ligands. The HSC is then influenced by both positive and negative regulatory growth factors. (CAM: cell adhesion molecule; SCF: stem cell factor; FL: Flt3-ligand; IFN: interferon; TNF: tumor necrosis factor; TGFβ transforming growth factor β; MIP-1α: macrophage inflammatory protein-1α (stem cell inhibitor); G-CSF: granulocyte-colony stimulating factor; GM-CSF: granulocyte-monocyte CSF; IL-: interleukin-).

cytes and loss of adhesion to ECM mediates release of mature granulocytes to the circulation. Adhesive interactions between the SC, PC, and the ECM function to help hold the hematopoietic precursor cells in microenvironmental niches, bringing cells into close proximity with growth regulatory cytokines that are also bound and held by the ECM.[51]

It has also been suggested that the quiescent state of stem cells is controlled by their localization in niches that block their responsiveness to differentiation-inducing signals (Figure 2-13 ■). Stromal cells produce cell-surface associated factors that restrain SC differentiation (TGF-β, MIP-1α). Any manipulation that removed SC from their niche would result in a cascade of differentiation events. It thus may be that a major role of the stromal tissue in the regulation of hematopoiesis may be to safeguard and ensure stem cell maintenance. This may explain the observation that bone marrow cells removed from their marrow environment do not retain their "stemness" for more than a few weeks when cultured in the absence of stromal cells. Inevitably, they differentiate into progenitor cells and mature cells of the various lineages, and thus undergo death by differentiation.

▶ ONCOGENES AND TUMOR SUPPRESSOR GENES

In recent years there has been an explosive growth in our knowledge of cancer cell biology. Of significance is the recognition that scattered throughout our own genome are genes that have the potential to cause cancer (**proto-oncogenes**)[52,53] and other genes that have the power to block it (**antioncogenes** or *tumor suppressor genes*).[54] As researchers have worked to understand the function of these oncogenes and tumor suppressor genes, they have found that many of them are components that regulate normal cell growth and differentiation and/or apoptosis.[55,56]

Cancer is a genetic disease: most tumors are clonally derived from a single common progenitor cancer cell that divides incessantly to generate a tumor of identical sibling cells. Cancer is stably inherited during cell division. This implies that the disease phenotype is determined by the tumor cell DNA. Researchers found that certain viruses, when inoculated into animals, were capable of causing tumors. In an effort to discover the particular genes capable of inducing malignant transformation, it was shown that tumor viruses carry discrete genetic elements, **oncogenes,** that are responsible for their ability to transform cells. The proteins encoded by these oncogenes play important roles in the cell cycle, such as initiation of DNA replication and transcriptional control of genes. Importantly, many viral oncogenes have counterparts in the normal human genome, now called cellular proto-oncogenes. The identification of cellular proto-oncogenes verified that the human genome carries genes with the potential to dramatically alter cell growth and even to kill.

ONCOGENES

One of the defining features of cancer cells is their ability to proliferate under conditions where normal cells do not.[57] The proteins encoded by proto-oncogenes function in the signaling pathways by which cells receive and execute growth instructions. The mutations that convert these proto-oncogenes to active oncogenes are usually either structural mutations resulting in the constitutive activity of a protein without an incoming signal, or regulatory mutations that lead to the production of the protein at the wrong place or time. The result in either case is a persistent internal growth signal uncoupled from environmental controls. It is possible that any gene playing a key role in cellular growth can become an oncogene if mutated in the appropriate way.

Generally, the proto-oncogenes that have been identified serve one of the following functions in normal growth control:

- Some encode growth factors, the molecules that are themselves the signals to grow; when activated to an oncogene, they result in an autocrine growth stimulation.
- Other proto-oncogenes encode growth factor receptors; when activated to an oncogene they are capable of triggering growth-promoting signals even in the absence of ligand (cytokine) binding.
- The largest class of proto-oncogenes encode proteins that associate with growth factor receptors inside the plasma

membrane and function to pass their signals to downstream targets. Many of these proto-oncogenes encode protein-tyrosine kinases found on the inner surface of the membrane. Often the oncogenic form of these genes produces signaling molecules that exist in a constantly activated state, in the absence of growth factor/receptor interaction and signaling.

- Some proto-oncogenes are transcription factors, proteins that bind DNA and function to control the expression of cellular genes required for proliferation.

Thus, proto-oncogenes are genes that regulate the initiation of DNA replication, cell division, and/or the commitment to cellular differentiation. As such, they are obvious targets for processes that damage the growth-control apparatus of the cell. Damage to these regulatory genes, referred to as activation of the proto-oncogene (resulting in the creation of an oncogene) occurs by one of three mechanisms: genetic mutation, genetic rearrangement, or genetic amplification. The result is either a qualitative change in function of the protein product of the gene, resulting in enhanced activity; a protein that is no longer subject to the control of regulatory factors; or a quantitative change (increased production) of an otherwise normal oncogene protein.

TUMOR SUPPRESSOR GENES

It is now widely accepted that cancer is a multihit phenomenon, resulting from several independent events occuring sequentially within a single cell. There are specific tumor suppressor genes, or antioncogenes in normal cells, that function to inhibit cell growth. Thus, in addition to mutations of oncogenes resulting in a growth-promoting activity, tumor cells often have inactivating mutations of growth-suppressing genes that also contribute to tumor development. Mutations in tumor suppressor genes behave differently from oncogene mutations (Table 2-12 ✪). Oncogene mutations tend to be activating mutations, which functionally are dominant to wild-type gene products; they produce proliferation signals even when a single copy of the oncogene is present. Tumor suppressor mutations, on the other hand, are recessive, loss-of-function mutations. Mutation in one gene copy usually has

no effect, as long as a reasonable amount of normally functioning wild-type protein remains.

Understanding the function of tumor suppressor genes has been greatly aided by studies of rare cancers that run in families. Members of affected families appear to inherit susceptibility to cancer and develop certain kinds of tumors at rates much higher than the normal population. The first of these to be explained at the molecular level was the inherited susceptibility to retinoblastoma (a tumor of the eye) seen in certain families.[58,59] Although retinoblastoma can occur sporadically, about one-third of the cases occur in related siblings, suggesting an inherited susceptibility to the disease. The development of retinoblastoma requires two mutations resulting in the inactivation of both of the *RB* loci on the chromosome 13 pair members. In the familial form of the disease, the affected children inherit one mutant *RB* allele and one normal allele. Retinoblastoma (or other malignancies) develops when acquired mutations eliminate the function of the remaining normal (wild-type) allele. Thus the *RB* gene acts as a tumor suppressor gene (antioncogene) that normally functions to arrest the growth of cells. As is typically true of tumor suppressor genes, even one copy is sufficient to keep growth in check. However, loss of both copies of *RB* eliminates the block and a tumor develops. As discussed above, the protein product of the *RB* gene is not specific to retinal tissue but rather serves as a universal cell-cycle brake in most cells. Acquired mutations of *RB* (i.e., nonfamilial) are found in about 25% of sporadic tumors.

Inactivation of the p53 gene, also a tumor suppressor antioncogene, is seen in over half of all human cancers, making it the most common genetic defect detectable in human tumors.[60,61] Interestingly, a damaged p53 gene can also be inherited, the Li-Fraumeini syndrome, resulting (like familial retinoblastoma) in an inherited susceptibility to a variety of tumors.[62,63] In affected individuals, 50% develop cancer by age 30 and 90% by age 70. The function of p53 in cell cycle regulation is to block cell cycle progression in the event of altered DNA or to trigger apoptosis if the damaged DNA cannot be repaired. P53 is a leader in the body's antitumor army, serving as a "molecular policeman" monitoring the integrity of the genome. Loss of function of the p53 gene facilitates tumor formation by allowing damaged cells to proceed through the cell cycle.

Although all of the Cdk inhibitors could potentially act as tumor suppressors,[64] the one that seems to have the strongest link to malignancy is p16.[65] Loss-of-function mutations of p16 have been described in a wide variety of human cancers. To date, there is much less information on the involvement of other Cdk inhibitors, although it is likely they could also function as tumor suppressors and thus play a role in tumorigenesis. In addition, there are tumor suppressor genes that tend to show tissue preference in terms of site of malignancy. These include the WT-1 gene, mutated in Wilms' tumor; the APC gene, mutated in adenomatous polyposis; the DCC

✪ TABLE 2-12

Properties of Oncogenes and Tumor Suppressor Genes

Property	Oncogenes	Tumor suppressor gene
Nature of mutation	Dominant	Recessive
	Gain of function	Loss of function
Inherited mutant allele	Never observed	Common—basis for inherited predisposition in cancers
Somatic mutations in cancers	Yes	Yes

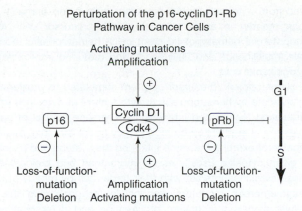

Perturbation of the p16-cyclinD1-Rb
Pathway in Cancer Cells

■ FIGURE 2-14 Alterations of the G1 checkpoint that can lead to malignancy. Loss-of-function alterations of negative regulators of the cell cycle (i.e., Cdk inhibitor p16 or cell cycle inhibitor Rb protein) may contribute to uncontrolled proliferation. Similarly, gain-of-function mutations of positive regulators of proliferation (i.e., Cyclin D, Cdk4) may contribute to uncontrolled proliferation. Inhibitory regulatory proteins with the potential to influence malignant transformation are called tumor suppressor genes, while positive regulatory proteins are called proto-oncogenes. ↓ indicates stimulation of the pathway; ⊥ indicates inhibition of the pathway. (+) indicates a mutation that increases activity of the indicated proteins; (-) indicates a mutation that decreases activity of the indicated proteins.

gene, deleted in colon carcinomas; and BRCA-1 and BRCA-2, mutated in breast cancers.

CELL CYCLE CHECKPOINTS AND CANCER

A common feature of many cancer cells is the loss of regulation of cell cycle checkpoints, either by aberrant expression of positive regulators (for example, cyclins and Cdks) or the loss of negative regulators (the Cdk inhibitors, p53, or Rb).[66,67] Cyclin D, cyclin E, and cyclin A are deregulated (overexpressed) in a variety of human cancers and function as oncogenes in their mutated configuration. Often, specific chromosomal translocations activate the expression of the cyclin gene by placing it under the influence of other transcriptional control elements (e.g., the t[11;14] translocation seen in some B-cell neoplasms places the cyclin D gene locus under the control of the immunoglobulin H [heavy] chain locus, resulting in activation of cyclin D expression). The Bcl-1 oncogene defined by the t(11;14) translocation is now known to represent a translocated cyclin D locus. Mutations of Cdk4 have also been reported in a number of human tumors, contributing to the excessive growth characteristics of the diseases. The p16-cyclin D-Rb pathway, which controls the G_1 checkpoint in cell cycle regulation, is believed to play a pivotal role in tumorigenesis (Figure 2-14 ■). Some investigators have proposed that a mutation involving at least one member of this checkpoint must occur in order for a malignant phenotype to be established.[68]

APOPTOSIS AND CANCER

The accumulation of excess numbers of cells characteristic of malignancies may be due to increased cell proliferation (see above), and/or to decreased cell death (apoptosis).[69] Thus, mutations of genes important in regulating apoptosis have also been identified as oncogenes and tumor suppressor genes. These include loss-of-function mutations of initiators of apoptosis such as p53, Bax, and other proapoptotic Bcl-2 family members, as well as overexpression of Bcl-2 and other Bcl-2 family members that function to inhibit apoptosis. Bcl-2 is overexpressed in most cases of B-cell follicular lymphoma, many cases of B-cell chronic lymphocytic leukemia (CLL), and some cases of acute myelocytic leukemia (AML). Mutations of Bax (resulting in loss of proapoptotic function) have been reported in about 20% of leukemic cell lines. The result is production of cells with an extended life span, increased proliferation capacity, and diminished cell death.

 Checkpoint! #6

Mutations of proto-oncogenes predisposing to malignancy are said to be dominant mutations, while mutations of antioncogenes are said to behave as recessive mutations, requiring loss of both alleles. Explain this difference in behavior of the gene products.

SUMMARY

The cell is an intricate, complex structure bound by a membrane. The membrane is a phospholipid bilayer with integral proteins throughout and containing receptors that bind extracellular molecules and transmit messages to the cell's nucleus. Within the cell is the cytoplasm, with numerous organelles, and the nucleus. The cellular organelles include ribosomes, endoplasmic reticulum, the Golgi apparatus, lysosomes, mitochondria, microfilaments, and

microtubules. The nucleus contains the genetic material, DNA, that regulates all cell functions.

The cell cycle is a highly ordered process that results in the accurate duplication and transmission of genetic information from one cell generation to the next. The cell cycle is divided into four stages: M phase (in which cell division or mitosis takes place), S phase (during which DNA synthesis occurs), and two gap phases, G_1 and G_2. G_0

refers to quiescent cells that are temporarily or permanently out of cycle. The normal cell is dependent on external stimuli (growth factors) to move it out of G_0 and through G_1. The cell cycle is regulated by a series of protein kinases, (Cdks) whose activity is controlled by complexing with a regulatory partner (cyclin). Different cyclins, with their associated (and activated) Cdks, function at specific stages of the cell cycle. Kinase activity is further modulated by both activating and inactivating phorphorylation of kinase subunits and by specific cell cycle kinase (Cdk) inhibitors. A series of checkpoint controls or surveillance systems functions to ensure the integrity of the process.

Cells utilize the process of programmed cell death, or apoptosis, as well as proliferation, to maintain tissue homeostasis. Apoptosis is a unique form of cell death that can be morphologically and biochemically distinguished from necrosis. Apoptosis plays important roles in the development of the organism, in controlling the number of various types of cells, and as a defense mechanism to eliminate unwanted and potentially dangerous cells. Apoptosis is an active process, initiated by the cell, resulting in the orderly dismantling of cellular constituents. It is directed by cysteine proteases called caspases. Proapoptotic and antiapoptotic proteins (Bcl-2 family members) and specific protein inhibitors (IAPs, or inhibitors of apoptosis) regulate this process. Apoptosis is triggered by loss of survival factors (survival cytokines or extracellular matrix components), presence of death cytokines, or cell damaging stress.

Hematopoiesis is the production of the various types or lineages of blood cells. Mature, terminally differentiated blood cells are derived from mitotically active precursor cells found primarily in the bone marrow in adults. Hematopoietic precursor cells include pluripotential hematopoietic stem cells, hematopoietic progenitor cells (multilineage and unilineage), and maturing (morphologically recognizable) cells.

Hematopoietic precursor cells are stimulated to proliferate and differentiate by hematopoietic growth factors or cytokines (colony-stimulating factors and interleukins). Cytokine control of hematopoiesis is characterized by redundancy (more than one cytokine is capable of exerting the same effect on the system) and pleiotrophy (a given cytokine usually exerts more than one biologic effect). These cytokines interact with their target cell by means of unique transmembrane receptors responsible for generating the intracellular signals that govern proliferation and differentiation. Hematopoiesis takes place in a unique microenvironment in the marrow consisting of stromal cells and extracellular matrix, which plays a vital role in controlling hematopoiesis.

The various processes that govern tissue homeostasis—proliferation, differentiation, cytokine regulation, and apoptosis—are highly ordered and tightly regulated. When the regulation of these processes malfunctions, the result can be deregulated cell production and malignant transformation. Oncogenes and tumor suppressor genes are genes whose normal transcription products regulate the processes that govern tissue homeostasis. Mutations that alter the structure or function of these genes may result in uncontrolled cell growth and malignancy.

REVIEW QUESTIONS

LEVEL I

1. Selective cellular permeability and structural stability is provided by: (Checklist #1)
   a. membrane lipids
   b. membrane proteins
   c. ribosomes
   d. the nucleus

2. Rough endoplasmic reticulum is important in: (Checklist #1)
   a. synthesizing lipid
   b. synthesizing hormones
   c. synthesizing and assembling proteins
   d. phagocytosis

3. The fundamental subunit of chromatin composed of ~180 base pairs of DNA wrapped around a histone protein is called: (Checklist #1)
   a. nucleolus
   b. genome
   c. heterochromatin
   d. nucleosome

4. Condensation of chromosomes occurs during which phase of mitosis? (Checklist #2)
   a. anaphase
   b. telophase
   c. prophase
   d. metaphase

LEVEL II

1. The kinase complex responsible for passage through and exit from mitosis is composed of: (Checklist #1)
   a. cyclin A/Cdk2
   b. cyclin D/Cdk4
   c. cyclin B/Cdk1
   d. cyclin E/Cdk2

2. CAK, the kinase activity responsible for the activating phosphorylations of Cdks, consists of: (Checklist #2)
   a. cyclin A/Cdk1
   b. cyclin H/Cdk7
   c. cyclin F/Cdk6
   d. cyclin C/Cdk2

3. Overexpression of the p21 protein would have what effect on the cell cycle of proliferating cells? (Checklist #2)
   a. no effect
   b. increase cell cycle progression
   c. decrease cell cycle progression
   d. trigger apoptosis

4. Apoptotic cell death is characterized by all of the following EXCEPT: (Checklist #6)
   a. triggering an inflammatory response
   b. condensation of the nucleus
   c. cleavage of chromatin into discrete fragments (multiples of 185 base pairs)
   d. condensation of the cytoplasm and cell shrinkage

REVIEW QUESTIONS (continued)

LEVEL I

5. Cells that have exited the cell cycle and entered a non-proliferative phase are said to be in: (Checklist #2)
   a. quiescence
   b. interphase
   c. G_1
   d. G_2

6. The regulatory subunit of the active enzyme complex responsible for regulating passage through the various phases of the cell cycle is: (Checklist #3)
   a. cyclin
   b. Cdk
   c. Cdk inhibitor
   d. p21

7. Self-renewal and pluripotential differentiation potential are characteristics of: (Checklist #8)
   a. mature cells
   b. stem cells
   c. progenitor cells
   d. maturing cells

8. All hematopoietic cells are derived from the CFU-GEMM EXCEPT: (Checklist #9)
   a. lymphocytes
   b. platelets
   c. eosinophils
   d. erythrocytes

9. The following cell is most sensitive to erythropoietin: (Checklist #10)
   a. reticulocyte
   b. CFU-GEMM
   c. BFU-E
   d. CFU-E

10. All of the following are thought to be negative regulators of hematopoiesis EXCEPT: (Checklist #11)
    a. TGFβ
    b. SCF
    c. TNF
    d. MIP-1α

LEVEL II

5. The components of apoptosis directly responsible for the dismantling of the cell during the programmed cell death process are: (Checklist #7)
   a. Bcl-2 family members
   b. IAPs
   c. initiator caspases
   d. effector caspases

6. A predominance of Bax-Bax homodimers has what effect on apoptosis? (Checklist #8)
   a. inhibits initiator caspases
   b. promotes activation of effector caspases
   c. activates death receptors on the cell surface
   d. neutralizes IAPs

7. All of the following are important regulators of granulopoiesis EXCEPT: (Checklist #13)
   a. GM-CSF
   b. FL
   c. IL-2
   d. IL-3

8. Which of the following growth factor receptors share a common β chain? (Checklist #14)
   a. IL-2 and IL-3
   b. TPO and EPO
   c. IL-3 and GM-CSF
   d. G-CSF and GM-CSF

9. The stromal elements of the hematopoietic microenvironment include all of the following EXCEPT: (Checklist #16)
   a. B-lymphocytes
   b. adipocytes
   c. fibroblasts
   d. macrophages

10. All of the following are considered characteristics of tumor suppressor genes EXCEPT: (Checklist #18)
    a. normally function as negative regulators of the cell cycle
    b. undergo gain-of-function mutations resulting in malignant transformation
    c. mutated forms of the genes often found in inherited predispositions to malignancy
    d. characteristic mutations are recessive in expression patterns.

www.prenhall.com/mckenzie

Use the above address to access the free, interactive Companion Web site created for this textbook. Get hints, instant feedback, and textbook references to chapter-related multiple choice questions.

REFERENCES

1. Singer SJ, Nicholson GL. The fluid mosaic model of the structure of cell membranes. *Science* 175:720–31, 1972.

2. Nasmyth K. Viewpoint. Putting the cell cycle in order. *Science* 1996; 274:1643–45.

3. Pardee AB. G_1 events and regulation of cell proliferation. *Science* 1989; 246:603–8.

4. Sherr CJ. G_1 phase progression: Cycling on cue. *Cell* 1994; 79:551–55.

5. King RW, Deshaies RJ, Peters JM, Kirschner MW. How proteolysis drives the cell cycle. *Science* 1996; 274:1652–59.

6. Morgan DO. Principles of Cdk regulation. *Nature* 1995; 374:131–34.

7. Sherr CJ, Roberts JM. Inhibitors of mammalian G-1 cyclin dependent kinases. *Genes Develop* 1995; 9:1149–63.

8. Murray AW. Creative blocks: Cell cycle checkpoints and feedback controls. *Nature* 1992; 359:599–604.

9. Gorbsky GJ. Cell cycle checkpoints: Arresting progress in mitosis. *BioEssays* 1997; 19:193–97.

10. Nurse P. Checkpoint pathways come of age. *Cell* 1997; 91:865–67.

11. Weinberg RA. The retinoblastoma protein and cell cycle control. Cell 1995; 81:323–30.

12. Herwig S, Strauss M. The retinoblastoma protein: A master regulator of cell cycle, differentiation, and apoptosis. *Eur J Biochem* 1997; 246:581–601.

13. Sidransky D, Hollstein M. Clinical implications of the p53 gene. *Ann Rev Med* 1996; 47:285–301.

14. Kerr JFR, Harmon BV. Definition and incidence of apoptosis: An historical perspective. In: *Apoptosis: The Molecular Basis of Cell Death.* New York: Cold Spring Harbor Laboratory Press; 1991: 5–25.

15. Steller H. Mechanisms and genes of cellular suicide. *Science* 1995; 267:1445–49.

16. Thompson CB. Apoptosis in the pathogenesis and treatment of disease. *Science* 1995; 267:1456–62.

17. Hetts SW. To die or not to die: An overview of apoptosis and its role in disease. *JAMA* 1998; 279:300–7.

18. Thornberry NA, Lazebik Y. Caspases: Enemies within. *Science* 1998; 281:1312–16.

19. Earnshaw WC, Martins LM, Kaufmann SH. Mammalian caspases: Structure, activation, substrates, and functions during apoptosis. *Ann Rev Biochem* 1999; 68:383–424.

20. Adams JM, Cory S. The Bcl-2 protein family: Arbiters of cell survival. *Science* 1998; 281:1322–26.

21. Chao DT, Korsmeyer SJ. Bcl-2 family: Regulators of cell death. *Ann Rev Immunol* 1998; 16:395–419.

22. Salvesen GS, Dixit VM. Caspase activation: The induced proximity model. *Proc Natl Acad Sci USA* 1999; 96:10, 964–67.

23. Susin SA, Zamzami N, Kroemer G. Mitochondria as regulators of apoptosis: Doubt no more. *Biochem Biophys Acta* 1998; 1366:151–65.

24. Green DR, Reed JC. Mitochondria and apoptossis. *Science* 1998; 281:1309–12.

25. Nagata S, Golstein P. The Fas death factor. *Science* 1995; 267: 1449–56.

26. Ashkenazi A, Dixit VM. Death receptors: Signaling and modulation. *Science* 1998; 281:1305–8.

27. Bessis M. *Blood Smears Reinterpreted.* Trans. G Brecher. Berlin-Heidelberg-New York: Springer-Verlag; 1977: 17.

28. Williams DA. Stem cell model of hematopoiesis. In: *Hematology: Basic Principles and Procedures,* 3rd ed. Edited by R Hoffman, EJ Benz, SJ Shattil, B Furie, HJ Cohen, LE Silberstein, P McGlave. New York: Churchill Livingstone; 2000: 126–38.

29. Lord BI, Testa NG. The hemopoietic system: Structure and regulation. In: *Hematopoiesis: Long-Term Effects of Chemotherapy and Radiation.* Edited by NG Testa and RP Gale. New York: Marcel Dekker; 1988: 1–25.

30. Bagby GC Jr. Hematopoiesis. In: *The Molecular Basis of Blood Diseases,* 2nd ed. Edited by G Stamatoyannopoulos, AW Nienhuis, PW Majerus, H Varmus. Philadelphia: W B Saunders; 1994.

31. Prchal JT et al. A common progenitor for human myeloid and lymphoid cells. *Nature* 1978; 197:590–1.

32. Bhatia M, Wang JCY, Kapp U, Bonnet D, Dick JE. Purification of primitive human hematopoietic cells capable of repopulating immune-deficient mice. *Proc Natl Acad Sci USA* 1997; 94:5320–5.

33. Berenson RJ, Andrews RG, Bensinger WI, Kalamasz D, Knitter G, Buckner CD, Bernstein ID. Antigen CD34$^+$ marrow cells engraft lethally irradiated baboons. *J Clin Invest* 1988; 81:951–55.

34. Nakahata T, Ogawa M. Identification in culture of a new class of hemopoietic colony forming units with extensive ability to self-renew and generate multipotential colonies. *Proc Natl Acad Sci USA* 1982; 79:3843–47.

35. Bradley TR, Hodgson GS. Detection of primitive macrophage progenitor cells in mouse bone marrow. *Blood* 1979; 54:1446–50.

36. Magli MC, Iscove NN, Odartchenko V. Transient nature of early haematopoietic spleen colonies. *Nature:* 1982; 295:527–29.

37. Sutherland HJ, Lannsdorp PM, Henkelman DH, et al. Functional characterization of individual human haematopoietic stem cells cultured at limiting dilution on supportive marrow stromal layers. *Proc Natl Acad Sci USA* 1990; 87:3584–88.

38. Quesenberry PJ. Hemopoietic stem cells, progenitor cells and cytokines. *In: Williams Hematology,* 5th ed. Edited by E Beutler, MA Lichtman, BS Coller, TJ Kipps. New York: McGraw-Hill; 1995: 211–28.

39. Long MW, Gragowski LL, Heffner CH, et al. Phorbol diesters stimulate the development of an early murine progenitor cell: The burst forming unit-megakaryocyte. *J Clin Invest* 76: 1985; 431–38.

40. Veiby OP, Jacobsen FW, Cui L, et al. The Flt3 ligand promotes the survival of primitive hemopoietic progenitor cells with myeloid as well as B lymphoid potential: Suppression of apoptosis and counteraction by TNF-alpha and TGF-beta. *J Immunol* 1996; 157: 2953–60.

41. Flanagan JG, Chan DC, Leder P. Transmembrane form of the kit ligand growth factor is determined by alternative splicing and is missing in the Sld mutant. *Cell* 1991; 64:1025–35.

42. Kopf M, Ramsay A, Brombacher F et al. Pleiotropic defects of IL-6 deficient mice including early hematopoiesis, T and B cell function, and acute-phase responses. *Ann NY Acad Sci* 762: 1995; 308–18.

43. Musashi M, Clark SC, Sudo T, et al. Synergistic interactions between interleukin-11 and interleukin-4 in support of proliferation of primitive hematopoietic progenitors of mice. *Blood* 1991; 778:1448–51.

44. Du XX, Neven T, Goldman S, Williams DA. Effects of recombinant human interleukin-11 on hematopoietic reconstitution in transplant mice: Acceleration of recovery of peripheral blood neutrophils and platelets. *Blood* 1993; 81:27–34.

45. Toombs CF, Young CH, Glaspy JA, Varnum BC. Megakaryocyte growth and development factor (MGDF) moderately enhances in-vitro platelet aggregation. *Thromb Res* 1995; 80:23–33.

46. Graham GJ, Wright EG, Hewick R, et al. Identification and characterization of an inhibitor of haemopoietic stem cell proliferation. *Nature* 1990; 344:442–44.

47. Dong F, Hoefsloot LH, Schelen AM, et al. Identification of a nonsense mutation in the granulocyte-colony-stimulating factor receptor in severe congenital neutropenia. *Proc Natl Acad Sci USA* 1994; 91:4480–4.

48. de la Chapelle H, Traskelin AL, Jubonen E. Truncated erythropoietin receptor causes dominantly inherited benign human erythrocytosis. *Proc Natl Acad Sci USA* 1993; 90:4495–99.

49. Gordon MS, Sosman JA. Clinical application of cytokines and biologic response modifiers. In: *Hematology: Basic Principles and Procedures,* 3rd ed. Edited by R Hoffman, EJ Benz, SJ Shattil, B Furie, HJ Cohen, LE Silberstein, P McGlave. New York: Churchill Livingstone; 2000: 939–78.

50. Verfaillie CM. Anatomy and physiology of hematopoiesis. In *Hematology: Basic Principles and Procedures,* 3rd ed. Edited by R Hoffman, EJ Benz, SJ Shattil, B Furie, HJ Cohen, LE Silberstein, P McGlave. New York: Churchill Livingstone; 2000: 139–53.

51. Quesenberry PF, Crittenden RB, Lowry P, et al. In vitro and in vivo studies of stromal niches. *Blood Cells* 1994; 2:97–104.

52. Prochownik E. Protooncogenes and cell differentiation. *Trans Med Rev* 1989; 3:24–38.

53. Studzinski GP. Oncogenes, growth, and the cell cycle: An overview. *Cell Tissue Kinet* 1989; 22:405–24.

54. Carbone DP, Minna JD. Antioncogenes and human cancer. *Ann Rev Med* 1993; 44:451–64.

55. Marx J. How cells cycle toward cancer. *Science* 1994; 263:319–21.

56. Marx J. Learning how to suppress cancer. *Science* 1993; 261:1385–87.

57. Sherr CJ. Cancer cell cycles. *Science* 1996; 274:1672–77.

58. Benedict WF, Xu HJ, Hu SX, Takahashi R. Role of the retinoblastoma gene in the initiation and progression of human cancer. *J Clin Invest* 1990; 85:988–93.

59. Bartek J, Bartkova J, Lukas J. The retinoblastoma protein pathway in cell cycle control and cancer. *Exp Cell Res* 1997; 237:1–6.

60. Levine AJ, Momand J, Finlay CA. The p53 tumour suppressor gene. *Nature* 1991; 351:453–56.

61. Greenblatt MS, Bennett WP, Hollstein M, Harris CC. Mutations in the p53 tumor suppressor gene: Clues to cancer etiology and molecular pathogenesis. *Cancer Res* 1994; 54:4855–78.

62. Srivastava S, Zou ZQ, Pirollo K, et al. Germ-line transmission of a mutated p53 gene in a cancer-prone family with Li-Fraumeini syndrome. *Nature* 1990; 348:747–79.

63. Malkin D, Li FP, Strong LC, Fraumeini JF et al. Germline p53 mutations in a familial syndrome of breast cancer, sarcomas and other neoplasms. *Science* 1990; 250:1233–38.

64. Tsihlias J, Kapusta L, Slingerland J. The prognostic significance of altered cyclin-dependent kinase inhibitors in human cancer. *Ann Rev Med* 1999; 50:401–23.

65. Nobori T, Miura K, Wu DJ, et al. Deletions of the cyclin-dependent kinase-4 inhibitor gene in multiple human cancers. *Nature* 1994; 368:753–36.

66. Hall M, Peters G. Genetic alterations of cyclins, cyclin-dependent kinases, and Cdk inhibitors in human cancer. *Adv Cancer Res* 1996; 68:67–108.

67. Bartek J, Lukas J, Bartkove J. Perspective: Defects in cell cycle control and cancer. *J Pathol* 1999; 187:95–99.

68. Rosenberg N, Krantiris RG. Molecular basis of neoplasia. In *Hematology: Basic Principles and Procedures,* 3rd ed. Edited by R Hoffman, EJ Benz, SJ Shattil, B Furie, HJ Cohen, LE Silberstein, P McGlave. New York: Churchill Livingstone; 2000:870–84.

69. Rinkenberger JL, Korsmeyer SJ. Errors of homeostasis and deregulated apoptosis. *Curr Opin Genet Dev* 1997; 7:589–96.

SECTION TWO • THE HEMATOPOIETIC SYSTEM

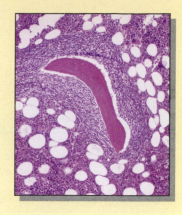

3

Structure and Function of Hematopoietic Organs

Annette I. Schlueter, M.D., Ph.D.

■ CHECKLIST - LEVEL I

At the end of this unit of study the student should be able to:

1. Identify the sites of hematopoiesis during embryonic and fetal development as well as in childhood and adulthood.
2. Identify organ/tissue sites in which each hematopoietic cell type differentiates.
3. Explain the difference between primary and secondary lymphoid tissue.
4. Describe the function of bone marrow, spleen, lymph nodes, and thymus.

■ CHECKLIST - LEVEL II

At the end of this unit of study the student should be able to:

1. Associate physical findings (hypersplenism, lymphadenopathy) with the presence of hematologic disease.
2. Describe the pathophysiologic changes that lead to bone marrow hyperplasia or extramedullary hematopoiesis.
3. Identify sites of extramedullary hematopoiesis.
4. Describe the structure of bone marrow, spleen, lymph nodes, and thymus.

CHAPTER OUTLINE

KEY TERMS

Adipocyte
Culling
Erythroblastic island
Extramedullary hematopoiesis
Germinal center
Hyperplasia
Lymphoid follicle
Medullary hematopoiesis
Osteoblast
Osteoclast
Pitting
Stroma
Trabecula

BACKGROUND BASICS

The information in this chapter will build on the concepts learned in the first two chapters. A basic anatomy and physiology course may also be helpful. To maximize your learning experience you should review these concepts before starting this unit of study:

Level I
▶ Define *microenvironment* as related to hematopoietic cell development. (∞ Chapter 2)
▶ Summarize the process of cell maturation in the bone marrow. (∞ Chapter 2)

Level II
▶ Summarize the mechanisms of positive and negative regulators of hematopoietic cell development. (∞ Chapter 2)
▶ Describe the details of hematopoiesis and the role of cytokines/growth factors in blood cell development. (∞ Chapter 2)

CASE STUDY

We will refer to this case throughout this chapter.
Francine, a 40-year-old female, saw her physician for complaints of fatigue and shortness of breath. Physical examination revealed splenomegaly and lymphadenopathy. A complete blood count was ordered with the following results: Hb 8 gL/d; WBC 6.5 × 10⁹/L; Platelets 21 × 10⁹/L.

1. Refer to the tables on the front inside cover of the book and determine which blood cell parameters are abnormal, if any.

OVERVIEW

This chapter includes a description of the tissues involved in the production and maturation of blood cells. It begins with a sequential look at blood cell production from the embryo to the adult. The histologic structure of each tissue and its function in hematopoiesis are discussed. Abnormalities in hematopoiesis that are associated with histologic and functional changes in these tissues are briefly described.

INTRODUCTION

Cellular proliferation, differentiation, and maturation of blood cells takes place in the hematopoietic tissue, which in the adult consists primarily of bone marrow. Mature cells are released to the peripheral blood. The link between the bone marrow and blood cell production was not established until it was recognized that blood formation was a continuous process. Before 1850, it was believed that blood cells formed in the fetus were viable until death of the host and that there was no need for a continuous source of new elements.

DEVELOPMENT OF HEMATOPOIESIS

Hematopoiesis begins as early as the nineteenth day after fertilization in an extraembryonic location, the yolk sac of the human embryo. The cells made in the yolk sac include erythrocytes and a few macrophages.[1] The ability to make erythrocytes is important since the embryo must be able to transport oxygen to developing tissue early in gestation. Shortly thereafter, intraembryonic hematopoiesis begins in a site known as the aorta-gonads-mesonephros (AGM) region, located along the developing aorta. This region has the ability to make a wider range of hematopoietic cells, including lymphocytes.[2] Cell production at this time is called primitive erythropoiesis because the hemoglobin is not typical of that seen in later developing erythroblasts. The primitive embryonic erythroblasts in the yolk sac arise from clusters of cells in the mesenchyme called blood islands and are closely related to development of endothelium, the cells lining blood vessels.[3] Embryonic red cells have a megaloblastic appearance with coarse clumped chromatin (∞ Chapter 14). The hemoglobin in these cells consists of the embryonic varieties, Gower 1, Gower 2, and Portland (∞ Chapter 13).[4]

At about the third month of fetal life, the liver becomes the chief site of blood cell production, and the yolk sac and AGM discontinue their role in hematopoiesis. The liver continues to produce a high proportion of erythroid cells, but myeloid and lymphoid cells begin to appear in greater numbers.[5] This is the beginning of a transition to adult patterns of hematopoiesis in which myeloid differentiation predominates over erythroid differentiation.

As fetal development progresses, hematopoiesis also begins to a lesser degree in the spleen, kidney, thymus, and

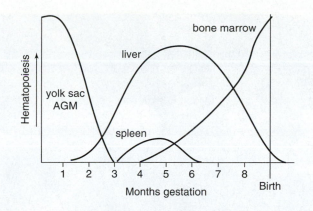

■ **FIGURE 3-1** Location of hematopoiesis during fetal development. At birth most blood cell production is limited to the marrow.

HEMATOPOIETIC TISSUE

The adult hematopoietic system includes tissues and organs involved in the proliferation, maturation, and destruction of blood cells. These organs and tissues include the bone mar-

lymph nodes. Erythroid and myeloid cell production, as well as early B cell (lymphocyte) development, gradually shifts from these sites to bone marrow during late fetal and neonatal life. The bone marrow becomes the primary site of hematopoiesis at about the sixth month of gestation and continues as the primary source of blood production after birth and throughout adult life (Figure 3-1 ■). The thymus becomes the major site of T cell (lymphocyte) production during fetal development and continues to be active throughout the neonatal period and childhood. As is true for erythrocytes in the yolk sac, the first T cells to develop are different than their adult counterparts. They use a different set of genes to make the T cell receptor, which is used by the T cell to recognize and react to foreign substances.[6] Lymph nodes and spleen continue as an important site of late B cell differentiation throughout life.

row, thymus, spleen, and lymph nodes. Bone marrow is the site of myeloid, erythroid, and megakaryocytic, as well as lymphoid, cell development. Thymus, spleen, and lymph nodes are primarily sites of lymphoid cell development. Tissues where lymphoid cell development occurs are divided into primary and secondary lymphoid tissue. Primary lymphoid tissues (bone marrow and thymus) are those where T and B cells develop from nonfunctional precursors into cells that are capable of responding to foreign antigens (immunocompetent cells). Secondary lymphoid tissues (spleen and lymph nodes) are those where immunocompetent T and B cells further differentiate and divide in response to antigen.

BONE MARROW

Blood-forming tissue located between the **trabeculae** of spongy bone is known as bone marrow. (Trabecula refers to a projection of calcified bone extending from cortical bone into the marrow space; it provides support for marrow cells.) This major hematopoietic organ is a cellular, highly vascularized, loose connective tissue. It is composed of two major compartments: the hematopoietic compartment and the vascular compartment. The hematopoietic compartment is the site of formation and maturation of blood cells (Figure 3-2 ■). This compartment includes both hematopoietic cells and stromal cells. The vascular compartment is composed of the nutrient artery, periosteal arteries, central longitudinal vein, arterioles, and sinuses.

Hematopoietic Cells

There is a pattern to the arrangement of hematopoietic cells within the marrow cavity. Erythroblasts constitute 25–30% of the marrow cells and are produced near the sinuses. A common finding among these developing cells is the **erythroblastic island.** The island is a composite of a single macrophage surrounded by erythroblasts in varying states of maturation. The macrophage cytoplasm extends out to sur-

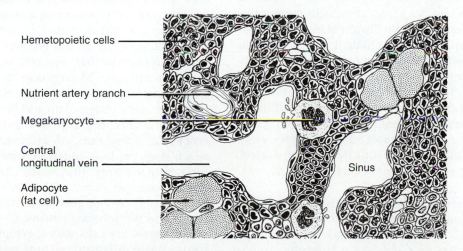

Hemetopoietic cells

Nutrient artery branch

Megakaryocyte

Central longitudinal vein

Adipocyte (fat cell)

Sinus

■ **FIGURE 3-2** Schematic drawing of a section of bone marrow.

round the erythroblasts. During this close association, the macrophages regulate erythropoiesis by secreting various cytokines.[7] The least mature cells are closest to the center of the island, and the more mature cells are at the periphery.

Leukocyte location differs depending on the type of leukocyte. Granulocytes are produced in nests close to the trabeculae and arterioles. These nests are not quite as apparent morphologically as erythroblastic islands. Lymphocytes are produced in lymphoid aggregates that are randomly dispersed throughout the marrow space. Lymphoid progenitor cells may leave the bone marrow and travel to the thymus where they mature into T lymphocytes. Some remain in the bone marrow where they mature into B lymphocytes. Some B cells return to the bone marrow after being activated in the spleen or lymph node. Activated B cells transform into plasma cells. These plasma cells may reside in the bone marrow and produce antibody.

Megakaryocytes are very large, multinucleated cells that produce platelets from their cytoplasm. Cytoplasmic processes of the megakaryocyte form long proplatelet processes. Pieces of these proplatelets pinch off to form platelets (Figure 3-3 ■).

Mast cells (tissue basophils) are large cells with numerous coarse granules that stain deeply basophilic and completely fill the cytoplasm of the cell. These cells are normally quite rare in the bone marrow but may be increased in certain conditions including aplastic anemia, chronic blood loss, and tumors of the lymphoid tissue involving bone marrow.[8]

When bone marrow is aspirated or biopsied for examination, the specimens may contain at least two other types of cells normally associated with bone: *osteoblasts* and *osteoclasts*. These cells are dislodged during puncturing of the bone by the needle in collection of the marrow specimen.

Osteoblasts are cells involved in formation of calcified bone. They are large cells (up to 30 μm in diameter) that resemble plasma cells, except that the perinuclear halo (Golgi apparatus) is detached from the nuclear membrane and, in Wright stained specimens, appears as a light area away from the nucleus. In addition, the cytoplasm may be less basophilic, and the nucleus has a finer chromatin pattern than plasma cells. Osteoblasts are normally found in groups. These cells are more commonly seen in children and in metabolic bone diseases. The cells are alkaline phosphatase positive.

Osteoclasts are cells involved in resorption and remodeling of calcified bone. They are even larger than osteoblasts and may reach up to 100 μm in diameter. The cells are multinucleated and have granular cytoplasm that may be either acidophilic or basophilic. They resemble megakaryocytes, except that the nuclei are usually discrete and often contain nucleoli.

Stroma

The bone marrow **stroma** (supporting tissue) forms a favorable microenvironment for sustained proliferation of hematopoietic cells.[9] It forms a meshwork of long, highly anastomosing branches that provides a three-dimensional scaffolding for hematopoietic cells. Stromal components also

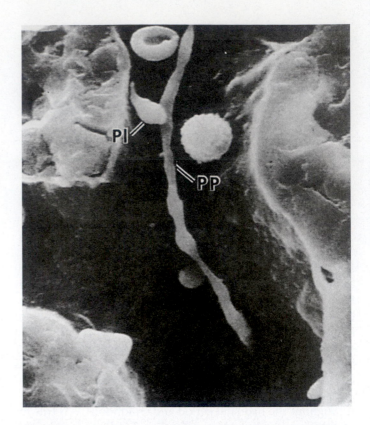

■ **FIGURE 3-3** Scanning electron micrograph of the luminal face of the myeloid sinus wall with an intraluminal segment of a proplatelet process (PP) showing periodic constriction along its length. Pl: platelet displaying tear-drop shape. (Reprinted, with permission, from: DeBruyn PPH: Structural substrates of bone marrow function. *Semin. Hematol* 1981; 18:179.)

provide cytokines that regulate hematopoiesis. The stroma is composed of three major cell types: macrophages, reticular cells (also referred to as fibroblasts), and **adipocytes.**

Macrophages serve two major functions in the bone marrow: phagocytosis and secretion of hematopoietic cytokines. Macrophages phagocytose the extruded nuclei of maturing erythrocytes and phagocytose abnormal cells such as B cells that have not differentiated properly. Some macrophages serve as the center of the erythroblastic islands discussed above. It is believed that these cells supply the developing erythroblasts with iron. Macrophages also provide many colony-stimulating factors needed for development of myeloid lineage cells. Macrophages stain acid phosphatase positive.

Reticular cells are groups of cells that form a reticulum or syncytium. These cells are associated with reticular fibers, which they produce and which form a three-dimensional supporting network that holds the vascular sinuses and hematopoietic elements. The fibers can be visualized with light microscopy and after silver staining. The reticular cells are alkaline phosphatase positive.

Adipocytes are cells whose cytoplasm is largely replaced with a single fat vacuole. These cells mechanically control the volume of bone marrow in which active hematopoiesis takes place. They also provide steroids that influence erythropoiesis and maintain osseous bone integrity.[10,11]

The proportion of bone marrow composed of adipocytes changes with age. For the first four years of life nearly all the marrow cavities are composed of hematopoietic cells, or red marrow. After 4 years of age, the red marrow in shafts of long bones is gradually replaced by adipocytes, or yellow marrow. By the age of 25 years, hematopoiesis is limited to the marrow of the skull, ribs, sternum, scapulae, clavicles, vertebrae, pelvis, upper half of the sacrum, and proximal ends of the long bones. The distribution of red:yellow marrow in these bones is about 1:1. The fraction of red marrow in these areas may decrease after age 70.

Bone forms a rigid compartment for the marrow. Thus, any change in volume of the hematopoietic elements, as occurs in many anemias and leukemias, must be compensated for by a change in the space-occupying adipocytes. Normal red marrow can respond to stimuli and increase its activity to several times the normal rate. As a result, the red marrow becomes hyperplastic and replaces portions of the fatty marrow. **Hyperplasia** (an excessive proliferation of normal cells within an organ) accompanies all conditions with increased or ineffective hematopoiesis.

The degree of hyperplasia is related to the severity and duration of the pathologic state. Acute blood loss may cause erythropoietic tissue to temporarily replace fatty tissue, whereas severe chronic anemia may cause erythropoiesis to be so intense that it not only replaces fatty marrow but also erodes the internal surface of the bone. In malignant diseases that invade or originate in the bone marrow such as leukemia, proliferating abnormal cells may replace both normal hematopoietic tissue and fat.

In contrast, the hematopoietic tissue may become inactive or hypoplastic. Fat cells then increase, providing a cushion for the marrow. Environmental factors such as chemicals and toxins may suppress hematopoiesis, whereas other types of hypoplasia may be genetically determined. Myeloproliferative disease, which begins as a hypercellular disease, frequently terminates in a state of aplasia in which hematopoietic tissue is replaced by fibrous tissue.

ℰ CASE STUDY *(continued from page 42)*

Microscopic examination of a stained blood smear from Francine revealed a predominance of very young blood cells (blasts) in the peripheral blood. These cells are normally found only in the bone marrow. Subsequently, she had a bone marrow aspirated for examination. This revealed 100% cellularity (red marrow) with a predominance of the same type of blasts as those found in the peripheral blood.

2. Describe Francine's bone marrow as normal, hyperplastic, or hypoplastic.

3. What conditions can cause this bone marrow finding?

Marrow Vasculature

The vascular supply of bone marrow is served by two arterial sources, a nutrient artery and a periosteal artery that enter the bone through small holes, the bone foramina. Blood is drained from the marrow via the central vein (Figure 3-4 ■). The nutrient artery branches and coils around the central longitudinal vein that spans the marrow cavity. It supplies blood only to the marrow and not to osseous bone. Arterioles radiate outward from the nutrient artery to endosteum (the inner lining of the cortical bone), giving rise to endosteal beds of interconnecting sinuses. Periosteal arteries supply both osseous bone and marrow. Periosteal capillaries and the capillary branches of the nutrient artery form a juncture with the venous sinuses. The sinuses, lined by single endothelial cells, gather into wider collecting sinuses, which open into the central longitudinal vein.[12] The central longitudinal vein continues through the length of the marrow and exits through the foramina where the nutrient artery entered.

Blood Cell Egress

The mechanism by which the mature hematopoietic cell navigates its passage from the hematopoietic compartment past the venous sinus wall barrier to the blood is only partially understood. Special properties of the maturing cell, as well as of the sinus wall, have been suggested as central features in the cell's interaction with the sinus wall.[13] The adventitial cell, a reticular cell, creates a discontinuous layer on the abluminal side of the sinus wall (marrow side), while endothelial cells line the luminal side of the sinus in a continuous layer. A basement membrane separates these two cell types. The adventitial cell extends its long cytoplasmic processes deep into the marrow cords, forming a part of the reticular meshwork that supports hematopoietic cells. As cell traffic across the sinus increases, the adventitial cells contract creating a less continuous layer over the abluminal sinus wall. This provides the mature hematopoietic cells with more interaction sites on the sinus endothelial surface. In areas where the adventitial layer contracts creating spaces between adventitial cells, it also retracts from the endothelium creating a subcompartment between the adventitial layer and the endothelial layer where mature cells accumulate.

The new blood cell interacts with the abluminal endothelial membrane by a receptor-mediated process, forcing it into contact with the luminal endothelial membrane. The two membranes fuse. Then under pressure from the passing cell, the membranes separate, creating a pore through which the remainder of the hematopoietic cell enters the lumen of the sinus. These pores are only 2–3 μm in diameter.

Because of the small size of the endothelial cell pores, blood cells must have the ability to deform so that they can pass through the sinusoidal lining. Progressive increases in deformability and motility have been noted as granulocytes mature from the myeloblast to the segmented granulocyte. This facilitates the movement of cells into the sinus lumen.

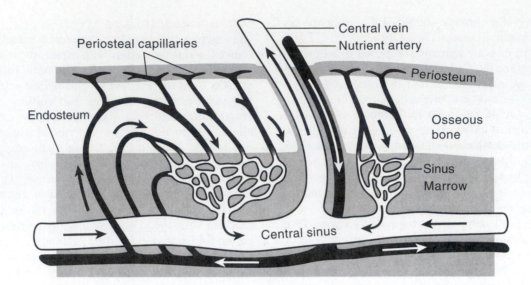

■ FIGURE 3-4 Diagram of the microcirculation of bone marrow. The major arterial supply to the marrow is from periosteal capillaries and from capillary branches of the nutrient artery, which have traversed the bony enclosure of the marrow through the bone foramina. The capillaries join with the venous sinuses as they reenter the marrow. The sinuses gather into wider collecting sinuses which then open into the central longitudinal vein (central sinus). (Adapted, with permission, from: DeBruyn PPH: Structural substrates of bone marrow function. *Semin. Hematol* 18:179, 1981.)

 Checkpoint! #1

Describe the process by which a blood cell moves from the marrow to the vascular space.

Extramedullary Hematopoiesis

Hematopoiesis in the bone marrow is called **medullary hematopoiesis. Extramedullary hematopoiesis** denotes blood cell production in hematopoietic tissue other than bone marrow. In certain hematologic disorders when hyperplasia of the marrow cannot meet the physiologic blood needs of the tissues, extramedullary hematopoiesis may occur in the hematopoietic organs that were active in the fetus, principally the liver and spleen. Organomegaly frequently accompanies significant hematopoietic activity at these sites. This extramedullary hematopoiesis in postnatal life may reflect the ability of inert hematopoietic cells to become active, functional cells if the need arises.

THYMUS

The thymus is a lymphopoietic organ located in the upper part of the anterior mediastinum. It is a bilobular organ demarcated into an outer cortex and central medulla. The cortex is densely packed with small lymphocytes (thymocytes), cortical epithelial cells, and a few macrophages. The medulla is less cellular, containing more mature thymocytes mixed with medullary epithelial cells, dendritic cells, and macrophages (Figure 3-5 ■).

The primary purpose of the thymus is to serve as a compartment for maturation of T lymphocytes.[14] Precursor T cells leave the bone marrow and enter the thymus through arterioles in the cortex. As they travel through the cortex and the medulla, they interact with epithelial cells and dendritic cells, which provide signals for differentiation. They also undergo rapid proliferation. Only about 3% of the cells generated in the thymus exit the medulla as mature T cells. The rest die by apoptosis and are removed by thymic macrophages. The thymus is responsible for supplying the T-dependent areas of lymph nodes, spleen, and other peripheral lymphoid tissue with immunocompetent T lymphocytes.

The thymus is a well-developed organ at birth and continues to increase in size until puberty. After puberty, however, it begins to atrophy, until in old age it becomes barely recognizable. This atrophy may be driven by increased steroid levels in puberty and adulthood. The atrophied thymus is still capable of producing new T cells if the peripheral pool becomes depleted, as occurs after the lymphoid irradiation that accompanies bone marrow transplantation.[15]

SPLEEN

The spleen is located in the upper left quadrant of the abdomen, beneath the diaphragm and to the left of the stomach. After several emergency splenectomies were performed

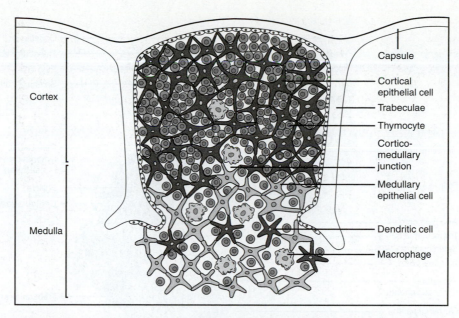

Cortex

Medulla

Capsule

Cortical epithelial cell

Trabeculae

Thymocyte

Cortico-medullary junction

Medullary epithelial cell

Dendritic cell

Macrophage

■ **FIGURE 3-5** A schematic drawing of the thymus. (Copyright 1999 from *Immunobiology* by Janeway et al. Reproduced by permission of Routledge, Inc., part of the Taylor & Francis Group.)

without causing permanent harm to the patients, it was recognized that the spleen was not essential to life. The removal of the spleen has also led to clarification of splenic function as a discriminatory filter. Splenic functions can be better understood after a brief description of the splenic architecture and blood flow.

Architecture

The spleen, enclosed by a capsule of connective tissue, contains the largest collection of lymphocytes and mononuclear phagocytes in the body (Figure 3-6 ■). These cells, together with a reticular meshwork, are concentrated in different areas of the spleen, contributing to the formation of three zones of tissue within the capsule: white pulp, red pulp, and the marginal zone.

The white pulp, a visible grayish white zone, is composed of lymphocytes and located around a central artery. The area closest to the artery, containing many T cells, as well as macrophages and dendritic cells, is termed the periarterial lymphatic sheath. Peripheral to this area are B cells arranged into follicles (a sphere of B cells within lymphatic tissue). Activated B cells are found in specialized follicular areas called **germinal centers.** Germinal centers appear as lightly stained areas in the center of a **lymphoid follicle.** They consist of a mixture of B lymphocytes, follicular dendritic cells, and phagocytic macrophages. The white pulp is where the immune response is initiated. In some cases of heightened immunologic activity the white pulp may increase to occupy half the volume of the spleen (normally 20% or less).

White pulp is surrounded by the marginal zone, a reticular meshwork containing blood vessels, macrophages, and specialized B cells. This zone lies at the junction of the white pulp and red pulp and is important in initiating certain

types of immune responses as well as performing functions similar to the red pulp (see below).

The red pulp contains sinuses and cords. The sinuses are dilated vascular spaces for venous blood. The red color of the pulp is caused by the presence of erythrocytes in the sinuses. The cords are composed of masses of reticular tissue and macrophages that lie between the sinuses. The cords of the red pulp provide zones for platelet storage and destruction of damaged blood cells.

Blood Flow

The spleen is richly supplied with blood. It receives 5% of the total cardiac output, a blood volume of 300 mL/minute. Blood enters the spleen through the splenic artery, which branches into many vessels in the trabeculae. Vessel branches may terminate in the white pulp, red pulp, or marginal zone. Blood entering the spleen may follow either the rapid transit pathway (closed circulation) or the slow transit pathway (open circulation). The rapid transit pathway is a relatively unobstructed route whereby blood enters the sinuses in red pulp from arteries and passes directly to the venous collecting system. In contrast, blood entering the slow transit pathway moves sluggishly through a circuitous route of macrophage-lined cords before it gains access to the sinuses. Plasma in the cords freely enters the sinuses, but erythrocytes meet resistance at the sinus wall as they squeeze through the tiny openings. This skimming of the plasma from blood in the cords to the sinuses sharply increases the hematocrit in the cords. Sluggish blood flow and continued erythrocyte metabolic activity in cords results in a splenic environment that is hypoxic, acidic, and hypoglycemic. Hypoxia and hypoglycemia occur as erythrocytes utilize available oxygen and glucose. Metabolic byproducts create the acidic environment.

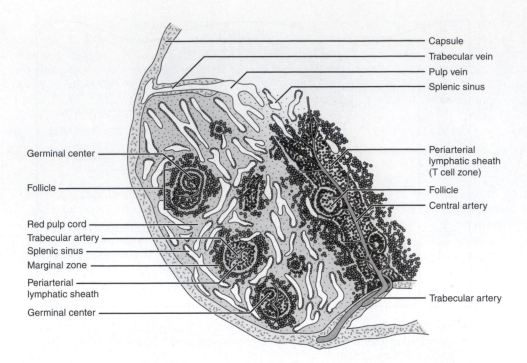

■ **FIGURE 3-6** A schematic drawing of splenic tissue. (Adapted from *Seminars in Hematology*, V7(4), Weiss L et al: "Anatomical hazards to the passage of erythrocytes through the spleen," p. 373, 1970, with permission from Elsevier.)

Functions

Blood that empties into the cords of the red pulp as well as the white pulp and marginal zone takes the slow transit pathway. The slow transit pathway is very important to splenic function, which includes culling, pitting, immune defense, and storage. The discriminatory filtering and destruction of senescent or damaged red cells by the spleen is termed **culling.** Cells entering the spleen through the slow transit pathway become concentrated in the hypoglycemic, hypoxic cords of the red pulp, a hazardous environment for aged or damaged erythrocytes. Slow passage through a macrophage-rich route allows the phagocytic cells to remove these old or damaged erythrocytes before or during their squeeze through the 3 μm pores to cords and sinuses. Normal erythrocytes withstand this adverse environment and eventually reenter the circulation.

Pitting refers to the spleen's ability to "pluck out" particles from intact erythrocytes without destroying them. Blood cells coated with antibody are also susceptible to pitting by macrophages. The macrophage removes the antigen-antibody complex and the attached membrane. The pinched-off cell membrane can reseal itself, but the cell cannot synthesize lipids and proteins for new membrane due to its lack of cellular organelles. Therefore, extensive pitting causes a reduced surface-area-to-volume ratio, resulting in the formation of spherocytes (erythrocytes that have no central area of pallor on stained blood smears). The presence of spherocytes on a blood film is evidence that the erythrocyte has undergone membrane assault in the spleen.

 Checkpoint! #2

Describe how old or damaged erythrocytes are removed from the circulation by the spleen.

The white pulp and marginal zones of the spleen are important lines of defense in blood-borne infections because of their rich supply of lymphocytes and phagocytic cells, as well as the slow transit circulation through these areas. Blood-borne antigens are forced into close contact with phagocytes (antigen-presenting cells) and lymphocytes, which allows for recognition of the antigen as foreign and leads to phagocytosis and antibody formation.

The immunologic function of the spleen is probably less important in the well-developed immune system of the adult than in the less-developed immune system of the child. Young children who undergo splenectomy may develop overwhelming, often fatal, infections with encapsulated organisms such as *S. pneumoniae* or *H. influenzae*. This may also be a rare complication of splenectomy in adults. The loss of the marginal zone may be especially important in this regard.[16]

Sequestering approximately one-third of the platelet mass, the red pulp cords of the spleen act as a reservoir for platelets. Massive splenomegaly may result in a pooling of 80–90% of the platelets, producing peripheral blood thrombocytopenia. Conditions associated with an enlargement of the spleen also are frequently accompanied by leukopenia and anemia, the result of splenic pooling and sequestration. Removal of the spleen results in a transient thrombocytosis, with a return to normal platelet concentrations in about l0 days.

Although the spleen is not essential to life, splenectomy does result in characteristic erythrocyte abnormalities easily noted on blood smears by experienced clinical laboratory professionals. After splenectomy, the normally agranular erythrocytes contain granular inclusions. Abnormal shapes may also be seen (∞ Chapter 10).

The lifespan of healthy erythrocytes is not increased after splenectomy. The culling function is assumed by other organs, primarily the liver. Blood flow through the liver also is slowed by passage through sinusoids, which are lined with specialized macrophages called Kupffer cells. These macrophages can perform functions similar to the phagocytes in the splenic cords and marginal zone. Even when a spleen is present, the liver, because of its larger blood flow, is responsible for removing most of the particulate matter of the blood. The liver, however, is not as effective as the spleen in filtering abnormal erythrocytes. This is probably because of the relatively rapid flow of blood past hepatic macrophages.

Hypersplenism

In a number of conditions the spleen may become enlarged and, through exaggeration of its normal activities of filtering and phagocytosing, cause anemia, leukopenia, thrombocytopenia, or combinations of cytopenias. A diagnosis of hypersplenism is made when four conditions are met: (1) the presence of anemia, leukopenia, or thrombocytopenia in the peripheral blood; (2) the existence of a cellular or hyperplastic bone marrow corresponding to the peripheral blood cytopenias; (3) the occurrence of splenomegaly; (4) the correction of cytopenias following splenectomy.

Hypersplenism has been categorized into two types: primary and secondary. The primary type is said to occur when no underlying disease can be identified. The spleen functions abnormally and causes the disease. This type of hypersplenism is very rare.

Secondary hypersplenism occurs in those cases where an underlying disorder causes the splenic abnormalities. The causes of secondary hypersplenism are many and varied. Hypersplenism may occur secondary to compensatory (or workload) hypertrophy of this organ. Inflammatory and infectious diseases are thought to cause splenomegaly by an increase in the defensive functions of the spleen. For example, an increase in the clearing of particulate matter may lead to an increase in the number of macrophages, or hyperplasia of lymphoid cells may result from prolonged infection. Several blood disorders may cause splenomegaly. In these disorders, the blood cells may be intrinsically abnormal or coated with antibody, and they are removed from circulation in large numbers (e.g., hereditary spherocytosis, immune thrombocytopenic purpura). Disorders in which the macrophages accumulate large quantities of undigestible substances are characterized by splenomegaly; some of these disorders, such as Gaucher's disease, will be discussed in ∞ Chapter 21.

Neoplasms or benign tumors in which the malignant cells occupy much of the splenic volume may cause splenomegaly, as may liver disease. The tumor cells, however, may incapacitate the spleen. In these cases the peripheral blood will show evidence of hyposplenism (similar to the findings after splenectomy). An outstanding feature of myelofibrosis, a disorder in which the bone marrow is progressively replaced with fibrous tissue, is splenomegaly. In these cases the spleen contains foci of extramedullary hematopoiesis. Congestive splenomegaly may occur following liver cirrhosis with portal hypertension, when blood that does not flow easily through the liver is rerouted through the spleen.

The effects of hypersplenism may be relieved by splenectomy; however, this procedure is not always advisable, especially when the spleen is performing a constructive role, such as antibody production or filtering of protozoa or bacteria. Splenectomy appears to be most beneficial in patients with hereditary or acquired conditions in which erythrocytes or platelets undergo increased destruction, such as hemolytic disorders or idiopathic thrombocytopenic purpura. The blood cells are still abnormal after splenectomy, but the site of their destruction is removed. Consequently, the cells have a more normal life span.

CASE STUDY (continued from page 45)

Francine was diagnosed as having leukemia.

4. What do you think is the cause of the splenomegaly?

5. Why might the peripheral blood reveal changes associated with hyposplenism when the spleen is enlarged?

► LYMPH NODES

The lymphatic system is composed of lymph nodes and lymphatic vessels that drain into the left and right lymphatic duct. The vessels originate in connective tissue spaces. They carry lymph toward the ducts near the neck, where lymph enters the blood. Lymph is formed from blood fluid that escapes into connective tissue. The bean-shaped lymph nodes occur in groups or chains along the larger lymphatic vessels. Lymph nodes contain an outer area called the cortex and an inner area called the medulla (Figure 3-7 ■). Fibrous trabeculae extend inward from the capsule to form irregular communicating compartments within the parenchyma. The cortex contains B cell follicles surrounded by T lymphocytes and macrophages. Within the follicles are areas of B cells known as germinal centers. A stimulated node may have many germinal centers filled with proliferating B lymphocytes, whereas a resting node contains follicles with small resting lymphocytes and macrophages. The medulla, which surrounds the efferent lymphatics, consists of cords of plasma cells that lie between sinusoids.

Lymph nodes act as filters removing foreign particles from lymph by phagocytic cells; thus, they are extremely important in immune defense. As antigens pass through the nodes, they contact and stimulate immunocompetent lymphocytes to proliferate and differentiate into effector cells. Stimulated B

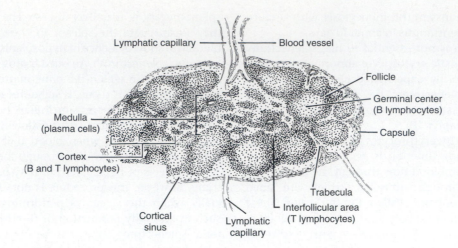

■ **FIGURE 3-7** A schematic drawing of a lymph node. Note the location of T and B lymphocyte populations.

cells move from the germinal centers to the medulla, where they reside as plasma cells and secrete antibody.

MUCOSA-ASSOCIATED LYMPHOID TISSUE (MALT)

MALT is a collection of loosely organized aggregates of lymphocytes found throughout the body in association with mucosal surfaces. Its basic organization is similar to that of lymph nodes in that T- and B-cell-rich areas can be identified, but they are not as clearly demarcated as in lymph nodes. The medulla is not present as a separate structure, and no fibrous capsule can be identified. In the intestine, some of these aggregates are known as Peyer's patches. The function of MALT is to trap antigens that are crossing mucosal surfaces and initiate immune responses rapidly.

LYMPHADENOPATHY

Lymph nodes may become enlarged by expansion of the tissue within the node due to inflammation, prolonged immune response to infectious agents, or malignant transformation of lymphocytes or macrophages. Alternatively, lymph node enlargement may occur because of metastatic tumors that originate in extranodal sites.

 CASE STUDY *(continued from page 49)*

Francine had lymphadenopathy. The leukemia was diagnosed as a leukemia of the lymphocytic cells.

6. What might explain the lymphadenopathy?

SUMMARY

Hematopoiesis occurs in several different locations during development. The major locations include the yolk sac, aorta-gonads-mesonephros (AGM) region, liver, bone marrow, and thymus. Further differentiation of lymphocytes also occurs in the spleen and lymph nodes. In the adult, the bone marrow is the location of the most primitive stem cells and thus is ultimately responsible for initiating all hematopoiesis. Myeloid cells, platelets, and erythrocytes essentially complete their differentiation in the bone marrow. T cells finish most of their differentiation in the thymus. B cells are able to respond to antigens by the time they leave the bone marrow, but differentiate further into antibody-secreting plasma cells in the spleen and lymph nodes. The spleen removes senescent or abnormal erythrocytes and removes particulate matter from erythrocytes. Lymph nodes are important in immune defense, removing foreign particles from lymph.

REVIEW QUESTIONS

LEVEL I

1. B cells develop or differentiate in all of the following tissues *EXCEPT:* (Checklist #2)
   a. thymus
   b. bone marrow
   c. spleen
   d. lymph nodes

LEVEL II

1. A common site of adult extramedullary hematopoiesis is the: (Checklist #3)
   a. liver
   b. thymus
   c. lymph node
   d. yolk sac

REVIEW QUESTIONS *(continued)*

LEVEL I

2. Lack of a spleen results in: (Checklist #4)
   a. younger circulating erythrocytes
   b. granular inclusions in erythrocytes
   c. pitting of erythrocytes
   d. spherocytes

3. Peyer's patches are most closely related to the: (Checklist #3)
   a. lymph node
   b. spleen
   c. thymus
   d. liver

4. All of the following are functions of bone marrow stroma *EXCEPT:* (Checklist #4)
   a. controls the volume of marrow available for hematopoiesis
   b. provides structural support for marrow elements
   c. secretes growth factors for hematopoiesis
   d. provides an exit route from marrow for mature blood cells

5. Which site of early hematopoiesis is extraembryonic? (Checklist #1)
   a. yolk sac
   b. liver
   c. AGM
   d. spleen

LEVEL II

2. Which of the following is a criterion for a diagnosis of hypersplenism? (Checklist #1)
   a. presence of a high WBC count in the blood
   b. low cell counts in the bone marrow
   c. circulating antibody-coated platelets
   d. correction of blood counts after splenectomy

3. Hypersplenism can result from increased: (Checklist #1)
   a. splenic macrophages
   b. B cell proliferation
   c. abnormal erythrocytes
   d. all of the above

4. Extramedullary hematopoiesis in the adult is often accompanied by: (Checklist #1, 2, 3)
   a. splenomegaly
   b. liver atrophy
   c. leukocytosis
   d. hyposplenism

5. Hypersplenism associated with compensatory hypertrophy of the spleen may be found: (Checklist #1, 4)
   a. in neoplasms when malignant cells occupy much of the splenic space
   b. when there are intrinsically abnormal erythrocytes
   c. in liver cirrhosis with portal hypertension
   d. when splenic macrophages accumulate large amounts of undigestible substances

www.prenhall.com/mckenzie

Use the above address to access the free, interactive Companion Web site created for this textbook. Get hints, instant feedback, and textbook references to chapter-related multiple choice questions.

REFERENCES

1. Gordon S, Fraser I, Nath D, Hughes D, Clarke S. Macrophages in tissues and in vitro. *Curr Opin Immunol.* 1992; 4:25–32.

2. Marcos MA, Godin I, Cumano A, Morales S, Garc a-Porrero JA, Dieterlen-Livre F, et al. Developmental events from hemopoietic stem cells to B-cell populations and Ig repertoires. *Immunol Rev.* 1994; 137:155–71.

3. Pardanaud L, Luton D, Prigent M, Bourcheix LM, Catala M, Dieterlen-Livre F. Two distinct endothelial lineages in ontogeny, one of them related to hemopoiesis. *Development.* 1996; 122:1363–71.

4. Farace MG, Brown BA, Raschella G, Alexander J, Gambari R, Fantoni A, et al. The mouse beta h1 gene codes for the z chain of embryonic hemoglobin. *J Biol Chem.* 1984; 259:7123–28.

5. Chang Y, Paige CJ, Wu GE. Enumeration and characterization of DJH structures in mouse fetal liver. *EMBO J.* 1992; 11:1891–99.

6. Elliott JF, Rock EP, Patten PA, Davis MM, Chien YH. The adult T-cell receptor delta-chain is diverse and distinct from that of fetal thymocytes. *Nature.* 1988; 331:627–31.

7. Sadahira Y, Mori M. Role of the macrophage in erythropoiesis. *Pathol Int.* 1999; 49(10):841–48.

8. Yoo D, Lessin LS, Jensen WN. Bone marrow mast cells in lymphoproliferative disorders. *Ann Intern Med.* 1978; 88:753–57.

9. Mayani H, Guilbert LJ, Janowska-Wieczorek A. Biology of the hemopoietic microenvironment. *Eur J Haematol.* 1992; 49:225–33.

10. Rickard DJ, Subramaniam M, Spelsberg TC. Molecular and cellular mechanisms of estrogen action on the skeleton. *J Cell Biochem.* 1999; Suppl 32–33:123–32.

11. Moriyama Y, Fisher JW. Effects of testosterone and erythropoietin on erythroid colony formation in human bone marrow cultures. *Blood.* 1975; 45:665–70.

12. Iversen PO. Blood flow to the haemopoietic bone marrow. *Acta Physiol Scand.* 1997; 159:269–76.

13. Lichtman MA, Packman CH, Costine LS. Molecular and cellular traffic across the marrow sinus wall. In: *Blood Cell Formation: The role of the hematopoietic microenvironment.* Edited by M. Tavassol; Clifton, NJ, Humana Press, 1989.

14. Shortman K, Egerton M, Spangrude GJ, Scollay R. The generation and fate of thymocytes. *Semin Immunol.* 1990; 2:3–12.

15. Douek DC, Koup RA. Evidence for thymic function in the elderly. *Vaccine.* 2000; 18(16):1638–41.

16. Kraal, G. Cells in the marginal zone of the spleen. *Int Rev Cytol.* 1992; 132:31–74.

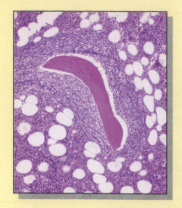

4

The Erythrocyte

Joel Hubbard, Ph.D.

CHAPTER OUTLINE

■ CHECKLIST - LEVEL I

At the end of this unit of study, the student should be able to:

1. List the stages of erythrocyte maturation in the marrow from youngest to most mature cell and describe each stage.
2. Explain the maturation process of reticulocytes and the cellular changes that take place.
3. Identify the normal range for reticulocytes.
4. Explain the function of erythropoietin; include the origin of production, bone marrow effects, and normal values.
5. Describe the function of the erythrocyte membrane.
6. Name the sole energy substrate of the erythrocyte.
7. Diagram the mechanism of extravascular erythrocyte destruction and hemoglobin catabolism.
8. Diagram the mechanism of intravascular erythrocyte destruction and hemoglobin catabolism.
9. State the average dimensions and life span of the normal erythrocyte.
10. Describe the function of 2,3-DPG and its relationship to the erythrocyte.

■ CHECKLIST - LEVEL II

At the end of this unit of study the student should be able to:

1. Differentiate the erythropoietic maturation stages in the proper chronological order and compare each stage on the basis of morphological appearance.
2. Summarize the mechanisms involved in the regulation of erythrocyte production.
3. Build a structure of the erythrocyte membrane, including general dimensions and features; assess the function of membrane components.
4. Compare and contrast three pathways of erythrocyte metabolism and identify key intermediates as well as the relationship of each to erythrocyte survival and longevity.
5. Generalize the metabolic and catabolic changes within the erythrocyte that occur with time that "label" the erythrocyte for removal by the spleen.
6. Compare and contrast erythrocyte extravascular destruction with intravascular destruction and differentiate which process is dominant given laboratory results.
7. Predict the effects of increased and decreased erythropoietin levels in the blood.

KEY TERMS

Bilirubin
Cyanosis
Erythropoiesis
Glycolysis
Haptoglobin
Heinz bodies
Hemopexin
Hemosiderin
Hemosiderinuria
Hypoxic
Normoblast
Polychromatophilic erythrocyte
Reticulocyte

BACKGROUND BASICS

The information in this chapter will build on the concepts learned in previous chapters. To maximize your learning experience you should review these concepts before starting this unit of study.

Level I

▶ Describe the process of cell differentiation and maturation, regulation, and the function of growth factors; describe cell organelles and their function. (Chapter 2)
▶ Give the functional description of erythroid marrow. (Chapter 3)

Level II

▶ List and describe the function of specific growth factors in erythrocyte development. (Chapter 2)
▶ Describe the structure and function of the spleen and bone marrow. (Chapter 3)

ⓔ CASE STUDY

We will address this case study throughout the chapter.
Stephen, a 28-year-old Caucasian male of Italian descent, became progressively ill following a safari vacation to West Africa. The patient arrived at the ER for evaluation following several days of fever, chills, and malaise. The advent of hemoglobinuria prompted the patient to seek emergency aid. A clinical history and physical examination supported a diagnosis of anemia. Since Stephen had recently returned from a malarial endemic area, the physician first suspected malaria, even though the patient had been on primaquine preventive drug therapy while traveling abroad. Blood smears examined for malaria, however, resulted in a negative diagnosis.

▶ OVERVIEW

This chapter is a study of the erythrocyte. It begins with a description of erythrocyte production and maturation. This is followed by an account of the erythrocyte membrane composition and function, cell metabolism, and kinetics of cell production. The chapter concludes with a description of destruction of the senescent cell.

▶ INTRODUCTION

The erythrocyte (red blood cell, RBC) was one of the first microscopic elements recognized and described after the discovery of the microscope. For centuries these corpuscles were considered inert particles with no function. In 1817, Francois Magendie diluted blood with water, found no microscopic corpuscles, and erroneously surmised that the red blood cells seen by others were probably air bubbles.[1] We now know that erythrocytes suspended in water will burst, which explains Magendie's negative findings. Magendie eventually recognized his mistake and later provided a morphologic description of the erythrocyte. It was not until 1865, however, when Felix Hoppe-Seyler discovered the oxygen-carrying capacity of the red pigment (hemoglobin) within the red blood cells, that the function of these "globules" began to be understood. Today, we recognize the erythrocyte as being one of the most highly specialized cells in the body.

▶ MATURATION

Erythropoiesis is normally an orderly process through which the peripheral concentration of erythrocytes is maintained in a steady state. Production begins with the hematopoietic stem cell (HSC) (∞ Chapter 2). Stem cell differentiation is induced by certain microenvironmental influences to become a committed erythroid progenitor cell. The committed erythroid progenitor cell compartment consists of two compartments as defined by their behavior in cell culture systems: the burst-forming unit-erythroid (BFU-E) and colony-forming unit-erythroid (CFU-E). The BFU-E stem cells maintain a cell cycle through the action of a burst-promoting factor (BPF), now known to be IL-3 or GM-CSF, that is released by the local microenvironment. BFU-E cells have a low concentration of erythropoietin (EPO) receptors and are relatively insensitive to EPO except in high concentrations. Differentiation of the BFU-E cell gives rise to the unipotential CFU-E stem cell. CFU-E have a high concentration of EPO membrane receptors, hence, they respond to lower EPO concentrations than BFU-E. EPO stimulation transforms CFU-E into the earliest recognizable erythroid precursor, the pronormoblast.

Nucleated erythrocyte precursors in the bone marrow are collectively called **normoblasts** or erythroblasts. Young erythrocytes with residual RNA, but without a nucleus, are referred to as **reticulocytes.** Bone marrow normoblast maturation occurs in an orderly and well-defined sequence. The process involves a gradual decrease in cell size together with condensation and eventual expulsion of the nucleus. The cytoplasm in the younger normoblasts stains deeply basophilic due to the predominance of RNA (Figure 4-1 ■). As the cell matures there is an increase in hemoglobin production, which is acidophilic, and the cytoplasm takes on a gray to orange appearance (Figures 4-1 ■, 4-2 ■). There are two terminology systems in use to describe erythrocyte precursors. One uses the term normoblast and the other rubriblast. In this text we will use the normoblast terminology. The stages, in order from most immature to mature cell, are: pronormoblast (rubriblast), basophilic normoblast (prorubricyte), polychromatophilic normoblast (rubricyte), orthochromatic normoblast (metarubricyte), reticulocyte, and erythrocyte (Table 4-1 ✪).

The normoblasts generally spend from 5 to 7 days in the proliferating and maturing compartment of the bone marrow. After maturation to the reticulocyte stage, the cell is released to the peripheral blood. The mature circulating erthrocyte has a lifespan of 100–120 days. This lengthy lifespan accounts for the relatively small amount of erythroid marrow in comparison to the large circulating erythrocyte mass.

CHARACTERISTICS OF CELL MATURATION

Although the stages of erythrocyte maturation are usually described in step-like fashion, the actual maturation is a gradual process (Table 4-1 ✪). Some normoblasts may not

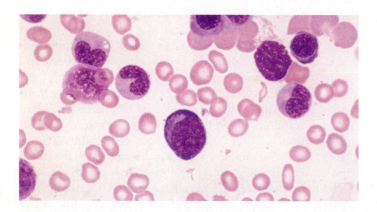

■ FIGURE 4-1 There is a pronormoblast in the center. Note the large N:C ratio, presence of nucleoli, and lacy chromatin. The cytoplasm is deep blue with a lighter pinkish area next to the nucleus. Also note above at about one o'clock the polychromatophilic normoblast. (Bone marrow; Wright-Giemsa stain, 1000X magnification)

conform to all the criteria of a particular stage and a judgment must be made. The more experience one has in examining the blood and bone marrow, the easier it becomes to make these judgments.

Pronormoblast
This is the earliest recognizable erythrocyte precursor. Each pronormoblast produces between 8 and 32 mature erythrocytes. The cell is the largest of the normoblast series, from 14–20 μm in diameter with a high nuclear:cytoplasmic (N:C) ratio. The nucleus occupies 80% or more of the cell. This cell is rather rare in the bone marrow and difficult to find.

Cytoplasm. The cytoplasm contains a large number of basophilic ribosomes and stains deeply basophilic. A larger pale area next to the nucleus is sometimes apparent. This represents the Golgi apparatus. Small amounts of hemoglobin are present, but its visible presence is obscured due to the large number of ribosomes.

Nucleus. The nucleus is large, taking up most of the cell volume, and stains bluish purple. The chromatin is in a fine linear network often described as lacy. The pronormoblast chromatin has a coarser appearance and stains darker than the chromatin of a white cell blast. The nucleus contains from 1 to 3 faint nucleoli.

Basophilic Normoblast
This cell is similar to the pronormoblast except that it is usually smaller (10–16 μm in diameter) and has a decreased N:C ratio. The nucleus occupies more than three-fourths of the cell volume.

Cytoplasm. The cytoplasm is still deeply basophilic, often more so than that of the previous stage, due to the increased number of ribosomes. However, in late basophilic normoblasts, the presence of varying amounts of hemoglobin may cause the cell to take on a lighter blue hue or show pink areas. A pale area surrounding the nucleus, the perinuclear halo, is sometimes seen. This halo represents the mitochondria, which do not stain.

Nucleus. The chromatin is coarser than that of the pronormoblast. The dark violet heterochromatin interspersed with the pink-staining euchromatin may give the chromatin a wheel-spoke appearance. A few small masses of clumped chromatin may be seen along the rim of the nuclear membrane. Nucleoli usually are not apparent.

Polychromatophilic Normoblast
The cell is about 10–12 μm in diameter with a decreased N:C ratio due to condensation of the nuclear chromatin. This is the last stage capable of mitosis.

✪ TABLE 4-1

Morphologic Characteristics of Erythroid Precursors

Cell Type (% of nucleated cells in BM)	Image (Wright stain)	Size	N/C Ratio	Cytoplasmic Characteristics	Nuclear Characteristics
Pronormoblast (Rubriblast) (1%)		14–20 μm	High (8:1)	Small to moderate amount of deep blue cytoplasm; pale area next to nucleus may be seen	1–3 faint nucleoli; reddish purple color; homogeneous, lacy chromatin
Basophilic Normoblast (Prorubricyte) (1–3%)		10–16 μm	Moderate (6:1)	Deep blue-purple; occasionally patches of pink; irregular cell borders may be present; perinuclear halo may be apparent	Indistinct nucleoli; coarsening chromatin; deep purplish-blue color
Polychromatic Normoblast (Rubricyte) (13–30%)		10–12 μm	Low (4:1)	Abundant gray-blue	Chromatin irregular and coarsely clumped, eccentric
Orthochromic Normoblast (Metarubricyte) (1-4%)		8–10 μm	Low (1:2)	Pink–orange; may have varying degrees of basophilia	Small; dense; round or bizarre shape; eccentric
Reticulocyte (new methylene blue stain)		7–10 μm	—	Polychromatophilic	No nucleus
Mature RBC		7–9 μm	—	Pink	No nucleus

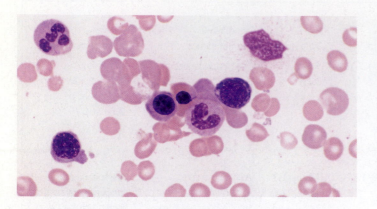

■ **FIGURE 4-2** Developing normoblasts. Starting at nine o'clock there is an early polychromatophilic normoblast, in the center from left to right are an early orthochromatic normoblast, late orthochromatic normoblast, band neutrophil, and a basophilic normoblast. (Bone marrow; Wright-Giemsa stain, 1000X magnification)

Cytoplasm. The most characteristic change in the cell at this stage is the presence of abundant gray blue cytoplasm. The staining properties of the cytoplasm are due to the synthesis of large amounts of hemoglobin and decreasing numbers of ribosomes. The cell derives its name, polychromatophilic, from this characteristic cytoplasmic feature.

Nucleus. The nuclear chromatin is irregular and coarsely clumped.

Orthochromatic Normoblast
This cell is about 8–10 μm in diameter with a low N:C ratio.

Cytoplasm. The cytoplasm is predominantly pink or orange-pink with only a tinge of blue.

Nucleus. The nuclear chromatin is heavily condensed. In late stages, the nucleus is structureless (pyknotic) or fragmented. The nucleus is often eccentric or even partially extruded.

Reticulocyte
After the nucleus is extruded, the cell is known as a reticulocyte. It has residual RNA and mitochondria in the cytoplasm. The residual RNA gives the young cell a bluish tinge with Wright's stain; thus, the cell is appropriately described as a **polychromatophilic erythrocyte.** About 65% of the cell's hemoglobin is made during the normoblast stages. The remaining 35% of cellular hemoglobin is made during the reticulocyte stage. The reticulocyte is slightly larger, 8–10 μm, than a mature erythrocyte. After 2 to 2½ days in the bone marrow, the reticulocyte is released

into the vascular sinuses of the marrow. From here, it gains access to the peripheral blood. Reticulocyte maturation continues in the peripheral blood for another day. These cells may be identified in vitro by reaction with supravital stains, new methylene blue N or brilliant cresyl blue, which cause precipitation of the RNA. In this method, the reticulocytes are identified by the presence of punctate purplish blue inclusions (∞ Chapter 7). Normally, reticulocytes comprise 0.5–2% (absolute concentration is 18–158 × 10^9/L) of peripheral blood erythrocytes in a nonanemic adult. The actual reference value varies between laboratories. The absolute concentration of reticulocytes is calculated by multiplying the percent of reticulocytes times the RBC count. When reticulocytes are increased, there is an increased number of polychromatophilic erythrocytes (polychromasia) seen on the Romanowsky stained peripheral blood smear.

Reticulocytes may contain small amounts of iron dispersed throughout the cytoplasm. The iron can be identified with Perl's Prussian blue stain. Erythrocytes with identified iron are called siderocytes. The spleen is responsible for removal of these excess granules and the normal mature cell is devoid of granular inclusions.

✔ **Checkpoint! #1**

What is the first stage of red cell maturation that has visible cytoplasmic evidence of hemoglobin production on a Romanowsky stained smear?

 CASE STUDY *(continued from page 53)*

In addition to malaria screening, the ER physician also ordered a CBC with the following results:

WBC:	14×10^9/L	Differential:	
RBC:	3.10×10^{12}/L	SEGS	70 %
HGB:	9.2 gm/dL	BANDS	11 %
HCT:	0.28 L/L	META	2 %
MCV:	93 fL	LYMPH	13 %
MCH:	30.6 pg/dL	MONO	2 %
MCHC:	32.5 gm/dL	EOS	2 %
PLT:	230×10^9/L	NRBCs/100 WBCs	18
		RBC Morphology:	
		Anisocytosis	3+
		Poikilocytosis	2+
		Spherocytosis	1+
		Schiztocytes	1+
		Polychromasia	2+

1. Predict Stephen's reticulocyte count: low, normal, or increased.

Erythrocyte

The mature erythrocyte is a biconcave disc about 7–8 μm in diameter, 80–100 fL in volume. It stains pink to orange because of the large amount of the intracellular acidophilic protein, hemoglobin. The cell has lost its residual RNA and mitochondria as well as important enzymes; therefore, it is incapable of synthesizing new protein or lipid.

▶ ERYTHROCYTE MEMBRANE

Around the beginning of the twentieth century, investigations began that established the complexity of the erythrocyte membrane. Steven Hedin performed experiments that demonstrated the osmotic properties and selective permeability of the erythrocyte.[2] He found that erythrocyte volume increased in hypotonic solutions (solutions having a lower osmotic pressure than the erythrocyte) as well as in solutions such as urea or glycerol. Other solutions, however, caused shrinking of the cell. Antigenic properties of the membrane were recognized several years later by Karl Landsteiner. He discovered that human sera caused clumping of the erythrocytes in different individuals. He originally divided these individuals into three groups, A, B, and C, according to their erythrocyte agglutination patterns with human sera.[3] Today, we identify these blood types as groups A, B, and O. Hundreds of other erythrocyte antigens have been identified.

A normal intact membrane is absolutely essential for normal erythrocyte function and survival. Studies of blood circulation have determined that the 7 μm erythrocyte must be a flexible (deformable) corpuscle to squeeze through the tiny 3 μm fenestrations of the capillaries of the spleen. The cell's deformability is not only a property of the erythrocyte membrane but also of the fluidity and concentration of the cell's content, mainly hemoglobin. Reversible deformability of the membrane occurs when the cell changes geometric shape but the surface area remains constant. Any decrease in deformability of membrane or fluidity of content or increased concentration of hemoglobin results in decreased erythrocyte deformability. Decreased deformability leads to trapping in the splenic cords or fragmentation of the cell under the normal stress of circulation.

MEMBRANE COMPOSITION

The erythrocyte membrane is a biphospholipid protein complex composed of 52% protein, 40% lipid, and 8% carbohydrate (Table 4-2✪).[5] This chemical structure and composition control the membrane functions of transport and flexibility and determine the membrane's antigenic proper-

✪ TABLE 4-2

Erythrocyte Membrane Composition

Lipids	Unesterified cholesterol
	Phospholipids
	cephalin
	lecithin
	sphingomylelin
	phosphatidylserine
	Glycolipids
Proteins	Integral proteins
	glycophorins A, B, C (carry antigens on exterior of membrane)
	band 3 (attaches skeletal lattice to membrane lipid bilayer)
	Peripheral proteins (form membrane skeletal lattice and attach it to membrane)
	spectrin
	actin
	ankyrin (band 2.1)
	band 4.2
	band 4.1
	adducin
	band 4.9 (dematin)
	tropomyosin

ties. Any defect in structure or alteration in chemical composition may alter any or all functions and lead to premature death of the cell (∞ Chapter 17). Mature erythrocytes lack the cellular organelles (nucleus and mitochondria) and enzymes necessary to synthesize new lipid and protein; thus, extensive damage to the membrane cannot be repaired, and the damaged cell will be culled from the circulation by the spleen.

Lipid Composition

Approximately 95% of the lipid content of the membrane consists of equal amounts of unesterified cholesterol and phospholipids. The remaining lipids are free fatty acids and glycolipids. Cholesterol affects the surface area of the cell and is responsible for the passive cation permeability of the membrane. It appears that membrane cholesterol exists in free equilibrium with plasma cholesterol. Thus, it is not surprising that increases in free plasma cholesterol, such as occurs in lecithin-cholesterol acyl transferase (LCAT) deficiency, result in accumulation of cholesterol on erythrocyte membranes. Studies on the effects of cholesterol in model membranes indicate that an increase in the cholesterol-to-phospholipid ratio increases the microviscosity of the membrane. Reticulocytes normally contain more membrane cholesterol than older erythrocytes. This excess cholesterol is removed from the reticulocytes during maturation by the spleen. Splenectomized patients usually have an abnormal accumulation of cholesterol on the membrane and presence of target cells on the blood smear. (Target cells are described in ∞ Chapter 10.)

Exchange between phospholipids of the membrane and plasma also may occur, especially with lecithin. The phospholipid molecules are arranged with polar heads directed to the inside and outside of the cell and the hydrophobic tails directed to the interior of the bilayer. Considerable evidence exists that the mobility of phospholipids within the membrane contributes to membrane fluidity. It is interesting to note that lipid associated with penetrating proteins appears to diffuse as a unit with the proteins. The function of these lipid-associated proteins is intimately involved with the lipid. Membrane enzymes associated with lipid require the presence of the lipid for full enzymatic activity.

A small portion of membrane lipids are glycolipids in the form of glycosphingolipid. Glycolipids are responsible for some antigenic properties of the membrane.

Protein Composition

Erythrocyte membrane proteins are of two types: integral proteins and peripheral proteins (Figure 4-3 ■). Integral proteins are firmly entrenched in the lipid bilayer, whereas peripheral proteins are outside the lipid framework on the cytoplasmic side of the membrane but attached to the membrane lipids or integral proteins by ionic and hydrogen bonds. Both types of membrane protein are synthesized during cell development. The proteins are usually identified by a number according to their separation by polyacrylamide gel electrophoresis in sodium dodecyl sulfate.

Integral proteins consist of two types: glycophorins and band 3 protein. The three major glycophorins—glycophorins A, B, and C—are made up of three domains: the cytoplasmic domain; the hydrophobic domain, which spans the bilayer; and the extracellular domain on the exterior surface of the membrane.[4] The extracellular domain is glycosylated and carries cell antigens. Glycophorin C also plays a role in attaching the skeletal protein network on the cytoplasmic side to the bilipid layer. The COOH group of sialic

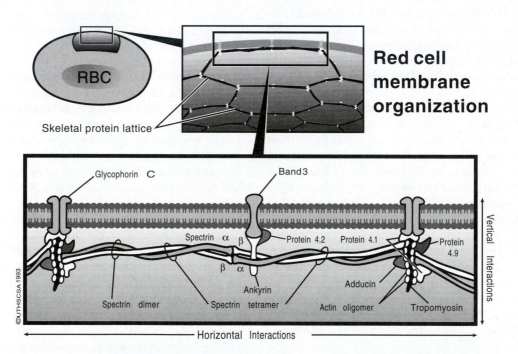

■ FIGURE 4-3 A model of the organization of the erythrocyte membrane showing the peripheral and integral proteins and lipids. Spectrin is the predominant protein of the skeletal protein lattice. Spectrin dimers join head to head to form spectrin tetramers. At the tail end, spectrin tetramers come together at the junctional complex. This complex is composed of actin oligomer and stabilized by tropomyosin, which sits in the groove of the actin filaments. Band 4.9 protein (dematin) binds to actin and bundles actin filaments. Spectrin is attached to actin by protein 4.1, which also attaches the skeletal lattice to the lipid membrane via its interaction with glycophorin C. Adducin binds to two spectrin heterodimers. Ankyrin links the skeletal protein network to the inner side of the lipid bilayer via band 3. Protein 4.2 interacts with ankyrin and band 3.

acid that is attached to the membrane glycophorins imparts a strong negative charge to the exterior of the cell. This charge is important in reducing erythrocyte interaction with one another. Band 3 is important in attaching the skeletal protein network to the lipid bilayer.

Peripheral membrane proteins are organized into a two-dimensional lattice network directly laminating the inner side of the membrane lipid bilayer.[5] The horizontal interactions of this lattice are parallel to the plane of the membrane and serve as a skeletal support for the membrane lipid layer. The vertical interactions of the lattice are perpendicular to the plane of the membrane and serve to attach the skeletal lattice network to the lipid layer of the membrane. The skeletal proteins give membranes their viscoelastic properties and contribute to cell shape, deformability, and membrane stability. It is not unusual to find that defects in this erythrocyte cytoskeleton are associated with abnormal cell shape, decreased stability, and hemolytic anemia (∞ Chapter 17).

The peripheral proteins include spectrin, actin, ankyrin (band 2.1), band 4.2, band 4.1, adducin, band 4.9 (dematin), and tropomyosin. Spectrin is the predominant skeletal protein composed of dimeric chains (α and β) that associate head to head to form tetramers. The tails of tetramers come together to form hexagons at junctional complexes. The junctional complexes are composed of spectrin, short actin oligomers, band 4.1, adducin, band 4.9 and tropomyosin. This skeletal lattice is attached to the inner side of the membrane lipid bilayer near the center of the spectrin tetramers by the association of the integral protein band 3, and peripheral proteins band 4.2, and ankyrin.

The skeletal proteins are not static but rather are in a continuous disassociation–association equilibrium with each other and with attachment sites. This occurs in response to various physical and chemical stimuli that affect the erythrocytes' journey while moving throughout the body.

Another membrane component that deserves mention because of its affect on the membrane is calcium. Most intracellular calcium (80%) is found in association with the erythrocyte membrane. Calcium is maintained at an extremely low intracellular concentration by the activity of an ATP-fueled pump. Conditions that allow accumulation of this cation in the erythrocyte result in rigid, shrunken cells with membrane protusions (echinocytes) and reduced deformability. The abnormal erythrocyte shape is assumed to be produced by calcium-induced irreversible cross-linking and alteration of the cytoskeletal proteins.

✓ Checkpoint! #2

Compare placement in the membrane and function of peripheral and integral erythrocyte membrane proteins.

► ERYTHROCYTE METABOLISM

The metabolism of the erythrocyte is limited because of the absence of a nucleus, mitochondria, and other subcellular organelles. Although the binding, transport, and release of O_2 and CO_2 is a passive process not requiring energy, a variety of energy-dependent metabolic processes occur that are essential to cell viability. The most important metabolic pathways in the mature erythrocyte require glucose as a substrate. These pathways include: (l) Embden-Meyerhof pathway, (2) hexose-monophosphate shunt, (3) methemoglobin reductase pathway, and (4) Rapoport-Luebering shunt. These pathways contribute energy for maintaining: (l) high intracellular K^+, low intracellular Na^+, and very low intracellular Ca^{++} (cation pump); (2) hemoglobin in reduced form; (3) high levels of reduced glutathione; and (4) membrane integrity and deformability (Table 4-3 ✪).

EMBDEN-MEYERHOF PATHWAY

The erythrocyte obtains its energy in the form of ATP, from glucose breakdown in the Embden-Meyerhof pathway (Figure 4-4 ■). About 90–95% of the cell's glucose consumption is utilized by this pathway. Normal erythrocytes have no glycogen deposits. They depend entirely upon environmental glucose for **glycolysis.** Glucose enters the cell by facilitated diffusion, an energy-free process. The glucose is metabolized to lactate, producing a net gain of two moles of ATP per mole of glucose.

Adequate amounts of ATP are necessary to maintain erythrocyte shape, flexibility, and membrane integrity through regulation of intracellular cation concentration. The cations, Na^+, K^+, Ca^{++}, and Mg^{++} are maintained in the erythrocyte at levels much different than in plasma (Table 4-4 ✪). Normally erythrocyte osmotic equilibrium is maintained both by the selective permeability of the membrane and by the cation pumps located in the cell membrane. The Na^+, K^+ cation pump hydrolyzes one mole of ATP in the expulsion of $3Na^+$ and the uptake of $2K^+$. Calcium plays a role in maintaining low membrane permeability to Na^+ and K^+. An increase in intracellular calcium is associated with excess K^+ leakage from the cell. Magnesium is another major intracellular cation. This divalent cation reacts with ATP to form the substrate complex Mg-ATP, for Ca^{++}, Mg^{++}-ATPase (calcium cation pump). Although Mg^{++} itself is necessary for active extrusion of Ca^{++} from the cell through this complex formation, Mg^{++} is not moved out of the cell in the process.

Enormous amounts of ATP are needed to maintain normal levels of these intracellular cations against their concentration gradients. Increased osmotic fragility is noted in cells with abnormally permeable membranes and/or decreased production of ATP. Upon the exhaustion of glucose, the fuel (i.e., ATP) for the cation pumps is no longer available. Cells

⊕ TABLE 4-3

Role of Metabolic Pathways in the Erythrocyte

Metabolic pathway	Key enzymes	Function	Hemopathology
Embden-Meyerhof	Phosphofructokinase Pyruvate kinase (PK)	Produces ATP accounting for 90% of glucose consumption in RBC	Hemolytic anemia - Hereditary PK deficiency
Hexose-monophosphate shunt	Glutathione reductase Glucose-6-phosphate dehydrogenase (G6PD)	Provides NADPH and glutathione to reduce oxidants that would shift the balance of oxyhemoglobin to methemoglobin	Hemolytic anemia - Hereditary G6PD deficiency - Glutathione reductase deficiency - Hemoglobinopathies
Rapoport-Leubering	DPG-Synthetase	Controls the amount of 2,3-DPG produced, which in turn affects the oxygen affinity of hemoglobin	Hypoxia
Methemoglobin Reductase	Methemoglobin reductase	Protects hemoglobin from oxidation via NADH (from E-M pathway) and methemoglobin reductase	Hemolytic anemia Hypoxia

cannot maintain normal intracellular cation concentrations without ATP, which leads to cell death.

HEXOSE MONOPHOSPHATE SHUNT

Five percent of cellular glucose enters the oxidative HMP shunt, an ancillary system for producing reducing substances (Figure 4-4 ■). This pathway produces reduced nicotinamide adenine dinucleotidephosphate (NADPH) and reduced glutathione (GSH) necessary for maintaining hemoglobin in the reduced functional state. The HMP shunt is functionally dependent on G6PD. Reduced GSH protects the cell from permanent oxidant injury by reducing oxidants. This reduction oxidizes glutathione (GSSG), which in turn is reduced back to GSH for recycling by adequate levels of NADPH. The erythrocyte normally maintains a large ratio of NADPH to NADP⁺. When this pathway is defective, hemoglobin sulfhydryl groups (-SH) are oxidized, which leads to denaturation and precipitation of hemoglobin in the form of **Heinz bodies.** Heinz bodies attach to the inner surface of the cell membrane, decreasing cell flexibility. Heinz bodies are removed from the cell together with a portion of the membrane by macrophages in the spleen. These bodies can be visualized with supravital stains. If large portions of the membrane are damaged in this manner, the whole cell may be removed. This commonly occurs in patients with sex-linked G6PD deficiency.

Reduced GSH is also responsible for maintaining reduced-SH groups at the membrane level. Decreases in GSH lead to oxidant injury of membrane SH groups resulting in leaky cell membranes. Cellular depletion of ATP may then occur due to increased consumption of energy by the cation pump.

Ascorbic acid, or vitamin C, is also an important antioxidant in the erythrocyte where it consumes oxygen free radicals and helps preserve alpha-tocopherol (vitamin E) in membrane lipoproteins. Erythrocytes have a high capacity to regenerate the vitamin C from its oxidized form, dehydroascorbic acid (DHA) by GSH in a direct chemical reaction. This is believed to be an important mechanism for preventing lipid peroxidative damage in areas of inflammation in a vascular bed.[6]

METHEMOGLOBIN REDUCTASE PATHWAY

The methemoglobin reductase pathway, an offshoot of the Embden-Meyerhof pathway, is essential to maintain heme iron in the reduced state, Fe⁺⁺ (Figure 4-4 ■). Hemoglobin with iron in the oxidized ferric state, Fe⁺⁺⁺, is known as methemoglobin. This form of hemoglobin cannot combine with oxygen. Methemoglobin reductase, together with NADH produced by the Embden-Meyerhof pathway, protects the heme iron from oxidation. In the absence of this system, the 2% of methemoglobin formed daily will eventually build up to 20–40%, severely limiting the oxygen-carrying capacity of the blood. Challenges by oxidant drugs can interfere with methemoglobin reductase and cause even higher levels of methemoglobin. This results in cyanosis. **Cyanosis** is a bluish discoloration of the skin due to an increased concentration of deoxyhemoglobin in the blood.

RAPOPORT-LEUBERING SHUNT

The Rapoport-Leubering shunt is a part of the Embden-Meyerhof pathway (Figure 4-4 ■). This pathway bypasses the formation of 3-phosphoglycerate and ATP from l,3-diphosphoglycerate (1,3 DPG). Instead, 1,3-DPG forms 2,3-DPG (more accurately known as 2,3-biphosphoglycerate, 2,3-BPG) catalyzed by a mutase and DPG synthase. Therefore, the ery-

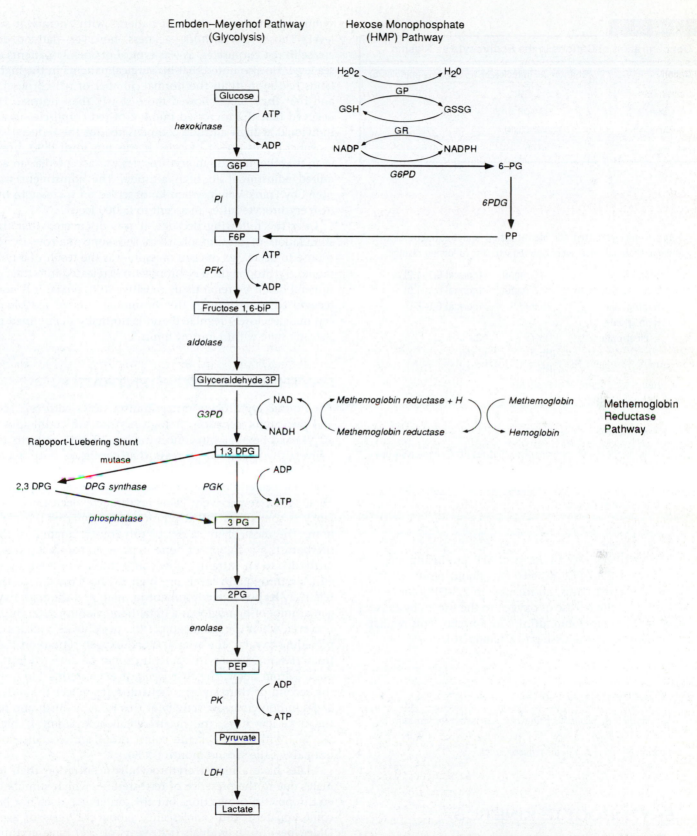

FIGURE 4-4 The erythrocyte metabolic pathways. The Embden-Meyerhof pathway is the major source of energy for the erythrocyte through production of ATP. The hexose-monophosphate pathway is important for reducing oxidants by coupling oxidative metabolism with pyridine nucleotide (NADP) and glutathione (GSSG) reduction. The methemoglobin reductase pathway supports methemoglobin reduction. The Rapoport-Luebering shunt produces 2,3-DPG, which alters hemoglobin-oxygen affinity.

TABLE 4-4

Concentration of Cations in the Erythrocyte vs Plasma

Cation	Erythrocyte (mmoles/L)	Plasma (mmoles/L)
Sodium (Na⁺)	5.4–7.0	135–145
Potassium (K⁺)	98–106	3.6–5.0
Calcium (Ca⁺)	0.0059–0.019	21.0–26.5
Magnesium (Mg⁺⁺)	3.06	0.65–1.05

CASE STUDY (continued from page 56)

Stephen was admitted for identification and treatment of the anemia. More lab tests were ordered with the following results:

Total bilirubin:	4.8 mg/dL	(normal 0.1–1.2)
Direct bilirubin:	1.6 mg/dL	(normal 0.1–1.0)
Haptoglobin:	25 mg/dL	(normal 60–270)
Hemoglobin		
electrophoresis:	Hb-A	98%
	Hb-F	1%
	Hb-A2	1%
Heinz body stain:	Positive	
Fluorescent spot		
test for G6PD		
deficiency:	Positive	

2. What is the cellular mechanism that results in hemolysis due to a deficiency in G6PD?

3. Explain how Heinz body inclusions cause damage to the erythrocyte membrane.

throcyte sacrifices one of its two ATP producing steps in order to form 2,3-DPG. When hemoglobin binds 2,3-DPG, oxygen is released. Thus, an increase in 2,3-DPG concentration facilitates the release of oxygen to the tissues by causing a decrease in hemoglobin affinity for oxygen. This regulates oxygen delivery to the tissues (∞ Chapter 10).

✔ Checkpoint! #3

Which erythrocyte metabolic pathway is responsible for providing the majority of cellular energy? For regulating oxygen affinity? For maintaining hemoglobin in the reduced state?

► ERYTHROCYTE KINETICS

In the middle of the nineteenth century, Dr. Dennis Jourdanet, a French physician practicing in the highlands of Mexico, noted that patients with altitude sickness exhibited symptoms similar to those of patients with anemia at sea level.[7] Those with altitude sickness, however, had no decrease in red corpuscles, as was typical of anemic patients at sea level. He also noted that his surgical patients in the highlands had more than the normal number of red corpuscles and that their blood flowed more slowly than normal. He believed that the increased number of red corpuscles in an individual at high altitude compensated for the reduced atmospheric pressure of oxygen. It was not until 1890, however, that the increase in erythrocytes was accepted as an acquired adjustment to high altitude. The adjustment was noted by Frank Viault, when he observed an increase in his own erythrocytes after an ascent to 15,000 feet.[7]

Over the following decades, it was discovered that the stimulation of erythropoiesis in the bone marrow in response to decreased oxygen pressure was the result of a hormone, erythropoietin. Erythropoietin is released into the peripheral blood by renal tissue sensitive to hypoxia. It is now recognized that through this hormonal control red blood cell mass is closely regulated and is normally maintained in a steady state within narrow limits.

ERYTHROCYTE CONCENTRATION

The normal erythrocyte concentration varies with sex, age, and geographic location. A high erythrocyte count (5.2 × 10^{12}/L) and hemoglobin concentration (19 g/dL) at birth are followed by a gradual decrease that continues until about the second or third month of extrauterine life. At this time, red blood cell and hemoglobin values fall to $3.5 × 10^{12}$/L and 10–11 g/dL, respectively.[8] This erythrocyte decrease in infancy is sometimes called physiologic anemia of the newborn. The most likely cause for physiologic anemia of the newborn is a cessation of bone marrow erythropoiesis after birth, due to an extremely low concentration of erythropoietin. Erythropoietin levels are high in the fetus due to the relatively **hypoxic** environment in utero and the high oxygen affinity of hemoglobin F (fetal hemoglobin). After birth, however, when the lungs replace the placenta as a means of providing oxygen, the arterial blood oxygen saturation rises from 45% to 95%. Erythropoietin cannot be detected in the plasma from about the first week of extrauterine life until the second or third month. Reticulocytes reflect the differences in bone marrow activity at this time. At birth and for the next few days, the mean reticulocyte count is high (4–7%). Within a week the count drops and remains low until about the second month (<1%).

Males have a higher erythrocyte concentration than females due to the presence of testosterone, which stimulates erythropoietin production, but this difference does not become apparent until adolescence (about 12 years of age). Older, healthy individuals (>70 years of age) have erythrocyte concentrations within the reference range.[9,10]

Individuals living at high altitudes have a higher mean erythrocyte concentration than those living at sea level.

Decreases in the partial pressure of atmospheric oxygen at high altitudes result in a physiologic increase in erythrocytes. This is an attempt by the body to provide adequate tissue oxygenation.

✓ Checkpoint! #4

Why are there different reference ranges for hemoglobin concentration in male and female adults but not in male and female children?

REGULATION OF ERYTHROCYTE PRODUCTION

The body can regulate the number of circulating erythrocytes by changing either the rate of cell production in the marrow or the rate of cell release from the marrow. This regulation is normally well balanced because the rate of erythrocyte destruction does not vary significantly. Impaired oxygen transport to the tissues and low intracellular oxygen tension (PO_2) triggers erythrocyte production in the marrow. Conditions that stimulate erythropoiesis include anemia, cardiac or pulmonary disorders, and high altitude.

Erythropoietin (EPO) is a thermostable, nondialyzable, glycoprotein renal hormone with an MW of about 34,000 daltons. It stimulates erythropoiesis in the bone marrow.[11] EPO is secreted by the kidney in response to cellular hypoxia. The hypoxic signal is detected by oxygen sensors located in the kidneys. This feedback control of erythropoiesis is the mechanism by which the body maintains optimal erythrocyte mass for tissue oxygenation. There may be additional sensor mechanisms for stimulation of EPO production, as plasma levels of erythropoietin are constant when the hemoglobin concentration is within the normal range but increases steeply when the hemoglobin decreases below 12 g/dL.[12]

EPO has been defined in biologic terms to have an activity of 7,000 units (U) per mg of the protein.[11] Normal plasma contains from 3 to 8 mU of EPO per mL of plasma. EPO may also be found in the urine at concentrations proportional to that found in the plasma, normally about l–4 mU/mL (Table 4-5 ✪).

In anemia, the actual titer of EPO is related to both hemoglobin concentration and the pathophysiology of the anemia. For example, patients with pure erythrocyte aplasia show EPO titers four times greater than patients with iron deficiency anemia and ten times greater than those with megaloblastic anemia even though hemoglobin concentration in all three types of anemia may be similar. Serum EPO levels are significant because they reflect not only EPO production but also its disappearance from the blood or utilization by the bone marrow. From 3–8 mU/mL can maintain normal steady-state erythropoiesis, whereas it takes 2,000–5,000 mU/mL EPO to increase erythropoiesis to ten times normal as is needed in

severe bleeding or hemolytic anemia. The reason for this steep increase in EPO is unknown (∞ Chapter 10).

Patients with renal disease and nephrectomized patients are usually anemic, but they continue to make erythrocytes and produce limited amounts of EPO in response to hypoxia. Anephric individuals have a plasma EPO titer of 2.8–6.0 mU/mL. These findings suggest that an extrarenal source of erythropoietin exists, most probably the liver; however, studies of anemic rats have demonstrated that the ability of the extrarenal tissue in rats to produce EPO is limited to about 20% of the total EPO concentration. In addition, the adult liver appears to require a more severe hypoxic stimulus for EPO production than the kidney. The role of the liver in EPO production is probably associated with its role in EPO production during the fetal and neonatal periods.[13,14]

The most important action of EPO is stimulation of committed stem cells, BFU-E and CFU-E, to proliferate and differentiate. Erythropoietin receptors on the cell membrane increase as the BFU-E matures to the CFU-E. These receptors decrease as normoblasts mature and are absent on the reticulocyte. The activity of the more immature BFU-E is also influenced by other growth factors, IL-3, SCF, and GM-CSF. The CFU-E, however, appear to be primarily controlled by EPO. Other effects of EPO include decreasing normoblast maturation time, increasing rate of hemoglobin synthesis, and stimulating early release of bone marrow reticulocytes (stress or shift reticulocytes). In addition, it has been recently suggested that EPO may play a unique role in protecting the erythrocyte membrane from oxidative damage.[15]

The normal bone marrow can increase erythropoiesis 5- to l0-fold in response to the appropriate EPO stimulation if sufficient iron is available. In hemolytic anemia there is a readily available supply of iron recycled from erythrocytes destroyed in vivo that results in a sustained increase in erythropoiesis.

TABLE 4-5

Characteristics of Erythropoietin

General Characteristics

Composition:	glycoprotein
Stimulus for synthesis:	cellular hypoxia
Origin:	kidneys 80%
	liver 20%
Normal Range:	plasma 3–8 mU/mL
	urine 1–4 mU/mL

Functions

Stimulates BFU-E and CFU-E to divide and mature

Decreases normoblast maturation time

Increases rate of hemoglobin synthesis

Stimulates early release of bone marrow reticulocytes (Shift reticulocytes)

Response to Anemia

Generally increased except in anemia of renal disease

The rate of erythropoiesis in blood loss anemia, where iron is lost from the body, however, is dependent upon preexisting iron stores. In this case the rate of erythropoiesis usually does not exceed 2.5 times normal, unless large parenteral or oral doses of iron are administered.

In addition to oxygen, other factors may have an influence on EPO production and erythropoietic activity. Plasma hemoglobin may provide feedback stimulation on erythrocyte production or cause increased EPO production as hemolytic anemias result in a higher reticulocyte count than other anemias. As mentioned previously it is well documented that testosterone stimulates erythropoiesis, which partially explains the difference in hemoglobin concentrations according to sex and age. Research has shown, however, that testosterone is unable to stimulate erythropoiesis in nephrectomized mice. It is probable that testosterone stimulates EPO production by the kidney rather than by directly stimulating the bone marrow unipotent stem cell.

Hormones from the pituitary, thyroid, and adrenals also affect erythropoiesis. Anemic patients with hypopituitarism, hypothyroidism, and adrenocortical insufficiency show an increase in erythrocyte concentration when the appropriate deficient hormone is administered. The reduction of EPO in hypothyroidism is probably the result of the reduced demand for cellular oxygen by metabolically inactive or hypoactive tissue.

A number of tumors have been reported to cause an increase in erythropoietin production. Hypothalmus stimulation may cause an increase in release of EPO from the kidney, which could explain the association of polycythemia and cerebellar tumors. The serum EPO level increases dramatically for patients undergoing chemotherapy for leukemia, as well as other cancers that are not marrow related. These changes are thought to be due to the suppression of erythroid marrow by chemotherapeutic agents.[16]

The production of synthetic hematopoietic growth factors using recombinant DNA technology has revolutionized the management of patients with some anemias. A recombinant form of EPO known as Epoetin alfa, is produced by mammalian cells transfected with the human genomic DNA for EPO. Epoetin alfa is identical to human urinary EPO in regard to amino acid sequence, but the recombinant version lacks several amino acid linkages present in the native hormone. The biological activity of Epoetin alfa is almost three times greater than that of purified human urinary EPO. Recombinant EPO is commonly used for treatment of the anemia associated with end-stage renal disease, anemia associated with chemotherapy and for HIV-related anemia.[17,18]

CASE STUDY *(continued from page 62)*

4. Would you predict Stephen's serum erythropoietin levels to be low, normal, or increased? Why?

 Checkpoint! #5

What would the predicted serum EPO levels be in a patient with an anemia due to end-stage kidney disease?

► ERTHROCYTE DESTRUCTION

Red blood cell destruction is normally the result of senescence. Erythrocyte aging is characterized by a decline in cellular enzyme systems, especially of those in the glycolytic pathway, which in turn leads to decreased ATP production and a loss of adequate reducing systems. Consequently, the cell loses the ability to maintain its shape and its deformability, as well as its membrane integrity. About 90% of aged erythrocyte destruction is extravascular, taking place in the histiocytic cells of the spleen, liver, and bone marrow. The remaining 10% is catabolized intravascularly, whereby the erythrocyte releases hemoglobin directly into the bloodstream.

EXTRAVASCULAR DESTRUCTION

Erythrocyte removal by the spleen, bone marrow, and liver is referred to as extravascular destruction. This pathway is the most efficient method of cell removal and conserves and recycles essential erythrocyte components such as amino acids and iron (Figure 4-5 ■). Most extravascular destruction of erythrocytes takes place in the macrophages of the spleen. Aged erythrocytes have more rigid, leaky membranes, and move slowly and with difficulty through the small apertures of the macrophage-lined cords of the spleen. In addition, the glucose supply in the spleen is low, limiting the energy producing process of glycolysis within the erythrocyte. Aged erythrocytes with leaky membranes quickly deplete their cellular level of ATP as attempts are made to maintain osmotic equilibrium by pumping excess cations out of the cells. Thus, the splenic environment is well suited for culling aged erythrocytes.

Hemoglobin is composed of a porphyrin ring, heme, complexed with iron and bonded to protein chains called globin (∞ Chapter 5). Within the macrophage, the hemoglobin molecule is broken down into heme, iron, and globin. The essential elements, iron and globin (a protein), are conserved and reused for new hemoglobin or other protein synthesis. Heme iron may be stored as ferritin or hemosiderin within the macrophage, but most is released to the transport protein, transferrin. If released to transferrin, the iron is delivered to developing normoblasts in the bone marrow. This endogenous iron exchange is responsible for about 80% of the iron passing through the transferrin pool. Thus, iron from the normal erythrocyte aging process is conserved and reutilized. The globin portion of the hemoglobin molecule is broken down and recycled into the amino acid pool.

Heme is further catabolized and excreted in the feces. The α-methane bridge of the porphyrin ring is cleaved producing

EXTRAVASCULAR HEMOGLOBIN DEGRADATION

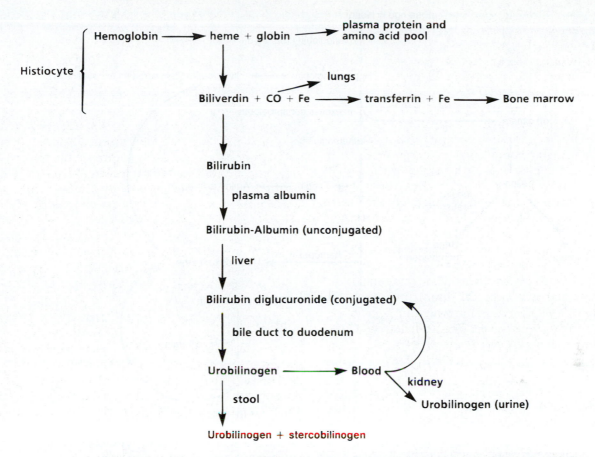

■ **FIGURE 4-5** Most hemoglobin degradation occurs within the macrophages of the spleen. The globin and iron portions are conserved and reutilized. Heme is reduced to bilirubin, eventually degraded to urobilinogen, and excreted in the feces. Thus, indirect indicators of erythrocyte destruction include the blood bilirubin level and urobilinogen concentration in the urine.

a mole of carbon monoxide and biliverdin. Carbon monoxide is released to the blood stream, where it is carried by erythrocytes as carboxyhemoglobin to the lungs and expired. The remaining portion of the porphyrin ring, biliverdin, is rapidly reduced within the cell to bilirubin. **Bilirubin,** released from the macrophage, is complexed with plasma albumin and carried to the liver. Upon uptake by the liver, bilirubin is conjugated to bilirubin glucuronide by the enzyme bilirubin UDP-glucuronyltransferase present in the endoplasmic reticulum of the liver. Once conjugated, bilirubin becomes polar and lipid insoluble. Bilirubin glucuronide is excreted into the bile and reaches the intestinal tract, where it is converted into urobilinogen by intestinal bacterial flora. Most urobilinogen is excreted in the feces, where it is quickly oxidized to urobilin or stercobilin. Ten to twenty percent of urobilinogen is reabsorbed from the gut. The reabsorbed urobilinogen is either excreted in urine or returned to the gut via an enterohepatic cycle. In liver disease, the enterohepatic cycle is impaired and an increased amount of urobilinogen is excreted in the urine.

INTRAVASCULAR DESTRUCTION

The small amount of hemoglobin released into the peripheral blood stream through intravascular erythrocyte breakdown undergoes dissociation into α–β dimers (Figure 4-6 ■). These dimers are quickly bound to the plasma glycoprotein **haptoglobin** (Hp) in a l:l ratio. This haptoglobin-hemoglobin (HpHb) complex is too large to be filtered by the kidney. Haptoglobin is an α2-globulin present in plasma at a concentration of 40–208 mg/dL. The haptoglobin carries hemoglobin dimers to the liver, where hemoglobin is processed within the hepatocyte in a manner similar to that of hemoglobin in extravascular destruction (∞ Chapter 16).

The HpHb complex is cleared very rapidly from the bloodstream, with a T½ disappearance rate of l0–30 minutes. The haptoglobin concentration may be depleted very rapidly in acute hemolytic states because the liver fails to synthesize haptoglobin in compensatory levels. Haptoglobin, however, is an acute-phase reactant, and increased concentrations may

INTRAVASCULAR HEMOGLOBIN DEGRADATION

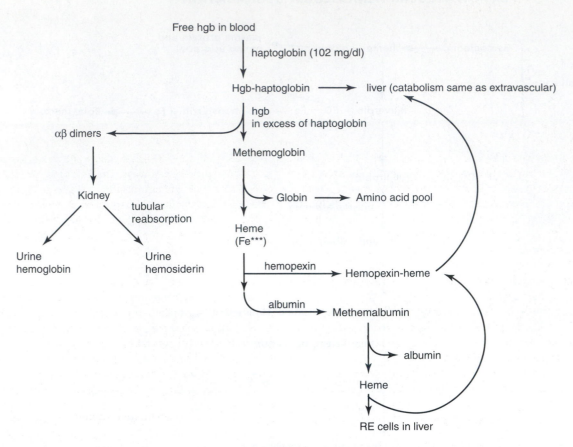

■ **FIGURE 4-6** When the erythrocyte is destroyed within the vascular system, hemoglobin is released directly into the blood. Normally, the free hemoglobin quickly complexes with haptoglobin, and the complex is degraded in the liver. In severe hemolytic states haptoglobin may become depleted, and free hemoglobin dimers are filtered by the kidney. Additionally, with haptoglobin depletion, some hemoglobin is quickly oxidized to methemoglobin and bound to either hemopexin or albumin for eventual degradation in the liver.

be found in inflammatory, infectious, or neoplastic conditions. Therefore, patients with hemolytic anemia accompanied by an underlying infectious or inflammatory process may have normal haptoglobin levels.

When haptoglobin is depleted, as in severe hemolysis, free α–β dimers may be filtered by the kidney and reabsorbed by the proximal tubular cells at a maximum rate of l.4 mg/minute. Dimers passing through the kidney in excess of the reabsorption capabilities of the tubular cells will appear in the urine as free hemoglobin. Dimers reabsorbed by the tubular cells are catabolized to bilirubin and iron, both of which eventually enter the plasma pool. However, some iron remains in the tubular cell and is complexed to storage proteins forming ferritin and **hemosiderin.** Eventually the iron loaded tubular cells are sloughed off and excreted in the urine. The iron inclusions can be visualized with the Prussian blue stain (∞ Chapter 9). Thus, the presence of iron in the urine (**hemosiderinuria**) is a sign of recent increased intravascular hemolysis.

Hemoglobin not excreted by the kidney or bound to haptoglobin is either cleared directly by hepatic uptake or may be oxidized to methemoglobin. Heme dissociates from methemoglobin and avidly binds to a β-globulin glycoprotein, **hemopexin.** Hemopexin is synthesized in the liver and combines with heme in a l:l ratio. The hemopexin–heme complex is cleared from the plasma slowly with a T½ disappearance of 7–8 hours. When hemopexin becomes depleted, the dissociated oxidized heme combines with plasma albumin in a l:l ratio to form methemalbumin. Methemalbumin clearance by the liver is also very slow. In fact, methemalbumin may only be a temporary combining form for heme until more hemopexin or haptoglobin becomes available. Heme is probably transferred from methemalbumin to hemopexin for clearance by the liver as it becomes available. When present in large quantity, methemalbumin and hemopexin-heme complexes impart a brownish color to the plasma. Schumm's test is designed to detect these abnormal compounds spectrophotometrically.

@ **CASE STUDY** *(continued from page 64)*

5. Stephen's haptoglobin level is 25 mg/dL. Explain why Stephen has a low haptoglobin value.

SUMMARY

Erythrocytes are derived from the unipotent committed stem cells BFU-E and CFU-E. Morphologic developmental stages of the erythroid cell include (in order of increasing maturity) the pronormoblast, basophilic normoblast, polychromatophilic normoblast, orthochromatic normoblast, reticulocyte, and erythrocyte. Erythropoietin, a hormone produced in renal tissues, stimulates erythropoiesis and is responsible for maintaining a steady-state erythrocyte mass. Erythropoietin stimulates differentiation of erythroid stem cells, increases the rate of erythropoiesis, and effects an early release of reticulocytes from the marrow.

The erythrocyte concentration varies with sex, age, and geographic location. Higher concentrations are found in males and newborns and at high altitudes. Decreases below the reference range result in a condition called anemia.

The erythrocyte membrane is a bilipid-protein complex that is important in maintaining cellular deformability and selective permeability. As the cell ages, the membrane becomes rigid and leaky, and the cell is culled in the spleen. The normal erythrocyte life span is 100–120 days.

The erythrocyte derives its energy and reducing power from glycolysis and ancillary pathways. The Embden-Meyerhof pathway provides ATP to help the cell maintain erythrocyte shape, flexibility, and membrane integrity through regulation of intracellular cation permeability. The HMP shunt provides reducing power to protect the cell from permanent oxidant injury. The methemoglobin reductase pathway helps protect heme from oxidation. The Rapoport-Leubering shunt facilitates oxygen delivery to the tissue.

Destruction of aged erythrocytes occurs in the macrophages of the spleen and liver through processes known as extravascular and intravascular destruction. Extravascular destruction of the erythrocyte is the physiologically preferred pathway of aged or abnormal erythrocyte removal and occurs primarily in the spleen and liver macrophage. Intravascular destruction of erythrocytes results in release of hemoglobin into the peripheral blood stream. Hemoglobin combines with albumin, haptoglobin, and/or hemopexin and is transported to the liver, where it is catabolized. Free hemoglobin may be filtered by the kidney and some reabsorbed by renal tubular cells. Free hemoglobin in the urine is a sign of acute intravascular hemolysis.

REVIEW QUESTIONS

LEVEL I

1. The earliest recognizable erythroid precursor on a Wright-stained smear of the bone marrow is: (Checklist # 1)
   a. pronormoblast
   b. basophilic normoblast
   c. CFU-E
   d. BFU-E

2. This renal hormone stimulates erythropoiesis in the bone marrow: (Checklist # 4)
   a. IL-1
   b. erythropoietin
   c. granulopoietin
   d. thrombopoietin

3. Haptoglobin may become depleted in: (Checklist # 8)
   a. inflammatory conditions
   b. intervascular hemolysis
   c. infectious diseases
   d. kidney disease

LEVEL II

1. This is the last stage of erythrocyte maturation that can undergo mitosis. (Checklist # 1)
   a. basophilic normoblast
   b. orthochromic normoblast
   c. pronormoblast
   d. polychromatophilic normoblast

2. Spherocytes are erythrocytes with an increase in cell hemoglobin concentration. This could result in: (Checklist # 3)
   a. an increase in membrane permeability
   b. increased cell elasticity
   c. an absence of the MN antigens
   d. decreased cell deformability

3. As a person ascends to high altitudes the increased activity of the Rapoport-Leubering pathway: (Checklist # 4)
   a. causes precipitation of hemoglobin as Heinz bodies
   b. has no effect on oxygen delivery to tissues
   c. causes increased release of oxygen to tissues
   d. causes decreased release of oxygen to tissues

LEVEL I

4. Which of the following characteristics most directly determines the erythrocyte life span? (Checklist # 5)
   a. spleen size
   b. serum haptoglobin levels
   c. membrane deformability
   d. cell size and shape

5. Which of the following depicts the normal sequence of erythroid maturation? (Checklist # 1)
   a. pronormoblast → basophilic normoblast → polychromatic normoblast → orthochromic normoblast → reticulocyte
   b. pronormoblast → polychromatic normoblast → orthochromic normoblast → basophilic normoblast → reticulocyte
   c. basophilic normoblast → polychromatic normoblast → reticulocyte → orthochromic normoblast → pronormoblast
   d. orthochromic normoblast → basophilic normoblast → reticulocyte → polychromatic normoblast → pronormoblast

6. The primary effector (cause) of increased erythrocyte production, or erythropoiesis, is: (Checklist # 4)
   a. supply of iron
   b. rate of bilirubin production
   c. tissue hypoxia
   d. rate of EPO excretion

7. An increase in the reticulocyte count should be accompanied by: (Checklist # 2)
   a. a shift-to-the-left in the Hb-O_2 dissociation curve
   b. abnormal maturation of normoblasts in the bone marrow
   c. an increase in total and direct serum bilirubin
   d. polychromasia on the Wright's stained blood smear

8. What property of the normal erythrocyte membrane allows the 7 μm cell to squeeze through 3 μm fenestrations in the spleen? (Checklist # 5)
   a. fluidity
   b. elasticity
   c. permeability
   d. deformability

9. An increase of erythrocyte membrane rigidity would be predicted to have what effect? (Checklist # 5)
   a. increase in erythropoietin production
   b. increase in cell volume
   c. decrease in cell life span
   d. decrease in reticulocytosis

10. A patient with an anemia due to increased intravascular hemolysis would likely present with which of the following lab results? (Checklist # 7, 8)
    a. increased haptoglobin
    b. increased serum bilirubin
    c. normal hemoglobin and hematocrit
    d. decreased serum bilirubin

LEVEL II

4. A newborn has a hemoglobin level of 160 g/dL at birth. Two months later a CBC is performed and the hemoglobin is 11.0 g/dL. The difference in hemoglobin concentration is most likely due to: (Checklist # 2)
   a. chronic blood loss
   b. presence of an inherited anemia
   c. increased intravascular hemolysis
   d. physiologic anemia of the newborn

5. Compared to sea level, at high altitudes an individual's erythrocyte level is: (Checklist # 2)
   a. produced at a lower rate
   b. larger than normal
   c. destroyed at an increased rate
   d. at a higher concentration

6. Which of the following is necessary to maintain reduced levels of methemoglobin in the erythrocyte? (Checklist # 4)
   a. vitamin B_6
   b. NADH
   c. 2,3-DPG
   d. lactate

7. A patient lost about 1500 mL of blood during surgery but was not given blood transfusions. His hemoglobin before surgery was in the normal range. What would be the most likely finding 3 days later. (Checklist # 2, 6)
   a. increase in total bilirubin
   b. increase in indirect bilirubin
   c. increase in erythropoietin
   d. increased haptoglobin

8. An anemic patient has hemosidinurea, increased serum bilirubin, and decreased haptoglobin. This is an indication that there is: (Checklist # 6)
   a. increased intravascular hemolysis
   b. decreased extravascular hemolysis
   c. hemolysis accompanied by renal disease
   d. a defect in the Rapoport-Leubering pathway

9. A laboratory professional finds evidence of Heinz bodies in the erythrocytes of a 30-year-old male. This is evidence of: (Checklist # 4)
   a. increased oxidant concentration in the cell
   b. decreased hemoglobin-oxygen affinity
   c. decreased production of ATP
   d. decreased stability of the cell membrane

10. A 65-year-old female presents with an anemia of 3 weeks duration. In addition to a decrease in her hemoglobin and hematocrit, she has an increased serum bilirubin, a decrease in serum haptoglobin, and 3+ polychromasia on her blood smear. Based on these preliminary findings, what serum erythropoietin result is expected? (Checklist # 6, 7)
    a. decreased
    b. normal
    c. increased
    d. no correlation

www.prenhall.com/mckenzie
Use the above address to access the free, interactive Companion Web site created for this textbook. Get hints, instant feedback, and textbook references to chapter-related multiple choice questions.

REFERENCES

1. Beutler E. The red cell: A tiny dynamo. In: Wintrobe, MM ed. *Blood, Pure and Eloquent*. New York: McGraw-Hill; 1980:141–68.

2. Hedin SG. Uber die Permeabilitaet der Blutkorperchen. *Pflugers Arch*. 1897; 68:229–338.

3. Landsteiner K. Uber Agglutinationserscheinungen normalen menschlichen Blutes. *Wien Klin Wochenschr*. 1902; 14:1132–34.

4. Mohandas N. The red cell membrane. *In:* Hoffman R, Benz Jr. EJ, Shattil SF, Furie B, Cohen HJ, eds. *Hematology Basic Principles and Practice*. New York: Churchill Livingstone; 1995:264–69.

5. Platt OS. Inherited disorders of red cell membrane proteins. *In:* Nagel RL, ed. *Genetically Abnormal Red Cells*. Boca Raton, Florida: CRC Press; 1988.

6. May JM. Ascorbate function and metabolism in the human erythrocyte. *Frontiers in Bio*. 1998; 3(1):1–10.

7. Viault F. Sur l'augmentation considerable du nombre des globules ranges dans le sang chez les habitants des haute plateaux de l'amerique du sud. *CR Acad Sci* (Paris). 1890; 119:917–18.

8. Bao W, et. al. Normative distribution of complete blood count from early childhood through adolelscence: The Bogalusa Heart Study. *Prev Med*. 1993; 22:825–37.

9. Cavalieri TA, Chopra A, Bryman PN. When outside the norm is normal: interpreting lab data in the aged. *Geriat*. 1992; 47:66–70.

10. Kosower NS. Altered properties of erythrocytes in the aged. *Am J Hematol*. 1993; 42:241–47.

11. Wang FF, Kung CK, Goldwasser E. Some chemical properties of human erythropoietin. *Endocrinology*. 1985; 116: 2286–92.

12. Gabrilove J. Overview: Erythropoiesis, anemia, and the impact of erythropoietin. *Sem Hematol*. 2000; 37(4), suppl6:1–3.

13. Zanjani ED, Ascensao JL, McGlave PB, Banisadre M, and Ash RC. Studies on the liver to kidney switch of erythropoietin production. *J Clin Invest*. 1981; 67:1183–88.

14. Zanjani ED and Ascensao JL. Erythropoietin. *Transfusion*. 1989; 29:46–57.

15. Chattopaohyay A, Choudhury TD, Bandyopadhyay D, Datta AG. Protective effect of erythropoietin on the oxidative damage of erythrocyte membrane by hydroxyl radical. *Biol Phar*. 2000; 59(4):419–25.

16. Swabe Y, Takiguchi Y, Kikuno K, et. al. Changes in levels of serum erythropoietin, serum iron, and unsaturated iron binding capacity during chemotherapy for lung cancer. *J Clin Onc*. 1998; 28(3):182–86.

17. MacDougall DS. Treatment with recombinant human erythropoietin is associated with increased survival and improved quality of life in persons with HIV-related anemia. *JIAPAC*. 1998; 10(1):H5–16.

18. Kimmel PL, Greer JW, Milam RA, Thamer M. Trends in erythropoietin therapy in the U.S. dialysis population. *Semin Nephrol*. 2000; 20(4):335–44.

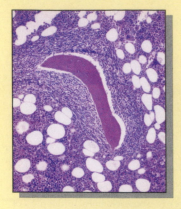

5

Hemoglobin

Shirlyn B. McKenzie, Ph.D.

■ CHECKLIST - LEVEL I

At the end of this unit of study the student should be able to:

1. Diagram the quaternary structure of a molecule of hemoglobin, identifying the heme ring, globin chains, and iron.

2. Assemble fetal, and adult hemoglobin molecules with appropriate globin chains.

3. Explain how pH, temperature, 2,3-DPG, and PO_2 affect the oxygen dissociation curve (ODC).

4. List the types of hemoglobin normally found in adults and newborns and give their approximate concentration.

5. Summarize hemoglobin's function in gaseous transport.

6. Define *normal hemoglobin values.*

7. Explain how the fine balance of hemoglobin concentration is maintained.

8. Compare HbA with HbA1c and explain what an increased concentration of HbA1c means.

■ CHECKLIST - LEVEL II

At the end of this unit of study the student should be able to:

1. Construct a diagram to show the synthesis of a hemoglobin molecule.

2. Describe the ontogeny of hemoglobin types; contrast differences in oxygen affinity of HbF and HbA and relate to structure of the molecule.

3. Explain the molecular control of heme synthesis.

4. Given information on pH, 2,3-DPG, CO_2, temperature and Hb F concentration, interpret the ODC and translate it into the physiologic effect on oxygen delivery.

5. Contrast the structures and functions of relaxed and tense hemoglobin and propose how these structures affect gaseous transport.

6. Describe how abnormal hemoglobins are acquired and select a method by which they can be detected in the laboratory.

7. Assess the oxygen affinity of abnormal acquired hemoglobins and reason as to how this affects oxygen transport.

8. Compare and contrast the exchange of O_2, CO_2, H^+, and Cl^- at the level of capillaries and the lungs.

KEY TERMS

Bohr effect
Carboxyhemoglobin
Chloride shift
Cyanosis
Deoxyhemoglobin
Glycosylated hemoglobin
Heme
Hypoxia
IRE-BP
Oxygen affinity
Oxyhemoglobin
Methemoglobin
(R) structure
Sulfhemoglobin
(T) structure

BACKGROUND BASICS

The information in this chapter will build on the concepts learned in previous chapters. To maximize your learning experience you should review these concepts before starting this unit of study.

Level I

▶ List and describe the stages of erythrocyte maturation. (Chapter 4)
▶ Summarize the role of erythropoietin in erythropoiesis. (Chapter 4)
▶ Describe the site of erythropoiesis. (Chapter 3)

Level II

▶ Describe the metabolic pathways present in the mature erythrocyte and explain their role in maintaining viability of the erythrocyte. (Chapter 4)
▶ Describe the appearance of the bone marrow when erythropoiesis is decreased or increased. (Chapter 4)
▶ Summarize the development of hematopoiesis from the embryonic stage to the adult. (Chapter 3)

⊚ CASE STUDY

We will address this case study throughout the chapter.
Jerry, a 44-year-old male, arrived in the emergency room by ambulance after a bicycle accident. Examination revealed multiple fractures of the femur. He was otherwise healthy. The next day he was taken to surgery for repair of the fractures. After surgery his hemoglobin was 7 gm/dL. He refused blood transfusions and was discharged 6 days later. Jerry called his doctor within days of being discharged and told him that he had difficulty walking around the house on crutches due to shortness of breath and lack of stamina. Consider why Jerry's hemoglobin was decreased after surgery and how this may be related to his symptoms now.

▶ OVERVIEW

This chapter describes the synthesis and structure of hemoglobin and factors that regulate its production. The different types of hemoglobin produced according to developmental stage are compared. The function of hemoglobin in gaseous exchange is considered, and factors that affect this function are analyzed. Structure, formation, and laboratory detection of abnormal hemoglobins are discussed also.

▶ INTRODUCTION

Hemoglobin is a highly specialized intracellular erythrocyte protein responsible for transporting oxygen from the lungs to tissue and carbon dioxide from the tissue to the lungs. Each gram of hemoglobin can carry 1.34 mL of oxygen.

Hemoglobin occupies approximately 33% of the volume of the erythrocyte and accounts for 90% of the cell's dry weight. Each cell contains between 27 and 32 pg of hemoglobin. This concentration is measured by cell analyzers and reported as mean corpuscular hemoglobin (MCH). In anemic states, the erythrocyte may contain less hemoglobin (decreased MCH) and/or there may be fewer erythrocytes present, which results in a decrease of the oxygen carrying capacity of the blood.

The erythrocyte's membrane and its metabolic pathways are responsible for protecting and maintaining the hemoglobin molecule in its functional state. Abnormalities in the membrane that alter its permeability or alterations of the cell's enzyme systems may lead to changes in the structure and/or function of the hemoglobin molecule and affect the capacity of this protein to deliver oxygen.

Although hemoglobin is synthesized as early as the pronormoblast stage, most hemoglobin synthesized in the developing normoblasts occurs at the polychromatophilic stage. All together 65% of the cell's hemoglobin is made before the extrusion of the nucleus. Since the reticulocyte does not have a nucleus, it cannot program the cell to make new RNA for protein synthesis. However, residual RNA and mitochondria in the reticulocyte enable the cell to make the remaining 35% of the cell's hemoglobin. The mature erythrocyte contains no nucleus or mitochondria and is unable to program or synthesize new protein.

Hemoglobin concentration in the body is the result of a fine balance between production and destruction of erythrocytes. The normal hemoglobin concentration in an adult male is about 15 g/dL, with a total blood volume of about 5000 mL. Therefore, the total body mass of hemoglobin is approximately 750 g:

$$15 \text{ g/dL} \times 5000 \text{ mL} \times 1 \text{ dL}/100 \text{ mL} = 750 \text{ g}$$

Since the normal erythrocyte life span is 120 days, $\frac{1}{120}$ of the total amount of hemoglobin is lost each day. Thus, the same amount must be synthesized each day to maintain a steady-state concentration. This amounts to approximately 6 g of new hemoglobin:

$$\frac{750\ g}{120\ days} = 6.25\ g/day\ \text{(amount of hemoglobin lost and synthesized each day)}$$

If we divide the total amount of hemoglobin synthesized each day (6.25 g) by the mean amount of hemoglobin in a red cell (MCH, which is about 30 pg), we can calculate how many new red cells must be synthesized each day:

$$\frac{6.25\ g/day}{30\ pg/cell} \times 10^{12}\ pg/g = 2 \times 10^{11}\ cells/day$$

This figure amounts to a turnover of approximately 4% of the total erythrocyte population per day. Since new erythrocytes enter the blood as reticulocytes, this 4% turnover is reflected by the reference range of the reticulocyte count, 0.8–2.5% for males and 0.8–4.0% for females.

► HEMOGLOBIN STRUCTURE

A molecule of hemoglobin is composed of four globular protein subunits (Figure 5-1 ■). Thus, the hemoglobin molecule is referred to as a tetramer. Each of the four subunits con-

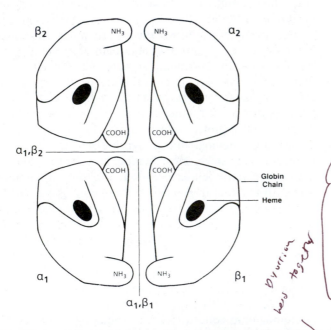

■ **FIGURE 5-1** Hemoglobin is a molecule composed of four subunits. Each subunit has a globin chain with a heme nestled in a hydrophobic crevice that protects the iron from being oxidized. Four different types of globin chains—α, β, δ, γ— occur in pairs. The types of globin chains present determine the type of hemoglobin. Depicted here is hemoglobin A consisting of 2 α and 2 β chains. The contacts between the α,β chains in a dimer (i.e., $\alpha_1\beta_1$) are extensive and allow little movement. The contacts between the dimer pairs (i.e., $\alpha_1\beta_2$ and $\alpha_2\beta_1$), however, are smaller and allow conformational change of the molecule as it goes from the oxyhemoglobin to deoxyhemoglobin.

★ TABLE 5-1	
The Structure of Hemoglobin	
Structure	**Conformational Description**
Primary	Sequencing of individual amino acids in the globin chains; critical to stability and function of molecule and determines the structure
Secondary	Three-dimensional arrangement resulting from the folding of the protein (75% α-helix; 25% β-pleat)
Tertiary	Folding superimposed on the helical and pleated forms; forms the heme hydrophobic pocket within globin chains; this tertiary structure changes upon ligand binding
Quaternary	Relationship of four protein subunits to one another; quaternary structure changes upon ligand binding are linked to the tertiary changes

tains a heme group and a globin chain. Heme, the prosthetic group of hemoglobin, is a tetrapyrrole ring with a ferrous iron located in the center of the ring. Hemoglobin structure is described in Table 5-1 ★.

The folding of the globin chains places the heme in a hydrophobic pocket near the exterior of the chain between the chain's E and F helices, where it is readily accessible to oxygen. The heme is between two histidines of the globin chain, the proximal and distal histidines. The proximal histidine (F8) is bonded with the heme iron. The iron is protected in the reduced ferrous state in this hydrophobic pocket. The exterior of the chain is hydrophilic, which makes the molecule soluble. Each heme can carry one molecule of oxygen bound to the central iron, thus each hemoglobin molecule can carry four molecules of oxygen.

The composition of the globin chains is responsible for the different functional and physical properties of hemoglobin. In adults, four types of globin chains are produced: alpha, beta, delta, and gamma (α, β, δ, γ). They combine in identical pairs (αα, ββ, δδ, γγ). A pair of α-chains combines with a pair of β, δ, or γ-chains to form one of three types of hemoglobin: hemoglobin A ($\alpha_2\beta_2$,), hemoglobin A_2 ($\alpha_2\delta_2$), and hemoglobin F ($\alpha_2\gamma_2$) (Table 5-2 ★). The arrangement of each globin chain is similar. The α-chain has 141 amino acids while the β-, δ-, or γ-chains have 146 amino acids. Each chain is wound up into 8 spiral or helical segments and attached by 7 short, nonhelical segments. The helical segments are lettered A–H, starting at the amino end.

The four globin chains are held together by salt bonds, hydrophobic contacts, and hydrogen bonds in a tetrahedral formation giving the hemoglobin molecule a nearly spherical shape. When ligands, such as oxygen, bind to hemoglobin, the number and strigency of intersubunit contacts changes. Mutations in the globin chains may affect subunit or dimer pair interactions and thus alter hemoglobin-oxygen affinity or stability of the molecule.

⭐ TABLE 5-2

Normal Types of Hemoglobin According to Developmental Stage

Developmental Stage	Type	Globin Chains	Reference Range
Embryonic	Gower I	$\zeta_2\varepsilon_2$	-
	Gower II	$\alpha_2\varepsilon_2$	-
	Portland	$\zeta_2\gamma_2$	-
Fetal	HbF	$\alpha_2\gamma_2$	90–95% before birth
			50–85% at birth
	HbA	$\alpha_2\beta_2$	10–40% at birth
	HbA$_2$	$\alpha_2\delta_2$	<1% at birth
>1 year old	HbF	$\alpha_2\gamma_2$	>95%
	HbA	$\alpha_2\beta_2$	<2%
	HbA$_2$	$\alpha_2\delta_2$	<3.5%
Adult	HbA	$\alpha_2\beta_2$	97%
	HbA$_2$	$\alpha_2\delta_2$	1.5–3.5%
	HbF	$\alpha_2\gamma_2$	<2%

✔ Checkpoint! #1

Describe the quaternary structure of a molecule of hemoglobin. How may a mutation in one of the globin chains at the subunit interaction site, $\alpha_1\beta_2$, affect hemoglobin function?

► HEMOGLOBIN SYNTHESIS

HEME

Heme is an iron-chelated porphyrin ring that always functions as a prosthetic group (nonamino acid component) of a protein. The porphyrin ring is composed of a flat tetrapyrrole ring with iron (Fe^{++}) inserted into the center. (Porphyrins are metabolically active only when chelated.)

Heme synthesis begins in the mitochondria with the condensation of glycine and succinyl coenzyme A (CoA) to form 5-aminolevulinic acid (ALA). This reaction occurs in the presence of pyridoxal phosphate, CoA, iron, and 5-aminolevulinate synthetase (ALAS). This first reaction is an important control site in the synthesis of heme. Synthesis continues through a series of steps in the cytoplasm to form coproporphyrinogen. Coproporphyrinogen enters the mitochondria to form the protoporphyrin ring (Figure 5-2 ■). The final step in the mitochondria, is the chelation of iron with the protoporphyrin ring catalyzed by ferrochelatase to form heme (Figure 5-3 ■). Heme then leaves the mitochondria to combine with globin chains in the cytoplasm. See Web Figure 5-1 ■ for detailed molecular structures of intermediates in heme synthesis.

GLOBIN

Globin chain synthesis is directed by eight genetic loci per haploid genome (Figure 5-4 ■). These genes produce 7 different types of globin chains: zeta, epsilon, gamma-A,

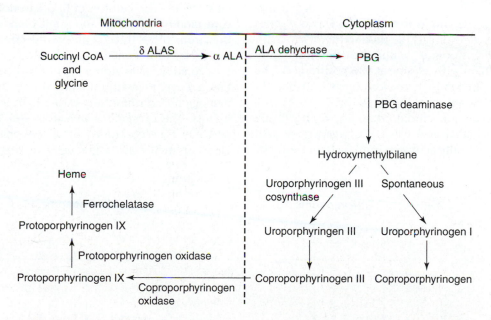

■ FIGURE 5-2 Synthesis of heme begins in the mitochondria with the condensation of glycine and succinyl CoA. The product, δ-aminolevulinate, leaves the mitochondria to form the pyrrole ring, porphobilinogen. The combination of four pyrroles to form a linear tetrapyrrole (hydroxymethylbilane), the cyclizing of the linear form to uroporphyrinogen, and the decarboxylation of the side chains to form coproporphyrinogen all occur in the cytoplasm. The final reactions, the formation of protoporphyrin IX, and the insertion of iron into the protoporphyrin ring, occur in the mitochondria.

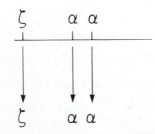

■ **FIGURE 5-3** Heme molecule. Heme is composed of a flat tetrapyrrole ring with iron inserted into the center. (p = propionic acid; v = vinyl; m = methyl)

gamma-G, delta, beta, and alpha (ζ, ε, γ^A, γ^G, δ, β, α). Two are found only in embryonic hemoglobin (ζ, ε). The genes for the ζ-chain, the fetal equivalent of the α chain, and α chains are located on chromosome 16. The ζ-chain is synthesized very early in embryonic development. After 8–12 weeks, ζ-chain synthesis is replaced by α-chain synthesis. All other globin genes are arranged in linear fashion in order of activation on chromosome 11. The ε-gene is located at one end of chromosome 11, and as it switches off, two γ-genes are activated. One γ-gene directs the production of a γ-chain with glycine at 136 position, γ^G, while the other directs the production of a γ-chain with alanine at 136 position, γ^A. The γ^G-chain synthesis predominates before birth (3:l) but γ^G- and γ^A-chain synthesis are equal (l:l) in adults.

The next two genes on chromosome 11, δ and β, are switched on to a small degree when the γ-genes are activated, but they are not fully activated until γ-chain synthesis

diminishes at about 35 weeks of gestation. The rate of synthesis of the δ chain is only $\frac{1}{40}$ that of the β-chain.

The synthesis of globin peptide chains occurs on polyribosomes in the cytoplasm (Figure 5-5 ■). Heme is inserted into the hydrophobic pocket near the surface of each globin chain. An α chain and non–α chain combine spontaneously, facilitated by electrostatic attraction, to form dimers. Two dimers combine to form the tetramer. After birth, most cells produce α and β chains for the formation of HbA, the major adult hemoglobin.

✓ **Checkpoint! #2**

What globin chains are produced in the adult?

▶ **ONTOGENY OF HEMOGLOBIN**

Hemoglobin type is determined by the makeup of its globin chains (Table 5-2 ✿). Some hemoglobins (Gower I, Gower II, and Portland) occur only in the embryonic stage of development. HbF is the predominant hemoglobin in the fetus and newborn while hemoglobin A is the predominant hemoglobin after 1 year of age.

Studies have suggested that the synthesis of different globin chains occurs in sequence dependent upon developmental stage. In vitro cultures of BFU-E from fetal liver, umbilical cord blood (neonatal), and adult blood show HbF production from these three sources to decrease in concentration from fetal to neonatal to adult. Moreover, the switch from fetal to adult hemoglobin synthesis is closely related to gestational age. Premature infants do not switch over to adult hemoglobin synthesis any earlier than if they were full-term infants. The perinatal switch from HbF to HbA synthesis is probably time controlled by a developmental clock.[1,2] The clone of stem cells is gradually reprogrammed during the

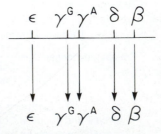

■ **FIGURE 5-4** The genes for the globin chains are located on chromosomes 11 and 16. The ζ chain appears to be the embryonic equivalent of the α chain, both of which are located on chromosome 16. Note the α gene is duplicated. The other globin genes are located on chromosome 11.

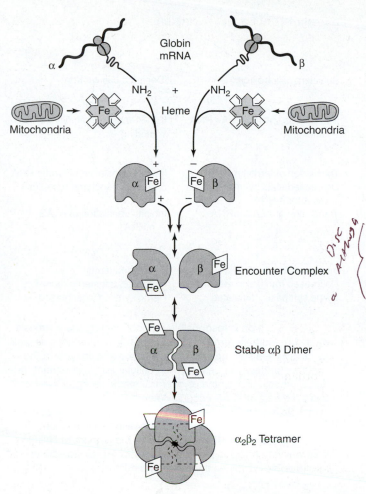

and are not usually detectable after the third month of gestation.

FETAL HEMOGLOBIN

Hemoglobin F (HbF; $\alpha_2\gamma_2$) is the predominant hemoglobin formed during liver and bone marrow erythropoiesis in the fetus. HbF composes 90–95% of the total hemoglobin production in the fetus until 34–36 weeks of gestation. At birth the infant has 50–85% HbF.

ADULT HEMOGLOBINS

In adults, hemoglobin A (HbA; $\alpha_2\beta_2$) is the major hemoglobin. Although HbA is found as early as 9 weeks gestation, β-chain synthesis does not exceed γ-chain synthesis until after birth. After birth, the percentage of HbA increases with the age of the infant until normal adult levels (>95%) are reached by the end of the first year of life.

HbF production constitutes less than 2% of the total hemoglobin of adults. Most, if not all HbF in adults is restricted to a few erythrocytes sometimes referred to as F cells (less than 8% RBC). From 13% to 25% of the hemoglobin in these F cells is HbF. The switch from HbF to HbA after birth is incomplete and in part reversible. For example, patients with hemoglobinopathies or anemia may have increased levels of HbF, often proportionate to the decrease in HbA. In bone marrow recovering from suppression, HbF levels often rise.

HbA$_2$, appears late in fetal life, composes less than 1% of the total hemoglobin at birth, and reaches normal adult values (1.5–3.5%) after one year.

> ### ✓ Checkpoint! #3
> *What are the names and globin composition of the embryonic, fetal, and adult hemoglobins?*

■ **FIGURE 5-5** Assembly of hemoglobin. The α and β globin polypeptides are translated on their respective mRNAs. On binding of heme, the protein folds into its native three-dimensional structure. The binding of α and β hemoglobin subunits to each other is facilitated by electrostatic attraction. An unstable intermediate encounter complex can rearrange to form the stable $\alpha\beta$ dimer. Two dimers combine to form the functional $\alpha_2\beta_2$ tetramer. (Adapted, with permission, from Bunn HF: Subunit assembly of hemoglobin: An important determinant of hematologic phenotype. *Blood.* 69:1, 1987.)

GLYCOSYLATED HEMOGLOBIN

HbA$_1$ on chromatography is a minor component of normal adult hemoglobin (HbA) that has been modified posttranslationally (HbA$_3$ on starch block electrophoresis). Usually a component has been added to the N terminus of the β chain. The most important subgroup of HbA$_1$ is HbA$_{1C}$, which has glucose irreversibly attached. This hemoglobin is referred to as **glycosylated hemoglobin.** HbA$_{1C}$ is produced throughout the life of the erythrocyte, its synthesis dependent on the time-averaged concentration of blood glucose. Thus, older erythrocytes contain more HbA$_{1C}$ than younger erythrocytes. However, if young cells are exposed to extremely high concentrations of glucose (>400 mg/dL) for several hours, the concentration of HbA$_{1C}$ increases both with concentration and time of exposure.

perinatal period leading to a switching from γ chain production to β chain production.

EMBRYONIC HEMOGLOBINS

Intrauterine erythropoiesis is associated with the production of the embryonic hemoglobins, Gower 1, Gower 2, and Portland, in the first trimester of gestation. The embryonic hemoglobins are made from the combination of pairs of embryonic globin chains, ζ and ε in pairs or embryonic chains in combination with α- and γ-chains. These primitive hemoglobins are detectable during hematopoiesis in the yolk sac

Measurement of HbA_{1C} is routinely used as an indicator of control of blood glucose levels in diabetics because it is proportional to the average blood glucose level over the last two to three months. Average levels of HbA_{1C} are 7.5% in diabetics and 3.5% in the normal individuals.

 Checkpoint! #4

A patient has an anemia caused by a shortened RBC lifespan (hemolysis); how would this affect the HbA_{1C} measurement?

► REGULATION OF HEMOGLOBIN SYNTHESIS

Hemoglobin synthesis is regulated by several mechanisms including:

- Activity of the enzyme ALAS
- Negative feedback of heme
- Concentration of iron
- Regulation of globin chain synthesis

The first enzyme in the heme synthetic pathway, ALAS, catalyzes the initial reaction of glycine and succinyl-CoA to form δ-ALA and is the rate-limiting enzyme in heme synthesis. As mentioned previously, this reaction takes place in the mitochondria. Since ALAS is synthesized on ribosomes in the cytosol, it must be imported into the mitochondria to catalyze the reaction. This mitochondrial import can be inhibited by high concentrations of heme.[3]

Iron entering the cell can be in either the utilization pool for metabolic processes (heme synthesis) or the storage pool (ferritin and hemosiderin). An iron responsive element-binding protein (**IRE-BP**) plays an important role in regulating the iron in these pools by affecting heme synthesis and formation of ferritin and transferrin receptors. The IRE-BP binds to the iron responsive element (IRE) of mRNA. The binding affinity of IRE-BP for the IRE is determined by the amount of cellular iron. When iron is scarce there is a high binding affinity, whereas when the cell is replete with iron there is a low binding affinity. When bound to the IRE, the IRE-BP modulates the translation of the mRNA.[4] The function modulated is determined by the context of the IRE.

There is an IRE in the ferritin gene, the ALAS gene, and the transferrin receptor gene. In the absence of iron, IRE-BP binds to the IRE of these mRNAs. Binding inhibits translation of ALAS and ferritin and enhances synthesis of transferrin receptor. When cellular iron is abundant, IRE-BP has a low affinity for IRE and translation of ALAS and ferritin mRNA proceeds, while translation of transferrin receptor mRNA decreases.[3,4,5,6,7] Since ALAS is the rate-limiting enzyme in heme synthesis, IRE-BP plays an important role in regulating heme synthesis.

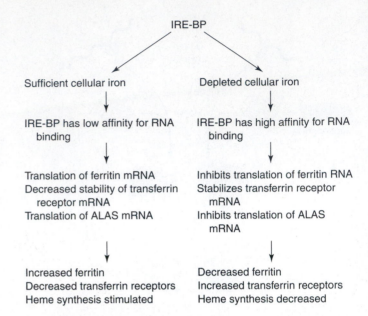

■ **FIGURE 5-6** Iron is responsible for coordinating the synthesis of ferritin and transferrin receptor in opposite directions as well as the synthesis of the enzyme ALAS, the first enzyme in the synthetic pathway of heme. When cellular iron is abundant, ferritin synthesis predominates over transferrin receptor synthesis and synthesis of ALAS occurs. When cellular iron is absent, synthesis of transferrin receptors increases and synthesis of ALAS and ferritin decreases. The iron responsive element-binding protein (IRE-BP) is sensitive to the amount of cellular iron, which controls the binding affinity of IRE-BP for IRE of mRNA and determines the fate of the mRNA.

The IRE-BP also regulates cellular iron by coordinating synthesis of ferritin and transferrin receptor in opposite directions (Figure 5-6 ■). Transferrin is the iron transport protein. The transferrin-iron complex combines with transferrin receptors on the cell and the iron is internalized. Ferritin is a cellular storage form of iron when iron is in excess of that needed for hemoglobin synthesis. The level of transferrin receptor expression reflects the need of the cell for iron and is an important factor in hemoglobin synthesis. When the cell needs more iron, transferrin receptors increase to maximize the amount of iron incorporated into the cell and formation of ferritin decreases. When cells have adequate iron, however, the ferritin levels rise and transferrin receptors decrease. Through this mechanism iron plays a central role in regulation of hemoglobin synthesis.

The rate of globin synthesis is governed primarily by the rate at which the DNA code is transcribed to mRNA, but it is also modified by processing of globin mRNA, by the translational events of mRNA, and by the stability of globin mRNA. Heme plays an important role in controlling the synthesis of globin chains. It stimulates globin synthesis by inactivating an inhibitor of translation.

CASE STUDY *(continued from page 71)*

Jerry's doctor gave him iron supplements to take every day.

1. If Jerry is iron deficient, what is the effect of this deficient state on synthesis of ALAS, transferrin receptor, and ferritin?

2. What was the rationale for giving Jerry the iron?

Discussion

► HEMOGLOBIN FUNCTION

The function of hemoglobin is to transport and exchange respiratory gases. The air we breathe is a mixture of nitrogen (78.6%), oxygen (20.8%), water, and carbon dioxide (CO_2). The sea level atmospheric pressure is 760 mm Hg. Each of the gases in the air contributes to this pressure in proportion to its concentration. The partial pressure each gas exerts is referred to as P. Thus, the partial pressure of oxygen in the atmosphere is 20.8% $\times$ 760 = 159 mm Hg.

It is the partial pressure gradient of a gas (in this case, oxygen) that determines the rate of diffusion of that gas across the alveolar-capillary membrane. When air is inspired, water vapor is added to the incoming gas to bring its relative humidity up to 100% at body temperature. This amounts to a relatively constant water vapor pressure of 47 mm Hg. Therefore, the PO_2 of inspired air is (760 − 47) $\times$ 20.8% = 148 mm Hg. As the inspired air mixes with alveolar gas, the PO_2 is diluted further by the presence of carbon dioxide given off at the lung as a byproduct of metabolism. The now arterialized blood leaves the lungs with a PO_2 of 100 mm Hg and a PCO_2 of 40 mm Hg. In comparison, the PO_2 of interstitial fluid is about 40 mm Hg and the PCO_2 is about 45 mm Hg. Thus, when blood reaches the tissues, oxygen diffuses out of the blood (because PO_2 in blood is more than in tissues) and CO_2 diffuses into the blood (because PCO_2 is more in tissues than in blood). The plasma is limited in the amount of O_2 and CO_2 it can absorb. Most O_2 and CO_2 diffuse into the erythrocyte to be transported to tissue or lungs.

OXYGEN TRANSPORT

Hemoglobin with oxygen is called **oxyhemoglobin;** hemoglobin without oxygen is called **deoxyhemoglobin.** The amount of oxygen bound to hemoglobin and released to tissue is not only dependent on PO_2 and PCO_2 but also is dependent on the affinity of Hb for O_2. The ease with which hemoglobin binds and releases oxygen is known as **oxygen affinity.** Hemoglobin affinity for oxygen determines the proportion of oxygen that is released to the tissues or loaded onto the cell at a given oxygen pressure (PO_2). Increased oxygen affinity means the hemoglobin has a high affinity for oxygen and does not readily give up its oxygen, whereas decreased oxygen affinity means the hemoglobin has a low affinity for oxygen and releases its oxygen more readily.

Oxygen affinity of hemoglobin is usually expressed as the PO_2 at which 50% of the hemoglobin is saturated with oxy-

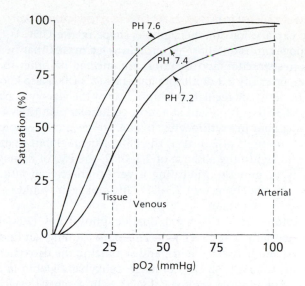

■ **FIGURE 5-7** The oxygen affinity of hemoglobin is depicted by the oxygen dissociaton curve (ODC). At a pH of 7.4 and an oxygen tension (PO_2) of 26 mm Hg hemoglobin is 50% saturated with oxygen. If the pH increases to 7.6, the curve is shifted left, indicating increased oxygen affinity. Conversely, if the pH drops to 7.2, the curve is shifted right, indicating decreased oxygen affinity. The curve also shifts in response to temperature, CO_2, O_2, and 2,3-DPG concentration.

gen (P_{50}). The P_{50} in humans is normally about 26 mm Hg. If hemoglobin-oxygen saturation is plotted versus the partial pressure of oxygen (PO_2), a sigmoid-shaped curve results. This is referred to as the oxygen dissociation curve (ODC) (Figure 5-7 ■). The sigmoid shape of the ODC indicates that there is a release of large quantities of oxygen from hemoglobin during small physiologic changes in PO_2. Note that the steepest part of the curve occurs at oxygen tensions found in tissues. This is physiologically of great importance for it allows the transfer of oxygen from the lungs to the tissues with only small changes in PO_2. The ODC shows that the oxygen saturation of hemoglobin drops from 100% in the arteries, where the PO_2 is about 100 mm Hg, to 75% in the veins, where the PO_2 is about 40 mm Hg. This indicates hemoglobin gives up about 25% of its oxygen to the tissues (5 mL of O_2 per 100 mL blood). When the curve is shifted to the right, it indicates that oxygen affinity is decreased. This results in release of more oxygen to the tissues. When the curve is shifted to the left, it indicates that oxygen affinity is increased. In this case, less oxygen is released to the tissues.

CASE STUDY *(continued from page 77)*

Jerry was lethargic and pale. He was having problems with activities of daily living.

3. Explain why Jerry may have these symptoms.

The Allosteric Property of Hemoglobin

The explanation for the sigmoid shape of the ODC is that hemoglobin is an allosteric protein. This means that hemoglobin's structure and function are affected by other molecules, primarily 2,3-diphosphoglycerate (2,3-DPG) also known as the allosteric regulator. A biproduct of the glycolytic pathway, 2,3-DPG, is present at almost equimolar quantities with hemoglobin in erythrocytes. In the presence of physiologic concentrations of 2,3-DPG, the P50 of hemoglobin is about 26 mm Hg. In the absence of 2,3-DPG, the P50 of hemoglobin is 10 mm Hg, indicating a very high oxygen affinity. Thus, in the absence of 2,3-DPG little oxygen would be released to the tissues.

Protons (H^+), CO_2, and organic phosphates (2,3-DPG) preferentially bind to deoxyhemoglobin forming salt bridges within and between chains, and stabilizing the deoxyhemoglobin structure. 2,3-DPG binds to deoxyhemoglobin in a l:l ratio. The binding site for 2,3-DPG is in a central cavity of the hemoglobin tetramer structure between the β globin chains. It binds to the positive charges on both β-chains, thereby crosslinking the chains and stabilizing the quaternary structure of deoxyhemoglobin.

Oxygen binds to oxyhemoglobin in a 4:1 ratio because it binds to the four heme portions of the molecule. The binding of oxygen by a hemoglobin molecule depends upon the interaction of the four heme groups, sometimes referred to as heme–heme interaction. The interaction of the heme groups is the result of movements within the molecule or tetramer triggered by the uptake of a single molecule of oxygen by one heme group. In the deoxy form, heme iron is 0.4–0.6Å out of the plane of the porphyrin ring, as the iron atom is too large to align in the plane of the porphyrin ring. Thus iron is displaced toward the proximal histidine of the globin chain to which it is linked by a coordinate bond. Upon uptake of oxygen by a heme subunit, the atomic diameter of iron becomes smaller due to changes in the distribution of electrons, and iron moves into the plane of the porphyrin ring pulling the histidine of the globin chain with it. These small changes in the tertiary structure of the molecule near the heme group result in a large shift in the quaternary structure, altering the bonds and contacts between chains, pulling the β-chains together and altering the deoxyhemoglobin structure. Consequently, the size of the central cavity decreases and 2,3-DPG is expelled. This structural change facilitates the binding of oxygen by the other three heme subunits because fewer subunit crosslinks need to be broken to bind each subsequent oxygen molecule. This cooperative binding of oxygen makes hemoglobin a very efficient oxygen transporter.

Oxygen interacts weakly with heme iron, and the two can dissociate easily. As O_2 is released by hemoglobin in the tissues, the heme pockets narrow and restrict entry of O_2 while the space between the β-chains widens and 2,3-DPG binds again in the central cavity. Thus, as 2,3-DPG concentration increases, the oxygen affinity decreases.

The conformational changes that occur as the hemoglobin molecule takes up and releases O_2 give rise to the names of the tense **(T) structure** for deoxygenated form and relaxed **(R) structure** for the oxygenated form. The salt bonds hold the deoxyhemoglobin in a high-energy or tense state, and energy is released when these salt bonds break as the molecule goes to the relaxed oxyhemoglobin state.

Adjustments in Hemoglobin-Oxygen Affinity

Variations in environmental conditions or physiological demand for oxygen result in changes in erythrocyte and plasma parameters that directly affect hemoglobin-oxygen affinity. In particular, PO_2, pH (H+), PCO_2, 2,3-DPG, and temperature affect hemoglobin-oxygen affinity (Table 5-3 ⊙).

Several physiologic mechanisms of oxygen delivery can be explained by the hemoglobin–2,3-DPG interaction. When a person goes from sea level to high altitudes, the body adapts to the decreased atmospheric pressure of oxygen by releasing more oxygen to the tissues. This adaptation is mediated by increases of 2,3-DPG in the erythrocyte, usually noted within 36 hours of ascent. EPO and erythrocyte mass also increase as a part of the adaptive mechanism to decreased PO_2.[8]

Fetal hemoglobin (HbF) has a high oxygen affinity compared to adult hemoglobin, HbA. Fetal blood's higher oxygen affinity is primarily due to the fact that hemoglobin F does not readily bind 2,3-DPG. The more efficient binding of 2,3-DPG to HbA facilitates the transfer of oxygen from the maternal (HbA) to the fetal circulation (HbF).

Rapidly metabolizing tissue, such as occurs during exercise, produces CO_2 and acid (H^+) as well as heat. These factors decrease oxygen affinity and promote the release of oxygen from hemoglobin to the tissue. However, in the alveolar capillaries of the lungs the high PO_2 and low PCO_2 drives off the CO_2 in the blood and reduces H^+ concentration, promoting the uptake of O_2 by hemoglobin (increasing oxygen affinity). Thus, PO_2, PCO_2, and H^+ facilitate the transport and exchange of respiratory gases.

The effect of pH on hemoglobin-oxygen affinity is known as the **Bohr effect.** The Bohr effect, an example of the acid-base equilibrium of hemoglobin, is one of the most important buffer systems of the body. A molecule of hemoglobin can accept H^+ when it releases a molecule of oxygen. Deoxy-

⊙ TABLE 5-3

Factors That Affect Oxygen-Hemoglobin Affinity

Increase Affinity	Decrease Affinity
↑O_2	↑CO_2
	↑ H^+
	↑ Temperature
	↑ 2,3-DPG

Key: ↑ = increased

hemoglobin accepts and holds on to the H^+ better than oxyhemoglobin. In the tissues, the H^+ concentration is higher because of the presence of lactic acid and CO_2. When blood reaches tissue, the affinity of hemoglobin for oxygen is decreased by the high H^+ concentration, thereby permitting the more efficient unloading of oxygen at these sites.

$$Hb(O_2) + H^+ \longrightarrow HHb + O_2$$

Thus, proton binding facilitates O_2 release and helps minimize changes in the hydrogen ion concentration of the blood when tissue metabolism is releasing CO_2 and lactic acid. Up to 75% of the hemoglobin oxygen can be released if needed (as in strenuous exercise) as the erythrocytes pass through the capillaries.

✔ Checkpoint! #5

What factors influence an increase in the amount of oxygen delivered to tissue during an aerobic workout?

✪ TABLE 5-4

Carbon Dioxide Transport in Blood

Mechanism	% of Transportation
Dissolved in plasma	7
Formation of carbonic acid, H_2CO_3	70
Bound to Hb	23

CARBON DIOXIDE TRANSPORT

After diffusing into the blood from tissue, carbon dioxide is carried to the lungs by three separate mechanisms: dissolution in the plasma, formation of bicarbonic acid, and binding to the N-terminus groups of hemoglobin (carbaminohemoglobin) (Table 5-4 ✪; Figure 5-8 ■).

Plasma Transport

A small amount of carbon dioxide is dissolved in the plasma and carried to the lungs. There it diffuses out of the plasma and is expired.

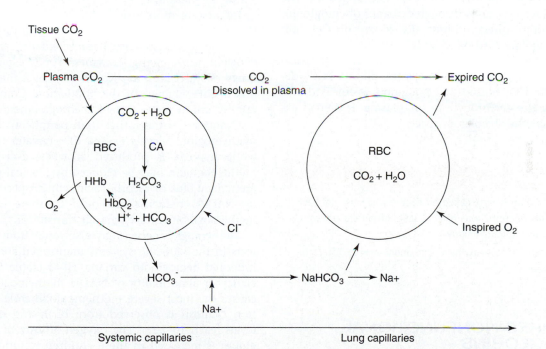

■ **FIGURE 5-8** Interrelations of oxygen and carbon dioxide transport in the erythrocyte are depicted. In the tissue, CO_2 diffuses into the erythrocyte and reacts with water to form bicarbonic acid, H_2CO_3. The bicarbonic acid dissociates into bicarbonate (HCO_3^-) and a proton (H^+). The HCO_3^- in the red cell is exchanged for chloride (Cl^-) in the cytoplasm (chloride shift) and then combines with Na to form $NaHCO_3$ in the cytoplasm. The proton is accepted by oxyhemoglobin (HbO_2), which through the Bohr effect, facilitates the dissociation of oxygen. In the lungs, the HCO_3^- dissociates from Na and enters the red cell. Here the HCO_3^- combines with H+ to form H_2CO_3, which dissociates into H_2O and CO_2, which are expired.

Bicarbonic Acid

Most of the carbon dioxide transported by the blood is in the form of bicarbonic acid, which is produced when carbon dioxide diffuses from the plasma into the erythrocyte. In the presence of the erythrocyte enzyme, carbonic anhydrase (CA), CO_2 reacts with water to form bicarbonic acid:

$$H_2O + CO_2 \xleftarrow{\quad} CA \xrightarrow{\quad} H_2CO_3$$

Subsequently, hydrogen ion and bicarbonate are liberated from carbonic acid and the H+ is accepted by deoxyhemoglobin:

$$H_2CO_3 \xleftarrow{\quad} CA \xrightarrow{\quad} \overset{\displaystyle \underset{\displaystyle \text{HHb}}{\uparrow}}{H^+} + HCO_3^-$$

The free bicarbonate diffuses out of the erythrocyte into the plasma in exchange for plasma Cl^- that diffuses into the cell, a phenomenon called the **chloride shift.** The bicarbonate combines with Na^+ ($NaHCO_3$) in the plasma and is carried to the lungs, where the PCO_2 is low. Here the bicarbonate diffuses back into the erythrocyte, is rapidly converted back into CO_2 and H_2O, and expired.

Hemoglobin Binding

Approximately 23% of the total CO_2 exchanged by the erythrocyte in respiration is through carbaminohemoglobin. Deoxyhemoglobin directly binds 0.4 moles of CO_2 per mole of hemoglobin. Carbon dioxide reacts with uncharged N-terminal amino groups of the four globin chains to form carbamino hemoglobin. At the lungs, the plasma PCO_2 decreases and the CO_2 bound to hemoglobin is released and diffuses out of the erythrocyte to the plasma. It then is expired as it enters the alveolar air space.

 CASE STUDY *(continued from page 77)*

After a week at home, Jerry called his doctor, who sent him back to the hospital, where he was given 2 units of packed red cells. Within a day, he had more energy.

4. Explain why Jerry may have had more energy after the transfusions.

▶ ACQUIRED NONFUNCTIONAL HEMOGLOBINS

The acquired, nonfunctional hemoglobins are hemoglobins that have been altered posttranslationally to produce molecules with compromised oxygen transport, thereby causing *hypoxia* and/or *cyanosis* (Table 5-5 ✪). **Hypoxia** is a condition whereby there is an inadequate amount of oxygen at the tissue level. (Hypoxemia is an inadequate amount of oxygen in the blood, arterial $PO_2 < 80$ mm Hg.) **Cyanosis** refers to a bluish color of the skin due to the presence of more than 5 g/dL of deoxyhemoglobin in the blood.

METHEMOGLOBIN

Methemoglobin is hemoglobin with iron in the ferric (Fe^{+++}) state. It is incapable of combining with oxygen. Methemoglobin not only decreases the oxygen-carrying capacity of blood, but it also results in an increase in oxygen affinity of the remaining normal hemoglobin. This results in an even higher deficit of O_2 delivery. Normally less than 1.5% methemoglobin is formed by auto-oxidation of hemoglobin per day. At this concentration the abnormal pigment is not harmful as the reduction in oxygen carrying capacity of the blood is insignificant. The accumulation of higher concentrations is held in control by several reducing systems (Table 5-6 ✪). Of these reducing systems the most important, accounting for over 60% of the reduction of methemoglobin, is NADH methemoglobin reductase.

Increased levels of methemoglobin are formed when an individual is exposed to certain oxidizing chemicals or drugs. Even small amounts of these chemicals and drugs may cause oxidation of large amounts of hemoglobin. If the offending agent is removed, methemoglobinemia disappears within 24–48 hours.

Infants are more susceptible to methemoglobin production than adults because HbF is more readily converted to methemoglobin and also because infants' erythrocytes are deficient in reducing enzymes. Foods (spinach, carrots), drugs, or water high in nitrates may cause methemoglobinemia in this segment of the population. Color crayons containing aniline may cause methemoglobinemia if ingested.

Cyanosis (central rather than peripheral) develops when methemoglobin levels exceed l0% (greater than 1.5 g/dL), while hypoxia is produced at levels exceeding 30–40%. Methemoglobin may be reduced by medical treatment with methylene blue or ascorbic acid, which speeds up reduction by NADPH reducing enzymes. In some cases of severe methemoglobinemia, exchange transfusions are helpful.

Methemoglobinemia may also result from congenital defects in the reducing systems mentioned above or from an inherited hemoglobin variant, HbM (Table 5-7 ✪). A deficiency or abnormality of NADH methemoglobin reductase causes the most severe methemoglobinemia. In this condition cyanosis is observed from birth and methemoglobin levels reach 10–20%. The oxygen affinity of normal hemoglobin is increased in these children resulting in increased erythropoiesis and subsequently higher than normal hemoglobin levels. The hereditary structural hemoglobin variant, HbM, also results in methemoglobinemia. HbM is characterized by amino acid substitutions in the globin chains near the heme pocket that stabilize the iron in the oxidized, Fe^{+++}, state. Methemoglobinemia caused by these hereditary defects cannot be reduced by treatment with methylene blue or ascorbic acid.

⊕ TABLE 5-5

Abnormal Acquired Hemoglobins

Hemoglobin	Acquired Change	Abnormal Function	Lab Detection
Methemoglobin	Hb iron in ferric state	Cannot combine with oxygen	Demonstration of maximal band at wavelength of 630 nm; chocolate color blood
Sulfhemoglobin	Sulfur combined with hemoglobin	1/100 oxygen affinity of HbA	Absorption band at 620 nm
Carboxyhemoglobin	Carbon monoxide combined with hemoglobin	Affinity for carbon monoxide is 200 times greater than for oxygen	Absorption band at 541 nm

⊕ TABLE 5-6

Erythrocyte Systems Responsible for Methemoglobin Reduction

Rank in Order of Decreasing Methemoglobin Reduction	System
First	NADH methemoglobin reductase (also known as cytochrome b5 methemoglobin reductase, diaphorase I, DPNH-diaphorase, DPNH dehydrogenase I, NADH dehydrogenase, NADH methemoglobin-ferrocyanide reductase)
Second	Ascorbic acid
Third	Glutathione
Fourth	NADPH methemoglobin reductase

Laboratory diagnosis of methemoglobinemia involves demonstration of a maximum absorbance band at a wavelength of 630 nm at pH 7.0–7.4. The blood sample may be chocolate brown in color when compared to a normal blood specimen. Differentiation of acquired types from hereditary types of methemoglobin requires assay of NADH-methemoglobin reductase and hemoglobin electrophoresis (Table 5-7 ⊕). Enzyme activity is only reduced in hereditary NADH-methemoglobin reductase deficiency, and hemoglobin electrophoresis is only abnormal in HbM disease. The acquired types of methemoglobinemia show normal enzyme activity and a normal electrophoresis pattern.

In the presence of methemoglobinemia, oxygen saturation obtained by a cutaneous pulse oximeter (fractional oxyhemoglobin, $FhbO_2$) may be lower than the oxygen saturation reported from a blood–gas analysis. This is because $FhbO_2$ is calculated as the amount of oxyhemoglobin compared to the total hemoglobin (oxyhemoglobin, deoxyhemoglobin, methemoglobin, and other inactive hemoglobin forms), whereas oxygen saturation in a blood–gas analysis is the amount of oxyhemoglobin compared to the total amount of hemoglobin able to combine with oxygen (oxyhemoglobin plus deoxyhemoglobin). $FhbO_2$ and oxygen saturation are the same if there is no abnormal hemoglobin present.[9]

Sulfhemoglobin

Sulfhemoglobin is a stable compound formed when a sulfur atom combines with each of the four heme groups of hemoglobin. Although the heme iron is in the ferrous state, sulfhemoglobin binds to oxygen with an affinity only one-hundredth that of normal hemoglobin. Thus, oxygen delivery to the tissues may be compromised if there is an increase in this abnormal hemoglobin. The bright green sulfhemoglobin compound is so stable that the erythrocyte carries it until the cell is removed from circulation. Ascorbic acid or methylene blue cannot reduce it; however, sulfhemoglobin can combine with carbon monoxide to form carboxysulfhemoglobin. Normal levels of sulfhemoglobin do not exceed 2.2%. Cyanosis is produced at levels exceeding 3–4%.

Sulfhemoglobinemia is formed during the oxidative denaturation of hemoglobin and accompanies methemoglobinemia, which usually precedes it. Sulfhemoglobin is formed upon exposure of blood to trinitroluene, acetanilid,

⊕ TABLE 5-7

Differentiation of Types of Methemoglobinemia

Cause of Methemoglobinemia	Inherited/Acquired	Enzyme Activity	Hb Electrophoresis
Exposure to oxidants	Acquired	Normal	Normal
Decreased enzyme activity	Inherited	Decreased	Normal
Presence of hemoglobin M	Inherited	Normal	Abnormal

phenacetin, and sulfonamides. It also is found to be elevated in severe constipation and in bacteremia with *Clostridium welchii*. Diagnosis of sulfhemoglobinemia is made spectrophotometrically by demonstrating an absorption band at 620 nm. Confirmation testing is done by isoelectric focusing. This is the only abnormal hemoglobin pigment not measured by the cyanmethemoglobin method, which is used to measure hemoglobin concentration.

Carboxyhemoglobin

Carboxyhemoglobin is formed when hemoglobin is exposed to carbon monoxide. Hemoglobin's affinity for carbon monoxide is more than 200 times greater than its affinity for oxygen. Carboxyhemoglobin is incapable of transporting oxygen. As is the case with methemoglobinemia, carboxyhemoglobin has a great impact on oxygen delivery because it destroys the molecule's cooperativity. High levels of carboxyhemoglobin impart a cherry-red color to the blood and skin. However, high levels of carboxyhemoglobin together with high levels of deoxyhemoglobin may give blood a purple pink color.

Normally blood carries small amounts of carboxyhemoglobin formed from the carbon monoxide produced during heme catabolism. The normal level of carboxyhemoglobin varies depending upon individuals' smoking habits and their environment. City dwellers have higher levels than country dwellers due to the carbon monoxide produced from automobiles and industrial pollutants.

Acute carboxyhemoglobinemia causes irreversible tissue damage and death from anoxia. Chronic carboxyhemoglobinemia is accompanied by increased oxygen affinity and polycythemia. In severe cases of carbon monoxide poisoning, patients may be treated in hyperbaric oxygen chambers.

Carboxyhemoglobin is commonly measured in whole blood by a spectrophotometric method. Sodium hydrosulfite reduces hemoglobin to deoxyhemoglobin and the absorbances of the hemolysate are measured at 555 nm and 541 nm. Carboxyhemoglobin has a greater absorbance at 541 nm.

 Checkpoint! #6

A 2-year-old child was found to have 15% methemoglobin by spectral absorbance at 630 nm. What tests would you suggest to help differentiate whether this is an inherited or acquired methemoglobinemia, and what results would you expect with each diagnosis?

SUMMARY

Hemoglobin is the intracellular protein of erythrocytes responsible for transport of oxygen from the lungs to the tissues. A fine balance between production and destruction of erythrocytes serves to maintain a steady-state concentration.

Hemoglobin is a globular protein composed of four subunits. Each subunit contains a porphyrin ring with an iron molecule (heme) and a globin chain. The four globin chains are arranged in identical pairs, each composed of two different globin chains. Hemoglobin synthesis is controlled by iron concentration within the cell, negative heme feedback, and activity and synthesis of the first enzyme in the heme synthetic pathway, ALAS.

The oxygen affinity of hemoglobin is dependent on PO_2, pH, PCO_2, 2,3-DPG, and temperature. Hemoglobin-oxygen affinity can be graphically depicted by the ODC. When the curve is shifted to the right, oxygen affinity is decreased, and when shifted to the left, oxygen affinity is increased. Increased CO_2, heat, and acid decrease oxygen affinity while high O_2 concentrations increase oxygen affinity.

Hemoglobin is an allosteric protein, which means that hemoglobin structure and function are affected by other molecules. In particular, the uptake of 2,3-DPG or oxygen can cause conformational changes in the molecule. The structure of deoxyhemoglobin is known as the T structure, and that of oxyhemoglobin is known as the R structure.

When hemoglobin is exposed to oxidants or other compounds, the molecule can be altered, which compromises its ability to carry oxygen. High concentrations of these abnormal hemoglobins can cause hypoxia and cyanosis. They can be detected by spectrophotometric methods.

REVIEW QUESTIONS

LEVEL I

1. Which of the following types of hemoglobin is the major component of adult hemoglobin? (Checklist #4)
   a. HbA
   b. HbF
   c. HbA_2
   d. Hb Portland

LEVEL II

1. Which of the following hemoglobins is not found in the normal adult? (Checklist #2)
   a. $\alpha_2\beta_2$
   b. $\alpha_2\gamma_2$
   c. $\alpha_2\delta_2$
   d. $\alpha_2\epsilon_2$

REVIEW QUESTIONS (continued)

LEVEL I

2. One of the most important buffer systems of the body is the: (Checklist #5)
   a. chloride shift
   b. Bohr effect
   c. heme–heme interaction
   d. ODC

3. When iron is depleted from the developing erythrocyte: (Checklist #8)
   a. the synthesis of heme is increased
   b. the activity of ALAS is decreased
   c. the formation of globin chains stops
   d. heme synthesis is not affected

4. When the H^+ concentration in blood increases, the oxygen affinity of hemoglobin: (Checklist #3)
   a. increases
   b. is unaffected
   c. decreases
   d. cannot be measured

5. Which of the following is the correct molecular structure of hemoglobin? (Checklist #1)
   a. four heme groups, two iron, two globin chains
   b. two heme groups, two iron, four globin chains
   c. two heme groups, four iron, four globin chains
   d. four heme groups, four iron, four globin chains

6. 2,3-DPG combines with which type of hemoglobin? (Checklist #3, 5)
   a. oxyhemoglobin
   b. relaxed structure of hemoglobin
   c. deoxyhemoglobin
   d. $\alpha\beta$ dimer

7. During exercise, the oxygen affinity of hemoglobin is: (Checklist #3)
   a. increased in males but not females
   b. decreased due to production of heat and lactic acid
   c. unaffected in those who are physically fit
   d. affected only if the duration is greater than 1 hour

8. Which of the following hemoglobins is *not* normally found in adults? (Checklist #4)
   a. hemoglobin A
   b. hemoglobin A_2
   c. hemoglobin F
   d. hemoglobin Portland

9. Which of the following is considered a normal hemoglobin concentration in an adult male? (Checklist #6)
   a. 110 g/L
   b. 210 g/L
   c. 150 g/L
   d. 90 g/L

LEVEL II

2. Which of the following is the major hemoglobin in the newborn? (Checklist #2)
   a. $\alpha_2\beta_2$
   b. $\alpha_2\gamma_2$
   c. $\alpha_2\delta_2$
   d. $\alpha_2\varepsilon_2$

3. A 2-year-old child was found to have 15% methemoglobin by spectral absorbance at 630 nm. What test would you suggest to help differentiate whether this is an inherited or acquired state? (Checklist #6)
   a. hemoglobin electrophoresis and NADPH reductase determination
   b. bone marrow aspiration and examination
   c. haptoglobin and sulfhemoglobin determination
   d. glycosylated hemoglobin measurement by column chromatography

4. A 25-year-old male was found unconscious in a car with the motor running. Blood was drawn and sent to the chemistry lab for spectral analysis. The blood was cherry-red in color. What hemoglobin should be tested for? (Checklist #6)
   a. sulfhemoglobin
   b. methemoglobin
   c. carboxyhemoglobin
   d. oxyhemoglobin

5. The oxygen dissociation curve in a case of chronic carboxyhemoglobin poisoning would show: (Checklist #7)
   a. shift to the right
   b. shift to the left
   c. normal curve
   d. decreased oxygen affinity

6. A college student from Louisiana vacationed in Colorado for spring break. He arrived at Keystone Resort area on the first day. The second day he was nauseated and had a headache. He went to the medical clinic at the resort and was told he had altitude sickness. The doctor told him to rest for another 24 hours before participating in any activities. What is the most likely reason he will overcome this condition in the next 24 hours? (Checklist #4)
   a. His level of HbF will increase to help release more oxygen to the tissues.
   b. The amount of carboxyhemoglobin will decrease to normal levels.
   c. The levels of ATP in his blood will reach maximal levels.
   d. The level of 2,3-DPG will increase and, in turn, decrease oxygen affinity.

7. A patient has iron deficiency anemia. How does this affect hemoglobin synthesis at the molecular level? (Checklist #3)
   a. Translation of mRNA for ALA is decreased.
   b. Transcription of mRNA for ALAS is decreased.
   c. Translation of mRNA for ALAS is decreased.
   d. Translation of globin chains is decreased.

REVIEW QUESTIONS *(continued)*

LEVEL I

10. Which of the following plays an important role in hemoglobin-oxygen affinity? (Checklist #3)
    a. 2,3-DPG
    b. NADPH reductase
    c. $NaHCO_3$
    d. Cl

LEVEL II

8. An aerobics instructor just finished an hour of instruction. Blood is drawn from her for a research study and the oxygen dissociation is measured. What would you expect to find? (Checklist #4)
    a. shift to the left
    b. shift to the right
    c. no shift
    d. increased oxygen affinity

9. In the lungs a hemoglobin molecule takes up one molecule of oxygen. What effect will this have on the hemoglobin molecule? (Checklist #5, 8)
    a. It will increase oxygen affinity.
    b. It will narrow the heme pockets blocking entry of additional oxygen.
    c. The hemoglobin molecule will take on the tense structure.
    d. The center cavity will expand and 2,3-DPG will enter.

10. A patient with emphysema would be expected to have (Checklist #4):
    a. increased in blood pH
    b. decreased in blood pH
    c. increased oxygen affinity
    d. decreased 2,3-DPG level

www.prenhall.com/mckenzie

Use the above address to access the free, interactive Companion Web site created for this textbook. Get hints, instant feedback, and textbook references to chapter-related multiple choice questions.

REFERENCES

1. Peschle C, Migliaccio AR, Migliaccio G, Lettieri F, Maguire YP, Condorelli M, et al. Regulation of Hb synthesis in ontogenesis and erythropoietic differentiation: In vitro studies on fetal liver, cord blood, normal adult blood or marrow, and blood from HPFH patients. In: Stamatoyannopoulos G, Nienhuis AW, eds. *Hemoglobins in Development and Differentiation.* New York: Alan R. Liss; 1980:359–71.

2. Papayannopoulou T, Nakamoto B, Agostinelli F, Manna M, Lucarelli G, Stamatoyannopoulos G, et al. Fetal to adult hemopoietic cell transplantation in humans: Insights into hemoglobin switching. *Blood.* 1986;67:99–104.

3. Ferreira GC, Gong J. 5-aminolevulinate synthase and the first step of heme biosynthesis. *J Bioenerg Biomembr.* 1995;27:151–59.

4. Klausner RD, Rouault TA, Harford JB. Regulating the fate of mRNA: The control of cellular iron metabolism. *Cell.* 1993;72:19–28.

5. Kawasaki N, Morimoto K, Tanimoto T, Hayakawa T. Control of hemoglobin synthesis in erythroid differentiating K562 cells. I. Role of iron in erythroid cell heme synthesis. *Arch Biochem Biophys.* 1996;328:289–94.

6. Kawasaki N, Morimoto K, Hayakawa T. Control of hemoglobin synthesis in erythroid differentiating K562 cells. II. Studies of iron mobilization in erythroid cells by high-performance liquid chromatography-electrochemical detection. *J Chromatogr B Biomed Sci Appl.* 1998;705:193–201.

7. Rouault TA, Klausner RD. Iron-sulfur clusters as biosensors of oxidants and iron. *Trends Biochem Sci.* 1996;21:174–77.

8. Boning D, Maassen N, Jochum F, Steinacker J, Halder A, Thomas A, et al. Aftereffects of a high altitude expedition on blood. *Int J Sports Med.* 1997;18:179–85.

9. Wentworth P, Roy M, Wilson B, Padusenko J, Smeaton A, Burchell. Clinical pathology rounds: Toxic methemoglobinemia in a 2-year-old child. *Lab Med.* 1999;30:311–15.

6

The Leukocyte

Mary Coleman, M.S.

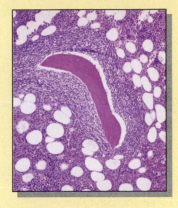

■ CHECKLIST - LEVEL I

At the end of this unit of study the student should be able to:

1. Define terms listed in the key term list.
2. Differentiate morphologically and immunologically the precursors found in the proliferative compartment of the bone marrow.
3. Compare and contrast the development, including distinguishing maturation and cell features, of the granulocytic, monocytic-macrophage, and the lymphocytic cell lines.
4. Compare and contrast the morphologic and other distinguishing cell features of each of the leukocytes found in the peripheral blood.
5. Compare and contrast the function of each of the leukocytes found in the peripheral blood.
6. Summarize the process of neutrophil migration and phagocytosis.
7. List the adult reference ranges for the leukocytes found in the peripheral blood.
8. Calculate absolute cell counts from data provided.
9. Differentiate absolute values and relative values of cell count data.
10. List causes/conditions that increase or decrease absolute numbers of individual leukocytes found in the peripheral blood.
11. Compare and contrast pediatric and newborn reference values and adult reference ranges.
12. Explain immunoglobulin diversity.

■ CHECKLIST - LEVEL II

At the end of this unit of study the student should be able to:

1. Summarize the kinetics of the granulocytic, monocytic-macrophage, and the lymphocytic cell lines.
2. Describe the processes that permit neutrophils to leave the peripheral blood circulation and move to a site of infection and propose how defects in these processes affect the body's defense mechanism.
3. Compare and contrast the immunologic features and functions of each of the leukocytes found in the peripheral blood.
4. Summarize lymphocyte membrane characteristics used to differentiate subtypes.
5. Differentiate between polyclonal and monoclonal antibodies.
6. Compare and discriminate morphological features of Russell bodies, Mott cells, and flame cells.
7. Design systems to evaluate laboratory data of leukocytes for error detection.
8. Formulate pathways to correlate laboratory data of leukocytes with clinical knowledge of the patient.

CHAPTER OUTLINE

KEY TERMS

Agranulocytosis
Azurophilic granules
Cell mediated immunity
Chemotaxis
Dutcher bodies
Erythrophagocytosis
Flame cell
Granulocytosis
Humoral immunity
Immune response
Immunoblast
Immunoglobulin
Large granular lymphocyte
Leukocytosis
Leukopenia
Monoclonal gammopathies
Monocyte-macrophage system
Mott cell
Natural killer cell
Neutrophilia
Null cell (null lymphocyte)
Phagocytosis
Plasma cell
Reactive lymphocyte
Russell bodies

BACKGROUND BASICS

In addition to the basics from previous chapters, it is helpful to have a basic understanding of immunology (immune system and function), biochemistry (proteins, carbohydrates, and lipids), algebra, the use of percentages, ratios and proportions, and the metric system.

To maximize your learning experience you should review these concepts from previous chapters before starting this unit of study:

Level I

▶ Identify components of the cell and describe their function. (Chapter 2)
▶ Summarize the function of growth factors and the heirarchy of hematopoiesis. (Chapter 2)
▶ Describe the structure and function of the hematopoietic organs. (Chapter 3)

Level II

▶ List the growth factors and identify their function in leukocyte differentiation and maturation. (Chapter 2)

CASE STUDY

We will refer to this case study throughout the chapter.
Mr. Mertzig, a 30-year-old male in good physical condition, had a routine physical examination as a requirement for purchasing a life insurance policy. A CBC was ordered with the following results: Hb 155 g/L; hct 0.47 L/L; RBC count 5.2×10^{12}/L; platelet count 175×10^9/L; and WBC count 12×10^9/L. Consider how you could explain these results in a healthy male.

▶ OVERVIEW

Leukocytes develop from the pluripotential hematopoietic stem cell in the bone marrow. Leukocytes are involved in defense against foreign antigens. In the presence of infection or inflammation, there may be an increase in the number of these cells, and they may show morphologic changes. Thus, an important screening test for a wide variety of conditions is the leukocyte (WBC) count. This chapter is a study of the normal differentiation and maturation of leukocytes. Each type of leukocyte is discussed including cell morphology, concentration, and function. The lymphocyte section is divided into T and B cell development and function. The synthesis and structure of immunoglobulins and lymphocyte receptors and cell antigens are described with attention to the use of these markers in identifying lymphocyte types.

▶ INTRODUCTION

Leukocytes (white blood cells, WBC) are essential cellular components of peripheral blood circulation. Leukocyte precursors originate in the bone marrow and are released into the peripheral blood, where they circulate until they move into the tissues in response to stimulation. The neutrophil, band neutrophil, eosinophil, basophil, monocyte, and lymphocyte are the leukocytes, also called white blood cells, normally found in the peripheral blood of children and adults.

The era of morphologic hematology began in 1877 with Paul Ehrlich's discovery of a triacidic stain.[1] The stain allowed differentiation of leukocytes on fixed blood smears via different staining properties of the components of the cells. Wright stain, a Romanowsky-type stain, is used to stain the cellular components of blood and bone marrow that is smeared on glass slides. Methylene blue and eosin are the major components of the Wright stain. Basic cellular elements react with the acidic dye, eosin, and acidic cellular elements react with the basic dye, methylene blue. One type of leukocyte, the eosinophil, contains much basic protein in its granules. Its granules react with the eosin dye, hence the name *eosinophil*. Another type of leukocyte, the basophil, has granules that are acidic. Its granules react with the basic dye, methylene blue, hence the name *basophil*. The neutrophil granules react with both acid and basic portions of the stain, giving the cell cytoplasm a neutral to pinkish appearance. The nuclear DNA and cytoplasmic RNA of cells are acidic and pick up the basic stain, methylene blue. Hemoglobin is a basic cellular component of red blood cells and reacts with the acid dye, eosin, and stains orange red to salmon pink.[2] The eosinophil, basophil, and neutrophil are polymorphonuclear and contain many granules. They are classified as granulocytes. Monocytes and lymphocytes are mononuclear cells and contain fine, small numbers of granules or no granules.

Leukocytes were first observed by William Hewson, the father of hematology, in the eighteenth century. In the nineteenth century, the studies of inflammation and bacterial infection intensified interest in leukocytes.[3] Many researchers studied the similarity of pus cells in areas of inflammation and the leukocytes of the blood. One researcher, Ilya Metchnikov, observed the presence of nucleated blood cells surrounding a thorn introduced beneath the skin of a larval starfish.[1] Many of Ehrlich's observations and Metchnikov's experiments provided the groundwork for understanding the leukocytes as defenders against infection. Ehrlich recognized that variations in numbers of leukocytes accompanied specific pathologic conditions, such as eosinophilia in allergies, parasitic infections, and dermatitis, as well as neutrophilia in bacterial infections.

It is now recognized that the leukocyte function of fighting infection includes two separate but interrelated events: phagocytosis and the subsequent development of the immune response. Granulocytes and monocytes are responsible for phagocytosis, while monocytes and lymphocytes interact to produce an effective immune response. More research is needed on the role of eosinophils and basophils.

▶ LEUKOCYTE CONCENTRATION IN THE PERIPHERAL BLOOD

Leukocytes develop from primitive pluripotential stem cells in the bone marrow. Upon specific hematopoietic growth hormone stimulation, the stem cell proliferates and differentiates into the various types of leukocytes: granulocytes, monocytes, and lymphocytes. Upon maturation, these cells may be released into the peripheral blood or may remain in the bone marrow storage pool until needed.

The total peripheral blood leukocyte count is high at birth, $9–30 \times 10^9/L$. A few immature granulocytic cells (myelocytes, metamyelocytes) may be seen in the first few days of life; however, immature leukocytes are not present in the peripheral blood after this age except in disease. In a week, the leukocyte count drops to $5–21 \times 10^9/L$. A gradual decline occurs until the age of 8 years, at which time the leukocyte concentration averages $8 \times 10^9/L$. The Bogalusa Heart Study found that in children between the ages of 5 and 17, females

had, on the average, leukocyte counts $0.5 \times 10^9/L$ higher than males.[4] Adult values average from 3.5 to $11.0 \times 10^9/L$. There are conflicting reports on the reference range for older adults. Some hematologists do not believe the reference range for older adults is different from that of other adults, while others believe the range is somewhat lower ($3–9 \times 10^9/L$). It is, however, generally accepted that the lymphocyte count is lower in older adults and that this decrease is due primarily to a decrease in T lymphocytes. Decreased leukocyte counts in the elderly may be due to drugs.[5]

Physiologic and pathological variations affect the concentrations of leukocytes. Pregnancy, time of day, activity level, and race affect the concentration. Ethiopian Jews and black Africans have significantly lower neutrophil and monocyte counts. However, black Americans or Africans eating a Western diet do not have evidence of lower concentrations. Infections and immune regulated responses cause changes in leukocytes. Many other pathologic disorders can cause quantitative and/or qualitative changes in white cells.

Thus, when evaluating cell count data it is helpful to know the age and sex of the patient as well as previous cell counts on the same patient. It also is helpful to assess the accuracy of cell counts by correlating them with the clinical history of the patient. Additional testing may be done as a result of abnormalities in the WBC count. Changes associated with diseases will be discussed in subsequent chapters on leukocytes.

ⓔ CASE STUDY *(continued from page 86)*

The CBC results on Mr. Mertzig were: Hb 155 g/L; hct 0.47 L/L; RBC count $5.2 \times 10^{12}/L$; platelet count $175 \times 10^9/L$; and WBC count $12 \times 10^9/L$.

1. Are any of these results outside the reference range? If yes, which one(s)?

2. If this were a newborn would you change your evaluation? Why?

ABSOLUTE CONCENTRATION VS RELATIVE CONCENTRATION

An increase or decrease in the total number of leukocytes may be caused by an altered concentration of all leukocyte types or, more commonly, is limited to an alteration in one specific type of leukocyte. For this reason, an abnormal total WBC count should be followed by a leukocyte differential count. A leukocyte differential count enumerates each leukocyte type among a total of 100 leukocytes. The differential results are reported in the percentage of each type counted. To accurately interpret whether an increase or decrease in cell types exists, however, it is necessary to calculate the absolute concentration using the results of the WBC count and the differential (relative concentration) in the following manner:

$$\text{Differential count (in decimal form)} \times \text{WBC count} \times (10^9/L) = \text{absolute cell count} \times (10^9/L)$$

The usefulness of this calculation is emphasized in the following example. Two different blood specimens both had a relative lymphocyte concentration of 60%. One had a total leukocyte count of $3 \times 10^9/L$ and the other a total leukocyte count of $9 \times 10^9/L$. The relative lymphocyte concentation on both specimens appears elevated (reference range is 20–40%); however, calculation of the absolute concentration (reference range 1.5 to $4.0 \times 10^9/L$) shows that only one specimen has an absolute increase in lymphocytes; the other is within reference range:

$$0.6 \times (3 \times 10^9/L) = 1.8 \times 10^9/L \text{ (reference range)}$$

$$0.6 \times (9 \times 10^9/L) = 5.4 \times 10^9/L \text{ (increased)}$$

NEUTROPHILS

The neutrophil is the most numerous leukocyte in the adult peripheral blood, 54–62% (2–$7 \times 10^9/L$). At birth, neutrophil concentration is about 60%; this level drops to 30% by 4–6 months of age. After 4 years of life, the concentration of neutrophils gradually increases until adult values are reached at 6 years of age. Most peripheral blood neutrophils are mature segmented forms; however, a few nonsegmented forms (bands) may be seen in normal specimens. Most variations in the total leukocyte count are due to an increase or decrease in neutrophils.

EOSINOPHILS

Eosinophil concentrations are maintained at 1–3% (up to $0.45 \times 10^9/L$) throughout life. It is possible that no eosinophils may be seen on a 100-cell differential; however, careful scanning of the entire smear should reveal an occasional eosinophil.

BASOPHILS

Basophils are the least plentiful cells in the peripheral blood, 0–1% (up to $0.2 \times 10^9/L$). It is common not to find basophils on a 100-cell differential; the finding of an absolute basophilia, however, is very important since it may indicate the presence of a hematologic malignancy.

MONOCYTES

Monocytes usually compose 4–10% (0.2–$0.8 \times 10^9/L$) of leukocytes. Occasionally, reactive lymphocytes may resemble monocytes. This gives even the experienced clinical laboratory scientist difficulty in the differential.

LYMPHOCYTES

The lymphocyte concentration varies with the age of the individual. About 30% of the leukocytes at birth are lymphocytes. This increases to 60% at about 4–6 months and remains at this level until 4 years of age. Then a gradual decline occurs until a mean level of 34% at 21 years is reached. The concentration in adults ranges from 20% to 40% (1.5–$4.0 \times 10^9/L$). After age 65, lymphocytes decrease in both sexes.

▶ LEUKOCYTE SURFACE MARKERS

Leukocytes, as well as other cells, can express a variety of molecules on their surface. These surface molecules can be used as markers to help identify the lineage of a cell as well as subsets. These markers can be identified by specific monoclonal antibodies. A nomenclature system was developed to identify antibodies with similar characteristics. The system uses CD (cluster designation) and a number. The CD designation is now used to name the molecule recognized by the monoclonal antibody as well as the antibody itself. In addition to using CD markers to identify cell lineage, some surface markers are used to identify stages of maturation as they are transiently expressed at a certain developing stage. Other markers are expressed only after the cell is stimulated and thus can be used as a marker of cell activation. Cell markers are very helpful in differentiating neoplastic hematologic disorders (∞ Chapter 26). These surface markers can be identified by flow cytometry or cytochemical stains (∞ Chapter 23).

🌀 CASE STUDY (continued from page 87)

A leukocyte differential was performed with the following results:

Neutrophils	58%
Lymphocytes	32%
Monocytes	6%
Eosinophils	3%
Basophils	1%

3. Are any of the WBC concentrations outside the reference interval (relative or absolute)?

▶ NEUTROPHILS

Neutrophils are the most numerous leukocyte in the peripheral blood. They are easily identified on Romanowsky stained peripheral blood smears as cells with a segmented nucleus and fine pinkish granules.

DIFFERENTIATION, MATURATION, AND MORPHOLOGY

Leukocytes develop from hematopoietic stem cells in the bone marrow. Differentiation is discussed in ∞ Chapter 2. Once differentiation has occurred maturation begins. Myeloid, monocytoid, and lymphoid elements go through the maturation process. The myeloid elements include the granulocytes and their precursors. The monocytoid elements include monocytes and their precursors. The lymphoid elements include the lymphocytes and their precursors.

The neutrophil undergoes six morphologically identifiable stages in the process of maturation. The stages from the first morphologically identifiable cell to the functional segmented neutrophil include: (1) myeloblast; (2) promyelocyte (progranulocyte); (3) myelocyte; (4) metamyelocyte; (5) band, or stab, neutrophil or unsegmented neutrophil; and (6) polymorphonuclear neutrophil (PMN), or segmented neutrophil.

During the maturation process, there is an obvious progressive change in the nucleus. The nucleoli disappear, the chromatin condenses, and the once round mass indents and eventually segments. These nuclear changes are accompanied by distinct cytoplasmic changes. The scanty, agranular, basophilic cytoplasm of the earliest stage is gradually replaced by pink to neutral-staining granular cytoplasm in the mature differentiated stage (Figures 6-1 and 6-2 ■, Table 6-1 ✪). Leukopoiesis is an amazing process generating $1–5 \times 10^9$ cells per hour or 10^{11} cells per day.[6] The morphology of the stages of maturation is discussed below.

Myeloblast

The myeloblast (Table 6-1 ✪, Figures 6-1a, 6-3 ■) is the earliest recognizable neutrophil precursor. The myeloblast size varies from 14 to 20 μm in diameter and has a high nuclear to cytoplasmic (N:C) ratio. The nucleus is usually round or oval and contains a delicate, lacy, evenly stained chromatin. There are from three to five large nucleoli. The small amount of cytoplasm is agranular, staining from deep blue to a lighter blue. A distinct unstained area adjacent to the nucleus representing the Golgi apparatus may be seen. These cells may stain positive for peroxidase and esterase enzymes, even though granules are not evident by light microscopy. When positive, peroxidase and esterase help differentiate myeloblasts from lymphoblasts. CD markers may also aid in differentiating the blasts. The myeloblast CD markers include CD33 and CD38.[7]

Promyelocyte

The promyelocyte/progranulocyte (Table 6-1 ✪, Figures 6-1b and 6-2 ■) varies in size from 15 to 21 μm. With the nucleus being quite large, the N:C ratio is high. The nuclear chromatin structure, although coarser than that of the blast, is still open and rather lacy, staining purple to dark blue. The color of the nucleus will vary somewhat depending on the stain product used. Several nucleoli may be visible at this stage. The basophilic cytoplasm is similar to that of the blast, but is differentiated from the blast by the presence of large, blue purple primary granules, also called nonspecific or **azurophilic granules.** The granules can be shown by cytochemical techniques to contain a number of enzymes and other substances. Contents of primary granules are listed in Table 6-2 ✪.

Myelocyte

The myelocyte (Table 6-1 ✪, Figures 6-1c, 6-2, and 6-3 ■) varies in size from 12 to 18 μm. The nucleus is reduced in size. The nuclear chromatin appears more condensed and more darkly stained than the chromatin in the promyelocyte. Nucleoli may be seen in the early myelocyte but are usually indistinct. Traditionally, we have thought of the myelocyte nucleus as round or oval, but recent evidence shows the nucleus sometimes assumes a markedly indented shape that may subsequently revert to an oval configuration.[8,9] Later stages of the myelocyte may show a flattening of one side of the nucleus. A clear light area is visible next to the nucleus, which represents the Golgi apparatus. The myelocyte goes through two to three divisions; this is the last stage capable of mitotic division. The early myelocyte will have a more bluish cytoplasm; the later stage has a more neutral to pink cytoplasm, and the N:C ratio is decreased. The hallmark for the myelocyte stage is the appearance of specific or secondary granules. The secondary granules are detected first near the nucleus in the Golgi apparatus. This has sometimes been referred to as the dawn of neutrophilia. These neutrophilic granules are small, sand-like granules, with a pink red to pink violet tint. The secondary granules, like the primary granules, are surrounded by a phospholipid membrane that stains with Sudan black B. Large primary azurophilic granules may still be apparent, but their synthesis has ceased. Their concentration and their ability to pick up stain decrease with mitotic divisions. Secondary granule contents are listed in Table 6-2 ✪.[8] Secretory vesicles are scattered throughout the cytoplasm and the plasma membrane of myelocytes, metamyelocytes, band neutrophils, and segmented neutrophils (Table 6-2 ✪).[10–13] Tertiary or gelatinase granules are synthesized mainly during the band and segmented neutrophil stages.[8]

Metamyelocyte

The metamyelocyte (Table 6-1 ✪, Figures 6-1d and 6-3 ■) varies in size from 10 to 18 μm in diameter. Traditionally, its most apparent differentiating characteristic from the myelocyte was nuclear indentation, giving the nucleus a kidney-bean shape. As discussed above, new research may dispute that differentiating feature. The nuclear chromatin is coarse and clumped and stains dark purple. Nucleoli are not visible. The cytoplasm is a neutral pink flesh-tone color with a predominance of secondary and secretory granules.

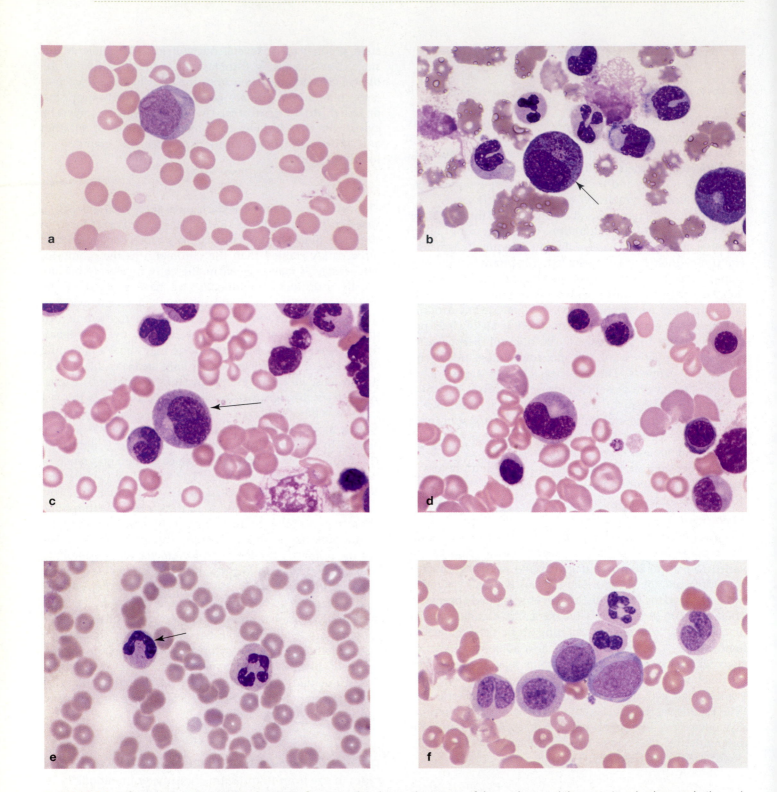

■ **FIGURE 6-1** Stages of neutrophil development. Compare the chromatin pattern of the nucleus and the cytoplasmic changes in the various stages. a. myeloblast: nucleus has fine chromatin and nucleoli; cytoplasm is agranular; b. promyelocyte: nucleus has coarser chromatin, nucleoli are still visible and there are primary granules in the cytoplasm; c. myelocyte: nuclear chromatin is condensed and nucleoli are not visible; secondary granules give the cytoplasm a pinkish color; d. metamyelocyte: nucleus is kidney-shaped and cytoplasm is pinkish; e. band (left) and segmented neutrophil: the nuclear chromatin is condensed and the cytoplasm is pinkish. f. Compare the nuclear and cytoplasmic features of these maturing neutrophilic cells. From left are a band, myelocyte, promyelocyte, myeloblast and band. Above the myeloblast are 2 segmented neutrophils. (Bone marrow; Wright-Giemsa stain; 1000× magnification)

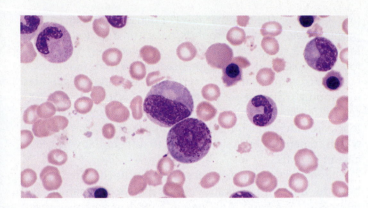

■ **FIGURE 6-2** In the center are a myelocyte (top) and a promyelocyte (bottom). Note the changes in the nucleus and cytoplasm. The myelocyte has a clear area next to the nucleus, which represents the Golgi apparatus. Note the azurophilic granules in the promyelocyte. Also present are two bands and a metamyelocyte in the top right corner. Orthochromatic normoblasts are present. (Bone marrow, Wright-Giemsa stain, 1000× magnification)

✪ TABLE 6-1

Characteristics of Cells in the Maturation Stages of the Neutrophil

Cell Stage (% in bone marrow)	Image	Size (μm)	Nucleus	Cytoplasm	N:C ratio	Granules	CD Markers
Myeloblast (0.2–1.5)	6-1a	14–20	Round or oval; delicate, lacy chromatin; nucleoli	Deep blue	High	Absent	CD33 CD38
Promyelocyte (2–4)	6-1b	15–21	Round or oval, chromatin lacy but more condensed than blast; nucleoli present	Deep blue	High but less than myeloblast	Large, blue purple, called azurophilic, primary or non-specific granules	CD33 CD38
Myelocyte (8–6)	6-1c	12–18	Round; chromatin more condensed than blast; nucleoli usually absent	Light pink but may have patches of blue	Decreased from promyelocyte	Small pinkish red specific granules; some azurophilic granules present	
Metamyelocyte (9–25)	6-1d	10–18	Chromatin condensed; stains dark purple; kidney bean shape	Pink	Decreased	Predominance of small pinkish red specific granules; some azurophilic granules present	
Band (nonsegmented) (9–15)	6-1e	9–15	Chromatin is pyknotic at ends of horseshoe shaped nucleus. Stains dark purple	Pink	Decreased	Abundant small, pinkish red; specific granules; some azurophilic granules present	
Polymorphonuclear (segmented) (6–12)	6-1f	9–15	Nucleus is segmented into 2–4 lobes; chromatin condensed; stains dark purple	Pink	Decreased	As in band	CD13

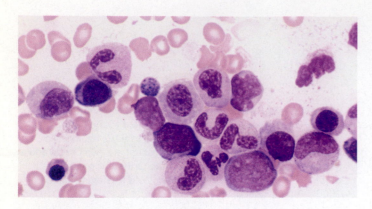

■ **FIGURE 6-3** At about nine o'clock in the central group of cells there is a pronormoblast. At about five o'clock is a myeloblast. Note that the myeloblast has a more lacy, lighter staining chromatin with distinct nucleoli and blue cytoplasm. The normoblast chromatin is more smudged with indistinct nucleoli and very deep blue purple cytoplasm. Also pictured are bands, metamyelocyte, myelocytes, basophilic normoblast, polychromatophilic normoblast, and orthochromatic normoblast. (Bone marrow, Wright-Giemsa stain, 1000× magnification)

Band Neutrophil

The band neutrophil, also called nonsegmented or stab neutrophil, is slightly smaller in diameter, 9–15 μm, than the metamyelocyte. The metamyelocyte becomes a band when the indentation of the nucleus is more than half the diameter of the hypothetical round nucleus (Table 6-1 ✪, Figure 6-1e ■). The indentation gives the nucleus a horseshoe shape. The chromatin displays degenerative changes with pyknosis at either end of the nucleus. The cytoplasm appears pinkish as in the previous stage. This is the first stage that may be normally found in the peripheral blood. All four forms of granules can be found in these cells (primary, secondary, secretory, and tertiary), but the primary granules are usually not visible by Wright's stain.

Segmented Neutrophil

Although similar in size to the band form, 9–15 μm, the polymorphonuclear neutrophil (PMN) is recognized, as its name implies, by a segmented nucleus with two or more lobes connected by a thin nuclear filament (Table 6-1 ✪, Fig-

ures 6-1e, f ■). The chromatin is condensed and stains a deep purple black. Most neutrophils have three or four nuclear lobes, but a range of two to five is given. Less than three lobes is considered hyposegmented. More than five lobes is considered abnormal and referred to as a hypersegmented neutrophil. Three or more five-lobed neutrophils in a 100-cell differential is also considered hypersegmented. The lobes are often touching or superimposed on one another, which sometimes makes it difficult to differentiate the cell as a band or PMN.

Different labs and agencies have outlined criteria as to how to differentiate bands from PMNs in manual differentials.[14,15] A band is defined as a nucleus with a connecting strip or isthmus with parallel sides and wide enough to reveal two distinct margins with nuclear chromatin material visible between the margins. If a margin of a given lobe can be traced as a definite and continuing line from one side across the isthmus to the other side, it is assumed that a filament is present even though it is not visible. If an examiner is not sure whether a neutrophil is a band form or a segmented form, it is arbitrarily classified as a segmented neutrophil. From a traditional clinical viewpoint, it has been useful to determine whether young forms of neutrophils (band forms and younger) are increased.[8] However, differentials performed by automated hematology instruments do not differentiate between band and segmented neutrophils. Band neutrophils are fully functional phagocytes and often are included with the total neutrophil count.[10]

The cytoplasm of the mature PMN stains a pink color. It contains many secondary granules, tertiary granules and secretory granules. Primary granules may be present but because of their scarcity and loss of staining quality, may not be readily identified.

Besides the protein material found in neutrophilic granules, lipids and carbohydrates also can be found. About one-third of the lipids in neutrophils is present in phospholipids. Much of the phospholipid is present in the plasma membrane, secretory granules, or specific granules. Cholesterol and triglycerides constitute most of the nonphospholipid neutrophil lipid. Cytoplasmic nonmembrane lipid bodies have also been found in neutrophils; their role in cell function is unclear. Lipid material also has been found in neutrophilic precursors. A cytochemical stain for lipids, Sudan

✪ TABLE 6-2

Granulocyte Granule Contents

Primary Granules	Secondary Granules	Secretory Vesicles	Tertiary Granules
esterase N	lactoferrin	alkaline phosphatase	lysozyme
cathespin G, B, and D	histaminase	complement receptor 1	gelatinase
defensins (group of cationic proteins)	collagenase	cytochrome b$_{558}$	
myeloperoxidase (gives pus its greenish color)			

black B, has been used to differentiate myeloid precursors from lymphoid precursors (∞ Chapter 26). Glycogen is also found in neutrophils and some myeloid precursors. Neutrophils sometimes have to function in hypoxic conditions, as at an abscess site, and can obtain energy by glycolysis, utilizing glycogen. A periodic acid-Schiff stain (PAS) has been used to detect glycogen in cells. CD markers on the neutrophil include CD16 and CD11.

In females with two X chromosomes or males with XXY chromosomes (Klinefelter syndrome), one X chromosome is randomly inactivated in each somatic cell of the embryo and remains inactive in all daughter cells. This inactive X chromosome appears as an appendage of the neutrophil nucleus and is called a drumstick, or an X chromatin body (Figure 6-4 ■). The number of chromatin bodies detected in the neutrophil is one less than the number of X chromosomes present, but keep in mind that chromatin bodies are not detected in every neutrophil. The X chromatin bodies may be identified in 2–3% of the circulating PMNs of 46, XX females and Klinefelter males.[8]

 Checkpoint! #1

An adult patient's peripheral blood smear revealed many myelocytes, metamyelocytes, and band forms of neutrophils. Is this a normal finding?

CONCENTRATION, DISTRIBUTION, AND DESTRUCTION

The kinetics of a group of cells—the production, distribution, and destruction of the cells—has also been described as the cell turnover rate.

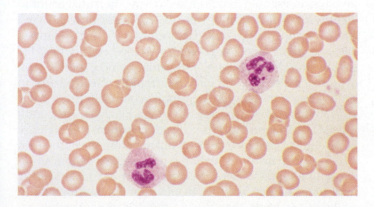

■ **FIGURE 6-4** The segmented neutrophil on the right has an X chromatin body. (Peripheral blood, Wright-Giemsa stain, 1000× magnification)

Bone Marrow

Neutrophils in the bone marrow can be divided into two pools: the mitotic pool and the postmitotic pool (Figure 6-5 ■). The mitotic pool, also called the proliferating pool, includes cells capable of DNA synthesis: myeloblasts, promyelocytes, and myelocytes. Cells spend about 3–6 days in this proliferating pool, undergoing 4 or 5 cell divisions. Three of these divisions occur in the myelocyte stage, but the number of divisions is probably not constant. The postmitotic pool, also known as the maturation storage pool, includes metamyelocytes, bands, and segmented neutrophils. Cells spend about 5–7 days in this compartment before they are released to the peripheral blood. The postmitotic storage pool is almost three times the size of the mitotic pool.[10]

The largest compartment of PMNs is found within the bone marrow. The blood compartment is about one-third the size of the bone marrow compartment, and only one-half of the blood compartment PMNs are in the bloodstream, while the other half are attached to the endothelium.[10]

Once the precursor cells have matured in the bone marrow they are released into the peripheral blood (∞ Chapter 3). Normally, input of neutrophils from the bone marrow to the peripheral blood equals output of the neutrophils from the blood to the tissues, maintaining a relative steady-state concentration in the peripheral blood. However, when the demand for neutrophils is increased such as in infectious states, the neutrophil concentration in the peripheral blood can increase almost immediately as neutrophils from the bone marrow storage pool are released. Depending on the strength and duration of the stimulus, the bone marrow stem cells also may be induced to proliferate and differentiate to form additional neutrophils. Transit time between development in bone marrow and release to peripheral blood can be decreased as a result of several mechanisms: (1) acceleration of maturation, (2) skipped cellular divisions, and (3) early release of cells from the marrow.

The mechanism regulating the production and release of neutrophils from the bone marrow to the peripheral blood is not completely understood, but it most likely includes a feedback loop between the circulating neutrophils and the bone marrow. GM-CSF is probably the primary humoral feedback substance in the normal steady-state. The most potent producers of GM-CSF are T lymphocytes. Inflammatory cytokines such as IL-1 and tumor necrosis factor (TNF) are probably important in causing an increase in the neutrophil concentration in pathologic conditions. The vascular endothelial cell that forms the inner lining of blood vessels also generates cytokines that govern activation and recruitment of leukocytes. Thus endothelial cells may be important in recruiting neutrophils in the earliest phases of inflammation and injury.

The release mechanism of the bone marrow storage pool is selective in normal, steady-state kinetics, releasing only segmented neutrophils and a few band neutrophils. The

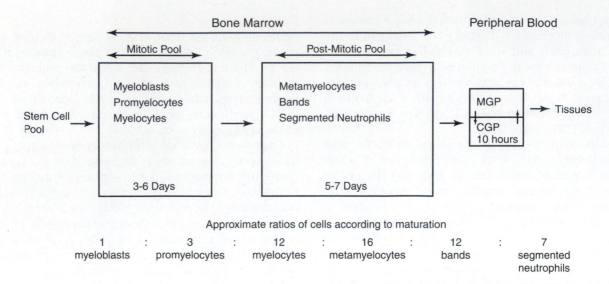

Bone Marrow | Peripheral Blood

Mitotic Pool | Post-Mitotic Pool

Stem Cell Pool

Myeloblasts	Metamyelocytes		MGP	→ Tissues
Promyelocytes	Bands			
Myelocytes	Segmented Neutrophils		CGP 10 hours	

3-6 Days | 5-7 Days

Approximate ratios of cells according to maturation

| 1 | : | 3 | : | 12 | : | 16 | : | 12 | : | 7 |
| myeloblasts | | promyelocytes | | myelocytes | | metamyelocytes | | bands | | segmented neutrophils |

■ **FIGURE 6-5** Neutrophils are produced from stem cells in the bone marrow and spend about 1–2 weeks in this maturation compartment. Most neutrophils are released to the peripheral blood as segmented forms. When the demand for these cells is increased, more immature forms may be released. One-half the neutrophils in the perpheral blood are in the marginating pool; the other half are in the circulating pool. Neutrophils spend about 10 hours in the blood before marginating and exiting randomly to tissue. (Adapted from Boggs DR, Winkelstein A. *White Cell Manual.* 4th ed. Philadelphia: FA Davis Co.; 1983)

mechanisms controlling this regulated release are not fully understood. The release is partially regulated by the small pore size in the vascular endothelium of bone marrow sinusoids and by the ability of the mature segmented neutrophil to deform enough to squeeze through the narrow opening. Immature cells are less deformable and cannot penetrate the small pores; however, when an increased demand for neutrophils exists, a greater proportion of less mature neutrophils are released into the peripheral blood.

Peripheral Blood

Neutrophils are released from the bone marrow to the peripheral blood, but not all neutrophils are circulating freely at the same time. About half the total blood neutrophil concentration is temporarily marginated along the vessel walls (marginating pool), while the other half is circulating (circulating pool). Thus, if all marginated neutrophils were to circulate freely, the total neutrophil count would double. Marginating neutrophils roll on the endothelial surface at a slow rate. This is caused by a loose binding interaction between selectin adhesion proteins on neutrophils and endothelial cells. The two pools, because they are in equilibrium, rapidly and freely exchange neutrophils. Margination occurs selectively in liver, lungs, and spleen and can be reversed by stimulants such as exercise, induced epinephrine release, β-agonists, and interleukin-6, temporarily increasing the circulating pool.

Most neutrophils move into the tissues from the marginal pool in response to antigenic stimulation. The average neutrophil circulates approximately 10 hours in the blood before diapedesing (transendothelial migration) to the tissues, although a few die of senescence.

Neutrophils constitute the majority of circulating leukocytes. The absolute number varies between 2.0 and 7.0 × 10^9/L. There are a number of physiologic and pathologic variations that will affect the numerical values of leukocytes. Physiologic variations are discussed at the end of the chapter. Pathologic causes in changes in leukocyte numbers will be discussed in subsequent chapters on white cell disorders, including ∞ Chapters 21–30.

Alteration in the concentration of peripheral blood leukocytes is often the first sign of underlying pathology (Table 6-3 ✪). A normal leukocyte count does not rule out the presence of disease, but **leukocytosis** (an increase in leukocytes) or **leukopenia** (a decrease in leukocytes) is an important clue to disease processes and deserves further investigation. This investigation should include a leukocyte differential count to identify the concentration of different types of leukocytes. Granulocytopenia (granulocytes below 2 × 10^9/L) defines a decrease in all types of granulocytes (i.e., eosinophils, basophils, and neutrophils). Neutropenia is a more specific term denoting a decrease in only neutrophils. Neutropenia in adults exists if the absolute neutrophil count falls below 2.0 × 10^9/L. When there is an absence of granulocytes, the condition is called **agranulocytosis,** and the patient is at high risk of developing an infection if not isolated from the normal environment. **Granulocytosis** is a term used to denote an increase in all granulocytes. **Neutrophilia** is a more specific term indicating an increase in neutrophils. Neutrophilia in adults occurs when the absolute number of neutrophils exceeds 7 × 10^9/L. This condition is most often a result of the body's reactive response to bacterial infection, metabolic intoxication, drug intoxication, or tissue necrosis.

✪ TABLE 6-3

Terms Associated with Abnormal Concentrations of Leukocytes

Terms Associated with Increases of Cells	Types of Cells Affected
Leukocytosis	General increase in total leukocyte concentration
Granulocytosis	Neutrophils, eosinophils, and/or basophils
Neutrophilia	Neutrophils
Eosinophilia	Eosinophils
Basophilia	Basophils
Monocytosis	Monocytes
Lymphocytosis	Lymphocytes
Terms Associated with Decreases of Cells	
Leukopenia	General decrease in total leukocyte concentration
Granulocytopenia	Neutrophils, eosinophils, basophils
Agranulocytosis	Neutrophils, eosinophils, basophils
Neutropenia	Neutrophils
Monocytopenia	Monocytes
Lymphocytopenia	Lymphocytes

The neutrophil will either be destroyed by trauma (cell necrosis), or live until programmed cell death, apoptosis, occurs (∞ Chapter 2).

✓ Checkpoint! #2

An adult patient's WBC count is 10×10^9/L, and there are 90% neutrophils. What is the absolute number of neutrophils? Is this in the reference range for neutrophils, and if not what term would be used to describe it?

FUNCTION

Neutrophils' primary function is to protect the host from infectious agents. The innate system (natural), along with the acquired (adaptive) or specific immune system, is a major defense system for the body. The neutrophils and macrophages, play a major role in the innate immune system. The lymphoid cells play the major role in the adaptive system and will be discussed later. The neutrophil must move to the site of the foreign agent, engulf it, and destroy it. Monocytes-macrophages help in this process, but they are slower to arrive at the site. The three steps in the innate immune response can be described as adherence, migration, and phagocytosis.

Adherence and Migration

Neutrophil adherence and migration to the site of infection begin with a series of interactions between the neutrophils and vascular endothelial cells (VEC). Several different families of adhesion molecules and their ligands play a major role in this process. Adhesion molecules are the selectins and their ligands, intercellular adhesion molecules (ICAMs), and the β_2 (CD18) family of leukocyte integrins (Table 6-4 ✪). Adhesion molecules and their receptors located on the leukocytes and VEC act together to induce activation dependent adhesion events. They are critical for every step of cell recruitment to sites of tissue injury, including marginating along vessel walls, diapedesis, and **chemotaxis.** Adhesion receptors are transmembrane proteins with three domains: extracellular, transmembrane, and intracellular. Binding of a ligand to the extracellular domain sends a signal across the membrane to the cell's interior. These signals activate secondary messengers within the cell. These secondary messengers affect calcium flux, NADPH oxidase activity, cytoskeleton assembly, and phagocytosis.

Neutrophils and endothelial cells are transformed from a basal state to an activated state by involvement of adhesion molecules. A model of the neutrophil-endothelial cell adhesion process has been proposed by Springer.[16] The process can be divided into at least four stages: (1) activation stages of VEC, (2) activation of neutrophils, (3) binding of neutrophils to inner vessel linings, and (4) transendothelial migration phase (Figure 6-6 ■).

Stage one involves the activation stage of VEC, which mediates a loose association of VECs with neutrophils. Inflammatory cytokines (IL-1, tumor necrosis factor-α [TNF-α], or interferon-γ [IFN-γ]) activate VEC to express E selectin. E selectin molecules on the VEC surface interact with a counterreceptor (ligand) on the neutrophil, causing the neutrophil flow to slow down. This interaction between the VEC and neutrophil causes the neutrophil to roll on the VEC surface.[10] The rolling neutrophils are in a state of readiness, waiting for a command from the chemoattractants (chemical messengers that cause migration of cells in one direction).

Stage two is the activation of neutrophils. Chemokines (chemoattractants) released by tissue cells and bound to the endothelial cell surface activate the bound leukocytes. This activates the leukocyte integrins. Chemoattractants also are called specific and nonspecific proinflammatory mediators. The neutrophil activation-dependent adhesion receptors include the β_2 integrin molecules, Mac-1 (also known as the CR3 or iC3b receptor) and leukocyte function associated antigen-1 (LFA-1). The neutrophil L selectin molecule is lost at this time. A lack of E and L selectins is seen in leukocyte adhesion deficiency type 2 (LAD-2) and results in reoccurring infections.[17]

Stage three involves arrest of the neutrophil rolling as activated neutrophils are more tightly bound to inner vessel linings near the infectious site. Expression of the neu-

⊛ TABLE 6-4

Adhesion Molecules Important in Leukocyte-Endothelial Cell Interactions (LFA = Leukocyte Function-Related Antigen; CD =Cluster of Differentiation; EC = Endothelial Cell; ICAM = intercellular adhesion molecules)

Molecules	CD Designation	Expressed By	Counter-Receptor/Ligand
1. β_2-integrins/Neutrophils			
$\alpha_L\beta_2$, LFA-1	CD11a-CD18	Activated leukocytes	ICAM-1 on EC (CD54)
			ICAM-2 on EC (CD102)
			ICAM-3 (CD50)
$\alpha_M\beta_2$, Mac-1	CD11b-CD18	Activated leukocytes	ICAM-1 on EC
			iC3b, fibrinogen, factor X
$\alpha_x\beta_2$, p150,95	CD11c-CD18	Activated leukocytes	iC3b, fibrinogen
2. Selectins			
L-selectin	CD62L	Leukocytes	Sialylated carbohydrates
E-selectin	CD62E	Activated ECs	Sialylated carbohydrates
P-selectin	CD62P	Activated ECs and platelets	Sialylated carbohydrates
3. Immunoglobulin			
supergene family			
ICAM-1	CD54	EC	LFA-1 (CD11a-CD18)
PECAM-1	CD31	?EC	CD31, $\alpha_v\beta_3$
ICAM-2	CD102	EC	LFA-1 (CD11a-CD18)
LFA-2	CD2	T lymphocytes	LFA-3 (CD58) on EC
LFA-3	CD58	EC	CD2 on T lymphocytes
VCAM-1	CD106	EC	VLA-4(CD49d) on monocytes,
			lymphocytes, eosinophils, basophils
T cell receptor	CD3	T lymphocytes	Antigen
CD4	CD4	T_H lymphocytes	MHC Class II
CD8		T_S lymphocytes	MHC Class I
MHC Class II	–	B lymphocytes	
		Activated T lymphocytes	
		Monocytes	
MHC Class I	–	Nucleated cells	CD8 on T_S lymphocytes
ICAM-3	CD50	Neutrophils	EC

trophils' activation-dependent adhesion receptors mediates firm adherence of neutrophils to intracellular adhesion molecules expressed by activated VEC. This results in a change from the loose selectin-mediated adherence to endothelium to a stronger β_2 integrin binding to ICAMs, which are immunoglobulin family-like receptors. The integrin receptors' intracellular domains react with the neutrophil's cytoskeleton, thus providing a transmembrane link between the extracellular ligand and the cytoskeleton. This can trigger a rapid cytoskeletal rearrangement in the neutrophil, characterized by elongation and formation of a posterior tail (uropod).

The β_2 integrins were the first adhesion molecules described. There are at least three β_2-integrins in the leukocyte plasma membranes: CD11a/CD18 (LFA-1), CD11b/CD18 (Mac-1), and CD11c/CD18. Each has an α subunit (CD11a, CD11b, and CD11c) noncovalently linked to a β subunit

(CD18). An autosomal recessive disorder, leukocyte adhesion deficiency type-I (LAD-I), has partial or total absence of expression of the β_2 integrins on leukocyte membranes. This results in absence of leukocyte adhesion to the VEC, as well as lack of motility or migration, and can result in life-threatening bacterial infections. Stage three ends with a strong, sustained attachment of the leukocyte to the VEC. At this time, leukocyte NADPH oxidase membrane complexes are assembled and activated, which will be discussed later. Aggregation of neutrophils also occurs, which is a Mac-1 dependent event.

Stage four involves the transendothelial migration phase that occurs when neutrophils move through endothelial cells in a process discussed previously, called diapedesis. The neutrophils use pseudopods to squeeze through endothelial cells. The neutrophils leave the vascular space and pass through the subendothelial basement membranes and pe-

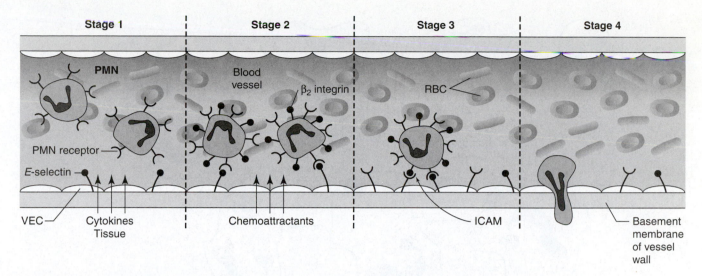

■ **FIGURE 6-6** Adhesion of neutrophils to the vascular endothelium and eventual migration of neutrophils into the tissue occurs as a result of activation of endothelial cells (EC) and neutrophils by exposure to chemoattractants. When the cells are activated they are induced to express adhesion molecules. These transmembrane molecules send a signal across the membrane to the interior of the cell when they attach to their receptor. The process occurs in 4 stages. (1) Expression of E-selectin on activated EC. The neutrophil receptor for E-selectin causes the neutrophil to attach loosely to the EC and roll along the endothelium. (2) Neutrophils are activated by the presence of chemoattractants in the local environment and express the β2-integrins. These chemoattractants also activate the ECs. (3) The neutrophils attach to the activated ECs via their attachment of the β2-integrins to ICAMs of the EC. This is a firmer attachment than in Stage 1 and halts the rolling of the neutrophil. (4) The neutrophil migrates through the endothelium (transendothelial) and basement membrane to the area of inflammation. They move in the direction of the chemoattractants (chemotaxis).

riendothelial cells, often causing vascular injury in the process. Subendothelial basement membranes are eroded, presumably by secretion of neutrophil gelatinase B and elastase. Migration is enhanced when the VEC is activated by IL-1 and/or TNF.

The neutrophils then respond to even higher concentrations of chemotactic agents in the tissues and continue their migration through the extracellular tissue matrices, moving by directed ameboid motion toward the infected site. **Chemotaxis** is induced by a variety of chemoattractant molecules including formyl peptides (FMLP), a cleavage product of the fifth component of complement ($C5_a$), leukotriene β_4(LTB$_4$), IL-8, and platelet activating factor (PAF).

 Checkpoint! #3

A patient with life-threatening recurrent infections is found to have a chromosomal mutation that results in a loss of active integrin molecules on the neutrophil surface. Why would this result in life threatening infections?

Phagocytosis

The monocytes and macrophages, which are the professional phagocytes, arrive at the site of injury after the neutrophils. They must recognize the pathogen as foreign before attachment occurs and phagocytosis begins (Figure 6-7 ■). **Phagocytosis** is an active process that requires a large expenditure of energy by the cells. The required energy can be provided by anaerobic glycolysis or aerobic processes.

The principal factor in determining whether or not phagocytosis can occur is the physical nature of the surfaces of both the foreign particle and the phagocytic cell. Phagocytes recognize unique molecular characteristics of the pathogen's surface and bind to the invading organism. Some pathogens may be recognized without surface modification, whereas others must be opsonized (the coating of a particle with a soluble factor). Enhancement of phagocytosis through the process of opsonization speeds the ingestion of particles.

Two opsonins are well-defined, immunoglobulin G (IgG) and complement component C3b. The antibody, IgG, binds to the microorganism/particle by means of its Fab region, while the Fc region of the antibody attaches to the Fc receptor on the neutrophil membrane. Thus, the antibody forms a connecting link between the microorganism/particle and the neutrophil. The neutrophil also has receptors for activated complement. (Some bacteria with polysaccharide capsules avoid recognition, thus reducing the effectiveness of phagocytosis.) Following recognition and attachment, the particle is surrounded by extended pseudopods of the neutrophil (Figure 6-7 ■). As the pseudopods touch, they fuse and pinch off, forming a phagosome that is bound by the cytoplasmic membrane turned inside out. A plasma mem-

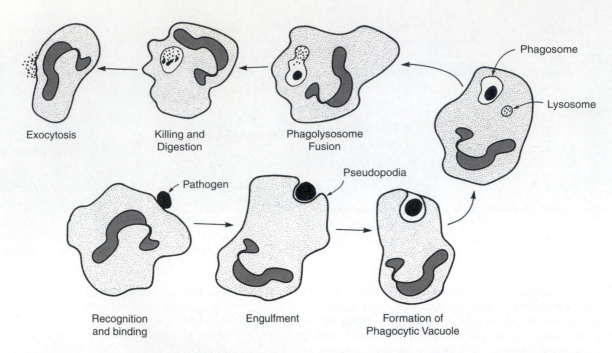

■ FIGURE 6-7 Phagocytosis begins with recognition and attachment of the pathogen to the neutrophil (or macrophage). The pathogen is then internalized, forming a phagocytic vacuole. Next, the lysosome fuses with the vacuole, forming a phagolysosome, and releases its contents into the vacuole to help kill and digest the microbe. This is followed by extrusion of the vacuole contents from the neutrophil (exocytosis). (Courtesy Denise Miller.)

brane-bound oxidase is activated during ingestion. This oxidase causes enzymatic reduction of oxygen, resulting in the formation of microbactericidal metabolites.

Digestion follows ingestion of particles. Degranulation of the PMN starts with the onset of phagocytosis. The phagosome fuses with one or more lysosomal granules that contain various lytic enzymes. This phagocytic vacuole is called the phagolysosome. Microbicidal mechanisms that follow ingestion can be divided into oxygen dependent/oxidative or oxygen independent/nonoxidative activities (Table 6-5 ✿). Oxygen dependent microbicidal activity is most important and depends on products of oxygen reduction. Phagocytosis is accompanied by an energy-dependent respiratory burst that generates oxidizing compounds produced from partial oxygen reduction. The oxidizing compounds are important agents in killing ingested organisms. In resting cells, the enzyme needed to generate oxygen reduction products, NADPH-dependent oxidase, also known as respiratory burst oxidase (RBO), is found in components in the plasma membrane (gp^{91phox}, p^{22phox}, and Rap^1) and intracellular stores (p^{47phox}, and p^{67phox}). When the resting cell is exposed to any of a wide variety of stimuli, activated NADPH oxidase is assembled from these components at the plasma membrane. Once assembled, the oxidase produces O_2^- and $NADP^+$. The $NADP^+$ activates the HMP shunt.

$$\overset{\text{oxidase}}{2O_2 + 2NADPH \rightarrow 2O_2^- + 2NADP^+ + 2H^+ \rightarrow H_2O_2 +}$$
$$O_2 + 2NADP^+$$

H_2O_2 is either generated from superoxide or is catalyzed by superoxide dismutase. When phagocytosis takes place, the plasma membrane is internalized as the wall of the phagocytic vesicle. Therefore, the outer plasma membrane surface now faces the interior of the phagosome. From this location, the NADPH oxidase pours O_2^- into the phagosome. The activated oxidase can be detected in the laboratory by a nitroblue tetrazolium test (NBT), cytochrome reduction, or chemiluminescence test. Through the enzyme myeloperoxidase, some of the products of oxygen metabolism give rise to oxidized halogens such as hypochlorous acid (HOCl), which increase bacterial killing.[18]

$$H_2O_2 + Cl^- \rightarrow OCl^- + H_2O$$

✿ TABLE 6-5

Neutrophil Antimicrobial Systems

Oxygen-dependent	Oxygen-independent
a. Myeloperoxidase-independent	–Acid pH of phagosome
–Hydrogen peroxide (H_2O_2)	–Lysozyme (primary granules)
–Superoxide anion (O_2^-)	–Lactoferrin (secondary granules)
–Hydroxyl radicals (OH^-)	–Cationic proteins (primary granules)
–Singlet oxygen ($^1O_2$)	
b. Myeloperoxidase-dependent	
(forms oxidized halogens)	

During particle ingestion, phagocytes show a twofold to threefold increase of O_2 consumption, a twofold to tenfold increase of glucose oxidation via the hexose monophosphate shunt, and the generation of hydrogen peroxide. This combination of metabolic activities is known as the respiratory burst. It was discovered in 1933.[18]

The oxidants generated by the respiratory burst have potent microbicidal activity against a wide variety of microorganisms such as bacteria, fungi, and multicellular and unicellular parasites. However, the phagocyte and surrounding tissues are also susceptible to damage. Phagocytes use a variety of mechanisms to detoxify the oxidant radicals, such as the superoxide, dismutase, catalase, and a variety of antioxidants.

Oxygen-independent granular proteins, present in primary, gelatinase, and specific granules of neutrophils can successfully kill and degrade many strains of both gram-negative and gram-positive bacteria. The most important antimicrobial proteins of PMNs are defensins, serprocidins, including cathepsin G and azurocidin (GAP 37), and bacterial permeability-increasing protein (BPI). Initially, the pH within the phagolysosome decreases, inhibiting bacterial growth, but this alone is insufficient to kill most microbes. Acidic conditions, however, may enhance the activity of some granular proteins such as hydrolases and lactoferrin, which perform optimally at low pH. In the extracellular environment, microorganisms that escape phagocytosis are also subject to killing by reactive oxygen metabolites such as H_2O_2 that forms from the O_2^- secreted by active plasma membrane NADPH complexes into the tissue matrices. Neutrophils themselves are not immune to the toxic effects of the oxidants they secrete, and thus have high mortality during any sustained inflammatory response.[19]

In patients with chronic granulomatous disease, neutrophils are missing a component of NADPH complex and therefore fail to produce the oxidative burst but are still capable of eliminating infection caused by strains of bacteria susceptible to killing by oxygen-independent mechanisms. Often, however, these patients eventually die of multiple infections with bacteria that are resistant to the killing actions of these granular proteins alone.

In addition to their primary functions of phagocytosis and killing of microorganisms, neutrophils interact in other physiologic processes. Neutrophils stimulate coagulation by releasing a substance that triggers prekallikrein to become kallikrein. Kallikrein activates the first contact factor of coagulation, thus initiating the extrinsic coagulation pathway. Kallikrein also converts kininogen to kinin. Kinins are responsible for vascular dilation and increased vessel permeability. Kinins, chemotactic for neutrophils, attract them to sites of inflammation. Neutrophils initially activate kinin production, but as the cells accumulate, they break down kinins. Neutrophils also contain pyrogen, a substance that acts on the hypothalamus to produce fever. This endogenous pyrogen is now known as interleukin-1 (IL-1).

✓ Checkpoint! #4

A patient has a compromised ability to utilize the oxygen dependent pathway in neutrophils. What two important microbial killing mechanisms could be affected?

► EOSINOPHILS

The eosinophil originates from the IL-5–responsive CD34$^+$ myeloid progenitor cells. The factors that influence the proliferation and the differentiation of the eosinophil lineage include GM-CSF and IL-3 and IL-5. The precise delineation of factors is the subject of ongoing studies. It is now recognized that IL-5 has lineage specificity for eosinophils and is the major cytokine required for eosinophil production.[20]

DIFFERENTIATION, MATURATION, MORPHOLOGY

The eosinophil undergoes a morphologic maturation similar to the neutrophil. It is not possible to morphologically differentiate eosinophilic precursors from neutrophilic precursors with the light microscope until the myelocyte stage, when the typical acidophilic crystalloid granules of the eosinophil appear. Granule formation begins in the promyelocyte, with small coreless granules.

Eosinophilic Myelocyte to Eosinophil

The myelocyte eosinophil contains large, eosin-staining, crystalloid granules. Maturation from the myelocyte to the metamyelocyte, band, and segmented neutrophil stage is similar to that described for the neutrophils, with gradual nuclear indentation and segmentation. There is no appreciable change in the cytoplasm in these latter stages of development. The reddish orange spherical granules are uniform in size and evenly distributed throughout the cell. Because of the low percentage of eosinophils in the bone marrow, no useful purpose is served by differentiating the eosinophil into its maturational stages (e.g., eosinophilic myelocyte) when the count is normal. Bone marrow maturation and storage time is about 9 days.

The mature eosinophil (Figure 6-8 ■) is from 12 to 15 μm in diameter. The nucleus usually has no more than two or three lobes, and the cytoplasm is completely filled with granules. The eosinophil contains three types of granules: primary granules; granules called small granules, which contain the enzymes acid phosphatase and aryl-sulphatase; and other granules called the eosinophil-specific, or crystalloid, granules that are bound by a phospholipid membrane and have a central crystalloid core surrounded by a matrix. The eosinophil specific granules contain four major proteins: major basic protein (MBP), eosinophil cationic protein (ECP), eosinophil peroxidase (EPO), and eosinophil-derived neurotoxin (EDN), also known as protein x (EPX) (Table 6-6 ✿). The MBP is located in

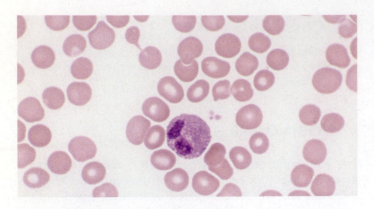

■ **FIGURE 6-8** Eosinophil (Peripheral blood, Wright-Giemsa stain, 1000× magnification)

the crystalloid core, while the other three proteins are found in the granule matrix. The crystalloid core also appears to store a number of proinflammatory cytokines such as IL-2, IL-4, and GM-CSF, while the matrix contains IL-5 and TNF-α. The eosinophil has the capacity to synthesize and elaborate a number of other cytokines. The capacity of the eosinophil to produce cytokines has led to increased interest and research into the eosinophil's role as an effector cell in allergic inflammation. The eosinophil, like the neutrophil, contains a number of lipid bodies; these lipid bodies increase during eosinophil activation in vitro.[20,21] Eosinophils express the CD9, CD11a, and CD13 molecule.

Tissue Eosinophils

In smears of bone marrow, one may find large cells with a well-defined reticular chromatin pattern in the nucleus, nucleoli present, an irregular cytoplasmic outline, and cyto-plasmic granules similar to the orange red granules of blood eosinophils. It is thought that these cells are fixed tissue variants of the more motile eosinophils of the peripheral blood, and are called tissue eosinophils.

CONCENTRATION, DISTRIBUTION, AND DESTRUCTION

Eosinophils in adults have a concentration in peripheral blood equal to or less than 0.45×10^9/L. The cell shows a diurnal variation of highest concentrations at 7 A.M. and the lowest concentrations at 10 A.M.[22] Blood eosinophil concentrations are somewhat higher in neonates, peaking at a mean level of 0.52×10^9/L at 6–7 weeks of age.[20]

Eosinophilia in adults is defined as $>0.45 \times 10^9$/L and has been associated with allergies, parasitic infections, and drug interactions. (∞ Chapter 21 for a complete list.)

Very little is known about the kinetics of eosinophils. Most of the body's eosinophil population is below the epithelial layer in tissues that are exposed to the external environment such as the nasal passages, skin, and the urinary tract. These cells spend very little time in the peripheral blood (1–8 hours) before migrating to the tissues, where they may live for several weeks.

FUNCTION

Eosinophils have multiple biologic functions and contribute to a variety of immune defense mechanisms. Their production and function are influenced by the cellular arm of the immune system.[20] Eosinophils are associated with allergic reactions, parasitic infections, and chronic inflammation. Their major defensive role is host defense against helminth

✪ **TABLE 6-6**

Major Proteins of Eosinophil Granules

Protein	Abbreviation	Characteristics
Major basic protein	(MBP)	Cytotoxic for protozoans and helminth parasites
		Stimulates release of histamine from mast cells and basophils
Eosinophil cationic protein	(ECP)	Capable of killing mammalian and nonmammalian cells
		Stimulates release of histamine from mast cells and basophils
		Inhibits T lymphocyte proliferation
		Preactivates plasminogen
		Enhances mucus production in the bronchi
		Stimulation of glycosaminoglycan production by fibroblasts
Eosinophil-derived neurotoxin	(EDN)	Ability to provoke cerebral and cerebellar dysfunction in animals
		Inhibitor of T cell responses
Eosinophil peroxidase	(EPO)	Combines with H_2O_2 and halide ions to produce a potent bactericidal and helminthicidal action
		Cytotoxic for tumor and host cells
		Stimulates histamine release and degranulation of mast cells
		Diminishes roles of other inflammatory cells by inactivating leukotrines

parasites via a complex interaction of the eosinophils, immune system, and parasite. They also are capable of phagocytosing bacteria.

The eosinophils are proinflammatory cells that are capable of either protecting or damaging the host, depending on the situation. Eosinophils respond weakly to IL-3, IL-5, and GM-CSF as chemotaxins, but IL-5, made by T lymphocytes, has been shown to prime eosinophils for a better chemotactic response to platelet activating factor (PAF), 5S-12R-dihydroxy-6,14-cis-8,10–trans-eicosatetraenoic acid (LTB$_4$), or IL-8. Especially chemotactic for eosinophils are products released from basophils and mast cells, lymphokines from sensitized lymphocytes, and antigen/antibody reactions of allergy. Eosinophils express Fc receptors for IgE, which is prevalent in the response to parasitic infections and mediates activation of eosinophil killing mechanisms. The cytokines IL-3, IL-5, and GM-CSF promote the adherence of eosinophils and induce weak chemoattractant-induced adhesion. These cytokines also prolong the survival of eosinophils in culture. Transendothelial migration is also ten times greater in the presence of these cytokines.

Eosinophils have a β_2 integrin-independent mechanism for recruitment into the tissues. This was first suggested when eosinophils and mononuclear leukocytes, but not neutrophils, were found at sites of infection in children with congenital β_2-integrin deficiency (LAD-1). Eosinophil recruitment appears to be modulated by the eosinophil adhesion receptor, very late activation antigen-4 (VLA-4), and its ligand on VEC, vascular cell adhesion molecule-1 (VCAM-1). VCAM-1 has been shown to be expressed on VEC when the vascular endothelium is activated with IL-1, TNF, or IL-4. Changes in eosinophil adhesion molecule expression occur during eosinophil migration. This implies that dynamic changes in cell adhesion molecules are involved in cell recruitment to areas of inflammation.

The eosinophil liberates substances that can neutralize mast cell and basophil products, thereby modulating the allergic response. Increasing evidence suggests a direct correlation between the degree of eosinophilia and severity of inflammatory diseases such as asthma. In these conditions, the cytotoxic potential of eosinophils is turned against the host's own tissue.[23]

► BASOPHILS

Basophils (Figure 6-9 ■) originate from the CD34$^+$ myeloid progenitors in the bone marrow. IL-3 is the main cytokine involved in human basophil growth and differentiation, but it is believed that GM-CSF, SCF, IL-4, and IL-5 may have a role.[24,25]

DIFFERENTIATION, MATURATION, AND MORPHOLOGY

Basophils undergo a maturation process similar to that described for the neutrophil. The first recognizable stage is the promyelocyte, although this stage is very difficult to differ-

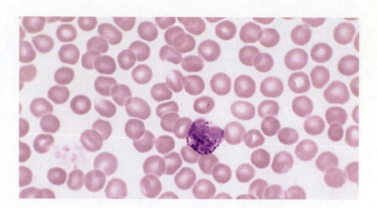

■ **FIGURE 6-9** Basophil. (Peripheral blood, Wright-Giemsa stain, 1000× magnification)

entiate from the promyelocyte of the neutrophil or eosinophil. The basophilic promyelocyte is smaller (12 μm) with a higher N:C ratio than the promyelocyte of neutrophils or eosinophils. As with the eosinophils, the various stages of the maturing basophil are characterized by a gradual indentation and segmentation of the nucleus.

Basophilic Myelocyte to Basophil

The basophilic myelocyte, metamyelocyte, band, and segmented form are easily differentiated from other granulocytes by the presence of the large purple black granules unevenly distributed throughout the cytoplasm. The granules are metachromatic. They contain histamine, heparin, cathepsin G, major basic protein, and lysophospholipase.[24] The mature basophil ranges in size from 10 to 15 μm and has a segmented nucleus and many purple granules obscuring the background of the cytoplasm. Basophil granules contain peroxidase and are positive with the periodic acid-Schiff (PAS) reaction. Basophils have an antigen profile similar to that of other granulocytes. Basophil granules are water soluble and may become washed out on a well rinsed Wright stained smear. Usually a few deep-purple staining granules remain to aid in the identification of the cell. Basophils express the CD9, CD11a, and CD13 molecule.

Mast Cell (Tissue Basophil)

The relationship between basophils and mast cells continues to be investigated. Research shows that mast cells and basophils represent distinct, terminally differentiated cells derived from the CD34$^+$ myeloid stem cells. The mast cells are found in the bone marrow and leave the bone marrow to mature in the tissue. Mast cells are not found in peripheral blood. Mast cells have proliferative potential and live weeks to months. At times, it is difficult to differentiate the mast cell and the basophil precursors in the bone marrow, although there are some differences (Table 6-7 ✪). The mast cell nucleus is round and surrounded by a dense population of granules. The mast cell granules contain acid phos-

⊕ TABLE 6-7

Comparison of the Characteristics of Basophils and Mast Cells

Characteristics	Basophils	Mast Cells
Origin	Hematopoietic stem cell	Hematopoietic stem cell
Site maturation	Bone marrow	Connective or mucosal tissue
Proliferative potential	No	Yes
Life span	Days	Weeks to months
Size	Small	Large
Nucleus	Segmented	Round
Granules	Few, small (peroxidase positive)	Many, large (acid phosphatase, alkaline phosphatase positive)
Key cytokine regulating development	IL-3	Stem cell factor (SCF)
Surface receptors:		
IL-3	Present	Absent
c-kit (receptor for SCF)	Absent	Present
IgE receptor	Present	Present

phatase, protease, and alkaline phosphatase. Mast cells have an antigen profile similar to that of macrophages.

CONCENTRATION, DISTRIBUTION, AND DESTRUCTION

Basophils' maturation in the bone marrow requires 2.5–7 days before they are released into circulation. In the peripheral blood, they number less than 0.2×10^9/L of the total leukocytes. Basophilia in adults is defined as >0.2×10^9/L in the peripheral blood. Basophils are end-stage cells incapable of proliferation and spend only hours in the peripheral blood.

FUNCTION

The basophil and mast cell function as mediators of inflammatory responses, especially those of immediate hypersensitivity reactions such as asthma, urticaria, allergic rhinitis, and anaphylaxis. These cells have membrane receptors for IgE. When IgE attaches to the receptor, the cell is activated and degranulation is initiated. Degranulation releases enzymes that are vasoactive, bronchoconstrictive, and chemotactic (especially for eosinophils). This release of mediators initiates the classic clinical signs of immediate hypersensitivity. These cells can synthesize more granules after degranulation occurs. Basophils and mast cells express CD40L, the ligand for CD40, an antigen on B lymphocytes. The interaction of B lymphocyte CD40 and basophil CD40L in conjunction with IL-4 can induce IgE synthesis by B lymphocytes. Thus, basophils may play an important role in inducing and maintaining allergic reactions.

Recruitment of basophils into sites of inflammation in tissues is mediated by adhesion molecules present on both eosinophils and basophils. Some of these molecules are not present on neutrophils (i.e., VLA-4). This may help explain the preferential recruitment of eosinophils and basophils into extravascular inflammatory sites associated with hypersensitivity and allergic responses.

 Checkpoint! #5

Indicate which of the granulocytes will be increased in the following conditions: a bacterial infection, an immediate hypersensitivity reaction, an asthmatic reaction.

▶ MONOCYTES

The monocyte is produced in the bone marrow from a bipotential stem cell (CFU-GM) that is capable of maturing into either a monocyte or a granulocyte. The differentiation and growth of CFU-GM into monocytes are dependent on the action of GM-CSF, IL-3, and monocyte stimulating factor (M-CSF). Monocytes transform to macrophages in the tissue. Monocytes and macrophages can be stimulated by T lymphocytes and endotoxin to liberate M-CSF. This may be one mechanism for the monocytosis associated with some infections. The M-CSF also activates the secretory and phagocytic activity of monocytes and macrophages.

DIFFERENTIATION, MATURATION, AND MORPHOLOGY

The monocyte precursors in the bone marrow are the monoblast and the promonocyte. These cells are found in abundance only in leukemic processes of the monocyte system. The monoblast of the marrow cannot be morphologically distinguished from the myeloblast by light microscopy

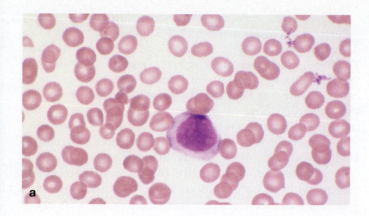

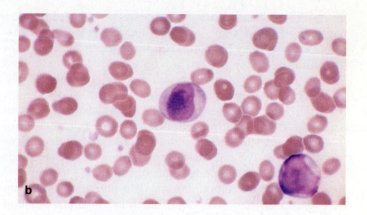

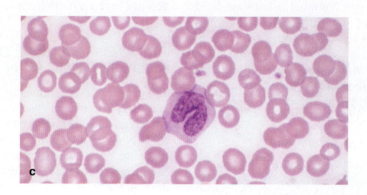

■ **FIGURE 6-10** Stages of monocyte maturation: a. monoblast—note lacey chromatin, nucleoli, and high N:C ratio; b. promonocyte—the chromatin is somewhat more coarse and the amount of cytoplasm is increased; c. monocyte—the nucleus is more lacey than that of a neutrophil or lymphocyte and is irregular in shape. (a, b: Bone marrow, Wright-Giemsa stain, 1000× magnification; c: Peripheral blood, Wright-Giemsa stain, 1000× magnification)

unless there is marked proliferation of the monocytic series, as occurs in monocytic leukemia. It is not known whether the leukemic process of maturation simulates normal monocytopoiesis. Cytochemical stains frequently are used to help differentiate myeloblasts and monoblasts.

The promonocyte is usually the first stage to develop morphologic characteristics that allow it to be differentiated as a monocyte precursor by light microscopy. The identification of early monocyte precursors is aided by observing folds or indentations in the nucleus and by their association with mature monocytes.

Monoblast

The monoblast's (Figure 6-10a ■) nucleus is most often ovoid or round but may be folded or indented. The light blue purple nuclear chromatin is finely dispersed (lacy) and several nucleoli are easily identified. The monoblast has abundant agranular blue gray cytoplasm. Differentiation of the monoblast from the myeloblast may be possible with special cytochemical stains (∞ Chapter 26). The monoblast has nonspecific esterase activity demonstrated by reaction with the substrates α-naphthyl butyrate or naphthol AS-D

acetate (NASDA). The NASDA activity is inhibited by sodium fluoride. The myeloblast has both specific esterase activity (demonstrated by reaction with the substrate naphthol AS-D chloroacetate) and nonspecific esterase activity, but the nonspecific esterases are not inhibited by sodium fluoride.

Promonocyte

The promonocyte (Figure 6-10b ■) is an intermediate form between the monoblast and the monocyte. The cell is large, 12–20 μm in diameter. The nucleus is most often irregular and deeply indented with a fine chromatin network. Chromatin filaments are coarser than the monoblast. Nucleoli may be present. The promonocyte's cytoplasm is abundant with a blue gray color. Azurophilic granules may be present. Cytochemical stains for nonspecific esterase, peroxidase, acid phosphatase, and arylsulfatase are positive. The CD14 marker is found on monocytic cells.

Monocyte

The mature monocytes (Figure 6-10c ■) range in size from 12 to 20 μm with an average of 18 μm, making them the largest mature cells in peripheral blood. The nucleus is frequently horseshoe- or bean-shaped and possesses numerous folds, giving it the appearance of brain-like convolutions. Sometimes nucleoli may be seen. The chromatin is loose and linear, forming a lacy pattern in comparison to the clumped dense chromatin of mature lymphocytes or granulocytes. Monocytes, however, are sometimes difficult to distinguish from large lymphocytes, especially in reactive states when there are many reactive lymphocytes. The monocyte cytoplasm has variable morphologic characteristics dependent on its activity. The cell adheres to glass and spreads or sends out numerous pseudopods resulting in a wide variation of size and shape on blood smears. The blue gray cytoplasm is evenly dispersed with fine, dust-like, membrane-bound granules, which give the cell cytoplasm the appearance of ground glass. Electron-microscopic cytochemistry reveals two types of granules. One type contains peroxidase, acid phosphatase, and arylsulfatase, suggesting that these granules are similar to the lysosomes (azurophilic granules) of neutrophils. Less is known about the content of the other type of granule, except that it does not contain alkaline phosphatase. The lipid membrane of the granules stain with Sudan black B. Many CD markers are found on monocytes including CD11, CD12, CD13, CD14, and CD15.

Macrophage

The monocyte eventually leaves the blood and enters the tissues, where it matures into a macrophage (Figure 6-11 ■). The transition from monocyte to macrophage is characterized by progressive cellular enlargement. Its size may range from 15 to 80 μm. The nucleus becomes round with a reticular (net-like) appearance, nucleoli appear, and the cytoplasm appears blue gray with ragged edges and many vacuoles present. As it matures, the macrophage loses peroxidase, but increases are seen in the amount of endoplasmic reticulum (ER), lysosomes, and mitochondria. Also, granules are noted in the maturing macrophage. These cells can live for months in the tissues. Macrophages do not normally reenter the blood, but in areas of inflammation, some may gain access to the lymph, eventually entering the blood.

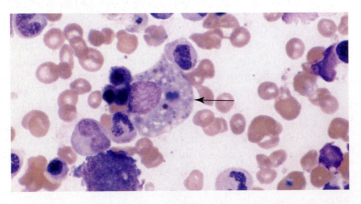

■ **FIGURE 6-11** A macrophage. Note the numerous vacuoles and cellular debris. (Bone marrow, Wright-Giemsa stain, 1000× magnification)

Macrophages, collectively known as histiocytes, develop different cytochemical and morphologic characteristics that depend on the site of maturation and habitation in tissue. These cells are given more specific names, depending on their location in the body. For example, macrophages in the liver are known as Kupffer cells, those in the lung as alveolar macrophages, those in the skin as Langerhans cells, and those in the brain as microglial cells.

Macrophages may proliferate in the tissue, especially in areas of inflammation, thereby increasing the number of cells at these sites. Occasionally, two or more macrophages fuse to produce giant multinucleated cells. This occurs in granulomatous lesions, where many macrophages are tightly packed together. Fusion also occurs when particulate matter is too large for one cell to ingest or when two cells simultaneously ingest a particle.

CONCENTRATION, DISTRIBUTION, AND DESTRUCTION

The promonocyte undergoes two or three divisions before maturing into monocytes. Bone marrow transit time is about 60 hours. In contrast to the large neutrophil storage pool, there is no reserve pool of monocytes in the bone marrow; most are released within a day after their derivation from promonocytes. Monocytes diapedese into the tissue in a random manner after an average transit time in the vascular space, reported at about 12 hours.[26]

The total vascular monocyte pool consists of a marginal pool and a circulating pool. The marginating pool is about three times the size of the circulating pool. Monocytes in the circulating peripheral blood number about $0.2–0.8 \times 10^9/L$ in the normal adult, or about 4% to 10% of the total leukocytes. Children have a slightly higher concentration. Monocytosis (increase in monocytes) in adults occurs when the absolute monocyte count is $>0.8 \times 10^9/L$.

FUNCTION

Monocytes and macrophages along with neutrophils are included in the innate, or natural, immune system. These cells are the first to respond in an infection. In addition to their phagocytic function, they secrete a variety of substances that affect the function of other cells, especially that of lymphocytes. Lymphocytes, in turn, secrete soluble products, lymphokines, that modulate monocytic functions.

Monocytes and macrophages ingest and kill microorganisms. They are especially important in inhibiting the growth of intracellular microorganisms. This inhibition requires cellular activation (enhancement of function) of monocytes by soluble products of T-lymphocytes. Killing by activated monocytes is nonspecific (i.e., the secretions from Listeria-sensitized T cells will activate a killing mechanism in monocytes not only to Listeria but to other microorganisms). Activation also may occur as the result of the actions of other substances on monocytes such as endotoxins and naturally occurring opsonins. Activation results in the production of many large granules, enhanced phagocytosis, and an increase in the HMP shunt.

Monocytes/macrophages have some ability to bind directly to microorganisms, but binding is enhanced if the microorganism has been opsonized by complement or immunoglobulin (Web Figure 6-1 ■). Macrophages possess receptors for the Fc component of IgG and for the complement component C3b. Following attachment, the opsonized organism is ingested in a manner similar to that for neutrophils (Figure 6-7 ■). Primary lysosomes fuse with the phagosome, releasing hydrolytic enzymes and other microbicidal substances. The most powerful microbicidal substances of monocytes and macrophages are products of oxygen metabolism: superoxide (O_2^-), hydroxy radical (OH^-), singlet oxygen ($^1O_2$), and hydrogen peroxide (H_2O_2).

Activated macrophages attach to tumor cells and kill them by a direct cytologic effect. If the tumor cell has immunoglobulin attached, the macrophage Fc receptor attaches to the Fc portion of the immunoglobulin and exerts a lytic effect on the tumor cell.

Macrophages are important scavengers, phagocytosing cellular debris, effete cells, and other particulate matter. Monocytes in the blood ingest activated clotting factors, thus limiting the coagulation process. They also ingest denatured protein and antigen–antibody complexes. Macrophages lining the blood vessels remove toxic substances from the blood, preventing their escape into tissues. The macrophages of the spleen are important in removing aged erythrocytes from the blood; they conserve the iron of hemoglobin by either storing it for future use or by releasing it to transferrin for use by developing normoblasts in the bone marrow. The splenic macrophages, by virtue of their Fc receptor, also remove cells sensitized with antibody. In autoimmune hemolytic anemias or in autoimmune thrombocytopenia, the spleen is sometimes removed to prevent premature destruction of these antibody-coated cells and alleviate the resulting cytopenias.

In some pathologic conditions, for unknown reasons, erythrocytes are randomly phagocytosed and destroyed by monocytes and macrophages in the blood and bone marrow (erythrophagocytosis) (Figure 6-12 ■). **Erythrophagocytosis** is readily identified when the ingested erythrocytes still contain hemoglobin. At times, erythrocyte digestion can be inferred by the finding of ghost spheres within the macrophage.

The **monocyte-macrophage system,** sometimes called the mononuclear phagocyte system or the misnomered reticuloendothelial system, plays a major role in initiating and regulating the **immune response**.[26] Macrophages phagocytize and degrade both soluble and particulate substances that are foreign to the host. Through unknown mechanisms, they spare critical portions of these antigens known as antigenic

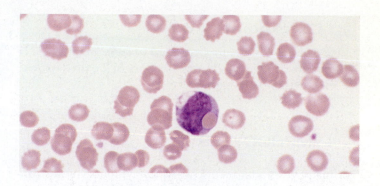

■ **FIGURE 6-12** Erythrophagocytosis by a monocyte. (Peripheral blood, Wright-Giemsa stain, 1000× magnification)

determinant sites, or epitopes. These antigenic determinants on the macrophage membrane are presented to antigen-dependent T lymphocytes. Thus monocytes/macrophages are known as antigen presenting cells (APC). In addition to antigen presentation, the APC provides cell surface molecules known as major histocompatibility complex (MHC) antigens and a secretory product, IL-1. Antigen-specific T lymphocyte proliferation requires antigen presentation in context with cell surface MHC antigens, and stimulation with soluble mediators such as IL-1 and IL-2. T lymphocytes will only respond to foreign antigens when the antigens are displayed on APCs that have the same MHC phenotype as the lymphocyte itself.

Macrophages stimulate the proliferation and differentiation of lymphocytes through secretion of cytokines. They secrete IL-1, which stimulates T lymphocytes to secrete interleukin-2 (IL-2). IL-2 is a growth factor that stimulates the proliferation of other T lymphocytes. In addition, IL-2 acts as in synergy with interferon (IFN) to activate macrophages. Arachidonic metabolites, when released from macrophages, inhibit the function of activated lymphocytes. Activated lymphocytes in turn, secrete lymphokines that regulate the function of macrophages. For these interdependent reactions to occur between the macrophage and lymphocyte, the two cell populations must express compatible MHC antigens.

Macrophages release a variety of substances that are involved in host defense or that may affect the function of other cells in addition to IL-1. Other secretory products that are involved in host defense include lysozymes, complement components, and IFN (an antiviral compound). Secreted substances that modulate other cells include: hematopoietic growth factors (G-CSF, M-CSF, GM-CSF), factors that stimulate the growth of new capillaries, factors that stimulate and suppress the activity of lymphocytes, chemotactic substances for neutrophils, and a substance that stimulates the hepatocyte to secrete fibrinogen. Activated macrophages also release, after death, enzymes such as collagenase, elastase, and neutral proteinase that hydrolyze tissue components.

✔ Checkpoint! #6

An adult patient's neutrophil count and monocyte count are extremely low (<0.50 × 10⁹/L and <0.050 × 10⁹/L, respectively). What body defense mechanism is at risk?

▶ LYMPHOCYTES

For many years after its discovery, the lymphocyte was considered an insignificant component of blood and lymph. Since 1960, major advances in immunology have targeted the lymphocyte as directing the activities of all other cells in the immune response. The lymphocyte's primary function is to react with antigen and, together with monocytes, modulate the immune response.

DIFFERENTIATION AND MATURATION

The lymphoid cell line arises from the pluripotential hematopoietic stem cell found in the bone marrow. This stem cell gives rise to committed cells: the lymphoid progenitor cell and the myeloid (CFU-GEMM) progenitor cell. The lymphoid progenitor cell differentiates and matures under the inductive influence of selective microenvironments into two types of morphologically identical but immunologically and functionally diverse lymphocytes, T lymphocytes and B lymphocytes (∞ Chapter 2). A third type of lymphocyte, the natural killer (NK) cell has characteristics distinctly different from those of T and B lymphocytes.

Lymphopoiesis can be divided into two different phases: antigen independent lymphopoiesis and antigen dependent lymphopoiesis (Figure 6-13 ■). Antigen-independent lymphopoiesis takes place within the primary lymphoid tissue (bone marrow, thymus, fetal liver, yolk sac, paraaortic region). This type of lymphopoiesis begins with the committed lymphoid stem cell and results in the formation of immunocompetent T lymphocytes and B lymphocytes (nicknamed virgin lymphocytes because they have not yet reacted with antigen). Antigen-dependent lymphopoiesis occurs in the secondary lymphoid tissue (adult bone marrow, spleen, lymph nodes, gut-associated lymphoid tissue). It begins with antigenic stimulation of the immunocompetent T and B lymphocytes through binding of antigen to specific antigen surface receptors on the cell. This type of lymphopoiesis results in the formation of effector (T and B) lymphocytes. They mediate the immune response through the

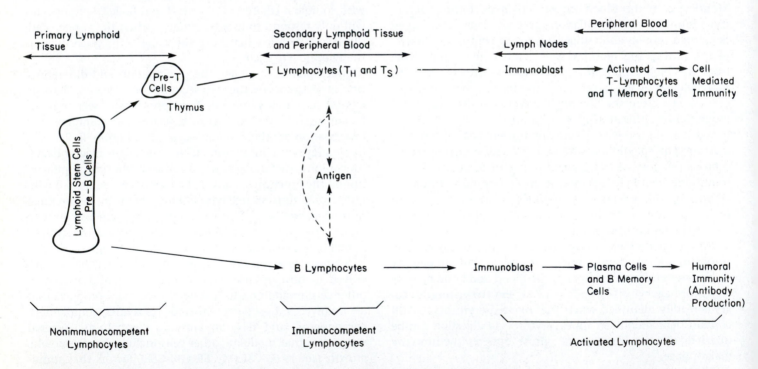

■ **FIGURE 6-13** Lymphocytes originate from the lymphoid stem cell (derived from the pluripotential stem cell) in the bone marrow. Lymphocytes that mature in the thymus become T lymphocytes, and those that mature in the bone marrow become B lymphocytes. Three morphologic stages can be identified in this development to T and B cells: lymphoblast, prolymphocyte, and lymphocyte. Upon encounter with antigen, these immunocompetent T and B lymphocytes undergo blast transformation, usually in the lymph nodes, to form effector lymphocytes. The B lymphocytes eventually emerge as plasma cells. Effector T lymphocytes, however, are morphologically indistinguishable from the original T lymphocytes. The recognizable morphologic stages of blast transformation include activated lymphocytes, immunoblasts, plasmacytoid lymphocytes (B cells), and plasma cells (B cells). Flow cytometry indicates that some morphologic stages may represent several stages of immunologic maturation.

production of lymphokines by T lymphocytes and antibodies by B lymphocytes.

Morphologic criteria cannot be used to differentiate between T and B lymphocyte categories. When there is a need to distinguish between the T and B lymphocytes, monoclonal antibodies and flow cytometry are most often used.

A third population of lymphocytes that develops from the lymphoid progenitor cell but that does not express antigen receptors is called natural killer (NK) cells. They can lyse tumor cells without prior sensitization.

Antigen-Independent Lymphopoiesis

Three stages of bone marrow morphologic maturation are recognized: lymphoblast, prolymphocyte, and lymphocyte.

Lymphoblast.   The lymphoblast (Figure 6-14a ■) is about 10–18 μm in diameter with a high N:C ratio. The nuclear chromatin is lacy and fine, but it appears more smudged or heavy than that of myeloblasts. One or two well-defined pale blue nucleoli are visible. The nuclear membrane is dense, and a perinuclear clear zone can be seen. The agranular cytoplasm is more scanty than in other white cell blasts and stains deep blue. There are more subtle differences, but lymphoblasts are usually morphologically indistinguishable

from myeloblasts. Cytochemical stains can be used to help identify their lymphoid origin (∞ Chapter 26). Unlike myeloblasts, the lymphoblasts have no peroxidase, lipid, or esterase but contain acid phosphatase and sometimes deposits of glycogen. Both T and B lymphoblasts contain a DNA polymerase, terminal deoxynucleotidyl transferase (TdT). It is believed that this enzyme is a specific marker for immature lymphoid cells that are in an intermediate developmental stage between the stem cell and differentiated T and B lymphocytes. CD markers and cytochemical stains may be used to help differentiate T and B cell precursors. Markers for B cell precursors include CD10, CD19, and cytoplasmic CD22. Markers for T cell precursors include CD1, CD2, CD3, CD5, and CD7. Lymphoblasts of T lymphocyte potential contain alpha naphthyl acid esterase, whereas B lymphoblasts may contain small amounts of immunoglobulin or the μ heavy chain immunoglobulin. The immunoglobulin can be detected by using immunofluorescent techniques.

Prolymphocyte.   The prolymphocyte is very difficult to distinguish in normal bone marrow specimens (Figure 6-14b ■). The prolymphocyte is slightly smaller than the lymphoblast with a lower N:C ratio. The nuclear chromatin

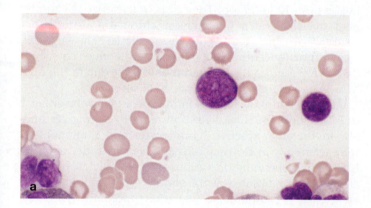
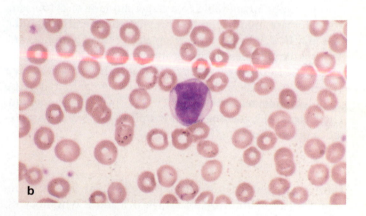
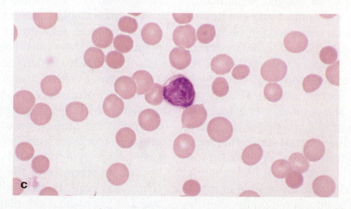

■ **FIGURE 6-14** Stages of antigen-independent lymphocyte maturation. **a.** lymphoblast—note the lacy chromatin and high N:C ratio, **b.** prolymphocyte—note the increased amount of cytoplasm; **c.** lymphocyte—the nuclear chromatin is coarse and smudged. (a, b: Bone marrow, Wright-Giemsa stain, 1000× magnification; c: Peripheral blood, Wright-Giemsa stain, 1000× magnification)

is clumped but more finely dispersed than that of the lymphocyte. Nucleoli are usually present. The cytoplasm is light blue and agranular.

Lymphocyte. The mature lymphocyte has extreme size variability, 7–16 μm, which is primarily dependent on the amount of cytoplasm present (Figure 6-14c ■). Small lymphocytes range in size from 7 to 10 μm. In these cells, the nucleus is about the size of an erythrocyte and occupies about 90% of the cell area. The chromatin is deeply condensed and lumpy, staining a deep, dark purple. Nucleoli, although always present, are only occasionally visible with the light microscope as small, light areas within the nucleus. The nucleus is surrounded by a small amount of sky-blue cytoplasm. A few azurophilic granules and vacuoles may be present. Lymphocytes are motile and may present a peculiar hand-mirror shape on stained blood smears. These cells have the nucleus in the rounded anterior portion trailed by an elongated section of cytoplasm known as the uropod. Small lymphocytes include a diversity of functional subsets including resting, immunocompetent T and B lymphocytes, differentiated T effector, and T and B memory lymphocytes.

Large lymphocytes are heterogeneous and range in size from 11 to 16 μm in diameter. The nucleus may be slightly larger than in the small lymphocyte, but the difference in cell size is mainly attributable to a larger amount of cytoplasm. The cytoplasm may be lighter blue with peripheral basophilia, or it may be darker than the cytoplasm of small lymphocytes. Azurophilic granules may be prominent. These granules differ from those of the myelocytic cells in that they are peroxidase negative. The nuclear chromatin appears similar to that of the small lymphocyte, and the nucleus may be slightly indented. These large cells, like the small lymphocytes, probably represent a diversity of functional subsets.

Antigen-dependent Lymphopoiesis

During development into immunocompetent (ability to respond to stimulation by an antigen) T and B lymphocytes, the cells acquire specific receptors for antigen, which commit them to an antigen specificity. Contact and binding of this specific antigen to receptors on immunocompetent lymphocytes begins a complex sequence of cellular events known as blast transformation (blastogenesis). The end result is a clonal amplification of cells responsible for the overt expression of immunity to the specific antigen. Usually occurring within the lymph node, this series of events includes cell enlargement, an increase in DNA synthesis, enlargement of the nucleolus, an increase in the rough endoplasmic reticulum (RER), and mitosis. These transformed cells, called immunoblasts, apparently have the option of differentiating into memory cells or effector cells that are capable of mediating the immune response. The morphologically identifiable forms of antigen-dependent lymphocytes include the reactive lymphocyte, reactive immunoblast, plasmacytoid lymphocyte, and plasma cell.

Reactive Lymphocyte. One form of antigen stimulated lymphocyte is the **reactive lymphocyte** (Figure 6-15a ■). Although this cell's place in the blast transformation process is not certain, it may be a precursor to the immunoblast. The reactive lymphocyte exhibits a variety of morphologic features. The cell may have one or more of the following features. It may increase in size (16–30 μm) and have a decreased N:C ratio. The nucleus may be round but is more frequently elongated, stretched, or irregular. The chromatin becomes more dispersed, staining lighter than the chromatin of a resting lymphocyte. Nucleoli may be seen when the chromatin pattern is more dispersed. There usually is an increase in diffuse or localized basophilia of the cytoplasm, and azurophilic granules and/or vacuoles may be present. The cytoplasmic membrane may be indented by surrounded erythrocytes, which sometimes gives the cell a scallop shape.

The reactive lymphocyte is also referred to as a stimulated, transformed, atypical, activated, or variant lymphocyte. A few reactive lymphocytes may be seen in the blood of healthy individuals, but they are found in increased concentrations in viral infections. For this reason, the reactive lymphocyte has also been called a virocyte.

Immunoblast. The **immunoblast** (Figure 6-15b ■) is the next stage in blast transformation. The cell is large, ranging in size from 12 to 25 μm. The cell is characterized by prominent nucleoli and a fine nuclear chromatin pattern (but coarser than that of other leukocyte blasts). The large nucleus is usually central and stains a purple blue. The abundant cytoplasm stains an intense blue color due to the high density of polyribosomes.

Reactive lymphocytes and immunoblasts may be either T or B lymphocytes. Final definition requires cell marker studies. In the past, reactive lymphocytes and immunoblasts were referred to as Downey cells and were classified as Types I, II, or III, depending on various morphologic criteria. This classification is obsolete as the various types of Downey cells are actually morphologic variations accompanying the process of blast transformation.

The immunoblast proliferates, increasing the pool of cells programmed to respond to the initial antigen. These programmed daughter cells (effector lymphocytes) mature into cells that mediate the effector arm of the immune response. The daughter cells of the B immunoblasts, which mediate **humoral immunity,** are plasmacytoid lymphocytes (Figure 6-15c ■) and plasma cells (Figure 6-15d ■). Humoral immunity is the production of antibodies by activated B-lymphocytes that were stimulated by antigen. The plasmacytoid lymphocyte (lymphocytoid plasma cell) is believed to be an immediate precursor of the plasma cell. It gains its descriptive name from its morphologic similarity to the lymphocyte but has marked cytoplasmic basophila similar to that of plasma cells.

The **plasma cell** has an eccentric nucleus with clumped chromatin, abundant deeply basophilic cytoplasm, and a

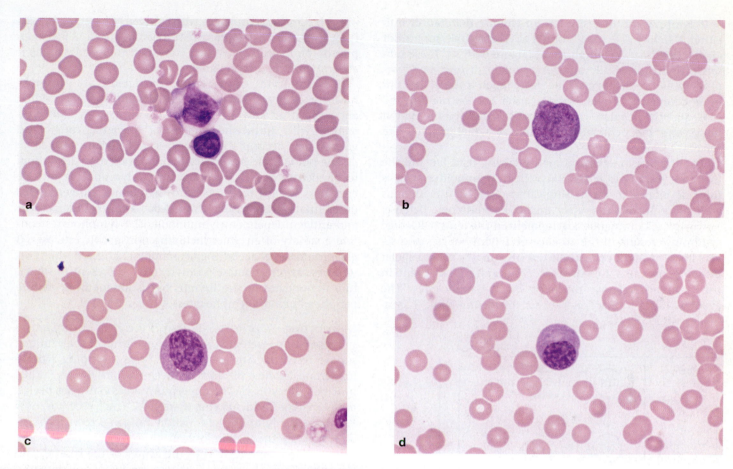

■ **FIGURE 6-15** Stages of antigen-dependent lymphocyte maturation. **a.** reactive lymphocyte—the cell is large with an increased amount of basophilic cytoplasm. Note the normal lymphocyte below the reactive lymphocyte; **b.** immunoblast—the N:C ratio is high. The nucleus has a lacy chromatin pattern and nucleoli are visible. The cytoplasm is deep blue; **c.** Plasmacytoid lymphocyte—the nuclear chromatin is coarse; there is a moderate amount of blue cytoplasm; **d.** plasma cell—the fully differentiated B cell. The nucleus is eccentric and there is a large amount of basophilic cytoplasm. (Peripheral blood, Wright-Giemsa stain, 1000× magnification)

prominent paranuclear unstained area (Golgi complex). Plasmacytoid lymphs and plasma cells will be discussed in more detail in the section on B lymphocytes.

In contrast to the progeny of the B immunoblast, the daughter cells produced from the T immunoblast, T effector lymphocytes, are morphologically indistinguishable from the original unsensitized lymphocytes. A number of the T and B immunoblast daughter cells alternatively form T and B memory cells. Memory cells are morphologically similar to the resting lymphocytes. They retain the memory of the stimulating antigen and are capable of eliciting a secondary immune response when challenged again by the same antigen.

The reactive lymphocyte is commonly found in the blood during viral infection; the immunoblast, plasmacytoid lymphocyte, and plasma cell are usually only found in lymph nodes and other secondary lymphoid tissue. During intense stimulation of the immune system, however, these transformed cells may be found in the peripheral blood due to recirculation.

✔ **Checkpoint! #7**

How would you morphologically differentiate a reactive lymphocyte from a plasma cell on a peripheral blood smear?

T Lymphocytes

Some of the bone marrow lymphoid precursor cells migrate to the thymus (primary lymphoid organ) where they proliferate and differentiate to acquire cellular characteristics of T lymphocytes. Lymphopoiesis, at this stage, is independent of antigen stimulation.

T Lymphocyte Development. It is believed that the hormone thymosin, synthesized and secreted by epithelial cells in the thymus, has an influence on T lymphocyte maturation. Intrathymic death for potential T lymphocytes is high, about 95%; consequently, only a small portion leave the thymus as immunocompetent T lymphocytes.

T lymphocytes diversify late in thymic maturation into either T helper (T_H, $CD4^+$, or T_4) or T cytotoxic/suppressor (T_C/T_S, $CD8^+$, or T_8) lymphocytes (Figure 6-16 ■). These subsets are phenotypically and functionally distinct but morphologically indistinguishable from each other. The immunocompetent T lymphocytes enter the circulation and subsequently populate the paracortical areas of the lymph nodes and the periarteriolar region of white pulp in the spleen.

The thymus functions primarily during fetal life and the first few years after birth; thus, the T lymphoid system is fully developed at birth. Surgical removal of the thymus after birth does not severely impair immunologic defense; however, lack of thymus development in the fetus (DiGeorge syndrome) results in the absence of T lymphocytes and severe impairment of **cell mediated immunity** or the cellular immune response. Cell-mediated immunity is an event in the immune response mediated by T lymphocytes. The event requires interaction between histocompatible T lymphocytes and macrophages with antigen. There are at least three important T lymphocyte subsets involved: helper, suppressor, and cytotoxic. When activated, these cells proliferate and produce lymphokines.

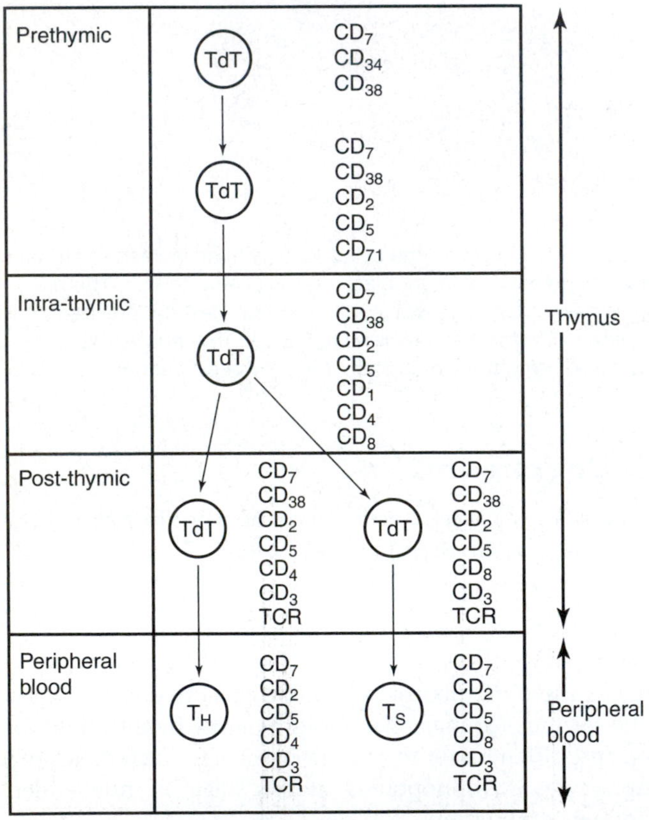

■ FIGURE 6-16 Immunologic maturation of the T lymphocyte from the committed lymphocyte progenitor cell to the peripheral blood T helper and T suppressor lymphocytes. Monoclonal antibodies have identified at least three intrathymic stages of maturation before the cells are released to the peripheral blood as mature T lymphocytes. Differentiation into either helper or suppressor lymphocytes occurs at the last intrathymic stage of maturation. (CD = cluster of differentiation; TCR = T cell receptor)

T lymphocytes confer protection against antigens that have the ability to avoid contact with antibody by residing and replicating within the cells of the host; thus, serious infection with intracellular parasites (bacteria, fungi, and viruses) may occur if T lymphocytes are deficient.

The phenotypic features of lymphocytes that allow them to be identified as T lymphocyte or B lymphocyte include enzymes, surface receptors, and membrane antigens. This differentiation is possible throughout antigen independent and antigen dependent lymphopoiesis. T lymphocytes contain a variety of enzymes including nonspecific esterases, β glucuronidase, N acetyl β glucosamidase, and a dotlike pattern of acid phosphatase positivity. TdT is present in immature thymocytes in the thymus but is absent from mature peripheral blood T lymphocytes.

Membrane Markers—T Lymphocyte. Lymphocyte subpopulations were first identified by virtue of their unique surface receptors. Surface receptors have a binding affinity for certain ligands. Binding of sheep red blood cells (SRBC) by T lymphocytes via the E receptor traditionally has been a useful marker for identifying these cells. The E receptor, now known as the lymphocyte function antigen-3 receptor (LFA-3) (CD2) on the T lymphocyte binds SRBC and forms a rosette. The lymphocyte is in the center of the rosette, and the SRBCs form the petals. The receptor is present primarily on mature thymocytes and peripheral blood T lymphocytes. T lymphocytes also possess receptors for the Fc portion of IgM and IgG (CD16). T lymphocytes can change the specificity of their Fc receptor upon antigenic stimulation.

It is possible to define distinct stages of intrathymic differentiation of T lymphocytes using monoclonal probes to identify the presence of CD antigens on the cell surface. Some antigenic determinants appear in a very early developmental stage of the cell and disappear with maturity; other unique determinants appear on more mature cells. Using these probes, it was found that developing T lymphocytes may be divided into three discrete intrathymic stages: prethymic, intrathymic, and postthymic (Figure 6-16 ■).

As the T lymphocyte matures it loses some CD antigens and expresses new ones (Figure 6-16 ■).[27] Although early thymocytes have markers of both helper and suppressor cells, later stages of maturation express one or the other. The CD4 lymphocytes are helper lymphocytes, while those with CD8 are suppressor lymphocytes. CD4 and CD8 are members of the immunoglobulin supergene family of adhesion molecules. Mature peripheral T lymphocytes lose CD38, but this antigen can be reexpressed when the cell is activated.[28] The CD25 antigen is associated with the IL-2 receptor and is present on activated T lymphocytes.

About 60–80% of peripheral blood T lymphocytes are CD4 cells (T_4). They are also the predominant T lymphocytes of the lymph nodes. CD8 cells (T$_8$) make up only 35% of peripheral blood T lymphocytes but are the predominant T lymphocyte found in the bone marrow. The normal T$_4$:T$_8$ ratio in circulating blood is 2:1. The balance between T$_4$ and T$_8$ must be maintained for normal activity of the immune system. This ratio may be depressed in viral infections, immune deficiency states, and acquired immune deficiency syndrome (AIDS). The ratio may be increased in other disorders, such as acute graft versus host disease, scleroderma, and multiple sclerosis.

T Lymphocyte Antigen Receptor. The T lymphocyte has an antigen receptor on its surface that is responsible for initiating the cellular immune response. The receptor, T cell receptor (TCR), is a heterodimer of two peptide chains linked by a disulfide bond near the membrane (Figure 6-17 ■). This receptor is a member of the immunoglobulin supergene family of adhesion molecules. There are two lineages of T cells defined by their utilization of distinct T cell receptor genes and by the nature of the heterodimer chains, TCR gamma and delta chains (TCR γ/δ) and TCR-alpha and beta chains (TCR α/β). Greater than 90% of T lymphocytes express the TCR α/β.[29,30] The organization of the TCR chains is similar to that of the immunoglobulin chains. Each TCR chain is composed of a variable region that binds antigen and a constant region that anchors the TCR to the cell membrane. The variable (V) gene is made from three DNA segments, variable (V), diversity (D), and joining (J), in the beta and delta genes but only two segments, V and J, in the alpha and gamma genes. A complete V gene is translocated to a constant (C) gene to form the TCR chains. Before synthesis, there is a rearrangement of the gene coding for this receptor. Rearrangement and recombination of the V, D, and J segments and subsequent joining with a C gene provide a diversity of TCR chains. This diversity allows the T lymphocyte to recognize many different antigens.

The TCR is expressed in a molecular complex with three other polypeptide chains on the cell membrane. The three chains are not covalently linked, but each chain is a transmembrane peptide. These three chains comprise the CD3 subunit. It is believed that the CD3 complex mediates extracellular to intracellular signal transduction when antigen in the context of major histocompatibility complex (MHC) molecules bind to the TCR. Since antigenic stimulation of T lymphocytes is MHC restricted, T lymphocytes will only respond to foreign antigens that are displayed on antigen presenting cells (APCs) that have the same MHC phenotype. The different subsets of T lymphocytes recognize different classes of MHC molecules. CD8$^+$ lymphocytes recognize Class I MHC molecules whereas CD4$^+$ lymphocytes recognize Class II MHC molecules.

B Lymphocytes

Potential B lymphocytes, produced from the committed lymphoid stem cell, mature in the bone marrow. As described previously, this maturation is independent of anti-

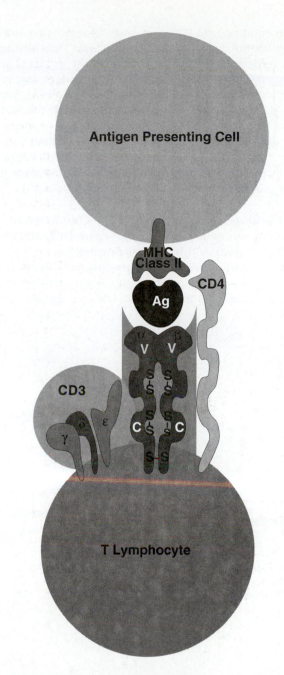

■ **FIGURE 6-17** The T lymphocyte has an antigen receptor (TCR) on its surface that is composed of two peptide chains linked by a disulfide bond. This receptor is expressed in a complex with CD3. This TCR is probably in close proximity to an MHC restricted receptor (CD4 or CD8) that recognizes the appropriate molecule on antigen presenting cells (APCs). The helper T lymphocyte receptor (CD4), shown here, recognizes Class II MHC molecules while the suppressor T lymphocytes receptor (CD8) recognizes Class I MHC molecules.

gen stimulation. The immunocompetent, mature B lymphocytes then enter the blood and migrate to the germinal centers (follicles) and medullary cords of lymph nodes, to the germinal centers of the spleen, and to other secondary lymphoid tissue. Antigenic stimulation causes the B lymphocytes to undergo proliferation and differentiation into immunoglobulin (antibody) secreting plasma cells in the germinal centers of the secondary lymphoid tissues. The immunoglobulin recognizes and binds to foreign antigen. B lymphocytes compose 15–30% of peripheral blood lymphocytes. B lymphocytes possess certain phenotypic features, distinct from those of T lymphocytes, that allow these cells to be identified. The enzyme TdT may be found on very young B cells but is not present on subsequent stages. The esterase and acid phosphatase stains are either negative or appear positive in a scattered granular pattern.

B Lymphocyte Development.

A uniform terminology for naming stages of B cells has not been designated. In the terminology used in this book, the earliest committed B cell precursor is the pro-B cell (Figure 6-18 ■).[31] Its immediate progeny is the pre-B lymphocyte, which synthesizes the heavy chain of IgM, the μ chain. At this stage, the μ chain

remains in the cytoplasm and is not combined with the light chain of IgM to form a complete immunoglobulin molecule. The next stage of development, the immature lymphocyte, is characterized by the disappearance of the cytoplasmic μ heavy chains, and the subsequent appearance of the surface membrane IgM that contains the normal immunoglobulin structure of two light and two heavy chains. This IgM is different from the IgM secreted and found in the blood in that it has several additional amino acids on its heavy chains that serve as an anchor to the membrane. Membrane IgD can be identified after the appearance of IgM on mature B cells. B lymphocytes are not capable of reacting with antigen until they develop both IgM and IgD on their surface. A dramatic decrease in membrane IgD is noted after cell stimulation. Two more immunoglobulin classes, IgG and IgA, may develop on the cell surface later in ontogeny. Most mature B lymphocytes possess only one class of immunoglobulin on their membrane, although a small percentage may express

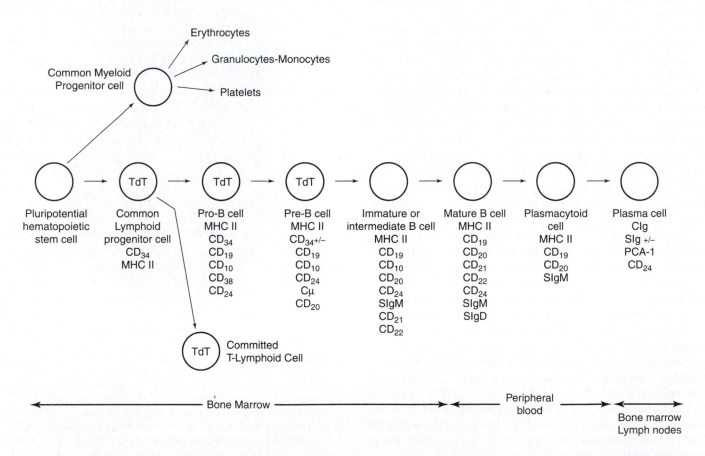

■ **FIGURE 6-18** Immunologic maturation of the B lymphocyte from the pluripotential hematopoietic stem cell to the plasma cell. Each stage of maturation can be defined by specific antigens (CD) that appear sequentially on the developing cell. Stem cells, pro-B lymphocyte, pre-B lymphocytes, and intermediate B lymphocytes are normally found in the bone marrow. The mature B lymphocyte is found in the peripheral blood. When stimulated by antigen, the B lymphocytes undergo maturation to plasma cells in the lymph nodes or bone marrow. (C μ = cytoplasmic μ chains; Sig = surface membrane immunoglobulin; Cig = cytoplasmic immunoglobulin; MHC II = Class II HLA antigens; CD = cluster of differentiation.)

IgG and IgA together with IgM and IgD. Surface-bound immunoglobulin serves as a receptor for a particular antigen.

When stimulated by antigen, mature B lymphocytes undergo proliferation and transformation into plasma cells. This phase is the antigen-dependent phase of lymphopoiesis for B lymphocytes. Plasma cells are the fully activated form of B lymphocyte maturation. Their primary function is formation and secretion of immunoglobulin that recognizes a particular antigen. Each plasma cell is committed to secreting large amounts of specific, single class immunoglobulin. Each plasma cell produces only one of the five classes of immunoglobulin. Plasma cells are rich in cytoplasmic immunoglobulin but contain little or no surface immunoglobulin.

Membrane markers. In addition to immunoglobulin, other membrane markers are present at various stages in B lymphocyte development. Some surface antigens appear on the B lymphocyte before immunoglobulin can be detected. Identification of B lymphocytes is now done using flow cytometry and a panel of antibodies to surface antigens. Monoclonal antibodies have defined specific B lymphocyte antigens that correspond to the stage of differentiation of the cell (Figure 6-18 ■).

CD markers expressed by pro-B lymphocytes include CD34, CD10, CD19, CD24, and CD38. CD34 is a hematopoietic stem cell antigen and may be present on a variety of stem cells already committed to a particular lineage. The CD19 antigen is the earliest B lymphocyte specific antigen and is retained until the latest stages of activation. Thus, it defines most cells of B lymphocyte lineage. This is followed by the appearance of CD10. The CD10 antigen, common acute lymphoblastic leukemia antigen (CALLA), was originally believed to be a specific marker of leukemia cells in acute lymphoblastic leukemia. It is now known that CALLA is present on a small percentage (less than 3%) of normal bone marrow cells. The CALLA antigen is found only on early B lymphocytes; the antigen disappears with cell maturity. CD24 is expressed at low levels from the late pro-B lymphocyte stage until plasma cell differentiation. Heavy chains of IgM can be found in the cytoplasm of pre-B lymphocytes. Pre-B lymphocytes express the CD10, CD19, CD20, and CD24 markers and lose the CD34 and CD38 markers.

Surface membrane IgM (SIgM) marks the next stage of the immature B lymphocyte. Surface membrane bound IgD appears at the mature stage. The CD 20 marker is lost upon differentiation into plasma cells. CD21 is the receptor for the Epstein-Barr virus, which remains with the cell to the mature lymphocyte stage. CD22 is first detected in the cytoplasm of pre-B cells and later is expressed on the surface of a subset of B cells. Fc receptors capable of binding the Fc component of IgG, IgM, IgA, and IgE, are also present on B lymphocyte membranes. Additional B lymphocyte antigens are continually being identified; therefore, the antigenic description here should not be considered complete and final.[31,32]

B lymphocytes may be identified in vitro by virtue of complement receptors and surface membrane immunoglob-ulin as well as CD antigens/markers. Mice erythrocytes form rosettes with B lymphocytes, as do sheep erythrocytes that are coated with antibody and complement (EAC). EAC attaches to B lymphocytes by means of the B lymphocyte complement receptors. Another technique for B lymphocyte identification involves demonstration of surface membrane immunoglobulin by fluorescein conjugated antisera to the different classes of immunoglobulins.

Plasma cell development. Stimulated B lymphocytes, cells that have encountered antigen to which they have been programmed to respond, undergo transformation from reactive lymphocytes to immunoblasts, to plasmacytoid lymphocytes, and finally to plasma cells in the lymph nodes. Plasma cells, the progeny of B immunoblasts, represent the fully activated mature B lymphocyte.

The intermediate stage in this transformation, the plasmacytoid lymphocyte (also called lymphocytoid plasma cell, intermediate form, Turk cell) may be identified. The plasmacytoid lymphocyte ranges in size from 15 to 20 μm. The nuclear chromatin is less clumped (more immature) than that of a plasma cell, and there may be a single visible nucleolus. The nucleus is central or slightly eccentric, and the cytoplasm is deeply basophilic. The cell has some cytoplasmic immunoglobulin as well as surface membrane immunoglobulin. This cell is occasionally seen in the peripheral blood of patients with viral infection.

Plasma cells are round or slightly oval with a diameter from 9 to 20 μm. The nucleus is off to one side (eccentrically placed) and contains blocklike radial masses of chromatin, often referred to as the cartwheel or spoke wheel arrangement. Nucleoli are not present. The paranuclear Golgi complex is obvious and surrounded by deeply basophilic cytoplasm. The cytoplasm stains red with pyronine (pyroninophilic) because of the high RNA content. The rough endoplasmic reticulum (RER) is well developed, and the cytoplasm expands because of production of large amounts of immunoglobulin. With an increase in cytoplasmic immunoglobulin, the secretory capacity of the cell is increased. Surface membrane immunoglobulin is usually absent. Azurophilic granules may be present as well as rodlike crystal inclusions. The plasma cell has lost the CD19 and CD20 antigens, but the PCA-1 antigen, the most limited membrane antigen, is present on the terminally differentiated B lymphocytes, the plasma cells.

Plasma cells are not normally present in the peripheral blood or lymph and constitute less than 4% of the cells in the bone marrow. Most plasma cells are found in the medullary cores of lymph nodes, although intense stimulation of the immune system may cause them to be found in the peripheral blood. Plasma cells may be noted in the blood in rubeola, infectious mononucleosis, toxoplasmosis, syphilis, tuberculosis, and multiple myeloma.

Morphologic variations of plasma cells include *flame cells* and *Mott cells* (Figure 6-19 ■). **Flame cells** are named for their reddish purple cytoplasm. The red tinge is caused by a glycoprotein produced in the RER, and the purple tinge is caused by the

SECTION THREE • HEMATOLOGY PROCEDURES

7

Routine Hematology Procedures

Cheryl Burns, M.S.

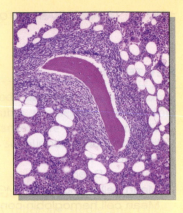

■ CHECKLIST - LEVEL I

At the end of this unit of study the student should be able to:

1. Identify the three anticoagulants used in the hematology laboratory and give examples of laboratory tests that should be performed on blood anticoagulated with each.

2. Explain the mechanism of preventing coagulation for each anticoagulant.

3. Identify equipment and supplies required for phlebotomy.

4. Describe OSHA standards related to phlebotomy.

5. List factors affecting the collection of a blood specimen.

6. Correlate the collection technique of a blood specimen with potential problems in specimen analysis.

7. Describe proper disposal of contaminated equipment and supplies.

8. Identify the component parts of a microscope and explain their functions.

9. Discuss the microscope's preventative maintenance procedures.

10. For each test discussed in this chapter:
    a. state the principle.
    b. describe the procedure.
    c. explain potential sources of error.

11. Calculate the erythrocyte indices.

12. Correlate erythrocyte indices with CBC data and peripheral blood smear examination.

13. Calculate the reticulocyte count.

14. Identify reference ranges for each test in terms of gender and age.

■ CHECKLIST - LEVEL II

At the end of this unit of study, the student should be able to:

1. Describe factors that influence brightfield microscopy.

2. Explain the principle of phase contrast microscopy.

3. Interpret test results and correlate abnormal values with clinical conditions.

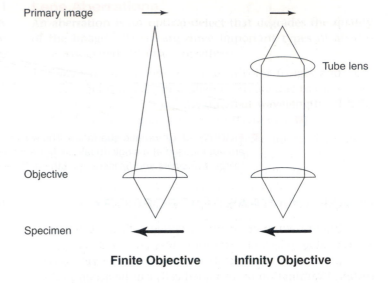

■ FIGURE 7-5 Finite objective *vs* infinity objective. In the finite objective, light rays projected from the objective converge to form the primary image within the optical tube. For the infinity objective, light is projected as parallel rays from the objective. These rays converge to form the primary image only after they pass through the tube lens. The infinity space as defined by the distance between the objective and the tube lens can vary from 160 mm to 200 mm.

 Checkpoint! #4

How does the examination of a specimen by phase-contrast microscopy differ from bright-field microscopy?

▶ CELL ENUMERATION BY HEMACYTOMETER

Cell counts are performed manually by diluting blood with a diluent, loading a small amount of the diluted specimen on a ruled device (hemacytometer), and counting the cells microscopically. The hemacytometer consists of two side-by-side identically ruled glass platforms mounted in a glass holder. Each platform contains a ruled square measuring 3×3 mm (9 mm^2), and is subdivided according to the improved Neubauer ruling (Figure 7-7 ■). This ruling subdivides the ruled square into 9 large squares, each measuring 1×1 mm (1 mm^2). The four corner squares labeled W are used for leukocyte counts; each corner square is further divided into 16 smaller squares. The center large square (1 mm^2) is used for platelet and erythrocyte counts. This square is divided into 25 smaller squares, each with an area of 0.04 mm^2. Each of the 25 squares is further divided into 16 smaller squares. The five squares labeled R are used in performing the erythrocyte count, whereas the entire center square is used in performing the platelet count.

■ FIGURE 7-6 Phase contrast light pathway. The annular ring within the condenser diaphragm creates a hollow cone of light that illuminates the specimen. Transmitted light is shifted one-quarter wavelength by the phase shifting element in the objective. This creates maximum contrast between a cell and its surroundings. (Reprinted, with permission, from Molecular Expressions' World Wide Web pages.)

On either side of the two ruled glass platforms, there is a raised ridge. The coverglass is placed on top of the ridge. The distance between the coverglass and the surface of the ruled area (depth) is exactly 0.1 mm. Thus the ruled area on each side of the hemacytometer holds a volume of 0.9 mm^3 ($3 \times 3 \times 0.1$).

The unopette system is a fast and accurate method for collecting and diluting blood for cell counts. For each laboratory determination performed, the unopette consists of the following elements: the reservoir, the pipet, and the pipet shield (Figure 7-8 ■). The reservoir contains a premeasured volume of diluting fluid that is specific for the cell count to be performed.

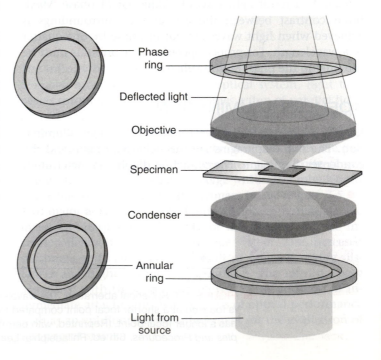

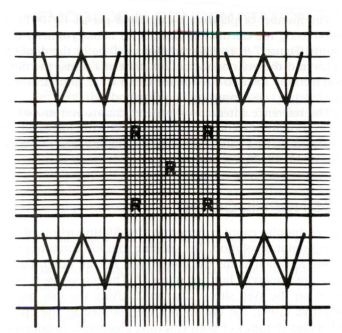

■ FIGURE 7-7 Neubauer hemacytometer counting area. W indicates the squares used for leukocyte counts, while R indicates the squares used for erythrocyte counts. The entire center square is used for platelet counts. (Reprinted, with permission, from Brown, BA. *Hematology: Principles and Procedures.* 6th ed. Philadelphia: Lea & Febiger, 1993.)

MANUAL LEUKOCYTE COUNT

Whole blood is diluted with a 3% acetic acid solution, which hemolyzes mature erythrocytes and facilitates leukocyte (white blood cell, WBC) counting.[14] The standard dilution for leukocyte counts is 1:20. The detailed procedure for the manual leukocyte count is provided on the Web site ∞ Chapter 7. With proper light adjustment, the leukocytes should appear as dark dots. The number of leukocytes in the four

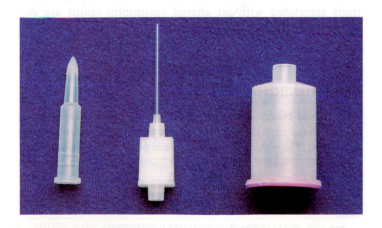

■ FIGURE 7-8 Unopette system (from left to right): pipet shield, pipet, and reservoir.

Total number of cells counted • dilution factor • 1/volume factor = cells/mm³

Example:	Total number of cells (one side of hemacytometer)	200 cells
	Dilution	1:20
	Area counted	4 mm²
	Depth	0.1 mm
	Volume factor (area × depth)	0.4 mm³

$200 \cdot 20 \cdot 1/0.4 \text{ mm}^3 = 10{,}000/\text{mm}^3 \text{ (}\mu\text{L) or } 10.0 \times 10^9/\text{L}$

■ FIGURE 7-9 Calculation formula for hemacytometer cell counts.

corner squares are counted using the 10× objective. Potential sources of error in performing hemacytometer cell counts are provided in Web Table 7-4 ✪.

The number of leukocytes are calculated per μL (×10⁹/L) of blood. To make this determination, the total number of cells counted must be corrected for the initial dilution of blood and the volume of blood used for counting (Figure 7-9 ■). The typical dilution of blood for leukocyte counts is 1:20; therefore, the dilution factor is 20. The volume of blood used is based on the area and depth of the counting area. The area counted is 4 mm² and the depth is 0.1 mm; therefore, the volume factor (area × depth) is 0.4 mm³. Thus, the number of leukocytes counted in 4 mm² is multiplied by 50 (20/0.4) and reported as number of leukocytes per 10⁹/L.

Reference intervals for leukocyte counts in adult males and females can be found in Table B ✪ on the inside cover. The reference intervals will vary in children as shown in Table B ✪ in the appendix. Conditions commonly associated with increased or decreased leukocyte counts are shown in Table 7-2 ✪ (∞ Chapters 6, 21, 22, 27, 29, 30, 31).

MANUAL ERYTHROCYTE COUNT

Whole blood is diluted with a 0.85% saline solution which prevents erythrocyte (red blood cell) lysis and facilitates erythrocyte counting.[15] The standard dilution for erythrocyte counts is 1:200. This procedure is provided on the Web site ∞ Chapter 7. For the manual erythrocyte count, erythrocytes are counted in five of the smaller squares within the large center square (R, Figure 7-7 ■) using the high dry objective (40 ×). Potential sources of error are listed in Web Table 7-4 ✪.

The number of erythrocytes is calculated per μL (×10¹²/L) of blood using the calculation formula for hemacytometer cell counts (Figure 7-9 ■). The variations will be in the dilution factor and the volume factor. For erythrocyte counts, the dilution factor is 200, and the volume factor is 0.04 mm³ (area = 0.4 mm²; depth = 0.1 mm).

The reference intervals for erythrocyte counts in adult males and adult females can be found in Table A ✪ on the inside cover. The reference intervals will vary with age as

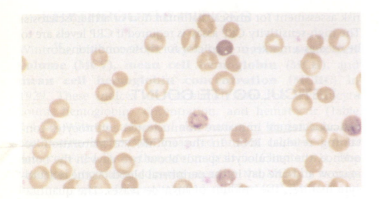

■ **FIGURE 7-12** Reticulocytes identified by new methylene blue stain. The reticulocytes are the cells containing bluish purple particulate inclusions. (1000× original magnification)

erythrocyte. Howell-Jolly bodies are usually one or two round, deep-purple staining inclusions and are also visible on Romanowsky stains. Pappenheimer bodies are indistiguishable from reticulum of reticulocytes. If Pappenheimer bodies are suspected, a Prussian-blue iron stain (∞ Chapter 9) should be performed to verify their presence. Reticulum will not stain with the Prussian-blue iron stain.

Misinterpretations may result when reporting only the percentage of reticulocytes present in the peripheral blood, because the reticulocyte result is dependent on the total number of erythrocytes present in the peripheral blood. If the total erythrocyte count is decreased, the reticulocyte percentage does not accurately reflect the bone marrow's production of new erythrocytes. The corrected reticulocyte count and the reticulocyte production index may be used to avoid interpretation errors due to the total erythrocyte count and increased bone marrow stimulation. These calculations are discussed in ∞ Chapter 10.

Automation is becoming a more popular method for the determination of the reticulocyte count. The new generation of automated hematology instruments is capable of performing absolute reticulocyte counts and other useful parameters. A thorough discussion can be found in ∞ Chapter 41.

 Checkpoint! #8

Morphologic evaluation of a Wright-stained peripheral blood smear reveals the presence of Pappenheimer bodies. How will this affect a reticulocyte count to be performed on the same blood sample? How would you confirm the presence of Pappenheimer bodies?

SOLUBILITY TEST FOR HEMOGLOBIN S

The solubility test is the most commonly used screening test for the presence of hemoglobin S (∞ Chapters 5, 12). It is based on the relative insolubility of hemoglobin S when combined with a reducing agent (sodium dithionite).[32] When anticoagulated whole blood is mixed with the reducing agent, erythrocytes will lyse due to the presence of saponin, and hemoglobin will be released (see Web site ∞ Chapter 7 for the detailed procedure). If hemoglobin S is present, it will form liquid crystals and give a turbid appearance to the solution (Figure 7–13 ■). A transparent solution is seen with other hemoglobins that are more soluble in the reducing agent.

The solubility test does not differentiate hemoglobin S disease from hemoglobin S trait. A hemoglobin electrophoresis procedure should be performed to differentiate these two states (∞ Chapter 40). In addition, there are several abnormal hemoglobin variants that cause sickling and will give a positive solubility test. These variants include HbC Harlem, HbS Travis, and HbC Ziguinchor. The **isoelectric focusing** procedure is used in the differentiation of these variants from HbS.

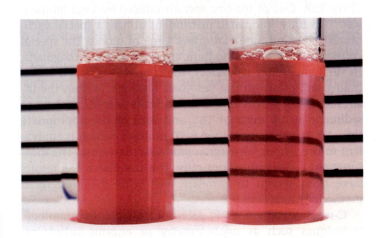

■ **FIGURE 7-13** Sodium dithionite tube test. Negative results are indicated by the clear solution, where the black lines on the reader scale are visible through the test solution. Positive results are shown as a turbid solution, where the reader scale is not visible through the test solution.

SUMMARY

This chapter reviewed the procedures that are performed daily within the hematology laboratory. The accuracy and reliability of the results will depend on the clinical laboratory personnel's knowledge of the test procedure and its application, as well as the possible problems that may arise in the performance of the test. Although all but one of these procedures are typically performed by automated instrumentation, the basic principles, applications, and potential sources of error will hold true for the automated adaptation of each procedure. The results obtained from these procedures are utilized in the diagnosis, prognosis, and therapeutic monitoring of a variety of disorders. For detailed procedures for each of these tests, the reader is referred to the Web site.

REVIEW QUESTIONS

LEVEL I

1. Which anticoagulant prevents coagulation by chelating calcium? (Checklist #2)
   a. lithium heparin
   b. sodium citrate
   c. EDTA
   d. sodium fluoride

2. What is the appropriate sequence to fill specimen collection tubes? (Checklist #6)
   a. red top, lavender top, blue top, green top
   b. lavender top, blue top, red top, green top
   c. blue top, red top, lavender top, green top
   d. red top, blue top, green top, lavender top

3. The 1999 OSHA directive on occupational exposure to blood-borne pathogens requires laboratory facilities to: (Checklist #4)
   a. supply phlebotomists with gloves
   b. implement the use of safe needle systems
   c. mandate vaccination for HBV
   d. provide training in proper handwashing technique

4. What is the function of a microscope's condenser? (Checklist #8)
   a. magnify the light beam prior to the specimen
   b. collect the diffracted light from the specimen
   c. direct the light beam onto the specimen
   d. project diffracted light to the objective

5. An apochromat lens will correct: (Checklist #8)
   a. chromatic aberrations at two colors and field curvature
   b. spherical aberrations at one color and chromatic aberrations at two colors
   c. chromatic aberrations at three colors and spherical aberrations at two colors
   d. spherical aberrations at three colors and field curvature

6. A manual leukocyte count was performed on an EDTA-anticoagulated specimen. The specimen was diluted 1:20, and a total of 165 leukocytes were counted in the four corner squares of the hemacytometer. What is the leukocyte count? (Checklist #10)
   a. 1.3×10^9/L
   b. 3.3×10^9/L
   c. 4.1×10^9/L
   d. 8.3×10^9L

7. Any turbidity in a peripheral blood specimen will result in a falsely elevated hemoglobin determination. Which of the following is NOT a potential source of turbidity? (Checklist #10)
   a. lipemia
   b. increased leukocyte count (60×10^9/L)
   c. increased levels of carboxyhemoglobin
   d. presence of hemoglobin S

LEVEL I (continued)

8. The following erythrocyte data were obtained from an EDTA-anticoagulated specimen: erythrocyte count = 2.84×10^{12}/L, hemoglobin = 7.2 g/dL, hematocrit = 26% (.26 L/L). Calculate the MCV. (Checklist #11)
   a. 25.3 fL
   b. 27.7 fL
   c. 65.9 fL
   d. 91.5 fL

9. Which of the following is NOT a condition associated with an elevated ESR? (Checklist #10)
   a. rheumatoid arthritis
   b. polycythemia vera
   c. multiple myeloma
   d. chronic infection

10. A reticulocyte count was performed using a Miller disk, and 65 reticulocytes (square A) were observed in 350 erythrocytes (square B). What is the reticulocyte count? (Checklist #13)
    a. 1.9%
    b. 2.1%
    c. 3.4%
    d. 6.5%

11. Which of the following will be observed if a purple-top collection tube is underfilled? (Checklist #6)
    a. falsely elevated erythrocyte count
    b. falsely decreased microhematocrit
    c. falsely elevated platelet count
    d. falsely decreased hemoglobin

12. Why is it important to perform the venipuncture within one minute after applying the tourniquet? (Checklist #6)
    a. Falsely elevated hemoglobin will occur if tourniquet is on for more than one minute.
    b. Excess tissue fluids will dilute the sample when the tourniquet is left on for extended periods.
    c. Falsely increased platelet count will occur due to platelet activation associated with prolonged tourniquet application.
    d. Although blood flow is decreased to the venipuncture site, the blood sample will be unaffected.

13. In performing a reticulocyte count, the clinical laboratory professional observes suspicious light bluish-green bodies at the periphery of some erythrocytes. What is the appropriate course of action? (Checklist #10)
    a. These bodies are aggregated reticulum, and erythrocytes containing them should be tabulated as reticulocytes.
    b. These bodies are iron-containing bodies and should be confirmed using the Prussian-blue stain.
    c. These bodies are aggregated DNA, and erythrocytes containing them should not be tabulated as reticulocytes.
    d. These bodies are denatured hemoglobin, and erythrocytes containing them should not be tabulated as reticulocytes.

REVIEW QUESTIONS *(continued)*

LEVEL I

14. The laboratory is experiencing problems with the air conditioning system and it is unusually warm. What effect will this temperature change have on the ESRs performed during this time period? (Checklist #10)
    a. ESRs will be falsely elevated since higher temperature will promote sedimentation.
    b. ESRs will be falsely decreased since erythrocytes will have a higher zeta potential.
    c. ESRs will be unaffected since erythrocyte sedimentation is not temperature-dependent.
    d. ESRs will be falsely elevated since erythrocytes will become swollen.

15. The following erythrocyte data were obtained from an EDTA-anticoagulated specimen: erythrocyte count = 2.63×10^{12}/L, hemoglobin = 9.7 g/dL, hematocrit = 30% (.30 L/L). What would you expect to observe on a Wright-stained peripheral blood smear? (Checklist #12)
    a. normochromic, normocytic erythrocytes
    b. hypochromic, microcytic erythrocytes
    c. normochromic, macrocytic erythrocytes
    d. hypochromic, normocytic erythrocytes

LEVEL II

1. In performing a manual platelet count using phase contrast microscopy, identification of the platelets is very difficult. What should be done to improve the identification of the platelets? (Checklist #2)
   a. lower the condenser to increase the depth of field
   b. align the annulus with the phase shifting element
   c. perform Koehler illumination with the 100× objective
   d. decrease the brightness dial to increase resolution

2. As the clinical laboratory professional removed the hemacytometer from the microscope stage, it was observed that the diluted sample had begun to evaporate from the edges. What effect would this have on the hemacytometer cell count? (Checklist #10)
   a. result would be unaffected
   b. result would be falsely decreased
   c. result would be falsely increased
   d. result would be equivocal

3. A clinical laboratory professional noticed a patient's blood specimen was lipemic. Which of the following parameters would be affected? (Checklist #3)
   a. MCV
   b. MCH
   c. RDW
   d. Hct

4. A manual platelet count was performed using the unopette system. A total of 526 platelets were counted on one side of the hemacytometer. Which of the following conditions is associated with this result? (Checklist #3)
   a. immune thrombocytopenic purpura
   b. megaloblastic anemia
   c. acute leukemia
   d. iron deficiency anemia

5. If the solubility test for hemoglobin S is positive, what is the appropriate reflex test? (Checklist #3)
   a. hemoglobin electrophoresis using cellulose acetate
   b. hemoglobin A_2 by column chromatography
   c. isoelectric focusing with SDS gel
   d. hemoglobin F determination

www.prenhall.com/mckenzie
Use the above address to access the free, interactive Companion Web site created for this textbook. Get hints, instant feedback, and textbook references to chapter-related multiple choice questions.

REFERENCES

1. National Committee for Clinical Laboratory Standards. *Evacuated Tubes and Additives for Blood Specimen Collection.* 4th ed. H1-A4. Villanova, PA: NCCLS; 1996.

2. National Committee for Clinical Laboratory Standards. *Collection, Transport, and Processing of Blood Specimens for Coagulation Testing and Performance of Coagulation Assays.* 3rd ed. H21-A3. Villanova, PA: NCCLS; 1998.

3. National Committee for Clinical Laboratory Standards. *Procedure for the Collection of Diagnostic Blood Specimens by Venipuncture.* 4th ed. H3-A4. Villanova, PA: NCCLS; 1998.

4. National Committee for Clinical Laboratory Standards. *Procedures for the Collection of Diagnostic Blood Specimens by Skin Puncture.* 4th ed. H4-A4. Villanova, PA: NCCLS; 1999.

5. Occupational Safety and Health Administration. *Occupational Exposure to Bloodborne Pathogens Standard.* 29 CFR 1910.1030. March 6, 1992.

6. Occupational Safety and Health Administration. Occupational Safety and Health Administration Instruction, CPL 2-2.44D. Enforcement Procedures for the Occupational Exposure to Bloodborne Pathogens Standard. 29 CFR 1910.1030. November 5, 1999.

7. Nikon, Inc. *Instructions for the Labophot-2.* Garden City, NY: Nikon, Inc.

8. Nikon, Inc. *Introduction to the Microscope: Operation and Preventive Maintenance Using the Nikon Labophot.* Garden City, NY: Nikon, Inc.

9. Locquin M, Langeron M. *Handbook of Microscopy.* Boston: Butterworths; 1983.

10. Nikon, Inc. *CF160 Optics Overview.* Garden City, NY: Nikon, Inc.; 2000.

11. Keller E. Light microscopy and cell structure. In *Cells: A Laboratory Manual.* Vol. 2. Edited by DL Spector, RD Goldman, and LA Leinwand. Cold Spring Harbor: Cold Spring Harbor Laboratory Press; 1997.

12. Barch MJ, Lawce HJ. Microscopy and imaging. In: *The AGT Cytogenetics Laboratory Manual.* 3rd ed. Edited by MJ Barch, T Knutsen, and JL Spurbeck. Philadelphia, PA: Lippincott-Raven; 1997.

13. Koenig AS, Day JC, Sodeman TM, Alpert NL. *Laboratory Instrument Verification and Verification Maintenance Manual.* 3rd ed. Skokie, IL: College of American Pathologists; 1982.

14. *Unopette WBC Determination for Manual Methods.* Rutherford, NJ: Becton, Dickinson, and Company; 1995.

15. *Unopette Erythrocyte Determination for Manual Methods.* Rutherford, NJ: Becton, Dickinson, and Company; 1995.

16. *Unopette WBC/Platelet Determination for Manual Methods.* Rutherford, NJ: Becton, Dickinson, and Company; 1996.

17. *Unopette Eosinophil Determination for Manual Methods.* Rutherford, NJ: Becton, Dickinson, and Company; 1995.

18. National Committee for Clinical Standards. *Reference and Selected Procedures for the Quantitative Determination of Hemoglobin in Blood.* 2nd ed. H15-A2. Villanova, PA: NCCLS; 1994.

19. Recommendations for reference method for haemoglobinometry in human blood (ICSH standard 1986) and specifications for international haemiglobincyanide reference preparation: 3rd ed. International Committee for Standardization in Haematology; Expert Panel on Haemoglobinometry. *Clin Lab Haematol.* 1987; 9(1):73–79.

20. National Committee for Clinical Laboratory Standards. *Procedure for Determining Packed Cell Volume by the Microhematocrit Method.* 2nd ed. H7-A2. Villanova, PA: NCCLS; 1993.

21. International Committee for Standardization in Hematology. Selected methods for the determination of packed cell volume. In: *Advances in Hematologic Methods: The Blood Count.* Edited by OW van Assendelft and JM England. Bocan Raton, FL: CRC Press; 1982.

22. National Committee for Clinical Standards. *Reference Procedure for Erythrocyte Sedimentaion Rate (ESR) Test.* 3rd ed. H2-A3. Villanova, PA: NCCLS; 1993.

23. International Committee for Standardization in Hematology. Recommendation for Measurement of Erythrocyte Sedimentation Rate of Human Blood. *Am J Clin Pathol.* 1977;68:505.

24. Comparison of automated systems for erythrocyte sedimentation rate. *Am J Clin Pathol.* 1998;110(3):334–40.

25. Gambino R. C-reactive protein—undervalued, underutilized. *Clin Chem.* 1997; 43(11):2017–18.

26. Ziegenhagen G, Drahovsky D. Klinishe Bedeutung des C-reaktiven Proteins. *Med Klin.* 1983; 78:45–50.

27. Rifai N, Ridker PM. High-Sensitivity C-Reactive Protein: A Novel and Promising Marker of Coronary Heart Disease. *Clin Chem.* 2001; 47(3):403–11.

28. Serke S, Riess H, Oettle H, Huhn D. Elevated reticulocyte count: A clue to the diagnosis of haemolytic-uraemic syndrome (HUS) associated with gemcitabine therapy for metastatic duodenal papillary carcinoma, a case report. *Br J Cancer.* 1999;79:1519–21.

29. Meidlinger P, et al. Granulocyte colony-stimulating factor-supported combined immunosuppressive therapy in patients with aplastic anemia: Tolerability, efficacy, and changes in the progenitor cell compartment. *Ann of Hematol.* 1999; 78(7):299–304.

30. Bhandari S, Norfolk D, Brownjohn A, Turney J: Evaluation of RBC ferritin and reticulocyte measurements in monitoring response to intravenous iron therapy. *Am J Kid Dis.* 1997; 30(6):814–21.

31. National Committee for Clinical Laboratory Standards. *Methods for Reticulocyte Counting (Flow Cytometry and Supravital Dyes).* H44-A. Villanova, PA: NCCLS; 1997.

32. National Committee for Clinical Laboratory Standards. *Solubility Test to Confirm the Presence of Sickling Hemoglobins.* 2nd ed. H10-A2. Villanova, PA: NCCLS; 1995.

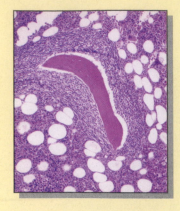

8

Peripheral Blood Smear

Cheryl Burns, M.S.

■ CHECKLIST - LEVEL I

At the end of this unit of study the student should be able to:

1. Describe the peripheral blood smear preparation methods.
2. Identify the characteristics of an optimally prepared peripheral blood smear.
3. Describe the Romanowsky staining technique.
4. Recognize characteristics of a properly stained peripheral blood smear.
5. Discuss potential causes of improperly stained peripheral blood smears.
6. List the components of a complete peripheral blood smear examination.
7. Correlate erythrocyte indices, leukocyte count, and platelet count with peripheral blood smear observations.
8. Determine the corrected leukocyte count based on the presence of nucleated erythrocytes.

■ CHECKLIST - LEVEL II

At the end of this unit of study the student should be able to:

1. Choose corrective actions for an improperly prepared or stained peripheral blood smear.
2. Detect abnormalities on peripheral blood smear examination, assess how they may alter cell count results (i.e., presence of nucleated erythrocytes or platelet satellitism), and recommend corrective action to assure valid results.

KEY TERMS

- Anemia
- Cold agglutinin disease
- Coverglass smear
- Multiple myeloma
- Optimal counting area
- Platelet clump
- Platelet satellitism
- Polycythemia
- Romanowsky-type stain
- Rouleaux
- Smudge cell
- Wedge smear

BACKGROUND BASICS

The information in this chapter will build on the concepts learned in previous chapters. To maximize your learning experience you should review these concepts before starting this unit of study.

Levels: I and II

▶ Outline the basics of specimen collection and describe the problems associated with improper collection and processing of a specimen. (Chapter 7)

▶ Describe the methodology used to perform a leukocyte count and platelet count and list potential sources of error in each. (Chapter 7)

▶ Calculate the erythrocyte indices and describe the erythrocytes based on the indices. (Chapter 7)

▶ Recognize the erythrocytic morphologic changes associated with size, shape, inclusions, and patterns of distribution. (Chapters 4, 10)

▶ Recognize neutrophil and monocyte morphology and the reactive changes associated with lymphocytes. (Chapter 6)

▶ Recognize and describe the morphologic characteristics of the developing erythrocytes and leukocytes. (Chapters 4, 6)

▶ OVERVIEW

Although automated leukocyte differentials have become a powerful tool in the hematology laboratory for screening and diagnosis of disease and monitoring therapy, they have limited ability to detect abnormal cells and identify specific erythrocyte morphology. For this reason, clinical laboratory personnel must be adept not only in the performance of standard techniques for blood smear preparation, staining, and examination, but also in the identification and correction of potential problems. This chapter will review those standard techniques and discuss potential sources of error and their resolution.

▶ PERIPHERAL BLOOD SMEAR PREPARATION

The morphologic evaluation of hematopoietic cells by light microscopy requires the preparation of a well-stained blood smear.[1–5] The accuracy of the morphologic evaluation depends in part on the quality of the blood smear.

MANUAL METHOD

There are two manual methods for preparing blood smears: the **coverglass smear** and the **wedge smear**. The coverglass smear method provides a smear with even distribution of the leukocytes. The disadvantages of this method are the difficulty in mastering the technique, the fragility of the coverglass, and the difficulty in staining the coverglass. The wedge smear is the method most commonly used in routine laboratory practice. This method is subject to poor leukocyte distribution, with monocytes and neutrophils being drawn out of the **optimal counting area** to the feather edge. Although the leukocyte distribution is poor, the technique is easily mastered, the smears are less fragile, and they may be stored for extended periods of time. An advantage of the leukocyte distribution in a wedge smear is that it allows for the identification of abnormal cells that tend to locate on the edges of the smear.

Either EDTA-anticoagulated venous blood or capillary blood (∞ Chapter 7) is acceptable for the preparation of a blood smear (see Web Table 8-1 ✪ for this procedure). An optimal blood smear will have the characteristics listed in Table 8-1 ✪. A common problem associated with blood smears is failure to dry the blood smear in a timely manner. This results in contraction artifacts of the cells, especially with increased humidity. In certain physiological conditions including **anemia, polycythemia, multiple myeloma,** and **cold agglutinin disease,** it is difficult to make good blood smears due to the abnormal composition of the blood (Table 8-2 ✪). The thickness or thinness of the blood smear may be regulated by:

- Adjusting the amount of blood used to make the drop
- Altering the speed with which the drop is smeared
- Altering the angle at which the spreader slide is used

✪ TABLE 8-1

Optimal Blood Smear Characteristics

- Minimum length 2.5 cm
- Gradual transition in thickness from thick to thin
- Straight feather edge
- Margins narrower than slide
- No streaks, waves, or troughs

✪ TABLE 9-1

Conditions for Which a Bone Marrow Evaluation Is Indicated

1. Primary diagnosis of hematolymphoid malignancies
   Acute leukemias
   Chronic myeloproliferative disorders
   Chronic lymphoproliferative disorders
   Myelodysplastic syndromes
   Hodgkin's and non-Hodgkin lymphomas
   Multiple myeloma
2. Staging of lymphoid malignancies and solid tumors
3. Post treatment follow-up
   Post chemotherapy and radiation therapy
   Post bone-marrow transplant
4. Detection of infection and/or source of fever of unknown origin
   Mycobacterium and fungal infections
   Granulomas
   Unknown infectious agents using cultures and special stains
   Hemophagocytic syndrome
5. Primary diagnosis of systemic diseases
   Metabolic disorders (Gaucher's disease, etc.)
   Systemic mastocytosis
6. Miscellaneous
   Evaluation of storage iron
   Evaluation of unexplained cytopenias

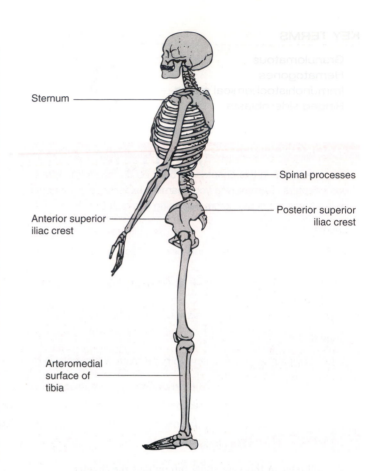

■ **FIGURE 9-1** Sites used for aspiration and biopsy of bone marrow.

▶ BONE MARROW PROCEDURE

Both bone marrow aspiration and core biopsy are obtained for optimal marrow examination. Most marrow specimens are taken from the posterior superior iliac crest (Figure 9-1 ■). The sternum and anterior iliac crest are occasionally used in adult patients. The anteromedial surface of the tibia is sometimes used in children less than two years of age. Occasionally the spines of the lumbar vertebral bodies L1 and L2 are used in older children.

The bone marrow aspirates and biopsies are obtained using disposable needles that are modifications of the needle first introduced by Jamshidi.[1] A sterile technique is always used. The skin over the biopsy site is first cleaned with a disinfectant solution, and then 1–2% lidocaine (local anesthetic) is infiltrated into the skin, subcutaneous tissue, and periosteum. Some patients require additional sedation with intravenous or intramuscular medications. A small skin incision is made with a blade to facilitate penetration of the needle. It is recommended to perform the biopsy first and then the aspirate to avoid distortion of the marrow architecture in the biopsy specimen. In adults, an 11-gauge cutting needle is commonly used to obtain a core of marrow tissue (this is known as a trephine core biopsy). This is followed by aspiration of about 2 mL of marrow using an 18-gauge needle.

In experienced hands, complications of bone marrow biopsy and aspirate are very rare (<0.1%). The most common complications are localized bleeding or infection. Most patients experience discomfort during the aspiration procedure even with adequate infiltration of local anesthetic. If not carefully performed, it is possible to go through the entire thickness of the bone and damage the underlying tissues. This risk is higher with a sternal aspiration. After the procedure, the patient is advised to lie on the biopsy site. The site should be reevaluated in 15–30 minutes for any bleeding or oozing. The actual procedure usually is performed with the assistance of a clinical laboratorian. It is the laboratorian's responsibility to assure adequacy of the samples.

Bone marrow aspiration and biopsy can be performed on patients with severe thrombocytopenia, coagulation factor deficiencies (however, over 50% factor activity is required), and in those receiving anticoagulant therapy. Applying pressure at the biopsy site and lying on the back for 20–30 minutes can control local bleeding in thrombocytopenic patients. Correction of severe coagulation factor deficiencies before the procedure is indicated in hemophiliacs because intense local bleeding can occur in these patients. The only time a bone marrow biopsy should not be performed is when a bone marrow will not assist in the diagnosis or evaluation of the patient's condition. The indication criteria for a bone marrow examination are listed in Table 9-1 .

> ✔ ## Checkpoint! #1
>
> *A 25-year-old male was recently diagnosed with ALL and received chemotherapy. It is 21 days after the chemotherapy. A bone marrow biopsy has been scheduled to determine if residual leukemia is present. His platelet count is $10 \times 10^9/L$. Does this patient have a significant risk of bleeding? Is it necessary to cancel the procedure until the platelet count is over $50 \times 10^9/L$?*

► PROCESSING OF BONE MARROW FOR EXAMINATION

A laboratorian with experience in bone marrow preparation accompanies the physician performing the bone marrow aspirate and biopsy.

BONE MARROW ASPIRATE SMEARS, PARTICLE PREPARATION, AND CLOT SECTIONS

Approximately 1.0–1.5 mL of aspirate is needed for evaluating bone marrow morphology. Each laboratory has its own preferences for processing the aspirate. Described here is a commonly used procedure. Depending upon the clinical setting, additional aspirate can be obtained for cytogenetics, flow cytometry, molecular studies, and cultures. Direct smears of bone marrow aspirate are prepared at the bedside using a technique similar to that for preparing peripheral blood smears.[2] Bone marrow particle crush smears can be prepared by pouring a small amount of marrow aspirate onto a watch glass. Using a glass pipette, the marrow particles are transferred onto several glass slides. A second slide is placed gently on top of the drop containing the particles. The top slide is pulled apart to evenly distribute the marrow particles. Cell morphology is better appreciated on the aspirate smears, while the architecture and cellularity are assessed on the trephine core biopsy and particle preparation. The clinical laboratory professional usually prepares several smears. These are used to do special stains necessary for the classification of acute leukemias and myelodysplastic syndromes and for evaluation of storage iron. The remaining bone marrow particles can be used for histologic evaluation.

Tissue particles admixed with blood may be left to clot, then fixed in 10% buffered formalin and processed for histologic sectioning (clot sections). However, better results are obtained if the blood and particles are transferred to an EDTA tube before clotting begins. The blood and particles are filtered through histo-wrap filter paper, and the concentrated particles on the paper are fixed in 10% buffered formalin. In the histology laboratory, these particles are collected by scraping the paper and then embedding the particles in paraffin for further processing.[3]

Some laboratories mix a portion of the marrow aspirate with EDTA. This anticoagulated marrow is placed in a Wintrobe tube and centrifuged. The marrow is separated into four layers: fat and perivascular cells, plasma, buffy coat, and red cells. The ratio between the fat/perivascular and the erythroid/myeloid layers reflects the overall marrow cellularity. Concentrate smears can be prepared from the buffy coat. The direct, concentrate, and particle crush smears are stained with Wright's stain.

TOUCH IMPRINTS AND CORE BIOPSY

Immediately after obtaining the bone marrow core biopsy, touch imprints of the biopsy can be made by gently touching the tissue several times on 2–4 glass slides. Some of these slides are stained with Wright's stain and the rest can be used for special stains in case a good aspirate is not available. The trephine core biopsy specimen is immersed without delay in B-5 or 10% buffered formalin fixative. After fixation, the trephine core biopsy, particle, and clot preparations undergo standard histologic processing including decalcifying, dehydrating, embedding in paraffin blocks, sectioning of 2–3 μm thick sections, and histologic staining with hematoxylin and eosin.

Trephine core biopsies are performed for primary diagnosis as well as for disease staging purposes. When performed for clinical staging of lymphoma, multiple myeloma, and carcinoma, bilateral biopsies are recommended.

► MORPHOLOGIC INTERPRETATION OF BONE MARROW

Morphologic review of bone marrow includes cytologic assessment of hematopoietic cells on the aspirate smear as well as histologic assessment of the clot, particle preparation, and core biopsy.

BONE MARROW ASPIRATE

It is good practice to review the complete blood count (CBC) data and the corresponding peripheral blood smear in conjunction with the bone marrow. The quantity and appearance of the blood cells will guide the morphologist to a differential diagnosis. The bone marrow aspirate is used to evaluate the quantity, morphology, and maturation process of erythroid and myeloid precursors and megakaryocytes (Figure 9-2 ■).

The examination of the bone marrow aspirate smears should start at low magnification with a 10× dry objective (100× magnification). Scanning the slide at this magnifica-

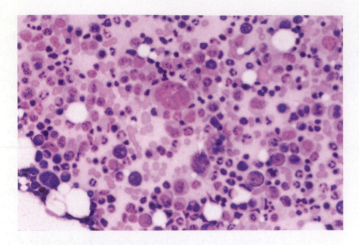

■ **FIGURE 9-2** Bone marrow aspirate smear showing normal maturing trilineage hematopoiesis. (Bone marrow; Wright-Giemsa stain; 200× magnification)

tion permits selection of a suitable area for examination and the differential count. Areas where the marrow cells are destroyed due to squashing or stripping of their cytoplasm by fibrin thread should be avoided. These areas are characterized by the presence of bare nuclei. An area is selected where the cells are well spread, intact, and not diluted by sinusoidal blood. At this low magnification, marrow cellularity is also evaluated. The number and the distribution of the megakaryocytes are usually noted adjacent to a spicule (particle). (Spicules are bone particles seen on the marrow aspirate smears.) They have hematopoietic precursors within them. An optimal aspirate usually has some spicules.

After the initial scan, immersion oil is applied on the slide and the examination continues on high magnification (500× and/or 1000×). This magnification provides detailed images of nuclear and cytoplasmic maturation. Evaluation of maturation is an important step when reviewing the marrow aspirate. Abnormal maturation can be seen in any of the three cell lines. For example, abnormal maturation is a diagnostic criteria in the myelodysplastic syndromes (MDS). In MDS, abnormalities of the red cell precursors include multinucleation and nuclear/cytoplasmic dysynchrony (nuclear maturation is delayed compared to cytoplasmic maturation). Myeloid precursors may show abnormal granule development, and megakaryocytes may reveal hypolobulation of the nucleus. Abnormalities in bone marrow that are characteristic of a specific pathology are discussed in subsequent chapters on anemia and neoplastic disorders.

Bone Marrow Differential Count

A 500 to 1000 cell differential is usually performed with the oil immersion objective on the direct smear or the crush particle preparation (the morphology is better preserved on these preparations).[4] The concentrate and/or touch imprints are a useful source when the bone marrow is very hypocellular or aspirate could not be obtained (dry tap), although the morphology is not as good as that on direct smears and

crush particle preparations. Overall marrow cellularity can be estimated on the particle preparation.

Since the bone marrow composition changes with age, it is important to know the age of the patient when evaluating bone marrow specimens. In infants during the first month after birth, dramatic alterations occur in the distribution of the different marrow compartments. At birth there is a predominance of granulocyte precursors. Within a month this changes to a predominance of lymphoid elements. In early infancy many lymphocytes have fine chromatin, a high nuclear-to-cytoplasmic ratio, and absence of distinct nucleoli. These cells are called **hematogones** and represent normal lymphoid *progenitor* cells (precursor B cells).[5] These hematogones can be misinterpreted as blasts if the observer is unfamiliar with these characteristics. In children up to 3 years old, one-third or more of the marrow cellularity is made up of lymphocytes. The lymphocyte number gradually declines to the normal adult level thereafter.

In adult marrow the lymphocytes are distributed randomly among the hematopoietic cells and in lymphoid follicles. Lymphoid follicles are collections or aggregations of lymphocytes. These lymphocytes can be malignant or benign (see section on benign vs malignant lymphoid aggregates). Depending on the placement of the bone marrow needle, the cells in the follicle may be aspirated. This can give an estimate of markedly increased lymphocytes in the marrow and introduce significant variation in the differential count from sample to sample in the same patient. The greatest mass of the adult marrow is composed of granulopoietic and erythropoietic precursors. For the purpose of the differential count, these hematopoietic cells are enumerated within different categories according to their stage of maturation.

Myeloid to Erythroid Ratio

When adequate numbers of cells are counted and differentiated, the percentage of each category is calculated. The ratio between all granulocytes and their precursors and all nucleated red cell precursors represents the myeloid to erythroid ratio (M:E ratio). The normal M:E ratio ranges between 2:1 and 4:1. The granulocytic tissue occupies two to four times more marrow space than the erythrocytic precursors, owing to the shorter survival of the granulocytes in the circulation (i.e., neutrophils' 6–10 hours versus erythrocytes' 120 days). Changes in the survival time of granulocytes and erythrocytes are reflected in changes in the M:E ratio. Normal, increased, or decreased M:E ratios are associated with certain disease entities. For example, patients with chronic myelogenous leukemia usually have an increased ratio; in contrast, patients with myelodysplastic syndrome usually have a decreased ratio. Megakaryocytes are unevenly distributed in the marrow, and a differential count is a poor means for their evaluation. Megakaryocytes are not included in the differential count. Usually 5–10 megakaryocytes are seen per microscopic field at 100× magnification.

✔ **Checkpoint! #2**

A 60-year-old male complained to his local physician of abdominal fullness. The CBC showed an elevated leukocyte count with absolute neutrophilia and basophilia. The peripheral blood smear revealed numerous myelocytes. A bone marrow biopsy was performed. The bone marrow differential was reported as follows: blasts 1%, myelocytes 35%, metamyelocytes 20%, bands 10%, segmented neutrophils 20%, eosinophils 1%, basophils 3%, pronormoblasts 1%, basophilic normoblasts 3%, polychromatophilic normoblasts 2%, orthochromatic normoblasts 4%, lymphocytes 0%, and monocytes 0%. What is the M:E ratio?

TOUCH IMPRINTS

When the bone marrow is a dry tap secondary to underlying fibrosis (myelofibrosis, hairy cell leukemia) or when the marrow aspirate lacks spicules and is hemodiluted, the touch imprints of the bone marrow biopsy may be the only source for study of cellular detail and the maturation sequence of the sample. Sometimes the touch preparations contain enough cells for performing a differential count and cytochemical stains (Figure 9-3 ■).

BONE MARROW PARTICLE PREPARATION, CLOT AND CORE BIOPSY

The leftover marrow particles obtained during the aspiration procedure and the biopsy specimen can be processed for histologic examination. The advantage of bone marrow biopsy is that it represents a large sample of marrow and bone structures in their natural relationship.

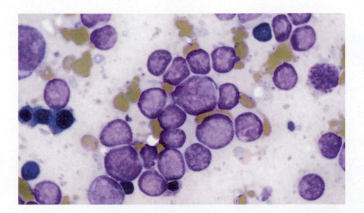

■ **FIGURE 9-3** Touch imprint from a case with ALL showing many lymphoblasts. Marrow was inaspirable and therefore was not available for the morphologic review. Cytochemical stains were performed on these imprints, and blasts were negative for all stains. (BM touch imprints; Wright-Giemsa stain; 500× magnification)

A variety of different stains can be used. Iron stain can be performed to evaluate storage iron; however, because of decalcification, the core biopsy may not be good to study marrow iron stores. Iron stores should be evaluated on aspirate smears, particle preparations, or clot sections. Reticulin and trichrome stains are used to evaluate the presence of fibrosis. Acid-fast organisms and fungi in **granulomatous** (a distinctive pattern of chronic reaction in which the predominant cell type is an activated macrophage with an epithelial-like appearance) diseases may be detected quickly with specific stains, offering great advantages in diagnosing these infections. When metastatic tumors and lymphomas are found in the bone marrow, **immunohistochemical stains** can be used on histologic sections to demonstrate specific tumor markers. Immunohistochemical stains use labeled antibodies to identify specific markers (antigens) on cells. Thus, a very precise diagnosis of the origin of a tumor can be made without elaborate, expensive, and more invasive techniques.

A disadvantage of the bone marrow biopsy is that fine cellular details are lost in the processing; therefore, it is of little value in the diagnosis of leukemias and some refractory anemias. In these situations, the touch preparation from the biopsy may supply the missing morphologic details.

Molecular studies may be done on marrow specimens to aid in diagnosis and management of some diseases. Polymerase chain reaction (PCR) can be performed on paraffin embedded formalin fixed marrow biopsy. PCR technology may be used to detect B cell or T cell gene rearrangements, various leukemias, and minimal residual disease and to diagnose infectious diseases (∞ Chapter 25).

Bone Marrow Cellularity

The overall bone marrow cellularity is estimated by comparing the amount of hematopoietic tissue with the amount of adipose tissue. An easy way to determine the normal expected cellularity range in an adult is to subtract the age of the patient from 100% and add and subtract (+/−) 10%. For example, a normal 70-year-old adult has an overall cellularity between 20% and 40%. The cellularity may vary from area to area, with subcortical and paratrabecular areas of bone marrow being more hypocellular than the deeper medullary area. Therefore, estimated cellularity should represent the average percentage. On the other hand, if hypercellular and hypocellular areas are seen in the medullary area, this should be mentioned descriptively in the report because an average cellularity may be difficult to estimate.

The bone marrow biopsy is the most reliable specimen for assessment of cellularity because it offers a large amount of tissue for evaluation. However, evaluation of cellularity can also be done on good aspirate smears or marrow particle preparations. The ratio of hematopoietic cells to fat is evaluated at low magnification using the 10× objective, so that larger areas are included in the field of observation. The term *decreased* or *increased* cellularity is applied when less than or more than the expected normal number of hematopoietic cells is seen. Precise evaluation can be achieved with experience, and good reproducibility can be attained among several observers (Figure 9-4 ■).

BENIGN LYMPHOID AGGREGATES VS MALIGNANT LYMPHOMA

Benign lymphoid aggregates can usually be seen in bone marrow of elderly patients. When the patient has a history of lymphoma, the distinction between benign lymphoid aggregates and malignant lymphoma is important. Benign lymphoid aggregates are usually small, well demarcated, nonparatrabecular, and comprised predominantly of small round lymphocytes with plasma cells at the periphery and blood vessels present within the aggregate (Figure 9-5 ■). The malignant lymphoid aggregates, on the contrary, are usually large with ill-defined borders, paratrabecular, comprised of atypical lymphocytes, and lack plasma cells at the periphery (Figure 9-6 ■). However, the lymphoid infiltrate of lymphoma can also be interstitial, diffuse, and patchy. Immunohistochemical stains and/or PCR can be performed on the marrow biopsy to differentiate between benign lymphoid aggregates and malignant lymphoma. In benign lymphoid aggregates there is an absence of clonal B cell and T cell rearrangements. On the other hand, clonal B cell or T cell rearrangements are often seen in malignant lymphomas.

BONE MARROW IRON STORES

Iron is stored as ferritin (iron complexed with apoferritin protein) and hemosiderin in reticuloendothelial cells and erythroblasts. The storage iron of the bone marrow that can be visualized is in the form of hemosiderin. Hemosiderin can

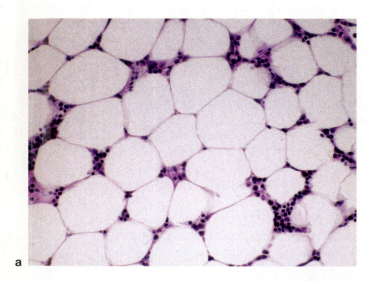

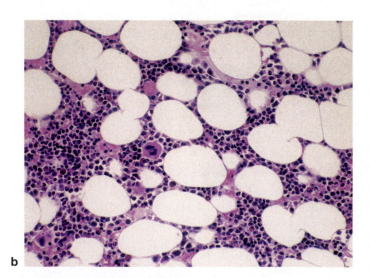

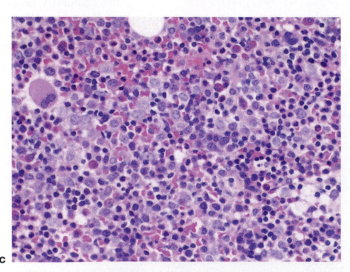

■ **FIGURE 9-4** If these bone marrow biopsies are from a 40-year-old patient then **a.** is a hypocellular marrow, **b.** is a normocellular marrow, and **c.** is a hypercellular marrow. (Bone marrow; paraffin section, hematoxylin-eosin stain; 100× magnification)

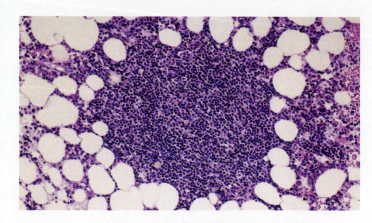

■ **FIGURE 9-5** Bone marrow biopsy showing a well circumscribed lymphoid aggregate indicating a benign lymphoid aggregate. (Bone marrow; paraffin section, hematoxylin-eosin stain; 100× magnification)

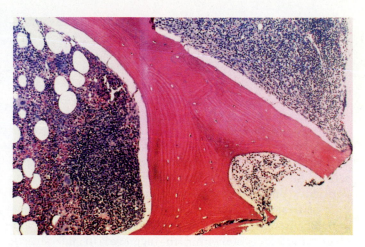

■ **FIGURE 9-6** Bone marrow biopsy showing two paratrabecular lymphoid infiltrates suggesting involvement of marrow by a follicle center cell lymphoma. (Bone marrow; paraffin section, hematoxylin-eosin stain; 100× magnification)

be seen on unstained smears as golden-yellow granules. On Wright-Giemsa-stained smears, it appears as brownish blue granules. However, for more precise evaluation, the Prussian blue reaction is used to demonstrate the intracytoplasmic iron.

Prussian-Blue Iron Stain

The Prussian-blue stain provides the most direct means for assessing body iron stores. It is designed to demonstrate the presence of hemosiderin in histiocytes, erythroblasts (sideroblasts), and/or erythrocytes (siderocytes). The EDTA chelating method should be used to decalcify the bone marrow biopsies if iron studies are being performed. Rapid acid decalcifying solutions extract iron, and therefore, these specimens must not be used.

In this staining procedure, a weak acid solution is needed to free the iron from the loose protein bonds present in the hemosiderin molecule. The freed iron combines with potassium ferrocyanide to produce ferric ferrocyanide. Freed iron will appear greenish blue.

Normal marrow iron is seen as fine cytoplasmic granules in histiocytes. From 30% to 50% of marrow erythroblasts contain iron specks and are called sideroblasts (Figure 9-7 ■). Clumps of iron easily seen at 100× magnification indicate increased storage, while only a few specks of iron found after searching several microscopic fields at 500× or 1000× magnification indicates decreased iron storage. When no stainable iron is detected in the bone marrow smear or tissue sections, iron is depleted or absent. The storage iron may be reported as absent, decreased, adequate, moderately increased, or markedly increased, or it can be given corresponding numerical values from 0 to 4, where 2 represents the normal (adequate) iron stores in an adult.

Iron is also stored as intracellular ferritin. All developing normoblasts and reticulocytes contain dispersed ferritin but may not stain with Prussian blue. Small amounts of ferritin

enter the blood and can be measured as serum ferritin. The amount of circulating ferritin parallels the concentration of storage iron in the body. Nonspecific increases are associated with chronic infection and inflammation, liver disease, and malignancy. Thus it is not as accurate an indicator of iron sufficiency as hemosiderin in these cases.

Use of Bone Marrow Iron Evaluation

The evaluation of marrow iron stores is essential in the diagnosis of anemias, especially in refractory and dyserythropoietic anemias. When the morphologic characteristic of the iron particles in the histiocytes and red cell precursors is an

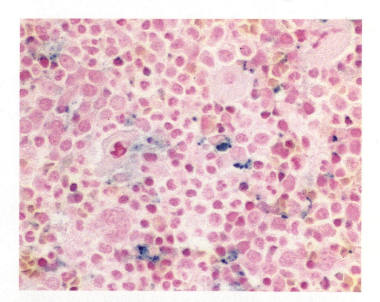

■ **FIGURE 9-7** Bone marrow clot section stained with Prussian blue. The bluish granules indicate the presence of iron. (Bone marrow; clot section, Prussian blue stain; 400× magnification)

important diagnostic consideration (such as in myelodysplastic syndrome), an iron stain is performed on a particle smear. If the overall distribution of the amount of iron is of clinical importance (iron deficiency anemia, anemia of chronic diseases), then histologic sections of bone marrow particles and marrow clotted particles are stained for iron.

The determination of bone marrow storage iron is useful in the classification of anemias associated with defective hemoglobin synthesis. Storage iron is markedly decreased or absent in iron deficiency anemia. When storage iron is present in the bone marrow, anemia cannot be a result of iron deficiency unless the patient has been transfused with red cells or treated with iron supplements. Iron stores are normal or increased in anemia of chronic disease and thalassemias. Iron stores are also increased in sideroblastic anemia. The presence of **ringed sideroblasts** is diagnostic for sideroblastic anemia and/or myelodysplastic syndrome. However, ringed sideroblasts can also be seen in myeloproliferative disorders, megaloblastic anemia, alcoholism, and following chemotherapy. Ringed sideroblasts are erythroid precursors that have a deposition of excess iron around the nucleus arranged like a necklace. This iron is located within the mitochondria that surround the nucleus.

 Checkpoint! #3

A pathologist is evaluating a bone marrow biopsy from a patient suspected of having a myelodysplastic syndrome. Evaluation of the peripheral blood reveals both hypochromic and normochromic red cells. The bone marrow aspirate shows dysplastic (abnormal cell development) changes in the red cell precursors. The pathologist ordered an iron stain on the particle crush preparation. Why is the iron stain useful in this case?

▶ CYTOCHEMICAL STAINS

In hematology, cytochemistry refers to in vitro staining of cells that allows microscopic examination of the cells' chemical composition. Cells of different lineage have different cytochemical composition. Cell morphology is not significantly altered in the staining process. Cytochemical stains are usually performed on specimens from patients who have a neoplasm of hematopoietic cells. These stains help differentiate the lineage of immature cells so that an accurate diagnosis of the type of neoplasm can be made.

Smears are usually made from peripheral blood and bone marrow. Although bone marrow aspirate is usually used to make smears for cytochemical stains, the touch imprints from the biopsy can be used if there is insufficient aspirate. The smears are incubated with substrates that react with specific cellular constituents (organelle-associated enzymes, carbohydrates, and proteins). If the specific constituent is present in the cell, its reaction with the substrate is confirmed by the formation of a colored product within the cell. The stained slides are evaluated with an ordinary light microscope. Most stains can be performed on air-dried smears. All cytochemical stains should be performed on recently prepared slides. Some cellular constituents are sensitive to heat, light, storage, and processing technique. If stains cannot be performed on recently prepared slides, then the unstained smears can be protected from light in the refrigerator. However, a fresh smear is preferred for the myeloperoxidase (MPO) stain. These stains are discussed in ∞ Chapter 26.

▶ ANCILLARY STUDIES

In most cases, a thorough examination of a well-stained bone marrow aspirate smear and core biopsy provide enough information by which diagnoses of hematopoietic disorders are made. However, several ancillary studies can provide additional information that help support or confirm the morphologic diagnosis. These studies can also provide prognostic information and in some cases can predict response to therapy. The most commonly used ancillary studies are flow cytometry, conventional cytogenetics, fluorescent in situ hybridization (FISH), and molecular genetic studies.

Flow cytometry allows analyzing simultaneously multiple characteristics of cells in suspension as they pass through a laser light beam. The size and internal complexity of the cells can be estimated, and with the use of fluorochrome labeled antibodies, the presence of specific cell markers can be determined. Flow cytometry has a wide range of uses in the evaluation of hematologic disorders. It is commonly used to establish the presence of clonality, diagnose and classify malignant lymphomas and leukemias, and detect minimal residual disease after use of chemotherapy. The immunophenotyping of peripheral blood, bone marrow, lymph node (and other) tissues, and body fluids is performed only on fresh samples (Table 9-2 ✪). These techniques are discussed in ∞ Chapter 23.

Chromosome analysis (cytogenetics) is frequently used in the study of hematopoietic disorders since certain malignancies have characteristic chromosomal alterations. In addition, the presence of some specific chromosomal abnormalities has prognostic implications. It is routinely used in the primary diagnosis of acute leukemias, myelodysplastic syndromes, and myeloproliferative disorders. Although a large number of malignant lymphomas also have characteristic abnormalities, cytogenetics is less frequently used in the diagnosis of lymphomas since lymphoma cells are more difficult to grow. Analysis is performed on fresh samples (Table 9-2 ✪). More recent techniques such as FISH have allowed specific cytogenetic questions to be answered more quickly.

Although molecular genetic techniques were initially used in research laboratories, they are now performed in

⊕ TABLE 9-2

Specimen Requirements for Ancillary Studies

Specimen	Flow Cytometry	Cytogenetics	Molecular Studies
Blood	5 mL in heparin sodium, EDTA or ACD	5 mL in heparin sodium	1–3 mL in EDTA (preferable over heparin)
Bone marrow	1 mL in heparin sodium, EDTA or ACD	1–3 mL in heparin sodium; bone marrow preferable over blood	1–3 mL in EDTA (preferable over heparin)
Fluids	As much as possible, anticoagulated if contaminated with blood	As much as possible, anticoagulated if contaminated with blood	5–10 mL
Tissue	0.5 cm^2 fresh in transport media or saline	1 cm^2 fresh in transport media	3–5 mm^2 fresh or frozen; fixed specimens good for PCR analysis
Storage	Should be kept at room temperature and analyzed within 24 hours; up to 72 hours may be acceptable in some cases. Should be refrigerated if analysis will not occur within 24 hours. Frozen or fixed specimens are unacceptable.	Should be kept at RT and transported to the laboratory within 24 hours. Frozen or fixed samples are unacceptable.	If samples are not analyzed within 24 hours, they should be refrigerated (2–8°C) for up to 1 week. Samples frozen at −20°C or −70°C can be stored for 2 weeks or 2 years, respectively.

EDTA = ethylenediaminetetraacetic acid, ACD = acid citrate dextrose, RT = room temperature

clinical laboratories. For hematolymphoid disorders both Southern blot hybridization and polymerase chain reaction (PCR) have emerged as leading adjunctive technologies. Both analyses are used to demonstrate cell clonality and lineage and to identify specific genetic rearrangements. Additionally, PCR can be used for the detection of minimal residual disease (∞ Chapters 25, 26). Fresh and frozen samples are required for Southern blot analysis and are preferable for PCR; however, samples fixed in formalin and embedded in paraffin are also acceptable for PCR analysis (Table 9-2 ⊕). Negative PCR results are often followed by Southern blot analysis.

data, clinical differential diagnosis, and relevant therapeutic information. The morphology and interpretation by the pathologist and laboratorian must include types of sample obtained, differential counts from both peripheral blood and bone marrow, and morphologic abnormalities in any cell lines in the patient's peripheral blood or bone marrow. The results must be interpreted in conjunction with any ancillary studies (special stains, flow cytometry, cytogenetics, molecular studies). If the ancillary studies are significant in establishing the diagnosis but are unavailable when the bone marrow report is written, an addendum report should mention the significance of these studies. The comparison of the current marrow specimen to the previous tissue samples (marrow or other nonmarrow biopsies) is essential in some situations.

Finally, the diagnostic interpretation by the pathologist should be rendered within a reasonable period of time. For example, if 50% blasts were present in the blood or in the bone marrow, it would be reasonable to call the clinician about the preliminary diagnosis of acute leukemia. However, the final diagnosis can be made only after special stains and flow cytometry studies are completed. Comments, if needed, should be concise and relevant to the case and may include a recommendation for additional tests and a possible differential diagnosis.

⊘ **CASE STUDY** *(continued from page 149)*

A bone marrow procedure was performed. The marrow was difficult to aspirate, but the physician was able to obtain some hemodiluted marrow. Bilateral marrow biopsy was also performed. Review of the aspirate smears showed a very hemodiluted sample but the pathologist was able to see an increased number of blasts. There was not enough aspirate sample to do flow cytometry, cytogenetic, and cytochemical stains.

2. How should you proceed with the marrow evaluation?

▶ BONE MARROW REPORT

The bone marrow report must contain all relevant information. An optimum bone marrow report is comprised of two components: clinical information and morphologic interpretation. The clinician should provide the patient's biographic

⊘ **CASE STUDY** *(continued from page 149)*

Processing of bone marrow biopsy usually is done overnight.

3. Can a diagnosis be made from tests on the aspirate rather than waiting for the biopsy slides?

SUMMARY

The bone marrow is the primary site of blood cell production after birth. Evaluation of bone marrow is indicated in diagnosis, management, and follow-up of a variety of disorders. Bone marrow specimens may include aspirates and biopsy. The marrow is processed and evaluated in the laboratory.

Differentiation and classification of acute leukemias depend on accurate identification of the blasts. Since the lineage of the cells is difficult to differentiate using only morphologic characteristics, cytochemical analysis and flow cytometry are used routinely to help identify blast lineage.

REVIEW QUESTIONS

LEVEL I

1. What is the site for bone marrow collection in children under 2 years of age? (Checklist #1)
   a. spleen
   b. sternum
   c. tibia
   d. lumbar vertebral bodies

2. Which of the following is an indication for a bone marrow biopsy? (Checklist # 2)
   a. 20-year-old male with suspected leukemia
   b. 60-year-old female who has been diagnosed with megaloblastic anemia
   c. 30-year-old male who has been diagnosed with HIV
   d. 20-year-old pregnant woman who is diagnosed with iron deficiency anemia

3. What site is most commonly used in adults for bone marrow biopsies? (Checklist # 1)
   a. sternum
   b. posterior iliac crest
   c. anterior iliac crest
   d. tibia

4. This marrow specimen is best for preserving the architecture of the bone marrow. (Checklist # 3)
   a. aspirate
   b. clot section
   c. particle smear
   d. biopsy

5. Which of the following is the best specimen to evaluate the morphology of the hematopoietic precursors? (Checklist #3, #4)
   a. bone marrow aspirate
   b. clot preparation
   c. iliac crest biopsy
   d. none of the above

6. In which of the following diseases are you more likely to find a decreased M:E ratio? (Checklist # 5)
   a. chronic blood loss
   b. granulocytic leukemia
   c. lymphocytic leukemia
   d. chronic infection

LEVEL II

1. The following is characteristic of a benign lymphoid aggregate. (Checklist # 1)
   a. patient history of lymphoma
   b. comprised predominantly of small lymphocytes
   c. large with ill-defined borders
   d. paratrabecular and lacks plasma cells at the periphery

2. A hypercellular bone marrow M:E ratio is 10:1. This indicates: (Checklist #3)
   a. decreased erythropoiesis
   b. increased erythropoiesis
   c. increased leukopoiesis
   d. decreased leukopoiesis

3. The following is the differential that you obtained in a patient with a diagnosis of AML: blasts 65%, myelocytes 4%, metamyelocytes 4%, bands 1%, segmented neutrophils 8%, pronormoblasts 2%, basophilic normoblasts 3%, polychromatic normoblasts 3%, orthochromatic normoblasts 3%, lymphocytes 4%, and monocytes 3%. What is the M:E ratio? (Checklist # 3)
   a. 10:1
   b. 5.4:1
   c. 7.4:1
   d. 1:7.4

4. When you evaluate bone marrow biopsy for estimating the marrow cellularity, which ratio are you trying to estimate? (Checklist # 4)
   a. cells to fat
   b. cells to bony trabeculae
   c. cells to vessels
   d. granulocytes to fat

5. A pathologist is evaluating a bone marrow biopsy in a patient recently diagnosed with lymphoma. Which of the following should be looked for in the bone marrow evaluation? (Checklist #1)
   a. malignant lymphoid aggregate
   b. granulomatous lesions
   c. iron stores
   d. presence of parasites

REVIEW QUESTIONS (continued)

LEVEL I

7. What is the expected overall cellularity in a bone marrow biopsy of a normal 50-year-old male? (Checklist # 6)
   a. 80% ±10
   b. 100% ±10
   c. 50% ±10
   d. 30% ±10

8. Which of the following stains is used to evaluate the presence of storage iron? (Checklist # 6)
   a. Wright-Giemsa
   b. Prussian blue
   c. PAS
   d. reticulin

9. Why would special stains be performed on a bone marrow specimen? (Checklist # 8)
   a. to differentiate leukemias
   b. to determine the M:E ratio
   c. to estimate bone marrow cellularity
   d. to identify hematogones

10. The hematology laboratory's role in bone marrow evaluation is to do the following: (Checklist #7)
    a. make direct bone marrow smears
    b. perform the bone marrow aspirate procedure
    c. administer the anesthetic before the procedure
    d. determine the appropriate therapy

LEVEL II

6. A pathologist is evaluating a bone marrow biopsy in a patient recently diagnosed with Hodgkin lymphoma. Inadvertently, the lab did an iron stain on a particle crush preparation. The pathologist saw a few ringed sideroblasts; however, he did not see any dysplastic changes suggestive of myelodysplastic syndrome. In which of the following conditions might you see ringed sideroblasts? (Checklist # 5)
   a. iron deficiency anemia
   b. thalassemia
   c. alcoholism
   d. Hodgkin's disease

7. A pathologist is evaluating the bone marrow particle preparation of a patient suspected of having acute leukemia. He identifies a large number of undifferentiated blasts. What ancillary test should be done? (Checklist #2)
   a. molecular diagnostics
   b. cytochemical stains
   c. fluorescent in situ hybridization
   d. HIV testing

8. A physician performs a bone marrow biopsy and aspirate on a 65-year-old male. The cellularity is estimated at 80% and the M:E ratio is .5 to 1. The correct description of this marrow is: (Checklist #3, 4)
   a. hypercellular with a decreased M:E ratio
   b. hypercellular with an increased M:E ratio
   c. hypocellular with a decreased M:E ratio
   d. hypocellular with an increased M:E ratio

9. You are assisting a physician during bone marrow biopsy in a patient with possible diagnosis of acute leukemia. The doctor is unable to obtain any aspirate; however, he was able to obtain two core biopsies. What is the best way to use the material obtained? (Checklist # 2, 6)
   a. Place both core biopsies in formalin and process one immediately; save the other for ancillary tests.
   b. Place one core biopsy in formalin and freeze the second one at −70°C.
   c. Place one core biopsy in formalin after making touch imprints; put the second in saline.
   d. Place both core biopsies in saline; freeze one at 0°C and process the other immediately.

10. A 20-year-old patient presented with severe headache. Lumbar puncture performed showed a marked increase in atypical mononuclear cells. The differential diagnosis is acute leukemia vs malignant lymphoma. What would be most helpful in distinguishing the two diagnoses? (Checklist #2)
    a. molecular diagnostic tests
    b. flow cytometry
    c. cytogenetics tests
    d. cytochemical stains

REFERENCES

1. Jamshidi K, Swaim WR. Bone marrow biopsy with unaltered architecture: A new biopsy device. *J Lab Clin Med.* 1971;77:335–42.

2. Rywlin AM, Marvan P, Robinson MJ. A simple technique for the preparation of bone marrow smears and sections. *Am J Clin Pathol.* 1970;53:389–93.

3. Peterson LC, Brunning RD. Bone marrow specimen processing. In: Knowles D, ed. *Neoplastic hematopathology,* 2nd ed. Philadelphia: Lippincott Williams & Wilkins; 2001.

4. Nelson DA, Davey FD. Hematopoiesis. In: Henry SB, ed. *Clinical diagnosis and management by laboratory methods.* 19th ed. Philadelphia: W.B. Saunders; 1996.

5. Longacre TA, Foucar K, Crago S, Chen IM, Griffith B, Dressler L, et al. Hematogones: A multiparameter analysis of bone marrow precursor cells. *Blood.* 1989;73:543–52.

SECTION FOUR • THE ANEMIAS

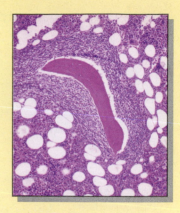

10

Introduction to Anemia

Shirlyn B. McKenzie, Ph.D.

■ CHECKLIST - LEVEL I

Upon completion of this chapter the student should be able to:

1. Describe and identify specific poikilocytes and anisocytes.
2. Classify erythrocytes based on erythrocyte indices.
3. Calculate absolute reticulocyte count and reticulocyte production index from reticulocyte results, hematocrit, and RBC count.
4. Describe and identify erythrocyte inclusions.
5. Recognize abnormal variation in erythrocyte distribution on stained smears.
6. Identify laboratory tests to evaluate erythrocyte destruction.
7. Given CBC results, categorize an anemia according to morphologic classification.
8. Correlate polychromatophilia on a blood smear with other laboratory results of erythrocyte production and destruction.

■ CHECKLIST - LEVEL II

Upon completion of this chapter, the student should be able to:

1. Relate adaptations to anemia with patient symptoms.
2. Correlate patient history and clinical symptoms with laboratory results in anemia.
3. Interpret RDW results.
4. Assess bone marrow response to anemia given CBC and reticulocyte results.
5. Correlate poikilocytes with mechanism of formation and assess clinical significance.
6. Correlate CBC results with findings on a blood smear and troubleshoot discrepancies.
7. Determine the clinical significance of erythrocyte inclusions and select methods to differentiate the inclusions.
8. Evaluate distribution of erythrocytes on stained smears and determine clinical significance.
9. Assess and interpret bone marrow findings in the presence of anemia.
10. Compare the sensitivity and specificity of tests used to screen and confirm a diagnosis of anemia.
11. Compare the morphologic and functional classification of anemia.
12. Given laboratory results, classify an anemia in terms of morphology and function.
13. Choose appropriate follow-up tests to determine anemia classification and evaluate results.

KEY TERMS

- Acanthocyte
- Anisocytosis
- Basophilic stippling
- Cabot rings
- Codocytes
- Echinocytes
- Elliptocytes
- Heinz bodies
- Helmet cells
- Howell-Jolly bodies
- Immature reticulocyte fraction (IRF)
- Knizocytes
- Leptocytes
- Macrocytes
- Megaloblastic
- Microcytes
- Pancytopenia
- Pappenheimer bodies
- Poikilocytosis
- Reticulocyte production index (RPI)
- Schistocytes
- Sickle cells
- Spherocytes
- Stomatocytes
- Target cells
- Teardrops

BACKGROUND BASICS

The information in this chapter will build on the concepts learned in previous chapters. To maximize your learning experience you should review these concepts before starting this unit of study.

Level I

▶ Describe the production, maturation, and destruction of blood cells and explain how the balance between erythrocyte production and destruction is maintained; describe the normal concentration and appearance of an erythrocyte. (Chapters 2, 4)

▶ Summarize the role of hemoglobin in gaseous transport; explain how 2,3-DPG, and H^+ affect oxygen affinity. (Chapter 5)

▶ Discuss the appearance of a normal bone marrow and list reasons why a bone marrow examination may be necessary. (Chapter 9)

▶ Discuss the principle and normal results of the following tests: hemoglobin, hematocrit, reticulocyte count, erythrocyte count, erythrocyte indices; calculate indices. (Chapter 7)

Level II

▶ Identify the stains that may be helpful in assessing bone marrow; correlate peripheral blood findings with bone marrow appearance. (Chapter 9)

▶ Correlate CBC results with findings on the peripheral blood smear and other laboratory test results; determine the validity and accuracy of CBC results and suggest corrective action when necessary. (Chapter 7)

CASE STUDY

We will address this case study throughout the chapter.

George, a 50-year-old male, visited his doctor when he noted the whites of his eyes appeared yellow and that he had dark urine. His CBC revealed a hemoglobin of 31 g/L. Given this clinical description, consider what laboratory tests should be ordered to assist in diagnosis.

▶ OVERVIEW

This chapter serves as a general introduction to anemia. It begins with a description of how anemia develops and the body's adaptations to a decrease in hemoglobin. The emphasis of the chapter is on the laboratory investigation of anemia. This includes discussion of screening tests used to diagnose anemia and other more specific tests used to identify the etiology and pathophysiology of the anemia. Identification of abnormal erythrocyte morphology and its association with anemia is discussed in depth. The chapter concludes with a description of the morphologic and functional classification schemes of anemia and the use of laboratory tests to correctly classify an anemia.

▶ INTRODUCTION

Anemia is functionally defined as a decrease in the competence of blood to carry oxygen to tissues, thereby causing tissue hypoxia. In clinical medicine it refers to a decrease in the normal concentration of hemoglobin or erythrocytes. It is one of the most common problems encountered in clinical medicine. However, anemia is not a disease but rather the expression of an underlying disorder or disease; it is an important clinical marker of a disorder that may be basic or sometimes more complex. Therefore, once the diagnosis of anemia is made, the physician must determine its exact cause.

Treating anemia without identifying its cause may not only be ineffective but could lead to more serious problems. For example, if a patient experiencing iron deficiency anemia due to chronic blood loss were given iron or a blood transfusion, the hemoglobin level might temporarily rise; however, if the cause of the deficiency is not isolated and treated, serious complications of the primary disease may develop, and the anemia would probably return after cessation of treatment. Thus it is necessary to identify and understand the etiology and pathogenesis of an anemia to institute correct treatment.

▶ HOW DOES ANEMIA DEVELOP?

To understand how anemia develops, it is necessary to understand normal erythrocyte kinetics. Total erythrocyte mass (M) in the steady state is equal to the number of new erythrocytes produced per day (P) times the erythrocyte life span (S), which is normally about 100–120 days.

$$M = P \times S$$

Mass   Production   Survival

Thus, the average 70 kg man with 2 liters of erythrocytes must produce 20 mL of new erythrocytes each day to replace the 20 mL normally lost due to cell senescence.[1]

$$\frac{2,000 \text{ mL (M)}}{100 \text{ days (S)}} = 20 \text{ mL/day (P)}$$

From this formula it can be seen that if the survival time of the erythrocyte is decreased by one-half, such as may occur in hemolysis or hemorrhage, the bone marrow must double production to maintain mass at 2,000 mL.

$$\frac{2,000 \text{ mL (M)}}{50 \text{ days (S)}} = 40 \text{ mL/day (P)}$$

New erythrocytes are released as reticulocytes. Thus, the increased production of cells is reflected by the absolute reticulocyte count in the peripheral blood. The marrow can compensate for decreased survival in this manner until production is increased to a level 5–10 times normal, which is the maximal functional capacity of the marrow. Thus, if all necessary raw products for cell synthesis are readily available, erythrocyte life span may decrease to about 18 days before marrow compensation is inadequate and anemia develops. If, however, bone marrow production of erythrocytes does not increase when the erythrocyte survival is decreased, the erythrocyte mass cannot be maintained and anemia develops. There is no mechanism for increasing erythrocyte life span to help accommodate an inadequate bone marrow response.

Thus anemia may develop if: (1) erythrocyte loss or destruction exceeds the maximal capacity of bone marrow erythrocyte production; (2) the bone marrow erythrocyte production is impaired.

▶ INTERPRETATION OF ABNORMAL HEMOGLOBIN CONCENTRATIONS

Diagnosis of anemia is usually made after discovery of a decreased hemoglobin concentration. Hemoglobin is the carrier protein of oxygen; thus, it is expected that a decrease in its concentration is accompanied by a decrease in oxygen delivery to tissues (functional anemia).

Screening for anemia generally relies on the relative hemoglobin and hematocrit. However, there are a few instances when the hemoglobin or hematocrit concentration may be misleading (Table 10-1 ✪).

- In *hypervolemia* the total blood volume increases. This is primarily caused by a plasma volume increase while the erythrocyte mass remains stable. In this case the relative

---

✪ TABLE 10-1

Nonanemic Conditions Associated with Abnormal Hemoglobin/Hematocrit

Conditions in which the hemoglobin or hematocrit may be misleading and require further investigation or interpretation in light of other factors

1. Hematocrit disproportionately low (relative increase in plasma volume):
   - Hydremia of pregnancy
   - Overhydration in oliguric renal failure
   - Congestive heart failure
   - Congestive splenomegaly
   - Chronic diseases
   - Hypoalbuminemia
   - Recumbency
2. Hematocrit disproportionately high (relative decrease in plasma volume):
   - Dehydration
   - Stress erythrocytosis
3. Higher reference range:
   - High altitudes
   - Smokers
4. Presence of abnormal hemoglobins

(Adapted, with permission, from *Wintrobe's Clinical Hematology*, 9th ed. Edited by GH Lee, TC Bithell, J Foerster, JW Athens, JN Lukens. Philadelphia: Lea & Febiger; 1993.)

---

hemoglobin/hematocrit concentration will appear falsely decreased.

- In *hypovolemia*, such as occurs in dehydration, there is a relative decrease in plasma volume resulting in a falsely elevated hemoglobin/hematocrit.

Diagnosis of anemia requires an upward adjustment of hemoglobin and hematocrit values dependent on the altitude.[2] The hemoglobin reference range at high altitudes is higher than the reference range at lower altitude. Therefore, signs of anemia at high altitudes may occur at higher hemoglobin levels than at sea level. Cigarette smoking has a similar effect. The hemoglobin reference range for cigarette smokers is higher than in nonsmokers.[3]

In most cases, the patient's clinical findings are integrated with laboratory test results by the physician to correctly diagnose the illness. The examples mentioned serve to emphasize the fact that the physician, when making a diagnosis of anemia, cannot depend solely on laboratory test results but also must consider patient history, physical examination, and symptoms.

▶ ADAPTATIONS TO ANEMIA

Signs and symptoms of anemia range from slight fatigue or barely noticeable physiologic changes to life-threatening reactions depending on:

- Rate of onset
- Severity of blood loss
- Ability of the body to adapt

With rapid loss of blood as occurs in acute hemorrhage, clinical manifestations are related to hypovolemia and vary with the amount of blood lost. A normal person may lose up to 1,000 mL or 20% of total blood volume and not exhibit clinical signs of the loss at rest, but with mild exercise, tachycardia is common.[4] Severe blood loss of 1,500–2,000 mL or 30–40% of total blood volume leads to circulatory collapse and shock. Death is imminent if the acute loss reaches 50% of total blood volume (2,500 mL).

Slow developing anemias may show an equally severe drop in hemoglobin, as is seen in acute blood loss, but the threat of shock or death is not usually present. The reason for this apparent discrepancy is that in slow developing anemias the body has several adaptive mechanisms that allow organs to function at hemoglobin levels of up to 50% less than normal. The adaptive mechanisms are of two types: an increase in the oxygenated blood flow to the tissues and an increase in oxygen utilization by the tissues (Table 10-2 ✪).

INCREASE IN OXYGENATED BLOOD FLOW

Oxygenated blood flow to the tissues may be increased by increasing the cardiac rate, the cardiac output, and the circulation rate. Oxygen uptake by hemoglobin in the alveoli of the lungs is increased by deepening the amount of inspiration and increasing the respiration rate. In anemia, decreased blood viscosity due to the decrease in erythrocytes and decreased peripheral resistance help to increase the circulation rate, delivering oxygen to tissues at an increased rate. Blood flow to the vital organs, the heart and brain, may preferentially increase while flow to tissues with low oxygen requirements and normally high blood supply such as skin and the kidneys is decreased.

INCREASE IN OXYGEN UTILIZATION BY TISSUE

An important compensatory mechanism at the cellular level that allows the tissue to extract more oxygen from hemoglobin involves an increase in 2,3-DPG (2,3-diphosphoglycer-ate) within the erythrocytes (∞ Chapter 5). An increase in erythrocyte 2,3-DPG is accompanied by a shift to the right in the oxygen dissociation curve, permitting the tissues to extract more oxygen from the blood even though the PO_2 remains constant. It is not clear exactly how anemia stimulates this increase in cellular 2,3-DPG.

Another adaptive mechanism at the cellular level involves the Bohr effect. The scarcity of oxygen causes anaerobic glycolysis by muscles and other tissue, which produces a buildup of lactic acid. This tissue acidosis decreases hemoglobin's affinity for oxygen in the capillaries, thus causing release of more oxygen to the tissues.

Even with these physiologic adaptations, different anemic patients respond differently to similar changes in hemoglobin levels. The extent of the physiologic adaptations is influenced by:

1. Severity of the anemia
2. Competency of the cardiovascular and respiratory systems
3. Oxygen requirements of the individual (physical and metabolic activity)
4. Duration of the anemia
5. Disease or condition that caused the anemia
6. Presence and severity of coexisting disease

▶ DIAGNOSIS OF ANEMIA

Anemia may impair an individual's ability to carry on activities of daily living and decrease the individual's quality of life (QOL). Thus, accurate diagnosis and treatment are essential to improve patient outcomes. The diagnosis of anemia and determination of its cause are made through a combination of information received from the patient history, the physical examination, and the laboratory investigation (Table 10-3 ✪).

HISTORY

The patient's history including symptoms may reveal some important clues as to the cause of the anemia. Information solicited by the physician should include dietary habits, medication taken, possible exposure to chemicals or toxins, and description and duration of the symptoms. The most common complaint is tiredness. Muscle weakness and fatigue develop when there is not enough oxygen available to burn fuel for production of energy.

Severe drops in hemoglobin may lead to a variety of additional symptoms. When oxygen to the brain is decreased, headache, vertigo, and syncope may occur. Dyspnea and palpitations from exertion, or occasionally while at rest, are not uncommon complaints. The patient should be questioned as to any overt signs of blood loss, such as hematuria, hematemesis, and bloody or black stools. Family history may help define the rarer hereditary types of hematologic disor-

✪ **TABLE 10-2**

Adaptations to Anemia

I. Increase in oxygenated blood flow
—Increase in cardiac rate
—Increase in cardiac output
—Increase in circulation rate
—Preferential increase in blood flow to vital organs

II. Increase in oxygen utilization by tissues
—Increase in 2,3-DPG in erythrocytes
—Decreased oxygen affinity of hemoglobin in tissues due to Bohr effect

TABLE 10-3

Important Information for Evaluating a Patient for Anemia

Diagnosis of anemia and determination of its cause requires information obtained from the patient history, physical examination, and laboratory data

I. Patient history
   Dietary habits
   Medications
   Exposure to chemicals and toxins
   Symptoms and their duration:
   a. Fatigue
   b. Muscle weakness
   c. Headache
   d. Vertigo
   e. Syncope
   f. Dyspnea
   g. Palpitations
   Previous record of abnormal blood examination
   Family history of abnormal blood examination

II. Signs of anemia obtained by physical examination
   a. Splenomegaly
   b. Hepatomegaly
   c. Skin pallor
   d. Pale conjunctiva
   e. Hypotension
   f. Jaundice
   g. Koilonychia
   h. Bone deformities in congenital anemias
   i. Smooth tongue
   j. Neurological dysfunction

III. Laboratory investigation
   a. Erythrocyte count
   b. Hematocrit
   c. Hemoglobin
   d. Erythrocyte indices: MCV, MCH, MCHC
   e. Reticulocyte count and reticulocyte production index
   f. Blood smear examination
   g. Leukocyte and platelet quantitative and qualitative examination
   h. Bone marrow examination (depending upon results of other laboratory tests and patient clinical data)
   i. Tests to measure erythrocyte destruction depending upon other information available: serum billrubin, urine hemosiderin, haptoglobin, methalbumin, lactate dehydrogenase (LDH)

- Organomegaly of the spleen and liver are of primary importance in establishing the extent of involvement of the hematopoietic system in production and destruction of erythrocytes. Massive splenomegaly is characteristic of some hereditary chronic anemias. The spleen may also become enlarged in some autoimmune hemolytic anemias when it is the primary site of destruction of antibody sensitized erythrocytes.
- Heart abnormalities may occur as a result of the increased cardiac workload associated with the physiologic adaptations to anemia. Usually cardiac problems occur only with chronic or severe anemias.
- Changes in epithelial tissue from oxygen deprivation will be noted in some patients. Skin pallor is easily noted in most Caucasian patients, but because of variability in natural skin tone, pale conjunctiva is a more reliable indicator of anemia. The presence of pallor, particularly conjunctival pallor, has been shown to be a cost-effective and feasible method to screen for anemia in a variety of settings.[5,6]
- Anemia may also occur secondary to a defect in hemostasis. The presence of bruises, ecchymoses, and petechiae indicates that the platelets may be involved in the disorder that is producing the anemia.
- Hypotension may accompany significant decreases in blood volume.

In addition to these general physical findings associated with anemia, there may be findings associated with a particular type of anemia. These include jaundice in hemolytic anemias, koilonychia in iron deficiency, bone deformities and extramedullary hematopoietic tissue masses in the hereditary hemoglobinopathies, a smooth tongue in megaloblastic anemia, and neurological dysfunction in pernicious anemia.

In addition to determining the extent of anemic manifestations, physical examination helps to establish the underlying disease process causing the anemia. Some disorders associated with anemia include chronic diseases such as rheumatoid arthritis, as well as malignancies, gastrointestinal lesions, kidney disease, parasitic infection, and liver dysfunction.

LABORATORY INVESTIGATION

After the physical examination and patient history, the physician will order laboratory tests if he suspects the patient has anemia. Initially, screening tests are performed to determine if anemia is present and to evaluate erythrocyte production and destruction/loss. The initial screening test is the complete blood count (CBC), which includes hemoglobin, and hematocrit, red blood cell (RBC) count, RBC indices, white blood cell (WBC) count, and platelet count. Depending on these test results, additional tests may be suggested such as the reticulocyte count, bilirubin, and review of the blood smear. In addition, the urine and stool

ders. For example, sickle cell anemia and thalassemia are frequently manifest to some degree in several members of the immediate family.

PHYSICAL EXAMINATION

Physical examination of the patient helps the physician detect the adverse effects of a long-standing anemia (Table 10-3).

may be examined for the presence of blood. These routine tests are followed by a protocol of specific diagnostic tests that help establish the etiology and pathophysiology of the anemia. These specific tests will be discussed in the appropriate chapters on anemia.

Erythrocyte Count, Hematocrit, and Hemoglobin

Determination of the erythrocyte count, hematocrit, and hemoglobin are routine laboratory tests used to screen for the presence of anemia. Generally, concentrations for these parameters parallel each other. Thus, in a clinic or physician's office with limited resources, screening may be limited to either the hematocrit or hemoglobin. Erythrocyte counts are usually performed only if automated instruments are available. If one of the three screening tests is abnormal, it is helpful to have the results of the other two so that the red cell indices can be calculated.

A decreased concentration in one or more of these parameters based on the age and sex of the individual should be followed by other laboratory tests to help establish criteria for diagnosis. The Centers for Disease Control (CDC) recommended cutoff values for a diagnosis of anemia according to age and sex are provided in Table 10-4 ✪. Upward adjustments for these cutoff values should be utilized for individuals living at high altitudes and for those who smoke. There is a direct dose–response relationship between the amount smoked and the hemoglobin level.[3] The CDC recommended

✪ TABLE 10-4

Hemoglobin (Hb) and Hematocrit (Hct) Cutoffs for a Diagnosis of Anemia in Children, Nonpregnant Females, and Males

Age (yrs)/Sex	Hb (g/dL)	Hct (%)
Both sexes		
1–1.9	11.0	33.0
2–4.9	11.2	34.0
5–7.9	11.4	34.5
8–11.9	11.6	35.0
Female		
12–14.9	11.8	35.5
15–17.9	12.0	36.0
≥18	12.0	36.0
Male		
12–14.9	12.3	37.0
15–17.9	12.6	38.0
≥18	13.6	41.0

*Based on fifth percentile values from the Second National Health and Nutrition Examination Survey after excluding persons with a higher likelihood of iron deficiency.

(From: Centers for Disease Control. *Morbidity and Mortality Weekly Report,* 38 (22), June 8, 1989.)

✪ TABLE 10-5

Altitude Adjustments for Hemoglobin (Hb) and Hematocrit (hct) Cutoffs for a Diagnosis of Anemia

Altitude (ft)	Hb (g/dL)	Hct (%)
<3000	0.0	0.0
3000–3999	+0.2	+0.5
4000–4999	+0.3	+1.0
5000–5999	+0.5	+1.5
6000–6999	+0.7	+2.0
7000–7999	+1.0	+3.0
8000–8999	+1.3	+4.0
9000–9999	+1.6	+5.0
>10,000	+2.0	+6.0

(From: Centers for Disease Control. *Morbidity and Mortality Weekly Report,* 38 (22), June 8, 1989.)

adjustments are included in Tables 10-5 ✪ and 10-6 ✪. Hemoglobin and hematocrit values also vary in pregnancy with a gradual decrease in the first two trimesters and a rise during the third trimester (Table 10-7 ✪).

The highest normal hemoglobin, hematocrit, and erythrocyte counts are seen at birth. In the neonate, erythrocytes are macrocytic and the reticulocyte count is 2–6%. From 3 to 10 nucleated erythrocytes per 100 leukocytes may be observed in the peripheral blood during the first week of life. A gradual decrease in these parameters occurs for 2 months after birth. This decline is followed by a gradual increase until normal adult values are reached at about 14 years of age. A difference in erythrocyte values between sexes is noted at puberty, females having lower values than males. The values change very little in normal older adults and increase slightly after menopause.[7] Normal reference ranges for elderly ambulatory clinic patients are given in Table 10-8 ✪. There is a diurnal variation in hemoglobin, hematocrit, and erythrocyte values. Highest values occur in the morning and lowest values occur in the evening.

✪ TABLE 10-6

Adjustments for Hemoglobin (Hb) and Hematocrit (Hct) in Smokers

Characteristic	Hb (gm/dL)	Hct (%)
Nonsmoker	0.0	0.0
Smoker (all)	+0.3	+1.0
½-1 pack/day	+0.3	+1.0
1–2 packs/day	+0.5	+1.5
>2 packs/day	+0.7	+2.0

(From Centers for Disease Control. *Morbidity and Mortality Weekly Report,* 38(22), June 8, 1989.)

⊛ TABLE 10-7

Hemoglobin Cutoffs for a Diagnosis of Anemia in Pregnancy by Month and Trimester*

Gestation (wks)	12	16	20	24	28	32	36	40
Trimester	1[†]	2	2[†]	2	3	3[†]	3	term
Mean Hb (g/dL)	12.2	11.8	11.6	11.6	11.8	12.1	12.5	12.9
5th percentile Hb values (g/dL)	11.0	10.6	10.5	10.5	10.7	11.0	11.4	11.9
§Equivalent 5th percentile hct values (%)	33.0	32.0	32.0	32.0	32.0	33.0	34.0	36.0

*Based on pooled data from four European surveys of healthy women taking iron supplements.
[†] Hb values adapted for the trimester-specific cutoffs.
§ Hematocrit
(From Centers for Disease Control. *Morbidity and Mortality Weekly Report*, 38 (22), June 8, 1989.)

Variations are also reported to occur as a result of blood drawing techniques. Hemoglobin values are about 7 g/L higher if the patient's blood is obtained while the individual is in an upright position rather than supine. Prolonged vasoconstriction by the tourniquet may cause hemoconcentration of the sample and elevate the hemoglobin.

Erythrocyte Indices

The erythrocyte indices help classify the erythrocytes as to their size and hemoglobin content (⊷ Chapter 7). Hemoglobin, hematocrit, and erythrocyte are used to calculate the three indices: mean corpuscular volume (MCV), mean corpuscular hemoglobin concentration (MCHC), and mean corpuscular hemoglobin (MCH). (The conversion factors in the formulas for the indices vary depending on if you use conventional units or Systeme International d Units [SI] units for the hemoglobin and hematocrit. Chapter 7 gives both conversion factors.) The indices give a clue as to what the erythrocytes should look like on the stained blood film. Since abnormal erythrocyte morphology is characteristic of distinct types of anemia, the indices are useful for classification of anemic states.

Mean Cell Volume   The MCV indicates the average volume of individual erythrocytes expressed in femtoliters (fL), (which is 10^{-15}L). It is measured directly on automated cell counters. It also may be manually calculated from the hematocrit and RBC count.

Example

A patient has a hematocrit of 0.45 L/L and an RBC count of 5×10^{12}/L.

$$MCV \ (fL) = \frac{0.45 L/L \ (hct)}{5 \times 10^{12}/L \ (RBC \ count)} \times 1000$$

$$= 90 \times 10^{-15}L \ or \ 90 \ fL$$

⊛ TABLE 10-8

Comparison of Red Blood Cell Measurements of Elderly (over 65 years) and Elderly Nonanemic with a General Population of Individuals

	Red Cell Count (10^{12}/L)	Hemoglobin (gm/dL)	Hematocrit (%)	MCV (fL)	MCH (pg)	MCHC (gm/dL)
Males						
All ages	5.40 ± 0.78	16.00 ± 1.96	47.00 ± .90	87.00 ± 4.90	29.00 ± 1.96	34.00 ± 1.96
Elderly (106)	4.68 ± 1.01	14.09 ± 3.43	42.18 ± 9.50	88.97 ± 16.88	30.32±6.19	33.54 ± 2.98
Elderly nonanemic (98)	4.72 ± 0.96	14.34 ± 2.84	42.82 ± 8.17	90.49 ± 14.44	30.54 ± 4.90	33.64 ± 2.53
Females						
All ages	4.80 ± 0.59	14.00 ± 1.96	42.00±4.90	87.00 ± 4.90	29.00 ± 1.96	34.00 ± .98
Elderly (186)	4.45 ± 1.12	13.37 ± 3.08	40.12 ± 8.92	90.26 ± 15.44	30.30±5.14	33.42 ± 2.49
Elderly nonanemic (177)	4.48 ± 1.03	13.54 ± 2.71	40.59±8.01	90.28 ± 13.72	30.35 ± 4.51	33.48 ± 2.43

MCV, MCH, MCHC = mean corpuscular volume, mean corpuscular hemoglobin, mean corpuscular hemoglobin concentration.
(From: Freedman, M.L. Anemias in the elderly: Physiologic or pathologic. *Hosp. Pract.* 17(5):121, 1982.)

...as a normal volume and

...ells as normocytic, micro-
... ✪). Abnormalities in the
...es of the hematopoietic sys-
...inary assessment of anemia

...s with the appearance of cells
on st... ..., cells with an increased MCV
appear larger [mac... ..., and cells with a decreased MCV
appear smaller [microcytes]). However, it must be remembered that MCV is a measurement of volume, whereas estimation of flattened cells on a blood smear is a measurement of cell diameter. Cell diameter and cell volume are not the same. Spherocytes usually have a normal or only slightly decreased volume (MCV), but on a stained smear they are unable to flatten as much as normal erythrocytes because of a decreased surface area and increased rigidity. Spherocytes, therefore, may appear to have a smaller diameter than normal cells. On the other hand, target cells may appear larger due to an increased diameter but the MCV is normal.

On instruments using hydrodynamic focusing technology, the MCV can change by up to 4 fL if the blood specimen is left uncapped for 4 hours or more due to oxygenation of the blood.[8] The MCV also can increase significantly if blood is stored for 24 hours at room temperature.

Mean Corpuscular Hemoglobin Concentration

The MCHC is the average concentration of hemoglobin in a deciliter of erythrocytes (g/dL). The MCHC is calculated from the hemoglobin and hematocrit.

Example

A patient has a hemoglobin concentration of 15 g/dL and a hematocrit of 0.45 L/L.

$$MCHC(g/dL) = \frac{15 \text{ g/dL (Hb)}}{.45 \text{ L/L (hct)}} = 33 \text{ pg}$$

The value, 33 pg, reveals that the cells contain a normal concentration of hemoglobin and are therefore normochromic.

This index indicates whether the general cell population is normochromic, hypochromic, or hyperchromic (Table 10-10 ✪). The normal MCHC is 32–36 g/dL. The term *hyperchromic* should be used sparingly. The only erythrocyte that is hyperchromic with an MCHC greater than 36 g/dL is the spherocyte. Spherocytes have a decreased surface-to-volume ratio

✪ TABLE 10-9

Classification of Erythrocytes Based on MCV	
Normocytic	80–100 fL
Microcytic	<80 fL
Macrocytic	>100 fL

✪ TABLE 10-10

Classification of Erythrocytes Based on MCHC	
Normochromic	32–36 g/dL
Hypochromic	<32 g/dL
Hyperchromic	>36 g/dL

due to a loss of membrane but have not lost an appreciable amount of their hemoglobin. The MCHC may be falsely increased with hemolysis, cold agglutinins, and/or insufficient blood in relation to EDTA in the collection tube. The erythrocyte's deformability and its viscosity affect the MCV and MCHC measurements using different automated technologies. The MCHC rarely changes using impedence analyzers and, therefore, its usefulness in classifying anemias may be limited.[8] The MCHC from analyzers using hydrodynamic focusing may be more clinically useful.

Mean Corpuscular Hemoglobin

The MCH is a measurement of the average weight of hemoglobin in individual erythrocytes. The MCH is calculated from the hemoglobin and erythrocyte count. The reference range of MCH for normocytic cells is 26–34 pg.

Example

A patient has a hemoglobin concentration of 15 g/dL and an RBC count of 5×10^{12}/L

$$MCH(pg) = \frac{15 \text{ g/dL (Hb)} \times 10}{5 \times 10^{12}/L \text{ (RBC count)}} = 30 \text{ pg}$$

The value 30 pg means the cell contains an average weight of hemoglobin.

The MCH does not take into account the size of a cell; it should not be interpreted without taking into consideration the MCV. It varies in a direct linear relationship with MCV. Smaller cells normally contain less hemoglobin, and larger cells normally contain more hemoglobin. In some anemias a decrease or increase in cell size (MCV) is associated with a proportional decrease or increase in the amount of hemoglobin within the cell (MCH), resulting in a normochromic cell (normal MCHC). In other anemias, however, the decrease in the amount of hemoglobin within the cell (MCH) is substantially more than the decrease in cell size, and the cell appears hypochromic (decreased MCHC). It is important to understand this concept because microcytic cells with an MCH <26 pg are not necessarily hypochromic, and macrocytes with an MCH >34 pg are not usually hyperchromic.

In certain conditions, the indices MCV, MCH, and MCHC may be falsely elevated. These are discussed in ∞ Chapters 7 and 42.

Developmental Changes in Erythrocyte Indices.

The MCV is increased to a mean of 108 fL at birth but decreases to a mean of 77 fL between the ages of 6 months and

2 years (Figure 10-1).[9] It increases to a mean of 80 fL by 5 years of age but does not reach the adult mean of 90 fL until about 18 years of age. The MCH changes in parallel to the MCV throughout infancy and childhood. The MCHC, however, remains constant within the adult range. Between the ages of 12 and 17 years, males have a higher MCHC and lower MCH and MCV than females.[10]

✔ Checkpoint! #1

Calculate the indices and describe the erythrocytes given the following information: Hb 7.1 g/dL, Hct 0.23L/L; RBC count 3.59 × 10¹²/L.

Calculate the indices and describe the erythrocytes given the following information: Hb 7.1 g/dL, Hct 0.23L/L; RBC count 3.59 × 10^{12}/L.

Red Cell Distribution Width   Since the MCV represents an average of erythrocyte volume, it is less reliable in describing the erythrocyte population when there is considerable variation in erythrocyte size (anisocytosis). The RDW is a calculated index provided by some hematology analyzers to help identify anisocytosis. The RDW is the coefficient of variation of erythrocyte volume distribution. It is calculated as follows:

$$\frac{\text{standard deviation of MCV} \times 100}{\text{mean MCV}} = \text{RDW}$$

The reference range for RDW is 11.5–14.5%. All abnormalities found to this time are on the high side, indicating an increase in the heterogeneity of erythrocyte size.

Caution must be used in interpreting the RDW since it is a reflection of the ratio of the standard deviation of cell size and the mean MCV. An increased standard deviation (heterogeneous cell population) with a high MCV may give a

normal RDW. Conversely, a normal standard deviation (homogeneous cell population) with a low MCV may give an increased RDW. Examination of the erythrocyte histogram/cytogram and stained blood smear will give clues as to the accuracy of the RDW in these cases. When the standard deviation is increased, indicating a true variability in cell size, the base of the erythrocyte histogram will be broader than usual.

⊘ CASE STUDY *(continued from page 162)*

George's only complaint was dark urine and the yellow color of his eyes. His CBC results were: Hemoglobin 3.1 g/dL; hematocrit 0.08 L/L; RBC count 0.71 × 10¹²/L; RDW 21.6; reticulocyte 22%. Calculate the erythrocyte indices. 1. Does the information given suggest acute or chronic blood loss? What is the significance of the RDW?

✔ Checkpoint! #2

A patient has an MCV of 130 fL and an RDW of 14.5. Review of the blood smear reveals anisocytosis. Explain the discrepancy between the blood smear finding and RDW.

Reticulocyte Count

Immature, anuclear erythrocytes containing organelles and an extensive ribosomal system for hemoglobin synthesis are known as reticulocytes (∞ Chapter 4). Reticulocytes usually spend 2–3 days in the bone marrow and an additional day in the peripheral blood before losing their RNA and becoming mature erythrocytes. The peripheral blood reticulocyte count indicates effective bone marrow activity and is one of the most useful and cost-effective laboratory tests in monitoring anemia and response to therapy (∞ Chapter 7). It is also helpful in classifying the pathophysiology of anemia. Reticulocytes may sometimes be identified as *polychromatophilic* erythrocytes (erythrocytes with a bluish tinge) on Romanowsky stained smears. The polychromatophilia is due to the presence of basophilic ribosomes (RNA) mixed with acidophilic hemoglobin (Figure 10-2 ■).

Methods for Counting Reticulocytes   The reticulocyte count is one of the few remaining common hematology tests to be performed manually (Figure 10-3 ■). Although automated methods are available on hematology analyzers, over half the laboratories still use the manual method[11] (∞ Chapter 41). Test results are expressed as a percentage of reticulocytes in relation to total RBC count or may be expressed as the absolute number (see next section). The reference range varies among laboratories and the procedure used, but it is about 0.8–4% or 18–158 × 10⁹/L. In the auto-

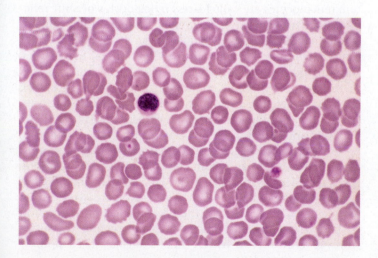

■ **FIGURE 10-1** Peripheral blood from a newborn; note the macrocytic erythrocytes. (Wright-Giemsa stain; 1000× magnification)

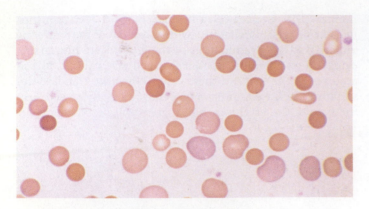

■ **FIGURE 10-2** The large erythrocytes with a bluish tinge are polychromatophilic erythrocytes. They are larger than the more mature erythrocytes. Note also the spherocytes. (Peripheral blood; Wright-Giemsa stain; 1000× magnification)

mated method, over 30,000 RBCs are assessed, so the method is more precise than the manual method (which assesses 1,000 RBCs) and is more accurate when the reticulocyte count is very low.

In the healthy aged, there appears to be a decrease in the lifespan of the erythrocyte.[12] This is compensated for by an active bone marrow, so that the hemoglobin and hematocrit remain in the reference range of other adults. There is, however, a slight reticulocytosis, reflecting the increased production of erythrocytes.

Absolute Reticulocyte Count   In anemia, a more informative index of erythropoietic activity is needed than the relative reticulocyte count. When reported in percentage, the reticulocyte count does not indicate the relationship between the peripheral blood erythrocyte mass and the number of reticulocytes being produced. The percentage can be increased due to either an increase in the number of reticu-

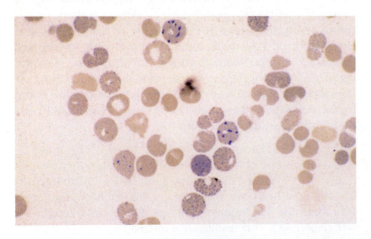

■ **FIGURE 10-3** The erythrocytes with the particulate inclusions are reticulocytes. The inclusions represent reticulum that stains with the supravital stain brilliant cresyl blue. (Peripheral blood; 1000 magnification)

locytes in circulation or a decrease in the number of total RBCs. Therefore, it is recommended that in addition to the percentage of reticulocytes, labs report the absolute reticulocyte count to provide a more useful estimate of reticulocyte production. The absolute count is provided by automated analyzers and can be calculated when using manual methods for reticulocytes:

$$\text{Absolute reticulocyte } (\times 10^9/\text{L}) = \text{RBC count} \\ (\times 10^{12}/\text{L}) \times \text{reticulocyte count (\%)}$$

For example in a patient with an RBC count of $3.5 \times 10^{12}/\text{L}$ and a 10% reticulocyte count, the absolute reticulocyte count is $(3.5 \times 10^{12}/\text{L}) \times 10\% = 350 \times 10^9/\text{L}$. The mean normal value is $90 \times 10^9/\text{L}$.

The corrected reticulocyte count is another means to adjust the reticulocyte count in proportion to the severity of anemia. In this procedure, the percentage of reticulocytes is multiplied by the ratio of the patient's hematocrit to an average normal hematocrit:

$$\text{Corrected reticulocyte count} = \frac{\text{patient hematocrit}}{\text{normal hematocrit}} \times \% \text{ reticulocyte}$$

It is recommended that the absolute count be used in place of the corrected reticulocyte count.[11,13]

✓ **Checkpoint! #3**

Is it possible to have an increased relative reticulocyte count but an absolute reticulocyte count in the normal range? Explain.

Quantitation of Reticulocyte Immaturity   When there is an increased need for reticulocytes, the bone marrow releases reticulocytes earlier than normal. These more immature reticulocytes are called stress reticulocytes or shift reticulocytes. They appear as large polychromatophilic cells on the Romanowsky stained blood smear. It takes longer for these reticulocytes to mature in the peripheral blood since the remainder of the bone marrow maturation time is added to the peripheral blood maturation time (Table 10-11). The more severe the anemia, the earlier the reticulocyte is released. In a stimulated marrow, hematocrit levels of 0.35L/L, 0.25 L/L, and 0.15 L/L are associated with early reticulocyte release and a prolongation of the reticulocyte maturation in peripheral blood to approximately 1.5, 2.0, and 2.5 days, respectively. This is similar to the left shift in granulocytes seen in peripheral blood when there is an increased need for granulocytes. To correct for the prolongation of maturation of these circulating shift reticulocytes and anemia, the **reticulocyte production index** (RPI) is calculated. The following formula is used:

$$\frac{\text{Patient's hematocrit}}{0.45 \text{ L/L}} \times \frac{\text{reticulocyte count (\%)}}{\text{reticulocyte maturation time (days)}}$$

✪ TABLE 10-11

Correlation of the Hematocrit with Reticulocyte Maturation Time in the Peripheral Blood

Hematocrit (L/L)	Reticulocyte Maturation Time (Days)
.35	1.5
.25	2.0
.15	2.5

For example, if a patient with a .25L/L hematocrit had a 15% reticulocyte count, the RPI would be:

$$\frac{.25 \text{ L/L}}{.45 \text{ L/L}} \times \frac{15\%}{2.5} = 3.3 \text{ RPI}$$

The RPI is a good indicator of the adequacy of the bone marrow response in anemia. Generally speaking, an RPI > 2 indicates an appropriate bone marrow response, whereas an RPI < 2 indicates an inadequate compensatory bone marrow response (hypoproliferation) or an ineffective bone marrow response. When utilized in this way, the reticulocyte count provides a direction for the course of investigation concerning anemia etiology and pathophysiology.

Reticulocyte maturity level also can be classified based on semiquantitative assessment of RNA concentration within the maturing erythrocyte. Younger reticulocytes contain more RNA than mature reticulocytes. Some automated hematology instruments not only provide a relative and absolute reticulocyte count but they also assess reticulocytes for maturity level based on RNA content level (assessed by intensity of staining) and report an index of maturity. The term used for this index varies by instrument manufacturer, but it is recommended that it be called the **immature reticulocyte fraction** (IRF).

The Miles H.3/Advia 120 System by Bayer Diagnostics uses a different method to classify reticulocyte maturity. It reports a reticulocyte hemoglobin content (CHr) and mean reticulocyte cell hemoglobin concentration (CHCMr) for reticulocyte maturity level.

The IRF may be helpful in evaluating bone marrow erythropoietic response to anemia, monitoring anemia, and evaluating response to therapy. In anemia, an increased IRF generally indicates an adequate erythropoietic response while a normal or subnormal IRF reflects an inadequate or nonresponse to the anemia.[14] (The normal range using the Cell-Dyn 3500 and 3700 systems with impedence technology is 0.29+/−0.6.)[8] When the bone marrow increases production of erythrocytes, there is an observable increase in the IRF *before* there is an increase in the reticulocyte count or an increase in hemoglobin, hematocrit, or RBC count. After bone marrow transplant, it is the first sign of a successful engraftment. In patients receiving human recombinant erythropoietin (rHuEPO) or iron therapy for anemia, an increased IRF predicts a successful outcome.

It is recommended by the National Committee for Clinical Laboratory Standards (NCCLS) that the IRF index replace the reticulocyte production index (RPI).[11] Laboratories that do not have instruments that measure this parameter may use the RPI.

CASE STUDY *(continued from page 169)*

George's RBC count is 0.7×10^{12}/L and his reticulocyte count is 22%.
2. Calculate his absolute reticulocyte count. Is this count increased, decreased, or normal?

Blood Smear Examination

The erythrocyte is sometimes called a discocyte because of its biconcave shape. On a Romanowsky stained blood smear, the erythrocyte appears as a 7 μm disc with a central area of pallor that is surrounded by a rim of pink staining hemoglobin. The area of pallor is caused by the closeness occurring between the two concave portions of the membrane when the cell becomes flattened on a glass slide. Normally the area of pallor occupies about one-third the diameter of the cell. The area of pallor is not seen in erythrocytes suspended in saline or plasma and viewed with the light microscope.

Although it is not always necessary, review of the stained blood smear assists in diagnosing the type of anemia in 25% of the cases.[15] The normal morphology of the erythrocyte may be altered by various pathological conditions intrinsic or extrinsic to the cell. Careful examination of a stained blood smear will reveal these morphologic aberrations. **Poikilocytosis** is the general term used to describe a nonspecific variation in the shape of erythrocytes (Figure 10-4 ■). **Anisocytosis** denotes a nonspecific variation in the size of the cells. Some variation in size is normal because of the variation in age of the erythrocytes, younger cells being larger and older cells smaller. Some shapes and sizes, however, are particularly characteristic of serious underlying hematologic disorders or malignancy. These include nucleated erythrocytes (except in newborns), schistocytes, teardrop erythrocytes, spherocytes, acanthocytes, and marked erythrocyte shape abnormalities in normocytic anemia without evidence of hemolysis. It is important to keep in mind that some abnormal morphology can be artifactual because of poorly made or improperly stained smears. If artifactual morphology is suspected, the erythrocytes should be examined in a wet preparation. If the abnormal morphology is present in this preparation, the possibility of artifacts can be eliminated.

Poikilocytosis   In the past, poikilocytosis was reported as slight, moderate, or marked (or 1+ to 4+). This practice is being replaced and many laboratories report only significant poikilocytosis. The stained smear should be reviewed keeping in mind the overall context of the laboratory results and

⭐ TABLE 10-12

Abnormalities in the Shape of Erythrocytes

Terminology	Synonyms	Description	Associated Disease States
Poikilocytosis	—	Increased variation in the shape of red cells	See disease states associated with specific poikilocytes on this table
Echinocyte (sea urchin)	Burr cell; crenated cell	Spiculated red cells with short equally spaced projections over the entire surface	Liver disease; uremia; pyruvate kinase deficiency; peptic ulcers; cancer of stomach; heparin therapy
Acanthocyte (spike)	Spur cell	Red cells with spicules of varying length irregularly distributed over the surface	Abetalipoproteinemia; alcoholic liver disease; disorders of lipid metabolism; post splenectomy; fat malabsorption; retinitis pigmentosa
Elliptocyte (oval)	Ovalocyte; pencil cell; cigar cell	Oval to elongated ellipsoid cell with central area of pallor and hemoglobin at both ends	Hereditary elliptocytosis; iron deficiency anemia; thalassemia; anemia associated with leukemia
Drepanocytes (sickle)	Sickle cells	Red cells containing polymerized HbS showing various shapes: sickle shaped, crescent, or boat shaped	Sickle cell disorders
Dacryocyte (tear)	Teardrop; tennis racquet cell	Round cell with a single elongated or pointed extremity; usually microcytic and/or hypochromic	Myelophthisic anemias; thalassemias
Codocyte (bell)	Target cell; Mexican hat cell	Thin bell-shaped cells with an increased surface-to-volume ratio; on stained blood smears they assume the appearance of a target with a bull's eye in the center, surrounded by an achromic zone and outer ring of hemoglobin; osmotic fragility is decreased	Hemoglobinopathies; thalassemias; obstructive liver disease; iron deficiency anemia; splenectomy; renal disease; LCAT deficiency
Schistocytes (cut)	Schizocyte; fragmented cell	Fragments of red cells; variety of shapes including triangles, comma shaped; microcytic	Microangiopathic hemolytic anemias; heart-valve hemolysis; DIC; severe burns; uremia
Keratocytes (horn)	Helmet cells; horn-shaped cells	Red cells with one or several notches with projections that look like horns on either end	Microangiopathic hemolytic anemias; heart-valve hemolysis; Heinz body hemolytic anemia; glomerulonephritis; cavernous hemangiomas
Spherocyte	—	Spherocytic red cells with dense hemoglobin content (hyperchromic); lack an area of central pallor; osmotic fragility is increased	Hereditary spherocytosis; immune hemolytic anemias; severe burns; ABO incompatibility; Heinz-body anemias
Stomatocytes (mouth)	Mouth cell; cup form; mushroom cap	Uniconcave red cells with the shape of a very thick cup; on stained blood smears cells have an oval or slit-like area of central pallor	Hereditary stomatocytosis; spherocytosis; alcoholic cirrhosis; anemia associated with Rh null disease; lead intoxication; neoplasms
Leptocytes (thin)	Thin cell	Thin, flat cell with hemoglobin at periphery; usually cup shaped, MCV is decreased but diameter of cell is normal	Thalassemia; iron deficiency anemia; hemoglobinopathies; liver disease
Knizocytes	—	Red cells with more than two concavities; on stained blood smears there is a dark stick of hemoglobin in center with a pale area on either end	Conditions in which spherocytes are found
Xerocytes	—	Dense, irregularly contracted cells; hemoglobin may be concentrated at periphery of the cell	Familial xerocytosis

and 10-7 ■). Upon staining, these cells exhibit a slit-like (mouth-like) area of pallor. Normal discocytes may be transformed under certain conditions to stomatocytes and, eventually, to spherostomatocytes. The stomatocyte shape is reversible, but the spherostomatocyte is not. Cationic drugs and low pH cause a gradual loss of biconcavity leading to the stomatocyte and eventually formation of a sphere. Stomatocytosis is the opposite of echinocytosis; the shape change in stomatocytosis is thought to be the result of an increase in the area of the inner bilayer of the lipid leaflet membrane.

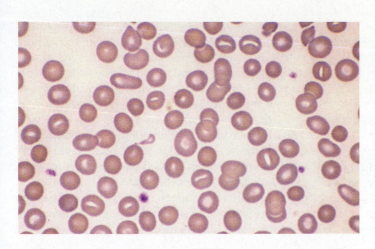

■ FIGURE 10-7 Stomatocytes. Note the slit-like area of pallor. (Peripheral blood; Wright-Giemsa stain; 1000× magnification)

Stomatocytes also may appear as an artifact on stained blood smears, and thus, care should be used in identifying them. Stomatocytes in vivo are characteristic of a rare autosomal dominant hemolytic anemia called hereditary stomatocytosis. Stomatocytes are also associated with a variety of other diseases (Table 10-12 ✪).

Spherocytes.   **Spherocytes** (Figures 10-5b and 10-6c ■) are erythrocytes that have lost their biconcavity due to a decreased surface-to-volume ratio. On stained blood smears the spherocyte appears as a densely stained sphere lacking a central area of pallor. Although the cell often appears microcytic on stained blood smears, the volume (MCV) is usually normal. The spherocyte is the only erythrocyte that may be called hyperchromic because of the increased MCHC. Spherocytes have increased osmotic fragility, with hemolysis beginning in NaCl concentrations of about 0.6% and complete at about 0.4%. Autohemolysis (in vitro suspension of patients' cells and serum) is increased. Spherocytes, which are less deformable than discocytes, have a decreased life span and are removed in the spleen. Spherocytes are seen in hereditary spherocytosis and a variety of other disorders (Table 10-12 ✪). They are a significant finding when associated with hemolytic anemia as it is an indication of immune hemolytic anemia.

Schistocytes.   **Schistocytes** are erythrocyte fragments caused by mechanical damage to the cell (Figures 10-5b and 10-6d ■, Table 10-12 ✪). They appear in a variety of shapes: triangular, comma-shaped, helmet-shaped, and others. Since schistocytes are fragments of erythrocytes they are usually microcytic. They maintain normal deformability, but their survival in the peripheral blood is reduced. The fragments may assume a spherical shape and hemolyze, or they may be removed in the spleen.

Schistocytes may be found whenever blood vessel pathology is present. Erythrocyte fragmentation is particularly as-

sociated with intravascular fibrin formation. Erythrocytes become hung-up on fibrin strands in the vessels (termed the clothes-line effect). The force of blood flow may release the distressed cell intact, or the cell may be fragmented by the fibrin strand, producing schistocytes. This mechanism of erythrocyte damage predominates in microangiopathic hemolytic anemias. Schistocytes may also be seen in valvular lesions, uremia, and march hemoglobinurea. Spheroschistocytes, seen in severe burn victims, are the result of heat damage to the spectrin in the membrane cytoskeleton.

Acanthocytes.   **Acanthocytes,** or spur cells, are small spherical cells with irregular thornlike projections (Figures 10-5b and 10-6e ■). Often the projections will have small bulblike tips. Acanthocytes do not have a central area of pallor. These cells have membranes with altered lipid content. Acanthocytes have a normal life span with a normal to slightly decreased osmotic fragility. Acanthocytes may be seen in liver disease, abetalipoproteinemia (congenital acanthocytosis), and other diseases (Table 10-12 ✪).

Leptocytes.   **Leptocytes** are thin, flat, cells with normal or greater than normal diameter. Although the diameter of the cell is normal or increased, the MCV is usually decreased. The cells have an increased surface-to-volume ratio either as a result of decreased hemoglobin content or increased surface area. The leptocyte is usually cup-shaped like stomatocytes, but the cup has little depth. Target cells may be formed from leptocytes when the depth of the cup increases. Leptocytes are seen in liver disease and in anemias characterized by hypochromic erythrocytes (Table 10-12 ✪).

Target Cells.   **Target cells,** also called Mexican hat cells or **codocytes,** are thin, bell-shaped cells with an increased surface-to-volume ratio (Figure 10-6f ■). On stained blood smears the cells have the appearance of a target with a bull's-eye in the center (Figure 10-8 ■). The bull's-eye is

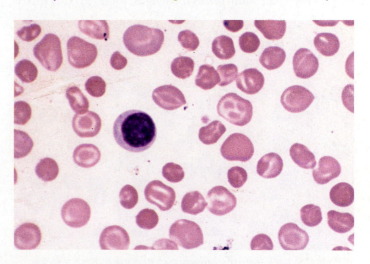

■ FIGURE 10-8 Target cells. (Peripheral blood; Wright-Giemsa stain; 1000× magnification)

surrounded by an achromic zone and a thin outer ring of pink staining hemoglobin. The typical appearance of these cells is only discernible in the area of the slide, where the cells are well separated, but not in the extreme outer feather edge, where all cells are flattened. Target cells may appear as artifacts when smears are made in a high-humidity environment or when a wet smear is blown dry rather than fan dried. Target cells have decreased osmotic fragility due to the increased surface-to-volume ratio of the cell.

Target cells may be seen in disorders in which there is an increase in membrane lipids, such as liver disease. Increased surface-to-volume ratio may also occur as a result of diminution of corpuscular hemoglobin as in iron deficiency anemia and thalassemia. Target cells may occur in some hemoglobinopathies, especially hemoglobin S and hemoglobin C disease (Table 10-12 ✪).

Teardrops.   **Teardrops,** also called dacryocytes, are erythrocytes that are elongated at one end to form a teardrop or pear-shaped cell (Figures 10-6G and 10-9 ■). Some teardrops may form after erythrocytes with cellular inclusions have transversed the spleen. Erythrocytes with inclusions are more rigid in the area of the inclusion, and this portion of the cell has more difficulty passing through the splenic filter than the rest of the cell. As a result, the cell is stretched into an abnormal shape. The teardrop cannot return to its original shape, because the cell either has been stretched beyond the limits of deformability of the membrane or has been in the abnormal shape for too long a time. This is most likely the mechanism of formation of teardrops observed in thalassemia when Heinz bodies are present. Teardrops are also observed in myelofibrosis with myeloid metaplasia and metastatic cancer to the bone marrow. The mechanism of formation of dacryocytes in these pathologic states is unknown (Table 10-12 ✪).

Sickle Cells.   **Sickle cells,** also called drepanocytes, are elongated, crescent-shaped erythrocytes with pointed ends (Figure 10-6h ■). Some forms have more rounded ends with a flat rather than concave side (Table 10-12 ✪). These modified forms of sickle shape may be capable of reversing to the normal discocyte. Sickle cell formation may be observed in wet preparations or in stained blood smears from patients with sickle cell anemia. The hemoglobin within the cell is abnormal and polymerizes into rods at decreased oxygen tension or decreased pH. The cell first transforms into a holly-leaf shape (Figure 10-6i ■). Then, as the hemoglobin polymerization continues, it transforms into a sickle-shaped cell. Some holly-leaf forms may be observed on stained blood smears in addition to the typical sickle shape. The sickle cell has decreased osmotic fragility but increased mechanical fragility. The irregular shape of the cell decreases the erythrocyte sedimentation rate by inhibiting rouleaux formation.

Elliptocytes.   **Elliptocytes,** also called pencil cells and cigar cells, vary from elongated oval shapes (ovalocytes) to elongated rod-like cells (Figures 10-6j and 10-10 ■). They have a central area of biconcavity with hemoglobin concentrated at both ends. Elliptocytes are formed after the erythrocyte matures and leaves the bone marrow, because reticulocytes in patients with elliptocytosis are normal in shape. The mechanism of formation is not known. The osmotic fragility of elliptocytes is normal except in hemolytic hereditary elliptocytosis, when osmotic fragility is increased. Autohemolysis at 48 hours is increased but is corrected by the addition of both glucose and ATP suggesting that elliptocytes have abnormal membrane permeability. Rouleaux formation is normal. Elliptocytes are the predominant shape of erythrocytes in hereditary elliptocytosis. These abnormal shapes also may occur in other diseases (Table 10-12 ✪). Megaloblastic anemia is associated with abnormally large oval erythrocytes called macroovalocytes.

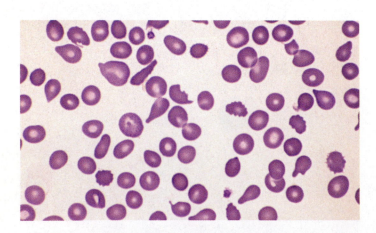

■ FIGURE 10-9 Note the presence of teardrops. Note also the echinocytes, acanthocytes and spherocytes. (Peripheral blood; Wright-Giemsa stain; 1000× magnification)

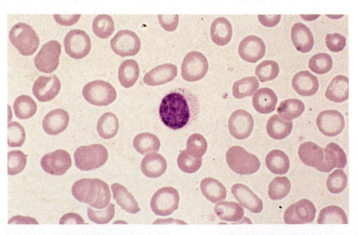

■ FIGURE 10-10 Microcytic, hypochromic erythrocytes. Compare the size of the erythrocytes with the nucleus of the lymphocyte. Normocytic cells are about the same size as the nucleus. There is only a thin rim of hemoglobin around the periphery of the cells indicating they are hypochromic. Note the elliptocytes. (Peripheral blood; Wright-Giemsa stain; 1000× magnification)

Helmet Cells. **Helmet cells,** also called keratocytes, are cells with a concavity on one side and two hornlike protrusions on either end (Figures 10.6k and 10.5b ■). They are produced by impalement on a fibrin strand. The two halves of the erythrocyte hang over the strand as saddlebags; the membranes of the touching sides fuse, producing a vacuole-like inclusion on one side. This cell with an eccentric vacuole is called a blister cell. The vacuole bursts leaving a notch with two spicules on the ends. It has also been suggested that these cells may result from repeated collisions in abnormalities of the circulation. Helmet cells are associated with microangiopathic hemolytic anemia (Table 10-12 ✪).

Knizocytes. **Knizocytes** are cells with more than two concavities (Figure 10-6l ■). The appearance of this cell on stained blood smears may vary depending upon how the cell comes to rest on the flat surface; however, most knizocytes have a dark staining stick in the center with a pale area on either side surrounded by a rim of pink staining hemoglobin. The mechanism of formation is unknown. Knizocytes are associated with spherocytosis. (Table 10-12 ✪).

same size as the lymphocyte nucleus. Figure 10-11 ■ shows erythrocytes with a marked degree of anisocytosis.

Macrocytes. **Macrocytes** are larger than normal erythrocytes, having a diameter greater than 8.0 μm and an MCV over l00 fL. The cell usually contains an adequate amount of hemoglobin resulting in a normal MCHC and normal to increased MCH. Macrocytes are associated with impaired DNA synthesis such as occurs in Vitamin B_{12}, or folate, deficiency as well as other diseases (Table 10-13 ✪). Young erythrocytes are normally larger than mature erythrocytes, but within a day of entering the blood stream they are groomed by the spleen to normal size. When the reticulocyte count is increased, the MCV may be increased.

Microcytes. **Microcytes** are erythrocytes with a diameter less than 7.0 μm and an MCV less than 80 fL. The cell is usually hypochromic but may be normochromic (Figure 10-10 ■). Microcytes in the shape of spheres (microspherocytes) are usually hyperchromic. Microcytes are usually associated with defective hemoglobin formation (Table 10-12 ✪).

@ **CASE STUDY** *(continued from page 171)*

George's blood smear revealed marked spherocytosis.

3. Explain the importance of this finding.

@ **CASE STUDY** *(continued from page 177)*

4. Explain George's abnormal indices.

Anisocytosis Anisocytosis, variation in cell size, may be detected by examining the blood smear and/or by reviewing the MCV and RDW. Normal erythrocytes have a diameter of about 7–8 μm and an MCV of 80–100 fL. If the majority of cells are larger than normal, the cells are macrocytic; if smaller than normal, they are microcytic (Table 10-13 ✪). If there is a significant variation in size with microcytic, normocytic, and macrocytic cells present, the MCV may be normal because it is an average of cell size. In this case, the RDW is helpful. An RDW more than 14.5 suggests that the erythrocytes are heterogeneous in size, which makes the MCV less reliable.[14] Microscopic examination of the cells is especially helpful when the RDW is elevated. To evaluate erythrocyte size microscopically, the cells are compared with the nucleus of a normal small lymphocyte. Normocytic erythrocytes are about the

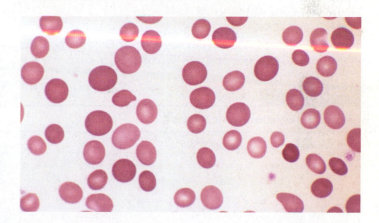

■ **FIGURE 10-11** These erythrocytes show marked anisocytosis. Note the spherocytes. (MCV 104 fL; RDW 30.2) (Peripheral blood; Wright-Giemsa stain; 1000× magnification)

✪ **TABLE 10-13**

Abnormalities in Erythrocyte Size

Terminology	Description	Associated Disease States
Anisocytosis	Increased variation in the range of red cell sizes	See disease states associated with microcytes and macrocytes below
Microcytosis	Red cells with a reduced volume (<80 fL)	Iron deficiency anemia; thalassemia; sideroblastic anemia
Macrocytosis	Red cells with an increased volume (>100 fL)	Megaloblastic anemias; hemolytic anemia; recovery from acute hemorrhage; liver disease; asplenia; aplastic anemia; myelodysplasia; endocrinopathies

✪ TABLE 10-14

Variations in Erythrocyte Color

Terminology	Description	Associated Disease States
Hypochromia	Decreased concentration of hemoglobin in the red cell; red cells have an increased area of central pallor (>1/3 diameter of cell)	Iron deficiency anemia; thalassemia; other anemias associated with a defect in hemoglobin production
Polychromasia	Young red cells containing residual RNA; stain a pinkish gray to pinkish blue color on Wright's stained blood smears; usually appear slightly larger than mature red cells	Hemolytic anemias; newborns; recovery from acute hemorrhage

Variation in Hemoglobin (Color). Normal erythrocytes have an MCH of approximately 30 pg. On stained smears, the erythrocyte has a central area of pallor approximately one-third the diameter of the cell. In certain conditions, the cells may contain less hemoglobin than normal. The only erythrocyte that contains more hemoglobin than normal in relation to its volume is the spherocyte. Spherocytes lack a central area of pallor and stain uniformly dense.

Hypochromic Cells. Hypochromic cells are poorly hemoglobinized erythrocytes with an exaggerated area of pallor (>1/3 the diameter of the cell) on Romanowsky stained blood smears. Hypochromic cells, although occasionally normocytic, are usually microcytic (Figure 10-10 ■). Hypochromic cells are the result of decreased or impaired hemoglobin synthesis (Table 10-14 ✪).

Polychromatophilic Erythrocytes. Polychromatophilic erythrocytes (reticulocytes) are usually larger than normal cells with a bluish tinge on Romanowsky stained blood smears. The bluish tinge is caused by the presence of residual RNA in the cytoplasm. Large numbers of these cells are associated with decreased erythrocyte survival or hemorrhage and an erythroid hyperplastic marrow (Table 10-14 ✪).

Erythrocyte Inclusions. Erythrocytes do not normally contain any particulate inclusions. When present, inclusions can help direct further investigation as they are associated with certain disease states. Diseases/conditions associated with these inclusions are listed in Table 10-15 ✪. The erythrocyte inclusions are described here as they appear on Romanowsky stained blood smears unless otherwise stated.

Basophilic Stippling. Erythrocytes with **basophilic stippling** are cells with bluish black granular inclusions distributed throughout their entire volume (Figure 10-12a ■). The granules may vary in size and distribution from small diffuse to coarse and punctate. The granules, which are composed

✪ TABLE 10-15

Abnormal Erythrocyte Inclusions

Terminology	Description	Associated Disease States
Howell-Jolly bodies	Small, round bodies composed of DNA usually located eccentrically in the red cell; usually occurs singly, rarely more than 2 per cell; stains dark purple with Wright's stain	Post splenectomy; megaloblastic anemias; some hemolytic anemias; functional asplenia; severe anemia
Basophilic stippling	Round or irregularly shaped granules of variable number and size distributed throughout the red cell; composed of aggregates of ribosomes (RNA); stain bluish black with Wright's stain	Lead poisoning; anemias associated with abnormal hemoglobin synthesis; thalassemia
Cabot rings	Appear as a figure-eight, ring, or incomplete ring; thought to be composed of the microtubules of the mitotic spindle; stain reddish violet with Wright's stain	Severe anemias; dyserythropoiesis
Pappenheimer bodies	Iron containing bodies usually found at the periphery of the cell; visible with Prussian blue stain, and with Wright's stain	Sideroblastic anemia; thalassemia; other severe anemias
Heinz bodies	Bodies composed of denatured or precipitated hemoglobin; not visible on Wright's stained blood smears; with supravital stain appear as purple shaped bodies of varying size, usually close to the cell membrane; can also be observed with phase microscopy on wet preparations	G6PD deficiency; unstable hemoglobin disorders; oxidizing drugs or toxins; post splenectomy
Reticulofilamentous substance	Artifactual aggregation of ribosomes; not visible on Wright's stained smears; supravital stain must be used (new methylene blue), appears as deep blue reticular network	Normal reticulocytes

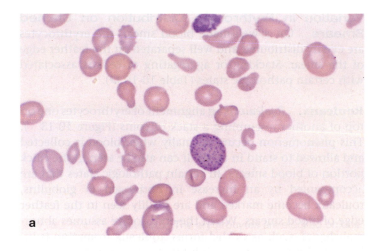

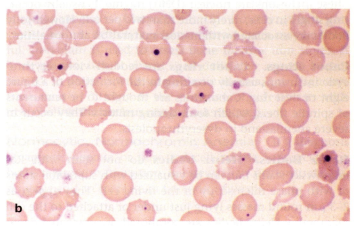

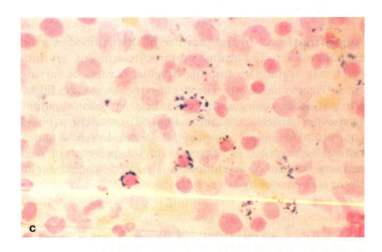

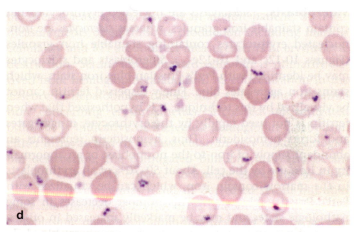

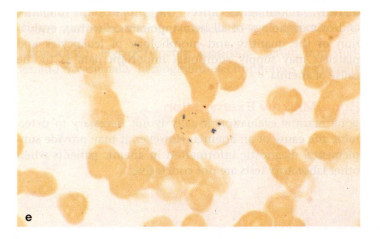

■ **FIGURE 10-12 a.** Erythrocyte with basophilic stippling. Note also the teardrop cells. **b.** Howell-Jolly bodies in erythrocytes. These bodies are the single round purple inclusions. Note echinocytes, acanthocytes, target cells, and spherocytes. **c.** The erythroblasts with blue inclusions (iron granules) are referred to as sideroblasts. These granules do not stain with Romanowsky stains. **d.** These erythrocytes contain iron granules called Pappenheimer bodies. These bodies will stain with both Romanowsky and Perl's Prussian blue stains. **e.** Siderocytes. (a. Peripheral blood; Wright-Giemsa stain; 1000× magnification; b. Peripheral blood; Wright-Giemsa stain; 1000× magnification c. Bone marrow, Perl's Prussian blue stain, 1000× magnification d. Peripheral blood; 1000× magnification; Wright-Giemsa stain e. Peripheral blood; Perl's Prussian blue stain; 1000× magnification)

of aggregated ribosomes, are sometimes associated with mitochondria and siderosomes. It is believed that basophilic stippling is not present in living cells; instead, stippling probably is produced during preparation of the blood smear or during the staining process. Electron microscopy has not shown an intracellular structure similar to basophilic stip-

pling. Cells dried slowly or stained rapidly may demonstrate fine, diffuse stippling as an artifact. Pathologic basophilic stippling is more coarse and punctate.

Howell-Jolly Bodies. **Howell-Jolly bodies** are dark purple or violet spherical granules in the erythrocyte (Figure 10-12b ■).

■ CHECKLIST - LEVEL II (continued)

7. Outline the classification of sideroblastic anemia and describe the differentiating feature of the hereditary type.

8. Describe the relationship of the anemias associated with alcoholism and malignant disease to sideroblastic anemia.

9. Describe the role of molecular diagnostics in hereditary sideroblastic anemia.

10. Explain the significance of finding microcytic anemia in the presence of lead poisoning and suggest reflex testing that would help define an accurate diagnosis.

11. Explain how lead poisoning and alcohol affect erythropoiesis, their relationship to sideroblastic anemia, and recognize the abnormal peripheral blood and clinical features that can be associated with these disorders.

12. Discuss the treatment for iron deficiency, sideroblastic anemia, and anemia of chronic disease and expected laboratory findings associated with successful therapy.

13. Differentiate primary (hereditary) and secondary hemochromatosis and summarize typical results of iron studies in this disease.

14. Describe the genetic abnormality associated with hereditary hemochromatosis and identify the screening and diagnostic tests for this disease.

15. Describe the basic defect in porphyria and its effect on the blood.

16. Develop a reflex testing pathway for an effective and cost-efficient diagnosis when microcytic and/or hypochromic cells are present.

17. Evaluate laboratory test results and use them to identify the etiology and pathophysiology of the anemias that have a defective heme component.

KEY TERMS

Apoferritin
Ferritin
Hemosiderin
Pappenheimer bodies
Percent saturation
Pica
Plumbism
Ropheocytosis
Sideroacrestic
Sideropenic
Total iron-binding capacity (TIBC)
Transferrin
Unsaturated iron-binding capacity (UIBC)

Level II

▶ Function, structure, and synthesis of hemoglobin: diagram the synthesis of heme and explain the role of iron in hemoglobin synthesis. (Chapter 5)

▶ Erythrocyte destruction: diagram degradation of hemoglobin when the erythrocyte is destroyed and interpret laboratory tests associated with erythrocyte destruction. (Chapter 4)

⊚ CASE STUDY

We will address this case study throughout the chapter.
Jose, an 83-year-old anemic male, was admitted to a local hospital with recurrent urinary tract bleeding and an infection associated with prostatitis. Consider how these conditions may affect the hematopoietic system.

BACKGROUND BASICS

The information in this chapter will build on the concepts learned in previous chapters. To maximize your learning experience you should review these concepts before starting this unit of study.

Level I

▶ Diagnosis of anemia: list the laboratory tests used to diagnose and classify anemias and identify abnormal values. (Chapter 10)

▶ Classification of anemia: outline the morphologic and functional classification of anemias. (Chapter 10)

▶ OVERVIEW

This chapter includes a discussion of a group of anemias associated with defective hemoglobin synthesis due to a lack of iron or abnormal utilization of iron. The discussion begins with a detailed description of iron metabolism and lab-

⊛ TABLE 11-1

Causes of Defective Hemoglobin Production That May Result in a Microcytic Hypochromic Anemia

1. Defects in heme synthesis
    - (a) abnormal iron metabolism
        - — iron deficiency
        - — defective iron utilization
    - (b) defective porphyrin metabolism
2. Defects in globin synthesis (thalassemias): deletion or mutation affecting globin genes

oratory tests used to assess the body's iron concentration. This is followed by a description of the specific anemias included in this group—iron deficiency anemia, anemia of chronic disease, and sideroblastic anemia. Hemochromatosis is also discussed even though it is not characterized by anemia. In this disease, iron studies are abnormal and results must be differentiated from sideroblastic anemia. Porphyrias are briefly discussed because porphyrin is an integral component in the synthesis of heme.

▶ INTRODUCTION

Defective hemoglobin production may be due to disturbances in either heme or globin synthesis (Table 11-1 ⊛). The result of these disturbances is a cytoplasmic maturation defect reflected by a microcytic, hypochromic anemia. Defective heme synthesis is caused by faulty iron metabolism (lack of iron or defective iron utilization) or, rarely, by defective porphyrin metabolism (Figure 11-1 ■). Defective globin synthesis is caused by a deletion or mutation of globin genes. These globin deletions and mutations are the result of a hereditary condition known as thalassemia. Thalassemias are discussed in ∞ Chapter 13.

The anemias discussed in this chapter are those defects in heme synthesis caused by faulty iron metabolism: *sideropenic* anemia and *sideroachrestic* anemia. **Sideropenic** anemia is characterized by a deficiency of iron for heme synthesis due to limited dietary intake of iron, malabsorption of iron, or increased iron loss. Sideropenic anemia is referred to as iron deficiency anemia (IDA).

Sideroachrestic anemias are characterized by adequate or excess stores of iron, but because of a block in the insertion of iron into the protoporphyrin ring, heme synthesis is decreased. This block may be the result of an acquired or inherited defect in porphyrin synthesis (sideroblastic anemia) or of defective reuse of iron from the macrophage (anemia of chronic disease).

For convenience, the rare erythropoietic porphyrias, congenital defects in porphyrin metabolism, are also included in this chapter. Except for the erythropoietic porphyria type, the porphyrias are not generally characterized by the presence of anemia.

▶ IRON METABOLISM

Iron is required by every cell in the body. It has vital roles in oxidative metabolism, in cellular growth and proliferation, and in oxygen transport and storage.[1] To serve in these functions, iron must be bound to protein compounds. Iron in inorganic compounds or in ionized forms is potentially dangerous. If the amount of iron exceeds the body's capacity to transport and store it in the protein-bound form, iron toxicity may develop, causing damage to cells. Conversely if too little iron is available, the synthesis of physiologically active iron compounds is limited, and critical metabolic processes are inhibited.

DISTRIBUTION

Iron-containing compounds in the body are one of two types: (1) functional compounds that serve in metabolic (hemoglobin) or enzymatic functions (iron responsive element-

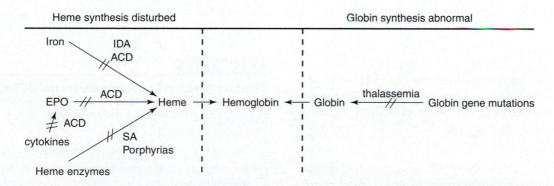

■ FIGURE 11-1 Sites of defective hemoglobin synthesis that can result in anemia. Some of these anemias are hereditary or congenital and others are acquired. (ACD = anemia of chronic disease; IDA = iron deficiency anemia; SA = sideroblastic anemia; EPO = erythropoietin)

⭑ TABLE 11-2

Composition and Distribution of Iron in Adults

Compound	Iron Content, Male (mg Iron/ Kg Body Weight)	Iron Content, Female (mg Iron/ Kg Body Weight)	Percent of Total Iron
Functional iron			
Hemoglobin	31	28	60–75
Myoglobin	5	4	10
Heme enzymes (cytochromes, catalases, peroxidases)	1	1	0.5
Nonheme enzymes (iron-sulfur proteins, metalloflavoproteins, ribonucleotide reductase)	1	1	0.5
Transport			
Transferrin	<1	<1	0.1
Storage			
Ferritin	8	4	10–20
Hemosiderin	4	2	5–10
Total iron	50	40	

binding protein); and (2) compounds that serve as transport (transferrin, transferrin receptor) or storage forms (ferritin and hemosiderin) for iron (Table 11-2 ⭑). The total iron concentration in the body is 40–50 mg of iron/kg of body weight. Men have higher amounts than women.

Hemoglobin constitutes the major fraction of body iron (functional iron) with a concentration of 1 gm iron/kg of erythrocytes or about 0.5 mg iron/mL blood. Iron in hemoglobin remains in the erythrocyte until the cell is removed from circulation. Hemoglobin released from the erythrocyte is then degraded in the macrophages of the spleen and liver, releasing iron. Approximately 85% of this iron is promptly recycled from the macrophage to the plasma where it is bound to the transport protein, **transferrin,** and delivered to developing normoblasts in the bone marrow for heme synthesis. This iron recycling provides most of the marrow's daily requirement for erythropoiesis (∞ Chapter 4).

ABSORPTION

Absorption occurs primarily in the mucosal cells of the proximal small intestine. The amount of iron absorbed is dependent on three important factors (Table 11-3 ⭑):

- The amount of iron absorbed
- Its bioavailability
- The iron balance of the individual

Absorption decreases progressively as iron passes farther down the gastrointestinal (GI) tract. Dietary iron must be exposed to the intestinal absorptive surface at sufficient intervals to permit adequate absorption by mucosal cells; thus,

increased motility of nutrients through the gastrointestinal tract or decreased absorptive surface area may result in decreased iron absorption.

Absorption depends not only upon the amount of iron present in the diet but also on the form of iron ingested and the food mixture eaten. Thus, the quantity of iron absorbed cannot be predicted from the amount of iron ingested.

Dietary iron exists in two different forms: nonheme iron (ferric form) present in vegetables and whole grains, and heme iron (ferrous form) present primarily in red meats in the form of hemoglobin. The ferric complexes are not easily absorbed. During digestion, ferric complexes are broken down; iron is reduced to the ferrous form and bound to high molecular weight chelators (an organic ligand that binds metal atoms). Chelators, gastric HCl, dietary lactic acid, and ascorbic acid help stabilize iron in the soluble, more easily absorbed ferrous form.

⭑ TABLE 11-3

Factors Affecting Iron Absorption in the GI Tract

1. Dietary iron intake: amount and forms ingested

2. Condition of mucosal cells in the GI tract

3. Intraluminal factors: parasites, toxins, intestinal motility

4. Hematopoietic activity of bone marrow: rate of activity directly related to the amount absorbed

5. Tissue iron stores: amount of storage iron inversely related to the amount absorbed

Heme iron is more readily absorbed than nonheme iron. Heme is split from the globin portion of hemoglobin in the intestine and is then assimilated directly by the mucosal cells. Once inside the mucosal cell, iron is believed to be released from heme by heme oxygenase. The iron then enters the same iron pool as nonheme iron.

There appears to be a predetermined set-point of iron stores that results in a negative correlation between the amount of iron absorbed and the amount of iron stored.[2] The efficiency of intestinal absorption of iron increases in response to accelerated erythropoietic activity and depletion of body iron stores. For instance, bleeding, hypoxia, or hemolysis results in accelerated erythrocyte production and enhanced absorption of iron. Increased iron uptake in extravascular hemolytic anemias, however, may lead to an excess of iron in various organs because the body does not actually lose the iron from erythrocytes hemolyzed in vivo. Conversely, diminished erythropoiesis, such as occurs in starvation, decreases the absorption of iron.

IDA due to a lack of dietary iron is usually treated with daily oral doses of ferrous salts. The efficiency of absorption of this therapeutic iron is greatest during initial treatment when body stores are depleted. Increased absorption occurs up to 6 months after hemoglobin values return to normal or until iron stores are replenished. Absorption is also increased 10–20% in early stages of developing ID.

TRANSPORT

Once in the mucosal cell, iron may combine with apoferritin, to form ferritin, or it may cross into the plasma and bind in the ferric form to the carrier protein, transferrin (Figure 11-2 ■).

Transferrin

Transferrin is a true plasma transport protein that mediates iron exchange between tissues (Table 11-4 ✪). It is not lost in delivering iron to the cells but returns to the plasma and is reused. Transferrin is a major serum protein. It is a single polypeptide chain composed of two homologous lobes, each of which contains a single iron binding site. The binding of a ferric iron to either site is random. If only one transferrin lobe binds an iron molecule it is termed monoferric transferrin, whereas if both sites are occupied it is diferric transferrin.

Each gram of transferrin will bind 1.4 mg of iron. Enough transferrin is present in plasma to bind 253–435 μg of iron per deciliter of plasma. This is referred to as the **total iron-binding capacity (TIBC).**

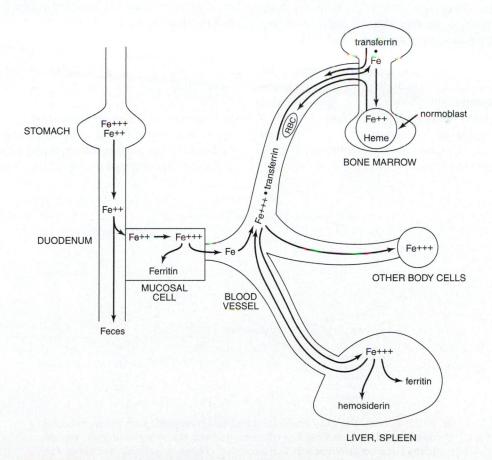

■ FIGURE 11-2 The supply, transport, and storage of iron.

✪ TABLE 11-4

Characteristics of Transferrin

- Function: responsible for transporting iron
- B_1-globulin
- MW 79,570 D
- Half-life: 18 days
- Synthesized in the liver

Serum iron concentration is about 70–201 µg/dL and almost all (95%) of this iron is complexed with transferrin; thus, transferrin is about one-third saturated with iron (serum iron/TIBC × 100 = % saturation of transferrin). The reserve iron-binding capacity of transferrin is referred to as the serum **unsaturated iron-binding capacity, UIBC** (TIBC − serum iron = UIBC).

The majority of transferrin-bound iron is delivered to the developing bone marrow normoblasts, where the iron is released for use in hemoglobin synthesis. Iron in excess of requirements is deposited in tissue for storage.

Only a small amount of transferrin-bound iron is derived from iron absorbed by mucosal cells. Most of the iron bound to this protein is recycled iron derived from the monocyte-macrophage system. The major flow of iron in the body is therefore undirectional, passing from transferrin to erythroid marrow, then to erythrocytes, and finally to macrophages when the senescent erythrocyte is removed and degraded by liver, bone marrow, and splenic macrophages. Released iron from hemoglobin catabolism in the monocyte-macrophage system enters the plasma and is again bound to transferrin for transfer to the bone marrow (Figure 11-3 ■).

In contrast to serum ferritin, transferrin is a negative acute phase reactant. Increased levels are found in pregnancy and in estrogen therapy.

Lactoferrin also functions as an iron transport protein but is found primarily in tissue fluid and cells. It is important in protecting the body from infection.

Transferrin Receptor (TfR)

Transferrin releases iron at specific receptor sites on the developing cell, referred to as the transferrin receptor (TfR). These receptors are expressed on virtually all cells, but the number per cell is a function of cellular iron requirements. Cells with high iron requirements have high numbers of TfR. Erythroid precursors, especially intermediate normoblasts that are rapidly synthesizing hemoglobin, have high numbers of transferrin receptors, about 800,000 per cell. The TfR is a transmembrane glycoprotein dimer with two identical subunits, each of which can bind a molecule of transferrin.

Iron enters the cell in an energy- and temperature-dependent process called **ropheocytosis.** After binding of transferrin to the receptor, the transferrin-receptor complex rapidly clusters with other transferrin-receptor complexes on the cell membrane, and the membrane invaginates and seals forming an endosome with the complex inside (Figure 11-4 ■). In the acidic endosome, iron is released from transferrin. The endosome with the transferrin and receptor is transported back to the surface of the cell. The transferrin is released to the plasma making both it and the receptor available for recycling. Cells release their transferrin receptors as they mature. Thus with increased erythropoiesis, there is an increase in transferrin receptors in the plasma.

STORAGE

The primary iron storage depot is the liver. The largest non-heme iron stores in the body are hemosiderin and ferritin (Table 11-5 ✪). Storage iron provides a readily available iron supply in the event of increased iron loss through bleeding.

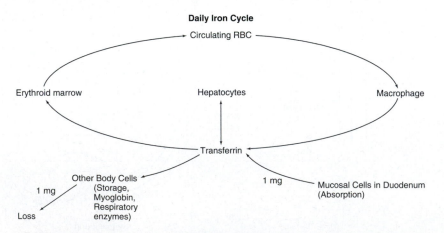

■ **FIGURE 11-3** The daily iron cycle. Most iron is recycled from the erythrocytes to the bone marrow. Only a small amount of iron is lost from the body through loss of iron containing cells. To maintain iron balance, a similar amount of iron is absorbed from the duodenum.

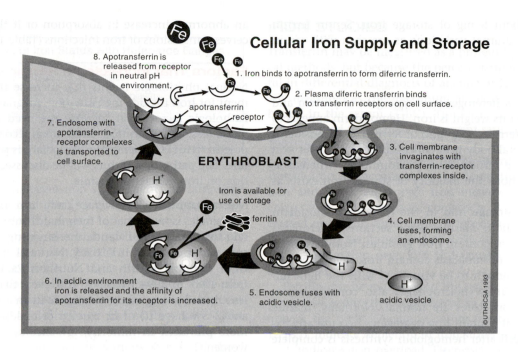

Cellular Iron Supply and Storage

8. Apotransferrin is released from receptor in neutral pH environment.

1. Iron binds to apotransferrin to form diferric transferrin.

apotransferrin receptor

2. Plasma diferric transferrin binds to transferrin receptors on cell surface.

7. Endosome with apotransferrin-receptor complexes is transported to cell surface.

ERYTHROBLAST

3. Cell membrane invaginates with transferrin-receptor complexes inside.

Iron is available for use or storage

ferritin

4. Cell membrane fuses, forming an endosome.

6. In acidic environment iron is released and the affinity of apotransferrin for its receptor is increased.

5. Endosome fuses with acidic vesicle.

acidic vesicle

©UTHSCSA 1993

■ **FIGURE 11-4** Iron binds to apotransferrin in the plasma forming monoferric or diferric transferrin. Transferrin binds to transferrin receptors on the cell surface. The transferrin-receptor complex enters the cell, where the iron is released. The apotransferrin-receptor complex is transported to the cell surface, where the apotransferrin is released to the plasma for reutilization. (Adapted from: Hoffman R, Benz EJ, Shattil SJ, Furie B, Cohen HJ, eds. *Hematology: Basic Principles and Procedures.* New York: Churchill Livingstone; 1991.)

Depletion of these storage compounds reflects an excess iron loss over that which is absorbed.

Ferritin

Ferritin consists of a spherical protein shell that can store up to 4,500 iron atoms. Ferritin is 17–33% iron by weight. Ferritin without iron in its shell is called **apoferritin.**

Isoferritins exist that are composed of various proportions of two polypeptides, heavy (H) and light (L). Isoferritins in the heart, placenta, and erythrocytes are rich in the H subunit, while isoferritins in the iron storage sites, such as the liver and spleen, are rich in the L subunits.

Ferritin acts as the primary storage compound for the body's iron needs and is readily available for erythropoiesis. It is found in the bone marrow, liver, and spleen. It is also an important antioxidant that protects cells against ferrous iron-catalyzed oxidative damage.

Ferritin is a water-soluble form of iron that cannot be visualized by microscopy and does not stain with iron stains. It is primarily an intracellular protein, but small amounts enter the blood through active secretion or cell lysis. The amount of circulating ferritin parallels the concentration of storage iron in the body. Therefore serum ferritin concentration is a reliable index of iron stores; 1 ng/mL of serum fer-

⭐ TABLE 11-5			
Storage Forms of Iron			
Iron Form	**Role**	**Laboratory Analysis**	**Reference Range**
Ferritin	Primary storage form of soluble iron; readily released for heme synthesis	Serum ferritin levels	100±60 µg/L
Hemosiderin	Major long-term storage form of iron; slow release	Bone marrow estimation using Prussian blue stain	40–60% sideroblasts in bone marrow

⊛ TABLE 11-9

Laboratory Test Profile of Fe Status

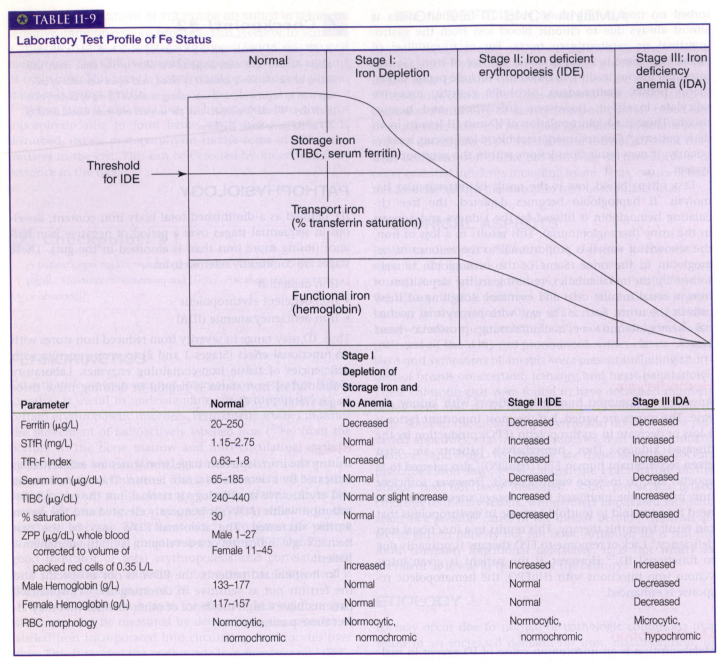

Parameter	Normal	Stage I Depletion of Storage Iron and No Anemia	Stage II IDE	Stage III IDA
Ferritin (µg/L)	20–250	Decreased	Decreased	Decreased
STfR (mg/L)	1.15–2.75	Normal	Increased	Increased
TfR-F Index	0.63–1.8	Increased	Increased	Increased
Serum iron (µg/dL)	65–185	Normal	Decreased	Decreased
TIBC (µg/dL)	240–440	Normal or slight increase	Increased	Increased
% saturation	30	Normal	Decreased	Decreased
ZPP (µg/dL) whole blood corrected to volume of packed red cells of 0.35 L/L	Male 1–27 Female 11–45	Increased	Increased	Increased
Male Hemoglobin (g/L)	133–177	Normal	Normal	Decreased
Female Hemoglobin (g/L)	117–157	Normal	Normal	Decreased
RBC morphology	Normocytic, normochromic	Normocytic, normochromic	Normocytic, normochromic	Microcytic, hypochromic

STfR = serum transferrin receptor; TfR-f = transferrin receptor-ferritin; zpp = zinc protoporphyrin

Stage 3

A long-standing negative iron flow eventually leads to the last stage of iron deficiency—IDA. Blood loss may significantly shorten the time for this stage to develop. All laboratory tests for iron status become markedly abnormal. The most significant finding is the classic microcytic hypochromic anemia.

It is apparent then, that when microcytic hypochromic anemia is present, the situation represents the advanced stage of severely deficient total body iron.

CLINICAL FEATURES

The onset of IDA is insidious, usually occuring over a period of months to years. Early stages of ID usually show no clinical manifestations, but as anemia develops, clinical symptoms appear. In addition to symptoms of anemia, a variety of other abnormalities may occur due to an absence of tissue iron in iron-containing enzymes. These include koilonychia (concavity of nails), glossitis, pharyngeal webs, muscle dysfunction, inability to regulate body temperature when cold or stressed, and gastritis.

A curious manifestation of ID is the *pica* syndrome. **Pica** is an unusual craving for ingesting unnatural items as food. The most common dysphagias described in patients with ID include ice-eating (phagophagia), dirt/clay-eating (geophagia), and starch-eating (amylophagia). In one study of 55 patients with IDA, 58% had pica, and of these 88% had phagophagia.[13] Among some cultural groups, pica is a practiced custom that may lead to the development of ID. A study in Kenya revealed that 56% of pregnant women ate soil regularly. There was a strong association with low hemoglobin and serum ferritin in these women.[14]

Iron deficient infants perform worse in tests of mental and motor development than do nonanemic infants.[15] There is speculation that untreated ID at this stage of human development has long-lasting effects on the central nervous system.[16] Symptoms reported to occur in iron deficient children include irritability, loss of memory, and difficulties in learning. Deficiencies of the immune system have been attributed to iron-related impairment of host defense mechanisms.

In the absence of iron in the gut, other metals are absorbed in increased amounts. This can be significant when an iron-deficient person is exposed to toxic metals such as lead, cadmium, and plutonium.

LABORATORY FEATURES

Laboratory tests are essential to an accurate diagnoses of ID and in evaluation of therapy.

Peripheral Blood

The blood picture in well-developed ID is microcytic (MCV 55–74 fL), hypochromic (MCHC 22–31 g/dL, MCH 14–26 pg) (Figure 11-5 ■). Because ID develops progressively, any gradation between the well-developed microcytic hypochromic

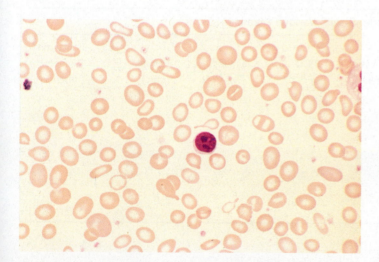

■ **FIGURE 11-5** Microcytic, hypochromic anemia of iron deficiency. (Peripheral blood; Wright-Giemsa stain; 1000× magnification)

iron-deficient picture and normal may occur. Microcytosis and anisocytosis, characterized by an increased RDW, are usually the first morphologic signs, developing even before anemia (∞ Chapter 10). The blood film demonstrates progressively abnormal poikilocytosis. The most frequent poikilocytes are target cells and elliptocytes or dacryocytes.

The typical blood picture may be masked if the iron deficient patient has a concurrent vitamin B_{12} or folate deficiency (causes of macrocytic anemia). In these cases microcytosis may become apparent only after vitamin B_{12}/folic acid replacement therapy.

Both the relative and absolute number of reticulocytes may be normal or even slightly increased, but the reticulocyte count is decreased in relation to the severity of the anemia, with an RPI less than two. A decreased CHr is an early indicator of iron-restricted erythropoiesis in nonanemic individuals and may be a promising alternative or adjunct to iron studies.[12] In patients on chronic hemodialysis, the CHr has been shown to be superior to the presence of hypochromic red cells in detecting iron deficiency. Using a cut-off of CHr <26 pg, the CHr has a sensitivity of 100% and a specificity of 73%.[17]

The leukocyte count is usually normal but may be increased due to chronic marrow stimulation in long standing cases or after hemorrhage. With concomitant hookworm infestation, eosinophilia may be present.

Platelets may be normal, increased, or decreased. Thrombocytopenia may occur in patients with severe or long-standing anemia, especially if accompanied by folate deficiency. Thrombocytosis frequently accompanies ID. It has been proposed that thrombocytosis is related to ID caused by chronic blood loss. Numeric changes seen in platelets are corrected with treatment that replenishes iron stores.

ⓒ **CASE STUDY** *(continued from page 190)*

Jose, our 83-year-old patient, had a CBC upon admission. The results were:

RBC:	4.15×10^{12}/L
Hb:	81 g/L
Hct:	0.26 L/L
Platelets:	174×10^9/L
WBC:	2.8×10^9/L

1. How would you describe his anemia morphologically?

Iron Studies

Iron studies on iron deficient patients will help establish the diagnosis. The serum iron is decreased, usually less than 30 μg/dL, the TIBC is increased, transferrin saturation is decreased to less than 16%. Serum iron concentration has a diurnal variation with highest levels in the morning, so sampling time is an important consideration.

⊕ TABLE 11-10

Serum Ferritin Cutoff Levels for Detecting Iron Deficiency in Patients with Other Diseases and Conditions

Disease	Upper Serum Ferritin Cut-Off Levels for a Diagnosis of ID
Chronic renal disease (absolute ID)	100 µg/L
*Chronic renal disease on EPO therapy (Functional ID)	100–800 µg/L
Anemia of chronic disease	50 µg/L
Rheumatoid arthritis	70 µg/L
Other medical problems	100 µg/L
Pregnancy	30 µg/L
Reference range:	
Males 20–250 µg/L	
Females 10–200 µg/L	

*Functional iron deficiency is present when iron saturation is 20–50%, serum ferritin 100–800 µg/L, and patient responds to intravenous iron therapy with an increase in hemoglobin and/or a decrease in requirement for EPO.

The serum ferritin level is decreased in all stages of ID and may be the first indication of a developing ID. Serum ferritin is generally considered the single best test to detect iron deficiency. Once serum ferritin levels fall below 12 µg/L, the levels may no longer correlate with storage iron because stores are exhausted. Serum ferritin is an important test to differentiate IDA from other microcytic hypochromic anemias. Levels are normal to increased in the anemia of chronic disease unless complicated by ID, and increased in sideroblastic anemia and thalassemia.

Since serum ferritin is an acute phase reactant, the lower limit of the reference range for this parameter may need to be reset to detect ID in some patient populations (Table 11-10 ⊕). It has been suggested that to detect ID in patients with concommitant anemia of chronic disease, inflammation, infection, pregnancy, and a wide range of concomitant medical problems the lower limit of serum ferritin should be raised from 12 g/L.[10, 18–21] It has also been suggested that the threshold level of serum ferritin for a diagnosis of ID in the aged subject be raised since serum ferritin levels rise with age.[22]

The serum transferrin receptor assay has proved useful in detecting and differentiating IDA and anemia of chronic disease. Patients with ID have a mean sTfR level over two times (13.91 + 4.63 mg/L) that of mean sTfR levels in normal individuals (5.36 + 0.82 mg/L). Conversely, patients with chronic disease and acute infection have mean levels almost identical to those of normal individuals (Table 11-11 ⊕). Receptor levels also parallel the reticulocyte count, suggesting that the receptor level may reflect the turnover of transferrin receptors as cells mature. Thus the sTfR level may provide an index of erythrocyte production in the marrow.

A combination of sTfR and serum ferritin can be used to calculate the TfR-F index.

$$TfR\text{-}F \text{ Index} = sTfR/\log \text{ferritin}$$

This index may improve detection of subclinical iron deficient states in healthy individuals.[23,24] An index of >1.8 indicates depletion of iron stores.

Combinations of serum ferritin, MCV, TIBC, percent saturation, and sTfR may eliminate the need for costly, inconve-

⊕ TABLE 11-11

Comparison of Iron Status Parameters Between Groups of Patients with Various Diseases

Patient Group	Hemoglobin (gm/L)*	MCV (fL)*	Serum Iron (µg/dL)*	TIBC (µg/dL)*	Saturation (%)*	Ferritin (µg/L)†	Transferrin Receptor (mg/L)
Normal controls (n = 17)	143 ± 12	93 ± 3	75 ± 28	377 ± 67	20 ± 8	43 (23–80)	5.36 ± 0.82
Iron-deficiency anemia (n = 17)	95 ± 12	74 ± 8	21 ± 15	428 ± 76	5 ± 4	7 (4–12)	13.91 ± 4.63
Acute infection (n = 15)	139 ± 12	88 ± 5	32 ± 23	302 ± 120	14 ± 15	252 (103–613)	5.11 ± 1.42
Anemia of chronic disease (n = 41)	102 ± 12	84 ± 7	35 ± 25	257 ± 87	14 ± 11	220 (86–559)	5.65 ± 1.91
Acute hepatitis (n = 5)	144 ± 8	94 ± 4	121 ± 72	400 ± 70	33 ± 24	2438 (1071–5552)	4.80 ± 1.19
Chronic liver disease with anemia (n = 10)	111 ± 13	97 ± 9	52 ± 32	193 ± 80	28 ± 19	280 (116–677)	5.98 ± 2.06

*Data expressed as mean ± S.D.
†Data expressed as geometric mean ± S.D.
MCV = mean cell volume
TIBC = total iron binding capacity
(With permission from: Ferguson BJ, et al.: Serum transferrin receptor distinguishes the anemia of chronic disease from iron deficiency anemia. *Journal of Laboratory and Clinical Medicine* 119: 385, 1992)

nient, and painful bone marrow examination to assess iron stores in patients with inflammation or chronic disease and in early stages of ID.[18,25,26]

CASE STUDY *(continued from page 201)*

Reflex testing for anemia followed on Jose based on the CBC results. The following test results were obtained:

Reticulocyte count:	2.6%
Serum iron:	18 μg/dL
TIBC:	425 μg/dL

2. Calculate % saturation.
3. Is this value normal, decreased, or increased?
4. What disease, if any, is suggested by this value?

Erythrocyte Protoporphyrin (EP) Studies

The evaluation of EP, using ZPP measurement, is useful when attempting to identify the etiology of microcytic hypochromic anemia. The concentration of ZPP is increased in iron deficient erythropoiesis and in anemias where heme synthesis is disturbed. Since ZPP persists throughout the lifespan of the cell, a measure of ZPP utilizing a hematofluorimeter provides a retrospective indicator of iron availability at the time of cell maturation. The ZPP measurement correlates inversely with serum ferritin concentration but is more cost-effective and diagnostically efficient.[27] It can detect iron depletion even before anemia develops and thus is a good screening tool for the early stages of ID. Since there is a significant number of nonanemic toddlers with iron depletion and ID has a detrimental effect on development in children, ZPP should be considered as a more sensitive test of ID than the hematocrit.[28] ZPP is also more diagnostically efficient than serum iron or serum ferritin in screening for ID in the presence of infection or inflammation and in hospitalized patients with microcytic anemia.[27,29] Thus, ZPP may be a valuable screening assay for these populations.

The level of ZPP is useful also as a screening test to differentiate ID and thalassemia, the two most common causes of microcytic hypochromic anemia. ZPP may be elevated in thalassemia but the increase in ID is 3–4 times higher than in thalasssemia.[30] When laboratory analysis reveals a high ZPP combined with a high RDW, ID is strongly suggested.[31] The RDW is normal or only slightly elevated in thalassemia trait. Table 11-12 lists other conditions associated with increased EP levels.

In patients with concurrent lead poisoning, the ZPP cannot be used to distinguish ID and thalassemia because lead inhibits ferrochelatase, the enzyme needed to incorporate iron into the protoporphyrin ring. Consequently, the free erythrocyte porphyrin complexes with zinc. Hence, ZPP is increased in lead poisoning whether or not iron is available.

★ TABLE 11-12

Conditions Associated with Increased Erythrocyte Protoporphyrin (EP)

Anemia of chronic disease

Iron deficiency anemia

Lead poisoning

Erythropoietic protoporphyria

Some sideroblastic anemias

Conditions with markedly increased levels of erythropoiesis

Thalassemia

Bone Marrow

The bone marrow shows mild to moderate erythroid hyperplasia with a decreased M:E ratio. Total cellularity is often moderately increased. This increase in marrow erythropoietic activity without a corresponding increase in peripheral blood reticulocytes suggests an ineffective erthropoietic component. With appropriate iron therapy the erythroid hyperplasia initially increases and then returns to normal. A common finding (not exclusive to IDA) is the presence of poorly hemoglobinized normoblasts with scanty irregular (ragged) cytoplasm. This change is most evident at the polychromatophilic stage. Erythroid nuclear abnormalities are sometimes present and may resemble the changes found in dyserythropoietic anemia. These changes include budding, karyorrhexis, nuclear fragmentation, and multinuclearity. Stains for iron reveal an absence of hemosiderin in the macrophages, an invariable characteristic of ID. Sideroblasts are markedly reduced or absent.

Evaluation of iron stores using serum iron studies eliminates the need for bone marrow examination in almost all cases.

THERAPY

Once the cause of the anemia has been established, the principles of treatment are to treat the underlying disorder (e.g., bleeding ulcer), administer iron, and observe the response. The anemia is usually corrected by the oral administration of ferrous sulfate. Parenteral iron therapy, which is more dangerous and expensive than oral iron therapy, may on rare occasion be indicated for unusual circumstances. Intravenous iron dextran is often required in patients with chronic renal disease who are receiving therapy with recombinant human EPO (rHuEPO).[32] To maintain a twofold to threefold increase in the rate of erythrocyte production in patients treated with epoetin alfa, enough iron should be given to maintain serum iron concentrations at 80–100 μg/dL.[33]

Iron deficient patients treated with iron experience a return of strength, appetite, and a feeling of well-being within 3–5 days, whereas the anemia is not alleviated for weeks.

The dysphagias also are corrected before the anemia is relieved.

A response to iron therapy is defined as an increase of 1 gm/hemoglobin in one month. Since reticulocytes are new red cells just released from the bone marrow, reticulocyte counts and the CHr or IRF give a snapshot of recent red cell production. Reticulocyte response to iron therapy begins at about the third day after the start of therapy, peaks at about the eighth to tenth day (4–10% reticulocytes), and declines thereafter. Increases in reticulocyte hemoglobin content (CHr) or the immature reticulocyte fraction (IRF) (∞ Chapter 10) are early indicators of a response to iron therapy and begin to increase well in advance of an increase in reticulocytes and hemoglobin.[17,34] If therapy is successful, the hemoglobin should rise until levels within normal limits are established, usually within 6–10 weeks. To restore iron stores, extended therapy with small amounts of iron salts may be required (usually 6 months) after the hemoglobin has returned to normal.

Due to the high prevalence of ID in toddlers, it is a well accepted practice to screen all one-year-olds for iron deficiency and/or anemia. It has been suggested that if the hemoglobin concentration is decreased, a therapeutic trial of iron be initiated in this population. If anemia persists after one month of therapy, further evaluation is necessary[35] (Web Figure 11-1 ■).

▶ ANEMIAS CAUSED BY ABNORMAL IRON METABOLISM

Anemias caused by abnormal iron metabolism are the result of either a block in the incorporation of iron into the protoporphyrin ring to form heme or defective iron reutilization (usually the result of a slow release of iron from macrophages). Although iron is absorbed at normal rates in these anemias, iron is used at less than normal rates for erythropoiesis. This results in a lack of iron for hemoglobin synthesis and a blood picture similar to that of IDA. In contrast to ID, however, the positive iron balance in these anemias may lead to an increase in iron stores predominantly in the spleen, liver, and bone marrow. Serum ferritin levels above 250 μg/L in the male or above 200 μg/L in the female indicate increased iron stores.

The anemias discussed in this section include sideroblastic anemia and the anemia of chronic disease. Lead poisoning also is included because of its pathophysiologic relationship to these anemias through a block in heme synthesis.

SIDEROBLASTIC ANEMIAS

Sideroblastic anemia (SA) is the result of diverse clinical and biochemical manifestations that reflect multiple underlying hereditary, congenital, or acquired pathogenic mechanisms. However, all types are characterized by: (1) an increase in total body iron, (2) the presence of ringed sideroblasts in the bone marrow, and (3) hypochromic anemia.

Classification

The classification of sideroblastic anemia is arbitrary at best, and one can find many different schemes of classification. The classification given in Table 11-13 ✪ is one of the most descriptive. There are two major groups, those that are inherited and those that are acquired.

Hereditary Form The most common form of hereditary sideroblastic anemia is due to a defective sex-linked recessive gene. Although carrier females often show a dimorphic population of morphologically abnormal and normal erythrocytes, they rarely have anemia. Affected males demonstrate the typical findings of sideroblastic anemia. In rare instances, both sexes are equally affected, implying that there is another hereditary form that is transmitted in an autosomal recessive manner. In the hereditary forms, anemia may become apparent in infancy but most commonly appears in young adulthood. Rarely, symptoms may not occur until age 60.

Acquired Form The acquired forms of sideroblastic anemia are more common than the hereditary forms. The acquired forms are classified according to whether the basis of the anemia is unknown (idiopathic type) or is secondary to an underlying disease or toxin (secondary type). The idiopathic form, *refractory anemia with ringed sideroblasts* (RARS), may affect either sex in adult life. RARS is included in a group of acquired stem cell disorders called myelodysplastic syndromes. These syndromes have a tendency to terminate in acute leukemia. This anemia is discussed in ∞ Chapter 28.

The acquired secondary type sideroblastic anemias are associated with malignancy, drugs, or other toxic substances. In this type, once the underlying disorder is effectively treated or the toxin removed, the anemia abates.

Pathophysiology

Studies of patients with sideroblastic anemia have shown disturbances of the enzymes regulating heme synthesis. Ringed sideroblasts are a specific finding for these heme enzyme abnormalities. Ringed sideroblasts are formed from an accumulation of nonferritin iron in the mitochondria that circle the normoblast nucleus. The mitochondria eventually

✪ **TABLE 11-13**

Classification of Sideroblastic Anemia

Hereditary	Acquired
Sex-linked	Idiopathic refractory sideroblastic anemia
Autosomal recessive	(IRSA) or refratory anemia with ringed sideroblasts (RARS)
	Secondary to drugs, toxins, lead
	Associated with malignancy

rupture as they become iron laden. When stained with Prussian blue, the iron appears as blue punctate deposits circling the nucleus. Normally iron within the normoblasts is deposited diffusely throughout the cytoplasm.

Hereditary Sideroblastic Anemia Defective heme synthesis appears to be involved in the pathogenesis of the hereditary form of sideroblastic anemia. The most common form of SA in this group is sex-linked and due to an abnormal δ-aminolevulinate synthase enzyme (ALAS).

There are two different forms of ALAS: the nonerythroid or hepatic form (ALAS1) and the erythroid form (ALAS2). The nonerythroid form, also known as the housekeeping form, is coded for by a gene expressed in all tissues and has been assigned to the chromosomal region 3p21. The erythroid form is coded for by a gene that has been assigned to the Xp21-q21 chromosomal region (female sex chromosome). ALAS2 is the first and rate-limiting enzyme in heme synthesis.

Sex-linked SA is due to an abnormal ALAS2 enzyme. The abnormal enzyme is the result of heterogeneous point mutations in the catalytic domain of the ALAS2 gene.[36] Over 22 different mutations have been described in this gene.[37] The mutations are located in exons 5–11 and all but one are missense (single base change) leading to substitution of a single amino acid in the protein.

Evidence indicates that the activity of ALAS2 is totally dependent on the presence of the cofactor, pyridoxal phosphate. This cofactor binds to the enzyme and is crucial for its stability, for maintaining a conformation that is optimal for substrate binding and product release, and for its catalytic activity. In 17 of the 22 ALAS2 mutations there is a partial to complete clinical response to pharmacologic doses of pyridoxine. Thus, it is possible that excess pyridoxine compensates for an abnormal enzyme. It has been demonstrated that in the pyridoxine-refractory sex-linked SA, the gene mutation results in an unstable ALAS2.[38]

Decreased heme synthesis due to a block in iron utilization is interpreted by the body as an increased need for iron. Increased iron absorption from the GI tract continues and results in iron overload as tissue sites are saturated with iron.

Other hereditary forms of sideroblastic anemia have been described but are less common than the sex-linked type.[39]

Acquired Sideroblastic Anemia The acquired SA may be categorized as refractory anemia with ringed sideroblasts (RARS) and those secondary to drugs or toxins.

RARS. This form of SA is considered to be the result of an acquired stem cell disorder. It is discussed in the chapter on myelodysplastic syndromes (∞ Chapter 28).

Secondary to Drugs or Toxins. Acquired sideroblastic anemia secondary to drugs/toxins is the result of the drugs' or toxins' interference with the activity of heme enzymes.

Lead and alcohol are the most common causes of this form of SA.

Lead Poisoning: Lead poisoning (**plumbism**) has been recognized for centuries. In children, it generally results from ingestion of flaked lead-based paint from painted items. Lead was removed from paint after 1978. Children from racial/minority groups and those in lower socioeconomic groups are at increased risk. Within these groups, children between 1 and 3 years of age are at greatest risk. Clinically, lead toxicity in children is associated with hyperactivity, low IQ, concentration disorders, hearing loss, and impaired growth and development. In adults, lead poisoning is primarily the result of inhalation of lead or lead compounds from industrial processes.

Many states require laboratories and physicians to report elevated blood lead levels to the state health department, which may report to the Centers for Disease Control (CDC). Twenty-seven states reported elevated blood levels to the CDC in 1998. Although average blood lead levels have dropped by 80% since the late 1970s, there were about 4,000 adult persons per quarter with blood lead levels >25 μg/dL in 1997–98.[40] There are still nearly one million children with increased blood lead levels.

Lead serves no physiological purpose. Although lead poisoning consistently shortens the erythrocyte life span, the anemia accompanying plumbism is not primarily the result of hemolysis but rather the result of a marked abnormality in heme synthesis. Once ingested, lead passes through the blood to the bone marrow, where it accumulates in the mitochondria of normoblasts and inhibits cellular enzymes involved in heme synthesis. The heme enzymes most sensitive to lead inhibition are δ-aminolevulinic acid dehydrase (δ-ALA-D) and ferrocheletase (heme synthase) (∞ Chapter 5). The effect of lead on ferrochelatase is competitive inhibition with iron. Other enzymes may be affected at higher lead concentrations. Thus, the synthesis of heme is primarily disturbed at the conversion of δ-ALA to porphobilinogen (δ-ALA-D), and at the incorporation of iron into protoporphyrin to form heme (ferrochelatase). As a result, there is an increase in urine excretion of δ-ALA. The erythrocyte protoporphyrin (ZPP) is also strikingly increased. Iron accumulates in the cell.

Studies have revealed that microcytic, hypochromic anemia is not characteristic of elevated lead levels in children. Evidence suggests that if a microcytic anemia is present, it is most likely due to complications of ID or to the coexistence of alpha-thalassemia trait.[41,42,43] In one study it was found that 33% of black children with lead poisoning and microcytosis had alpha-thalassemia trait.[41]

Coexistent ID and lead poisoning put children at a higher risk of developing even more serious lead poisoning because these children not only absorb larger portions of lead in iron deficient states, but the competitive inhibition of ferrochelatase by lead is even greater in the absence of iron. Thus, it is critical to make a diagnosis of ID when it coexists with lead poisoning.

substitutions in the globin protein chain. These mutations cause structural variation in one of the globin chain classes (structural hemoglobin variants). The nomenclature of these disorders is discussed in a later section. The most common clinical disorder of this type of mutation is sickle cell anemia.

The quantitative globin disorders are the result of various genetic defects that reduce synthesis of structurally normal globin chains. The quantitative disorders are known collectively as the **thalassemias.**

As a result of the globin chain defects, hemoglobinopathies are frequently, but not always, associated with a chronic hemolytic anemia. Clinical expression of the hemoglobinopathy varies depending upon the class of globin chain involved (α, β, δ, or γ), the severity of hemolysis, and the compensatory production of other normal globin chains. Some of the hemoglobinopathies produce no clinical signs or symptoms of disease and are identified only through population studies specifically designed to reveal "silent" carriers. As discovery of silent carriers increases, the incidence of these genetic disorders is proving to be much higher than originally thought. It is believed that hemoglobinopathies are the most common lethal hereditary diseases in humans.[1]

Hemoglobinopathies are found worldwide but occur most commonly in African blacks and ethnic groups from the Mediterranean basin and Southeast Asia. The geographic locations where the quantitative and qualitative hemoglobin disorders are found frequently overlap; thus, it is not uncommon for individuals to have a structural hemoglobin variant together with a form of thalassemia. This may partly explain the wide variety of clinical findings associated with hemoglobinopathies.

This chapter discusses the structural hemoglobin variants, and ∞ Chapter 13 discusses the thalassemias.

▶ STRUCTURAL HEMOGLOBIN VARIANTS

The largest group of hemoglobinopathies results from an inherited structural change in one of the globin chains; however, synthesis of the abnormal chain usually is not impaired. Any of the globin chain classes, α, β, δ, or γ, may be affected.

Sickle cell anemia, the most common structural hemoglobin variant, was recorded by James Herrick of Chicago in 1910.[2] Herrick described the typical crescent-shaped sickled erythrocytes in a young black student from the West Indies. Following this initial report, additional cases of the disease were described, and the clinical pattern of sickle cell anemia was established. The pathophysiologic aspects of the disease, however, remained a mystery until Linus Pauling in 1949 discovered the altered electrophoretic mobility of the hemoglobin in patients with sickle cell disease.[3] The altered elec-

trical charge of the molecule was ascribed to a molecular abnormality of the globin chain. More than 300 abnormal hemoglobins have since been discovered.

IDENTIFICATION OF HEMOGLOBIN VARIANTS

Most structural hemoglobin variants result from a single amino acid substitution or deletion in the non-α polypeptide globin chain. Substitutions and deletions, however, do not necessarily alter the physical (solubility and stability) or functional properties of the hemoglobin molecule. Only when the mutation affects these properties does clinical disease result. In fact, the majority of the structural variants result in no clinical or hematologic abnormality and have only been discovered by population studies or through family studies. Certain substitutions at critical interaction sites, however, may alter the structure of the hemoglobin molecule in such a way as to profoundly affect its function, solubility, or stability. These phenotypic variants produce both clinical and hematologic abnormalities of varying severity, depending on the nature and site of the mutation. Laboratory tests designed to detect hemoglobin variants are based on the altered structure or function of the molecule.

Hemoglobin Electrophoresis

Hemoglobin carries an electrical charge resulting from the presence of carboxyl (COOH) and protonated (H^+) nitrogen groups. The type and strength of the charge depend on both the amino acid sequence of the hemoglobin molecule and the pH of the surrounding medium. Many amino acid substitutions alter this electrophoretic charge of the molecule, enabling detection of a structural hemoglobin variant by **hemoglobin electrophoresis.** It is important to understand, however, that different substitutions may cause identical changes in the net charge of the molecule; thus, two different mutant hemoglobins may have identical electrophoretic mobility. By varying the medium and pH of the procedure, many clinically significant hemoglobins may be identified. Methods for performing hemoglobin electrophoresis, examples of electrophoretic patterns, and more complete discussions of the tests that follow are included in ∞ Chapter 40, Special Procedures in Hematology.

Other Tests

Most clinically symptomatic hemoglobinopathies involve abnormalities of the β globin chain, resulting in a decrease or absence of HbA ($\alpha_2\beta_2$) and an increase in HbF ($\alpha_2\gamma_2$) and/or HbA$_2$ ($\alpha_2\delta_2$). Typically, an elevation in HbF and/or HbA$_2$ is the clue to the presence of a hemoglobinopathy, although HbF is frequently elevated in other hematologic disorders. HbF concentrations >10% can be measured accurately by electrophoresis and densitometry. Smaller but significant increases in HbF can be measured more accurately by **alkali denaturation**. Its distribution among the erythrocyte population, however, is evaluated by the acid elution test. These tests are based on the fact that HbF is more resistant to alkali and acid treatment than other hemoglobins.

Other tests for abnormal hemoglobins are based on altered physical properties of the structural variants. These include solubility tests, heat precipitation tests, and tests for Heinz bodies. The uses of these tests are included in the following discussion of the corresponding specific structural variants. Procedures are included in ∞ Chapter 40.

Techniques are also available to identify the specific molecular defect of hemoglobin disorders.[4] These techniques are discussed in ∞ Chapter 25. The polymerase chain reaction (PCR) has been incorporated into all diagnostic procedures for identifying point mutations because it enhances sensitivity and reduces the amount of DNA required and time for analysis. Prenatal diagnosis may be carried out in the first trimester of pregnancy using DNA from chorionic villi. In hemoglobinopathies caused by a single mutation, such as sickle cell anemia, only the DNA of fetal origin needs to be studied, while in highly heterogeneous mutations, the DNA of the parents is studied first to identify the mutation.

✔ Checkpoint! #1

Why can't all structural hemoglobin variants be identified by hemoglobin electrophoresis? Can thalassemia be identified by hemoglobin electrophoresis?

CASE STUDY *(continued from page 221)*

1. Identify a laboratory test needed to determine Shane's hemoglobinopathy.

NOMENCLATURE

The first abnormal hemoglobin discovered was called hemoglobin S (HbS) because it was associated with crescent-shaped erythrocytes (S for sickle). Subsequently, other hemoglobin variants were discovered, and they were given successive letters of the alphabet according to electrophoretic mobility beginning with the letter C. The letter A was already used to describe the normal adult hemoglobin, HbA. The letter B was not used to avoid confusion with the ABO blood group system. The letter F had been designated to describe fetal hemoglobin, HbF. The letter M was given to those hemoglobins that tended to form methemoglobin (HbM).

As more and more variants were discovered, it was recognized that the alphabetical system was not sufficient and an-

other nomenclature system was needed. It also became apparent that some variants with the same letter designation (same electrophoretic mobility) had different structural variations. Thus, subsequent hemoglobins were given common names according to the geographic area in which they were discovered (e.g., Hb Ft. Worth). If the hemoglobin has the electrophoretic mobility of a previously lettered hemoglobin, that letter is used in addition to the geographic area (e.g., HbG Honolulu).

An international committee has attempted to create a semblance of order out of the confusion surrounding hemoglobin nomenclature. They recommend that all variants be given a scientific designation as well as a common name. The scientific designation includes the following: (1) the mutated chain, (2) the position of the affected amino acid, (3) the helical position of the mutation, and (4) the amino acid substitution. For example, HbS would be designated β6 (A3) Glu→Val. The mutation is in the β-chain affecting the amino acid in the sixth position of the chain located in the A3 helix position. The amino acid valine is substituted for glutamine. Hemoglobins with amino acid deletions include the word *missing* after the amino acid and helix designation (e.g., β56-59 [D7-E3] missing). The advantage of the helical designation is that amino acid substitutions in the same helix may lead to similar functional and structural alterations of the hemoglobin molecule, allowing a better understanding of the clinical manifestations of each.

Not all globin chain defects cause symptoms of disease, and thus, many go undetected. Only those that cause symptoms are likely to be brought to the attention of a physician. The majority of abnormal hemoglobins discovered have been those that affect the β-chain. One possible explanation for this greater frequency is that the β-chain is a constituent of the major adult hemoglobin, HbA. Thus, an alteration of this chain produces a quantity of abnormal hemoglobin that is sufficient to produce symptoms of disease.

Although the α-chain is also a constituent of HbA, fewer hemoglobin variants have been linked to an abnormality in this chain. This could be explained by the fact that four α-genes exist, two on each homologous chromosome. This means that from one to four genes may be mutated, producing varying amounts of the abnormal hemoglobin from 25% to 100%. It is unlikely, however, that all four genes would be mutated; thus, hemoglobins with α-chain defects usually constitute a smaller proportion of the total hemoglobin than those with β-chain defects. Symptoms of disease in α-chain defects, if present, may be mild and frequently go unnoticed. Those substitutions affecting the δ or γ chains are not clinically significant because these chains are constituents of the minor adult hemoglobins, HbA$_2$ and HbF. They are not likely to produce symptoms and therefore are not easily detected.

If an individual is homozygous for the gene coding for a structural globin mutant of the β chain, no HbA is produced and the term *disease* or *anemia* is used to describe the specific disorder (i.e., sickle cell anemia). If, however, one of the genes coding for the β chain is normal and the other β gene codes for a structural variant, both HbA and the abnormal hemoglobin are produced, and the term *trait* is used to describe the heterozygous disorder (i.e., sickle cell trait). The abnormal hemoglobin usually accounts for less than 50% of the total hemoglobin in the trait form, whereas, in the homozygous state of disease the abnormal hemoglobin constitutes more than 50% of the total hemoglobin. The lower concentration of abnormal hemoglobin in the heterozygous state probably occurs because the α chains have a stronger attraction to bind with normal β chains than with the abnormal β chains. If the variant hemoglobin constitutes greater than 50% of the total hemoglobin and the patient is known through family studies to be heterozygous for the mutant gene, then the patient has probably inherited two different abnormal hemoglobin genes (**compound heterozygote**). The possibility that the patient has inherited a form of thalassemia with the hemoglobin variant should also be considered.

 Checkpoint! #2

What is meant by the term silent carrier *when referring to a hemoglobinopathy?*

 CASE STUDY *(continued from page 223)*

Results of hemoglobin electrophoresis were: 90% HbS, 9% HbF, and 1% HbA$_2$.

2. What is the abnormal hemoglobin causing this patient's disease?

3. Is the patient heterozygous or homozygous for the disorder?

4. What is this disorder called?

PATHOPHYSIOLOGY

The structural hemoglobin variants cause symptoms if the amino acid substitution occurs at a critical site of the molecule. Most mutations cause clinical signs of disease because the mutation affects the solubility, function (oxygen-affinity), and/or stability of the hemoglobin molecule.

Altered Solubility

If a nonpolar amino acid is substituted for a polar residue near the surface of the chain, the solubility of the hemoglobin molecule may be affected. Hemoglobin S and hemoglobin C are examples of this type of substitution. In the deoxygenated state, the HbS molecule polymerizes into insoluble, rigid aggregates. The majority of surface substitutions, however, do not affect the tertiary structure, heme function, or subunit interactions and are therefore innocuous.

Altered Function

Polar amino acid substitutions for nonpolar residues near the hydrophobic crevice of the globin chain that contains the heme (heme pocket) may affect the oxygen affinity of hemoglobin by stabilizing heme iron in the ferric state (∞ Chapter 5). The normal nonpolar heme pocket helps maintain heme iron in the reduced ferrous state. Hemoglobins M and Chesapeake are examples. Most structural variants affecting the heme pocket are caused by a substitution of tyrosine for histidine near the heme iron, stabilizing the iron in the ferric state and producing permanent methemoglobinemia. Methemoglobin cannot combine with oxygen.

Mutations at the subunit interaction site, α_1, β_2, may affect the allosteric properties of the molecule leading to increased or decreased oxygen affinity. There is considerable movement in the α_1, β_2 contact region upon oxygenation, which triggers the allosteric interactions (∞ Chapter 5). Other substitutions affecting oxygen affinity occur in the binding site for 2,3-DPG and in the C-terminal end of the β chain, which are sites involved in the stability of the deoxygenated state. High oxygen affinity hemoglobin variants produce congenital erythrocytosis, whereas decreased oxygen affinity variants produce anemia and cyanosis.

Altered Stability

Amino acid substitutions in the internal residues may prevent the hemoglobin molecule from folding into its normal conformation. Normal folding of the molecule places the hydrophilic residues on the surface, whereas hydrophobic residues are oriented toward the interior of the molecule. Substitution of polar for nonpolar internal residues can disrupt this conformation. Other substitutions may alter the alpha-helix structure or subunit interaction sites. Mutations in the heme crevice may impair the binding of heme to globin. These various altered properties of the hemoglobin molecule cause hemoglobin instability.

Clinically, the unstable variants are known as **congenital Heinz body hemolytic anemias.** The unstable hemoglobin denatures in the form of Heinz bodies. Heinz bodies attach to the cell membrane causing membrane injury and premature cell destruction. In addition to altering the molecule's stability, disruption of normal conformation also may affect the molecule's function. The unstable hemoglobins have a tendency to spontaneously oxidize to methemoglobin.

 Checkpoint! #3

The mutation in HbJ-Capetown, α92, Arg→Gln, stabilizes hemoglobin in the R state (Chapter 5). What functional effect would this have on the hemoglobin molecule?

► SICKLE CELL ANEMIA

Worldwide, sickle cell anemia is the most common symptomatic hemoglobinopathy, with greatest prevalence in Africa (Table 12-1 ✪). Gene frequency in equatorial Africa may exceed 20%. The sickle cell gene is also common in areas around the Mediterranean, the Middle East, India, Nepal, and in geographic regions in which there has been migration from endemic areas, such as North, Central, and South America.[5] Sickle cell disease occurs in 0.3–1.3% and sickle cell trait occurs in 8–10% of African Americans.

It is interesting to note that geographic areas with the highest frequency of sickle cell genes are also areas where infection with *Plasmodium falciparum* is common. This correlation strongly suggests that HbS in heterozygotes confers a selective advantage against fatal malarial infections. By this mechanism the gene frequency builds up. Children with sickle cell trait are readily infected with the malarial parasite, but parasite counts remain low. It has been suggested that resistance to malaria occurs because parasitized cells sickle more readily, leading to sequestration and phagocytosis of the infected cell by the spleen. Other, as yet undefined, factors may also contribute to reduced malarial susceptibility in individuals with HbS.[6] Epidemiological data also suggest there may be similar selective advantages to HbE and HbC.[5]

PATHOPHYSIOLOGY

Hemoglobin S is the mutant hemoglobin produced when nonpolar valine is substituted for polar glutamine at the sixth position, in the A3 helix of the β chain (β6 [A3] Glu→Val). This substitution is on the surface of the molecule, producing a change in the net charge; hence, it changes the electrophoretic mobility of the molecule. The solubility of HbS in the deoxygenated state is markedly reduced, producing a tendency for deoxyhemoglobin S molecules to polymerize into rigid aggregates. Following polymerization, the cells assume a crescent shape.

There is a delay time between deoxygenation and the formation of HbS polymers. The length of delay is highly dependent on temperature, pH, ionic strength, and oxygen tension in the cell's environment. Hypoxia, acidosis, hypertonicity, and temperatures more than 37°C promote deoxygenation and the formation of HbS polymers. The spleen, kidney, retina, and bone marrow provide a sufficiently hypoxic, acidotic, and hypertonic microenvironment to promote HbS polymerization and sickling.

Sickling also depends on HbS concentration within the erythrocyte (MCHC) and intracellular hemoglobin composition (the proportion of HbA, HbS, HbA_2, and HbF present). HbA and oxyhemoglobin S are equally soluble at concentrations about the normal MCHC of 34%. The more concentrated the HbS is within the cell, however, the higher the MCHC and the greater the potential for HbS aggregates to form. Using this concept, attempts are made to treat the disease by hydrating the cells, which decreases the MCHC and prevents sickling. The presence of other hemoglobins such as HbA inhibits polymerization and decreases sickling.

Polymerization of deoxyhemoglobin S begins when the oxygen saturation of hemoglobin falls below 85% and is complete at about 38% oxygen saturation. The HbS aggregates cause the erythrocyte to become stiff and less deformable. The aggregates also damage the erythrocyte membrane leading to increased fragility of the cell.

Irreversibly Sickled Cells

The sickled erythrocyte may return to a normal biconcave shape upon reoxygenation of the hemoglobin; however, with repeated sickling events, the erythrocyte membrane undergoes changes that cause it to become leaky and rigid. After repeated sickling episodes, the cells become **irreversibly sickled cells** (ISC) and are removed by

---

✪ TABLE 12-1

Summary of the Most Common Hemoglobin Variants

Hb	Peripheral Blood	Electrophoresis	Mutation	Geographic Distribution
HbS	Normocytic, normochromic anemia; reticulocytosis; poikilocytosis with sickled and boat-shaped cells	Homozygous: HbS, F, A_2 Heterozygous: HbA, S, F, A_2	β6(A3)Glu→Val	Tropical Africa, Mediterranean, Middle East, India, Nepal
HbE	Microcytic, hypochromic anemia; target cells	Homozygous: HbE, F, A_2 Heterozygous: HbA, E, F, A_2	β26(B8)Glu→Lys	Burma, Thailand, Cambodia, Malaysia, Indonesia
HbC	Normocytic, normochromic anemia with reticulocytosis; poikilocytosis with folded, irregularly contracted cells; target cells	Homozygous: HbC, F, A_2 Heterozygous: HbA, C, F, A_2	β6(A3)Glu→Lys	West Africa

mononuclear phagocytes in the spleen, liver, or bone marrow. The ISC may also initiate or increase the severity of vaso-occlusive crises because of impaired cell deformability and increased cell adherence to vascular endothelium. The mechanism for this interaction between sickled cells and the endothelium is unknown but may be related to changes in the surface properties of sickled cells and endothelial cells as well as plasma factors.[7,8]

The ISC is the result of a permanent deformation of the submembrane skeletal lattice.[9] The spectrin dimer–dimer association is the primary site of skeletal rearrangement. The intracellular polymerization of HbS may also decouple the lipid bilayer from the membrane skeleton. From 5% to 50% of the circulating erythrocytes in sickle cell anemia are ISC. They have a very high MCHC and a low MCV. These cells are ovoid or boat-shaped with a smooth outline. They lack the spicules characteristic of deoxygenated sickled cells.

Sickled cells have difficulty changing their shape enough to squeeze through the small capillaries. Consequently, the rigid cells aggregate in the microvasculature. More erythrocytes behind the blockage release their oxygen to the surrounding hypoxic tissue and consequently form rigid intracellular inclusions increasing the size of the plug (Figure 12-1 ■). Erythrocytes from nearby capillaries are forced to give up more oxygen than they normally would to feed the oxygen-starved tissue around the blockage. These cells then form rigid aggregates of deoxyhemoglobin, expanding the blockaded region. Lack of oxygen, in turn, causes local tissue necrosis. Most of the signs and symptoms of the disease are related to this process of microvasculature blockage and tissue necrosis.

Cause of Anemia

The primary cause of anemia in sickle cell anemia is extravascular hemolysis. Erythrocyte survival depends on intracellular HbF concentration and degree of membrane damage.[10] Changes in the erythrocyte membrane, coupled with Heinz body formation from denatured HbS, lead to a decreased cell surface area and removal of the cell by the reticulendothelial system.[11] The lifespan of circulating HbS erythrocytes may decrease to as few as 14 days. The hypoglycemic, hypoxic environment of the spleen promotes blood sickling, slows blood circulation in the cords, and enhances phagocytosis of erythrocytes containing HbS. Early in childhood, however, the spleen loses its function as repeated ischemic crises lead to splenic tissue necrosis and atrophy. With splenic atrophy, other cells of the mononuclear phagocyte system in the liver and bone marrow take over the destruction of these abnormal cells.

Sickle Cell Trait

Sickle cell trait is not as severe a disorder as sickle cell anemia since the presence of HbA or other β-chain structural variant hemoglobin interferes with the process of HbS polymerization. Although hemoglobins other than HbS can be assembled into the polymer of deoxyhemoglobin S, the presence of alternate β chains of these hemoglobins with the β chains of HbS creates a weakened structure and decreases the degree of polymerization. The poorer the fit, the less polymerization of deoxyhemoglobin S. If, however, the alternate β chains from another β chain mutant increase the strength of the intertetramer bonds of the polymer, then sickling is enhanced.

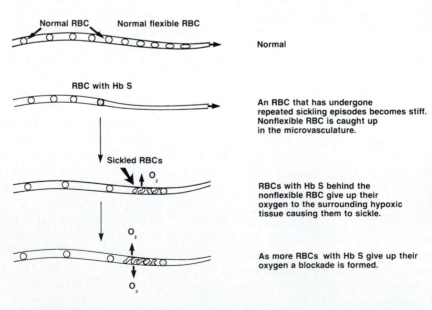

■ **FIGURE 12-1** How sickle cells block a vessel and precipitate a vaso-occlusive crisis.

Oxygen Affinity of HbS

The oxygen affinity of HbS differs from that of HbA, resulting in important physiologic changes in vivo. HbS has decreased oxygen affinity. The 2,3-DPG level of homozygotes is increased. This shift to the right in the oxygen dissociation curve facilitates the release of more oxygen to the tissues. On the other hand, this phenomenon also increases the concentration of deoxyhemoglobin S, promoting the formation of sickle cells.

CLINICAL FINDINGS

The first clinical signs of sickle cell anemia appear at about 6 months of age when the concentration of HbS predominates over HbF. Clinical manifestations result from chronic hemolytic anemia, vaso-occlusion of the microvasculature, overwhelming infections, and acute splenic sequestration.

Anemia

A moderate to severe chronic anemia as the result of extravascular hemolysis is characteristic of the disease. Gallstones, a complication of any chronic hemolytic disorder, are a common finding due to cholestasis and increased bilirubin turnover. Folate deficiency due to increased erythrocyte turnover may further exacerbate the anemia producing megaloblastosis.

Hemodynamic changes occur in an attempt to compensate for the tissue oxygen deficit; as a result, symptoms of cardiac overload, including cardiac hypertrophy, cardiac enlargement, and eventually congestive heart failure, are frequent complications of the disease.

Hyperplastic bone marrow caused by chronic hemolysis is accompanied by bone changes, such as thinning of cortices and hair-on-end appearance in x-rays of the skull. Hyperplasia results from a futile attempt by the marrow to compensate for premature erythrocyte destruction. Conversely, aplastic crises may accompany or follow viral, bacterial, and mycoplasmal infections. This temporary cessation of erythropoiesis in the face of chronic hemolysis leads to a worsening of the anemia. The aplasia may last from a few days to a week. Increasing evidence suggests that many cases of aplasia occur as a result of infection with parvovirus. Parvovirus will also cause a cessation of erythropoiesis in normal individuals, but normal blood cell production in these individuals is restored before any noticeable changes in erythrocyte concentration take place.

Vaso-Occlusive Crisis

The blockage of microvasculature by rigid sickled cells accounts for the majority of the clinical signs of sickle cell anemia. The occlusions do not occur continuously but, rather, spontaneously, causing acute signs of distress. These episodes are called **vaso-occlusive crises** and are the most frequent cause of hospitalization. The crises may be triggered by infection, decreased atmospheric oxygen pressure, dehydration, or slow blood flow, but frequently they occur without any known cause. The occlusions are accompanied by pain, low grade fever, organ dysfunction, and tissue necrosis. The episodes last for 1 to 2 weeks and subside spontaneously.

Recurrent occlusive episodes lead to infarctions of tissue of the genitourinary tract, liver, bone, lung, and spleen. The chronic organ damage is accompanied by organ dysfunction. Although splenomegaly is present in early childhood, repeated splenic infarctions eventually result in splenic fibrosis and calcifications (usually by age 4 or 5). This organ damage, secondary to infarction, is known as **autosplenectomy**. As a result, splenomegaly is rare in adults with this disease. Aseptic necrosis of the head of the femur is common. Dactylitis, a painful symmetrical swelling of the hands and feet (hand-foot syndrome) caused by infarction of the metacarpals and metatarsals, is often the first sign of the disease in infants. Recurrent priapism is a characteristic, painful complication that occasionally requires surgical intervention.

The slow flow of blood in occlusive areas may lead to thrombosis. Thrombosis of the cerebral arteries resulting in stroke is common. Magnetic resonance imaging shows evidence of subclinical cerebral infarction in 20–30% of children with sickle cell anemia. If the arterioles of the eye are affected, blindness can occur. Chronic leg ulcers, found also in other hemolytic anemias, may occur at any age. The ulcers appear without any known injury. These painful sores do not readily respond to treatment and may take months to heal.

Placental infarctions in pregnant women with sickle cell disease can be a hazard to the fetus. Anemia often becomes more severe during pregnancy. In addition, other clinical findings may be exacerbated during pregnancy, endangering the life of both the mother and the fetus.

Bacterial Infection

Overwhelming bacterial infection is a common cause of death in young patients. There is an extremely high risk of septicemia from encapsulated microorganisms. Bacterial pneumonia is the most common infection, but meningitis is also prevalent. Infections are primarily due to *Streptococcus pneumoniae* and *Hemophilus influenzae*. The reasons for this increased susceptibility to infection are not fully understood but may be related to functional asplenia, impaired opsonization, and abnormal complement activation.[12] The spleen is important to host defense in the young. There is also significant impairment of in-vivo neutrophil adherence to vascular endothelium in HbS disease. This may prevent neutrophils from rapidly relocating to areas of inflammation.[12] Prophylactic penicillin is now advocated for all children with sickle cell anemia to reduce morbidity and mortality from infection.

 Checkpoint! #4

Why don't newborns with sickle cell anemia experience episodes of vaso-occlusive crisis?

Acute Splenic Sequestration

In young children, sudden splenic pooling of sickled erythrocytes may cause a massive decrease in erythrocyte mass within a few hours. Thrombocytopenia may also occur. Hypovolemia and shock follow. At one time this was the leading cause of death in infants with sickle cell anemia. Early diagnosis, instruction of parents to detect an enlarging spleen, and rapid intervention with transfusion have served to decrease morbidity and mortality associated with splenic sequestration.

Acute Chest Syndrome

This illness resembling pneumonia is the most common cause of death in children with sickle cell disease and the second most common cause of hospitalization.[13] Clinical findings include cough, fever, chest pain, dyspnea, chills, wheezing, and pulmonary infiltrates. Hemoglobin concentration and oxygen saturation decreases.[14] The etiology of chest syndrome is not clear. In some cases an infectious agent can be identified. Other possible causes include pulmonary edema from overhydration, fat embolism from infarcted bone marrow, and hypoventilation due to pain from rib infarcts or from narcotic analgesics used to combat pain. The long-term effects of recurrent episodes of chest syndrome are unknown.

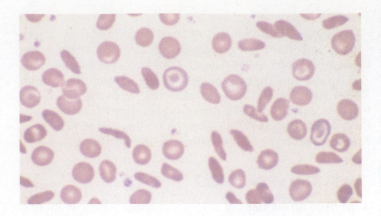

■ **FIGURE 12-2** Hemoglobin S disease (sickle cell anemia). Note abnormal boat-shaped, sickled, and ovoid erythrocytes. (Peripheral blood; Wright-Giemsa stain; 1000× magnification)

higher than normal. After the age of 40, the hemoglobin concentration, reticulocyte count, leukocyte count, and platelet count decrease.[16]

The blood smear shows variable anisocytosis with polychromatophilic macrocytes and variable poikilocytosis with the presence of sickled cells and target cells. Nucleated erythrocytes can usually be found. The RDW is increased. During hemolytic crisis the RDW increases linearly with increases in reticulocytes.[17] If the patient is not experiencing a crisis, sickled cells may not be present.

In older children and adults, signs of splenic hypofunction are apparent on the peripheral blood smear with the presence of basophilic stippling, Howell-Jolly bodies, siderocytes, and poikilocytes.

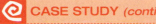 **CASE STUDY** *(continued from page 224)*

The chest radiograph showed consolidation in the left lower lobe, indicating that Shane has pneumonia.

5. What physiological conditions does this patient have that may lead to sickling of his erythrocytes?

6. What is the cause of this patient's pain and acute distress?

7. Why might Shane be more susceptible to pneumonia than an individual without sickle cell disease?

LABORATORY FINDINGS

Peripheral Blood

A normocytic, normochromic anemia is characteristic of sickle cell anemia; however, with marked reticulocytosis, the anemia may appear macrocytic (Figure 12-2 ■). Reticulocytosis from 10 to 20% is typical. The hemoglobin ranges from 6 to 10 g/dL and the hematocrit from 0.18 to 0.30 L/L. A calculated hematocrit from an electronic cell counter is more reliable than a centrifuged microhematocrit because excessive plasma trapped by sickled cells in centrifuged specimens falsely elevates the hematocrit.

The Cooperative Study of Sickle Cell Disease revealed that individuals homozygous for HbS have higher steady-state leukocyte counts than normal, especially in children less than 10 years of age.[15] Platelet counts are also frequently

CASE STUDY *(continued from page 228)*

Admission laboratory data on Shane included:

WBC:	16.4×10^9/L
RBC:	2.5×10^{12}/L
HGB:	7.8 g/dL
Hct:	0.24 L/L
PLT:	467×10^9/L

Differential: Segs 76%, Bands 10%, Lymphs 9%, Monos 3%, Eos 1%, Basos 1%

RBC morphology: Sickle cells, 3+ target cells, 1+ ovalocytes, 1+ polychromasia, 3 NRBC/100 WBCs, Howell-Jolly bodies

8. Which of the patient's hematologic test results are consistent with a diagnosis of sickle cell anemia?

9. What does the presence of polychromatophilic erythrocytes signify?

10. Why is the absolute neutrophil count elevated?

11. What is the significance of ovalocytes on the blood smear?

12. What is the significance of Howell-Jolly bodies on the smear?

Bone Marrow

Bone marrow aspiration shows erythroid hyperplasia, reflecting the attempt of the bone marrow to compensate for chronic hemolysis. Erythrocyte production increases to 4–5 times normal. If the patient is deficient in folic acid, megaloblastosis may be seen. Iron stores are most often increased but may be diminished if hematuria is excessive. Bone marrow examination is not usually performed because it yields no definitive diagnostic information.

Hemoglobin Electrophoresis

The presence of HbS is confirmed by hemoglobin electrophoresis. Electrophoresis on cellulose acetate at a pH of 8.4 shows 85–100% HbS. HbF is usually not greater than 15%. Higher levels of HbF (25–35%) may signify compound heterozygosity for HbS and hereditary persistence of fetal hemoglobin. HbA_2 is normal. Newborns have 60–80% HbF with the remainder HbS. In infants less than 3 months of age with small amounts of HbS, electrophoresis on citrate agar gel at a pH of 6.2 permits more reliable separation of HbF from both HbA and HbS. Citrate agar gel electrophoresis is also useful in separating HbD and HbG from HbS. Both of these nonsickling hemoglobins migrate with HbS on alkaline electrophoresis with paper or starch gel but migrate like HbA on agar gel electrophoresis at acid pH.

Solubility Test

The solubility test is a rapid test for HbS in the heterozygous or homozygous state. In severe anemia, the amount of HbS may be too low to be detected, and the procedure may need to be altered. This should not be used as a screening test for newborns because of the low concentration of HbS in this group. Unstable hemoglobins may give a false positive test if many Heinz bodies are present. Other rare hemoglobin variants may also give positive tests (e.g., HbC Harlem, HbI). False positive tests also occur with elevated plasma proteins and lipids.

Sickling Test

Another confirmatory test, performed less often, is the sodium metabisulfite slide test for sickling. This test is positive in both sickle cell anemia and sickle cell trait.

Other Diagnostic Tests

Isoelectric focusing in agar gels and high performance liquid chromatography are used to identify abnormal hemoglobins such as HbS. Preferred methods for prenatal screening and diagnosis use DNA-based analysis (polymerase chain reaction) to detect point mutation in globin gene sequences.[4] This DNA testing provides a genotype diagnosis and eliminates the need for later neonatal testing when the phenotype results may be inconclusive. The molecular techniques are discussed in ∞ Chapter 25.

Other Laboratory Findings

Other laboratory findings are less specific. The hemolytic nature of the disease causes indirect bilirubin to increase, haptoglobin to decrease, and uric acid and serum lactic dehydrogenase (LD) to increase. Osmotic fragility may be decreased due to the presence of target cells. These tests offer no diagnostic information on sickle cell anemia but may be performed to evaluate complicating conditions.

 CASE STUDY *(continued from page 228)*

The LD level was reported as 1260 U/L. (Reference interval 75–200 U/L)

13. What is the significance of the patient's elevated LD?

✔ Checkpoint! #5

A child's parents both have sickle cell trait. The physician orders a hemoglobin electrophoresis on the child. Results of electrophoresis on cellulose acetate at pH 8.4 show 65% HbS, 30% HbA, 3% HbF, 2% HbA_2. Explain these results and suggest further testing that may help in diagnosis.

THERAPY

Preventive therapy is aimed at eliminating conditions that are known to precipitate vaso-occlusion, such as dehydration and infection. Transfusion of packed erythrocytes or whole blood is required in aplastic crises or splenic sequestration. Preoperative transfusion is helpful in preventing the complications of anesthesia-induced sickling. Long-term transfusion therapy may be useful in preventing complications of sickle cell anemia. This therapy is aimed at suppressing the formation of new HbS by the patient's bone marrow. Complications of transfusion therapy include transmission of blood-borne diseases, alloimmunization, expense, inconvenience, and iron overload.

Hydroxyurea (HU), a pharmacological agent, is used to reduce intracellular sickling.[18] HU reactivates fetal genes and elevates HbF in most HbS containing erythrocytes. This decreases intracellular polymerization of HbS. Children respond well to HU, experiencing fewer vaso-occlusive crises and hospitalizations. The most frequent side effects are neutropenia, reticulocytopenia, and thrombocytopenia. HU does not seem to produce serious irreversible toxicity; however, long-term effects are unknown.[19]

Bone marrow transplantation (BMT) affords the potential for cure of sickle cell disease. Results of two multicenter case series showed cure rates ranging from 73 to 90%. Risk of complications, particularly neurological problems, is high for patients with sickle cell disease undergoing BMT. Because of a wide range of heterogeneity in clinical severity of sickle cell disease, it is difficult to predict which patients may benefit from BMT.[20] Furthermore, BMT is extremely expensive and beyond the means of many patients with sickle cell disease. Gene therapy, in which normal genes are inserted into a patient's defective cells, also holds a promise of cure but is not feasible at this time. Progress toward finding a stable gene vector capable of expressing therapeutic levels of normal globin β chains over time has been slow.[21]

 Checkpoint! #6

Outline the treatment options that might be used for a patient with HbS disease, pneumonia, and vaso-occlusive crisis. Discuss how each would affect his clinical condition.

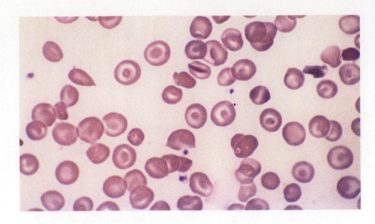

■ **FIGURE 12-3** Hemoglobin C disease. Note the cell in the center with HbC crystal, target cells, and folded cells. (Peripheral blood; Wright-Giemsa stain; 1000× magnification)

SICKLE CELL TRAIT

Sickle cell trait is the heterozygous β^S state. The patient has one normal β gene and one β^S gene. Since HbA constitutes more than 50% of the total hemoglobin in these individuals, there are no clinical symptoms, and results of physical examination appear normal. However, the condition is important to diagnose because, statistically, one of four children born to parents who each have the trait will have sickle cell anemia, and two of four will have the trait.

Complications of splenic infarction and renal papillary necrosis have been reported in affected individuals subjected to extreme and prolonged hypoxia such as after flying at high altitude in unpressurized aircraft or following general anesthesia.

Hematologic parameters are normal. No anemia or sickled cells are found in routine blood counts and differentials. Sickling can be induced with the sodium metabisulfite test, however, and the solubility test is also positive. Hemoglobin electrophoresis results show 50–65% HbA, 35–45% HbS, normal HbF, and normal or slightly increased HbA₂. If HbA constitutes less than 50% of the total hemoglobin in sickle cell trait, the patient is probably heterozygous for another hemoglobinopathy such as thalassemia.

▶ HEMOGLOBIN C DISEASE

Hemoglobin C, the second hemoglobinopathy to be recognized, is the third most prevalent hemoglobin variant. The first cases of HbC were discovered in the heterozygous state with HbS; this is not surprising because both hemoglobinopathies are prevalent in the same geographical area. It is found predominantly in West African blacks, where the incidence of the trait may reach 17–28% of the population. From 2–3% of African-Americans carry the trait, while 0.02% have the disease.

Hemoglobin C is produced when lysine is substituted for glutamine at the sixth position (A3) in the β chain (β6 [A3] Glu→Lys). Since the nonpolar lysine amino acid substitution is in the same β chain position as the substitution for HbS, a decrease in hemoglobin solubility can be expected. Deoxyhemoglobin C, like deoxyhemoglobin S, has a decreased solubility, forming intracellular crystals when cells are dehydrated or in hypertonic solutions. Erythrocytes with crystals become rigid and are trapped and destroyed in the spleen. Erythrocyte life span is decreased to 30–55 days.

Hemoglobin C disease (β^c/β^c) is usually asymptomatic, but patients may experience joint and abdominal pain. In contrast to sickle cell anemia, the spleen is most often enlarged. Variable hemolysis results in a mild to moderate anemia.

The hemoglobin ranges from 8 to 12 g/dL and the hematocrit from 0.25 to 0.35 L/L. The anemia is accompanied by a slight to moderate increase in reticulocytes. The stained blood smear contains small cells that appear to be folded and irregularly contracted and many target cells (Figure 12-3 ■). Intracellular hemoglobin crystals may be found if the smear has been dried slowly. Microspherocytes are occasionally present. Osmotic fragility is decreased.

Hemoglobin electrophoresis on citrate agar gel at acid pH demonstrates greater than 90% HbC with a slight increase in HbF (not more than 7%). On cellulose acetate at an alkaline pH, HbC migrates with HbA₂. HbE and HbO-Arab also migrate with HbC at alkaline pH but can be separated by agar gel electrophoresis at an acid pH.

Hemoglobin C trait (β^c/β) is symptomless. No hematologic abnormalities are produced except that target cells are readily noted on blood smears. Mild hypochromia may be present. About 60–70% of the hemoglobin is HbA and 30–40% is HbC. Higher levels of HbC and microcytosis are found when HbC is associated with β-thalassemia (β^c/β^thal) (Figure 12-4 ■).

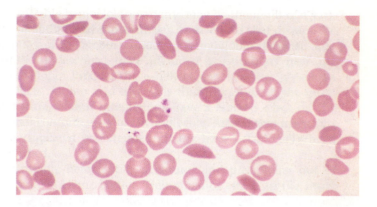

■ **FIGURE 12-4** Hemoglobin C/β-thalassemia. Note the microspherocytes and target cells. This patient had 94% HbC and 6% HbF. (Peripheral blood; Wright-Giemsa stain; 1000× magnification)

■ **FIGURE 12-5** Hemoglobin S/C disease. Notice the elongated cells and boat-shaped cells. The small contracted cells are typical of those seen in hemoglobin C disease. Target cells are also present. (Peripheral blood; Wright-Giemsa stain; 1000× magnification)

There is considerable heterogeneity in the clinical and hematological features of HbC/β^{thal}, which appears to be dependent on the particular variety of β thalassemia gene interacting with HbC. HbC/β^{+thal} is characterized by mild anemia similar to that found in heterozygous β thalassemia. There is 65–80% HbC, 2–5% HbF, and the remainder HbA. In HbC/β^{othal}, there is more severe anemia and an absence of HbA. Hemoglobin electrophoresis reveals only HbC, HbA$_2$, and HbF. HbF ranges from 3–10%.

▶ HEMOGLOBIN S/C DISEASE

In hemoglobin S/C disease, both β chains are abnormal. One β gene codes for β^s chains, and the other gene codes for β^c chains (β^{s}β^c). Thus, HbA is absent. This heterozygous state for HbS and HbC results in a disease almost as severe as homozygous HbS. The concentration of hemoglobin in individual erythrocytes (MCHC) is increased, and the concentration of HbS is greater than in sickle cell trait. The increased MCHC contributed by HbC makes the HbS/C cells more prone to sickling than cells that contain HbA/HbS. HbC also enhances the polymerization of HbS. Increased erythrocyte rigidity is noted at oxygen tensions less than 50 mm Hg. Additionally, there is evidence that cells containing HbS/C have intracellular HbC crystals.[21] Thus, in HbS/C disease, both sickling and crystal formation contribute to the pathophysiology of the disease.

The clinical signs and symptoms of the disease are similar to those of mild sickle cell anemia. Patients develop vaso-occlusive crises leading to the complications associated with this pathology. A notable difference from sickle cell anemia, however, is that in HbS/C disease splenomegaly is prominent.

Mild to moderate normocytic, normochromic anemia is present. The hematocrit is above 0.25 L/L, and the hemoglobin concentration is between l0 and l4 g/dL. The higher hemoglobin concentration does not necessarily mean that he-

molysis is less severe than in sickle cell anemia; it may be that the higher oxygen affinity of HbS/C cells stimulates higher erythropoietin levels. Peripheral blood smears reveal a large number of target cells (up to 85%), folded cells, boat-shaped cells, and sickled forms (Figure 12-5 ■). HbC crystals are found in some patients. Some erythrocytes contain a single eccentrically located, densely stained, round mass of hemoglobin that makes part of the cell appear empty. These cells have been referred to as billiard-ball cells.[22] Anisocytosis and poikilocytosis range from mild to severe. Small, dense, misshapen cells, some with crystals of various shapes jutting out at angles, have been referred to as HbSC poikilocytes.[23] Hemoglobin electrophoresis shows nearly equal amounts of HbS and HbC. HbF may be increased up to 7%. No HbA is found due to the absence of normal β chains.

 Checkpoint! #7

What is the functional abnormality of HbC and HbS? Why do these two abnormal hemoglobins have the same altered functions?

▶ HEMOGLOBIN D

Hemoglobin D has several variants, of which the identical variants HbD Punjab and HbD Los Angeles (β121 [GH4] Glu→Gln) are the most common in American blacks (<0.02%). The heterozygous and homozygous states are both asymptomatic. Although there are no hematologic abnormalities, the homozygous state may occasionally have an increase in target cells and a decrease in osmotic fragility. Although rare, the heterozygous state of HbD with HbS exists. HbD interacts with HbS, producing aggregates of deoxyhemoglobin (Figure 12-6 ■). This produces a relatively mild form of sickle cell anemia.

Acute hemolysis may also be accompanied by the excretion of dark urine due to the presence of dipyrroles in the urine.

LABORATORY FINDINGS

Peripheral Blood

The anemia of congenital Heinz body hemolytic anemia is usually normocytic and normochromic. It may occasionally have a slightly decreased MCH and MCHC because of the removal of hemoglobin from erythrocytes as Heinz bodies in the spleen. The reticulocyte count is typically increased. The blood film may show basophilic stippling, pitted cells (bite cells), and small contracted cells. Osmotic fragility is usually abnormal after 24 hours of incubation.

Heinz bodies formed in vivo may be demonstrated in the peripheral blood following splenectomy; however, this finding is not specific for unstable hemoglobin disorders. Heinz bodies can also be demonstrated in erythrocyte enzyme abnormalities that permit oxidation of hemoglobin, in thalassemia, and after administration of oxidant drugs in normal individuals. Heinz bodies of unstable hemoglobins can be generated in vitro by incubation of the erythrocytes with brilliant cresyl blue or other redox agent. These intracellular inclusions cannot be demonstrated with Wright's stain.

Other Laboratory Findings

Most unstable hemoglobins have the same charge and electrophoretic mobility as normal hemoglobin. Only about 45% can be diagnosed by electrophoresis. Hemoglobin A_2 and HbF are sometimes increased. This may provide a clue to the presence of an abnormal hemoglobin when it is not detected by its electrophoretic pattern. The heat instability test is always positive in unstable hemoglobin disorders. The unstable hemoglobin is precipitated in 20 minutes with the isopropanol stability test. Normal hemoglobin remains solvent 30–40 minutes.

 Checkpoint! #10

(a) *Explain why patients with an unstable hemoglobin variant usually experience acute hemolysis only after administration of certain drugs or with infections.*

(b) *A patient is suspected of having a congenital Heinz body hemolytic anemia but hemoglobin electrophoresis is normal. Why is it necessary to perform additional tests?*

THERAPY

Most patients with these disorders do not require any therapy. Splenectomy may be performed if hemolysis is severe. Patients are advised to avoid oxidizing drugs, which may precipitate a hemolytic episode.

► HEMOGLOBIN VARIANTS WITH ALTERED OXYGEN AFFINITY

Amino acid substitutions in the globin chains close to the heme pocket may affect the ability of hemoglobin to carry oxygen by preventing binding of heme to the globin chain or by stabilizing iron in the oxidized ferric state. Other substitutions that affect oxygen affinity include substitutions near the $\alpha\beta$ contacts, substitutions at the C terminal end of the β chain, and substitutions near the 2,3-DPG binding site. These are critical sites that are involved in the allosteric properties of hemoglobin and/or in the physiologic regulation of hemoglobin affinity for oxygen. Either the α or β chain may be affected, but most substitutions are associated with the β chain. Permanent methemoglobin formation and cyanosis characterize decreased hemoglobin affinity. Increased oxygen affinity results in congenital polycythemia, a compensatory mechanism for the inability of the hemoglobin to unload oxygen to the tissues.

DECREASED OXYGEN AFFINITY

Methemoglobin is hemoglobin with iron oxidized to the ferric state. Oxygen cannot be carried by methemoglobin, resulting in cyanosis. The amount of methemoglobin produced under normal physiologic conditions is maintained at concentrations less than 1% through the NADH dependent enzyme, methemoglobin reductase. This system is capable of reducing methemoglobin to deoxyhemoglobin at a rate 250 times the rate at which heme is normally oxidized.

Methemoglobinemia is a clinical condition, which occurs when methemoglobin encompasses more than 1% of the hemoglobin. This condition can occur when the methemoglobin reductase system is overwhelmed (acquired) or deficient (congenital) and when a structurally abnormal globin chain stabilizes methemoglobin by rendering the molecule poorly susceptible to reduction (congenital) (Table 12-2 ❂).

Acquired methemoglobinemia may occur in normal individuals when drugs or other toxic substances oxidize hemoglobin in circulation at a rate that exceeds the reducing capacity of the methemoglobin reductase system (∞ Chapter 5).

Congenital cyanosis caused by the presence of methemoglobin may be inherited as a dominant or recessive characteristic. Recessive inheritance is usually associated with a defect in the methemoglobin reduction system, NADH-diphorase (reductase, dehydrogenase) deficiency, rather than with an alteration in the structure of the hemoglobin molecule. With defects in the methemoglobin reduction system, the small amount of methemoglobin formed daily cannot be reduced and consequently accumulates within the cell. Dominant inheritance of methemoglobinemia is usually ascribed to the presence of a structural variant of hemoglobin called hemoglobin M (HbM). Many variants of HbM have been described; however, all variants have been found only in the heterozygous state. In the homozygous state the he-

⊛ **TABLE 12-2**

Causes and Characteristics of Methemoglobinemia

Type	Cause	Electrophoretic Pattern	NADH-Diaphorase Activity	Reduction with Methylene Blue
Acquired	Hb oxidized at a rate exceeding capacity of methemoglobin reductase system	Normal	Normal	Yes
Congenital				
Recessive	Defect in methemoglobin reductase system (recessive)	Normal	Decreased	Yes
Dominant	Structural abnormality of hemoglobin (HbM) (dominant)	HbM variant	Normal	No

moglobin could not deliver any oxygen to tissues; therefore, the homozygous condition is incompatible with life.

Most HbM variants are produced by a tyrosine substitution for the proximal or distal histidine in the heme pocket of the α or β chains. Tyrosine forms a covalent link with heme iron, stabilizing the iron in the ferric state. If the substitution occurs in the α chain, cyanosis is present from birth because the α chain is a component of HbF ($\alpha_2\gamma_2$), the major hemoglobin at birth. If the substitution occurs in the β chain, cyanosis does not occur until about the sixth month after birth when HbA ($\alpha_2\beta_2$) becomes the major hemoglobin.

The presence of methemoglobin imparts a brownish color to the blood. Aside from this abnormal color, no other hematologic abnormality is present.

Hemoglobin M will not always separate from HbA at an alkaline pH. Hemoglobin electrophoresis on agar gel at pH 7.1 of a blood sample containing HbM reveals a brown band (HbM) running anodal to a red band (HbA). The pattern may appear sharper with gel electrofocusing. Oxidizing the erythrocyte hemolysate with ferricyanide before electrophoresis reveals a sharp separation of congenital HbM and methemoglobin formed from HbA. Methemoglobin formed from HbA by oxidation of iron has no change in molecular charge and therefore has the same electrophoretic mobility as HbA.

Whereas HbM may be detected by spectral abnormalities of the hemoglobin, methemoglobin formed in NADH-diaphorase deficiency has a normal absorption spectrum. In addition, methemoglobin formed as the result of NADH-diaphorase deficiency can be readily reduced by incubation of blood with methylene blue, whereas methemoglobin caused by a structural hemoglobin variant such as HbM does not reduce with the methylene blue. To confirm NADH-diaphorase deficiency, a quantitative assay of the enzyme activity is necessary.

Congenital methemoglobinemia resulting from NADH-diaphorase deficiency and acquired toxic methemoglobinemia may be treated by administration of ascorbic acid or methylene blue. Conversely, there is no treatment for the HbM structural variants because the abnormal hemoglobin cannot be reduced.

INCREASED OXYGEN AFFINITY

High affinity hemoglobins are inherited as autosomal dominants. All such hemoglobins discovered have been in the heterozygous state. The variants result from amino acid substitutions that involve the $\alpha_1\beta_2$ contacts. These contacts are involved in considerable intramolecular movement as hemoglobin goes from the oxygenated to the deoxygenated state. Other substitutions affect the C-terminal end of the β chain, which is important in maintaining the stability of the deoxygenated form. A few substitutions affect the 2,3-DPG binding sites.

The abnormal hemoglobin results in a shift to the left of the oxygen dissociation curve. The P50 of the hemoglobin is decreased to 12–18 mm Hg. This means less oxygen is given up to tissues where the P50 is about 26 mm Hg. The resulting tissue hypoxia stimulates erythropoietin production and, subsequently, formation of a compensatory increased erythrocyte mass. In addition to the primary effect of increasing oxygen affinity, secondary effects of the mutations may also occur, including instability of the protein, reduced Bohr effect, and reduced cooperativity of the oxygen binding.[25]

Individuals with these hemoglobin variants are asymptomatic. A ruddy complexion may occasionally be apparent.

Erythrocyte counts and hematocrit levels are increased, and hemoglobin levels are increased to about 20 g/dL. Other hematologic parameters are normal. About half of the hemoglobin variants have an altered electrophoretic mobility enabling diagnosis by starch gel or cellulose acetate electrophoresis. Diagnosis is established by measuring oxygen affinity.

✓ **Checkpoint! #11**

Why should red cell enzymes measurement and hemoglobin electrophoresis both be performed on a patient with congenital cyanosis?

Thal

Tim R.

■ CHECKLIST - LEVEL II *(continued)*

6. Correlate clinical severities of both α- and β-thalassemia with their respective genotypes.
7. Compare and contrast other thalassemia and thalassemia-like conditions to include:
   a. δβ-thalassemia
   b. γδβ-thalassemia
   c. Hemoglobin Constant Spring
   d. Hereditary persistence of fetal hemoglobin (HPFH)
   e. Hemoglobin Lepore
   f. Thalassemia/hemoglobinopathy combination disorders
8. Differentiate iron deficiency anemia and HPFH from thalassemia based on results of laboratory tests and clinical findings.

KEY TERMS

Allele
Compression syndrome
Congenital
Crossover
Diploid
Double heterozygous
Extramedullary erythropoiesis
Functional hyposplenism
Gene cluster
Genotype
Haplotypes
Heterozygous
Homozygous
Ineffective erythropoiesis
P_{50} value
Phenotype
Zygosity

▶ Describe the extravascular destruction of erythrocytes. (Chapter 4)

Level II
▶ Summarize the synthesis and molecular structure of hemoglobin and correlate alterations in structure with function; describe globin chain synthesis in utero and throughout life. (Chapters 3, 5)
▶ Interpret hemoglobin migration patterns on electrophoresis, acid elution of fetal hemoglobins, hemoglobin solubility tests, and iron panels to distinguish iron metabolism disorders and hemoglobinopathies from thalassemias. (Chapter 39)

⊙ CASE STUDY

We will refer to this case throughout the chapter.
John is a 4-year-old boy who frequently complains of weakness, fatigue, and dyspnea. The family moved to the United States from Greece before the child's birth. Both parents experienced fatigue from time to time but never consulted a physician. Consider the types of anemia most often found at this age and the laboratory tests that could help establish a diagnosis. What is the significance, if any, of knowing the parents' background and medical history?

BACKGROUND BASICS

The information in this chapter will build upon concepts presented in previous chapters. To maximize your learning experience you should review the following concepts before beginning this unit of study.

Level I
▶ Describe the pathophysiology of hemoglobinopathies. (Chapter 12).
▶ Describe the morphologic and functional classification of anemias and the associated lab tests. (Chapter 10)
▶ Interpret routine laboratory tests, such as CBC and differential, and apply both normal and abnormal results in the diagnosis of anemias. (Chapters 7, 8, 10)
▶ Describe the basic structure and function of hemoglobin and identify the globin chain composition of normal hemoglobin types. (Chapter 5)

▶ OVERVIEW

This chapter discusses a group of hereditary anemias collectively called thalassemias. It begins with a general description of thalassemias including the genetic defects and types, pathophysiology, and clinical and laboratory findings. Subsequently, each type is discussed in the following format: pathophysiology, clinical findings, laboratory findings, treatment, and prognosis. Other thalassemia-like conditions are

---

REVIEW QUESTIONS *(continu...*

LEVEL I

www.prenhall.com/m...
Use the above address...
hints, instant feedback,...

REFERENCES

1. Weatherall DJ, Clegg JB. Genetic disord... *Hematol.* 1999; 36 (4 Suppl 7):24–37.
2. Herrick JB. Peculiar elongated and sickle-cles in a case of severe anemia. *Trans A:* 25:553–61.
3. Pauling L, Itano HA, Singer SJ, Wells IC. Si... ular disease. *Science.* 1949; ll0:543–48.
4. Cao A, Galanello R, Rosatelli MC. Prenatal... of the haemoglobinopathies. *Baillieres* 11:215–38.
5. Flint J, Harding RM, Boyce AJ, Clegg JB. Th... the haemoglobinopathies. *Baillieres Clin Ha...*
6. Bunyaratvej A, Butthep P, Sae-Ung N, Fuch... Reduced deformability of thalassemic erythr... with abnormal hemoglobins and relation... *Plasmodium falciparum* invasion. *Blood.* 1992...
7. Ballas SK, Smith ED. Red blood cell changes... the sickle cell painful crisis. *Blood.* 1992; 79:2...
8. Mackie LH, Hochmuth RM. The influence o... perature, and hemoglobin concentration on... ties of sickle erythrocytes. *Blood.* 1990; 76:12...
9. Liu SC, Derick LH, Palek J. Dependence of th... tion of red blood cell membranes on spectri... librium: Implication for permanent membran... versibly sickled cells. *Blood.* 1993; 81:522–28.
10. Steinberg MH. Pathophysiology of sickle cell... *Haematol.* 1998; 11:163–84.
11. Liu SC, Yi SJ, Mehta JR, Nichols PE, Ballas SK,... cell membrane remodeling in sickle cell anem... 97:29–36.
12. Boghossian SH, Nash G, Dormandy J, Bevan... trophil adhesion in sickle cell anaemia and c... blood rheology. *Br J Haematol.* 1991; 78:437–41...
13. Ballas SK. Sickle cell disease: Clinical manage... *Haematol.* 1998; 11:185–14.

described and compared and contrasted with thalassemia. The chapter concludes by describing the laboratory differential diagnosis of types of thalassemia and other disorders that have similar peripheral blood morphology.

INTRODUCTION

Thalassemia constitutes a family of **congenital** disorders in which mutations in one or more of the globin genes of hemoglobin cause decreased or absent synthesis of the corresponding globin chains. Consequences of the mutation depend on the particular chain affected and the amount of globin chain produced. Limited availability of globin chains results in a reduction in the assembly of hemoglobin. Patients with mild genetic defects are generally asymptomatic. Patients with more severe defects present with symptoms that result from one or more of the following: decreased production of normal hemoglobin; synthesis of abnormal hemoglobins; **ineffective erythropoiesis;** and disproportionate production of unaffected globin chains. Symptoms include anemia, hepatosplenomegaly, infections, gallstones, and bone deformities that alter facial features and result in pathologic fractures.

The most important thalassemias are alpha- (α) and beta- (β) thalassemia. Alpha-thalassemia results from a decreased or absent production of α-globin chains, while β-thalassemia is caused by a reduction or absence of β-globin chains. Defects in the α- and β-chains may cause anemia because approximately 97% of normal adult hemoglobin (HbA) is composed of α- and β-globin chains.

The first clinical description of thalassemia was offered by Thomas Cooley in Detroit in 1925.[1] At that time, thalassemia was thought to be a rare disorder restricted to the Mediterranean races. Dr. Cooley's work broadened our understanding of the nationalities that potentially could be affected by thalassemia and suggested that the disease was hemolytic in nature. By 1960, it was apparent that the thalassemias were a heterogeneous group of genetic disorders. With the advent of molecular biology, thalassemias have been widely studied by many groups of researchers. Methods developed in the last 25 years enable researchers to measure the quantity of globin chains synthesized and identify specific genetic mutations.

Thalassemia is now recognized as one of the most common genetic disorders affecting the world's population. It is estimated that between 100,000 and 200,000 individuals worldwide are born each year with severe forms of thalassemia. In North America about 20% of Southeast Asian immigrants and 6–11% of African Americans have detectable α-thalassemia. Many more are silent carriers. About 6% of individuals with Mediterranean ancestry, 5% of Southeast Asians, and 0.8% of African Americans have β-thalassemia.

Thalassemia is a major health problem in countries where these disorders are prevalent. Prevention is seen as an essential part in the management of the problem. Thus, many of these countries now have large screening and education programs to detect carriers. This has drastically reduced the number of individuals born with both homozygous and heterozygous forms of the disease.

THALASSEMIA VS HEMOGLOBINOPATHY

The system of categorizing thalassemias and hemoglobinopathies differs among hematologists. Some use hemoglobinopathy as a disease category that includes both structural variants of hemoglobin like sickle cell anemia, and thalassemias. Others categorize all structural variants as hemoglobinopathies and describe thalassemias as a separate disease entity. In this text we will refer to the two diseases separately.

In the preceding chapter, hemoglobinopathies were defined as qualitative defects in the structure of globin chains resulting in production of abnormal hemoglobin molecules. Thalassemias, on the other hand, are quantitative disorders of hemoglobin synthesis that produce reduced amounts of normal hemoglobin.

The different outcomes of hemoglobinopathies and thalassemia are a direct result of the types of mutations encountered in these disease states. Hemoglobinopathies result from a point mutation in the β-globin gene, predominantly, that is translated into a β-globin chain containing a single amino acid substitution. All hemoglobin containing β-chains are produced at normal levels but are structurally abnormal. In contrast, thalassemias result from both deletional and nondeletional mutations in globin genes that reduce or eliminate the synthesis of the corresponding globin chain. This results in the assembly of inadequate amounts of normal hemoglobin and a reduced oxygen carrying capacity of the blood. Unlike hemoglobinopathies, the amino acid sequence of the chain, if produced, is normal and is assembled into the appropriate hemoglobin as usual, albeit in reduced amounts. In some of the less common thalassemias, the globin chains may be lengthened or truncated (Table 13-1).

✓ Checkpoint! #1

Differentiate the etiology of thalassemias and hemoglobinopathies.

GENETIC DEFECTS IN THALASSEMIA

Nearly all thalassemic mutations fall into one of five categories of genetic lesions: gene deletion, promoter mutation, nonsense mutation, mutated termination (stop) codon, and splice site mutation (Table 13-2 ○). Regardless of the type of mutation encountered, the results are the same; the globin chain corresponding to the mutated globin gene will be

⊛ TABLE 13-1

Comparison of Hemoglobinopathies and Thalassemias

Disease	RBC Count	Indices	Erythrocyte Morphology	Abnormal Hb	Hb Solubility Test	Ancestry	Reticulocyte Count
Hemoglobinopathy	↓	Normocytic, normochromic	Target cells, Sickle cells (in HbS) HbC crystals (in HbC) Others	HbS HbC HbE, etc.	+ in HbS, Hb Bart's, and HbC^{Harlem}	African Mediterranean Middle East Southeast Asian	↑↑
Thalassemia	↑ Compared to what is expected for the Hb level	Microcytic, hypochromic	Target cells, Basophilic stippling	HbH (β^4) Hb Bart's (γ^4)	Negative	Mediterranean Southeast Asian African	↑

↓=slight decrease, ↑=slight increase, ↑↑=moderate increase, Hb=hemoglobin, RBC=red blood cell, +=positive

absent, reduced in concentration or, on occasion, somewhat longer or shorter than normal.

If all the globin genes of a single type of globin chain are deleted, the corresponding hemoglobin is absent. This scenario is most common in α-thalassemia. Reduction in globin chain production from nondeletional mutations is more common in the β-thalassemias. The degree of reduction in globin chain production is a direct reflection of the type of mutation encountered and parallels the severity of the clinical disorder (Table 13-2 ⊛).

✓ Checkpoint! #2:

What are the most common types of genetic mutations associated with α-thalassemia?

TYPES OF THALASSEMIA

Since there are six normal globin genes (α, β, γ, δ, ε, ζ), at least six versions of thalassemia are possible. In addition, deletions can occur to entire **gene clusters,** concurrently affecting more than one globin chain. Of the six normal globin genes, epsilon and zeta (ε, ζ) are normally synthesized only in utero, and gamma (γ) is produced in high quantities from approximately the third trimester of pregnancy until birth. After birth, γ-chain synthesis begins to decrease but can still be detected in low quantities in adult life. The three remaining globin chains (α, β, and δ), along with the γ-chains, are considered normal adult globin chains and combine to form hemoglobin A ($\alpha_2\beta_2$), hemoglobin A$_2$ ($\alpha_2\delta_2$), and hemoglobin F ($\alpha_2\gamma_2$), respectively. Since approximately 97% of normal adult hemoglobin is HbA, a deficiency of ei-

⊛ TABLE 13-2

Five Common Genetic Defects in Thalassemia

Mutation Type	Thalassemia Encountered	Effect on Gene	Effect on Globin Chain
Deletion	Predominantly α-thalassemia, some β-thalassemia	Loss of gene	Absence of production
Promoter	Predominantly β-thalassemia	Impaired transcription	Reduced or absent production
Nonsense	Predominantly β-thalassemia	In frame substitution	Amino acid change
		Frame shift	Amino acid changes distal to shift
			Longer or shorter globin chains
Stop codon	Predominantly β-thalassemia	Convert stop codons to amino acid codons	Slightly lengthened globin chain (retained)
			Significantly lengthened globin chain (degraded)
Splice site	Predominantly β-thalassemia	Create new splice sites	Slightly shortened globin chain (retained)
			Significantly shorthened globin chain (degraded)
		Loss of splice sites	Slightly lengthened globin chain (retained)
			Significantly lengthened globin chain (degraded)
			Unaltered globin chain

ther α- or β-chains will affect hemoglobin A assembly, reducing HbA concentration and thus affecting the oxygen-carrying capacity of the blood.

Two major types of classical thalassemia have been described, α-thalassemia and β-thalassemia. When synthesis of the α-chain is impaired, the disease is α-thalassemia. When synthesis of the β-chain is affected, the disease is β-thalassemia. A third type of thalassemia, δ-thalassemia, has been reported, but its occurrence is rare and it is not clinically significant because the δ-chain is a component of the minor hemoglobin HbA_2, which comprises only 2.5% of total hemoglobin. Rarely, combinations of gene deletions lead to δβ-thalassemia or γδβ-thalassemia. The affected chains are all synthesized at a reduced rate.

Occasionally, synthesis of a structural hemoglobin variant will decrease hemoglobin concentration, giving the clinical picture of thalassemia. These structural variants include those hemoglobins with abnormally long or short globin chains (hemoglobin Constant Spring). Hemoglobin Lepore is a hemoglobin variant in which the non–α-globin chains are not only structurally abnormal but are also ineffectively synthesized. Because of their clinical similarity to thalassemias, these particular structural variants will be discussed in this section.

A variant of β-thalassemia, known as hereditary persistence of fetal hemoglobin (HPFH), is characterized by continued production of HbF throughout life. In this disorder, there is a failure in the switch of γ-chain production to β-chain production after birth. In the homozygotes, 100% of circulating hemoglobin is HbF.

PATHOPHYSIOLOGY

Normally equal quantities of α- and β-chains are synthesized by the maturing erythrocyte, resulting in a β-chain to α-chain ratio of 1.0. In α- and β-thalassemia, synthesis of one of these chains is decreased or absent, resulting in an excess of the other chain. If the α-chain is affected, there is an excess of β-chains, and if the β-chain is affected, there is an excess of α-chains. This imbalanced synthesis of chains has several effects, all of which contribute to anemia: (1) a decrease in total erythrocyte hemoglobin production, (2) ineffective erythropoiesis, and (3) chronic hemolysis.

Excess α-chains are unstable and precipitate within the cell. The precipitates bind to the cell membrane, causing membrane damage and decreased erythrocyte deformability. The precipitate filled erythrocytes may be destroyed in the bone marrow by macrophages resulting in a large degree of ineffective erythropoiesis. Circulating erythrocytes with precipitates are pitted and/or removed by the spleen causing chronic hemolysis.

Excess β-chains can combine to form hemoglobin molecules with four β-chains, hemoglobin H (HbH). This hemoglobin has a high oxygen affinity and is also unstable. Thus, it is a poor transporter of oxygen. In the infant, excess γ-chains combine to form hemoglobin Bart's (Hb Bart's)

when α-chains are decreased. This hemoglobin also has a very high oxygen affinity.

In addition to α- and β-thalassemia, other thalassemias and thalassemia-like conditions may occur. Structural hemoglobin variants may result in decreased synthesis of globin chains, giving the clinical picture of thalassemia.

CLINICAL FINDINGS

Clinical findings are related to anemia, chronic hemolysis, and ineffective erythropoiesis (Table 13-3). The combination of reduced HbA synthesis, ineffective erythropoiesis, and hemolysis results in anemia. There is a wide variation in severity of anemia depending on the specific genetic mutation and number of genes affected. Hypoxia from anemia is exacerbated in some cases by the presence of abnormal hemoglobins that have a high oxygen affinity (HbH and Hb Bart's). These hemoglobins do not release oxygen readily to the tissues.

Chronic hemolysis has several adverse effects. Splenomegaly is frequently present as the spleen is a major site of extravascular hemolysis. Occasionally, the spleen may become overburdened by the process of erythrocyte destruction resulting in **functional hyposplenism**. In this case its function as a secondary lymphoid tissue is compromised leading to an increase in infections (∞ Chapter 3). Chronic hemolysis can also result in formation of gallstones.

The chronic demand for erythrocytes also has adverse effects. The bone marrow will respond by increasing erythropoiesis, resulting in erythroid hyperplasia. In some of the more severe thalassemias, this results in bone marrow expansion and thinning of calcified bone. Consequently, patients develop skeletal abnormalities and pathologic fractures. The increased iron demand needed to support the erythropoietic activity stimulates the absorption of more iron. This additional iron is not effectively incorporated into hemoglobin, so it accumulates in macrophages in the bone marrow, liver, and spleen. As this process continues, iron will eventually accumulate in parenchymal cells of various organs and adversely affect organ function. Ineffective erythropoiesis in the bone marrow may be accompanied by **extramedullary erythropoiesis** in the liver and spleen. Extramedullary erythropoiesis can produce masses large enough to cause **compression syndromes** (Table 13-3).

> ### ✓ Checkpoint! #3
>
> *Why do α- and β-thalassemia result in more clinically severe disease than other types of thalassemia?*

LABORATORY FINDINGS

Peripheral blood findings provide clues to the disease (Table 13-3). Thalassemias are characterized by microcytic, hypochromic anemia with a decrease in MCV, MCH, and

TABLE 13-3

Clinical and Laboratory Findings Associated with Thalassemia

Clinical Finding	Pathophysiology	Laboratory Finding
Anemia/hypoxia	Decreased hemoglobin production/erythropoiesis	↓ RBC count, hemoglobin, hematocrit
	Ineffective erythropoiesis	Microcytic/hypochromic RBCs
	Presence of high-affinity hemoglobins (HbH and Hb Bart's)	↓MCV, ↓MCH, ↓MCHC
	Increased extravascular hemolysis	↑ Reticulocyte count
		Anisocytosis and poikilocytosis
		Target cells, basophilic stippling, nucleated RBCs
		BM erythroid hyperplasia
		↑ RDW
		Abnormal hemoglobin electrophoresis
Splenomegaly/hemolysis	Splenic removal of abnormal erythrocytes	↑ Bilirubin
	Ineffective erythropoiesis	↓ Haptoglobin
Gallstones	Increased intravascular and extravascular hemolysis	↑ Bilirubin
Skeletal abnormalities	Expansion of bone marrow	BM erythroid hyperplasia
Pathologic fractures	Thinning of calcified bone	
Iron toxicity	Multiple transfusions	↑ Prussian blue staining in BM
		↑ Serum iron/ferritin and ↓ TIBC

usually MCHC. The erythrocyte count is often normal or increased for the degree of anemia. The RDW may be increased. Target cells and microcytosis usually are present even in cases without anemia or symptoms of anemia. Basophilic stippling and nucleated erythrocytes may be present. Anisocytosis and poikilocytosis are common. Precipitates of excess chains or unstable hemoglobin may be visualized with supravital stains. Reticulocytes and bilirubin are usually increased due to the chronic hemolysis. Haptoglobin, a protein that transports free plasma hemoglobin to the liver, may be decreased depending on the degree of hemolysis.

Hemoglobin electrophoresis is always indicated if thalassemia is suspected. HbA is usually decreased. HbF and HbA$_2$ are increased in β-thalassemia but decreased in α-thalassemia. Hemoglobin Bart's and HbH may also be present in α-thalassemia.

Bone marrow studies are not necessary for diagnosis but when performed show marked erythroid hyperplasia. Normoblasts appear abnormal with very little cytoplasm, uneven cytoplasmic membranes, and striking basophilic stippling. Prussian blue stain reveals an abundance of iron and occasionally a few ringed sideroblasts. Phagocytic "foam" cells similar to Gaucher cells have been reported in the more severe forms. The foam is probably the result of partially digested red cell membrane lipids associated with intense ineffective erythropoiesis.

Since the emphasis is now on screening programs to detect thalassemia carriers in areas of high prevalence and in certain populations, laboratorians must look for assays that are uncomplicated, time efficient, and accurate. The reverse dot blot procedure, a molecular technique, seems to be the most popular for this purpose as it is rapid and accurate. It allows for the screening of several mutations with a single hybridization reaction. In this procedure, mutant probes are fixed on a membrane. Since there are hundreds of different globin gene mutants leading to thalassemia, the probes selected are those commonly found in a particular geographic region. The patient's DNA is PCR-amplified, labeled, and added to the membrane with the probes. The patient's DNA will hybridize only to probes complementary to its sequence. The pattern of hybridization of the patient's DNA with the probes determines if a particular mutation is present.

α-THALASSEMIA

GENERAL CONSIDERATIONS

Alpha-thalassemia is a group of four disorders characterized by decreased synthesis of α-chains. Although each will be discussed separately, several features common to each type will be presented here.

Etiology

In the human genome, two α-genes are located on each of the two chromosome 16 structures, totaling four α-genes in the **diploid** state (Figure 13-1 ■). Mutations can affect one or more of the α-genes resulting in four discrete clinical severities that have been described. A patient in whom all four α-genes are mutated produces no α-chains, and the condition is referred to as hydrops fetalis. When three of the

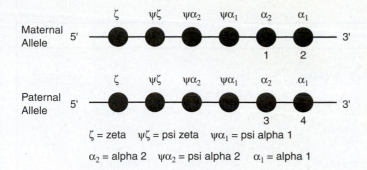

Maternal Allele

Paternal Allele

ζ = zeta   ψζ = psi zeta   ψα₁ = psi alpha 1

α₂ = alpha 2   ψα₂ = psi alpha 2   α₁ = alpha 1

■ **FIGURE 13-1** A short section of chromosome 16 showing the 5' to 3' orientation of three functional genes ζ, α_2, and α_1 along with three pseudogenes $\psi\zeta$, $\psi\alpha_2$, and $\psi\alpha_1$. Pseudogenes are the result of partial gene duplications but are not expressed. There are two α-genes on each allele; the α_2-gene expresses 2 to 3 times as much protein product as the α_1-gene.

four α-genes are deleted, the disorder is known as hemoglobin H (HbH) disease. The deletion of two α-genes is known as α-thalassemia minor, and the deletion of a single α-gene is known as silent carrier. Though less common, nondeletional mutations and mutations that produce unstable α-chains are also found in α-thalassemia. The outcome is usually the same as a deletion mutation, a reduction in α-chains and in the corresponding α-containing hemoglobins.

Affected Alleles

The quantity of α-chains synthesized is somewhat proportional to the number of affected **alleles**. In general, erythrocytes will produce higher concentrations of α-chains than the number of affected alleles predict. There are two main reasons for this phenomenon. First, the four α-genes can be described as two pairs of equally functioning genes designated as α_1 and α_2. Each chromosome 16 contains an α_1- and an α_2-gene oriented with the α_2-gene positioned upstream from the α_1-gene (Figure 13-1 ■). It has been shown that the α_2-gene produces two to three times the amount of mRNA as the α_1-gene.[2] Therefore, a deletion of the α_2-gene would reduce α-chain production to a greater degree than would a deletion of the α_1-gene. Second, the erythropoietic system has an internal mechanism designed to stimulate increased production of α-chains from the unaffected genes to compensate for deletions, thus minimizing the reduction of α-chains.

Affected Individuals

Alpha-thalassemia is concentrated in people of Mediterranean, Asian, and African ancestry. In particular, it is commonly seen in blacks, Indians, Chinese, and Middle Eastern people, with blacks expressing a milder version of the disease. The reason patients of African descent tend to present with a milder version of α-thalassemia is because the deletion usually involves the α_1-gene.

Genotypes

Three nomenclature systems have been developed—genotypic, genotypic description, and phenotypic—that classify the α-thalassemias into five discrete categories. The addition of the normal **genotype** produces a total of six possibilities. In the genotypic system, deleted genes are designated as $(-)$ and unaffected genes as (α). The genotypic description system combines the **zygosity** state, **homozygous** or **heterozygous,** with either a gene symbol (α^0 or α^+) or a nominal descriptor (thal-1 or thal-2) to designate the number of deleted α-genes on each chromosome. Both thal-1 and α^0 indicate the deletion of both α-genes on the same chromosome $(-,-)$. Likewise, thal-2 and α^+ refer to one deleted and one unaffected α-gene on a given allele $(-, \alpha)$. The phenotypic system describes four clinical types, hydrops fetalis, hemoglobin H disease, α-thalassemia minor, and silent carrier, with the α-thalassemia minor type exhibiting two clinical severities (Table 13-4 ✪).[2] Occasionally patients will bear a nondeletional mutation of the α-thalassemia gene, designated as α^T, that functions to reduce but not eliminate α-chain production from that gene.

α-THALASSEMIA MAJOR (α^0-THAL-1/α^0-THAL-1; HYDROPS FETALIS)

This is the most severe form of α-thalassemia, involving the deletion of all four α-genes. Both parents of the thalassemia patient must have α-thalassemia to have a child with hydrops fetalis because both α-genes on each parental allele inherited by the child are deleted.

Pathophysiology

Since all four α-genes are deleted in hydrops fetalis, no normal adult hemoglobins can be synthesized. Therefore, this disorder is incompatible with life, and infants are either stillborn or die within hours of birth. In the absence of α-chains, erythrocytes assemble hemoglobin using the γ-, δ-, and β-chains available. Therefore, abnormal hemoglobin tetramers involving γ-chains (Hb Bart's, γ_4) and β-chains (HbH, β_4) are produced. Hb Bart's has a very high oxygen affinity and no Bohr effect (∞ Chapter 5). Therefore, this hemoglobin cannot supply tissues with sufficient oxygen to sustain life, and the developing infant dies of hypoxia and congestive heart failure. Hemoglobin Portland, although normally absent following the first trimester, continues to be synthesized until birth in α-thalassemia since it does not contain α-chains.

Clinical Findings

Infants that survive until birth exhibit significant physical changes upon routine exam. The babies are underweight and edematous, with a distended abdomen. The liver and often the spleen are enlarged due to extramedullary hematopoiesis. There is massive bone marrow hyperplasia. He-

✪ TABLE 13-4

Characteristics of α-thalassemia

Genotype	Genotypic Description	Phenotype	Hematologic Findings	Severity	Hemoglobins Present
(−−/−−)	Homozygous α⁰-thalassemia-1	Hydrops fetalis	Marked anemia Microcytic/hypochromic RBCs ↑↑↑ anisopoikilocytosis ↑ NRBC	Fatal	Hb Bart's (80–90%) Hb Portland (10–20%)
(−−/−α)	Heterozygous α⁰-thalassemia-1/ α⁺-thalassemia-2	Hemoglobin H disease	Moderate to marked anemia Microcytic/hypochromic RBCs Target cells Basophilic stippling Poikilocytosis	Chronic, moderately severe hemolytic anemia	Birth=Hb Bart's Adult=HbH
(−−/αα)	Heterozygous α⁰-thalassemia-1	α-thalassemia-minor	Slight anemia Microcytic/hypochromic RBCs Target cells Basophilic stippling Poikilocytosis	Mild to moderate	Birth=Hb Bart's Adult=normal
(−α/−α)	Homozygous α⁺-thalassemia-2	α-thalassemia-minor	Slight anemia Microcytic/hypochromic RBCs Target cells Basophilic stippling Poikilocytosis	Mild	Birth=Hb Bart's Adult=normal
(−α/αα)	Heterozygous α⁺-thalassemia-2	Silent carrier	Normocytic or slightly microcytic RBCs	Normal	Normal
(αα/αα)	Normal	None	Normal	Normal	Normal

↑↑↑=marked increase, ↑=slight increase

molysis in the fetus is probably severe, as there is extensive deposition of hemosiderin.

Laboratory Results

Laboratory results can confirm the diagnosis. There is severe anemia with hemoglobin values ranging from 3 to 10 g/dL. Hemoglobin electrophoresis on cellulose acetate at alkaline pH shows 80–90% Hb Bart's and 10–20% Hb Portland, with HbH sometimes detectable. HbA, HbA₂ and HbF are absent due to the lack of α-chain production (Figure 13-2 ■).

Checkpoint! #4

Which of the three normal adult hemoglobins would be affected in hydrops fetalis?

HEMOGLOBIN H DISEASE (α⁰-THAL-1/α⁺-THAL-2)

HbH disease, a symptomatic but nonfatal type of α-thalassemia, was the first type to be described in 1956. It occurs when three of four α-genes are deleted. African Americans

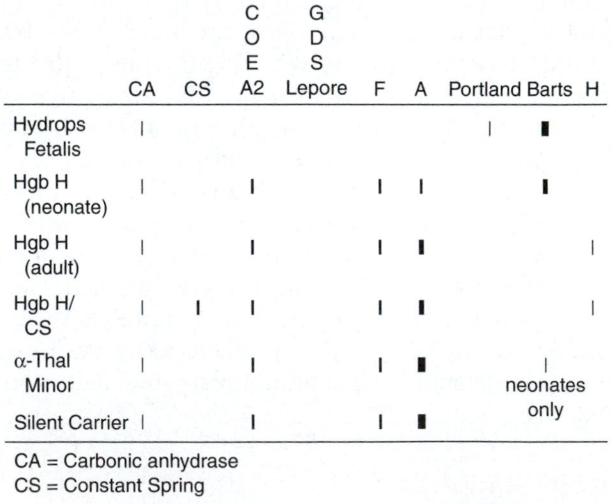

	CA	CS	C O E A2	Lepore	F	A	Portland	Barts	H
Hydrops Fetalis	I						I	■	
Hgb H (neonate)	I		I		I	I		■	
Hgb H (adult)	I		I		I	■			I
Hgb H/ CS	I	I	I		I	■			I
α-Thal Minor	I		I		I	■		I neonates only	
Silent Carrier	I		I		I	■			

CA = Carbonic anhydrase
CS = Constant Spring

■ **FIGURE 13-2** Hemoglobin electrophoresis on cellulose acetate at pH 8.4 is helpful in distinguishing the type of thalassemia and in differentiating thalassemias from hemoglobinopathies. In α-thalassemias, there is a reduction in α-containing hemoglobins (HbA, HbA₂, and HbF) proportional to the number of deleted α-genes and in the more severe cases, the emergence of non–α-containing hemoglobins (HbH and Hb Bart's).

seldom present with HbH disease because they rarely express a deletion of two α-genes on the same chromosome.[3]

This disorder usually results when two heterozygous parents, one with α^0-thal-1 $(--/\alpha\alpha)$ and the other expressing the α^+-thal-2 $(-\alpha/\alpha\alpha)$ genotype, bear children.[2] All children from a patient with HbH disease will have one of the four types of α-thalassemia, the severity of which depends on the genotype of the other parent.

Pathophysiology

The dramatic reduction in α-chain synthesis results in a decrease in the assembly of HbA, HbA$_2$, and HbF. In addition, a decrease in α-chains creates a relative excess of β-chains, which unite to form tetrads of four β-chains called HbH. γ-chains are also produced in excess of α-chains, especially at birth, and combine to form Hb Bart's.

HbH is thermolabile, unstable, and tends to precipitate inside erythrocytes triggering chronic hemolytic anemia. It also has an oxygen affinity 10 times that of HbA, which reduces oxygen delivery to the tissues. Its high oxygen affinity is attributed to the lack of heme–heme interaction and absence of the Bohr effect. This increased oxygen affinity is reflected in the lower **P$_{50}$ value** of HbH relative to HbA and myoglobin (Figure 13-3 ■).

Hemoglobin H also occurs as an acquired defect in erythroleukemia and other myeloproliferative disorders. However, the clinical manifestations and hematological abnormalities of these acquired disorders make it possible to distinguish them from HbH disease. Acquired HbH is probably due to a defect that prohibits the transcription of the α-gene.

Clinical Findings

Symptoms are related to anemia and chronic hemolysis. Hemoglobin H disease shows a wide variation in the degree of anemia, from mild to severe, that worsens during pregnancy, in infectious states, and during administration of oxidant drugs. Splenomegaly and, less often, hepatomegaly are present. Less than half of affected patients exhibit skeletal changes similar to those found in β-thalassemia major.

Laboratory Results

Hemoglobin H disease is characterized by a microcytic, hypochromic anemia with hemoglobin levels usually ranging from 8 to 10 g/dL. Reticulocytes are moderately increased from 5 to 10%, and nucleated red blood cells are observed on the peripheral blood smear (Figure 13-4a ■).

Hemoglobin electrophoresis of affected neonates shows about 25% Hb Bart's with decreased levels of HbA, HbA$_2$, and HbF. After birth, β-chains begin to replace γ-chains, and HbH eventually replaces Hb Bart's. Hemoglobin H, a fast-migrating hemoglobin at alkaline pH, makes up from 2 to 40% of the hemoglobin in adults with HbH disease. HbA$_2$ is decreased to a mean of 1.5%, but HbF is normal. A trace of Hb Bart's can be demonstrated in approximately 10% of affected adults, with the remainder of the hemoglobin being HbA (Figure 13-2 ■). Other laboratory tests are available to assess patients with HbH disease. Hemoglobin H inclusions are easily found upon incubation of blood with brilliant cresyl blue (Figure 13-4b ■). These inclusions tend to cover the inside of the plasma membrane, giving the appearance of a golf ball.

Treatment and Prognosis

Treatment for patients with HbH disease is variable but when indicated involves long-term transfusion therapy and splenectomy. Early treatment is necessary to prevent the typical clinical manifestations of thalassemia. With supportive and behavioral interventions, patients with HbH disease experience a normal life expectancy.

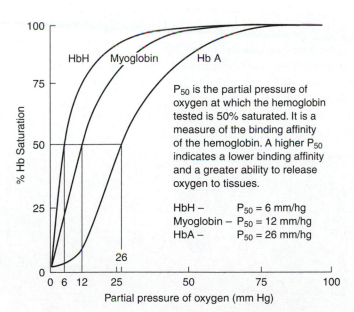

■ **FIGURE 13-3** The Hb dissociation curve illustrates the relative binding affinities of HbA, HbH and myoglobin using the P$_{50}$ value. The monomeric myoglobin molecule lacks heme/heme interactions causing it to bind oxygen tightly, decreasing the P$_{50}$ value relative to HbA. The P$_{50}$ value is even lower for HbH indicating an even stronger affinity for oxygen, estimated to be 10 times greater than the oxygen affinity of HbA.

P$_{50}$ is the partial pressure of oxygen at which the hemoglobin tested is 50% saturated. It is a measure of the binding affinity of the hemoglobin. A higher P$_{50}$ indicates a lower binding affinity and a greater ability to release oxygen to tissues.

HbH –   P$_{50}$ = 6 mm/hg
Myoglobin –   P$_{50}$ = 12 mm/hg
HbA –   P$_{50}$ = 26 mm/hg

α-THALASSEMIA MINOR (α$^+$-THAL-2/ α$^+$-THAL-2, OR α^0-THAL-1/NORMAL)

The α-thalassemia trait (homozygous α^+-thal-2 or α^0-thal-1 trait) occurs when two of the four α-genes, either on the same or on opposite chromosomes, are missing. The condi-

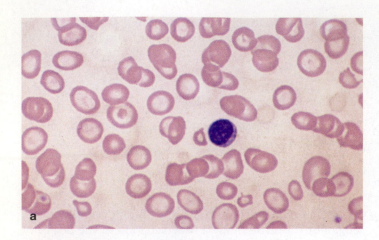
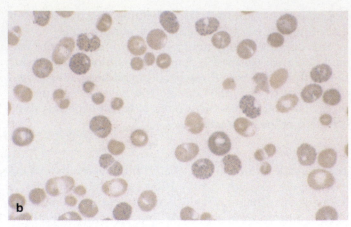

■ **FIGURE 13-4 a.** This peripheral blood smear is from a patient with HbH disease. Note the microcytic, hypochromic anemia with target cells. **b.** Peripheral blood from patient in Figure 13-4a after incubation with brilliant cresyl blue. Notice the cells that have dimples and look like golf balls. These are the cells with precipitated HbH. (a. Brilliant cresyl blue stain; 1000× magnification)

tion is found in all geographic locations.[4] In African Americans the homozygous α^+-thal-2 form is the most common. Genetic testing has identified at least nine **haplotypes**, representing different mutations that all result in the deletion of both α-genes on the same chromosome, which is more common in patients of Southeast Asian or Mediterranean descent.[5]

Pathophysiology

Although there is a measurable decrease in the production of α-containing hemoglobins, the unaffected globin genes are able to direct synthesis of globin chains faster than normal and therefore compensate for the affected genes. There are only minor changes in the erythrocyte count, indices, hemoglobin electrophoresis patterns, and red cell morphology.

Clinical Findings

Patients with α-thalassemia trait are asymptomatic with a mild anemia and are often diagnosed incidentally or when being evaluated for family studies. This mild **phenotype** is the reason this form is called thalassemia minor.

Laboratory Results

The most demonstrable laboratory abnormalities are observed in the newborn. The presence of 5–6% Hb Bart's in neonates may be helpful in diagnosing this condition.[6] Three months after birth, Hb Bart's decreases to undetectable levels and hemoglobin electrophoresis becomes normal. The only persistent hematological abnormality thereafter is microcytic, hypochromic anemia.

In adult patients, hemoglobin levels are above 10 g/dL and the erythrocyte count is above 5×10^{12}/L. The peripheral blood film demonstrates significant microcytosis with an MCV of 60–70 fL with few target cells (Figure 13-5 ■). Occasional cells may exhibit HbH inclusions after incubation with brilliant cresyl blue.

In some cases, α-thalassemia may be masked by iron deficiency anemia. Persistence of microcytes following successful treatment of iron deficiency is suggestive of thalassemia, but further investigation is suggested.

Treatment and Prognosis

These patients have a normal life span and do not require medical intervention for their thalassemia.

SILENT CARRIER (α^+-THAL-2/NORMAL)

The silent carrier version of α-thalassemia (α^+-thal-2 trait) is missing only one of four functioning α-genes. Greater than 25% of African Americans have been shown to express a deletion of one α-gene.[7–9]

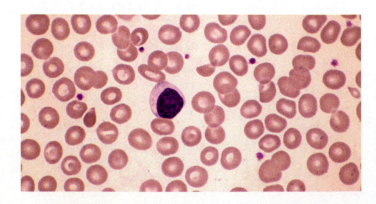

■ **FIGURE 13-5** This is a peripheral blood smear from a patient with α-thalassemia trait. The hemoglobin is 15 g/dL, RBC 6.4 × 10^{12}/L, MCV 69.4 fL. The high RBC count with microcytosis is typical of thalassemia minor or trait. (Peripheral blood; Wright-Giemsa stain; 1000× magnification)

Pathogenesis/Clinical Findings/Laboratory Results

In silent carrier disease the three remaining α-genes direct the synthesis of an adequate number of α-chains for normal hemoglobin synthesis. This carrier state is asymptomatic and totally benign, but adults often present with a borderline normal MCV of around 78–80 fL.[5] In affected infants, 1–2% Hb Bart's may be found at birth but cannot be detected after three months of age. The only definitive diagnostic test for thalassemias in adults with one or two gene deletions is globin gene analysis.

Treatment and Prognosis

Patients with silent carrier disease require no treatment and have a normal life span.

CASE STUDY *(continued from page 240)*

Below are the CBC and differential results for John, our 4-year-old Grecian patient.

CBC		Differential	
WBC:	11.4×10^9/L	Segs:	55%
RBC:	1.7×10^{12}/L	Bands:	1%
Hb:	8.3 g/dL	Lymphs:	36%
Hct:	0.24L/L	Mono:	7%
MCV:	69 fL	Eos:	1%
MCH:	21 pg	Moderate poikilocytosis,	
MCHC:	29.2 g/dL	polychromasia, and target	
Plt:	172×10^9/L	cells; few teardrop cells	

1. Based on the indices, classify the anemia morphologically.
2. Name the dominant poikilocyte observed in this peripheral blood smear.
3. Name three disorders that frequently present with the same poikilocyte that dominates in this peripheral blood smear.
4. List two additional lab tests that would help to confirm the diagnosis and predict the results of each.

β-THALASSEMIA

GENERAL CONSIDERATIONS

As with α-thalassemias, some features found in β-thalassemias are common to all forms of the disease. The genetics of β-thalassemia and the individuals affected with the disorder will be presented before the discussion of the various forms of β-thalassemia.

Genetics

Whereas there are a total of four α-globin genes resulting in four major genotypes of α-thalassemia, there are only two β-globin genes, one located on each chromosome 11 (Figure

13-6 ■). If the prominent type of mutation found in β-thalassemia were also deletional, one would expect two severities, the severe homozygote and the mild heterozygote. However, in β-thalassemia most mutations are nondeletional resulting in a near continuum of clinical severities. In an attempt to gain some control over nomenclature of this diverse group of diseases, two classification systems are currently in use. The genotypic system classifies β-thalassemia patients into six genotypes based on zygosity and the degree of alteration of the β-genes, while the phenotypic system divides patients into four categories based on the severity of clinical symptoms.

In the genotypic system, all β-gene mutations are categorized into two groups based on the impact of the mutation on β-globin production. The two gene varieties are termed β^+ and β^0. The β^+-gene mutation causes a partial block in β-chain synthesis. The β^0-gene mutation results in a complete absence of β-chain synthesis. In addition, a minimally affected β-allele called silent carrier has been identified. It is found only in the most benign version of β-thalassemia. When the two gene designations (β^0 and β^+) are combined with the normal allele (β) and the two possible zygosity patterns (homozygous and heterozygous), six possible genotypes emerge (β^0/β^0, β^0/β^+, β^+/β^+, β^0/β, β^+/β, β/β). When the silent carrier mutation is added, a total of seven β-genotypes can be described (Table 13-5 ❂).

β-thalassemia is the result of several different types of molecular defects. Over 180 mutations have been described that result in partial to complete absence of β-gene expression, but only 20 mutations account for 80% of the diagnosed β-thalassemias.[3] β-thalassemia is rarely due to deletion of the structural gene as is the case in the α-thalassemias. Most defects in β-thalassemia are point mutations in regions of the DNA that control β-gene expression. These types of mutations can affect gene expression ranging from minor reductions in β-globin production to complete absence of synthesis. Mutations may affect any step in the

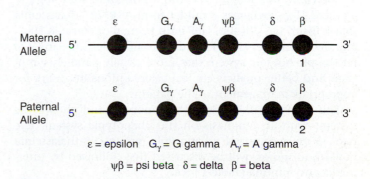

ε = epsilon G_γ = G gamma A_γ = A gamma

$\psi\beta$ = psi beta δ = delta β = beta

■ **FIGURE 13-6** Chromosome 11 is the location of four types of globin genes (ε, γ, δ, β). The 5' to 3' orientation of the genes is depicted. There is a gene for ε, δ, and β and two γ-genes. A β-pseudogene ($\psi\beta$) has been identified but does not express protein product.

✪ TABLE 13-5

Characteristics of β-thalassemia

Genotype	Zygosity	Phenotype	RBC Count	RBC Morphology	Hb Electrophoresis	Severity
β^0/β^0	Homozygous	Major	Relative ↑	↑↑↑ Target cells	No A, ↑A$_2$, ↑↑F	Severe
β^0/β^+	Double heterozygous	Major or intermedia	Relative ↑	↑↑↑ Target cells ↑↑ Target cells	↓A, ↑A$_2$, ↑↑F ↓A, ↑A$_2$, ↑↑F	Severe Moderate
β^+/β^+	Homozygous	Major or intermedia	Relative ↑	↑↑↑ Target cells ↑↑ Target cells	↓A, ↑A$_2$, ↑↑F ↓A, ↑A$_2$,↑↑F	Severe Moderate
β^0/β	Heterozygous	Intermedia or minor	Relative ↑	↑↑ Target cells ↑ Target cells	↓A, ↑A$_2$, ↑F ↓A, ↑A$_2$, ↑F	Moderate Mild
β^+/β	Heterozygous	Minor	Relative ↑	↑ Target cells	↓A, ↑A$_2$, ↑F	Mild
β^{SC}/β	Heterozygous	Minima	Normal	+/− Target cells	Normal	Normal
β/β	Homozygous	Normal	Normal	Normal	Normal	Normal

↑=Slight increase, ↑↑=Moderate increase, ↑↑↑=Marked increase, +/−=occasionally seen, ↓=Slight decrease, A=HbA, A$_2$=HbA$_2$, F=HbF, β^{SC}=silent carrier

pathway of globin gene expression including gene transcription, RNA processing, m-RNA translation and post-translational integrity of the protein.[10,11] Within a given population, a few genetic lesions account for most of the β-thalassemia mutations. For instance, in Greece, five mutations account for 87% of the gene defects.[11]

The phenotypic system recognizes four groups of patients categorized by the severity of symptoms, medical interventions, and prognoses. The four groups, listed in order from most severe to least severe, are β-thalassemia major, β-thalassemia intermedia, β-thalassemia minor, and β-thalassemia minima (Table 13-5 ✪).

One reason some prefer to organize β-thalassemias into a genotypic system is that phenotypic terms do not accurately reflect the genetic description of the disease. However, a disadvantage to the genotypic system is that patients with identical genotype designations may express β-thalassemia that is phenotypically diverse. For instance, a severe form of β^+/β^+-thalassemia (Mediterranean form) is characterized by an increase in HbF (50–90%) and a normal or only slightly elevated HbA$_2$, whereas a milder form of β^+/β^+-thalassemia (black form) has 20–40% HbF with normal or elevated HbA$_2$ and the remainder HbA. For this reason, some clinicians prefer the phenotypic system that more closely parallels symptoms and better predicts clinical interventions necessary for appropriate management of the patient.

This section will combine the genotypic and phenotypic systems with an emphasis on the phenotypic system. The two more recognized phenotypic groups, β-thalassemia major and minor, will be discussed first, followed by intermedia and minima (Table 13-5 ✪).

Affected Individuals

The most severe genotype (β^0) occurs more frequently in the Mediterranean regions—specifically in northern Italy, Greece, Algeria, Saudi Arabia—and Southeast Asia. Two severities of the β^+ mutation tend to originate in different ethnic populations. The more severe version is observed in the Mediterranean region, the Middle East, the Indian subcontinent, and Southeast Asia, while the milder version is localized to patients of African descent.[4]

β-THALASSEMIA MAJOR (β^0/β^0, β^0/β^+, $\beta^+\beta^+$)

Expected Genotypes

Beta-thalassemia major, also referred to as Cooley's anemia, is caused by a homozygous (β^0/β^0, $\beta^+\beta^+$), or **double heterozygous** (β^0/β^+) inheritance of abnormal β-genes resulting in marked reduction or absence of β-chain synthesis. As can be seen in Table 13-5 ✪, two of these three genotypes (β^0/β^+, β^+/β^+) can also present as the milder β-thalassemia intermedia that will be discussed later.

Pathophysiology

The dramatic reduction or absence of β-chain synthesis will affect the production of HbA. The symptoms that result from β-thalassemia major begin to manifest in infants approximately six months after birth. Other non–β-containing hemoglobins, HbA$_2$ and HbF, are increased in partial compensation for the decreased HbA levels.

The pathophysiologic mechanisms that result from a lack of β-chain production can be classified into four categories: reduced HbA, the compensatory production of abnormal hemoglobins, ineffective erythropoiesis with hemolysis, and erythroid hyperplasia (Figure 13-7 ■).

A dramatic reduction in HbA will compromise the oxygen carrying capacity of the blood. Other non–β-containing hemoglobins, HbF and HbA$_2$, are increased. HbF has a higher affinity for oxygen than HbA (∞ Chapter 5). The result is to exacerbate the already compromised oxygen delivery to tissues.

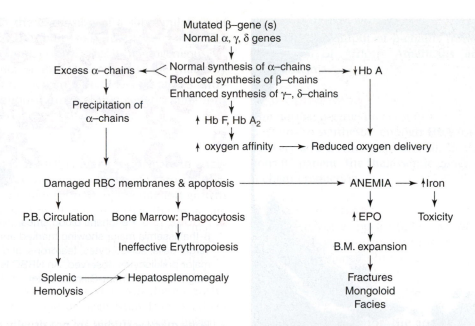

■ **FIGURE 13-7** In β-thalassemia major, the decreased synthesis of β-chains reduces the production of HbA and increases the production of non–β-chain containing hemoglobins (HbA₂ and HbF). Excess α-chains form insoluble precipitates inside erythrocytes damaging the membranes and reducing RBC lifespan through splenic sequestration and ineffective erythropoiesis. All these factors contribute to a reduced oxygen delivery to the tissues resulting in anemia and hypoxia. The compensatory erythroid hyperplasia in the bone marrow expands the marrow cavity resulting in pathologic fractures and mongoloid facial features.

In β-thalassemia major, reduced synthesis of β-chains results in an excess of free α-chains and a β-to-α chain ratio of less than 0.25. The free excess α-chains cannot form hemoglobin tetramers, so they precipitate within the cell, damaging the cell membrane, which leads to chronic hemolysis.[12] Many erythrocytes in the bone marrow are destroyed by marrow macrophages resulting in a large degree of ineffective erythropoiesis. Excess α-globin aggregates appear to activate apoptosis (∞ Chapter 2).[13] If the patient has inherited α-thalassemia with β-thalassemia, the symptoms associated with hemolysis may be lessened because the excess of α-chains is reduced by the α-thalassemia.

The combination of reduced HbA, increased HbF, ineffective erythropoiesis, and chronic hemolysis results in significant anemia. The body attempts to compensate by stimulating erythropoiesis. Erythroid hyperplasia results in bone marrow expansion and the thinning of calcified bone. Increased erythropoietic activity stimulates the absorption of more iron, leading to iron toxicity. Ineffective erythropoiesis in the bone marrow is accompanied by extramedullary hematopoiesis in the liver and spleen (Figure 13-7 ■).

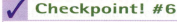 **Checkpoint! #6**

Why do symptoms of β-thalassemia major delay until approximately the sixth month of life?

Clinical Findings

Symptoms of β-thalassemia are first observed in infants as irritability, pallor, and a failure to thrive and gain weight. Diarrhea, fever, and an enlarged abdomen are also common findings. If therapy is not begun during early childhood, the clinical picture of thalassemia develops within a few years.

Severe anemia is the clinical condition responsible for many of the problems experienced by these children. The anemia places a tremendous burden on the cardiovascular system as it attempts to maintain tissue perfusion. Constant high output of blood usually results in cardiac failure in the first decade of life; this is the major cause of death in untreated children. Growth is retarded and a brown pigmentation of the skin is notable. Chronic hemolysis often produces gallstones, gout, and icterus.

Bone changes accompany the hyperplastic marrow. Marrow cavities enlarge in every bone, expanding the bone and producing characteristic bossing of the skull, facial deformities, and "hair-on-end" appearance of the skull on x-ray (Figure 13-8 ■). The thinning bone cortex in long bones may lead to pathologic fractures.

Extramedullary hematopoiesis is found in the liver and spleen and occasionally elsewhere in the body. The spleen may become massively enlarged and congested with abnormal erythrocytes.

Other clinical findings are associated with the body's attempt to increase erythrocyte production. Features that sug-

elevated reticulocyte count. Bone marrow shows slight erythroid hyperplasia and normoblasts poorly filled with hemoglobin.

Hemoglobin electrophoresis demonstrates an increase in HbA_2 from 3.5 to 7% with a mean of 5.5%. Newborns have a normal HbA_2 concentration of 0.27+/−0.02%.[16] HbF is normal in approximately half of the patients and increased in the other half (Figure 13-10 ■).[26,27] If HbF exceeds 5%, however, the individual has probably inherited an HPFH gene (discussed later) in addition to the β-thalassemia gene. Vital stains to detect Heinz bodies are usually negative.

DNA probing techniques can be performed to identify the type of mutation present and validate the heterozygous inheritance pattern, but this is of limited diagnostic value. Such information may be helpful in counseling prospective parents with β-thalassemia minor.

 Checkpoint! #7

In β-thalassemia, what erythrocyte parameter on the CBC differs significantly from that found in iron deficiency?

Treatment and Prognosis

Patients generally do not require treatment if they maintain good health and nutrition. They are generally asymptomatic except during periods of physiologic stress, and they have a normal life expectancy.

β-THALASSEMIA INTERMEDIA ($β^0/β^+$, $β^+/β^+$, $β^0/β$)

Expected Genotypes

All three patterns of inheritance, homozygous, double heterozygous, and heterozygous, can produce β-thalassemia intermedia (Table 13-5 ✪). The homozygous and double heterozygous forms represent a mutation in both β-alleles resulting in a moderate degree of reduction in β-chain synthesis. Occasionally, patients who inherit a deletion of one β-gene in conjunction with a normal β-gene exhibit symptoms significant enough to be classified as β-thalassemia intermedia rather than β-thalassemia minor.

Patients with β-thalassemia intermedia that co-express α-thalassemia or HPFH, may actually experience milder symptoms as compared to those with pure β-thalassemia. In both cases, α-chain accumulation and precipitation is lessened, which reduces the ineffective erythropoiesis and extravascular hemolysis responsible for much of the pathology. In the case of concomitant β-thalassemia intermedia and HPFH, the overexpressed γ-chains combine with the excessive α-chains to produce HbF, which reduces α-chain precipitation.

Clinical Findings

Patients with β-thalassemia intermedia can present with symptoms spanning the gap between severe β-thalassemia major to mild β-thalassemia minor. The $β^0/β^+$-genotype produces the greatest reduction in β-chain synthesis, and thus, patients have symptoms that can rival β-thalassemia major, while patients expressing the $β^0/β$-genotype generally express mild symptoms. The more severely affected patients develop moderate anemia that is transfusion dependent. Frequent transfusions curb developmental delays. Transfusion therapy, coupled with the increased intestinal absorption of iron may result in iron overload. Symptoms intensify during periods of physiological stress such as with pregnancy and infection.

Laboratory Results

The CBC reflects a moderate microcytic hypochromic anemia with a hemoglobin value ranging from 6 to 10 g/dL. In the milder versions, patients express only a slight reduction in hemoglobin values. The red blood cell count is disproportionately higher than the hemoglobin values, often approaching normal.

Target cells are the predominant poikilocytes observed. Basophilic stippling and nucleated red blood cells are also present. The bone marrow shows hypochromic normoblasts in the context of erythroid hyperplasia. However, bone marrow examination is not needed for diagnosis.

Hemoglobin electrophoresis patterns in patients with the more severe forms of β-thalassemia intermedia ($β^0β^+$ and $β^+β^+$) are nearly indistinguishable from those observed in the milder forms of β-thalassemia major ($β^+β^+$). Patients express elevated HbA_2 (5–10%) and HbF (30–75%) with the remainder being HbA. Milder versions of β-thalassemia intermedia produce lower HbA_2 (>3.2%) and HbF levels (1.5–12.0%), making them easily distinguishable from patients with β-thalassemia major (Figure 13-10 ■). Although hemoglobin electrophoresis is helpful in the diagnosis of β-thalassemia intermedia, differentiation from β-thalassemia major and minor is a clinical decision.

Treatment and Prognosis

Even in the most severe patient, hypertransfusion therapy is not required, but regular transfusions are administered in most patients. Splenomegaly is common. Functional hyposplenism leads to infections requiring regular interventions with antibiotic therapy. Chelation therapy is warranted to combat iron overload, which tends to develop later than in patients with β-thalassemia major. Most patients have a normal life span.

β-THALASSEMIA MINIMA ($β^{SC}/β$)

Beta-thalassemia minima is a form of β-thalassemia that is asymptomatic and exhibits no major laboratory abnormalities. The disorder is usually discovered serendipitously during family studies. The gene has been given the designation β^{SC} for silent carrier. The genotype used to describe a patient with β-thalassemia minima is β^{SC}/β.[28]

CASE STUDY *(continued from page 249)*

Additional tests were performed on John's blood to determine the cause of his anemia.

HEMOGLOBIN ELECTROPHORESIS		IRON PANEL	
HbA:	66%	Serum iron:	92 µg/dL
HbA$_2$:	1.0%	TIBC:	310 µg/dL
HbF:	1.0%	Serum ferritin:	88 ng/mL
Hb Bart's:	8%	Iron saturation:	33%
HbH:	24%		

5. Is the hemoglobin electrophoresis normal or abnormal?

6. If abnormal, list hemoglobins that are elevated, decreased, or abnormally present.

7. If abnormal, which globin chain(s) are decreased?

8. If abnormal, which globin chains are produced in excess?

9. Is the iron panel normal or abnormal?

10. If the iron tests are abnormal, list those tests outside the normal range and indicate if they are elevated or decreased.

11. If abnormal, state the disorder(s) consistent with the abnormal iron panel.

12. Given all the data supplied, what is the definitive diagnosis of John's anemia?

▶ OTHER THALASSEMIAS AND THALASSEMIA-LIKE CONDITIONS

In theory, any globin gene can be mutated resulting in a reduction in the synthesis of globin chains and the corresponding hemoglobin. Patients have been observed with deficiencies in each of the normal adult globin chains. However, the thalassemias that involve globin chains other than α and β are relatively benign in their clinical course because they are not a constituent of the major adult hemoglobin, HbA. Thalassemias have been observed involving more than one globin gene and in combination with structural hemoglobin disorders like sickle cell anemia and HbC disease (Table 13-6 ◯).

δβ-THALASSEMIA

Delta, beta-thalassemia is a rare thalassemia observed in patients of Greek, African, Italian, and Arabian ancestry in which production of both β- and δ-chains is affected. The δβ-mutation can be categorized into two genotypes, $\delta\beta^0$ and $\delta\beta^+$. The $\delta\beta^0$ designation indicates a lack of synthesis of both β- and

δ-chains, whereas the $\delta\beta^+$-genotype suggests a reduction in β- and δ-chain synthesis. The absence of β- and δ-chains is most often due to deletion of the structural β- and δ-gene complex. One or both of the γ-genes remain, resulting in 100% HbF.[22] However, increased γ-chain production fails to fully compensate for the loss of β-chain production.

It appears that in δβ-thalassemia, there is less compensation of γ-chain synthesis than in HPFH but more than in homozygous β-thalassemia. The clinical disease is classified as thalassemia intermedia and rarely requires blood transfusions except in cases of physiological stress such as in pregnancy or infection. Thus, most patients with δβ-thalassemia have a mild hypochromic, microcytic anemia. Patients have slight hepatosplenomegaly and some bone changes associated with chronic erythroid hyperplasia. Hemolysis probably contributes to the anemia since both reticulocytes and bilirubin are elevated.

The heterozygous form of δβ-thalassemia ($\delta\beta^0/\beta$) is not identified with any specific clinical findings. There is no anemia or splenomegaly. The hematological picture, however, is similar to that of β-thalassemia minor with microcytic, hypochromic erythrocytes. Hemoglobin A$_2$ is normal or slightly decreased while HbF is increased to 5–20%. HbA is usually less than 90% (Table 13-6 ◯).

γδβ-THALASSEMIA

This rare form of thalassemia has several variants and is characterized by deletion or inactivation of the entire β-gene complex.[17] Deletion of the γ-, δ-, and β-genes would result in the absence of all normal adult hemoglobins. Therefore, only the heterozygous state has been encountered, presumably because a homozygous condition would be incompatible with life. Although neonates have severe hemolytic anemia, as the child grows, the disease evolves to a mild form of β-thalassemia.

HEMOGLOBIN CONSTANT SPRING

Hemoglobin Constant Spring (HbCS) is hemoglobin formed from the combination of two structurally abnormal α-chains, each elongated by 31 amino acids at the carboxy-terminal end, and two normal β-chains. This genetic mutation is common in Thailand. The chromosome with the CS gene presumably carries one normal α-gene (remember that there are 2 α-genes) on each chromosome 16 for a total of 4 α-genes; thus, the homozygous HbCS carrier has two normal α-genes, one on each chromosome, and the heterozygous HbCS carrier has three normal α-genes.

The elongated α-chains of HbCS are probably the result of a mutation of the chain termination codon by a single base substitution.[29] The abnormal α-chains are inefficiently synthesized due to reduced stability of the mRNA translation apparatus. Synthesis of HbCS decreases significantly during maturation of the normoblasts in the bone marrow. The

HEMOGLOBIN LEPORE

Incidence and Affected Individuals

Hemoglobin Lepore was first described in 1958 as a structural hemoglobin variant with hematological changes and clinical manifestations resembling those of thalassemia.[31] The disorder is widely distributed throughout the world but is especially common in Middle and Eastern Europe.

Genetics

In Hb Lepore, the non–α-chain is a δ/β-globin hybrid in which the N-terminal end of a δ-chain is fused to the C-terminal end of a β-chain. The variant hybrid chains are thought to arise during meiosis from an aberrant **crossover** event resulting in recombination of misaligned δ- and β-genes on separate chromosomes. The result of the unequal crossover event is two fusion genes, the δ/β-Lepore and the β/δ–anti-Lepore fusion genes. The δ/β-Lepore fusion gene is transcribed and translated into the δ/β-fusion globin chain, two of which combine with two α-chains to form Hb Lepore. The β/δ–anti-Lepore fusion gene still contains intact β- and δ-genes that are synthesized normally to form HbA and A_2, respectively. Progeny will bear genes from the involved chromosome that are neither fully paternal nor fully maternal. Since the recombination event occurred in the germ cells, the newly formed chromosomes become a permanent part of the gene pool of the family. Hb Lepore is stable and has normal functional properties except for a slight increase in oxygen affinity.

Pathophysiology

The pathophysiology of hemoglobin Lepore is similar to that of β-thalassemia. The β-gene is nonfunctional, so β-chain synthesis is absent. The Hb Lepore gene is under the influence of the δ-gene promoter, which limits synthesis of the Lepore chain to approximately 2.5% of β-chain production. Thus, the abnormal Lepore chains are inadequately synthesized leading to an excess of α-chains. In the homozygous state, no β-chains would be synthesized to combine with the α-chains being produced. The more severely affected children may become transfusion dependent and develop complications of hemosiderosis. The combination of ineffective erythropoiesis, decreased HbA, increased affinity of HbF and chronic extravascular hemolysis produces a microcytic hypochromic anemia that is classified as β-thalassemia major in the more severe cases and as β-thalassemia intermedia in the remaining cases. As with β-thalassemia major, symptoms emerge within the first five years of life.

Patients with heterozygous Hb Lepore are asymptomatic and classified as β-thalassemia minor. The blood picture is similar to that seen in β-thalassemia minor.

Laboratory Results

In the homozygous state, hematologic findings are similar to β-thalassemia major. There is no detectable HbA or A_2 on hemoglobin electrophoresis, Hb Lepore ranges from 8–30%, and the remainder consists of HbF. Hemoglobin electrophoresis must be interpreted with caution because Hb Lepore comigrates with HbS on cellulose acetate at an alkaline pH and with HbA on citrate agar at an acid pH.

In the heterozygous state, hematologic findings are similar to thalassemia minor (Figure 13-12 ■): Hemoglobin electrophoresis reveals a mean Hb Lepore concentration of 10%; HbA_2 is decreased with a mean of 2%; HbF is usually slightly elevated to 2–3%; and HbA makes up the remainder (Table 13-6 ✪).

The severely anemic cases of Hb Lepore require a regular transfusion protocol from early childhood. Splenectomy is also performed in an attempt to lessen the degree of anemia.

COMBINATION DISORDERS

Occasionally an individual is doubly heterozygous for a structural hemoglobin variant and thalassemia, inheriting one of the two abnormalities from each parent. The most common structural hemoglobin variants involved in combination disorders are HbS, HbC, and HbE. When a structural variant is inherited with a β-thalassemia gene, the severity of the combination disorder is dependent on the type of β-gene mutation. Patients expressing the β^0-gene produce no HbA and experience moderate to severe symptoms. The β^+-gene produces some β-chains resulting in HbA synthesis and few to no symptoms. The most common example is HbS/β-thalassemia accounting for 1 in 1,667 births among African Americans.[32] This has also been reported in patients of Greek, Turkish, Indian, North American, Mediterranean, and Rumanian ancestry.[33] Three clinical severities have been identified: HbS/β^0-Type 1(severe), HbS/β^+-Type 1 (moderate), and HbS/β^+-Type 2 (asymptomatic). Differentiating this combination disorder from sickle cell disease, HbSS and HbAS, is difficult, but a comparison of β/α ratio is helpful (Web Table 13-1 ✪). In sickle cell disorders the β/α ratio is approximately 1/1, whereas it is closer to 0.5/1 in HbS/β-thalassemia.[34]

Combination disorders are more complex when the structural hemoglobin gene mutation is on the β-gene and the thalassemia mutation involves the α-gene, because different

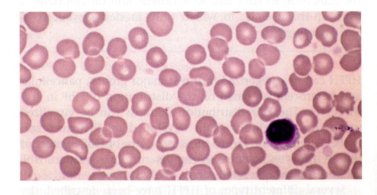

■ **FIGURE 13-12** Peripheral blood smear from a patient with hemoglobin Lepore. Note the anisocytosis, poikilocytosis, and microcytosis. (Wright-Giemsa stain; 1000× magnification)

chromosomes are involved. These patients can be either homozygous or heterozygous for the structural hemoglobin variant and coexpress any of the possible α-gene combinations.

The severity of the combination disorder is directly proportional to the total number of affected genes and ranges from moderate to asymptomatic.[35–37] Coexistent α-thalassemia decreases synthesis of α-chains resulting in fewer α-globin chains available to combine with the structurally abnormal β-chain. Thus, the concentration of the structural variant is decreased. HbF and HbA$_2$ will increase to compensate for the reduction in the structural hemoglobin variant allowing for better oxygen exchange. This reduces the abnormal pathophysiology associated with the particular structural hemoglobin variant inherited.

In HbS disease with α-thalassemia, lesser amounts of HbS in the cell decrease the tendency of HbS to polymerize and, thus, decreases cell hemolysis and the clinical symptoms associated with occlusion of the microvasculature (∞ Chapter 12). HbF has also been shown to decrease the sickling process.[4] The wide variety of clinical severities seen in sickle cell anemia may be related to the high incidence of α-thalassemia in the same population (Figure 13-13 ■).

Laboratory diagnosis is accomplished by applying the techniques used to identify each of the disorders individually. Patients will express a mild microcytic, hypochromic anemia with target cells and the poikilocytes associated with the structural hemoglobin variant inherited. Patients who inherit HbS may express sickle cells, and those with HbC will sometimes show HbC crystals. Hemoglobin electrophoresis is helpful in resolving the structural hemoglobin variant and will show the quantitative changes in normal and abnormal hemoglobins associated with α- and β-thalassemias. In HbS/α-thalassemia, the concentration of HbS is inversely proportional to the number α-gene deletions. HbS concentration is 35% with one α-gene deletion, 28% in two α-deletions, and 20% when three α-genes are missing.[38]

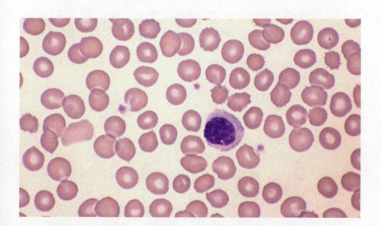

■ FIGURE 13-13 Peripheral blood smear from a patient with hemoglobin S and α-thalassemia. The cells are microcytic. There are acanthocytes and cells with pointed ends present. (Wright-Giemsa stain; 1000× magnification)

In cases where less common structural variants (HbE, HbO, HbD, etc.) are coexpressed with thalassemias, further testing may be necessary because they comigrate with HbS or HbC on hemoglobin electrophoresis (Figure 13-2). Molecular techniques, including automated sequencing, dot-blot analysis, or allele-specific amplification, can be used in these cases.[39]

Double heterozygotes for sickle cell and HPFH exhibit a mild form of sickle cell trait with no occurrence of crises or anemia. It has been suggested that the surprisingly favorable clinical picture is related to the distribution of HbF in erythrocytes. The peripheral blood smear shows anisocytosis and target cells, while the sodium metabisulfite and solubility tests are positive. Hemoglobin electrophoresis produces a pattern that is easily confused with that of sickle cell anemia. Only HbS, HbF, and HbA$_2$ are present, with HbF levels ranging from 15 to 35%. Hemoglobin A$_2$ is normal or reduced. Family studies are helpful in identifying double heterozygous states.

Due to the significant variations in clinical expression of the various hemoglobin structural variants and β-thalassemia alleles, it is suggested that identification of these conditions should go beyond hematologic analysis and hemoglobin electrophoresis.[39] A better defined diagnosis at the molecular level to identify the genetic mutation may lead to better clinical management of the disease. A summary of the differentiating characteristics of combination thalassemia and hemoglobinopathy disorders can be found in Table 13-1 ✪ on the Web site.

✓ Checkpoint! #9

In combination disorders of structural Hb variants and thalassemia, why is the severity less when α-thalassemia is inherited with sickle cell trait than when β-thalassemia is coexpressed with sickle cell trait?

▶ DIFFERENTIAL DIAGNOSIS OF THALASSEMIA

Signs, symptoms, and CBC results are strikingly similar in microcytic hypochromic anemias regardless of the etiology of the anemia, making the clinical diagnosis difficult. Differentiating the various thalassemias is even more difficult because they are all inherited and occur in similar nationalities. Additional laboratory tests are therefore crucial in making the differential diagnosis.[40,41] Table 13-2 ✪ on the Web site summarizes the tests used to differentiate thalassemia from other anemias.

✓ Checkpoint! #10

Which laboratory tests should be done first to differentiate thalassemia and iron deficiency?

SUMMARY

Thalassemias result from genetic defects that affect the production of globin chains. Any of the globin chains may be affected, but the most clinically significant are α- and β-chain defects. The clinical severity of the disease is related to the number of mutated genes and the type of genetic defect. There are normally four α-genes in the human diploid genome. In α-thalassemia, from one to four of the α-genes may be deleted. If only one gene is affected, the condition is not clinically or hematologically apparent, but if two or three are affected, there are both clinical and hematological abnormalities of moderate or marked severity, respectively. Deletion of all four α-genes is incompatable with life. There are two normal β-alleles and two β-thalassemia gene defects, one that causes a complete absence of β-chain production (β^0-thalassemia), and the other that causes decreased synthesis of β-chain production (β^+-thalassemia). This results in five potential β-thalassemia genotypes, ($\beta^0\beta^0$, $\beta^0\beta^+$, $\beta^+\beta^+$, $\beta^0\beta$, $\beta^+\beta$), that are categorized into four clinical severities, (β-thalassemia major, intermedia, minor, and silent carrier) ranging from severe to asymptomatic.

The thalassemias generally produce a microcytic, hypochromic anemia with changes in the concentrations of HbF, HbA_2 and HbA. HbF and HbA_2 are elevated in β-thalassemia and decreased in α-thalassemia, with decreased concentrations of HbA in both. In the more severe α-thalassemias, HbH and Hb Bart's may be detected. Erythrocyte morphology is similar in both major forms of thalassemia and in iron deficiency anemia; however, hemoglobin electrophoresis and iron studies will assist in differentiation of these two entities. Some structural hemoglobin variants are synthesized in decreased quantities (i.e., Hb Lepore) and have morphologic similarities to thalassemias. Molecular techniques are now available to identify the genetic mutation in the globin gene but are not always necessary for diagnostic purposes.

Current therapies are improving and medical access in underdeveloped countries is expanding. As a result of these advances, the general health and quality of life is improving for patients with thalassemia.

REVIEW QUESTIONS

LEVEL I

1. Select the statement that best defines thalassemia. (Checklist #1)
   a. A qualitative disorder of hemoglobin synthesis derived primarily from a genetic point mutation in one or more globin genes.
   b. A disorder of inappropriate iron metabolism due to abnormal transferrin.
   c. A quantitative disorder of hemoglobin synthesis resulting from deletional and nondeletional mutations of globin genes.
   d. A single amino acid substitution in a globin chain affecting the function of hemoglobin.

2. Which of the following statements is *false* for a patient with thalassemia but *true* in certain hemoglobinopathies? (Checklist #2)
   a. Abnormal hemoglobin will polymerize inside erythrocytes altering red cell shape.
   b. Novel hemoglobins composed of abnormal combinations of normal globin chains may be detected on hemoglobin electrophoresis.
   c. Elevations in embryonic and fetal hemoglobins may be observed.
   d. The amino acid sequence of the globin chains of the abnormal hemoglobins is normal.

3. What is the typical morphologic classification of erythrocytes in thalassemia? (Checklist #3)
   a. macrocytic, normochromic
   b. normocytic, normochromic
   c. microcytic, hyperchromic
   d. microcytic, hypochromic

LEVEL II

1. Alpha-thalassemia most commonly results from which of the following genetic lesions? (Checklist #1)
   a. gene deletion
   b. promoter mutation
   c. termination codon mutation
   d. splice site mutation

2. Why is hydrops fetalis incompatible with life? (Checklist #4b)
   a. Life cannot exist without HbA.
   b. Lack of embryonic hemoglobins precludes fetal development.
   c. All three normal adult hemoglobins contain α-chains.
   d. Fetal hemoglobin is essential to sustain life after birth.

3. Which pathophysiologic event is involved in the pathogenesis of HbH disease? (Checklist #4b)
   a. HbH has a higher affinity for oxygen that hampers oxygen release.
   b. HbH is an embryonic hemoglobin that is not present at birth.
   c. HbH cannot bind and transport oxygen.
   d. Polymerization of abnormal hemoglobin alters erythrocyte shape.

4. The genetic designation heterozygous α^0-thal-1/normal refers to: (Checklist #4a)
   a. α-thalassemia minor
   b. Cooley's anemia
   c. HbH disease
   d. silent carrier

REVIEW QUESTIONS (continued)

LEVEL I

4. Select the disorder that is an α-thalassemia. (Checklist #5a, b)
   a. HbH disease
   b. Cooley's anemia
   c. HPFH
   d. Hb Lepore

5. Alpha-thalassemia is characterized by: (Checklist #5c)
   a. deletion of β-genes
   b. amino acid substitutions in the α-chain
   c. excess α-chain production
   d. deletion of α-genes

6. Which nationality is *most* likely to be affected by thalassemia? (Checklist #5b, 6a)
   a. Chinese
   b. South American Indians
   c. Southeast Asians
   d. Europeans

7. Which of the following laboratory results would be expected in a patient with α-thalassemia? (Checklist #5e)
   a. MCH=32 pg
   b. MCV=70 fL
   c. stomatocytes
   d. increased HbA

8. The pathogenesis of β-thalassemia includes: (Checklist #6b)
   a. decreased production of β-chains
   b. abnormal structure of α-chains
   c. bone marrow hypoproliferation
   d. decreased synthesis of erythropoietin

9. In β-thalassemia major, hemoglobin electrophoresis will show: (Checklist #6d)
   a. reduced HbF
   b. reduced HbA₂
   c. reduced HbA
   d. increased HbH

10. Select the thalassemia type in which the patient presents with an abnormal hemoglobin that is sensitive to oxidation and precipitates in red cells after incubation with brilliant cresyl blue. (Checklist #6d)
    a. hydrops fetalis
    b. HbH disease
    c. β-thalassemia minor
    d. silent carrier

LEVEL II

5. The single best laboratory test to distinguish β-thalassemia minor from α-thalassemia, iron deficiency anemia, HPFH, and hemoglobinopathies is: (Checklist #8)
   a. hemoglobin solubility
   b. serum iron
   c. Heinz body stain
   d. HbA₂ level

6. Hemoglobin Constant Spring can best be described as: (Checklist #7c)
   a. deletion of three α-genes
   b. two normal β-chains and two elongated α-chains
   c. two normal α-chains and two β/γ-fusion chains
   d. continued synthesis of γ-chains throughout adult life

7. Select the statement that best describes hereditary persistence of fetal hemoglobin. (Checklist #7d)
   a. Homozygous state is incompatible with life.
   b. HbF is elevated in adults.
   c. It results from the deletion of the γ-gene.
   d. It is a form of β-thalassemia.

8. A 4-year-old male patient has a microcytic, hypochromic anemia. Hemoglobin electrophoresis shows: 46% HbS, 49% HbA, 3.5% HbA₂, 1.5% HbF. His parents have no symptoms of anemia. What is the most likely phenotype of his parents? (Checklist #5,7)
   a. sickle cell trait and β-thalassemia major
   b. sickle cell anemia and α-thalassemia
   c. sickle cell anemia and heterozygous β-thalassemia
   d. sickle cell trait and normal

9. Which combination disorder would exhibit more severe symptoms? (Checklist #7f)
   a. HbS and β-thalassemia minor
   b. HbC trait and α-thalassemia minor
   c. HPFH and β-thalassemia minor
   d. HbS and HPFH

10. A 28-year-old female from Laos was diagnosed with iron deficiency anemia and was given iron supplements. Her reticulocyte count increased to 5% after 6 days of treatment. Six months later she returned for a follow-up CBC. Her hemoglobin was 11.5 g/dL and the red cells were microcytic (75 fL), normochromic. What reflex test should be done? (Checklist #8)
    a. hemoglobin electrophoresis
    b. serum iron
    c. bone marrow
    d. serum ferritin

www.prenhall.com/mckenzie
Use the above address to access the free, interactive Companion Web site created for this textbook. Get hints, instant feedback, and textbook references to chapter-related multiple choice questions.

■ CHECKLIST - LEVEL II *(continued)*

4. Compare and contrast the various clinical forms and causes of a vitamin B_{12} and folate deficiency on the basis of clinical symptoms and laboratory results.

5. Categorize the causes and clinical variations of pernicious anemia.

6. Compare and contrast the various clinical forms and causes of a folic acid deficiency.

7. Demonstrate how a folate or vitamin B_{12} deficiency results in megaloblastic maturation.

8. Choose and briefly explain four laboratory tests used to identify the cause of a macrocytic anemia; give the expected results of these four tests in a patient with an autoantibody directed against intrinsic factor.

9. Assess Schilling's test results and provide a differential diagnosis.

10. Compare and contrast the causes of macrocytosis with a normoblastic marrow.

11. Construct an algorithm of laboratory testing to distinguish between a megaloblastic anemia and a macrocytic, normoblastic anemia.

12. Evaluate a case study from a patient with anemia. Determine, from the medical history and laboratory results, the most probable diagnosis.

KEY TERMS

Achlorhydria
Cobalamin
Demyelination
Dyspepsia
Glossitis
Intrinsic factor (IF)
Megaloblastic
Nuclear-cytoplasmic asynchrony
Pernicious anemia (PA)
Schilling test

The information in this chapter will build on the concepts learned in previous chapters. To maximize your learning experience you should review these concepts before starting this unit of study.

Level I

▶ Describe the maturation process of erythrocytes in the marrow. (Chapter 4)

▶ Outline the functional and morphologic classification of anemia and list the basic laboratory tests to diagnose anemia. (Chapter 10)

Level II

▶ Summarize the concepts of cell development, regulation, and the process of cell division. (Chapter 2)

▶ List and describe the laboratory tests used in differential diagnosis of anemia. (Chapter 10)

@ CASE STUDY

We will refer to this case study throughout the chapter.
Ms. Kathy Allison, a 36-year-old female, experienced a recent 35-pound weight loss. Her tongue was red and fissured. She also complained of chronic fatigue and shortness of breath upon exertion. Physical examination suggested signs of jaundice and decreased fibratory sensation of fingers and toes. She was hospitalized with the general diagnosis of moderate anemia, jaundice, and neurological symptoms. Her admitting CBC demonstrated the following laboratory results:

WBC:	4.5×10^9/L	Differential:	
RBC:	2.50×10^{12}/L	LY%	36.0
HGB:	10.0 g/dL	MO%	3.8
HCT:	0.31 L/L	GR%	59.4
MCV:	124.0 fL	EO%:	1.0
MCH:	40.5 pg/dL	BASO%:	0.0
MCHC:	32.7 gm/dL		
RDW:	21.2	NRBCs/100WBCs:	5
PLT:	155×10^9/L		

*Moderate hypersegmented neutrophils

The following abnormal erythrocyte morphology was reported:

Macrocytes:	2+
Anisocytosis:	3+
Poikilocytosis:	2+
Ovalocytes:	1+
Basophilic stippling:	1+
Occasional Howell-Jolly bodies	

1. What is the morphologic classification of the patient's anemia?

▶ OVERVIEW

This chapter is a study of the macrocytic anemias. These anemias can be megaloblastic or nonmegaloblastic. The experienced laboratorian can often identify diagnostic clues on review of a blood smear. The first part of the chapter discusses the megaloblastic anemias. This begins with a description of the clinical and laboratory findings. Since megaloblastic anemia is most often due to deficiencies or abnormal metabolism of folate or vitamin B_{12}, the metabolism of these vitamins is discussed in detail. The latter part of the chapter reviews the causes of nonmegaloblastic macrocytic anemia and compares the laboratory test results in nonmegaloblastic and megaloblastic anemia.

▶ INTRODUCTION

Macrocytic anemias are characterized by large erythrocytes (mean MCV >l00 fL) with a normal hemoglobin content (MCHC). This is an important group of anemias since macrocytosis is frequently a sign of a disease process that can result in significant morbidity if left untreated.

Macrocytosis is found in 2.5–4% of adults who have a routine complete blood count.[1] In up to 60% of cases, macrocytosis is not accompanied by anemia,[2] but isolated macrocytosis should always be investigated. Macrocytosis without anemia may be an indication of early folate or **cobalamin** (vitamin B_{12}) deficiency since macrocytosis precedes development of anemia.

Macrocytosis detected by automated cell counters may not always be apparent microscopically on stained blood smears. In some cases the erythrocyte size on automated counters is falsely elevated due to hyperglycemia, cold agglutinins, and extreme leukocytosis (Table 14-1 ✪). These causes of false macrocytosis need to be differentiated from true macrocytosis.

The most common cause of macrocytosis is alcoholism. Other causes include folate and cobalamin deficiencies, drugs including chemotherapy, reticulocytosis due to hemolysis or bleeding, myelodysplasia, liver disease, and hypothyroidism.[2]

Macrocytic anemias are generally classified as **megaloblastic** or nonmegaloblastic depending on morphologic characteristics of erythroid precursors in the bone marrow. The megaloblastic anemias are the result of abnormal DNA synthesis (a nuclear maturation defect). As a result, there is delayed nuclear development that prevents cell division. RNA synthesis and cytoplasmic maturation are not affected. The result is production of large cells with **nuclear cytoplasmic asynchrony**. The basis for the nonmegaloblastic anemias is not as well defined but may be related to an increase in membrane lipids. Often, in nonmegaloblastic macrocytic anemia the macrocytes are round while in megaloblastic anemia the macrocytes are oval. A flow chart for

✪ TABLE 14-1	
Conditions Associated with Megaloblastic and Nonmegaloblastic Macrocytic (Normoblastic) Anemias	
Megaloblastic	**Normoblastic**
Folate Deficiency	Alcoholism
Nutritional deficiency	Liver disease
Increased requirement	Shift reticulocytosis in hemolytic
(i.e., pregnancy)	anemia or hemorrhage
Intestinal malabsorption	Hypothroidism
Drug inhibition	Aplastic anemia
B_{12} Deficiency	Obstructive jaundice
Pernicious anemia	Splenectomy
Small bowel resection	Pregnancy
Gastrectomy	Artifactual
Intestinal malabsorption	
Nutritional deficiency	
Transcobalamin II deficiency	
Nitrous oxide abuse	
Other Causes	
Chemotherapy with metabolic	
inhibitors	
Orotic aciduria	
CDA	

laboratory analysis to help distinguish causes of macrocytic anemia is shown in Figure 14-1 ■.

▶ MEGALOBLASTIC ANEMIA

Although very little was known about the function or origin of blood cells before the twentieth century, some perceptive individuals began to make associations between anemia and other clinical signs of the patient. In 1822, J. S. Coombe, a Scottish physician, made the initial clinical description of a patient who appeared to have megaloblastic anemia. He was the first to suggest that this anemia might be related to **dyspepsia**.[3] In 1855, Thomas Addison reported his description of a macrocytic anemia, but he made no reference to the typical microscopic blood findings.[4] The discovery and description of the abnormal erythroid precursors in the bone marrow associated with this anemia were made possible by the advent of triacid stains. In 1891 Paul Ehrlich is credited with coining the term *megaloblast* to describe the large abnormal precursors in megaloblastic anemia.[5]

Megaloblastic anemia is classified as a nuclear maturation defect. Anemia is attributed primarily to a large degree of ineffective erythropoiesis resulting from disrupted DNA synthesis. The anemia was called megaloblastic in an attempt to describe the giant abnormal-appearing erythroid precursors (megaloblasts) in the bone marrow. Other nucleated cells of the marrow are also typically abnormal. About 95% of megaloblastic anemias are caused by deficiencies of either vitamin

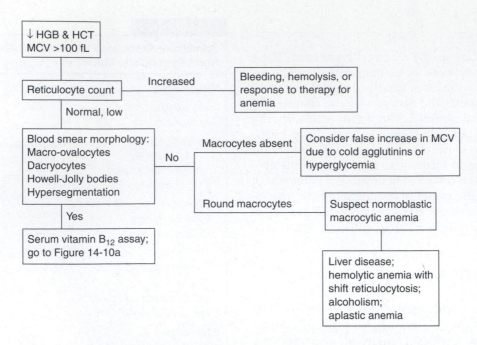

■ **FIGURE 14-1** Algorithm to the differential diagnosis of the megaloblastic anemias from other macrocytic anemias. (HGB = hemoglobin; HCT = hematocrit; MCV = mean cell volume

B_{12} or folic acid vitamins necessary as coenzymes for nucleic acid synthesis. In the majority of cases, vitamin B_{12} deficiency is secondary to a deficiency of **intrinsic factor**, a factor necessary for absorption of vitamin B_{12} rather than to a nutritional deficiency of the vitamin. Folic acid deficiency, on the other hand, is most often due to an inadequate dietary intake. Inherited disorders affecting DNA synthesis are a rare cause of megaloblastosis.

CLINICAL FINDINGS

The onset of megaloblastic anemia is usually insidious with typical anemic symptoms of lethargy, weakness, and a yellow or waxy pallor. Dyspeptic symptoms are common. **Glossitis** with a beefy red tongue or, more commonly, a smooth pale tongue is characteristic. Loss of weight and loss of appetite are common complaints. Atrophy of the gastric parietal cells causes decreased secretion of intrinsic factor and hydrochloric acid. Bouts of diarrhea may be the result of epithelial changes in the gastrointestinal tract.

Neurological disturbances occur only in vitamin B_{12} deficiency, not in folic acid deficiency. These are the most serious and dangerous clinical signs because neurological damage may be permanent if the deficiency is not treated promptly. Occasionally the patient's initial complaints are related to neurological dysfunction rather than to anemia. Neurological damage has been reported to occur even before anemia or macrocytosis in some cases. The bone marrow, however, always reveals megaloblastic changes even in the absence of anemia. Tingling, numbness, and weakness of the

extremities reflect peripheral neuropathy. Loss of vibratory and position (proprioceptive) sensibilities in the lower extremities may cause an abnormal gait in the patient. Mental disturbances such as loss of memory, depression, and irritability are sometimes noted by the patient's relatives. *Megaloblastic madness* is a term used to describe severe psychotic manifestations of vitamin B_{12} deficiency. Occasionally a patient with severe anemia may be asymptomatic, which is probably a reflection of a very slow developing anemia.

 Checkpoint! #1

Patients with megaloblastic anemia often present with a yellow or waxy pallor. What is the diagnostic significance of this clinical symptom?

LABORATORY FINDINGS

Laboratory tests are critical to a diagnosis of megaloblastic anemia. The routine CBC with a review of the blood smear will give important diagnostic clues and help in selecting reflex tests.

Peripheral Blood

Megaloblastic anemia is typically a macrocytic, normochromic anemia. The MCV is usually greater than 100 fL and may reach a volume of 140 fL. However, an increased MCV is not specific for megaloblastic anemia. The MCH is increased

tissue folate depletion. [...]
THF by vitamin B_{12}, ho[...]
nine, a precursor of S-ad[...]
tion requires methionin[...]
thought to be critical to [...]

Requirements

Folic acid is present in [...]
yeast, and liver, but is [...]
vegetables (from which [...]
sized by microorganisms.[...]
thus, when food is over[...]
stroyed. Ascorbate protect[...]
present, may protect folat[...]
dation. The recommende[...]
acid for adults is 200 µg, o[...]
in the intestine. This is a[...]
daily requirement of 50 µ[...]
metabolism. The liver sto[...]
which is enough to provid[...]
to six months if folic acid is[...]

Folate plays an importar[...]
Observations reveal that the[...]
late levels in women who [...]
tube defects (NTD) compar[...]
normal babies. Several studi[...]
tation of folate during pre[...]
birth defects by as much as [...]
tective effect is not clear, bu[...]
effect may be confined to a [...]
fective folate metabolism. In [...]
defects, the United States gov[...]
tions of grain products with [...]
of 1997.[13] The goal was to in[...]
100 µg per person. It has b[...]
women need an intake of abou[...]

Folic acid can become de[...]
with rapid cell turnover such [...]
molytic anemia. Thus, the d[...]
with these disorders is increase[...]

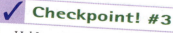

✓ Checkpoint! #3

*Hal Jones had small bowel resection [...]
he is at high risk for folate deficiency.[...]*

Pathophysiology of Folic [...]

Folate deficiency results in decr[...]
methylene THF, which is needed [...]
thesis. Consequently, there is a m[...]
thesis. In addition, the intermedi[...]
a cofactor for metabolism, homoc[...]

TABLE 14-2

Comparison of Common Laboratory Values in Megaloblastic and Nonmegaloblastic Macrocytosis

Laboratory Value	Megaloblastic Macrocytosis	Nonmegaloblastic Macrocytosis
WBC count	Decreased	Normal
Platelet count	Decreased	Normal
RBC count	Decreased	Decreased
Hemoglobin	Decreased	Decreased
Hematocrit	Decreased	Decreased
MCV	Usually >110 fL	>100 fL
RBC morphology	Ovalocytes, Howell-Jolly bodies, polychromasia	Polychromasia, target cells and stomatocytes (liver disease), schistocytes (hemolytic anemias)
Hypersegmentation of neutrophils	Present	Absent
Reticulocyte count	Normal to decreased	Normal, decreased, or increased
Serum B_{12}	Decreased in B_{12} deficiency	Usually normal
Serum folate	Decreased in folate deficiency	Normal (except in alcoholism where it may be decreased)
FIGLU	Increased in folate deficiency	Normal
MMA	Increased in B_{12} deficiency	Normal
Homocysteine	Increased	Normal
Serum bilirubin	Increased	Normal to increased
LD	Increased	Normal to increased

MCU = mean corpuscular volume; FIGLU = formiminoglutamic acid; MMA = methylmalonic acid; LD = lactic dehydrogenase

because of the large cell volume, but the MCHC is normal. In vitamin B_{12} deficiency a macrocytosis may precede the development of anemia by months to years.[6–8] On the other hand, the MCV may remain in the reference range. Epithelial changes in the gastrointestinal tract related to vitamin B_{12} deficiency may cause iron absorption to be impaired. If an iron deficiency, which characteristically produces a microcytic, hypochromic anemia, coexists with megaloblastic anemia, macrocytosis may be masked and the MCV may be in the normal range.[9] Other conditions that have been shown to coexist with megaloblastic anemia in the absence of an increased MCV include thalassemia, chronic renal insufficiency, and chronic inflammation or infection.[8] Sometimes these coexisting causes of anemia are not recognized until after the megaloblastic anemia has been treated.

Hematologic parameters vary considerably (Table 14-2 ✪). The hemoglobin and erythrocyte count range from normal to very low. Occasionally the erythrocyte count may be less than 1×10^{12}/L. However, anemia is not always evident. In one study of 100 patients with confirmed B_{12} deficiency, only 29% had a hemoglobin less than 12 g/dL.[10] This is significant because neurologic symptoms may be present even if the MCV and/or hematocrit are normal.[11] Unlike other anemias that typically involve only erythrocytes, the megaloblastic anemias involve all three blood cell lines: erythrocytes, leukocytes, and platelets. The leukocyte count may be decreased due to an absolute neutropenia. Platelets may also be decreased but do not usually fall below 100×10^9/L. The relative reticulocyte count

(percentage) is usually normal; however, because of the severe anemia, the RPI is less than 2 (∞ Chapter 10).

On the stained blood smear the distinguishing features of megaloblastic anemia include the triad of oval macrocytes (macroovalocytes), Howell-Jolly bodies, and hypersegmented neutrophils (Figure 14-2 ■). Anisocytosis is moderate to severe with normocytes, and with a few microcytes in addition to the macrocytes. Poikilocytosis may be striking and is usually more severe when the anemia is severe. Polychromatophilia and

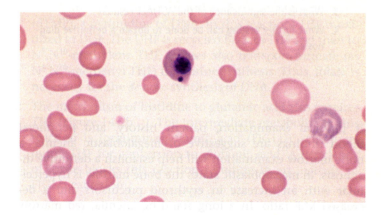

■ **FIGURE 14-2** Peripheral blood film from a patient with pernicious anemia. Note the anisocytosis with oval macrocytes and the nucleated red blood cell with a Howell-Jolly body. (Wright-Giemsa stain; 1000× magnification)

precipitate vitamin B_{12} deficiency. It is not clear as to whether the entire IF-B_{12} complex is absorbed into the cell or just the cobalamin portion of the complex.

Transport Vitamin B_{12} leaves the mucosal cell and is picked up by a group of transport proteins present in the blood. These transport proteins include transcobalamin I, transcobalamin II, and transcobalamin III. Transcobalamin I and III are R-binder proteins, but transcobalamin II is not. The disappearance of the vitamin from each of these transcobalamins is different. Transcobalamin II is an α-globulin, MW 40,000, produced in the liver, the ileum, and by macrophages. Although only about 5% saturated, it is the primary transport protein of vitamin B_{12}. Transcobalamin II binds 90% of the newly absorbed vitamin B_{12}. This transport complex disappears rapidly from blood (T 1/2 of 6–9 minutes) as it is taken up by cells in the liver, bone marrow, and by other dividing cells that have specific receptors for transcobalamin II. Inside the cell, vitamin B_{12} is released and utilized. The transcobalamin is degraded. Congenital deficiency of transcobalamin II produces a severe megaloblastic anemia in infancy. However, serum vitamin B_{12} concentration in this condition is normal.

The functions of transcobalamin I and transcobalamin III, are less well understood. Transcobalamin I has an electrophoretic mobility of α_1-globulin and is produced in part by granulocytes. Although it binds 75% of the recycled endogenous vitamin B_{12} in the body, it is only about 50% saturated, its turnover is slow (T 1/2 of 10 days), and its function is unknown. It has been suggested that it serves as a passive reservoir that is in equilibrium with liver stores of the vitamin. Lack of transcobalamin I produces no megaloblastosis or anemia but results in a decreased serum vitamin B_{12}. Transcobalamin III has an electrophoretic mobility of the α_2-globulins. It appears to be released from granulocytes during the clotting process and does not bind significant portions of cobalamin. Both transcobalamin I and III are increased in myeloproliferative disorders, presumably due to proliferation of granulocytes that produce the protein. Other vitamin B_{12} binder proteins are present in plasma, saliva, gastric juice, pancreatic juice, amniotic fluid, and milk.

Requirements

About 3–5 μg of vitamin B_{12} per day is needed to maintain normal biochemical functions. It is estimated that only about 70% of vitamin B_{12} intake is absorbed, which suggests that the diet should include from 5 to 7 μg of the vitamin per day. This amount is available in a regular mixed diet but will not be provided by strict vegetarian diets. Vitamin B_{12} stores (5000 μg) are sufficient to provide the normal daily requirement for about 1000 days. Therefore, it takes several years to develop a deficiency if no vitamin B_{12} is absorbed from the diet. About half of this storage vitamin is in the liver.[16] The rest is located in the heart and kidneys.

✓ Checkpoint! #6

Explain why there is a megaloblastic anemia in transcobalamin II deficiency when the serum vitamin B_{12} concentration is normal.

Pathophysiology of Vitamin B_{12} Deficiency

Deficiency of vitamin B_{12} is reflected by (1) impaired DNA synthesis, and (2) defective fatty acid degradation.

Impaired DNA Synthesis A deficiency in either vitamin B_{12} or folic acid will result in impaired production of THF and methionine. This leads to a defect in thymidylate synthesis and ultimately to a defect in DNA synthesis. This produces megaloblastic anemia and columnar and squamous epithelial cell abnormalities. All dividing cells are affected, including the hematopoietic cells in the bone marrow.

Homocysteine + methyltetrahydrofolate ⟶ methionine + tetrahydrofolate ⟶ DNA synthesis
(↑ Dietary folate; ↑ Vit B_{12})

Defective Fatty Acid Degradation Adenosylcobalamin is a cofactor in the conversion of methylmalonyl CoA to succinyl CoA. In vitamin B_{12} deficiency there is a defect in degradation of propionyl CoA to methylmalonyl CoA and, finally, to succinyl CoA. As propionyl CoA accumulates, it is used as a primer for fatty acid synthesis replacing the usual primer acetyl CoA. This results in fatty acids with an odd number of carbons. These odd-chain fatty acids are incorporated into neuronal membranes causing disruption of membrane function. It is probable that **demyelination** (destruction, removal, or loss of the lipid substance that forms a myelin sheath around the axons of nerve fibers), a characteristic finding in vitamin B_{12} deficiency, is a result of this erroneous fatty acid synthesis.

A critical feature of demyelination in vitamin B_{12} deficiency is neurological disease. Peripheral nerves are most often affected, presenting as motor and sensory neuropathy. The brain and spinal cord may also be affected leading to dementia, spastic paralysis, and other serious neurological disturbances. Occasionally demyelination has been known to occur without any sign of anemia or macrocytosis, making accurate diagnosis difficult but critical. The bone marrow, however, will always show megaloblastic hematopoiesis.[17] Neurological disease may not be totally reversible but, if treated early, may be partially resolved. Neurological disease does not usually occur in folic acid deficiency. Administration of synthetic folic acid will correct the anemia of vitamin B_{12} deficiency but will not halt or reverse neurological disease. This occurs because synthetic folic acid, unlike dietary folic acid, is reduced directly to THF without the requirement of vitamin B_{12} as a cofactor.[18] The THF can correct the megaloblastosis, but since there is a bypass of the vitamin B_{12} dependent reaction of conversion of homocysteine to methionine, S-adenosylmethionine, a metabolite considered critical to nervous system function, is not formed. Thus, it is essential to differentiate between folate deficiency and vitamin B_{12} deficiency so that appropriate treatment can be given.

Gastritis and abnormalities of the gastrointestinal epithelium secondary to vitamin B_{12} deficiency may interfere with the absorption of folic acid and iron, complicating the anemia.

Causes of Vitamin B_{12} Deficiency

There are many causes of vitamin B_{12} deficiency including lack of intrinsic factor (pernicious anemia), malabsorption, nutritional deficiency, and impaired utilization by tissues due to defective or absent transport proteins or enzyme deficiencies (Table 14-5 ✪).

Pernicious Anemia   **Pernicious anemia (PA)** is a specific term used to define the megaloblastic anemia caused by an absence of IF secondary to gastric atrophy. An absence of IF leads to vitamin B_{12} deficiency as the vitamin cannot be absorbed without it. This is the most common cause of vitamin B_{12} deficiency, accounting for 85% of all deficiencies. Total atrophy of gastric parietal cells is demonstrated by the finding of **achlorhydria** of gastric juice after histamine stimulation (these cells also produce HCl). It is a disease of older adults usually occurring after 40 years of age. This anemia is seen more commonly among people of Northern Europe, especially Great Britain and Scandinavia, but can be found in all racial groups. More women are affected than men. Although no particular genetic abnormality has been identified, some patients have premature graying or whitening of the hair. A positive family history of PA increases the risk of developing PA by 20 times. There is also an increased incidence of gastric carcinoma in these patients.[19]

Pernicious anemia frequently occurs with other autoimmune diseases such as Grave's disease and Hashimoto's thyroiditis. This association between pernicious anemia and autoimmune diseases has led researchers to suggest that perhaps pernicious anemia may develop as the result of a hereditary autoimmune disease. Indeed, up to 90% of pernicious anemia patients have antibodies against parietal cells.[20] However, these antibodies are not specific for pernicious anemia victims. They are also found in patients with gastritis, thyroid disease, and Addison's disease. On the other hand, serum antibodies against intrinsic factor are specific for pernicious anemia patients and can be found in 56% of these patients. Antibodies against IF have also been found in the gastric secretions of 75% of pernicious anemia patients. These specific antibodies are of two types: blocking and binding. Blocking antibodies prevent formation of the IF-vitamin B_{12} complex. Binding antibodies react with the IF-vitamin B_{12} binding sites, preventing absorption in the ileum. This raises the question of whether the IF antibodies are pathogenic or merely accompany the development of pernicious anemia.

Pernicious anemia is rare in children. *Juvenile pernicious anemia* is a term used to describe the anemia accompanying a congenital deficiency of IF. There are at least two types of juvenile pernicious anemia. The most common type is characterized by a lack of IF but otherwise normal gastric secretion and no antibodies against parietal cells. A less common type is more typical of the pernicious anemia found in adults. In this type there is absence of intrinsic factor together with gastric atrophy, decreased gastric secretion, and antibodies against IF and parietal cells.

Laboratory diagnosis of pernicious anemia usually involves gastric analysis and/or the Schilling test and serum vitamin B_{12} assay. The serum vitamin B_{12} assay establishes the fact that a deficiency exists but does not provide a distinction of pernicious anemia from other causes of vitamin B_{12} deficiency. Gastric analysis and the Schilling test are more useful in establishing the specific diagnosis of pernicious anemia.

Gastric Analysis   Since atrophy of the parietal cells is a universal feature of pernicious anemia, positive diagnosis

✪ TABLE 14-5

Causes of Vitamin B_{12} Deficiency and Associated Conditions

Cause	Associated Conditions
Malabsorption	Pernicious anemia (lack of IF)
	Gastrectomy or gastric bypass
	Crohn's disease
	Tropical sprue
	Celiac disease
	Surgical resection of the ileum
	Imerslund-Grasbeck disease
	Pancreatic insufficiency
	Drugs (colchicine, neomycin, p-aminosalicylic acid, or omiprazole)
	Blind loop syndrome
	Diverticulitis
	Intestinal parasite—*Diphyllobothrium latum*
Biologic competition	Intestinal parasite: i.e., *Diphyllobothrium latum*
	Bacterial overgrowth
Nutritional deficiency	Strict vegetarian diets
	Pregnant women on a poor diet
	Malnutrition
Impaired utilization	Transcobalamin II deficiency
	Nitrous oxide inhalation

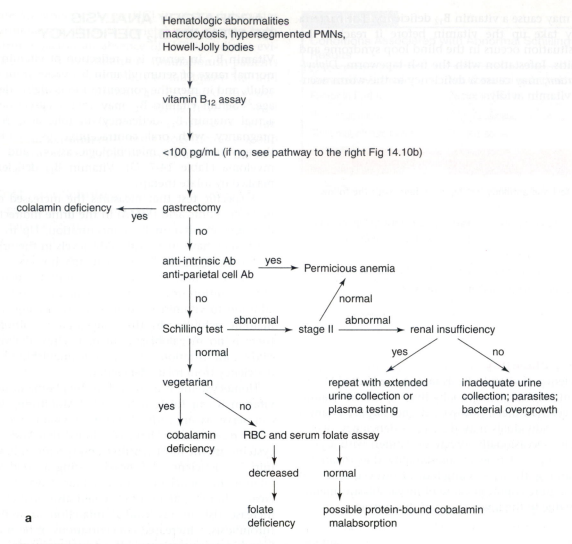

Hematologic abnormalities
macrocytosis, hypersegmented PMNs,
Howell-Jolly bodies

↓

vitamin B₁₂ assay

↓

<100 pg/mL (if no, see pathway to the right Fig 14.10b)

↓

colalamin deficiency ← yes — gastrectomy

│ no
↓

anti-intrinsic Ab   — yes → Pernicious anemia
anti-parietal cell Ab

│ no
↓   normal
                                           ↑
Schilling test — abnormal → stage II — abnormal → renal insufficiency

│ normal   yes   no

vegetarian   repeat with extended   inadequate urine
                               urine collection or   collection; parasites;
yes   no   plasma testing   bacterial overgrowth

cobalamin   RBC and serum folate assay
deficiency
                    decreased   normal

                    folate   possible protein-bound cobalamin
                    deficiency   malabsorption

a

■ **FIGURE 14-10** Algorithm of diagnosis of vitamin B₁₂ and folic acid deficiency using laboratory tests. The algorithm above (a) is followed if the serum vitamin B₁₂ level is <100 pg/mL. If higher, follow the algorithm to the right (b). Use this figure with Figure 14-1 to determine if macrocytosis is megaloblastic or nonmegaloblastic. (Adapted, with permission, from: Snow CF. Laboratory diagnosis of vitamin B₁₂ and folate deficiency. *Arch Intern Med.* 1999; 159:1289–98.) *(continues)*

measurements.[26] By contrast, some have found that MMA and homocysteine measurements are more sensitive tests of early pernicious anemia preceding hematologic abnormalities and decreased serum vitamin B₁₂ levels and recommend them as a superior testing regimen (Figure 14-10 ■).

Homocysteine and MMA tests are also helpful in determining a patient's response to treatment with vitamin B₁₂ and folate. The serum MMA level remains increased in vitamin B₁₂ deficient patients treated inappropriately with folate. In folate deficient patients treated inappropriately with cobalamin, the serum homocysteine level remains increased.

A new technology, electrospray tandem mass spectrometry, may make testing for serum levels of MMA and homocysteine easier and more practical.[27] The procedure does not require expensive immunodiagnostic reagents and chromatographic columns and can be performed in under five minutes.

THERAPY

Therapeutic trials in megaloblastic anemia using *physiologic* doses of either vitamin B₁₂ or folic acid will only produce a reticulocyte response if the specific vitamin that is deficient is being administered. For instance small doses (1 μg) of vitamin B₁₂ given daily will produce a reticulocyte response in vitamin B₁₂ deficiency but not in folic acid deficiency. On the other hand, large therapeutic doses of vitamin B₁₂ or folic acid may induce a partial response to the other vitamin deficiency, as well as the specific deficiency.

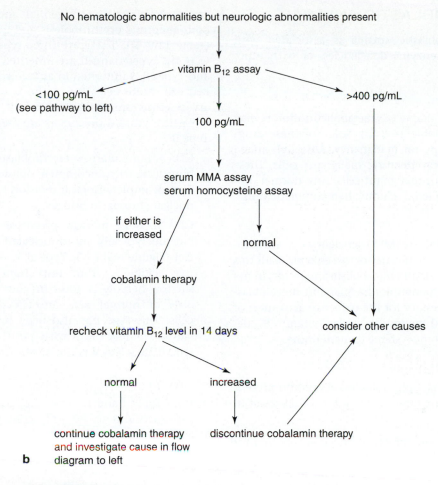

No hematologic abnormalities but neurologic abnormalities present

vitamin B_{12} assay

<100 pg/mL
(see pathway to left)

>400 pg/mL

100 pg/mL

serum MMA assay
serum homocysteine assay

if either is
increased

normal

cobalamin therapy

recheck vitamin B_{12} level in 14 days

consider other causes

normal

increased

continue cobalamin therapy
and investigate cause in flow
b diagram to left

discontinue cobalamin therapy

■ **FIGURE 14-10** (*continued*)

Generally, it is best to determine which deficiency exists and treat the patient with the specific deficient vitamin. Large doses of folic acid are proven to correct the anemia in vitamin B_{12} deficiency but will not correct or halt demyelination. This makes diagnosis and specific therapy critical in vitamin B_{12} deficiency. Specific therapy will cause a rise in the reticulocyte count after the fourth day of therapy. Reticulocytosis peaks at about five to eight days and returns to normal after two weeks. The degree of reticulocytosis is proportional to the severity of the anemia, with more striking reticulocytosis in patients with severe anemia. The hemoglobin rises about 2–3 g/dL every two weeks until normal levels are reached. The marrow responds quickly to therapy as evidenced by pronormoblasts (normal) appearing within 4–6 hours and nearly complete recovery of erythroid abnormalities within 2–4 days. Granulocyte abnormalities disappear more slowly. Hypersegmented neutrophils can usually be found for 12–14 days after therapy is begun.[16]

In vitamin B_{12} deficiency, specific therapy may reverse the peripheral neuropathy, but spinal cord damage is irreversible. Pernicious anemia must be treated with lifelong monthly parenteral doses of hydroxycobalamin because of the inability of these patients to absorb oral vitamin B_{12}. Recently it was reported that orally administered vitamin B_{12} therapy may be feasible if the patient is compliant.[20] The rationale behind oral therapy is that a small amount (from 1 to 3%) of the vitamin is absorbed without IF. The optimal dose has not been determined.

ⓔ CASE STUDY (*continued from page 277*)

6. How would the diagnosis change if the special testing results were as follows?

    Schilling test: Part I, before intrinsic factor: 1%
                       Part II, after intrinsic factor: 3%

Intrinsic-factor-blocking
       antibodies: Negative

7. What would you predict this patient's reticulocyte count to be?

OTHER MEGALOBLASTIC ANEMIAS

Occasionally, a megaloblastic anemia is associated with drugs, with congenital enzyme deficiencies, or with other hematopoietic diseases.

Drugs

A large number of drugs that act as metabolic inhibitors may cause megaloblastosis (Table 14-8 ✪). Some of these drugs are used in chemotherapy for malignancy. Although aimed at eliminating rapidly proliferating malignant cells, these drugs are not selective for malignant cells. Any normal proliferating cell is also affected, including hematopoietic cells.

Enzyme Deficiencies

Methionine synthase reductase (MSR) deficiency is a rare autosomal recessive disorder. A deficiency of this enzyme leads to a dysfunction of folate/cobalamin metabolism and results in hyperhomocysteinemia, hypomethioninemia, and megaloblastic anemia.[28] MSR is necessary for the reductive activation of methionine synthase and the resultant folate/vitamin B_{12} dependent conversion of homocysteine to methionine.

Congenital Deficiencies

A congenital deficiency is a physiological aberration present at birth. The following are deficiencies at birth that result in megaloblastosis.

Orotic Aciduria Inborn defects in enzymes required for pyrimidine synthesis or folate metabolism may result in megaloblastic anemia. Orotic aciduria is a rare autosomal recessive disorder in which there is a failure to convert orotic acid to uridylic acid. The result is excessive excretion of orotic acid. Children with this disorder also fail to grow and develop normally. The condition responds to treatment with oral uridine.

Congenital Dyserythropoietic Anemia Congenital dyserythropoietic anemia (CDA) is actually a heterogeneous group of refractory, congenital anemias characterized by both abnormal erythropoiesis and ineffective erythropoiesis (Table 14-9 ✪). There are three types: CDA I, CDA II, and CDA III. Types I and II are inherited as autosomal recessive, and Type III is inherited in an autosomal dominant fashion. Red cell multinuclearity in the bone marrow and secondary siderosis are recognized in all types; however, megaloblastic erythroid precursors are present only in Type I and Type III.

CDA I. Bone marrow erythroblasts are megaloblastic and binucleate with incomplete division of nuclear segments. The incomplete nuclear division is characterized by internuclear chromatin bridges.

CDA II. Bone marrow precursors are not megaloblastic but are typically multinucleated with up to seven nuclei (Figure 14-11 ■). Type II is distinguished by a positive acidified serum test (Ham test) but a negative sucrose hemolysis test. In the Ham test, only about 30% of normal sera are effective in lysing CDA II cells. This type has also been termed *hereditary erythroblastic multinuclearity* with positive acidified serum test (HEMPAS). CDA II is the most common of the three types of CDA.

CDA III. This type of CDA is morphologically distinct from Types I and II because of the presence of giant erythroblasts (up to 50 μm) containing up to 16 nuclei. Sometimes the erythrocytes are agglutinated by anti-I and anti-i antibodies.

Other Hematopoietic Diseases

The myelodysplastic syndromes are a group of stem cell disorders characterized by peripheral cytopenias and dyshematopoiesis. Erythroid precursors in the bone marrow frequently exhibit megaloblastic-like changes. Occasionally there is a nonmegaloblastic macrocytic anemia. These diseases will be discussed in ∞ Chapter 28.

✪ TABLE 14-8

Drugs That May Cause Megaloblastosis

DNA Base Inhibitors			
Pyrimidine	Purine	Antimetabolites	Other
Azauridine	Acyclovir	Cytosine arabinoside	Azacytidine
	Adenosine arabinoside	Fluorocytidine	Cyclophosphamide
	Azathioprine	Fluorouracil	Zidovudine
	Gancyclovir	Hydroxyurea	
	Mercaptopurine	Methotrexate	
	Thioguanine		
	Vidarabine		

○ **TABLE 14-9**

Comparison of Congenital Dyserythropoietic Anemia (CDA) Types

Characteristics	CDA I	CDA II	CDA III
Inheritance	Autosomal recessive	Autosomal recessive	Autosomal dominant
RBC multinuclearity	Present	Present	Present
Number of nuclear lobes	2	Up to 7	Up to 16
Siderosis	Present	Present	Present
Megaloblastosis	Present	Absent	Present
Other characteristics	Incomplete nuclear division	Positive Ham's test (HEMPAS)	RBC agglutination by anti-I and anti-i antibodies

▶ ## MACROCYTIC ANEMIA WITHOUT MEGALOBLASTOSIS

The typical findings of megaloblastic anemia are not evident in other macrocytic anemias (Table 14-10 ○). The macrocytes in macrocytic anemias without megaloblastosis are not usually as pronounced as the macrocytes in megaloblastic anemia. In addition, these macrocytes are usually round rather than oval as seen in megaloblastic anemia. Hypersegmented neutrophils are not present and leukocytes and platelets are quantitatively normal. There is an absence of jaundice, glossitis, and neuropathy, the typical clinical findings in megaloblastosis. The cause of the macrocytosis without megaloblastosis is unknown in most cases. It has been suggested that macrocytes may be due to an increase in membrane lipids or to a delay in blast maturation. Some diseases associated with nonmegaloblastic macrocytic anemia are listed in Table 14-1 ○. Three of the most common are discussed in this section: alcoholism, liver disease, and reticulocytosis (stimulated erythropoiesis).

ALCOHOLISM

Alcohol abuse is one of the most common causes of nonanemic macrocytosis. It has been suggested that all patients with macrocytosis should be questioned about their alcohol consumption.[29] The macrocytosis associated with alcoholism is usually multifactorial and may be megaloblastic. Macrocytosis is probably the result of one or more of four causes: (1) folate deficiency due to decreased dietary intake, (2) reticulocytosis associated with hemolysis or gastrointestinal bleeding, (3) associated liver disease, and (4) macrocytosis related to alcohol intoxication.

Folate deficiency associated with a megaloblastic anemia is the most common cause of the macrocytosis found in

○ **TABLE 14-10**

Conditions Associated with Nonmegaloblastic Macrocytosis

Condition	Cause of Macrocytosis
Alcoholism	Direct toxic effect of alcohol on erythroid precursors
	Reticulocytosis associated with hemolysis or GI bleeding
	Liver disease: abnormal RBC membrane lipid composition
	May also be megaloblastic due to folate deficiency
Liver disease	Reticulocytosis associated with stimulated erythropoiesis; increased RBC membrane lipids
Hemolysis or posthemorrhagic anemia	Reticulocytosis associated with stimulated erythropoiesis
Hypothroidism	Unknown
Aplastic anemia	Unknown
Artifactual	Cold agglutinin disease
	Severe hyperglycemia
	RBC clumping
	Swelling of RBCs

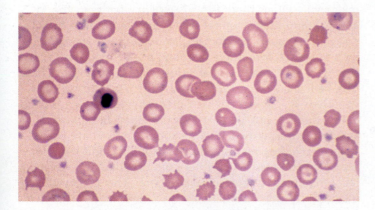

■ **FIGURE 14-11** Peripheral blood microphotograph of a case of congenital dyserythropoietic anemia type II (CDA-II). There is anisocytosis with microcytic, hypochromic cells as well as macrocytes and normocytes. Cabot's rings are visible. The nucleated cell is an orthochromic normoblast showing lobulation of the nucleus. (Wright-Giemsa stain; 1000× magnification)

hospitalized alcoholics. The deficiency probably results from poor dietary habits, although ethanol also appears to interfere with folate metabolism.

The reduced erythrocyte survival with a corresponding reticulocytosis has been associated with chronic gastrointestinal bleeding secondary to hepatic dysfunction (decreased coagulation proteins) or thrombocytopenia, hypersplenism from increased portal and splenic vein pressure, pooling of cells in splenomegaly, and altered erythrocyte membranes caused by abnormal blood lipid content in liver disease (∞ Chapter 17). Stomatocytes are associated with acute alcoholism, but there appear to be no cation leaks, and hemolysis of these cells is not significant.

Liver disease is common in alcoholics; typical hematologic findings associated with this disease are discussed in the following section. Even when anemia is absent, most alcoholics have a mild macrocytosis (100–110 fL) that is unrelated to liver disease or folate deficiency. This may be caused by a direct toxic effect of the ethanol on developing erythroblasts. Vacuolization of red cell precursors, similar to that seen in patients taking chloramphenicol, is a common finding after prolonged alcohol ingestion. If alcohol intake is eliminated, the cells gradually assume their normal size, and the bone marrow changes disappear. The association of a sideroblastic anemia and alcoholism is discussed in ∞ Chapter 11.

The multiple pathologies of this type of anemia result in the possibility of a variety of abnormal hematologic findings. Thus, it is possible to have a blood picture resembling that of megaloblastic anemia, of chronic hemolysis, of chronic or acute blood loss, of liver disease, or (more than likely) of a combination of these conditions. Alcohol may also cause disordered heme synthesis as discussed in ∞ Chapter 11.

LIVER DISEASE

The most common disease associated with a nonmegaloblastic macrocytic anemia is liver disease (including alcoholic cirrhosis). The causes of this anemia are multifactorial and include hemolysis, impaired bone marrow response, folate deficiency, and blood loss (Table 14-11 ✪). Although macrocytic anemia is the most common form of anemia in liver disease, occurring in over 50% of the patients, normochromic or microcytic anemia may also be found, depending on the predominant pathologic mechanism.

Erythrocyte survival appears to be significantly shortened in alcoholic liver disease, infectious hepatitis, biliary cirrhosis, and obstructive jaundice. The reason for this is unknown. Cross-transfusion studies in which patient cells are infused into normal individuals demonstrate an increase in patient cell survival. These studies suggest an extracorpuscular factor is probably responsible for cell hemolysis. The spleen is thought to play an important role in sequestration and hemolysis in individuals with splenomegaly or hypersplenism. In some cases, hemolysis is well compensated for by an increase in erythropoiesis, and there is no anemia. In some patients with alcoholic liver disease, a heavy drinking spree produces a brisk but transient hemolysis. These patients also show abnormal liver function and have markedly increased levels of plasma triglycerides.

Abnormalities in erythrocyte membrane lipid composition are a common finding in hepatitis, cirrhosis, and obstructive jaundice. There is an increase in both cholesterol and phospholipid, resulting in cells with an increased surface-to-volume ratio. This abnormality is not thought to cause decreased cell survival. In contrast, in severe hepatocellular disease, erythrocyte membranes have an excessive amount of cholesterol relative to phospholipid, which decreases the erythrocyte deformability. This is associated with the formation of spur cells in which the erythrocyte exhibits spike-like projections. These cells have a pronounced shortened life span leading to an anemia termed *spur cell anemia* (∞ Chapter 17).

Kinetic iron studies have revealed that the bone marrow response in liver disease may be impaired. It has been proposed that liver disease may affect the production of erythropoietin because this organ has been shown to be an important extrarenal source of the hormone in rats.[30] In alcoholic cirrhosis, the alcohol may have a direct suppressive effect on the bone marrow.

Clinical findings and symptoms in liver disease are secondary to the abnormalities in liver function. The liver is involved in many essential metabolic reactions and in the synthesis of many proteins and lipids. Therefore, the anemia is only a minor finding among the abnormalities associated with dysfunction of this organ.

The anemia is usually mild with an average hemoglobin concentration around 12 g/dL. With complications, the anemia may be severe. The erythrocytes may appear normocytic, macrocytic (usually not greater than 115 fL MCV), or microcytic. Often there is a discrepancy between the MCV and the appearance of the cells microscopically. In these cases, thin, round macrocytes (as determined by diameter) with target cell formation are found on the blood smear, but the MCV is within normal limits. The reticulocyte count may be increased but the RPI is usually less than two unless hemolysis is a significant factor. Thrombocytopenia is a frequent finding and platelet function may be abnormal. A variety of nonspecific leukocyte abnormalities have been described including neutropenia, neutrophilia, and lymphopenia. The bone marrow is either normocellular or hypercellular, often with erythroid hyperplasia. The precursors are qualitatively normal unless folic acid deficiency is present. In this case, megaloblastosis is apparent with the typical associated blood abnormalities.

Other laboratory tests of liver function are variably abnormal including increased serum bilirubin and increased hepatic enzymes. Tests for carbohydrate and lipid metabolites

⊛ TABLE 14-11

Causes and Characteristics of Anemia in Liver Disease

Causes	Anemia Type	Characteristics
Abnormal liver function	Macrocytic	MCV normal to increased
		Increased RBC membrane cholesterol results in target cells and acanthocytes
		Normal to slightly increased reticulocytes
Folic acid deficiency	Macrocytic	MCV increased
		Pancytopenia
		Ovalocytes and teardrop cells
		Normal to decreased retics
		Functional folate deficiency
Stimulated erythropoiesis	Macrocytic	MCV increased
		Slightly increased WBC count
		Normal platelet count
		Shift reticulocytosis
Hemolysis	Normocytic or macrocytic	MCV normal to increased
		Spur cells and schistocytes
		Increased reticulocytes
Hypersplenism	Normocytic	MCV normal
		Pancytopenia
		Increased reticulocytes
		Portal hypertension
Marrow hypoproliferation	Normocytic	MCV normal
		Pancytopenia
		Decreased reticulocytes
		Associated with renal disease or alcohol suppression
Chronic blood loss	Microcytic	MCV decreased
		Iron deficiency
		Slightly increased leukocyte and platelet counts
		Increased reticulocytes
		Commonly associated with gastrointestinal bleeding

are frequently abnormal depending on the degree of liver disease.

STIMULATED ERYTHROPOIESIS

Increased erythropoietin (stimulation) in the presence of an adequate iron supply (e.g., autoimmune hemolytic anemia) can result in the release of shift reticulocytes from the bone marrow. These cells are larger than normal with an MCV that may be as high as 130 fL. A reticulocyte count and examination of the blood smear will allow distinction of this macrocytic entity from megaloblastic anemia. In the presence of large numbers of shift reticulocytes, there is a marked increase in polychromasia. In addition, the oval macrocytes typical to megaloblastic anemia are not present in conditions associated with increased erythropoietin stimulation.

HYPOTHROIDISM

Anemia of hypothroidism presents as a mild to moderate anemia with a normal reticulocyte count. Thyroid hormone regulates cellular metabolic rate, and therefore tissue oxygen requirement. With a decrease in thyroid hormone (i.e., hypothyroidism) there is a smaller tissue oxygen requirement, which is interpreted by the kidneys as a more than adequate oxygen-tension. The net result is a decrease in the production of EPO. This type of anemia often presents as a macrocytic, normochromic anemia but can also be a normo-cytic, normochromic anemia. The anemia may be complicated by iron, folic acid, or B_{12} deficiency, and the blood picture may reflect these forms of anemia.

 Checkpoint! #8

What are three clinical or laboratory findings (besides assessing the bone marrow) that can distinguish a nonmegaloblastic macrocytic anemia from a megaloblastic anemia?

SUMMARY

Macrocytosis due to megaloblastic anemia must be differentiated from macrocytosis with a normoblastic marrow. The laboratory profile of a patient with megaloblastic anemia commonly presents with pancytopenia. The blood smear reveals macrocytes (i.e., ovalocytes), poikilocytosis, teardrop cells, and neutrophil hypersegmentation. The marrow is characterized by megaloblastosis of precursor cells due to a block in thymidine production. Because thymidine is one of the four DNA bases, the deficiency leads to a diminished capacity for DNA synthesis and a block in mitosis. The marrow is hypercellular but erythropoiesis is ineffective. Causes of megaloblastosis are nearly always due to vitamin B_{12} or folic acid deficiencies.

Folate is primarily acquired from the diet in such foods as eggs, milk, leafy vegetables, yeast, liver, and fruits. Liver tissue is the main storage site of folic acid. Clinically, symptoms from inadequate dietary folate can occur within months, as compared to years for a B_{12} deficiency.

Vitamin B_{12} (i.e., cyanocobalamin) metabolism occurs in the small intestine. Dietary vitamin B_{12} is released from digestion of animal proteins in meats and bound by gastric intrinsic factor (IF). Once absorbed, vitamin B_{12} is bound to specific plasma proteins known as transcobalamin-I, II, or III. Normal serum vitamin B_{12} values are highly variable on age and sex. B_{12} function is related to DNA synthesis because vitamin B_{12} is a vital cofactor in the conversion of methyl tetrahydrofolate (i.e., folic acid) to tetrahydrofolate.

This substrate is an important cofactor needed for the production of DNA thymidine.

Defective production of intrinsic factor is the most common cause of vitamin B_{12} deficiency. Pernicious anemia (PA) is a conditioned nutritional deficiency of vitamin B_{12}, caused by failure of the gastric mucosa to secrete IF. PA most commonly occurs in people after 40 years of age, with accompanying clinical symptoms of abdominal pain, constipation, diarrhea, and central nervous system symptoms such as numbness and tingling of the extremities, difficulty with balance and gait, loss of vibration sensation, weakness, and spasticity and personality changes in advanced cases. The Schilling test is a definitive test useful in the diagnosis of intrinsic factor deficiency. Other causes of vitamin B_{12} deficiency include gastrectomy, malabsorption diseases such as Crohn's disease, or drugs. Rarely, megaloblastic anemia results from chemotherapeutic drugs, congenital enzyme deficiencies, or with other hematopoietic diseases such as congenital dyserythropoietic anemia.

Macrocytosis due to megaloblastic anemia must be differentiated from macrocytosis with a normoblastic marrow. Normoblastic, macrocytic anemias can result from acute blood loss or hemolysis due to shift reticulocytosis from the marrow. Alcohol abuse is one of the most common causes of normoblastic macrocytosis. Liver disease, often resulting from alcohol abuse, is also commonly associated with macrocytosis without a megaloblastic marrow.

REVIEW QUESTIONS

LEVEL I

1. The most common cause of macrocytosis is: (Checklist #5)
   a. folate deficiency
   b. alcoholism
   c. liver disease
   d. pernicious anemia

2. In the majority of cases, B_{12} deficiency is due to a deficiency of: (Checklist #2)
   a. intrinsic factor
   b. vitamin B_6
   c. folate
   d. methylmalonic acid

LEVEL II

1. If a patient presented with anemia, macrocytosis, pancytopenia, and malnutrition, which of the following should be investigated first as a possible cause of the anemia? (Checklist #4, 12)
   a. pernicious anemia
   b. folic acid deficiency
   c. B_{12} deficiency
   d. celiac disease

2. The characteristic triad of distinguishing features on a megaloblastic anemia includes all of the following, *except:* (Checklist #2, 3)
   a. macroovalocytes
   b. hypersegmentation
   c. reticulocytosis
   d. Howell-Jolly bodies

REVIEW QUESTIONS (continued)

LEVEL I

3. Which of the following would be the best clue in diagnosing megaloblastic anemia? (Checklist #3)
   a. decreased hemoglobin and hematocrit
   b. leukocytosis
   c. hypersegmented neutrophils
   d. poikilocytosis

4. Increases in urinary excretion of formiminoglutamic acid (FIGLU) would most likely indicate which of the following? (Checklist #4)
   a. vitamin B_{12} deficiency
   b. autoantibodies to intrinsic factor
   c. folic acid deficiency
   d. hemolysis

5. The liver stores enough folate to meet daily requirement needs for how long? (Checklist #2)
   a. 1 month
   b. 6–8 weeks
   c. 2 years
   d. 3–6 months

6. Which of the following conditions increases the daily requirement for vitamin B_{12}? (Checklist #2)
   a. pregnancy
   b. aplastic anemia
   c. hypothyroidism
   d. splenectomy

7. A deficiency of vitamin B_{12} leads to impaired: (Checklist #1)
   a. Folic acid synthesis
   b. DNA synthesis
   c. intrinsic factor secretion
   d. absorption of folate

8. Laboratory diagnosis of pernicious anemia usually involves which of the following? (Checklist #3)
   a. urinary FIGLU
   b. WBC count
   c. Schilling test
   d. LDH

9. Alcoholics commonly develop a macrocytic anemia due to: (Checklist #8)
   a. folate deficiency
   b. increased blood cholesterol levels
   c. development of autoantibodies against intrinsic factor
   d. intestinal malabsorption of B_{12}

10. Anemia due to liver disease is often associated with which of the following RBC morphological forms? (Checklist #9)
    a. ovalocytes
    b. microcytes
    c. spur cells
    d. teardrop cells

LEVEL II

3. Which of the following can be found in a patient with megaloblastic anemia? (Checklist #2, 8, 11)
   a. giant metamyelocytes and hypolobated neutrophils
   b. Howell-Jolly bodies and Pappenheimer bodies
   c. hypersegmented neutrophils and oval macrocytes
   d. hypochromic macrocytes and thrombocytosis

4. The metabolic function of tetrahydrofolate is to: (Checklist #3)
   a. synthesize methionine
   b. transfer carbon units from donors to receptors
   c. serve as a cofactor with cobalamin in the synthesis of thymidylate
   d. synthesize intrinsic factor

5. Folic acid deficiency can be caused by: (Checklist #6)
   a. alcoholism
   b. chronic blood loss
   c. strict vegetarian diet
   d. vitamin B_6 deficiency

6. A lack of intrinsic factor may be due to: (Checklist #7)
   a. gastrectomy
   b. vitamin B_{12} deficiency
   c. folate deficiency
   d. large bowel resection

7. Which of the following is more typical of nonmegaloblastic than megaloblastic anemia? (Checklist #2, 3)
   a. oval macrocytes
   b. round macrocytes
   c. Howell-Jolly bodies
   d. hypersegmented PMN

8. If a patient excretes less than 7.5% of a radioactively tagged crystalline B_{12} dose after 24 hours, both before and after administration of a dose of oral intrinsic factor, which of the following is a possible diagnosis? (Checklist #9)
   a. pernicious anemia
   b. liver disease
   c. gastrectomy
   d. celiac disease

9. Which type of congenital dyserythropoietic anemia (CDA) presents with giant multinucleated erythrocytes in the marrow? (Checklist #10)
   a. CDA I
   b. CDA II
   c. CDA III
   d. CDA IV

REVIEW QUESTIONS (continued)

LEVEL I

LEVEL II

10. A 48-year-old Caucasian female was seen by her physician due to fatigue, loss of appetite, and weight loss over a period of three months. A medical history revealed she had a history of alcohol abuse. An initial laboratory workup demonstrated that she was anemic, had a leukocyte count of 3×10^9/L, and had an MCV of 119 fL. Macroovalocytes and neutrophil hypersegmentation was noted on her blood smear evaluation. Based on the initial laboratory test results, her physician obtained a serum vitamin B_{12} and folate workup. Results were as follows:

Serum vitamin B_{12}:	550 pg/mL
Serum folate:	4.0 ng/mL
RBC folate:	105 ng/mL

Based on her clinical history and laboratory results, the best possible diagnosis is which of the following? (Checklist #12)
   a. pernicious anemia
   b. folate deficiency
   c. primary B_{12} deficiency
   d. anemia of liver disease

www.prenhall.com/mckenzie
Use the above address to access the free, interactive Companion Web site created for this textbook. Get hints, instant feedback, and textbook references to chapter-related multiple choice questions.

REFERENCES

1. Hoggarth K. Macrocytic anaemias. *Practitioner.* 1993; 237(1525): 331–32, 335.

2. Colon-Otero G, Menke D, Hook CC. A practical approach to the differential diagnosis and evaluation of the adult patient with macrocytic anemia. *Med Clin North Am.* 1992; 76:581–97.

3. Kass L. Pernicious anemia. In: Smith LH Jr, editor. *Major Problems in Internal Medicine.* Vol. 7. Philadelphia: W.B. Saunders, Co; 1976: 1–62.

4. Addison T. *On the Constitutional and Local Effects of Disease of the Suprarenal Capsules.* London, England: Sam Highley; 1855:43.

5. Ehrlich P. *Farbenanalytische Untersuchungen zur Histologie und Klinik des Blutes.* Berlin, Germany: A. Hirschwald; 1891:137.

6. Carmel R. Macrocytosis, mild anemia, and delay in the diagnosis of pernicious anemia. *Arch Intern Med.* 1979; 139:47–50.

7. Hall CA. Vitamin B_{12} deficiency and early rise in mean corpuscular volume. *JAMA.* 1981; 245:1144–46.

8. Spivak JL. Masked megaloblastic anemia. *Arch Intern Med.* 1982; 142:2111–14.

9. Carmel R, Weiner JM, Johnson CS. Iron deficiency occurs frequently in patients with pernicious anemia. *JAMA.* 1987; 257: 1081–83.

10. Pruthi RK, Tafferi A. Pernicious anemia revisited. *Mayo Clin Pro.* 1994; 69:144–50.

11. Lindenbaum J, Healton EB, Savage DG, et al. Neuropsychiatric disorders caused by cobalamin deficiency in the absence of anemia or macrocytosis. *N Engl J Med.* 1988; 318:1720–28.

12. Klee GG. Cobalamin and folate evaluation: Measurement of methylmalonic acid and homocysteine vs vitamin B_{12} and folate. *Clin Chem.* 2000; 46(8 Pt 2):1277–83.

13. Jacques PF, Selhub J, Bostom AG, Wilson PWF, Rosenberg IH. The effect of folic acid fortification on plasma folate and total homocysteine concentrations. *N Engl J Med.* 1999; 340:1449–54.

14. MRC Vitamin Study Research Group. Prevention of neural tube defects: Results of the Medical Research Council Vitamin Study. *Lancet.* 1991; 338(8760):131–37.

15. Minot GR, Murphy W. Observations on patients with pernicious anemia partaking of a special diet. A. Clinical aspects. *Trans Assoc Am Physicians.* 1926; 41:72–75.

16. Chanarin I. Megaloblastic anaemia, cobalamin, and folate. *J Clin Pathol.* 1987; 40:978–84.

17. Hsing AW, et al. Pernicious anemia and subsequent cancer: A population-based cohort study. *Cancer.* 1993; 71:745–50.

18. Snow CF. Laboratory diagnosis of vitamin B_{12} and folate deficiency: A guide for the primary care physician. *Arch Intern Med.* 1999; 159:1289–98.

19. Lindgren A, Lindstedt G, Kilander AF. Advantages of serum pepsinogen A combined with gastrin or pepsinogen C as first-line

analytes in the evaluation of suspected cobalamin deficiency: A study in patients previously not subjected to gastrointestinal surgery. *J Intern Med.* 1998; 244:341–49.

20. Carmel R, Sinow RM, Siegel ME, Samloff IM. Food cobalamin malabsorption occurs frequently in patients with unexplained low serum cobalamin levels. *Arch Intern Med.* 1988; 148:1715–19.

21. Fairbanks VF, Elveback LR. Tests for pernicious anemia: Serum vitamin B_{12} assay. *Mayo Clin Proc.* 1983; 58:135–37.

22. Norman EJ, Morrison JA. Screening elderly populations for cobalamin (vitamin B_{12}) deficiency using the urinary methylmalonic acid assay by gas chromatography mass spectrometry. *Am J Med.* 1993; 94:589–94.

23. Welch GN, Loscalzo J. Homocysteine and atherothrombosis. *N Engl J Med.* 1998; 338:1042–50.

24. Bernard BA, Firdaus M, Nakonezny PA, Kashner TM. Urinary methylmalonic acid/creatinine ratio: A gold standard test for tissue vitamin B_{12} deficiency. *J Am Geriatr Soc.* 1999; 47:1158–59.

25. Ridker PM, Hennekens CH, Selhub J, Miletich JP, Malinow MR, Stampfer MF. Interrelation of hyperhomocyst(e)inemia, factor V Leiden, and risk of future venous thromboembolism. *Circulation.* 1997; 95:1777–82.

26. Holleland G, Schneede J, Ueland PM, Lund PK, Refsum H, Sandberg S. Cobalamin deficiency in general practice: Assessment of the diagnostic utility and cost-benefit analysis of methylmalonic acid determination in relation to current diagnostic strategies. *Clin Chem.* 1999; 45:189–98.

27. Magera MF, Lacey JM, Casetta B, Rinaldo P. Method for the determination of total homocysteine in plasma and urine by stable isotope dilution and electrospray tandem mass spectrometry. *Clin Chem.* 1999; 45:1517–22.

28. Wilson A, Leclerc D, Rosenblatt DS, Gravel RA. Molecular basis for methionine synthase reductase deficiency in patients belonging to the cblE complementation group of disorders in folate/cobalamin metabolism. *Hu Mol Gene.* 1999; 8:2009–16.

29. Seppa K, Sillanaukee P, Saarni M. Blood count and hematologic morphology in nonanemic macrocytosis: Differences between alcohol abuse and pernicious anemia. *Alcohol.* 1993; 10:343–47.

30. Katz R, et al. Studies on the site of production of erythropoietin. *Ann NY Acad Sci.* 1968; 149:120–27.

⊙ **TABLE 15-4**

Comparison of the Features of Diamond-Blackfan Anemia and Transient Erythroblastopenia of Childhood (TEC)

Feature	Diamond-Blackfan	TEC
PRCA	Present	Present
Fetal erythrocyte characteristics (I antigen, HbF increased)	Present	Absent (if child is >1 year old)
Etiology	Inherited	Follows viral infection (mechanism unknown)
MCV	May be increased	Normal
Age at onset	Birth to 1 year old	Up to 4 years old
Therapy	Corticosteroids, transfusions	None, spontaneous recovery

PRCA = pure red cell aplasia

and potentially harmful to children with TEC.[26] Patients with TEC recover within 2 months of diagnosis. Therapy involves only supportive care.

► **OTHER HYPOPROLIFERATIVE ANEMIAS**

Other hypoproliferative anemias, due primarily to defective hormonal stimulation of erythroid stem cells, include the anemia associated with chronic renal disease and the anemias associated with endocrine disorders. In most cases these anemias can be traced to a decrease in erythropoietin production.

RENAL DISEASE

Chronic renal disease is a common cause of anemia. Anemia, however, is only an incidental finding; the patient primarily seeks medical attention for symptoms related to renal failure. The hemoglobin begins to decrease when the blood urea nitrogen level increases to greater than 30 mg/dL. Anemia is slow developing and most patients tolerate the low hemoglobin levels well.

Pathophysiology

Due to the complexity of the clinical settings in uremia, anemia is frequently the result of several different pathophysiologies (Table 15-5 ⊙):

1. The most important and consistent factor is bone marrow hypoproliferation, attributed to a decrease in erythropoietin production by the diseased kidney.

2. In some cases, the erythropoietin level is normal but the bone marrow does not respond. The unresponsiveness may be caused by the presence of a low molecular weight dialyzable inhibitor of erythropoiesis present in the serum of uremic patients. Improvement in hemoglobin levels is seen after dialysis.

3. In addition to hypoproliferation, decreased erythrocyte survival compounds the anemia. One factor responsible for the shortened survival is related to an unknown extra-corpuscular cause—perhaps an unfavorable metabolic environment or mechanical trauma. Another cause of hemolysis may be related to an acquired abnormality in erythrocyte metabolism that involves the pentose phosphate shunt. This abnormality causes impaired generation of NADPH and reduced glutathione.[27] Thus, when exposed to oxidants, the erythrocytes develop Heinz bodies, inducing acute hemolysis. Hemolysis may also be related to a reversible defect in erythrocyte membrane sodium-potassium ATPase.

4. The anemia may be related to blood loss from the gastrointestinal tract because of a decrease in platelets and/or platelet dysfunction. Blood is also lost during priming for dialysis. Patients receiving dialysis lose about 5–6 mg of iron daily. Thus, an anemia associated with iron deficiency is common (∞ Chapter 11).

5. Patients on dialysis may become folate-deficient because folate is dialyzable. Without folate supplements the patient may develop a megaloblastic anemia.

Laboratory Findings

A normocytic and normochromic anemia is typical in renal disease except when the patient is deficient in folate or iron;

⊙ **TABLE 15-5**

Possible Causes of Anemia in Chronic Renal Disease

1. Decreased erythropoietin production
2. Presence of a dialyzable inhibitor of erythropoiesis
3. Decreased erythrocyte survival
4. Blood loss
5. Iron deficiency
6. Folate deficiency

then a macrocytic anemia or microcytic anemia prevails. Moderate anisocytosis with some degree of microcytosis may be present. Hemoglobin levels are reduced to 5–8 g/dL, and the reticulocyte production index is approximately 1. There is moderate to severe poikilocytosis with burr cells and schistocytes. The number of burr cells correlates roughly with the severity of azotemia. Spherocytes are associated with hypersplenism. Nucleated erythrocytes are noted in the peripheral blood. Leukocytes and platelets are usually normal. The bone marrow reveals erythroid hypoproliferation, especially when compared to the degree of anemia.

Other laboratory findings vary depending upon the severity of renal impairment. Blood urea nitrogen is >30 mg/dL, and serum creatinine is increased. Electrolytes are abnormal. Hemostatic abnormalities may be present. Serum ferritin levels are higher than normal in chronic renal failure, even if iron deficiency is present. Therefore, it has been suggested that if the serum ferritin level is below 40 ng/mL, iron deficiency should be considered. Increased iron-binding capacity may be a useful predictor of iron deficiency in these cases.

Therapy

Therapy for chronic renal disease includes renal transplantation, hemodialysis, and continuous ambulatory peritoneal dialysis. All treatments tend to ameliorate the anemia, but hemodialysis exposes the patient to additional causes of anemia. These additional causes include blood loss, iron and folate deficiency, and hemolysis. Thus, iron and folic acid supplements are frequently given in conjunction with hemodialysis. Intermittent doses of EPO three times a week cause improvement in 1–2 weeks. In some cases a normal hemoglobin is achieved, and in all cases the patients remain transfusion-independent.

ENDOCRINE ABNORMALITIES

Endocrine deficiencies are associated with a decrease in erythropoietin. The resulting anemia is usually normocytic, normochromic with normal erythrocyte morphology. The bone marrow findings suggest erythroid hypoproliferation.

A slow developing normocytic, normochromic anemia is characteristic of hypothyroidism. Erythrocyte survival is normal and reticulocytosis is absent. The anemia is most likely a physiologic response to a decrease in tissue demands for oxygen. With hormone replacement therapy, the anemia slowly remits.

Hypopituitarism is associated with an anemia more severe than that of hypothyroidism, and the leukocyte count may be decreased. However, anemia is a minor component of the other manifestations of hypopituitarism. The pituitary has an effect on multiple endocrine glands, including the thyroid and adrenals. In males, a decrease in androgens may be partly responsible for the anemia, since androgens stimulate erythropoiesis. In addition, a decrease in the growth hormone may have a trophic effect on the bone marrow.

SUMMARY

The hypoproliferative anemias include a group of acquired and constitutional disorders in which there is a chronic marrow hypocellularity. If only the erythrocytes are affected, the term *pure red cell aplasia* is appropriate. More commonly, there is a hypocellularity affecting all cell lines, and the diagnosis is aplastic anemia.

The hypocellularity in aplastic anemia may be due to immune suppression, defective or deficient stem cells, or rarely, a defective bone marrow microenvironment. Acquired aplastic anemia may be idiopathic or secondary to drugs, chemical agents, ionizing radiation, or infectious agents. Constitutional aplastic anemia has a congenital disposition and may be associated with other anomalies. Fanconi's anemia is a form of constitutional anemia with progressive bone marrow hypoplasia and other congenital defects. The disorder is characterized by chromosomal instability. A subset of Fanconi's anemia is familial aplastic anemia. This form does not have congenital abnormalities.

The laboratory findings in aplastic anemia reveal pancytopenia. The erythrocytes are usually normocytic, normochromic but may be macrocytic. The reticulocyte count is low and the RPI is less than 2. The bone marrow is less than 25% cellular.

Pure red cell aplasia is characterized by a selective decrease in erythroid cells. This disorder may be acquired or congenital. The acquired forms are seen in thymoma, with administration of certain drugs, in autoimmune disorders, and in infection, especially viral infections. Diamond-Blackfan syndrome is a congenital progressive erythrocyte aplasia occurring in young children. This congenital form of aplasia must be differentiated from TEC, a temporary aplasia occurring after viral infection.

Other hypoproliferative anemias are due primarily to defective hormonal stimulation of erythroid stem cells. These include anemia associated with renal disease and with endocrinopathies. The laboratory findings reflect not only anemia but also pathologies of the primary disorder.

Immunosuppressive therapy using antithymocyte globulin, antilymphocyte globulin, or cyclosporine A is the treatment of choice for the majority of patients who are not candidates for stem cell transplants. Transplantation is potentially curative but not without risks. Transplantation still remains unavailable for many patients due to the inability to find matched donors.

REVIEW QUESTIONS

LEVEL I

1. What is the typical morphologic classification of erythrocytes in aplastic anemia? (Checklist #7)
   a. hypochromic, microcytic
   b. normochromic, normocytic
   c. normochromic, microcytic
   d. hypochromic, macrocytic

2. The bone marrow in aplastic anemia is typically: (Checklist #7)
   a. hypocellular
   b. hypercellular
   c. dysplastic
   d. normal

3. Which of the following is (are) considered a cause of hypoproliferation in aplastic anemia? (Checklist #2)
   1. damage to stem cells
   2. depletion of stem cells
   3. inhibition of stem cells
   a. 1 only
   b. 1 and 2 only
   c. 2 and 3 only
   d. 1, 2, and 3

4. What term best describes the peripheral blood findings of a person with aplastic anemia? (Checklist #7)
   a. pancytopenia
   b. bicytopenia
   c. granulocytopenia only
   d. anemia only

5. Diagnostic criteria for aplastic anemia include: (Checklist #3)
   a. corrected reticulocyte count of greater than 1%
   b. platelet count less than 100×10^9/L
   c. granulocyte count less than 0.5×10^9/L
   d. bone marrow less than 50% cellular

6. What percentage of cases of aplastic anemia occurs in persons less than 20 years of age? (Checklist #4)
   a. 0
   b. 10
   c. 25
   d. 50

7. Exposure to drugs, radiation, or infectious agents may result in which type of aplastic anemia? (Checklist #8)
   a. idiopathic
   b. congenital
   c. constitutional
   d. acquired

8. If a patient with anemia had a decrease in only the red cells in the bone marrow, this might be: (Checklist #9)
   a. pure red cell aplasia
   b. acquired aplastic anemia
   c. megaloblastic anemia
   d. constitutional aplastic anemia

LEVEL II

1. What confirmatory test should be performed in suspected cases of aplastic anemia? (Checklist #4)
   a. serum iron and TIBC
   b. hemoglobin electrophoresis
   c. bone marrow examination
   d. direct antiglobulin test

2. A 3-year-old patient presents with severe normocytic, normochromic anemia. Platelet counts and leukocyte counts are normal. The mother reported that the child has been healthy since birth but recently had a cold. Which of the following laboratory test results would support a diagosis of TEC? (Checklist #1, 5, 6)
   a. decreased numbers of erythrocyte precursors on bone marrow examination
   b. a normal hemoglobin F level on hemoglobin electrophoresis
   c. abnormal karyotype
   d. i antigen on the patient's erythrocytes

3. A bone marrow from an anemic patient that demonstrates a marked erythroid hypoplasia but normal numbers of other cell lines is most consistent with a diagnosis of: (Checklist #5)
   a. Fanconi's anemia
   b. aplastic anemia
   c. pure red cell aplasia
   d. myelophthisic anemia

4. A male patient with previously diagnosed infectious mononucleosis infection has become suddenly anemic. A possible cause of the anemia is: (Checklist #1)
   a. iron deficiency
   b. folic acid deficiency
   c. anemia of chronic disease
   d. aplastic anemia

5. What is the standard treatment for patients with aplastic anemia? (Checklist #3)
   a. immunosuppressive therapy
   b. bone marrow transplant
   c. administration of growth factors
   d. blood transfusion

6. The peripheral blood finding that helps differentiate aplastic anemia from myelophthisic anemia is: (Checklist #5)
   a. leukoerythroblastic reaction in aplastic anemia
   b. fetal-like erythrocytes in aplastic anemia
   c. poikilocytosis in myelophthisic anemia
   d. microcytic anemia in myelophthisic anemia

7. Which patient with aplastic anemia may have the best prognosis for recovery? (Checklist #2)
   a. one associated with parvovirus infection
   b. one with idiopathic aplastic anemia
   c. one who has severe bone marrow hypoplasia
   d. one who has severe pancytopenia

REVIEW QUESTIONS (continued)

LEVEL I

9. Which of the following is most characteristic of the peripheral blood picture in pure red cell aplasia? (Checklist #9)
   a. pancytopenia
   b. granulocytopenia and thrombocytopenia
   c. leukocytosis
   d. decreased hemoglobin and hematocrit

10. Peripheral blood findings in patients with chronic renal disease include: (Checklist #10)
   a. a mild anemia with hemoglobin levels around 10 g/dL
   b. poikilocytosis with burr cells and schistocytes
   c. normally shaped erythrocytes
   d. decreased leukocytes and platelets

LEVEL II

8. A bone marrow biopsy is performed on an infant with severe congenital abnormalities and severe anemia. Results of the biopsy demonstrate marked hypoplasia of all cell lines. These findings are most consistent with a diagnosis of: (Checklist #4)
   a. transient erythroblastopenia of childhood
   b. familial aplastic anemia
   c. Diamond-Blackfan anemia
   d. Fanconi's anemia

9. Clinical signs and symptoms of aplastic anemia include: (Checklist #4)
   a. hepatomegaly
   b. bleeding
   c. splenomegaly
   d. lymphadenopathy

10. A 75-year-old male was diagnosed with aplastic anemia. He has no known living blood relatives. What treatment would most likely be initiated? (Checklist #3)
   a. none
   b. bone marrow transplant
   c. immunosuppressive therapy
   d. chemotherapy

www.prenhall.com/mckenzie

Use the above address to access the free, interactive Companion Web site created for this textbook. Get hints, instant feedback, and textbook references to chapter-related multiple choice questions.

REFERENCES

1. Gale RP, Champlin RE, Feig SA, Fitchen JH. Aplastic anemia: Biology and treatment. *Ann Intern Med*. 1981; 95:477–94.

2. Issaragrisil S, Leaverton PE, Chansung K, Thamprasit T, Porapakham Y, Vannasaeng S, et al. Regional patterns in the incidence of aplastic anemia in Thailand. The Aplastic Anemia Study Group. *Am J Hematol*. 1999; 61:164–68.

3. Guinan EC. Clinical aspects of aplastic anemia. *Hematol Oncol Clin North Am*. 1997; 11:1025–44.

4. Young NS. Hematopoietic cell destruction by immune mechanisms in acquired aplastic anemia. *Semin Hematol*. 2000; 37:3–14.

5. Marsh JC. Results of immunosuppression in aplastic anaemia. *Acta Haematol*. 2000; 103:26–32.

6. Stewart FM. Hypoplastic/aplastic anemia: Role of bone marrow transplantation. *Med Clin North Am*. 1992; 76:683–97.

7. Marsh JC, Chang J, Testa NG, Hows JM, Dexter TM. The hematopoietic defect in aplastic anemia assessed by long-term marrow culture. *Blood*. 1990; 76:1748–57.

8. Marsh JC, Chang J, Testa NG, Hows JM, Dexter TM. In vitro assessment of marrow "stem cell" and stromal cell function in aplastic anaemia. *Br J Haematol*. 1991; 78:258–67.

9. Levere RD, Ibraham NG. The bone marrow as a metabolic organ. *Am J Med*. 1982; 73:615–16.

10. Kasten MJ. Clindamycin, metronidazole, and chloramphenicol. *Mayo Clin Proc*. 1999; 74:825–33.

11. Brown KE, Tisdale J, Barrett AJ, Dunbar CE, Young NS. Hepatitis-associated aplastic anemia. *N Engl J Med*. 1997; 336(15):1059–64.

12. Tisdale JF, Dunn DE, Maciejewski J. Cyclophosphamide and other new agents for the treatment of severe aplastic anemia. *Semin Hematol*. 2000; 37:102–9.

13. Baker RI, Manoharan A, de Luca E, Begley CG. Pure red cell aplasia of pregnancy: A distinct clinical entity. *Br J Haematol*. 1993; 85:619–22.

14. Socie G, Rosenfeld S, Frickhofen N, Gluckman E, Tichelli A. Late clonal diseases of treated aplastic anemia. *Semin Hematol*. 2000; 37:91–101.

15. Garcia-Higuera I, Kuang Y, D'Andrea AD. The molecular and cellular biology of Fanconi anemia. *Curr Opin Hematol*. 1999; 6:83–88.

16. Kupfer GM, Naf D, D'Andrea AD. Molecular biology of Fanconi anemia. *Hematol Oncol Clin North Am*. 1997; 11:1045–60.

KEY TERMS

Compensated hemolytic disease
Hemoglobinemia
Hemoglobinuria
Hemolysis
Hemosidinuria

BACKGROUND BASICS

The information in this chapter will build on the concepts learned in previous chapters. To maximize your learning experience you should review these concepts before starting this unit of study.

Level I

▶ Diagram the process of intravascular and extravascular hemolysis. (Chapter 4)

▶ Identify and define types of poikilocytes. (Chapter 10)

▶ Explain the morphologic and functional classification of anemia. (Chapter 10)

▶ Identify laboratory tests used to assess anemia. (Chapters 7, 10)

Level II

▶ Classify an anemia based on laboratory findings. (Chapter 10)

▶ Interpret results of laboratory tests and clinical findings based on type of hemolysis and functional defect. (Chapters 7, 10)

▶ Review the erythrocyte membrane structure. (Chapter 4)

CASE STUDY

We will address this case study throughout the chapter.

Ms. Nummi is a 58-year-old female. Her amylase and lipase values were markedly increased. Her hemoglobin was 15.5 g/dL. Two months later she had surgery for a pancreatic pseudocyst. She received 3 units of packed red blood cells. Three days after surgery her hemoglobin was 5.2 g/dL, RBC 1.5×10^{12}/L, hematocrit 0.148 L/L. The physician is concerned about the possibility of internal bleeding. Consider what other laboratory tests may be helpful in defining the source of blood loss in this patient.

▶ OVERVIEW

The laboratory plays an important role in differentiating the etiology of hemolytic disease. This chapter serves as an introduction to the next three chapters on hemolytic anemia. It describes the classification schemes of hemolytic disease and gives the general laboratory and clinical findings found in this group of anemias. The use of laboratory tests in differentiating the intravascular or extravascular sites of ery-throcyte destruction and defining the source of defect intrinsic or extrinsic to the red cell is discussed.

▶ INTRODUCTION

The hemolytic anemias are a heterogeneous group of normocytic, normochromic anemias in which the erythrocyte is prematurely destroyed. This premature destruction is referred to as **hemolysis**. Hemolytic anemia may be classified according to the source of the defect causing the hemolysis (intrinsic or extrinsic to the erythrocyte), mode of onset (inherited or acquired), or location of hemolysis (intravascular or extravascular) (Table 16-1 ✪). Intrinsic abnormalities are generally genetically determined, while extrinsic abnormalities are acquired. Depending on the type and extent of injury, hemolysis may be intravascular or extravascular.

These anemias can also be classified by type of poikilocyte present on the blood smear: schistocytes or spherocytes (Figure 16-1 ■). Schistocytes are an indication of mechanical trauma to the erythrocyte and are characterized by intravascular hemolysis. Spherocytes are an indication that part of the cell's membrane has been removed by phagocytes. Membrane can be removed due to antigen/antibody complexes on the membrane, a defective membrane, or abnormal inclusions in the cell. Spherocytes are hemolyzed extravascularly.

The ultimate aim of any classification is to help identify the etiology of the anemia so that the appropriate treatment can be given and prognosis determined. Laboratory tests are a very important part of this process.

Reticulocytosis is a constant feature of all hemolytic anemias reflecting the increased activity of the bone marrow as it attempts to maintain erythrocyte mass in the peripheral blood. If the bone marrow is able to increase erythropoiesis enough to compensate for the decreased erythrocyte life span, anemia does not develop. In this case, cells are being produced at the same or nearly the same rate as they are hemolyzed. This condition is called **compensated hemolytic disease**. Compensated hemolytic disease may rapidly develop into anemia if one of the following occurs: (1) erythrocyte destruction accelerates beyond the compensatory capacity of the marrow (hemolytic crises); or (2) the marrow suddenly stops producing erythrocytes (aplastic anemia). Normal bone marrow can increase its production rate sixfold to eightfold if suf-

✪ TABLE 16-1

Possible Classifications of Hemolytic Anemia Based on Pathophysiology, Etiology, and/or Laboratory Findings

Source of Defect	Mode of Onset	Site of Hemolysis	Predominant Poikilocyte
Intrinsic to red cell	inherited	intravascular	spherocyte
Extrinsic to red cell	acquired	extravascular or intravascular	schistocyte/ spherocyte

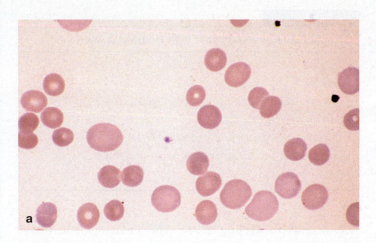

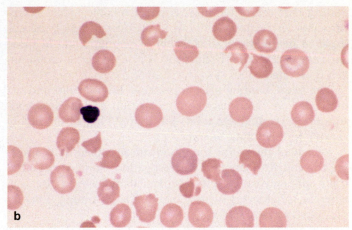

■ **FIGURE 16-1 a.** Peripheral blood smear from a patient with autoimmune hemolytic anemia. There is marked anisocytosis with numerous spherocytes and large polychromatophilic erythrocytes. **b.** Peripheral blood smear from a patient with thrombotic, thrombocytopenic purpura, a microangiopathic hemolytic anemia. There are many schistocytes present. There are also spherocytes present, but the predominant poikilocyte is the schistocyte (both: 1000× magnification; Wright-Giemsa stain).

ficient iron is mobilized. Thus, the erythrocyte life span can drop to one-eighth of normal, or about 15–18 days, without anemia developing. If the life span decreases to less than 15 days, anemia develops.

► LABORATORY FINDINGS

Hematologic characteristics of hemolytic anemia reflect the increased activity of the bone marrow and the increased erythrocyte destruction (Table 16-2 ✪). Erythroid hyperplasia of the bone marrow with decreased amounts of fat is more pronounced than in any of the nonhemolytic anemias. Consequently, the myeloid-to-erythroid ratio (M:E) is decreased. Increased plasma iron turnover reflects the increased erythrocyte destruction and increased utilization of iron by erythroid precursors in the bone marrow.

Peripheral blood reticulocytosis, increased immature reticulocyte fraction (IRF), marked polychromasia, and nucleated erythrocytes in the peripheral blood are clues to the presence of increased erythropoietic activity in the bone marrow. The hemolytic anemias are the only anemias with a reticulocyte production index (RPI) greater than 2 (except in acute hemorrhage). Thus, the RPI is useful in differentiating hemolytic anemias from other normocytic, normochromic anemias in which the bone marrow is not increasing effective erythropoiesis. Occasionally, the degree of reticulocytosis is great enough to cause an increased MCV. (Reticulocytes are larger than mature erythrocytes.)

Results of laboratory tests that are used to evaluate heme catabolism are usually abnormal. Unconjugated/indirect bilirubin is often increased, but the conjugated/direct fraction is usually normal unless hepatic or biliary dysfunction is present. However, a significant number of patients with hemolytic disease have normal serum bilirubin levels, sug-

✪ TABLE 16-2

Common Laboratory Findings Reflecting Increased Production and Destruction of Erythrocytes in Hemolytic Anemias

Increased Bone Marrow Production of Erythrocytes	Increased Erythrocyte Destruction
Reticulocytosis (RPI >2)	Anemia
Increased IRF	Presence of spherocytes, schistocytes, and/or other poikilocytes
Leukocytosis	
Nucleated erythrocytes in the peripheral blood	Positive AHG test
	Decreased haptoglobin and hemopexin
Polychromasia of erythrocytes on Romanowsky stained blood smears	Decreased glycosylated hemoglobin
	Increased fecal and urine urobilinogen
Normoblastic erythroid hyperplasia in the bone marrow	Increased bilirubin (unconjugated)
	Hemoglobinemia*
	Hemoglobinuria*
	Hemosidinuria*
	Methemoglobinemia*
	Increased serum LD
	Increased expired CO

*Associated only with intravascular hemolysis; AHG = antihuman globulin; IRF = immature reticulocyte fraction; LD = lactic dehydrogenase; RPI = reticulocyte production index; CO = carbon monoxide

gesting that serum bilirubin is not a reliable index of erythrocyte destruction. Bilirubin levels over 5 mg/dL are unusual in hemolytic disease except in neonates and in those with coexisting liver dysfunction. Urine and fecal urobilinogen is elevated.

The heme binding plasma proteins, haptoglobin and hemopexin, are often decreased as a result of increased consumption. Haptoglobin levels less than 25 mg/dL are highly specific for hemolytic anemia.

Review of the peripheral blood smear is helpful in directing the course of laboratory investigation. Poikilocytes other than spherocytes suggest mechanical damage to the cell, whereas spherocytes suggest membrane grooming (loss) by phagocytes in the spleen.

⊘ TABLE 16-3

Clinical Findings Associated with Hemolytic Anemia

- Jaundice
- Gallstones
- Dark or red urine
- Symptoms of anemia
- Thinning of cortical bone (in chronic hemolytic anemia)
- Extramedullary hematopoietic masses (in chronic hemolytic anemia)
- Splenomegaly

Ⓒ CASE STUDY *(continued from page 304)*

Ms. Nummi's reticulocyte count is 19%, total serum bilirubin 9.8 mg/dL, and haptoglobin <13mg/dL. The peripheral blood smear revealed many spherocytes.

1. What type of anemia is suggested by the laboratory results and clinical history?

 Checkpoint! #1

A patient is suspected of having a hemolytic disease. The reticulocyte count is increased, but the hemoglobin, serum bilirubin, and haptoglobin are within the normal range. Explain.

▶ CLINICAL FINDINGS

Clinical signs of hemolytic anemia are associated with increases in both heme catabolism (erythrocyte destruction) and erythropoiesis (Table 16-3 ⊘). Jaundice is a reflection of an increase in bilirubin production. Gallstones consisting primarily of bilirubin are common in congenital and other chronic hemolytic anemias. Dark or red urine due to excretion of plasma hemoglobin may be noted in intravascular hemolysis.

Chronic severe hemolytic anemias stimulate the expansion of bone marrow, consequently thinning cortical bone and widening spaces between inner and outer tables of bone. In children, this expansion is evident in skeletal abnormalities. These bone changes may result in spontaneous fractures and a type of arthritis termed *osteoarthropathy*.[1] Extramedullary hematopoietic masses may be found. Some of these masses are believed to represent extrusions of the marrow cavity through thinned bone cortex. Small colonies of erythrocytes also may be found in the spleen, liver, lymph nodes, and perinephric tissue. The hematopoietic tumor masses may cause pressure symptoms on adjacent organs.[1] In extravascular hemolysis, splenic hypertrophy is a constant finding.

Other clinical findings and the primary symptoms are those associated with anemia, including pallor, fatigue, and cardiac symptoms.

▶ SITES OF DESTRUCTION

Hemolysis may occur within the circulation (intravascular) or within the macrophages of the spleen, liver, or bone marrow (extravascular). In some cases, depending on the degree of damage to the cell, destruction may occur both intravascularly and extravascularly. The results of laboratory tests may provide important clues to the hemolytic process.[2] To correlate laboratory results with the etiology and pathophysiology of the anemia, an understanding of intravascular and extravascular hemolysis is essential (∞ Chapter 4).

INTRAVASCULAR HEMOLYSIS

In intravascular hemolysis the erythrocyte is destroyed within the blood vessels. When the erythrocyte is hemolyzed, free hemoglobin is released into the plasma. The hemoglobin is bound to the plasma protein haptoglobin; transported as a complex to the liver, where it is metabolized to bilirubin; and excreted to the intestinal tract via the bile duct. Normally the concentration of hemoglobin in plasma is less than 5 mg/dL. In severe intravascular hemolysis, synthesis of haptoglobin may not be sufficient to replace that being used, and free hemoglobin accumulates in the plasma. It should be remembered, however, that haptoglobin is an acute phase reactant and may be normal or even increased in individuals with concomitant infections, inflammation, or malignant disease despite an increase in intravascular hemolysis. Levels also may be decreased in liver disease due to decreased synthesis of the protein and in hereditary deficiency of haptoglobin. Although haptoglobin functions as an intravascular heme-binding protein, it also may be decreased in association with extravascular hemolytic diseases. Thus, by itself, the haptoglobin level cannot be used to differentiate intravascular and extravascular hemolysis.

Another plasma protein, hemopexin, complexes with heme when haptoglobin is depleted. This complex may also be cleared from the plasma by the liver faster than it can be synthesized and is quickly depleted. A decrease in hemopexin is secondary to a reduction in haptoglobin.

Hemoglobin bound to haptoglobin or hemopexin forms complexes that are too large to pass through the glomerulus of the kidney. When these two transport proteins are depleted, free hemoglobin circulates in the plasma (**hemoglobinemia**). Some of this hemoglobin is removed directly by the liver, but some dissociates into dimers small enough to be filtered by the glomerulus. Filtered hemoglobin may be reabsorbed in the proximal renal tubules, but when the rate of filtration exceeds the tubular reabsorption capabilities, free hemoglobin appears in the urine (**hemoglobinuria**). The presence of free hemoglobin in the urine is a sign of rapid and severe intravascular hemolysis.[3] Depending on the degree of hemolysis, the urine may be pink, red, or brownish black.

Some renal tubular cells may become laden with hemoglobin iron. When these tubular cells are sloughed off into the urine, hemosiderin granules may be visualized by staining the urine sediment with an iron stain and examining it microscopically. Hemosiderin in the urine (**hemosidinuria**) is a sign that the kidney has filtered a significant amount of hemoglobin.[3] In chronic intravascular hemolysis, hemosiderin granules may appear in the urine even in the absence of hemoglobinuria.

Free hemoglobin not bound to either of the two transport proteins or not excreted by the kidney is quickly oxidized to methemoglobin. Methemoglobin dissociates into hemin (oxidized form of heme) and globin. Hemin may bind to hemopexin if it is available or to albumin, forming methemalbumin. Methemalbumin is not excreted in the urine but can be detected in the plasma by Schumm's test.

Laboratory findings of intravascular hemolysis include hemoglobinemia, hemoglobinuria, hemosidinuria, methemoglobinemia, decreased haptoglobin, and decreased hemopexin. In addition, the serum lactic dehydrogenase (LD) may increase to as much as 800 IU/L (upper normal 207 IU/L). Lactic dehydrogenase, an exzyme present in high concentration in erythrocytes, is released from the erythrocyte into the plasma in intravascular hemolysis, and it is cleared from plasma even more slowly than hemoglobin.

Erythrocytes must be severely damaged to undergo intravascular destruction. Phagocytes in the spleen or liver remove minimally or moderately damaged erythrocytes. Intravascular hemolysis may be caused by: (1) activation of complement on the erythrocyte membrane, (2) physical or mechanical trauma to the erythrocyte, or (3) the presence of soluble toxic substances in the erythrocyte's environment (Table 16-4 ✪).

EXTRAVASCULAR HEMOLYSIS

If premature erythrocyte destruction is the result of extravascular hemolysis, the erythrocytes are removed from circulation by phagocytes in the tissues. This type of hemolysis is more common than intravascular hemolysis. There is no hemoglobinemia, hemoglobinuria, or hemosidinuria as hemoglobin is not released directly into the plasma. Instead, the hemoglobin is degraded within the phagocyte to heme and globin. The heme is further catabolized to iron, biliverdin, and carbon monoxide. The biliverdin then enters the plasma as bilirubin, binds to albumin, and is excreted by the liver.

Significant laboratory findings in hemolytic anemias associated with extravascular hemolysis are measurements of the products of heme catabolism. These findings include an increase in expired carbon monoxide, an increase in carboxyhemoglobin, an increase in serum bilirubin (especially in the unconjugated fraction), and an increase in both urine and fecal urobilinogen. In severe or chronic extravascular hemolysis, haptoglobin and hemopexin levels may also be decreased.

Extravascular hemolysis may occur in phagocytes of the spleen, liver, or bone marrow. The type and degree of erythrocyte damage determines the primary site of erythrocyte

---

✪ TABLE 16-4

Anemias Characterized by Intravascular Hemolysis

Activation of Complement on the Erythrocyte Membrane	Physical or Mechanical Trauma to the Erythrocyte	Toxic Microenvironment of the Erythrocyte
Paroxysmal nocturnal hemoglobinuria	Microangiopathic hemolytic anemia	Bacterial infections
Paroxysmal cold hemoglobinuria	Abnormalities of the heart and great vessels	*Plasmodium falciparum* infection
Some transfusion reactions	Disseminated intravascular coagulation	Venoms
Some autoimmune hemolytic anemias		Arsine poisoning
		Acute drug reaction in G6PD deficiency
		Intravenous administration of distilled water

REVIEW QUESTIONS (continued)

LEVEL I

LEVEL II

10. The function of C8 binding protein (C8bp) is to: (Checklist #3)
    a. induce erythrocyte aggregation
    b. interfere with the end stages of complement activation
    c. prevent production of an autoantibody
    d. all of the above

www.prenhall.com/mckenzie

Use the above address to access the free, interactive Companion Web site created for this textbook. Get hints, instant feedback, and textbook references to chapter-related multiple choice questions.

REFERENCES

1. Palek J, Jarolim P. Clinical expression and laboratory detection of red blood cell membrane protein mutations. *Sem Hematol.* 1993; 30:249–83.

2. Palek J. The red cell skeleton and haemolytic anaemias. *Br J Haematol.* 1992; 82:260–64.

3. Hassoun H, Vassiliadis JN, Murray J, et al. Characterization of the underlying molecular defect in hereditary spherocytosis associated with spectrin deficiency. *Blood.* 1997; 90:398–406.

4. Lanciotti M, Perutelli P, Valetto A, DiMartino D, Mori PG. Ankyrin deficiency is the most common defect in dominant and nondominant hereditary spherocytosis. *Haematologica.* 1997; 82:460–62.

5. Miraglia del Giudice E, Lombardi C, Francese M, et al. Frequent de novo monoallelic expression of beta-spectrin gene (SPTB) in children with hereditary spherocytosis and isolated spectrin deficiency. *Br J Haematol.* 1998; 101:251–54.

6. Basseres DS, Vincentim DL, Costa FF, Saad STO, Hassoun H. Beta-spectrin Promiss-ao: A translation initiation codon mutation of the beta-spectrin gene (ATG→GTG) associated with hereditary spherocytosis and spectrin deficiency in a Brazilian family. *Blood.* 1998; 91:368–69.

7. Jarolim P, Murray JL, Rubin HL, et al. Characterization of 13 novel band 3 gene defects in hereditary spherocytosis with band 3 deficiency. *Blood.* 1996; 88:4366–74.

8. DeFranceschi L, Olivieri O, Miraglia del Giudice E, et al. Membrane cation and anion transport activities in erythrocytes of hereditary spherocytosis: Effects of different membrane protein defects. *Am J Hematol.* 1997; 55:121–28.

9. Gilsanz F, Ricard MP, Millan I. Diagnosis of hereditary spherocytosis with dual-angle differential light scattering. *Am J Clin Pathol.* 1993; 100:119–22.

10. Gallagher P, Jarolim P. Red cell membrane disorders. In: Hoffman R, Benz EJ, Shattil SJ, Furie B, Cohen HJ, Silberstein LE, McGlave P, editors. *Hematology: Basic Principles and Practice.* 3rd ed. New York: Churchill Livingstone; 2000:576–610.

11. Bossi D, Russo M. Hemolytic anemias due to disorders of red cell membrane skeleton. *Mol Aspects Med.* 1996; 17:171–88.

12. Tse W, Lux S. Red blood cell membrane disorders. *Br J Haematol.* 1999; 104:2–13.

13. McMullin MF. The molecular basis of disorders of the red cell membrane. *J Clin Pathol.* 1999; 52:245–48.

14. Gallagher PG, Ferriera J. Molecular basis of erythrocyte membrane disorders. *Curr Opin Hematol.* 1997; 4:128–35.

15. Wang DN. Band 3 protein: Structure, flexibility, and function. *FEBS Lett.* 1994; 346:26–31.

16. Conboy JG. Structure, function, and molecular genetics of erythroid membrane skeletal protein 4.1 in normal and abnormal red blood cells. *Sem Hematol.* 1993; 30:58–73.

17. O'Donnell A, Allen SJ, Mgone CS, et al. Red cell morphology and malaria anaemia in children with Southeast-Asian ovalocytosis band 3 in Papua New Guinea. *Br J Haematol.* 1998; 101:407–12.

18. Silveira P, Cynober T, Dhermy D, Mohandas N, Tchernia G. Red blood cell abnormalities in hereditary elliptocytosis and their relevance to variable clinical expression. *Am J Clin Pathol.* 1997; 108:391–99.

19. DePalma L, Lubon NLC. Hereditary pyropoikilocytosis. *Am J Dis Child.* 1993; 147:93–95.

20. Kanzaki A, Kawata Y. Hereditary stomatocytosis: Phenotypical expressions of sodium transport and band 7 peptides in 44 cases. *Br J Haematol.* 1992; 82:133–41.

21. Cooper RA. Anemia with spur cells: A red cell defect acquired in serum and modified in the circulation. *J. Clin. Invest.* 1969; 48: 1820–31.

22. Doll DC, Doll NJ. Spur cell anemia. *South Med. J.* 1982; 75: 1205–10.

23. Rader DJ, Brewer HB. Abetalipoproteinemia. New insights into lipoprotein assembly and vitamin E metabolism from a rare genetic disease. *JAMA.* 1993; 270:865–69.

24. Gregg RE, Wetterau JR. The molecular basis of abetlipoproteinemia. *Curr. Opin. Lipidol.* 1994; 5:81–86.

25. Jarolim P. Sequencing of antigens of the Diego blood group system helps to characterize ectoplasmic loops of erythroid band 3 protein. *Br J Haematol.* 1998; 102:12.

26. Nicholson-Weller A, March JP, Rosenfeld SI, Austen KF. Affected erythrocytes of patients with paroxysmal nocturnal hemoglobin-

uria are deficient in the complement regulatory protein, decay-accelerating factor. *Proc Natl Acad Sci USA*. 1983; 80:5066–77.

27. Zalman LS, Wood LM, Frank MM, Muller-Eberhard HJ. Deficiency of the homologous restriction factor in paroxysmal nocturnal hemoglobinuria. *J Exp Med*. 1987; 165:572–77.

28. Taguchi R, Funahashi Y, Ikezawa H, et al. Analysis of PI (phosphatidylinositol)-anchoring antigens in a patient of paroxysmal nocturnal hemoglobinuria (PNH) reveals deficiency of 1F5 antigen (CD59), a new complement-regulatory factor. *FEBS Lett*. 1990; 261:142–46.

29. Yeh ET, Rosse WF. Paroxysmal nocturnal hemoglobinuria and the glycosylphosphatidylinositol anchor. *J Clin Invest*. 1994; 93: 2305–10.

30. Rotoli B, Bessler M, Alfinito F, del Vecchiu L. Membrane proteins in paroxysmal nocturnal haemoglobinuria. *Blood Reviews*. 1993; 7:75–86.

31. Schubert J, Ostendorf T, Schmidt RE. Biology of GPI anchors and pathogenesis of paroxysmal nocturnal hemoglobinuria. *Immunol Today*. 1994; 15:299–301.

32. Luzzatto L. Somatic mutation in paroxysmal nocturnal hemoglobinuria. *Hosp Pract* (Off Ed). 1997; 32:125–31, 135–36, 139–40.

33. Okuda K, Kanamaru A, Ueda E, Kitani T, Nagai K. Membrane expression of decay-accelerating factor on neutrophils from normal individuals and patients with paroxysmal nocturnal hemoglobinuria. *Blood*. 1990; 75:1186–91.

34. Graham DL, Gastineau DA. Paroxysmal nocturnal hemoglobinuria as a marker for clonal myelopathy. *Am J Med*. 1992; 93:671–74.

35. Rosse WF. Paroxysmal nocturnal hemoglobinuria. In: Hoffman R, Benz EJ, Shattil SJ, Furie B, Cohen HJ, Silberstein LE, McGlave P, editors. *Hematology: Basic Principles and Practice*. 3rd ed. New York: Churchill Livingstone; 2000:331–42.

36. Brodsky RA, Mukhina GL, Li S, et al. Improved detection and characterization of paroxysmal nocturnal hemoglobinuria using fluorescent aerolysin. *AJCP*. 2000; 114(3):459–66.

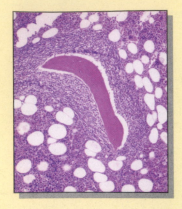

18

Hemolytic Anemia: Enzyme Deficiencies

Dan Bessmer, M.S.

■ CHECKLIST - LEVEL I

At the end of this unit of study the student should be able to:

1. Identify the two main pathways by which erythrocytes catabolize glucose.
2. Explain the role of enzymes in maintaining erythrocyte integrity and describe how deficiencies in these enzymes lead to anemia.
3. Identify the most common erythrocyte enzyme deficiency.
4. Describe the inheritance pattern for glucose-6-phosphate dehydrogenase (G6PD).
5. Explain how the diagnosis of G6PD deficiency is made.
6. List and describe the tests used to detect G6PD deficiency.
7. Recognize the erythrocyte morphology in a Romanowsky-stained blood smear associated with G6PD deficiency.
8. Identify common compounds that induce anemia in G6PD deficiency.

■ CHECKLIST - LEVEL II

At the end of this unit of study the student should be able to:

1. Recommend appropriate laboratory testing and interpret results for suspected G6PD deficiency following a hemolytic episode.
2. Explain the function of glutathione in maintaining cellular integrity.
3. Associate the mechanisms of hemolysis with defects in the Embden-Meyerhof and hexose-monophosphate shunt pathways.
4. Correlate clinical and laboratory findings with the common G6PD isoenzyme variants.
5. Diagram the reaction catalyzed by pyruvate kinase and explain how a defect of this enzyme can cause hemolysis.
6. Recognize erythrocyte morphology associated with pyruvate kinase deficiency.
7. Review and interpret laboratory findings in a case study presentation of G6PD deficiency.
8. Explain the mechanism of basophilic stippling formation in erythrocytes in the presence of increased lead levels.

KEY TERMS

Chronic nonspherocytic hemolytic anemia
Favism
Hypoxia
Lyonization

BACKGROUND BASICS

The information in this chapter will build on concepts learned in previous chapters. To maximize your learning experience, you should review the following concepts from previous chapters.

Level I and Level II

▶ Describe the normal erythrocyte metabolic processes. (Chapter 4)

▶ Recognize RBC morphology as it relates to hemolytic disease processes. (Chapter 16)

▶ Understand basic enzymology and techniques to measure enzyme activity. (from previous classes)

CASE STUDY

We will address this case study throughout the chapter. The patient, Henry, was a 25-year-old African American male soldier who was in the process of being deployed to West Africa for a 3-month temporary duty. Because of the high prevalence of malaria in the area, he was started on antimalarial prophylaxis (primaquine) 3 days prior to leaving to join his command. Twenty-four hours after starting the medication, he developed fever, chills, and general malaise. He subsequently reported to the emergency department and was admitted to the hospital for observation and additional testing.

Physical exam revealed a normal appearing well-nourished adult male, in no acute distress. His family history was noncontributory, and he had no known drug allergies.

Laboratory analysis yielded the following.

CBC

White blood cells:	12×10^9/L
Hemoglobin:	9.1 g/dL
Hematocrit:	27%
MCV:	90 fL
Platelet Count:	423×10^9/L
Total Bilirubin:	5.0 mg/dL
Direct:	0.2 mg/dL
Indirect:	4.8 mg/dL
Haptoglobin:	39 mg/dL

Based on the clinical history and these laboratory results, consider what may have precipitated this patient's condition.

▶ OVERVIEW

Intrinsic defects in the erythrocyte membrane, hemoglobin, or enzymes may lead to hemolysis. This chapter discusses defects of enzymes within the erythrocyte that lead to hemolytic anemia. The most common enzyme deficiencies are those associated with the hexose monophosphate shunt and the Embden-Meyerhof pathway. Thus, the chapter begins with a description of the role of these two pathways in erythrocyte metabolism and a general overview of the clinical and laboratory findings in enzyme deficiencies associated with the pathways. The two most common enzyme deficiencies, glucose-6-phosphate dehydrogenase and pyruvate kinase, are discussed in detail in the format of pathophysiology, clinical and laboratory findings, and therapy.

▶ INTRODUCTION

The erythrocyte life span can be shortened significantly if the cell is intrinsically abnormal. Although the enzymes in the erythrocyte are limited, those that are involved in processes that protect the cell from oxidant damage and provide the cell with energy through glycolysis are absolutely essential for cell survival. As reticulocytes mature, they lose their nucleus, mitochondria, and microsomes. Consequently, they also lose their ability to synthesize protein and undergo oxidative phosphorylation for ATP production. Thus, the mature erythrocyte is entirely dependent on anaerobic glucose metabolism for its energy needs. All erythrocyte enzymes are present in a fixed concentration and must remain active for the entire life span of the erythrocyte. An inherited deficiency in one of these enzymes may compromise the integrity of the cell membrane or hemoglobin and cause hemolysis. The more common hereditary enzyme deficiencies known to cause a hemolytic anemia are listed in Table 18-1 ⚙. Most are associated with the two erythrocyte metabolic pathways: hexose monophosphate (HMP) shunt and the Embden-Meyerhof (EM) pathway. To understand how defects in these two pathways can result in hemolysis, the pathways will be reviewed next. (For a more thorough discussion of each, review ∞ Chapter 5.)

HEXOSE MONOPHOSPHATE SHUNT

Glucose, the cell's primary metabolic substrate, enters the cell in a carrier-mediated, energy-free transport process and is catabolized via the EM pathway or the HMP shunt. Approximately 10% of the glucose is catabolized by the HMP shunt, which is essential for maintaining adequate concentrations of reduced glutathione (GSH). GSH levels are maintained by conversion of NADP to NADPH, a step catalyzed by glucose-6-phosphate dehydrogenase (G6PD) (Figure 18-1 ■). GSH protects the erythrocyte from oxidant damage; it maintains hemoglobin in the reduced functional state and preserves

⊕ TABLE 18-1

Eythrocyte Enzyme Deficiencies Associated with Congenital (Chronic) Nonspherocytic Hemolytic Anemia

Metabolic Pathway	Enzyme Deficiency
Embden-Meyerhof	Pyruvate kinase (PK)
	Glucose phosphate isomerase (GPI)
	Hexokinase (HK)
	Phosphoglyceratekinase (PGK)
	Triosephosphate isomerase (TPI)
Hexose-monophosphate	Glucose-6-phosphate dehydrogenase (G6PD)
	Glutathione synthetase
	Glutamylcysteine synthetase
Nucleotide	Pyrimidine 5′-nucleotidase (P5N)

vital cellular enzymes from oxidant damage. When the cell is exposed to an oxidizing agent, the production of NADPH increases. If enzymes in the HMP shunt are deficient, the reducing power of the cell is compromised, and oxidized hemoglobin accumulates, subsequently denaturing in the form of Heinz bodies. Heinz bodies aggregate at the cell membrane causing membrane damage. As the cells pass through the spleen, the macrophages attempt to remove the Heinz bodies. This leads to premature extravascular hemolysis. The most common enzyme deficiency of the HMP shunt is G6PD deficiency.

EMBDEN-MEYERHOF PATHWAY

Most of the energy of the cell is produced via glycolysis in the EM pathway. About 90% of the glucose is utilized by this pathway as one mole of glucose is catabolized to lactic acid with a net production of two moles of ATP. ATP is needed for active cation transport of Na^+, K^+, and Ca^{++}, for maintaining membrane deformability (ability of the membrane to

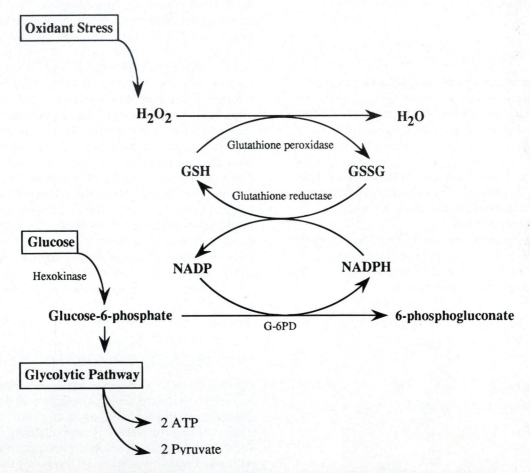

■ **FIGURE 18-1** G6PD is needed for maintaining adequate quantities of gultathione (GSH), an important buffer to oxidants within the erythrocyte. As GSH reduces H_2O_2 to H_2O, it is oxidized (GSSG). G6PD generates NADPH in the conversion of glucose-6-phosphate to 6-phosphogluconate. NADPH, in turn, serves to regenerate reduced glutathione from oxidized glutathione.

temporarily change shape in response to multiple forces in the cell's environment), and for maintaining normal erythrocyte biconcave disc shape in the resting or steady state. The ability of the erythrocyte to deform is an important determinant of its survival. Deficiencies in enzymes of the EM pathway decrease ATP production and lead to hemolysis. Heinz bodies are not formed since the reducing power of the cell is primarily linked to the HMP shunt. The mechanism of hemolysis is related to decreased ATP leading to impaired cation pumping. Membrane integrity is compromised and increased osmotic fragility results. The osmotically fragile cells are trapped in the hostile splenic environment and phagocytosed.

The Rapaport-Luebering shunt of the EM pathway provides the erythrocyte with 2,3-DPG. If this shunt is used, there is no net gain of ATP from glycolysis. The activity of this shunt is stimulated during **hypoxia.** (Hypoxia is a state of decreased oxygen tension and delivery to tissues. This is sometimes evidenced by a blue appearance of normally pink tissues, such as the fingernail beds.) When 2,3-DPG combines with hemoglobin, the oxygen affinity of hemoglobin is decreased, making more oxygen available to the tissues.

CLINICAL AND LABORATORY FINDINGS IN ERYTHROCYTE ENZYME DEFICIENCIES

Most erythrocyte enzyme deficiencies are inherited as autosomal recessive traits. However, the most common enzyme deficiency, G6PD deficiency, is inherited as an X-linked (sexlinked) disorder. Patients with the homozygous autosomal recessive enzyme deficiencies and males with X-linked G6PD deficiency have a chronic normocytic, normochromic anemia (sometimes no anemia is present or hemolysis is sporadic), reticulocytosis, hyperbilirubinemia, and neonatal jaundice. The direct antiglobulin test is negative, indicating an absence of autoantibodies, and there is no evidence to suggest a defect in either the erythrocyte membrane or hemoglobin. These anemias associated with inherited defects of erythrocyte metabolism are often collectively referred to as **chronic (or congenited) nonspherocytic hemolytic anemias.** Although the anemias are not life threatening, they can be disabling and lead to debilitating complications.[1]

DIAGNOSIS

Definitive diagnosis of enzyme deficiencies requires spectrophotometric measurement of the suspected deficient enzyme. The time of testing and interpretation of results is important to accurate diagnosis. Sometimes the abnormal cells are selectively removed from circulation in vivo, and the enzyme activity of the remaining cells is normal. Some abnormal enzymes have normal activity in the reticulocytes, but

enzyme activity decreases as the cell ages. Thus, depe.. upon the degree of reticulocytosis, the enzyme content may appear normal. For these reasons, it is important to delay testing of the patient immediately after a hemolytic attack when most of the enzyme deficient cells have been hemolyzed and there is a reticulocytosis. Sometimes it may be helpful to centrifuge the blood and test the erythrocytes at the bottom of the column. These cells are usually the older erthrocytes. If a patient has been transfused, testing should be delayed until the transfused cells have outlived their life span.[1]

> ✓ **Checkpoint! #1**
>
> *Transfusion of red blood cells in a patient with chronic nonspherocytic, hemolytic anemia due to an erythrocyte enzyme deficiency does not reverse or prevent the recipient's condition. If tests are performed to quantitate the enzyme after a transfusion, the results may be within the normal reference range. Explain.*

▶ GLUCOSE-6-PHOSPHATE DEHYDROGENASE DEFICIENCY

G6PD deficiency is the most common erythrocyte enzyme disorder. It was first recognized during the Korean War when 10% of African-American soldiers who were given the antimalarial drug primaquine developed a self-limited hemolytic anemia. G6PD deficiency is found worldwide in whites, blacks, and Asians. It occurs most frequently in the Mediterranean area, Africa, and China. The geographic distribution coincides with that of malaria, suggesting that G6PD deficient cells may be more resistant to malarial parasites than normal cells.

The disease is a sex-linked disorder carried by a gene on the X chromosome and therefore fully expressed only in males. However, it is not exclusively a male disorder. Heterozygote females appear to have two populations of cells, one deficient in G6PD and one normal. This occurs because of **lyonization** of an X chromosome (random inactivation of one set of X-linked genes in each cell). The degree to which females are affected depends upon the relative amount of deficient cells present. Web Figure 18-1 ■ illustrates the expected progeny from G6PD deficient males or females.

The disease is heterogenous with differences in severity among races and sexes. The majority of people with G6PD deficiency have no clinical expression of the deficiency unless they have neonatal jaundice, are exposed to chemicals or drug oxidants, or have severe infection. Compounds that have been associated with hemolytic anemia in G6PD deficiency are listed in Table 18-2 .

✪ TABLE 18-2

Compounds Associated with Hemolysis in G6PD Deficiency

Antimalarials	primaquine
	pamaquine
	pentaquine
	quinacrine (Atabrine)
Sulfonamides	sulfanilamide
	sulfacetamide
	sulfapyridine
	sulfamethoxazole (Gantonol)
	sulfasalazine (Azulfidine)
Sulfones	thiazosulfone
	diaphenylsulfone (DDS, Dapsone)
	sulfoxone (Diasone)
Nitrofurans	nitrofurantoin (Furadantin)
Analgesics	acetanilid
Miscellaneous	methylene blue
	naxidlic acid
	naphthalene (moth balls)
	niridazole
	phenylhydrazine
	toluidine blue
	trinitrotoluene (TNT)
	hydroxylamines
	fava beans

✓ Checkpoint! #2

Oxidant compounds are harmful because they result in production of harmful peroxides or other oxygen radicals that overwhelm the natural mechanisms to scavenge them. Why is the mechanism of protection against oxidants easily compromised in G6PD deficiency?

PATHOPHYSIOLOGY

G6PD is necessary for maintaining adequate levels of GSH for (Figure 18-1 ■) reducing cellular oxidants. In G6PD deficiency, the generation of GSH is impaired and cellular oxidants accumulate. The buildup of cellular oxidants leads to erythrocyte injury and hemolysis. Hemoglobin is oxidized to methemoglobin, which precipitates in the form of Heinz bodies. Heinz bodies attach to the erythrocyte membrane causing increased membrane permeability to cations, osmotic fragility, and cell rigidity. Heinz bodies are removed from the erthrocytes by splenic macrophages producing "bite" cells and blister cells. With progressive membrane loss, spherocytes may be formed. These cells, less deformable than normal, become trapped and hemolyzed in the spleen.

Heinz bodies require a supravital stain to be visualized, as they are not evident on Romanowsky-stained blood smear stains.

It is also likely that membrane damage may account for the acute intravascular hemolysis seen in G6PD deficiency. Oxidant stress may oxidize membrane lipids and proteins. This disruption of the membrane structural integrity results in removal of the cell from circulation by splenic macrophages.

Normally, G6PD activity is highest in young cells, decreasing as the cell ages. It has been shown that normal erythrocytes use only 0.1% of their maximum G6PD enzyme capacity.[2] Thus, even older cells retain enough G6PD activity to maintain adequate GSH levels. This also explains why even G6PD deficient cells can maintain normal function and hemolysis is sporadic. Only in situations that create excessive oxidant stress is G6PD activity inadequate to maintain normal metabolic function. Those cells that are most deficient undergo oxidant damage and are rapidly removed from circulation. This accounts for the sporadic hemolysis that accompanies oxidant stress in G6PD deficiency. In most G6PD variants, hemolysis is self-limited. (Self-limited refers to the fact that hemolysis stops after a time even if the oxidant stress continues.) This occurs because initially the older, most G6PD deficient erythrocytes are destroyed but the younger cells remain. The reticulocytes released from the bone marrow in response to the hemolytic episode have enough enzyme activity to maintain metabolic activity even under oxidant stress. It is also important to recognize that under the stress of severe oxidants (drugs, chemicals) even normal cells may experience oxidant damage and hemolyze.

✓ Checkpoint! #3

Erythrocyte morphology should always be examined carefully. The ability to pick up subtle clues to the cause of a disease process can be conveyed by a comprehensive evaluation of abnormal erythrocyte morphology. How is this likely to aid the diagnosis of G6PD deficiency?

G6PD VARIANTS

More than 350 variants (isoenzymes) of the G6PD enzyme have been identified.[1] Many of these variants differ in their activity, stability, and electrophoretic mobility (Table 18-3). G6PD is a 59 KDa protein that exists primarily as a dimer.[3] The mutant enzymes have been categorized into five classes according to the degree of deficiency and hemolysis (Table l8-4 ✪). Most variants have normal enzyme activity. Deficient enzyme variants tend to have mutations clustered in domains responsible for stable dimerization or the NADP binding site.[4] Only the most common variants will be discussed here. All

✪ TABLE 18-3

Characteristics of the Most Common Variants of G6PD Enzyme in Comparison to the Normal Isoenzyme (B)

G6PD Isoenzyme	Half-life	Clinical Severity	Favism	Class	Electrophoretic Mobility
G6PD-B	62 days	normal	−	IV	normal
G6PD-A$^+$	−	normal	−	IV	fast
G6PD-A$^-$	13 days	mod to severe hemolysis after oxidant exposure, self-limiting	−/+	III	fast (about same as A$^+$)
G6PD Mediterranean	hours	severe hemolysis after oxidant exposure, not self-limiting	+	II	normal
G6PD Canton	−	severe hemolysis after oxidant exposure, may not be self-limiting	?	III	fast

variants except G6PD-B, G6PD-A+, and G6PD-A– are given geographic names or other types of names.

- Class V: Increased activity. This class of variant enzymes is not associated with hemolysis.
- Class IV: Normal activity.
  - **G6PD-B:** This is the most common normal isoenzyme.
  - **G6PD-A$^+$:** The isoenzyme G6PD-A+ is found in about 20% of African American males. This isoenzyme has normal enzymatic activity and is not associated with disease. The A$^+$ isoenzyme, however, has a faster mobility on electrophoresis due to a single amino acid substitution of an asparagine for aspartate.
- Class III: Moderately to mildly deficient.
  - **G6PD-A$^-$:** G6PD-A– is found in 10% of African Americans. The minus sign denotes deficient enzyme activity. This variant has only 5–15% of the enzymatic activity of G6PD-B and the same electrophoretic mobility as G6PD-A+. Individuals with this variant are susceptible to hemolytic episodes after administration of oxidant drugs or during infections. In G6PD-A–, the older cells are markedly deficient in enzyme activity and are preferentially destroyed, but young cells have enough activity to

✪ TABLE 18-4

Classes of Mutant G6PD Isoenzymes

Class	G6PD Activity	Hemolysis
I	Severely deficient	Chronic (nonspherocytic hemolytic anemia)
II	Severely deficient (<10%)	Acute, episodic
III	Moderately to mildly deficient (10–60%)	Acute, episodic
IV	Normal (60–150%)	Absent
V	Increased	Absent

maintain GSH levels. The reticulocytosis that accompanies hemolytic episodes causes the hemolysis to be self-limited. However, when the drug is withdrawn or the infection subsides, older cells will once again accumulate and hemolysis could occur again if the cell is stressed with oxidants.
  - **G6PD Canton:** G6PD Canton is the most common abnormal variant among Asians. Its activity is similar to that of G6PD Mediterranean. Hemolysis is usually severe and may not be self-limited. Persons with this variant may be susceptible to a wider variety of drugs than those with G6PD-A–.
- Class II: severely deficient.
  - **G6PD Mediterranean:** G6PD Mediterranean is the most common abnormal variant in Caucasians, especially in those of the Mediterranean area. This isoenzyme has the same electrophoretic mobility as G6PD-B, but it has a marked decrease (<1%) in enzyme stability and activity. Thus, it was formerly referred to as G6PD-B–. All erythrocytes, even reticulocytes, are grossly deficient in enzyme activity; therefore, hemolysis is severe and not self-limited. In some cases hemolysis is chronic.
- Class I: Severely deficient hereditary nonspherocytic hemolytic anemia: This group of enzyme variants is associated with a chronic hemolytic anemia first noted during infancy or early childhood. The anemia may be mild to severe. This is in contrast to the other classes of variants in which hemolysis is precipitated by a drug, infection, or fava bean ingestion.

FEMALES WITH G6PD DEFICIENCY

Female heterozygotes for G6PD deficiency always contain two populations of cells; one normal and one with G6PD deficiency. By contrast, in affected males all cells are G6PD deficient. The dual population in females is caused by random inactivation of one X chromosome in a given stem cell. Depending on the proportion of abnormal erythrocytes, females may have no clinical expression of the deficiency or they may be affected as severely as males. Although rare, there are case reports of homozygous deficient females.[5]

CLINICAL FINDINGS

Most persons with G6PD deficiency have no clinical symptoms, and they are not anemic. Diagnosis usually occurs during or after infectious illnesses or following exposure to certain drugs because these conditions commonly precipitate hemolytic attacks. Hemolysis is variable and is dependent on the degree of oxidant stress, the G6PD isoenzyme, and sex of the patient. The symptoms are those of acute intravascular hemolytic anemia (∞ Chapter 16). Drug induced hemolysis usually occurs within 1 to 3 days after exposure to the drug. Sudden anemia develops with a 3–4 g/dL drop in hemoglobin. Jaundice is not prominent. The patient may experience abdominal and low back pain. Urine is dark or black because of hemoglobinuria. In one study of 35 G6PD deficient children in India, the most common important complication, occuring in more than 50% of the cases, was renal failure.[6] Hemoglobinemia is prominent. Often, however, hemolysis is less striking and is not accompanied by hemoglobinuria or conspicuous symptoms.

Favism is a peculiar disorder in which some idividuals with G6PD deficiency develop a sudden severe hemolytic episode after the ingestion of fava beans (broad beans). Hemolytic episodes occur in much the same way as drug induced episodes. The most likely components of the bean responsible for the sensitivity are isouramil and divicine. This complication is often thought to be associated with severe G6PD deficiency, especially the G6PD Mediterranean variant. It is now clear, however, that other forms of G6PD deficiency are also associated with favism, including G6PD-A– and G6PD Aures, a type identified in Algerian subjects.[7]

The hemolysis is similar to the acute hemolytic episodes that occur after primaquine administration in individuals with the G6PD-A– variant. Consumption of fava beans is widespread in the Mediterranean area and the Middle East. The first signs of favism are malaise, severe lethargy, nausea, vomiting, abdominal pain, chills, tremor, and fever.[1] Hemoglobinuria occurs a few hours after ingestion of the beans. Persistent hemoglobinuria usually prompts the individual to seek medical attention. Jaundice may be intense. Severe favism usually affects children between the ages of 2 and 5 years. The age distribution of favism is changing in some countries, however, due to neonatal screening and parental education. Even though favism occurs more often in males due to the X-linked nature of the disease, females may also be affected depending on the proportion of enzyme deficient erythrocytes present.

LABORATORY FINDINGS

There are no anemia or abnormal peripheral blood findings except during hemolytic attacks. Rarely patients may exhibit chronic hemolysis. During or immediately following a he-

molytic attack, polychromasia, occasional spherocytes, small hypochromic cells, erythrocyte fragments, and bite cells may be seen on the blood smear. Bite cells, which have a chunk of the cell removed from one side, are frequently thought to be typical of G6PD deficiency (Figure 18-2 ■). However, bite cells are more characteristic of drug-induced oxidant hemolysis in individuals with normal hemoglobin and enzyme activity.[8]

A peculiar cell referred to by a variety of descriptive terms (irregularly contracted cell, eccentrocyte, erythrocyte hemighost, double-colored erythrocyte, and cross-bonded erythrocyte) has been described in G6PD deficiency after oxidant-related hemolysis. These cells are rigid, with decreased volume and increased MCH. The hemoglobin is confined to one side of the cell while the other side is transparent. The transparent side often contains Heinz bodies. The transparent part of the cell has flattened membranes in which the opposing membrane sides are interconnected. This crossbonding of the membrane appears to decrease deformability and destine the cell for phagocytosis by macrophages.

A variety of abnormal laboratory findings related to hemolysis can be found after or during a hemolytic attack. Reticulocytosis is characteristic following a hemolytic episode.[9] Leukocytes may be increased during hemolytic attacks. Platelets are normal. Indirect bilirubin and serum LDH may be increased. Haptoglobin is commonly decreased during the acute hemolytic phase. Absence of haptoglobin in the recovery stage indicates chronic hemolysis.

Definitive diagnosis depends upon the demonstration of a decrease in erythrocyte G6PD enzyme activity. In blacks, the enzyme activity may appear normal during and for a time after a hemolytic attack because older cells with less G6PD are preferentially destroyed during the attack and

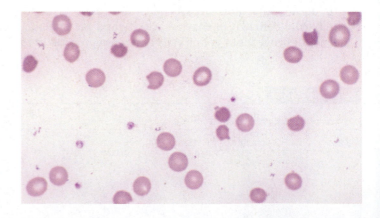

■ **FIGURE 18-2** Heinz body hemolytic anemia. Peripheral blood from a patient with G6PD deficiency during a hemolytic episode. There are erythrocytes with a portion of the cell missing. These are known as bite cells. The spleen pits the Heinz body with a portion of the cell producing these misshapen erythrocytes. Some of the cells reseal and become spherocytes. (Wright-Giemsa stain; 1000× magnification)

reticulocytes have normal activity. A reticulocytosis of greater than 7% is associated with a normal enzyme screen after hemolysis.[10] For this reason, assays for G6PD should be performed 2 to 3 months after a hemolytic episode in blacks. In G6PD Mediterranean, however, even young cells have gross deficiencies of G6PD, and enzyme activity appears abnormal even with reticulocytosis. Both severe and mild types of G6PD deficiency are detected with measurement of the enzyme if the patient is not undergoing hemolysis.

CASE STUDY (continued from page 333)

Because of the low hemoglobin, Henry was transfused with 2 units of packed red cells. Examination of the peripheral blood smear was remarkable for occasional spherocytes and bite cells. This blood smear finding, presentation of anemia, and the onset of illness coinciding with the initiation of primaquine, suggested shortened RBC life span due to oxidative damage.

1. What test should be considered after finding bite cells on a blood smear?

Fluorescent Spot Test

The fluorescent spot test is a reliable and sensitive screening test for G6PD deficiency. Whole blood is added to a mixture of glucose-6-phosphate (G6P), NADP, and saponin. A drop of this mixture is placed on a piece of filter paper and examined under ultraviolet light for fluorescence. Normally, the G6PD enzyme present in erythrocytes metabolizes G6P, producing NADPH. NADPH fluoresces but NADP does not, so lack of fluorescence indicates G6PD deficiency.

Dye Reduction Test

In the dye reduction screening test a hemolysate of patient's blood, G6P, NADP, and the dye brilliant cresyl blue are incubated together. If the hemolysate contains G6PD, the NADP will be reduced to NADPH, which in turn reduces the blue dye to its colorless form. The time it takes for this change to occur is inversely proportional to the amount of G6PD present. Normal blood is used in this test for comparison. The test is specific and is available in commercial kits.

Ascorbate Cyanide Test

The ascorbate cyanide test is the most sensitive screening test for detecting heterozygotes and for detecting G6PD deficiency during hemolytic attacks in blacks. The test is not specific for G6PD deficiency but also will detect other defects or deficiencies in the HMP shunt. The test is also positive in PNH, pyruvate kinase deficiency, and in unstable hemoglobin disorders. The principle of the test is based on the failure of G6PD-deficient cells to reduce hydrogen peroxide. Patient's blood is incubated with sodium ascorbate, sodium cyanide, and glucose. Hydrogen peroxide is generated by the interaction of ascorbate with hemoglobin. The sodium cyanide inhibits the activity of normal erythrocyte catalase, an inhibitor of the formation of hydrogen peroxide. With inhibition of catalase, hydrogen peroxide is formed. Erythrocytes deficient in G6PD cannot reduce the peroxide, and hemoglobin is oxidized to methemoglobin. Methemoglobin imparts a brown tint to the solution.

Definitive Test

The definitive test for G6PD deficiency requires quantitation of the enzyme. An erythrocyte hemolysate is incubated with G6P and NADP, and the rate of reduction of NADP to NADPH is measured at 340 nm in a spectrophotometer. In the case of heterozygotic females, when the quantitation of the enzyme may yield misleading results, especially during or after a hemolytic episode, it is best to perform polymerase chain reaction (PCR) tests to reveal the genetic abnormality.

CASE STUDY (continued from page 339)

A spectrophotometric assay for G6PD was performed on peripheral blood of the patient. The result was borderline normal. A preliminary diagnosis of G6PD deficiency was made. Primaquine usage was discontinued and the patient recovered without complications. Upon follow-up the patient was retested for G6PD deficiency and was found abnormal and confirmed the diagnosis.

2. Why were the initial G6PD test result normal and the repeat test abnormal?

THERAPY

The majority of patients with G6PD deficiency are asymptomatic and do not experience chronic hemolysis; thus, no therapy is indicated. However, patients should avoid exposure to the oxidant drugs and foods that may precipitate hemolytic episodes. In acute hemolytic episodes, supportive therapy including blood transfusions, treatment of infections, and removal of the precipitating agent is used. Exchange transfusion may be necessary in severe neonatal jaundice. Dialysis is indicated in patients with oliguria and severe azotemia.[6]

CASE STUDY (continued from page 339)

3. What was the precipitating cause of the patient's anemia?

► OTHER DEFECTS AND DEFICIENCIES OF THE HMP SHUNT AND GSH METABOLISM

Erythrocytes synthesize about 50% of their total glutathione every four days. Deficiencies in the enzymes needed for glutathione synthesis (glutathione synthetase and glutamylcysteine synthetase) have been reported to be associated with a decrease in GSH and a congenital nonspherocytic hemolytic anemia. Hemolysis increases during administration of certain drugs. Glutathione reductase is an enzyme that catalyzes the reduction of GSSG to GSH. Deficiencies in this enzyme are not associated with a hematologic disorder. Glutathione peroxidase catalyzes the detoxification of hydrogen peroxide by GSH. Deficiencies in this enzyme, although common, are not a cause of hemolysis. This might be explained by the fact that peroxide reduction by GSH occurs nonenzymatically at a significant rate.

► PYRUVATE KINASE (PK) DEFICIENCY

Pyruvate kinase deficiency is the most common enzyme deficiency in the Embden-Meyerhof pathway and the second most common erythrocyte enzyme deficiency. There are many pyruvate kinase enzyme mutants, which probably explains the variety of clinical manifestations of the disorder. The more severe types are noted in infancy, whereas the milder types may not be detected until adulthood. Inheritance is autosomal recessive. Clinically significant hemolytic anemias of PK deficiency are limited to the homozygous state or double heterozygosity for two mutant enzymes. Single heterozygotes are usually asymptomatic.[11] Acquired PK deficiency is seen in some leukemias and myelodysplastic disorders.

PATHOPHYSIOLOGY

A number of different mutations in the PK gene that affect the enzymes activity have been identified. PK catalyzes the conversion of phosphoenol pyruvate (PEP) to pyruvate concurrently with the conversion of ADP to ATP (Figure 18-3 ■). In PK deficiency this energy producing reaction is prevented, resulting in a loss of two ATP molecules per molecule of glucose catabolized. The inability of the cell to maintain normal ATP levels results in alterations of the erythrocyte membrane, causing potassium loss and dehydration (echinocytes). The decrease in echinocyte deformability enhances erythrocyte sequestration in splenic cords and phagocytosis by macrophages.

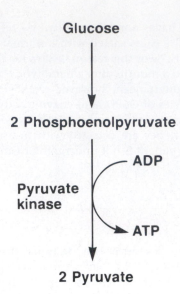

■ FIGURE 18-3 Glucose is metabolized to pyruvate in the Embden-Meyerhof pathway. ATP is generated as phosphoenolpyruvate is converted to pyruvate. There is a net gain of two ATP at this step. Two molecules of pyruvate are formed from one molecule of glucose. In pyruvate kinase deficiency, this reaction is slowed resulting in deficient production of ATP.

CLINICAL FINDINGS

There is a mild to moderate anemia with splenomegaly. The anemia is well tolerated because of the increase in 2,3-DPG that accompanies the distal block in glycolysis. The two to three times normal increase in 2,3-DPG enhances the release of oxygen to the tissues. Jaundice may occur with intermittant hemoglobinuria. Gallstones are a common complication.

LABORATORY FINDINGS

Patients with PK deficiency have a normocytic, normochromic anemia with hemoglobin levels of 6–12 g/dL. Reticulocytosis ranges from 2 to 15% and increases even more after splenectomy, often above 40%. The blood smear exhibits irregularly contracted cells and occasional echinocytes before splenectomy (Figure 18-4 ■). After splenectomy these abnormal cells are a more conspicuous finding. In contrast to G6PD deficiency, Heinz bodies and spherocytes are not found in PK deficiency. Serum indirect bilirubin and LDH are increased. Haptoglobin is decreased or absent. Osmotic fragility is normal, but cells demonstrate increased hemolysis when incubated at 37°C. Autohemolysis is increased at 48 hours, is not corrected with the addition of glucose, but is corrected with the addition of ATP.

In performing enzyme tests for PK, the erythrocytes are separated from leukocytes since leukocytes contain more PK

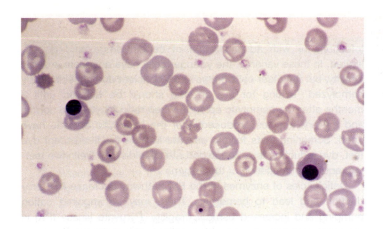

■ **FIGURE 18-4** Blood smear from a patient with pyruvate kinase deficiency. Note the echinocyte, acanthocyte, target cells, and irregularly contracted cells. There are also Howell-Jolly bodies present. (Wright-Giemsa stain; 1000× magnification)

than erythrocytes. In PK deficiency only the erythrocytes are deficient; leukocytes are normal. The screening procedure developed by Bentler is based on disappearance of fluorescence as erythrocytes are incubated with phosphoenol-pyruvate (PEP), LDH, ADP, and NADH.

$$PEP + ADP \xrightarrow{\quad PK \quad} pyruvate + ATP$$

$$Pyruvate + NADH + H^+ \xrightarrow{\quad LDH \quad} Lactate + NAD^+$$
$$\text{(fluoresces)} \qquad\qquad \text{(no fluorescence)}$$

Some mutant PK enzymes have normal activity at high substrate concentrations and abnormal activity at low substrate concentrations. A modification of this procedure has been developed to improve the interpretation of the endpoint.[12] In this modification, patient blood is frozen and thawed to ensure complete hemolysis of the specimen before testing.

In normal erythrocytes fluorescence disappears in 30 minutes. In PK deficiency fluorescence persists 45–60 minutes. The quantitative test for PK deficiency is performed in the same manner as the screening test except that the rate of disappearance of fluorescence is measured in a spectrophotometer at 340 nm. A rapid potentiometric method has also been developed in which enzymatic activity is measured by monitoring the change in pH in a reaction buffer during the conversion of the substrate to pyruvate.

THERAPY

There is no specific therapy for PK deficiency. Transfusions help maintain the hemoglobin above 8–10 g/dL. Splenectomy may improve the hemoglobin level and decrease the need for transfusions in some affected individuals; however, hemolysis continues.

✔ **Checkpoint! #4**

What are the differentiating characteristics of PK and G6PD deficiencies found on the peripheral blood smear?

▶ **OTHER ENZYME DEFICIENCIES IN THE EMBDEN-MEYERHOF PATHWAY**

When associated with anemia, other enzyme deficiencies in the Embden-Meyerhof pathway have clinical manifestations and laboratory findings that resemble those of PK deficiency.

Glucose Phosphate Isomerase Deficiency (GPI) This is the second most common disorder of the EM pathway. Almost all GPI mutants are unstable, causing hemolytic anemia. Affected individuals show a partial response to splenectomy.

Hexokinase (HK) Deficiency Hexokinase is the first enzyme in the glycolytic pathway and thus is responsible for priming the glycolytic pump. There are two types of HK deficiency. One is associated with hemolytic anemia that responds to splenectomy. The other is associated not only with hemolytic anemia but also with an array of other abnormalities. A deficiency in this enzyme interferes with production of 2,3-DPG and patients tolerate the anemia poorly.

Phosphoglyceratekinase (PGK) Deficiency This is a sex-linked disorder that causes hemolytic anemia and mental retardation in males. Females have a milder form of the disorder.

Triosephosphate Isomerase (TPI) Deficiency A deficiency of TPI causes severe abnormalities in erythrocytes resulting in severe hemolysis. Abnormalities are also noted in striated muscle and the central nervous system. Death in infancy is common.

▶ **ABNORMAL ERYTHROCYTE NUCLEOTIDE METABOLISM**

Pyrimidine 5′-nucleotidase (P5N) contributes to the degradation of nucleic acids by cleaving pyrimidine nucleotides into smaller nucleosides that can diffuse out of the cell. The buildup of pyrimidine nucleotides decreases the adenine nucleotide pool needed for normal function. P5N deficiency is an autosomal recessive disorder that leads to a severe hemolytic anemia unresponsive to splenectomy. Partially degraded mRNA and rRNA accumulate within the cell and are visualized as basophilic stippling in stained smears. Lead inhibits this enzyme, which may explain the similar coarse basophilic stippling seen in lead poisoning.

■ CHECKLIST - LEVEL II

7. Compare and contrast the pathophysiology and clinical findings of an immediate transfusion reaction with those of a delayed reaction.

8. List the causes of the secondary types of cold agglutinin syndrome and warm autoimmune hemolytic anemia and identify key laboratory results linking the cause and the autoimmune condition.

9. Compare the typical laboratory findings in immediate versus delayed transfusion reactions.

KEY TERMS

Alloimmune hemolytic anemia
Antihuman globulin (AHG)
Autoimmune hemolytic anemia (AIHA)
Direct antiglobulin test (DAT)
Donath-Landsteiner antibody
Drug-induced hemolytic anemia
Erythroblastosis fetalis
Hemolytic disease of the newborn
Hemolytic transfusion reaction
Immune hemolytic anemia (IHA)
Indirect antiglobulin test (IAT)
Kernicterus
Paroxysmal cold hemoglobinuria (PCH)

BACKGROUND BASICS

The information in this chapter will build on the concepts learned in previous chapters. Additionally, a basic understanding of immunology principles and an introduction to immunohematology will be helpful. To maximize your learning experience you should review these concepts before starting this unit of study.

Level I

▶ Summarize the normal production, lifespan, and destruction of erythrocytes. (Chapter 4)

▶ List the reference range for the hematology parameters: hemoglobin, hematocrit, erythrocyte count, and reticulocytes. (Chapters 4, 10)

▶ List the different intrinsic and extrinsic factors that may result in hemolytic anemia. (Chapter 16)

▶ Describe the basic structure of immunoglobulin and its normal physiologic role. (Chapter 6)

Level II

▶ Describe the role of erythropoietin and regulation of its production. (Chapter 4)

▶ Differentiate intravascular and extravascular destruction of erythrocytes and relate to laboratory parameters in the diagnosis of abnormal hemolysis. (Chapter 4)

▶ Choose laboratory tests used to assist in the diagnosis of anemia in a cost-efficient and effective manner. (Chapter 10)

▶ Identify clinical signs of hemolytic anemia and changes that occur in laboratory tests that signal possible hemolytic anemia. (Chapter 16)

℮ CASE STUDY

We will refer to this case study throughout the chapter.

Ms. Nelson, a 28-year-old female, makes an appointment with her physician because she is tired all the time and is short of breath with minor exertion. She indicates that the symptoms have been ongoing for about 3 weeks. She has no known history of chronic diseases. Consider the initial laboratory tests that should be done to evaluate this patient's condition based on clinical history and symptoms.

▶ OVERVIEW

This chapter compares the different types of immune mediated hemolytic anemias—autoimmune, alloimmune, and drug-induced. The underlying mechanism for each of these anemias involves the reaction of an antibody with erythrocyte antigens and subsequent cell destruction either by intravascular or extravascular processes. The mechanisms of intravascular and extravascular erythrocyte destruction are compared. The tests necessary to detect erythrocyte sensitization and identify the causative antibody are described.

The pathophysiology, clinical and laboratory findings, differential diagnosis, and therapy are discussed for each of the major types of autoimmune hemolytic anemia. Hemolytic transfusion reactions and hemolytic disease of the newborn are included as examples of alloimmune hemolytic anemia. The causative antibody and clinical presentation for acute and delayed transfusion reactions are compared and the laboratory tests required to confirm hemolytic transfusion reactions are described. In the section on hemolytic disease of the newborn (HDN), there is a comparison between ABO-HDN and Rh-HDN. The treatment of a fetus and the newborn with this condition as well as preventative measures are included.

▶ INTRODUCTION

When erythrocytes are destroyed prematurely by an immune mediated process (antibody and/or complement), the disorder is referred to as an **immune hemolytic anemia (IHA).** The individual, however, may or may not become anemic depending on the severity of hemolysis and the ability of the bone marrow to compensate for erythrocyte loss. Initial confirmation of the underlying immune mechanism is accomplished by demonstrating attachment of antibody or complement to the patient's erythrocytes. Diagnosis of anemia (and underlying hemolysis) is determined by laboratory findings such as low hemoglobin and hematocrit values, an increase in reticulocytes and/or indirect bilirubin, and a decrease in serum haptoglobin. Table 16-2 ✪ (∞ Chapter 16) summarizes some common laboratory values and clinical findings that are characteristically seen in hemolytic anemia.

▶ CLASSIFICATION OF IMMUNE HEMOLYTIC ANEMIAS

Determining the underlying process of immune hemolysis is important because each type requires a specific treatment regimen. Initially, IHA may be classified into three broad categories based on the stimulus for antibody production (Table 19-1 ✪): These are:

- Autoimmune hemolytic anemia
- Drug-induced hemolytic anemia
- Alloimmune hemolytic anemia

Autoimmune hemolytic anemia (AIHA) is a complex and incompletely understood process characterized by an immune reaction against self-antigens. Individuals produce antibodies against their own erythrocyte antigens (autoantibodies). These autoantibodies are directed against high-incidence antigens (antigens present on the erythrocytes of most people) such as the I antigen and certain antigens of the Rh system. The autoantibodies characteristically react not only with the erythrocytes of the individual but also with the erythrocytes of most people. The reactions that occur may include erythrocyte lysis, or sensitization (attachment of antibody or complement) or agglutination.

Autoimmune hemolytic anemias are further classified as warm or cold hemolytic anemia based on clinical symptoms and on the optimal temperature at which the antibody reacts (in vivo and in vitro) (Table 19-2 ✪). Some antibodies react best at body temperature (37°C), and the anemia they

✪ TABLE 19-1

Classification of Immune Hemolytic Anemias

Classification	Causes
Autoimmune	Warm-reactive antibodies
	Primary or idiopathic
	Secondary
	Autoimmune disorders (systemic lupus erythematosus, rheumatoid arthritis and others)
	Chronic lymphocytic leukemia
	Hodgkin's disease
	Viral infections
	Neoplastic disorders
	Chronic inflammatory diseases
	Cold-reactive antibodies
	Primary or idiopathic (cold hemagglutinin disease)
	Secondary
	Mycoplasma pneumoniae
	Viral infections
	Lymphoproliferative disorders
	Paroxysmal cold hemoglobinuria
	Mixed-type
Drug-induced	Drug adsorption
	Immune complex
	Autoantibody induction
	Membrane modification
Alloimmune	Hemolytic transfusion reaction
	Hemolytic disease of the newborn

produce is termed *warm autoimmune hemolytic anemia* (WAIHA). About 70% of the AIHAs are of the warm type. The majority of warm autoantibodies are of the IgG class (IgG1 most frequently) and cause extravascular hemolysis of the erythrocyte. A few warm-reacting autoantibodies of either the IgM class or the IgA class have been identified.[1,2] Cold hemolytic anemias on the other hand are usually due to the presence of an IgM antibody with an optimal thermal reactivity below 30°C. Hemolysis with cold reacting antibodies results from the binding and activation of complement by IgM. The IgM antibody attaches to erythrocytes in the cold and fixes complement. After warming, the antibody dissociates from the cell, but the complement remains, either causing direct cell lysis or initiating extravascular hemolysis. Included in the cold hemolytic anemia classification is a special condition, paroxysmal cold hemoglobinuria (PCH), which is characterized by a cold-reacting IgG class antibody.

A third major category, mixed-type autoimmune hemolytic anemia, demonstrates both warm-reacting (IgG) autoantibodies and cold-reacting (IgM) autoantibodies.

Drugs that attach to the erythrocyte membrane or alter it in some way may cause **drug-induced hemolytic anemia**. Historically several different mechanisms of hemolysis

is considered positive evidence for the presence of IgG and/or complement components on the cells.

A positive test with polyspecific AHG should be followed by a DAT with antiserum that reacts specifically with either immunoglobulin or complement (monospecific AHG to either IgG or complement) to determine the type of proteins bound to the erythrocyte. IgG antibodies may be found with or without complement attached. Therefore, if the DAT with anti-IgG is positive, the test with anticomplement (anti-C3d and anti-C4) may be positive or negative. If the anti-IgG test is positive, the antibody can be removed from the cell by an elution process. The resulting eluate (solution containing the antibody) is reacted with a panel of cells of known antigenic makeup to identify the specificity of the antibody.

If an autoantibody is IgM, only complement will be detected on the erythrocytes as the IgM dissociates from the cells in the warmer part of the circulation. The polyspecific and the anti-C3 monospecific DAT test will be positive; the anti-IgG will be negative. An elution procedure is not used if only complement is detected on the erythrocyte.

INDIRECT ANTIGLOBULIN TEST

The **indirect antiglobulin test (IAT)** is used to detect antibodies in a sample of the patient's serum. A positive IAT is indicative of either alloimmunization (immunization to antigens from another individual) or of the presence of free autoantibody in the patient's serum. Free autoantibody may be present when antigenic sites on the patient's cells are saturated with antibody or when there are large amounts of autoantibody with a low erythrocyte-binding affinity. In the IAT, free antibody is detected by incubating patient's serum with erythrocytes of known antigenic makeup. After a specified incubation period, the cells are washed free of excess serum, and the AHG antiserum is added. If antibody has attached to its corresponding erythrocyte antigen during the initial incubation period, the cells will agglutinate with AHG (Web Figure 19-2).

 Checkpoint! #4

Compare the purpose of the DAT and the IAT and state the type of specimen used for each test.

NEGATIVE DAT IN AIHA

In some cases, even though erythrocyte survival is markedly decreased, antibody cannot be detected on the cells. In this instance, antibody may be present on the cell, but there may be an insufficient number of antibody molecules to be detected by the DAT. The DAT will detect as few as 100–500 molecules of IgG per cell or 400–1100 molecules of complement per cell[3] but *in vivo* removal of sensitized cells by macrophages may occur when cells are coated with fewer

IgG molecules. Thus, the in vivo life span of the sensitized cell may be significantly shortened, as evidenced by the clinical findings of a typical hemolytic anemia, but the concentration of antibodies on the cell may be insufficient to give a positive DAT. Newer, more sensitive techniques, such as enzyme linked DAT, may detect lower concentrations of antibodies than the conventional DAT technique. In some cases IgA may coat the cell, activate the alternate complement pathway, and cause lysis. This process also cannot be detected by the DAT procedure.

POSITIVE DAT IN NORMAL INDIVIDUALS

In contrast, some patients with a positive DAT may not have shortened erythrocyte survival. The reason that some individuals have autoantibody coating their erythrocytes but have no evidence of hemolytic disease is not clear. Factors that may be responsible for this phenomenon include the following:

1. The individual's macrophages may not be as active in removing sensitized cells as the macrophages in individuals with hemolytic disease.

2. The amount of antibody bound to cells may not be sufficient to cause decreased erythrocyte life span.

3. The subclass of antibody sensitizing the cell may not be recognized by macrophages. Macrophage Fc receptors have low affinity for the IgG2 and IgG4 subclasses. Erythrocytes coated with these immunoglobulins will give a positive direct DAT but in vivo survival of the cells will be normal.

4. The thermal amplitude of the antibody may be less than 37°C.

5. The positive DAT may be due to the presence of complement on erythrocytes. Increased amounts of C3d may be found on the erythrocytes, but because this component is not detected by macrophage receptors, erythrocytes do not have decreased survival.

6. Patients with hypergammaglobulinemia or receiving high-dose intravenous gamma globulin (IVIG) may have a positive DAT because of nonspecific binding of immunoglobulins to the erythrocytes.

7. Patients taking certain drugs, (i.e., methyldopa) may have a positive DAT but normal erythrocyte survival.

CASE STUDY (continued from page 348)

When the laboratorian examined the peripheral blood smear of the patient, she noted that there were spherocytes present. The reticulocyte count was elevated. She called the blood bank and found that the DAT on Ms. Nelson was positive with polyspecific AHG, anti-IgG, but negative with anticomplement.

2. What is the significance of the spherocytes?

3. Based on these results what do you suspect is going on in this patient? Explain.

► AUTOIMMUNE HEMOLYTIC ANEMIAS (AIHA)

During fetal life a person's immune system recognizes self-antigens (those that appear on the individual's cells) and in turn does not usually mount an immune response to these antigens. The immune system normally prevents autoimmunization by ignoring self-antigenic determinants such as those that occur on an individual's erythrocytes. These antigens may, however, stimulate an immune response if injected into another individual because this person's immune system recognizes them as "foreign." The immune regulatory mechanisms that govern response to foreign or self-antigens are collectively known as *immune tolerance*.[5]

It is generally accepted that autoimmune diseases occur because of a defect in the mechanism regulating immune tolerance. Suppressor T lymphocytes normally induce tolerance to self-antigens by inhibiting the antibody producing activity of B lymphocytes to these antigens. Loss of this suppressor cell activity could result in the formation of antibodies against self. This loss of self tolerance and resulting AIHA may occur at any age. The mechanism of antibody formation in AIHA is unknown, but since many cases of AIHA are associated with microbial infection, neoplasia, or drug administration, these agents may be involved in alteration of self antigens and subsequent immune system response. Either warm or cold AIHA also can be categorized based on whether there is an underlying disease associated with it. The two categories are:

• Primary or idiopathic: no underlying disease
• Secondary: underlying disease present

WARM AUTOIMMUNE HEMOLYTIC ANEMIA

Warm autoimmune hemolytic anemia (WAIHA) is the most common form of AIHA (70% of cases).[6] It is mediated by IgG antibodies whose maximal reactivity is at 37°C. In a majority (90%) of WAIHA cases, erythrocytes are sensitized with IgG and complement or IgG alone. Only 7% of cases are sensitized with complement alone.[6] Most often, the antibody involved is IgG1 or IgG3. Rarely, the antibody involved may be IgM or IgA.

About 60% of the cases of warm AIHA are idiopathic. In acute idiopathic WAIHA, severe anemia develops over 2 to 3 days, but the hemolysis is self-limited with duration of several weeks to several years. In other instances, the hemolysis is chronic and unabating.

The underlying disorders most frequently associated with secondary AIHA are:

• Lymphoproliferative disease, including chronic lymphocytic leukemia, and Hodgkin's disease. Many children with idiopathic WAIHA will eventually develop a lymphoproliferative disease, especially Hodgkin's disease.[7] Chronic lymphocytic leukemia (CLL), found most frequently in older adults, is the disease most frequently associated with the development of secondary AIHA (∞ Chapter 30). WAIHA often develops late in the disease when the immune dysregulation is greatest.[8] In one study, greater than 60% of the cases of WAIHA were in patients with CLL.[9]

• Neoplastic diseases[10]
• Other autoimmune disorders, including systemic lupus erythematosus and rheumatoid arthritis[11,12]
• Certain viral and bacterial infections (e.g., viral hepatitis)
• Some chronic inflammatory diseases (e.g., ulcerative colitis).[13,14]

Presence of the underlying disorder may complicate diagnosis and treatment of hemolytic anemia. In many cases the AIHA is resolved with treatment of the underlying disease.

Pathophysiology

The warm autoantibody in AIHA is reactive with antigens on the patient's erythrocytes. Most often (70%), the specificity of the antibody is directed against antigens of the Rh system, although other antigen systems may be involved. When directed against the Rh system, the antibody may be specific for a single antigen (such as auto-anti-e) or, more commonly, the antibody will react with a complex Rh antigen found on all erythrocytes except Rh null cells.[9] The epitope against which these antibodies are directed has not been defined.[9] Recent research suggests that the antibody may be against a component of the erythrocyte membrane such as band protein 4.1.[15,16]

Most hemolysis in WAIHA is extravascular via splenic macrophages. Although complement is not needed for cell destruction, if both antibody and complement are on the cell membrane, phagocytosis is enhanced. If erythrocyte destruction exceeds the compensatory capacity of the bone marrow to produce new cells, anemia develops. Direct complement mediated intravascular hemolysis associated with IgM antibodies in warm AIHA is rare.

Clinical Findings

The most common presenting symptoms in idiopathic AIHA are related to anemia. Progressive weakness, dizziness, and jaundice are common. In secondary AIHA signs and symptoms of the underlying disorder can obscure the features of the hemolytic anemia. The patient may present with signs and symptoms of both the disease and hemolysis or just the underlying disease. While mild to modest hepatosplenomegaly may be present in AIHA, massive splenic enlargement is suggestive of an underlying lymphoproliferative disorder.

 Checkpoint! #5

What are the clinical findings and the immune stimuli for WAIHA?

Laboratory Findings

The most common laboratory findings associated with WAIHA are found in Table 19–4 ✪. Findings such as the positive DAT, autoantibody in the serum, and presence of spherocytes on the peripheral blood smear reflect the immune mediated destruction of the erythrocyte.

Peripheral Blood   Moderate to severe normocytic, normochromic anemia is typical. In well-compensated hemolytic disease, anemia may be mild or absent, and the only abnormal parameters may be a positive DAT and an increase in reticulocytes. Reticulocytes are invariably increased in uncomplicated hemolytic disease. The reticulocyte production index may be as high as 6 or 7. Depending on the degree of reticulocytosis, macrocytosis may be present.

The blood smear frequently shows erythrocyte abnormalities suggestive of a hemolytic process. Polychromasia, nucleated red blood cells, spherocytes, schistocytes, and other poikilocytes are characteristic (Figure 19–4 ■). The spherocytes of AIHA are usually more heterogeneous than the spherocytes associated with hereditary spherocytosis. This anisocytosis is readily noted when the blood smear is examined and is also indicated by an increase in red cell distribution width (RDW) on automated hematology analyzers. Erythrophagocytosis by monocytes may be seen. The engulfed erythrocyte is readily detected if the cell still contains its pink staining hemoglobin. If the hemoglobin has leaked out of the cell, however, only colorless vacuoles are seen. Leukocyte counts are normal or increased with neutrophilia. Platelet counts are usually normal or slightly decreased.

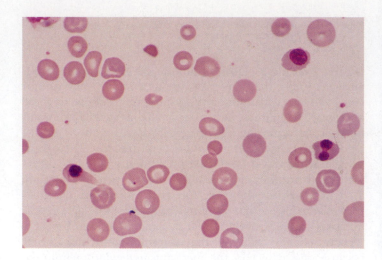

■ **FIGURE 19-4**   A blood smear from a patient with warm autoimmune hemolytic anemia (WAIHA). There is marked anisocytosis due to the presence of spherocytes and large polychromatophilic erythrocytes. The nucleated cells are normoblasts. (Wright stain; 1000× original magnification)

When severe thrombocytopenia accompanies warm AIHA, the disease is called *Evan's syndrome.*

Bone Marrow   Bone marrow examination is not necessary for the diagnosis of WAIHA. The bone marrow may show erythroid hyperplasia. Erythrophagocytosis by macrophages may be seen. Compensatory bone marrow response may be less than expected in concomitant folic acid deficiency. In chronic hemolysis, the folic acid requirement increases two to three times normal; without folic acid supplements, the stores of this vital nutrient are quickly depleted. If the patient contracts viral infections that are associated with bone marrow suppression, life-threatening anemia (aplastic crisis) may occur.

Other Laboratory Tests   The DAT is a useful test to distinguish the immune nature of this hemolytic anemia from non–immune-mediated hemolytic anemias. The test is usually positive with polyspecific AHG and anti-IgG monospecific antiserum. Only about 30% of the cases of WAIHA have a reaction with anti-C3, either with or without the concurrent presence of IgG.[6]

Reaction of patients' serum with screening cells typically shows no agglutination at room temperature or at 37°C, but agglutination with all cells is observed when AHG is added. The autocontrol (patient serum and patient erythrocytes) shows similar reactions. Other laboratory findings are nonspecific but reflect the hemolytic component of the condition (Table 19-4 ✪).

Differential Diagnosis

Warm AIHA, with the presence of spherocytes, may be differentiated from hereditary spherocytosis (HS) by the DAT. Antibodies are not responsible for the formation of sphero-

✪ TABLE 19-4

Laboratory Findings Associated with WAIHA	
Common findings	Positive DAT
	Normocytic, normochromic anemia
	Increased reticulocytes
	Spherocytes and other erythrocyte abnormalities
	Presence of autoantibody in the serum
	Increased serum bilirubin (total and unconjugated)
	Decreased serum haptoglobin
	Positive antibody screen
	Incompatible crossmatches with all donors
Other laboratory findings that may be associated with hemolysis in WAIHA.	Increased osmotic fragility
	Increased urine and fecal urobilinogen
	Hemoglobinemia,* hemoglobinuria, methemoglobinemia, hemosiderinurea

*Seen only in acute hemolytic episode

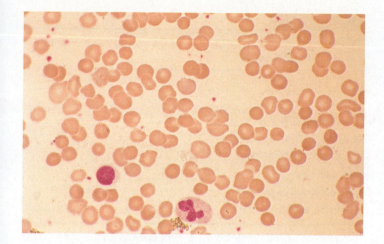

■ FIGURE 19-5 Cold autoimmune hemolytic anemia from a patient with chronic lymphocytic leukemia. Some of the erythrocytes are in small clumps. There are also spherocytes present. (Peripheral blood; Wright stain; 1000× original magnification)

tubes, blood is taken from each finger and the tubes are centrifuged in a microhematocrit centrifuge. The plasma layer is examined for hemolysis. A positive test shows hemolysis in blood from the finger incubated in cold water but no hemolysis in the finger incubated in warm water.

 Checkpoint! #8

Explain why the MCV, MCH, and MCHC may be falsely increased when blood from someone with CHD is tested using an automated cell counter.

Differentiation of CHD Agglutinins from Benign Cold Agglutinins

The serum of most normal individuals exhibits the presence of cold autoantibodies when the serum and cells are incubated at 4°C. These antibodies are termed *benign cold auto-*

agglutinins because their thermal amplitude and concentration are not high enough to cause clinical problems. Whenever pathologic cold agglutinins are suspected as the cause of anemia, laboratory tests should be performed to differentiate these pathologic ones from harmless cold agglutinins (Table 19-7). The DAT with polyspecific AHG and monospecific anticomplement antiserum is positive in pathologic cold agglutinin disease but negative or only weakly positive with benign cold agglutinins. The DAT, utilizing monospecific anti-IgG, is negative both in CHD and with benign cold agglutinins.

The cold agglutinin test should be performed whenever a diagnosis of cold AIHA is suspected. This test demonstrates the ability of the pathologic antibody to agglutinate the patient's cells at temperatures from 0°C to 20°C in saline and up to 32°C in albumin suspensions. The reaction is reversible with agglutinates dispersing at 37°C. With benign cold antibodies, agglutination occurs at 0–4°C and may occur up to 20°C. Agglutination is not enhanced, however, in albumin suspensions. Titers of benign cold agglutinins reach 1:64 in normal individuals; in cold agglutinin disease the titer is usually greater than 1:1000. Titers of 1:256 or more with a positive DAT using monospecific anti-C3 antisera and a negative DAT using monospecific anti-IgG antisera are highly suggestive of cold agglutinin disease.

 Checkpoint! #9

Compare the DAT findings and the antibody specificity in WAIHA and CHD.

Therapy

Effective relief is usually achieved by keeping the extremities warm. Difficult cases with chronic hemolysis may require more aggressive treatment such as chlorambucil or plasma exchange, but these will only decrease high titers for a short time. Neither steroids nor splenectomy are usually effective.

⊕ **TABLE 19-7**

Differentiation of Pathologic Cold Agglutinins Found in CHD from Benign Cold Agglutinins Found in Normal Individuals

	Pathologic Agglutinins	Benign Agglutinins
Antibody class	IgM	IgM
Antibody specificity	Usually anti-I but in secondary CHD may be anti-i	anti-I
Antibody clonality	Monoclonal in idiopathic type; polyclonal in secondary type	Polyclonal
Thermal amplitude	0–31°C	0–4°C
Agglutination at room temperature	Significant	Not present
Titer	Usually >1:1000	<1:64
DAT	Positive with polyspecific AHG and monospecific anticomplement	Negative

---

cytes in hereditary spherocytosis (HS); therefore, the DAT is negative. The autohemolysis test is abnormal in both HS and in AIHA with spherocytes. In HS, autohemolysis is significantly corrected by the addition of glucose; however, glucose does not correct hemolysis in AIHA. The peripheral blood smear also gives clues to diagnosis. The spherocytes in HS appear as a rather homogeneous population, while in AIHA there is a mixture of spherocytes, microspherocytes, and normocytes.

✓ **Checkpoint! #6**

What is the DAT pattern in WAIHA? Explain why spherocytes are commonly seen in WAIHA.

Therapy

In self-limiting hemolytic disorders without life-threatening anemia, transfusion therapy is not necessary. When transfusion is indicated, finding a suitable donor is difficult since the patient's autoantibody usually reacts with all donor cells in the crossmatch. If serologically compatible blood cannot be found, donor cells demonstrating the least incompatibility are usually chosen. The clinical problems, however, are twofold: donor cells are often destroyed as rapidly as the patient's own erythrocytes, and they may also stimulate the production of alloantibodies. If the autoantibody has an identifiable single specificity (such as autoanti-e), the donor blood chosen for the compatibility test should be negative for the antigen.[17]

The aims of other therapies in WAIHA are to decrease the production of autoantibodies and to slow the destruction of erythrocytes. Additional therapies include:

- Corticosteroids. Initial therapy of patients with AIHA is often a course of immunosuppressive drugs such as corticosteroids. These are used to produce immunosuppression by decreasing lymphocyte proliferation and suppressing macrophage sequestration of sensitized cells by affecting the Fc receptors. Less than 20% of patients undergo complete remission with this therapy, but over 80% of patients on these drugs will show a decrease in erythrocyte destruction.[18]

- Cytotoxic drugs. There are a number of alternative therapies for patients who do not respond to corticosteroids. Cytotoxic drugs such as cyclophosphamide and azathioprine are used to cause general suppression of the immune system, which decreases synthesis of autoantibody.[18]

- High-dose intravenous immunoglobulin (IVIG) may block Fc receptors on macrophages and affect T and B cell function by increasing T suppressor cells or reducing B cell function. It has a variable success rate and is most often used as an adjunct therapy along with corticosteroids.

- Plasma exchange and plasmapheresis may dilute or temporarily remove the autoantibody from the patient's circulation. It has been successful in reducing antibody load for a short time in some cases but is not a satisfactory long-term therapy.

- Splenectomy may be indicated when severe anemia is unresponsive to medical therapies including glucocorticoid therapy or other cytotoxic drugs. Removal of the spleen will decrease the destruction of IgG-coated erythrocytes that would normally adhere to Fc receptors on splenic macrophages. If, however, the antibody concentration remains high, the destruction of sensitized erythrocytes may continue in the liver. There is some evidence that splenectomy may be more beneficial in patients with idiopathic WAIHA than in those with the secondary type.[19]

In patients with secondary AIHA, treatment of the underlying disease is important.[18] Often resolution of the disease will lead to decreased production of the autoantibody.

COLD AUTOIMMUNE HEMOLYTIC ANEMIA

Cold AIHA, also termed *cold hemagglutinin disease* (CHD), is associated with an IgM (rarely IgG or IgA) antibody that fixes complement and is reactive below 37°C. This disorder is less common (occurring in up to a third of all immune hemolytic anemias) than anemia associated with warm antibodies.[6]

Cold AIHA, like warm AIHA, may be either idiopathic or secondary and may be acute as chronic (Table 19-5 ⊕). Idiopathic cold agglutinin disease is usually chronic, occurring after age 50.[20] The antibody is usually a monoclonal kappa light chain IgM antibody with autoanti-I specificity. The secondary type may have either an acute or a chronic presentation. The secondary acute form is usually self-limiting and associated with *Mycoplasma pneumoniae* infections, although a transient anti-i can be seen in infectious mononucleosis. The secondary chronic form, typically found in older individuals, is often associated with lymphoproliferative

⊕ **TABLE 19-5**

Autoimmune Hemolytic Anemia Caused by Cold-Reacting Antibodies

Cold hemagglutinin disease (CHD)	Primary (idiopathic)
	Secondary
	Mycoplasma pneumoniae
	Infectious mononucleosis
	Lymphoproliferative diseases
Paroxysmal cold hemoglobinuria	Primary (idiopathic)
	Secondary
	Viral infections
	Tertiary syphilis

disorders such as CLL or lymphoma. The antibody in secondary cold AIHA is usually a polyclonal IgM antibody with autoanti-I specificity.[9] A more severe type of cold AIHA, paroxysmal cold hemoglobinuria (PCH), is associated with a biphasic cold-reacting IgG antibody and is discussed in the next section.

Pathophysiology

The severity of CHD is related to the thermal range of the antibody. Those cold reacting antibodies with a wide range of activity (up to 32°C) can cause problems when the peripheral circulation cools to this temperature. Complement-mediated lysis accounts for most of the erythrocyte destruction.

The cold-reacting antibody is usually directed against the I antigen, which is expressed on erythrocytes of almost all adults. The I antigen specificity of the antibody may be defined by reactivity of the patient's serum with all adult erythrocytes but minimal or no reactivity with infant cells (which lack the I antigen). In CHD associated with infectious mononucleosis and lymphoproliferative disease, however, the antibody may have anti-i specificity. (This antigen is expressed on the erythrocytes of infants younger than 2 years old.)

The second most common specificity for cold autoagglutinins is the Pr antigens. The antigens are expressed on both adult and infant erythrocytes. Other specificities that have been reported include anti-A₁, anti-M-like, anti-Type II H, and anti-Gd.[9]

Clinical Findings

In some instances CHD may be associated with a chronic hemolytic anemia with or without jaundice. In others, hemolysis is episodic and associated only with chilling. Erythrocyte agglutination occurs in areas of the body that cool to the thermal range of the antibody and cause sludging of the blood flow within capillaries. The skin turns white, then blue, and on rewarming, red. Discoloration is frequently accompanied by numbness, tingling, and pain. These vascular changes are referred to as *acrocyanosis* or *Raynaud's phenomenon*. The condition primarily affects the extremities, especially the fingers and toes. Hemoglobinuria accompanies the acute hemolytic attacks. Splenomegaly may be present (Table 19-6 ✪).

 Checkpoint! #7

Describe the mechanism of cell destruction in CHD.

Laboratory Findings

Often, the first indication of the presence of unsuspected cold agglutinins is from blood counts performed on electronic cell counters. The erythrocyte count is inappropri-

✪ **TABLE 19-6**

Criteria for Clinical Diagnosis of Cold Hemagglutinin Disease (CHD)

Clinical history	Acrocyanosis
	Hemoglobinuria on exposure to cold
Laboratory findings	Serological
	DAT: Positive with polyspecific AHG
	Negative with anti-IgG
	Positive with anti-C3
	IAT: antibody showing characteristic reactions at <25°C
	Cold agglutinin titer >1000 at 4°C
	False increase in MCV, MCH, and MCHC
	False decrease in erythrocyte count
	Normocytic, normochromic anemia
	Reticulocytosis
	Spherocytes, agglutinated RBCs, rouleaux, nucleated RBCs on blood smear
	Increased bilirubin (total and unconjugated)
	Decreased haptoglobin
	Hemoglobinemia, hemoglobinuria in acute hemolysis
	Hemosiderinuria in chronic hemolysis

ately decreased for the hemoglobin content and the MCV is falsely elevated (Table 19-6 ✪). These erroneous values occur when erythrocyte agglutinates are sized and counted as individual cells. The hematocrit calculated from this erroneous erythrocyte count and MCV is falsely low. The MCH and MCHC, calculated from the erythrocyte count, and hematocrit are falsely elevated. The hemoglobin assay is accurate as the cells are lysed to determine this parameter. Accurate cell counts may be obtained by warming blood and diluting reagents to 37°C. Visible autoagglutination in tubes of anticoagulated blood can be observed as the blood cools to room temperature.

When blood counts are performed at 37°C, the results indicate a mild to moderate normocytic, normochromic anemia. The blood film shows polychromasia, some spherocytes, rouleaux, or clumps of erythrocytes, and sometimes, nucleated red cells (Figure 19-5 ■). Erythrophagocytosis may be seen but is more typical on smears made from buffy coats after the blood has incubated at room temperature. Leukocyte and platelet counts are usually normal. Leukocytosis may occur during acute hemolysis as the result of a bone marrow stress response. The bone marrow exhibits normoblastic hyperplasia.

The Ehrlich finger test is used to demonstrate hemolysis in the microcirculation at cold temperatures. The venous blood flow is stopped on two fingers (one on each hand) with a rubber band. One finger is immersed in cold water (20°C) and the other in warm water (37°C). Using capillary

---

PAROXYSMAL COLD HEMOGLOBINURIA

Paroxysmal cold hemoglobinuria (PCH) is a rare autoimmune hemolytic disorder that may occur at any age and is characterized by massive intermittent acute hemolysis and hemoglobinuria. Historically, PCH was associated with congenital or tertiary syphilis. It is now most often seen in children with viral infections (e.g., measles, mumps, influenza) and has been associated with non-Hodgkin lymphoma in adults.[20, 21] It is usually a transient disorder that resolves after recovery from the infectious process. The disease also may be idiopathic.

Pathophysiology

PCH was the first hemolytic anemia for which a mechanism of hemolysis was established. This hemolytic anemia is distinct from the other cold AIHA because of the nature of the antibody involved. It is caused by a biphasic complement-fixing IgG antibody, the **Donath-Landsteiner (D-L) antibody**. Biphasic refers to the two incubation temperatures necessary for optimal lysis of the erythrocytes. The antibody reacts with erythrocytes in the capillaries at temperatures less than 20°C and avidly binds the early-acting complement components. Upon warming to 37°C, the antibody molecule disperses from the cell, but the membrane attack complement components are activated on the cell membrane, causing cell lysis. The PCH antibody is specific for the P-antigen.

Clinical Findings

After exposure to the cold, the patient experiences sudden onset of chills, back and leg pain, and fever followed by hemoglobinuria. Raynaud's phenomenon may occur during acute episodes followed by jaundice.

Laboratory Findings

The degree of anemia depends upon the frequency and severity of hemolytic attacks. During the attack, there is a sharp drop in hemoglobin concentration accompanied by hemoglobinemia, methemalbuminemia, and hemoglobinuria. Leukopenia caused by abrupt neutropenia, a shift to the left, erythrophagocytosis, and spherocytes accompany erythrocyte lysis. Serum bilirubin is elevated. Serum complement and haptoglobin are decreased.

Antibodies on the cells are not usually detected by the DAT since the D-L antibody elutes at warm temperatures. A weakly positive DAT with anticomplement antisera may appear and persist for several days after the hemolytic episode. The IAT may be positive if performed in the cold. Normal erythrocytes incubated with patient serum react more positively in the IAT than patient cells.

D-L antibodies are not usually present in high titers, but their presence may be verified by the D-L test, which employs a biphasic reaction (Table 19-8 ✪). In this test the patient's blood is collected in two clot tubes; one is incubated at 4°C for 30 minutes and the other at 37°C for 30 minutes.

✪ **TABLE 19-8**

Donath-Landsteiner (D-L) Test for Detecting the Presence of D-L Antibodies*

	Control	Test
Incubate for 30 min at	37°C	4°
Incubate for 30 min at	37°C	37°C
Centrifuge. Observe plasma for presence of hemolysis		
Interpretation		
D-L antibodies present	No hemolysis	Hemolysis
No D-L antibodies present	No hemolysis	No hemolysis

*Two tubes of patient's whole blood are used, one tube serves as the control and the other as the test.

Both tubes are then incubated at 37°C. If the D-L antibody is present, it will cause intense hemolysis in the tube initially incubated at 4°C and then warmed to 37°C. No hemolysis is present in the tube kept at 37°C. Hemolysis in this test may also occur in cold hemagglutinin disease, but the hemolysis occurs very slowly. Table 19-9 ✪ compares PCH and CHD.

Therapy

PCH associated with acute infections terminates spontaneously upon recovery from the infection. Generally no transfusion is required unless severe anemia is present. The

✪ **TABLE 19-9**

Comparison of Cold Hemagglutinin Disease (CHD) and Paroxysmal Cold Hemoglobinuria (PCH)

	CHD	PCH
Patient	Usually children after viral infection	Usually adults >50 years of age
Clinical findings	Acrocyanosis	Chills, fever, hemoglobinuria
DAT	Positive with polyspecific AHG and monospecific C3	Positive with polyspecific AHG and monospecific C3
Donath-Landsteiner test	Negative	Positive
Antibody class	IgM	Biphasic IgG (D-L)
Antibody specificity	Anti-I	Anti-P
Thermal amplitude of antibody	Up to 31°C	Under 20°C
Hemolysis	Chronic extravascular/ intravascular	Acute intravascular
Therapy	Avoid the cold	Supportive; treatment of underlying illness

chronic form of the disease is best treated by avoiding exposure to the cold.

 Checkpoint! #10

Compare the antibody specificity and the confirmatory test for PCH and CHD.

MIXED-TYPE AIHA

Mixed-type AIHA is characterized by the presence of a warm-reacting IgG autoantibody and a cold-reacting IgM autoantibody.[22, 23] About 50% of the cases are idiopathic; most of the remainder are associated with collagen disease such as systemic lupus erythematosus. Less than 10% are associated with CLL or non-Hodgkin lymphoma.[22] Patients frequently present with an acute, severe anemia. The IgG class antibody mediates extravascular hemolysis while the IgM is responsible for complement fixation and intravascular hemolysis. Some patients may have a chronic course with intermittent exacerbations. Most patients respond to steroid therapy and require few or no transfusions.

In the DAT procedure both C3 and IgG can be detected on the erythrocyte. The cold autoantibody has a high thermal amplitude (reacts at >30°C) but is usually present in low concentrations (titer <1:64). The cold-reacting antibody often has an autoanti-I specificity but may have no apparent specificity. The warm-reacting autoantibody is similar to those found in classic WAIHA and has a complex specificity.

DRUG-INDUCED HEMOLYTIC ANEMIAS

Drug-induced immune hemolytic anemia is the result of an immune mediated hemolysis precipitated by ingestion of certain drugs. The drug by itself does not cause erythrocyte injury, and not all individuals taking the drug may develop this immune hemolytic anemia. Drugs may also cause immune destruction of other blood cells. Anemia, thrombocytopenia, and agranulocytosis may occur together or separately. It has been proposed that the ability of a drug to induce production of antibodies against different cell lines is related to the affinity of the drug to the cells.[24] The greater the affinity, the more likely sensitization against the drug-cell complex will occur.

Over 70 drugs have been found that induce a positive DAT or an immune mediated hemolytic anemia; some are listed in Web Table 19-2 ✪. This type of hemolysis must be distinguished from both drug-induced, nonimmune hemolysis that occurs secondary to erythrocyte metabolic defects such as G6PD deficiency (∞ Chapter 18) as well as from spontaneous autoimmune disorders. This is important because drug-induced, immune hemolytic anemias are the result of an immune response to drug-induced alteration of the erythrocyte antigenicity. The resolution for this group of anemias involves only withdrawal of the offending drug, and supportive treatment.

Three classic mechanisms have been hypothesized to explain drug-induced immune hemolysis (Table 19-10 ✪):

- Drug absorption
- Immune complex formation
- Autoantibody induction

A fourth mechanism, membrane modification, has not been associated with causing immune hemolytic anemia (Table 19-10 ✪). Regardless of the underlying mechanism, erythrocytes sensitized with either antibody and/or complement have a shortened life span. Each of these mechanisms will cause a positive DAT with polyspecific AHG and with one or more monospecific antiseras.

A new theory described at the end of this section proposes a unified approach to drug-induced autoantibody formation.[25–27]

✪ **TABLE 19-10**

Summary of Mechanisms Drug-Induced Immune Hemolytic Anemia

Type	Action	Direct Antiglobulin Test	Mechanism of Cell Destruction
Drug adsorption	Drug bound to cell → antibody binds to drug	Positive (reaction to Ig)	Extravascular adhesion to macrophages via Fc and phagocytosis
Immune complex	Forms immune complex (drug-antibody) → immune complex adsorbs to membrane → activates complement cascade	Positive (usually reaction to complement)	Intravascular complement-mediated lysis
Autoantibody induction	Drug adheres to cell membrane → alters membrane structure → forms neoantigen → stimulates production of autoantibody	Positive (reaction to Ig)	Extravascular adhesion to macrophages via Fc and phagocytosis
Membrane modification	Modification of cell membrane	Positive (variety of proteins)	No hemolysis

Drug Adsorption (Hapten-Type)

Some drugs such as penicillin are antigenic but lack the molecular size or complexity to initiate an immune response. In the hapten/drug adsorption mechanism, it is proposed that the drug or its metabolites bind to proteins on the erythrocyte membrane creating an immunogenic complex on the cell membrane. Antibodies are produced against the drug-cell complex and react with the complex on the erythrocyte membrane, coating the cell (Web Figure 19-3 ■). Only patients receiving high doses of intravenous penicillin develop the penicillin coating on their cells. Only a small portion of these individuals will have a positive DAT; even fewer develop hemolysis. The hemolytic anemia usually develops over a 7- to l0-day period. Hemolysis is extravascular, mediated by Fc receptors on splenic macrophages. Spherocytes may be present. The reticulocyte count is usually elevated. Hemoglobinemia and hemoglobinuria do not occur.

The DAT is usually positive. Although both IgG and IgM antibodies may be formed, only the IgG antibody causes hemolysis. Complement activation does not usually occur. Although the IAT is negative, a high titer of the IgG penicillin antibody is present in the serum. This can be detected by incubating the patient's serum with normal erythrocytes in the presence and absence of penicillin (indirect AHG test). If antibodies to the penicillin-protein membrane complex are present in the patient's serum, the AHG test with the "penicillinized" erythrocytes is positive and negative with cells without penicillin.

Immune Complex Formation

In this mechanism, a drug or drug metabolite with a low affinity for the cell membrane combines with a plasma protein forming a new antigenic complex in the plasma and stimulating either IgM or IgG antibodies. A drug/antidrug immune complex forms in the plasma, and this immune complex attaches to the erythrocyte in a nonspecific (non-immune) manner (Web Figure 19-4 ■). The attached immune complex usually has the ability to activate complement. After the immune complex activates complement on the cell membrane, it can dissociate from the membrane and attach to another cell. Complement-mediated hemolysis occurs as the C3b coated red cells are cleared from circulation by macrophages, or the cells may be lysed if the terminal complement components are activated. The immune complex may also bind to leukocytes and platelets and shorten the lifespan of these cells. Most often the hemolytic episode is acute with signs of intravascular hemolysis (hemoglobinuria, hemoglobinemia). Spherocytes may be present on the blood smear.

The DAT with anti-C3 is positive but negative with anti-IgG as the antibody complex has dissociated from the membrane. The anti-C3 DAT may remain positive for several months after the hemolytic episode because of the persistence of inactivated complement components (C3d) on the red cell. Unlike the hemolysis associated with penicillin, only small amounts of the drug are needed to induce immune hemolysis by immune complex formation. Quinidine is the classic drug associated with this mechanism. Although there are a large number of drugs that can cause this type of reaction, the incidence of drug induced immune hemolysis by this mechanism has been low. However, in recent years there have been increased reports of fatal intravascular hemolysis by this mechanism in patients receiving intravenous third-generation cephalosporins.[28,29]

In the laboratory, the antibody is detected only if the drug and complement are present in the test system. Diagnosis is confirmed by incubating the patient's serum with normal erythrocytes in the presence of the offending drug (indirect AHG test). If the antibody is present in the patient's serum, it will combine with the drug-protein complex and the erythrocytes. Subsequently, complement is activated. Specific antiserum to complement is utilized to demonstrate the deposition of complement on the cell membrane.

Autoantibody Induction

In approximately 10–20% of patients receiving the antihypertensive drug, Aldomet (α-methyldopa), a positive DAT develops after about 3–6 months. However, hemolytic anemia develops in only 1% of these patients. The mechanism by which antibody production is induced is unknown; however, evidence indicates the drug alters normal erythrocyte antigens so they are no longer recognized as self.[30] Erythrocyte destruction is extravascular, and anemia develops gradually. If the drug is withdrawn, the antibody production gradually stops, but the DAT may remain positive for years.

The DAT is dose dependent—the larger the dose of Aldomet, the more likely the patient is to have a positive DAT. The DAT using anti-IgG is positive but because complement is rarely activated, the DAT using anti-C3 is usually negative. Those in whom hemolytic anemia develops also have a positive IAT using patient serum and normal erythrocytes. This is because the drug induces the formation of IgG autoantibodies against native erythrocyte antigens.[31] The antibody, however, does not react with the drug itself in vitro. Serologically, the antibodies are indistinguishable from those of warm autoimmune hemolytic anemia.

Membrane Modification

In addition to causing a positive DAT and immune hemolysis due to the drug adsorption mechanism, cephalosporins are also capable of modifying the erythrocyte membrane so that normal plasma proteins (e.g., albumin, globulins) as well as IgG and complement bind to the membrane in a nonspecific manner. This adsorption of proteins is not the result of an immunologic mechanism and is not associated with a hemolytic anemia. The adsorbed antibodies are not specific to any drug or drug/cell complex. The DAT is positive with polyspecific antisera and can be positive or negative with anti-IgG and anti-C3. Monospecific reagents such as antifibrinogen, antiglobulin, and antialbumin may also react with the cell.

Checkpoint! #11

Compare the different types of drug induced hemolysis including the type of hemolysis, the drug usually associated with the mechanism, and the DAT profile.

Alternate Theory

A "unifying theory" proposes drug induced antibodies can be explained by a single mechanism.[26,27] The drug must first bind to the erythrocyte membrane. Then the body responds to this foreign antigen by producing a variety of antibodies directed against different epitopes of the drug-membrane complex. Some antibodies react only with antigens on the drug, others with antigenic complexes of drug and cell membrane, and others to the altered cell membrane only. Patients may make antibodies to only one of these epitopes or to several. For example a patient who makes antibodies only to altered erythrocyte antigens would have antibodies that are characterized as autoantibodies in the classic designation. Patients who make antibodies to the drug/membrane complex have antibodies that react with the characteristics described as the drug adsorption/hapten mechanism.

 CASE STUDY *(continued from page 352)*

Two days later Ms. Nelson's hemoglobin dropped to 50 gm/L. The physician ordered several more tests. She had a positive IAT, and the antibody reacted with all cells including her own. Other test results indicated that this patient had systemic lupus erythematosus.

4. What type of antibody appears to be present in this patient? Explain.

5. What is the relationship of the patient's primary disease, systemic lupus erythematosus, and her anemia?

► ALLOIMMUNE HEMOLYTIC ANEMIA

Hemolytic anemia induced by immunization of an individual with erythrocyte antigens on the infused cells of another individual is known as alloimmune hemolytic anemia. The patient's erythrocytes lack the antigen(s) present on infused cells. These transfused antigens are recognized as foreign and induce the recipient to form antibodies that, in turn, react with infused cells. This type of immunologic destruction of erythrocytes is characteristic of transfusion reactions and hemolytic disease of the newborn (HDN).

HEMOLYTIC TRANSFUSION REACTIONS

Transfusion of blood may cause a **hemolytic transfusion reaction** due to interaction of foreign (nonself) erythrocyte antigens and plasma antibodies. In contrast to AIHA, the antibodies produced in transfusion reactions cause immunologic destruction of donor cells but do not react with the erythrocytes of the person making the antibody. There are two types of transfusion reactions involving antibodies to erythrocyte antigens: immediate (within 24 hours) and delayed (occurring 2–14 days after transfusion) (Table 19-11 ✪). An acute or immediate hemolytic transfusion reaction results when the infused erythrocytes react with antibodies that already exist in the blood (for example, ABO system antibodies). This type of reaction is usually the result of clerical or other human error. For example, the patient is given the wrong unit of blood or is misidentified by the phlebotomist or nurse or laboratory personnel. Most errors occur in patient care areas and not in the transfusion service area.[32] Patients will exhibit classic clinical signs including changes in pulse rate, hypotension, chills and fever, pain, or difficulty in breathing. When an acute transfusion reaction is suspected, the transfusion must be stopped immediately because of the severity of the reaction. Laboratory investigation of the reaction must be performed.

The delayed hemolytic transfusion reaction is usually the result of an anamnestic response whereby the donor erythrocytes contain an antigen to which the patient has been previously sensitized. In these cases, the antibody was not detectable prior to transfusion but the infused erythrocytes restimulate antibody production. In cases of delayed transfusion reaction the patient may show no clinical signs, and the reaction is detected only by laboratory testing. Patients at highest risk for delayed reactions are those who must receive multiple transfusions over a lifetime.[33]

Pathophysiology

An acute hemolytic transfusion reaction is characterized by intravascular hemolysis with hemoglobinuria as a result of

✪ TABLE 19-11

Comparison of Acute and Delayed Hemolytic Transfusion Reactions

	Acute	Delayed
Timing	Immediate (within 24 hours)	2–14 days
Underlying cause	ABO antibodies (wrong unit of blood given)	Other antibodies—often Kidd system (anamnestic response)
Hemolysis	Intravascular	Extravascular
Symptoms	Fever, chills, back-pain, hypotension, pain at site of infusion	Uncommon (fever, hemoglobinuria)
Laboratory findings	Hemoglobinemia Positive DAT (transient)	Positive DAT Antibody in eluate

complete sequential activation of complement components. This type of hemolysis of donor cells is usually mediated by IgM antibodies, although IgG are rarely involved. This type of reaction is typical of an ABO incompatibility and begins very shortly after the infusion of the donor unit has begun. As cells are lysed, the release of thromboplastic-like substances from the erythrocyte membrane may activate the intrinsic and extrinsic coagulation cascade. The resulting consumptive coagulopathy (disseminated intravascular coagulation) may damage the kidney by deposition of fibrin in the microvasculature (∞ Chapter 37). Presence of increased tumor necrosis factor-alpha (TNF-α) and other interleukins mediate the clinical symptoms.[34] The usual antibodies involved in an acute hemolytic transfusion reaction are anti-A or anti-B. Other antibody specificities such as anti-I, anti-P_1, have been implicated only rarely. Mortality rates from ABO acute hemolytic transfusion reactions may range from 10 to 50%.[35]

Extravascular hemolysis is typical of a delayed hemolytic transfusion reaction. This occurs when erythrocytes are coated with IgG antibodies and removed via macrophage Fc receptors in the spleen. The speed of the removal depends on the amount of antibody on the cell. Complement is not usually involved but when present may enhance phagocytosis.

Delayed transfusion reactions occur 2–14 days after a transfusion. Although an antibody to this antigen may not be detected in pretransfusion testing because the antibody concentration is lower than sensitivity level of the test, antigens on infused donor cells induce a secondary antigenic stimulus. The antibody produced is usually IgG, and hemolysis is extravascular. The first indication of a delayed reaction is a sharp drop in the hemoglobin concentration several days after the transfusion. Intravascular hemolysis may also occur but is less pronounced than in acute reactions. Laboratory investigation reveals a positive DAT because of antibody-coated donor cells in the patient's circulation. Antibodies characteristically associated with a delayed transfusion reaction are in the Kidd System (anti-Jk[a], anti-Jk[b]). Antibodies to antigens in the Rh system (especially anti-E, anti-C, and anti-D), anti-Kell, and anti-Fya have also caused delayed reactions.

Clinical Findings

Symptoms of an immediate transfusion reaction begin within minutes to hours after the transfusion is begun. The reaction between antigen and antibody may trigger cytokine release, activation of the complement cascade and the coagulation cascade. A variety of nonspecific symptoms may occur including fever, low back pain, sensations of chest compression or burning at the site of infusion, hypotension, nausea, and vomiting. Unless the transfusion is immediately stopped, shock may occur. Anuria due to tubular necrosis secondary to inadequate renal blood flow and bleeding due to DIC are both common complications. The severity of the reaction and extent of organ damage are directly proportional to the amount of blood infused.

Most delayed transfusion reactions cause few signs or symptoms. The most common sign is unexplained fever several days after the transfusion. Some patients notice the presence of hemoglobin in the urine.

 Checkpoint! #12

Compare the underlying mechanisms, pathophysiology, and clinical symptoms of an acute hemolytic transfusion reaction and a delayed one.

Laboratory Findings

The laboratory findings will vary depending upon whether the transfusion reaction is acute or delayed. The acute reaction is usually accompanied by intravascular hemolysis, and the delayed reaction is usually accompanied by extravascular hemolysis. The DAT is usually positive in both types of reaction but may not be detected until 12 or more hours after transfusion in the delayed type of reaction.

Acute Transfusion Reaction If an acute transfusion reaction is suspected, the transfusion should be stopped immediately and blood samples should be drawn and sent to the laboratory. Three things must be done to determine if an immediate transfusion reaction has occurred:

- Check for clerical errors
- DAT
- Visual hemoglobin test

The clerical check will reveal any errors in patient or specimen identification. The visual hemoglobin test involves comparing the patient's pretransfusion plasma against the posttransfusion plasma to detect signs of posttransfusion hemolysis (hemoglobinemia). If there is hemolysis, the plasma may have pink, red, or brown discoloration. The pretransfusion and posttransfusion specimens should be compared side by side to detect subtle changes between the specimens. The DAT performed on the posttransfusion specimen will detect the presence of cell-bound immunoglobulin and/or complement. Often the DAT is only weakly or transiently positive because the antibody-coated cells are rapidly destroyed. If the DAT is positive and/or there is evidence of hemolysis and/or clerical error, a full transfusion reaction workup is indicated.

The pretransfusion and posttransfusion specimens are typed for ABO and Rh blood groups as well as tested for the presence of antibodies to assure that the pretranfusion specimen was correctly identified and tested. Compatibility tests are also repeated. Donor units are retyped. Despite the fact that posttransfusion specimens drawn several hours after the reaction may not contain free hemoglobin, hemoglobinuria in the first posttransfusion urine can usually be detected if intravascular hemolysis occurred. Free red cells (hematuria) in the urine, however, are not associated with intravascular or extravascular hemolysis.

Delayed Transfusion Reaction In many cases the clinical signs of a delayed transfusion reaction are so mild that the reaction is discovered only if the patient is crossmatched again several days later for another transfusion. In this case, the posttransfusion specimen will show a positive DAT. A mixed field positive DAT may be seen because only donor cells and not the patient's cells, are coated by immunoglobulin or complement and agglutinated by AHG.[36]

If the DAT is positive, an elution procedure should be performed to determine the specificity of the antibody. This procedure will release the antibody bound to the erythrocyte membrane so that the antibody can be identified. If, however, the antibody is only weakly positive, there may not be sufficient antibody on the erythrocytes to prepare an eluate. After several days, the antibody level may be increased enough to allow identification of its specificity. Hemoglobinemia and hemoglobinuria are not usually found. Other laboratory tests such as haptoglobin and bilirubin analyses may be helpful. If a reaction has occurred, the haptoglobin may be decreased and serum bilirubin increased.

 Checkpoint! #13

What are the required laboratory tests for investigating a suspected transfusion reaction? Compare the characteristic laboratory findings in acute hemolytic transfusion reactions and delayed transfusion reactions.

Therapy

The most important immediate action taken when an acute transfusion reaction occurs is prompt termination of the transfusion. A major effort is made to maintain urine flow to prevent renal damage. Shock and bleeding require immediate attention. In a delayed reaction, future units of blood given to the patient must lack the antigen to which the patient has made an antibody.

 CASE STUDY *(continued from page 361)*

The clinician wants to start Ms. Nelson on therapy and give her a transfusion.

6. How would knowing that the patient had not been transfused in the last several months help you make a decision on the underlying cause of the antibody?

7. What would you tell the clinician about giving a transfusion?

8. What kind of therapy might be used?

HEMOLYTIC DISEASE OF THE NEWBORN (HDN)

Hemolytic disease of the newborn (HDN) is an alloimmune disease associated with increased fetal erythrocyte destruction during fetal and neonatal life and is caused by fetomaternal blood group incompatibility. **Erythroblastosis fetalis,** another term used to describe this condition, reflects the presence of large numbers of nucleated erythrocytes found in the baby's peripheral blood in very severe cases. More than 95% of HDN cases are due to either Rh_o (D) or ABO antibodies. Although HDN caused by ABO antibodies is more common than HDN caused by Rh_o antibodies, Rh_o incompatibility causes more severe disease (Table 19-12 ✪). Other antibodies associated with the remaining 5% of HDN cases include anti-K, anti-c, anti-C, and anti-E.[37]

Pathophysiology

The pathophysiology of HDN involves initial sensitization and antibody production, in utero effects, and postnatal effects. Four conditions must be met for HDN to occur:

- The mother must be exposed (sensitized) to an erythrocyte antigen that she lacks.

- The fetus must possess the antigen to which the mother is sensitized.

- The mother must produce antibodies to the foreign antigens.

- The mother's antibody must be able to cross the placenta and enter the fetal circulation.

Sensitization   The mother may have been exposed to foreign (nonself) erythrocyte antigens by previous pregnancy or transfusion. Normally, the placenta does not allow free passage of erythrocytes from fetal to maternal circulation, but small amounts of erythrocytes may enter the maternal circulation during gestation. Additionally, during delivery small amounts of blood can also enter the mother's circulation. The risk of sensitization increases as the volume of the fetal bleed increases. If the fetal-maternal bleed is sufficient to stimulate the production of maternal antibodies, subsequent pregnancies may be at risk for HDN.

✪ **TABLE 19-12**

Comparison of Hemolytic Disease of the Newborn Caused by ABO and Rh_o

Feature	Rh	ABO
Antibody	Immune IgG	Nonimmune or immune IgG
Blood group	Mother Rh negative Baby Rh positive	Mother, group O; baby, group A or B
Obstetric history	Only pregnancies after the first are affected	First pregnancy and subsequent pregnancies may be affected
Clinical findings	Moderate to severe anemia and bilirubinemia	Mild anemia, if present; mild to moderate bilirubinemia with a peak 24–48 hours after birth
Laboratory findings	DAT positive No spherocytes	DAT weakly positive or negative Spherocytes present
Therapy	Exchange transfusion, if severe	Phototherapy

Three classes of immunoglobulins may be produced during immunization of the mother—IgG, IgM, IgA—but only IgG has the ability to cross the placenta and cause HDN. The IgG antibody is actively transported across the placenta and causes destruction of fetal erythrocytes. The fetus/newborn will have varying degrees of severity of anemia and bilirubinemia based on the strength of immune response.

Most ABO incompatibilities occur in Group A or Group B infants of Group O mothers. In ABO-HDN the mother already has the naturally occurring antibodies of the ABO system (anti-A and anti-B of IgG class), which may cross the placental barrier to destroy fetal cells. Stimulation and production of these antibodies does not require previous fetal erythrocyte sensitization. In contrast to Rh-HDN, in ABO-HDN the first baby may be affected because the mother has this IgG anti-A,B antibody in her circulation.

In Rh-HDN, the mother is Rh negative (D negative) and the baby is Rh positive (D positive). The firstborn is not usually affected, but babies in subsequent pregnancies are. The first pregnancy serves as a sensitizing event, and each successive pregnancy with an Rh positive fetus increases the antibody response.

Prenatal Period   If the destruction of fetal erythrocytes is severe enough in utero, the fetus becomes anemic and may develop complications as a result of the anemia. Extramedullary hematopoiesis occurs in the liver and spleen, causing enlargement of these organs. Because of hemolysis, the unconjugated (indirect) bilirubin concentration increases. In the fetus, this bilirubin traverses the placenta and is excreted by the mother. With procedures such as amniocentesis the amount of bilirubin in amniotic fluid can be measured to help determine the relative severity of hemolysis. The most serious complication is cardiac failure and hydrops fetalis, which occurs when the fetus is no longer able to produce sufficient erythrocytes.

Postnatal Period   Erythrocyte destruction persists after birth because of maternal antibody in the newborn's circulation. Now the newborn must conjugate and excrete the bilirubin on its own. In the neonate, albumin levels for bilirubin transport are limited, and liver glucuronidase for bilirubin conjugation is low; therefore, considerable amounts of toxic unconjugated bilirubin may accumulate in the baby after delivery. In the unconjugated state, bilirubin is toxic because it is lipid soluble and can easily cross cell membranes. This form of bilirubin has a high affinity for basal ganglia of the CNS. Thus, the excess unconjugated bilirubin may lead to **kernicterus,** an irreversible form of brain damage. The conjugated form of bilirubin will not cause this type of problem because it is water soluble but lipid insoluble and cannot cross cell membranes.

Clinical Findings

Anemia due to the increased cell destruction is the greatest risk to the infant with HDN both in utero and in the first 24 hours of life. Bilirubinemia is the greatest risk thereafter. In Rh incompatibility, the cord blood hemoglobin may be low normal at birth (normal hemoglobin at birth is 14–20 g/dL) and the baby does not appear jaundiced. However, significant hemolysis occurring in the first 24 hours of life outside the womb results in anemia with pallor and jaundice. In severe cases, hepatosplenomegaly may be present. Severe anemia may be accompanied by heart failure and edema. As the level of unconjugated bilirubin rises, kernicterus may occur. In Rh-HDN some infants with severe kernicterus may die.[37] With premature infants, the risks of hyperbilirubinemia are even greater because of the inability of the premature liver to excrete the excess bilirubin.

ABO incompatibility is not as severe as Rh incompatibility. Within 24–48 hours after birth, the infant appears jaundiced but kernicterus is extremely rare. Anemia is mild and pallor is uncommon. Hepatosplenomegaly, if present, is mild.

 Checkpoint! #14

Compare the pathophysiology and clinical findings of ABO-HDN and Rh-HDN.

Laboratory Findings

Laboratory tests are essential to identify the etiology of HDN, determine prognosis, and select appropriate treatment. The laboratorian must be able to interpret and evaluate results of these tests.

Rh Incompatibility   About 50% of affected infants have a cord blood hemoglobin concentration less than 14 g/dL. Because the capillary blood hemoglobin may be up to 4 g/dL higher due to placental transfer of blood at birth, the cord blood hemoglobin concentration is most useful as an indicator of anemia at birth and as a baseline to follow destruction of erythrocytes after birth. There is a direct relationship between the initial cord blood hemoglobin level and the severity of the disease. Lower cord hemoglobin levels at birth are associated with a more severe clinical course. After birth, hemoglobin levels may fall at the rate of 3 g/dL/day. Lowest hemoglobin values are present at 3–4 days. The erythrocytes are macrocytic and normochromic. Reticulocytes are markedly increased, sometimes reaching 60%. Nucleated red cells are markedly increased in the peripheral blood (10–100×10^9/L) reflecting the rapid formation of cells in response to erythrocyte destruction. Normal infants also have nucleated red cells in the peripheral blood, but their concentration is much lower (0.2–2.0×10^9/L).

The blood smear shows marked polychromasia, mild or absent poikilocytosis, and few, if any, spherocytes. The leukocyte count is increased to 30×10^9/L or more due to an increase in neutrophils reflecting the marrow response to stress. (The normal leukocyte count at birth is 15–20×10^9/L.) Often, there is a significant shift to the left. The platelet count is usually normal, but thrombocytopenia may develop with an increase in disease severity.

Cord blood bilirubin is elevated but is usually less than 5.5 mg/dL. However, cord blood bilirubin does not accurately reflect the severity of hemolysis since bilirubin produced before birth readily crosses the placenta. The serum bilirubin peaks on the third or fourth day and may reach 40–50 mg/dL if the baby is not treated. Most bilirubin is in the unconjugated form. Full-term infants with bilirubin concentrations more than 10 mg/dL are at increased risk for kernicterus. Premature infants may develop kernicterus with levels as low as 8–10 mg/dL.

Only the unconjugated bilirubin not bound to albumin is toxic to the CNS. Therefore the potential risks of bilirubin toxicity can be determined by measuring the amount of bilirubin binding reserve of albumin. One such test utilizes the ability of the infants' albumin to bind a dye, hydroxybenzeneazobenzoic acid (HBABA) or phenolsulfonphthalein (PSP). An inverse relationship between the dye binding capacity of albumin and serum bilirubin levels has been established.

The postnatal workup consists of laboratory tests on both the mother and the infant. The baby's blood and mother's blood are typed. An IAT is performed on the maternal serum. A DAT is performed on the infant's cells. Typically, the DAT is positive with polyspecific antiserum and monospecific anti-IgG sera. An elution is performed to remove antibody that is coating the cells, and the specificity of the antibody is determined. The erythrocyte-typing results of an infant's cells must be interpreted with care. Sometimes baby cells coated with a large amount of anti-D antibody will type as an Rh negative. This is due to the blocking of Rh antigenic sites by maternal antibody. In these cases, specific procedures must be performed to determine the Rh type of the infant.

ABO Incompatibility A weakly positive DAT is found in the cord blood, but it often becomes negative in 12 hours. The weak reaction is due to the small number of anti-A or anti-B antibody molecules attached to the erythrocyte. Eluates demonstrate the antibody specificity. Complement is not attached to the cells.

 Checkpoint! #15

Compare the laboratory findings including the peripheral blood smear findings and the DAT for infants born with ABO-HDN and those with Rh-HDN.

Therapy

The major efforts of therapy are prevention of hyperbilirubinemia and anemia. If the destruction of erythrocytes and degree of anemia appears to affect the viability of the fetus, an intrauterine transfusion may be given. Methods for detecting in utero hemolysis have allowed decisions to be made on whether an intrauterine transfusion with Group O Rh-negative, washed, irradiated cells should be given. The antigen-negative cells lack the specific binding site for antibody and therefore have a normal lifespan. This permits the fetus to remain in the womb longer to help ensure survival after delivery.

In mild cases postnatally, the infant is treated with phototherapy, which slowly lowers the toxic bilirubin level. Infusion of albumin to bind more unconjugated bilirubin is used less often. Although toxic levels of bilirubin are 19–20 mg/dL, exchange transfusion is usually performed before that level is reached. Exchange transfusions may also be indicated if the bilirubin is rising more than 1 mg/dL/hour or if there is significant anemia. The transfusion has several beneficial effects:

- Removes plasma containing maternal antibodies and dilutes the concentration of remaining antibodies
- Removes some of the antibody-coated erythrocytes
- Lowers the level of bilirubin
- Corrects the anemia

It also may reverse congestive heart failure in some hydropic infants.

Rh Immune Globulin (RhIG)

The passive injection of Rh immunoglobulin (RhIG) that contains increased levels of anti-D (Rh_o) prevents isoimmunization of the mother. About 7–8% of Rh-negative women develop antibodies to Rh positive cells after the birth of an Rh-positive ABO compatible infant. The routine use of RhIG in Rh-negative women during gestation (antepartum) and following the birth (postpartum) of an Rh positive child has decreased the incidence of HDN considerably. The majority of women (92%) who develop anti-D during pregnancy do so at 28 weeks or later. This antepartum administration of RhIG is given prophylactically between weeks 28 and 30 of gestation. The RhIG acts as an immunosuppressant, depressing the production of immune IgG. The RhIG binds to fetal cells in maternal circulation, mediating their removal in the spleen, thereby preventing the possibility of maternal sensitization to the Rh antigen.

Postnatally, a dose of RhIG protects against the consequences of a fetal-maternal bleed. If a fetus's Rh-positive erythrocytes enter the mother's circulation at birth, they can stimulate the mother's immune system to make antibodies. As in the antepartum administration of RhIG, RhIG given postnatally can bind fetal cells and mediate their removal in the spleen. The dose should be determined based on the number of fetal cells in the maternal circulation. Although the Kleihauer-Betke test is the traditional method employed for this count, newer methods such as flow cytometry use monoclonal antibody to fetal hemoglobin to determine the number of fetal cells present.[38]

SUMMARY

Immune hemolytic anemia (IHA) is mediated by antibodies and/or complement and may be classified as autoimmune, alloimmune, or drug-induced, depending on the underlying process. All of these will have a positive DAT due to the immunoglobulin or complement on the cell. The autoimmune hemolytic anemias (AIHA) are caused when the offending antibody reacts with an antigen on the patient's erythrocytes (self-antigen). These antibodies also have the ability to react with erythrocytes of most other persons. They are further classified as warm or cold, depending on the thermal reactivity of the causative antibody. WAIHA is most often caused by IgG antibodies that react at body temperature (37°C) and cause extravascular hemolysis. Patients with WAIHA often have spherocytes as a result of this hemolysis. Cold hemagglutinins are IgM antibodies that generally react at less than 20°C but are efficient complement activators and usually cause intravascular hemolysis. In both cases, the DAT is positive and the antibody can be detected by the IAT procedure. PCH, another type of cold autoimmune hemolytic condition, is mediated by an IgG biphasic antibody that binds complement in the cool peripheral circulation. As the coated cells reach warmer portions of the circulation, the complement cascade is activated and intravascular hemolysis occurs.

Drug-induced autoimmune hemolytic conditions are mediated by several mechanisms, depending on the causative drug. In drug adsorption the antibody adheres to the drug, which is attached to the erythrocyte membrane. In immune complex type the antibody and drug form a circulating immune complex that activates complement, resulting in intravascular hemolysis. In autoantibody formation, the drug appears to cause a change in the erythrocyte membrane that causes the body to recognize it as foreign and produce antibody against the cell. The membrane modification mechanism is associated only with adherence of immunoglobulins to the cell but has not been reported to cause an immune hemolysis.

Alloimmune hemolytic anemia has two presentations: transfusion reaction and hemolytic disease of the newborn. In both conditions the antibody is stimulated by infusion of erythrocytes containing foreign (nonself) antigens. This sensitization causes the production of antibodies to the foreign antigens, resulting in destruction of the cell. The antibody can be detected in the serum and will cause a positive DAT (often mixed field because the AHG used in the test reacts only with the antibody-coated cells).

REVIEW QUESTIONS

LEVEL I

1. The characteristic erythrocyte seen in a peripheral blood smear in WAIHA is a(n): (Checklist #3)
   a. macrocyte
   b. spherocyte
   c. dacrocyte
   d. elliptocyte

2. Which of the following might be observed on a peripheral blood smear in cases of cold autoimmune hemolytic anemia? (Checklist #3)
   a. helmet cells
   b. macrocytes
   c. agglutination
   d. spherocytes

3. When the complement cascade is activated, what molecule remains attached to the erythrocyte membrane and increases phagocytosis by liver macrophages? (Checklist #2)
   a. complement
   b. IgM
   c. IgG
   d. IgA

4. One purpose of the DAT is to: (Checklist #2)
   a. detect erythrocytes coated with immunoglobulin in vivo
   b. detect antibodies in the serum
   c. neutralize serum complement
   d. prevent agglutination by IgM antibodies

5. Intravascular hemolysis is characteristic of which of the following alloantibody situations? (Checklist #5)
   a. delayed hemolytic transfusion reaction
   b. ABO-HDN
   c. Rh-HDN
   d. acute hemolytic transfusion reaction

LEVEL II

1. The drug-induced mechanism that leads to intravascular hemolysis is: (Checklist #3)
   a. drug adsorption
   b. immune complex
   c. membrane modification
   d. autoantibody formation

2. A newborn shows evidence of jaundice and a workup for HDN is started. The baby has a weakly positive DAT with anti-IgG. The mother is Group O, Rh negative. The baby is Group A, Rh negative. The blood smear shows evidence of spherocytes. What is the most likely cause? (Checklist #6)
   a. Rh-HDN
   b. ABO-HDN
   c. combined ABO- and Rh-HDN
   d. normal results

3. Which autoimmune syndrome is characterized by the presence of a biphasic complement-fixing IgG antibody? (Checklist #4)
   a. PCH
   b. WAIHA
   c. cold hemagglutinin disease
   d. immune complex drug-induced

4. High-dose intravenous administration of what drug is characteristically associated with the drug adsorption mechanism? (Checklist #3)
   a. penicillin
   b. aldomet
   c. quinidine
   d. third-generation cephalosporins

5. Macrophages with receptors for the Fc portion of IgG are found in which organ? (Checklist #1)
   a. spleen
   b. bone marrow

LEVEL I

6. A patient with WAIHA would most likely have serum that reacts in which of these patterns? (Checklist #5)

   serum + own erythrocytes   serum + erythrocytes of others
   a. negative   negative
   b. negative   positive
   c. positive   positive
   d. positive   negative

7. Which of the following is *not* considered a condition caused by autoantibodies? (Checklist #5)
   a. PCH
   b. CHD
   c. delayed transfusion reaction
   d. drug-induced hemolytic anemia

8. A patient who is receiving a transfusion shows evidence of intravascular hemolysis. What antibody specificity and immunoglobulin class would most likely be involved? (Checklist #6)
   a. Rh/IgG
   b. ABO/IgM
   c. Kidd system/IgG
   d. I system/IgM

9. Which of the following is *not* part of the typical peripheral blood picture in Rh-HDN? (Checklist #4)
   a. macrocytes
   b. polychromasia
   c. spherocytes
   d. increased nucleated erythrocytes

10. Antibodies in WAIHA are usually directed against which of the following antigen systems? (Checklist #1)
    a. I
    b. P
    c. Kidd
    d. Rh

LEVEL II

   c. thymus
   d. liver

6. What is the *most* likely mechanism of hemolysis in WAIHA? (Checklist #1)
   a. increased sensitivity to complement
   b. fixing of complement by IgM antibody
   c. biphasic reactions by IgG antibodies
   d. phagocytosis of IgG coated erythrocytes

7. A patient who received a transfusion 6 days ago is suspected of having a delayed transfusion reaction. Which of the following would *not* be a characteristic finding? (Checklist #7)
   a. positive DAT
   b. presence of spherocytes on the peripheral smear
   c. hemoglobinuria
   d. decreased hemoglobin

8. How would you interpret the following results of a Donath-Landsteiner test? (Checklist #4)

   Patient incubated at 4°C and then 37°C: hemolysis
   Control incubated only at 37°C: no hemolysis

   a. positive
   b. negative
   c. invalid because of control reaction
   d. equivocal—repeat in 2 weeks

9. A 75-year-old man presents to the physician with complaints of weakness and fatigue. His leukocyte count is elevated, and his hemoglobin is 60 gm/L. The peripheral blood smear shows a majority of the cells are small, mature lymphocytes. The diagnosis is CLL. Spherocytes are present. The physician suspects hemolytic anemia, and laboratory tests suggest a hemolytic process with an increase in reticulocytes and bilirubin. Based on this information what is the *most* likely problem? (Checklist #8)
   a. secondary CHD
   b. secondary PCH
   c. secondary WAIHA
   d. secondary cold agglutinins

10. The following DAT results were seen in a 35-year-old female who was being investigated for a drug-induced hemolytic anemia. She had a hemoglobin of 70 gm/L, and her serum reacted with all cells against which it was tested. What drug is the *most* likely cause? (Checklist #3)

    DAT (polyspecific)   positive
    DAT anti-IgG   positive
    DAT anti-C3   negative

    a. penicillin
    b. quinidine
    c. cephalosporin
    d. aldomet

REFERENCES

1. Sokol RJ, Booker DJ, Stamps R, Booth JR, Hook V. IgA red cell autoantibodies and autoimmune hemolysis. *Transfusion.* 1997; 37: 175–81.

2. Friedmann AM, King KE, Shirey RS, Resar LM, Casella JF. Fatal autoimmune hemolytic anemia in a child due to warm-reactive immunoglobulin M antibody. *J. Ped. Hem. Onc.* 1998; 20:502–5.

3. Freedman J. The significance of complement on the red cell surface. *Transfus. Med. Rev.* 1987; 1:58–70.

4. Nielsen CH, Fischer EM, Leslie RGQ. The role of complement in the acquired immune response. *Immunology.* 2000; 100:4–12.

5. Schwartz RS, Berkman EM, Silberstein LE. The autoimmune hemolytic anemias. In Hoffman R, Benz EJ, Shattil SJ, Furie B, Cohen HJ, eds. *Hematology: Basic Principles and Practice.* New York: Churchill Livingstone; 1991.

6. Vengelen-Tyler V, ed. *Technical Manual.* 13th ed. Arlington, Virginia: American Association of Blood Banks; 1999.

7. Carpentieri U, Daeschner CW, Haggard ME. Immunohemolytic anemia and Hodgkin's disease. *Pediatrics.* 1982; 70:320–21.

8. Diehl LF, Ketchum LH. Autoimmune disease and chronic lymphocytic leukemia: Autoimmune hemolytic anemia, pure red cell aplasia, and autoimmune thrombocytopenia. *Sem. in Oncology.* 1998; 25:80–97.

9. Engelfriet CP, Overbeeke MAM, von dem Borne AEGK. Autoimmune hemolytic anemia. *Sem. Hematol.* 1992; 29:3–12.

10. Moleszewski, CR et al. Expression cloning of a human Fc receptor for IgA. *J. Exp. Med.* 1990; 172:1665.

11. Miescher PA, Tucci A, Beris P, Favre H. Autoimmune hemolytic anemia and/or thrombocytopenia associated with lupus parameters. *Sem. Hematol.* 1992; 29:13–17.

12. Kokori SIG, Ionnidis JPA, Voulgarelis M, Tzioufas AG, Moutsopoulos HM. Autoimmune hemolytic anemia in patients with systemic lupus erythematosus. *Am. J. Med.* 2000; 108:198–209.

13. Oliff IA, Compton CC. Weekly clinicopathological exercises: Case 7-2000, a 23-year-old man with hemolytic anemia and bloody diarrhea. *NEJM.* 2000; 342:722–28.

14. Giannadaki E, Potamianos S, Roussomoustakaki M, Kyriakou D, Fragkiadakis N, Manousos ON. Autoimmune hemolytic anemia and positive Coombs test associated with ulcerative colitis. *Am. J. Gastroenterol.* 1997; 92:1872–74.

15. DeAngelis V, DeMatteis MC, Cozzi MR, Florin F, Pradella P, Steffan A, et al. Abnormalities of membrane protein composition in patients with autoimmune haemolytic anaemia. *Br. J. Haem.* 1996; 95:273–77.

16. Leddy JP, Falany JL, Kissel GE, Passador ST, Rosenfield SI. Erythrocyte membrane proteins reactive with human (warm-reacting) anti-red cell autoantibodies. *J. Clin. Investig.* 1993; 91:1672–80.

17. Sokol RJ, Booker DJ, Stamps R. Investigation of patients with autoimmune haemolytic anaemia and provision of blood for transfusion. *J. Clin. Pathol.* 1995; 48:602–10.

18. Collins PW, Newland AC. Treatment modalities of autoimmune blood disorders. *Sem. Hematol.* 1992; 29:64–74.

19. Akpek G, McAneny D, Weintraub L. Comparative response to splenectomy in Coombs-positive autoimmune hemolytic anemia with or without associated disease. *Am. J. Hematol.* 1999; 61: 98–102.

20. Hadnagy C. Agewise distribution of idiopathic cold agglutinin disease. *Z. Gerontol.* 1993; 26:199–201.

21. Sharara AI, Hillsley RE, Wax TD, Rosse WF. Paroxysmal cold hemoglobinuria associated with non-Hodgkin lymphoma. *Southern Med. J.* 1994; 87:397–99.

22. Sivakumaran M, Murphy PT, Booker DJ, Wood JK, Stamps R, Sokol RJ. Paroxysmal cold haemoglobinuria caused by non-Hodgkin's lymphoma. *Br. J. Haematol.* 1999; 105:278–79.

23. Sokol RJ, Hewitt S, Stamps BK. Autoimmune haemolyis: Mixed warm and cold antibody type. *Acta Haematol.* 1983; 69:266–74.

24. Kaji E, Miura Y, Ikemoto S. Characterization of autoantibodies in mixed-type autoimmune hemolytic anemia. *Vox Sang.* 1991; 60: 45–52.

25. Salama A, Mueller-Eckhardt C. Immune-mediated blood cell dyscrasias related to drugs. *Sem. Hematol.* 1992; 29:54–63.

26. Muellar-Eckhart C, Salama A. Drug-induced immunocytopenias: A unifying pathogenic concept with special emphasis on the role of drug metabolites. *Trans. Med. Rev.* 1990; 4:69–77.

27. Habibi B. Drug-induced red blood cell autoantibodies co-developed with drug specific antibodies causing haemolytic anemias. *Brit. J. Haematol.* 1985; 61:139–43.

28. Scimea PG, Weinblatt ME, Boxer R. Hemolysis after treatment with ceftriaxone. (Letter) *J. Pediatr.* 1996; 128:163.

29. Chambers LA, Donovan LM, Kruskall MS. Ceftazidime-induced hemolysis in a patient with drug-dependent antibody reacting by immune complex and drug adsorption mechanisms. *Am J Cl Pathol.* 1991; 95:363–96.

30. Petz LD. Drug-induced autoimmune hemolytic anemia. *Transf Med Rev.* 1993; 7:242–54.

31. Garraty G, Arndt P, Prince HE, Shulman IA. The effect of methyldopa and procainamide on suppressor cell activity in relation to red cell autoantibody production. *Br. J. Haematol.* 1993; 84: 310–15.

32. Harrahill M, Boshkov L. ABO incompatible transfusion: What you need to know. *J. Emerg Nurs.* 2000; 26:387–89.

33. Syed SK, Sears DA, Werch JB, Udden MM, Milam JD. Delayed hemolytic transfusion reaction in sickle cell disease. *Am J Med Sci.* 1996; 312:175–81.

34. Winkelstein A, Kiss JE. Immunohematologic disorders. *JAMA.* 1997; 278:1982–92.

35. Linden JV, Kaplan HS. Transfusion errors: Causes and effects. *Transfus Med Rev.* 1994; 8:169–83.

36. Ness PM, Shirey RS, Thoman SK, Buck SA. The differentiation of delayed serologic and delayed hemolytic transfusion reactions: Incidence, long-term serologic findings, and clinical significance. *Transfusion.* 1990; 30:688–93.

37. Bowman JM, Pollock JM, Manning FA, Harman CR, Menticoglou S. Maternal Kell blood group alloimmunization. *Obstet Gynecol.* 1992; 79:239–44.

38. Davis BH, Olsen S, Bigelow NC, Chen JC. Detection of fetal red cells in fetomaternal hemorrhage using a fetal hemoglobin monoclonal antibody by flow cytometry. *Obstet Gynec Survey.* 1999; 54:153–54.

20

Hemolytic Anemia: Nonimmune Defects

Linda A. Smith, Ph.D.

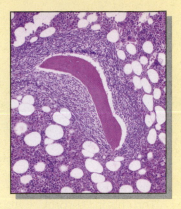

■ CHECKLIST - LEVEL I

At the end of this unit of study the student should be able to:

1. Define *microangiopathic hemolytic anemia* (MAHA); list several associated disorders and the age group most commonly affected.
2. Describe the general morphology and hematologic values associated with MAHA and criteria that distinguish disseminated intravascular coagulation (DIC); thrombotic thrombocytopenic purpura (TTP), and hemolytic uremic syndrome (HUS).
3. Recognize the characteristic erythrocyte morphology of MAHA on a stained blood film.
4. Identify several organisms that may cause erythrocyte hemolysis.

■ CHECKLIST - LEVEL II

At the end of this unit of study the student should be able to:

1. Summarize the general pathophysiology for MAHA.
2. Compare and contrast the clinical findings, underlying cause, treatment, and the characteristic findings for erythrocytes, platelet count, and coagulation tests for each of the following types of MAHA:
   a. Hemolytic uremic syndrome (HUS)
   b. Thrombotic thrombocytopenic purpura (TTP)
   c. Disseminated intravascular coagulation (DIC)
3. Define *march hemoglobinuria.*
4. Given a set of data and clinical history, determine whether MAHA is a probability, the possible etiology, and propose follow-up tests that should be performed.
5. Compare the cause of hemolysis by the following infectious agents:
   a. malaria
   b. babesiosis
   c. bartonellosis
   d. *Clostridium* infection

KEY TERMS

Cryosupernatant
Disseminated intravascular coagulation (DIC)
Fresh frozen plasma (FFP)
HELLP syndrome
Hemolytic uremic syndrome (HUS)
Microangiopathic hemolytic anemia (MAHA)
Plasma exchange
Thrombotic thrombocytopenic purpura (TTP)
von Willebrand factor (vWF)

BACKGROUND BASICS

The information in this chapter will build on concepts learned in previous chapters. To maximize your learning experience you should review the following concepts:

Level I

▶ Describe the normal production, life span, and destruction of the erythrocyte. (Chapter 4)
▶ List the normal reference ranges for basic hematology parameters. (Chapters 7, 10)
▶ Identify sources of defects that lead to hemolytic anemia. (Chapter 16)
▶ Review the immune hemolytic anemias and describe how they differ from other hemolytic anemias. (Chapter 19)
▶ Review the intrinsic hemolytic anemias and describe how they differ from extrinsic hemolytic anemias. (Chapters 16, 17, 18)

Level II

▶ Describe the structure and function of the major proteins of the erythrocyte membrane. (Chapter 4)
▶ Identify the key tests that may be used in diagnosis of anemia. Identify clinical signs of anemia. (Chapter 10)
▶ Describe the different nonimmune mechanisms of hemolysis and how they are detected. (Chapter 16)
▶ Identify the laboratory tests that differentiate immune from nonimmune anemia. (Chapter 16)

CASE STUDY

We will refer to this case study throughout the chapter.
Ms. Chang, a 35-year-old woman, was seen by her physician. She complained of weakness, low grade fever, periods of forgetfulness, and memory loss for the last week or so. She denied any viral illness prior to onset of symptoms. She was on oral contraceptives but was not taking any other drugs. Her initial laboratory tests showed:

Hemoglobin: 60 g/L
Hematocrit: 0.18 L/L
White blood cell count: 8.9×10^9/L

Consider reflex testing that may be helpful in identifying the cause of the anemia.

OVERVIEW

This chapter deals with the mechanisms of hemolysis that are not included in the chapters on membrane defects (∞ Chapter 17), metabolic deficiencies (∞ Chapter 18), or immune mechanisms (∞ Chapter 19). It includes conditions that result in microangiopathic hemolytic anemia such as hemolytic uremic syndrome (HUS) and thrombotic thrombocytopenic purpura (TTP), which are discussed in detail. For these conditions, topics include disease association, pathophysiology, clinical findings, and laboratory findings. Uncommon causes of hemolysis such as hypertension, mechanical heart devices, burns, and infectious agents are briefly discussed.

INTRODUCTION

Erythrocytes that have normal hemoglobin, enzymes, and membranes may be susceptible to premature destruction by factors that are extracorpuscular or extrinsic to the cell. This destruction may be immune mediated via antibodies and/or complement as was discussed in ∞ Chapter 19. However, a number of nonimmune factors may also cause either extravascular or intravascular hemolysis, depending on the type and extent of injury to the erythrocyte. This chapter will discuss the nonimmune acquired defects that lead to premature erythrocyte destruction. The causes for these defects can be clustered into several major categories: physical trauma to the erythrocyte, abnormalities of plasma and erythrocyte membrane lipids, which was discussed in ∞ Chapter 17 with intrinsic erythrocyte membrane disorders, and other types of antagonists in the blood (toxins, infectious agents) (Table 20-1 ⊛).

HEMOLYTIC ANEMIA CAUSED BY PHYSICAL INJURY TO THE ERYTHROCYTE

Hemolytic anemia caused by traumatic physical injury to the erythrocytes in the vascular circulation is characterized by intravascular and/or extravascular hemolysis and striking abnormal shapes of the circulating peripheral blood erythrocyte, including fragments (schistocytes) and helmet cells.

MICROANGIOPATHIC HEMOLYTIC ANEMIA

Microangiopathic hemolytic anemia (MAHA) is an inclusive term that describes a hemolytic process caused by microcirculatory lesions. Damage to the endothelial lining of the small vessels results in deposits of fibrin within the vessel. As the erythrocytes are forced through the fibrin strands, the membrane may be sliced open. In some cases

TABLE 20-1

Hemolytic Anemias Caused by Nonimmune Antagonists in the Erythrocyte Environment

Category	Antagonist	Mode of Hemolysis
Microangiopathic hemolytic anemia		
HUS, TTP, DIC	thrombi in microcirculation	physical damage to erythrocytes by microthrombi
Malignant hypertension	unknown	physical damage to erythrocytes
Other physical trauma		
March hemoglobinuria	external force	fragmentation of erythrocytes due to excessive external force as they pass through microcapillaries
Thermal injury	heat	thermal damage to erythrocyte membrane proteins
Traumatic cardiac	physical stress	erythrocyte fragmentation
Infectious agents	*Plasmodium* sp.	direct parasitization of erythrocyte; hypersplenism; acute intravascular hemolysis (*P. falciparum* infection)
	Babesia sp.	direct parasitization
	Bartonella sp.	attachment to erythrocyte membrane
	Clostridium sp.	hemolytic toxins
Animal venoms	snake bites	mechanical cell damage due to DIC
	spider bites	venom?
	bee stings	venom?
Chemicals and drugs	water	osmotic lysis
	oxidants	hemoglobin denaturation
	lead	erythrocyte membrane damage

the fragmented membrane seals itself, leading to abnormal erythrocyte shapes that are noted as schistocytes and keratocytes on the peripheral blood smear (∞ Chapter 10). These damaged cells are often removed in the spleen (extravascular hemolysis). Severely damaged erythrocytes may be destroyed intravascularly. Depending on the underlying pathology, leukocytes may be increased and platelets may be decreased. Evidence of intravascular coagulation and fibrinolysis may be present. The plasma concentration of markers of hemolysis (bilirubin and haptoglobin) will vary depending on the type and extent of hemolysis (∞ Chapter 16).

The underlying diseases and conditions responsible for microangiopathic hemolytic anemia include hemolytic uremic syndrome, thrombotic thrombocytopenic purpura, malignant hypertension, disseminated cancer, and pregnancy (eclampsia, preeclampsia). A severe form of preeclampsia that is characterized by **h**emolysis, **e**levated **l**iver enzymes and **l**ow **p**latelet counts (HELLP syndrome) may also cause MAHA. Hemolytic uremic syndrome (HUS) and thrombotic thrombocytopenic purpura (TTP) may present with similar initial clinical symptoms, but the underlying etiology, the age group affected, and the target organ(s) differ.

✓ **Checkpoint! #1**

Microangiopathic hemolytic anemia is characterized by what abnormal erythrocyte? How is this cell formed?

 CASE STUDY *(continued from page 370)*

Ms. Chang's peripheral blood smear showed moderate schistocytes and polychromasia.

1. What are some conditions that result in the presence of schistocytes?

Hemolytic Uremic Syndrome

Hemolytic uremic syndrome (HUS), first described in the mid-1950s, is characterized by a tetrad of clinical findings including hemolytic anemia with erythrocyte fragmentation, acute renal failure, thrombocytopenia, and variable central nervous system symptoms (Table 20-2 ✪). HUS is considered the most common cause of acute renal failure in children and may also result in chronic renal failure in some children. This syndrome begins a few days or weeks after an episode of gastroenteritis (especially with *Shigella* or *E. coli* 0157:H7). HUS has also been associated with an upper respiratory infection, urinary tract infection, or viral disease such as varicella or measles.[1]

The adult-onset HUS, which is less frequently seen, occurs in those over 16 years old. These cases may be primary (no identifiable cause) or secondary. Secondary HUS is associated with bacterial infections (classic HUS), connective tissue dis-

✪ TABLE 20-2

Comparison of Characteristics Associated with HUS and TTP

TTP	HUS
Adults ages 20–50	Children <5 years old
Hemolytic anemia with red cell fragmentation	Hemolytic anemia with red cell fragmentation
Renal dysfunction	Acute renal failure
Thrombocytopenia	Thrombocytopenia
Severe CNS symptoms	Mild CNS symptoms
Fever	

eases such as systemic lupus erythematosus, and cancer (especially stomach, colon, and breast).[2] The disease has been reported in young women with complications of pregnancy or after normal delivery or with the use of oral contraceptives. HUS also has been associated with the presence of lupus anticoagulant and immunosuppressive therapy used in renal and bone marrow transplantation.[3,4] HUS triggered by *E. coli* infection is rarely lethal and usually does not recur, while that associated with other secondary causes has a higher risk of recurrence and a lower survival rate.[2]

HUS can be subdivided into two groups based on the presence or absence of a bloody diarrheal prodrome[1] (Table 20-3 ✪). The diarrhea-associated (D+) HUS is the most common form and is responsible for acute renal failure in children. The D+ HUS is usually associated with verocytotoxin (Shiga-like toxin I and II) producing *Escherichia coli* infections. The most common serotype of enterohemorrhagic *E. coli* that produces this toxin is *E. coli* O157:H7. The organism is normally found in the gastrointestinal tract of cattle. The majority of human infections have been traced to the ingestion of incompletely cooked beef contaminated with

✪ TABLE 20-3

Types of HUS and Associated Conditions That May Precipitate Them

Type of HUS	Associated Condition
Diarrhea-related (classic) HUS (D+)	*Eschericia coli* O157:H7
	Shigella dysenteriae serotype I
Non–diarrhea-related HUS (D−)	Postinfectious
	S. pneumoniae
	Viral infections
	Immunosuppression-related
	Chemotherapy/cytotoxic drugs
	Renal and bone marrow transplantation
	Pregnancy or oral-contraceptive related
	Toxins
	Acute rhabdomyolysis

the organism. About 15% of individuals with this infection will develop HUS.[5] The other organism associated with D+ HUS is *Shigella dysenteriae* Type I (produces Shiga toxin I). Mild to moderately severe cases of D+ HUS have the best prognosis for recovery (more than 80%). Non–diarrhea-associated (D−) HUS has been reported in both children and adults. Various causes have been attributed to D− HUS[1] (Table 20-3 ✪). The onset of D+ HUS tends to occur between the ages of 6 months and 1 year, while D− HUS does not appear to show an age predilection.

✓ Checkpoint! #2

What are the two types of HUS, and what organisms or diseases are most commonly associated with each type?

Pathophysiology   More than 90% of the cases of HUS have been associated with damage to the renal glomerular capillary endothelium by verocytotoxins produced by bacterial pathogens *S. dysenteriae* type I and *E. coli* O157:H7. In these infections, damage to the intestinal mucosa allows the toxin and inflammatory mediators to enter the circulation[6] (Figure 20-1 ■). The toxins then attach to target glycolipid receptors on endothelial cells of capillaries and in the microvasculature of glomerulus.[5] Endothelial damage has been

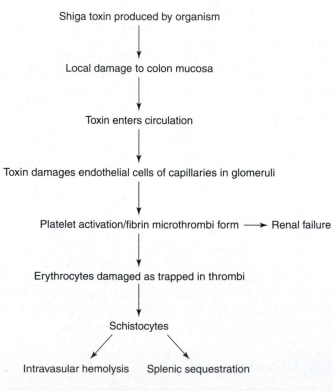

Shiga toxin produced by organism

↓

Local damage to colon mucosa

↓

Toxin enters circulation

↓

Toxin damages endothelial cells of capillaries in glomeruli

↓

Platelet activation/fibrin microthrombi form ⟶ Renal failure

↓

Erythrocytes damaged as trapped in thrombi

↓

Schistocytes

↙ ↘

Intravasular hemolysis   Splenic sequestration

■ **FIGURE 20-1** A possible mechanism for damage by Shiga-like toxin of *Escherichia coli* O157:H7.

linked to the release of vasoactive and platelet-aggregating substances causing platelet activation with subsequent formation of thrombi, primarily in the renal microvasculature, although other organ systems (central nervous system, heart, liver, gut) can be affected. This thrombotic microangiopathy, which traps erythrocytes and causes fragmentation, is responsible for the clinical findings associated with HUS. Shiga-like toxins may also stimulate production of cytokines such as interleukins and tumor necrosis factor that may result in a synergistic cytotoxic effect.[7]

HUS has also been linked to invasive *Streptococcus pneumoniae* infections.[8] It has been suggested that the enzyme neuraminidase, produced by the bacteria, is responsible for capillary damage. Neuraminidase cleaves cell membrane glycoproteins and glycolipids, facilitating tissue invasion by the bacteria and exposing the normally hidden T-antigen (Thomsen-Friedenreich antigen) on capillary walls, platelets, and erythrocytes. Naturally occurring anti-T antibodies cause agglutination of cells and platelets leading to thrombosis in the small vessels.[1] Catabolic enzymes (especially leukocyte elastase) and oxidative products released from the granules of activated neutrophils have been implicated in causing endothelial damage.

 Checkpoint! #3

Explain how infection with E. coli O157:H7 results in intravascular hemolysis.

Clinical Findings The disease occurs in previously healthy children, with the highest incidence in the first year of life. The onset is acute with sudden pallor, abdominal pain, vomiting, foul-smelling and bloody diarrhea, and macroscopic hematuria. Other symptoms may include a low-grade fever, hypertension, petechiae, bruising, and jaundice. The most important and/or serious complication of HUS is acute renal failure. The duration of oliguria and anuria is variable, with the longest reported period of anuria being 75 days.[3]

Regardless of what organ is affected in addition to the kidneys, the pathology is the same (i.e., thrombosis of the microcirculation). Central nervous system symptoms, which are less severe than those associated with TTP, may result directly from microangiopathy of the central nervous system or from hypertension. Lethargy and minor seizures are the most common symptoms. Hepatomegaly may be present; splenomegaly is less common. Hyperglycemia is common in children due to pancreatic damage secondary to HUS.

Laboratory Findings A moderate to severe normocytic, normochromic anemia is typical with hemoglobin levels as low as 3–4 g/dL (median values 7–9 g/dL) (Table 20-4 ✪). The peripheral blood smear shows fragmented and deformed

TABLE 20-4

Laboratory Findings in HUS and TTP

Evidence of hemolysis	Decreased hemoglobin/hematocrit
	Increased reticulocytes/polychromasia
	Thrombocytopenia
	Leukocytosis with shift to the left
	Presence of schistocytes
Evidence of intravascular hemolysis	Hemoglobinemia
	Hemoglobinuria
	Decreased haptoglobin
	Increased serum bilirubin
Evidence of thrombotic microangiopathy	Thrombocytopenia
	Fibrin degradation products (normal to slightly increased)
	PT and APTT (normal to slightly abnormal)
	Factors I, V, VIII (normal to increased)

cells (schistocytes, burr cells, helmet cells, spherocytes), with the degree of anemia correlated directly with the degree of morphologic change (Figure 20-2 ■). Polychromasia and an occasional nucleated erythrocyte may be seen. A leukocytosis with a shift to the left is common. Platelet counts vary from low normal to markedly decreased, with a median value of 50×10^9/L. The duration of thrombocytopenia is 1–2 weeks.

Hemoglobinemia with an increase in serum bilirubin (2–3 mg/dL) and a decrease in serum haptoglobin reflects chronic intravascular hemolysis. Serum lactate dehydrogenase is markedly elevated, and cardiac enzymes may be elevated due to myocardial damage. Blood urea nitrogen and creatinine levels are increased, reflecting renal failure. Metabolic acidosis, hyponatremia, and hypokalemia are common.

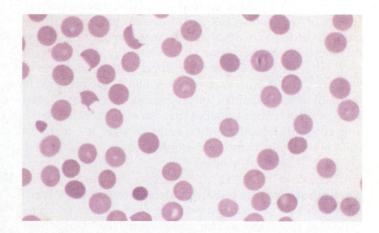

■ **FIGURE 20-2** A peripheral blood smear from a patient with hemolytic uremic syndrome (HUS). The platelets are markedly decreased. There are schistocytes and spherocytes present. (Wright-Giemsa stain; 1000× magnification)

Screening tests for coagulation abnormalities include the prothrombin time (PT) and activated partial thromboplastin time (APTT). In HUS, the PT may be normal or slightly prolonged but the APTT is usually normal. Fibrin split products (fragments of fibrin produced by plasmin degradation of fibrin) are elevated, although disseminated intravascular coagulation (DIC) is rare. In DIC there is an uncontrolled inappropriate formation of fibrin within the blood vessels and subsequent consumption of coagulation factors that causes abnormal results for coagulation screening tests. The direct and indirect antiglobulin tests (Coombs' tests) are usually negative (∞ Chapter 19); however, in some cases of HUS due to infection with *S. pneumoniae* there may be a positive result.[9]

Urinalysis reveals gross abnormalities including moderate to massive amounts of protein (1–2g/24 hours to 10g/24 hours), gross and microscopic hematuria, pyuria, and casts (hyaline, granular, and renal epithelial). The presence of hemosiderin in the urine sediment reflects chronic intravascular hemolysis.

 Checkpoint! #4

What are the typical erythrocyte morphology and coagulation test results in children with HUS?

Therapy   With improvement in early diagnosis and supportive care, especially during oliguric or anuric phase, the mortality of the disease has been reduced to 5–15%. Supportive care includes close observation, blood transfusion, control of electrolyte and water imbalances, control of hypertension, and peritoneal dialysis in anuria. Platelet transfusions may be required in some patients. The beneficial use of fresh frozen **plasma exchange** in HUS remains unclear. It has not been shown to be efficacious in patients with D+ HUS. In contrast, D− HUS patients may benefit from plasma exchange. Plasma infusions are contraindicated in patients with HUS who have a positive direct antiglobulin test or who are infected with *S. pneumoniae* due to the presence of naturally occurring anti-T in the plasma. Over the past few years, there has been evidence that the use of antimicrobials and antidiarrheal/antimotility drugs to treat the diarrheal prodrome may increase the risk of HUS.[10, 11]

Thrombotic Thrombocytopenic Purpura

Thrombotic thrombocytopenic purpura (TTP) is another relatively uncommon disorder in which platelet aggregation on the microvascular endothelium results in serious complications. In most cases, it is an acute disorder of unknown cause that affects young adults (ages 20–50, with a peak incidence in the third decade). TTP occurs more frequently in females than in males. It is characterized by the same tetrad of clinical findings as HUS (thrombocytopenia, microangiopathic hemolytic anemia, neurological abnormalities, and renal dysfunction), but with the addition of fever as a fifth clinical finding (Table 20-2 ✪). Neurological symptoms are more severe and more prominent in TTP than HUS. Because of the similarity in clinical symptoms, there has been considerable ongoing debate as to whether HUS and TTP are simply different clinical expressions of the same disease. However, the conditions respond differently to treatment and are still described as separate entities.[12]

Although it is primarily a disorder of unknown cause, a variety of clinical events have been identified as possible precipitating factors (Table 20-5 ✪). Infections are the most common precipitating factor (40%), followed by pregnancy (10–25%). Without treatment, TTP has a mortality rate in excess of 90% due to multiorgan failure.

✪ TABLE 20-5

Some Reported Clinical Conditions That May Be Precipitating Factors in TTP

- Infections

  Bacterial—enteric organisms

Shigella sp.	*E. coli*
Salmonella sp.	*Campylobacter* sp.
Yersinia sp.	

  Bacterial—other

  Streptococcus pneumoniae

  Legionella sp.

  Mycoplasma sp.

  Viral

HIV	EBV
Influenza	Herpes simplex

- Pregnancy or oral-contraceptive related
- Lymphomas and carcinomas
- Drugs

  Antimicrobials—penicillin

  Ticlopidine

  Chemotherapeutic agents

- Connective tissue diseases

  Systemic lupus erythematosus (SLE)

  Rheumatoid arthritis (RA)

  Ankylosing spondylitis

  Sjogren's syndrome

- Miscellaneous

  Bee sting

  Dog bite

  Carbon monoxide poisoning

Different variants of TTP have been recognized:

- Single episode
- Intermittent relapsing
- Chronic relapsing
- Childhood/familial[12]

Single-episode TTP is the most common presentation. In this type, there is no identifiable precipitating condition and no recurrence. In intermittent relapsing TTP (11–36% of cases), the patient has episodes of TTP that recur after healthy periods of months or years.[12] Chronic relapsing TTP, on the other hand, is characterized by very frequent recurrent episodes. These individuals have unusually large multimers of von Willebrand factor (ULvWF) in their plasma even between episodes. A number of cases of the chronic relapsing form have been associated with the presence of lupus anticoagulant.[13] In the few cases of childhood/familial TTP that have been reported, TTP begins very early in life (6 months of age) with multiple relapses continuing through adult life. Reports of families with multiple siblings with recurrent childhood TTP have been described. Cases of secondary TTP have been linked to drug therapy with cyclosporin or ticlopidine.[12,14] There is some indication that persons with HIV infection may be more susceptible to attacks of TTP.[12]

Pathophysiology Although the formation, structure, and function of **von Willebrand factor (vWF)** will be discussed in depth in the chapters on primary hemostasis (∞ Chapters 34 and 36), it is necessary to briefly explain its function now in order to understand TTP. vWF is a glycoprotein composed of identical subunits that combine to form molecules of varying sizes. The subunits are stored in Weibel-Palade bodies of the endothelial cells in blood vessels and are secreted after injury to the vessel. Subsequently the subunits form dimers and multimers in the plasma. vWF, along with glycoprotein Ib, serves as a "bridge" to help platelets adhere to collagen and initiate the platelet response that results in the primary hemostatic plug. It also participates in fibrin clot formation by serving as a carrier for Factor VIII, one of the hemostatic proteins. The vWF is degraded after hemostasis is complete.

TTP is characterized by multiple hyaline-like platelet microthrombi occluding capillaries and arterioles in a variety of organs, most frequently the kidneys, brain, pancreas, heart, spleen, and adrenal glands. Immunohistochemical stains have shown that the thrombi contain platelets and sometimes also contain immunoglobin and complement.[15] In comparison to the microthrombi in disseminated intravascular coagulation, DIC, (see later section), there is little fibrin present. There is also little inflammation or subendothelial exposure.[12]

The primary stimulus for the vascular deposits is unknown but is probably due either to damage of the endothelial lining of small blood vessel walls, resulting in enhanced platelet aggregation, or to platelet activation and subsequent

endothelial damage. Early investigations into TTP focused on several possible causes including:[15]

- Defect in prostaglandin $I_2(PGI_2)$ synthesis. PGI_2 has important thromboresistant properties because of its potent inhibition of platelet activation. It has been reported that plasma from patients with TTP depresses the synthesis of PGI_2 in the vessel wall and also rapidly degrades PGI_2 in the plasma.
- Depressed fibrinolysis (lysis of a fibrin clot). Fibrinolytic activity is depressed at the site of microthrombin formation. Decreased tissue plasminogen activator activity and decreased levels of protein C also have been seen in TTP plasma. Impaired fibrinolysis may contribute to the stability of the platelet plug and enhance tissue injury.
- von Willebrand Factor anomaly. One of the agents implicated is unusually large von Willebrand factor (ULvWF) multimers, not typically found in normal plasma or in TTP plasma during remission but found in plasma during TTP episodes.[16] These multimers are very effective in binding to glycoproteins (Ib and IIb/IIIa) on the endothelial cell surface and inducing platelet aggregation. These multimers may be the agents responsible for inducing platelet aggregation in TTP.
- In some patients, a deficiency in a protease that cleaves vWF or an antibody that inhibits this protease has been identified.[17–19] Most evidence now implicates the lack of vWF-cleaving protease as the major reason for TTP. In normal patients, when the vWF multimers attach to the endothelial lining, shear stress unfolds the molecules and enhances proteolysis by vWF-cleaving protein. In patients with TTP, the enzyme is lacking, and the unfolded multimers bind to platelets.[20] In acute cases there is evidence that an IgG antibody that inhibits the protease is present.[20] In other cases, no antibody can be identified and the cause of the deficiency in the protease is unknown.

Clinical Findings The clinical aspects of TTP are similar to those of HUS except that TTP occurs most often in young adults and involves more organ systems. Neurologic symptoms are more prominent, renal dysfunction is less severe, and the mortality rate is higher than in HUS.

The variety of manifestations present in TTP reflects damage to multiple organs. The widespread thrombotic process results in visual defects, heart failure, abdominal pain, and damage to the pancreas and adrenal glands. Central nervous system damage, however, is the most constant finding. Headaches, confusion, seizures, and coma reflect cerebral lesions. In HIV-associated TTP, the central nervous system abnormalities are more severe.[21,22]

Symptoms may be reversible if treated early, although some patients recovering from TTP may have permanent manifestations of hematuria, proteinuria, and increased blood urea nitrogen. Some patients require dialysis and in rare cases, chronic renal failure occurs. Jaundice reflects both hemolysis and liver damage.

Laboratory Findings Typical laboratory results are shown in Table 20-4 ✪. The hemoglobin is usually less than 10.5 g/dL (average, 8–9 g/dL). The MCV is variable. It may be normal or decreased if there is marked erythrocyte fragmentation or increased, depending on the degree of reticulocytosis. The MCH and MCHC are normal. Reticulocytes are increased as evidenced by the presence of increased polychromasia. Nucleated erythrocytes are found in the peripheral blood reflecting the bone marrow response to hemolysis. The most striking blood finding is the abundance of shistocytes. Leukocytosis with counts of over 20×10^9/L occurs in 50% of patients and is usually accompanied by a shift to the left. Thrombocytopenia is often severe ($8–44 \times 10^9$/L) due to consumption of platelets in the formation of microthrombi. Megakaryocytes are abundant in the bone marrow. The bleeding time may be prolonged if the platelet count is less than 100×10^9L.

Coagulation tests are usually normal or only mildly disturbed in TTP, which helps differentiate TTP from DIC, in which there is an increase in fibrin degradation products, as well as prolonged PT, APTT, and thrombin time.

Hemoglobinemia, hemoglobinuria, decreased haptoglobin levels, and increased serum bilirubin are direct evidence of intravascular hemolysis.

A biopsy of affected tissue to demonstrate the vascular lesion typical of TTP is sometimes done but is not considered necessary. Inguinal nodes have been recommended as the biopsy site because vessels in lymph node capsules contain typical lesions and bleeding can be controlled with pressure.

Therapy TTP is a relatively rare disorder, making the establishment of treatment protocols difficult. With early diagnosis and new modes of therapy, 80% or more of TTP patients survive. Although infusion with **fresh frozen plasma (FFP)** was once used as primary treatment for TTP, studies have shown that plasma exchange with FFP is more effective.[23,24] Patients undergoing plasma exchange have shown a higher response rate and lower mortality than those given only plasma infusions. With plasma exchange, the deficiency of vWF cleaving protease is reversed and the factors responsible for damaging the endothelium are removed. Recently, the use of **cryosupernatant** instead of FFP has been introduced. This product lacks the large vWF multimers present in FFP, yet still contains the vWF cleaving protease missing in TTP patients.[25–27] Platelet transfusions are contraindicated because of the increased risk of thrombosis.

Antiplatelet agents such as aspirin and dipyridamole have widespread use as platelet inhibitor drugs. In some patients intravenous administration of steroids has been used as adjunct therapy. Vincristine in combination with corticosteroids and plasma also has been used. Splenectomy is reported to have beneficial effects in patients who do not respond to plasma exchange or in patients with the chronic relapsing type.

Disseminated Intravascular Coagulation

Disseminated intravascular coagulation (DIC) is a complex condition in which the normal coagulation process is altered by an underlying condition, resulting in complications such as thrombotic occlusion of vessels, bleeding, and ultimately organ failure. The more common conditions that precipitate DIC include bacterial sepsis, neoplasms, immunologic disorders or trauma.[28] (Table 20-6 ✪). DIC is initiated by damage to the endothelial lining of vessels. This damage causes release of thromboplastic substances that activate the coagulation mechanism in vivo. As a result, there is deposition of fibrin in the microvasculature. As erythrocytes become entangled in the fibrin meshwork in the capillaries (clothesline effect) they fragment to form schistocytes. Hemolysis is not usually severe, but the effects of consumptive coagulopathy (consumption of various coagulation proteins and platelets) may cause thrombocytopenia and serious bleeding complications.

The typical findings on the blood smear include the presence of schistocytes and thrombocytopenia (Figure 20-3 ◼). However, it is the abnormal coagulation tests that help dis-

✪ TABLE 20-6

Causes of Disseminated Intravascular Coagulation

Bacterial sepsis	Endotoxins
	Exotoxins
Neoplasm	Solid tumors
	Myeloproliferative disorders
Serious trauma	
Immunologic disorders	Hemolytic transfusion reactions
	Transplant rejection
Miscellaneous	Venom—snake or insect
	Drugs

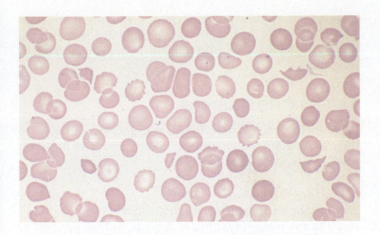

FIGURE 20-3 Peripheral blood from patient with disseminated intravascular coagulation. Notice the schistocytes and thrombocytopenia. (Wright stain; 1000× magnification)

tinguish this condition from others (TTP and HUS) that give a similar picture on a peripheral blood smear. Abnormal coagulation tests include:

- Prolonged prothrombin time (PT), activated partial thromboplastin time (APTT), and thrombin time (TT)
- Increase in fibrin degradation products (FDP)
- Decrease in fibrinogen

If the prothrombin time, fibrinogen, and platelet count are all abnormal, DIC may be diagnosed with greater than 90% certainty. If only two of the three are abnormal but the concentration (titer) of FDP is high, diagnostic accuracy remains greater than 90%. Treatment may include erythrocyte and platelet transfusions as well as infusion of fresh frozen plasma or factor concentrates to replace coagulation factors. Most important, however, is the treatment and resolution of the underlying disorder responsible for the DIC. The etiology, diagnosis, and treatment of DIC will be discussed further in ∞ Chapter 37.

 Checkpoint! #6

Explain how DIC can be differentiated from TTP and HUS based on coagulation tests.

HELLP Syndrome

The **HELLP syndrome** is an obstetric complication characterized by **h**emolysis, **e**levated **l**iver enzymes, and a **l**ow **p**latelet count. The etiology and pathogenesis are not well understood. As with TTP and HUS, the precipitating factor is unknown, but the clinical aspects are characterized by capillary endothelial damage and intravascular platelet activation.[29] HELLP shares some of the characteristics of preeclampsia and eclampsia such as hypertension and pro-

teinuria, but is distinguished from these by the three aspects that gave it its name. Approximately 10% of pregnancies with eclampsia develop HELLP syndrome, with a mortality rate of about 1%.[30,31]

The peripheral blood findings are similar to those found in TTP, HUS, or other microangiopathic conditions. Overall, however, the hemolysis and thrombocytopenia are less severe than that associated with TTP or HUS. Liver damage is due primarily to obstruction of hepatic sinusoids by fibrin and subsequent hemorrhage or necrosis.[29,30] The liver enzyme most frequently measured is aspartate aminotransferase (AST) and levels >70 IU/L are common. Coagulation tests such as the PT and APTT are usually normal until late in the course of the disease.[32] The platelet count is usually $<100,000 \times 10^9$/L. Although DIC infrequently occurs as a complication of HELLP, patients may have an undetectable underlying coagulopathy.[29]

Steroid therapy may be useful in controlling cell destruction if the fetus cannot be immediately delivered. Plasma exchange is rarely used as a treatment. The use of dexamethasone has eliminated the need for platelet transfusions in most patients with platelet counts $<50 \times 10^9$/L.[32]

 CASE STUDY *(continued from page 376)*

Ms. Chang's (PT and APTT) were only slightly prolonged. The fibrinogen levels were slightly decreased.

4. What do these findings indicate about the underlying problem?

Malignant Hypertension

The hemolytic anemia associated with malignant hypertension is characterized by a low platelet count and erythrocyte fragmentation. The mechanism of hemolysis is unknown. It has been suggested that it may be caused by fibrinoid necrosis of arterioles or deposition of fibrin fed by thromboplastic substances released from membranes of lysed erythrocytes. Hemolysis disappears when the blood pressure is lowered.

Traumatic Cardiac Hemolytic Anemia

This hemolytic anemia is an uncommon complication following surgical insertion of prosthetic heart valves. Excessive acceleration or turbulence of blood flow around the valve tears the erythrocytes apart from shear stress. The term *Waring blender syndrome* has been used to describe this disorder because of the localized turbulent blood flow. Many erythrocyte fragments are apparent on the blood smear. Some of the severely traumatized cells are removed by the spleen, but most undergo intravascular hemolysis. In severe anemia the patient must have the valve replaced.[33]

Thermal Injury

Hemolytic anemia occurs within the first 24–46 hours after extensive thermal burns, and the degree of hemolysis depends upon the percentage of body surface area burned. Hemolysis probably results from the direct effect of heat on spectrin in the erythrocyte membrane. (If erythrocytes are heated to 48°C in vitro, they lose elasticity and deformability due to degradation of spectrin.) Peripheral blood smears show erythrocyte budding, schistocytes, and spherocytes. After 48 hours, signs of hemolysis such as hemoglobinuria and hemoglobinemia are no longer prominent. Thermal injury to erythrocytes has also occurred during hemodialysis when the dialysate is overheated.

March Hemoglobinuria

March hemoglobinuria describes a transient hemolytic anemia occurring after strenuous exercise that involves contact with a hard surface (e.g., running, tennis). However, it is not seen in every individual participating in these activities. The hemolysis is probably due to physical injury to erythrocytes as they pass through the capillaries of the feet. At least two cases of March hemoglobinuria have been reported in individuals with varicosity of the long saphenous veins.[34] After crossectomy of the vein and resection of the convolutes, the episodes of hemoglobinuria ceased.

In contrast to the other hemolytic conditions discussed so far in this chapter, there are no erythrocyte fragments seen on the peripheral blood smear, but the hallmarks of intravascular hemolysis—hemoglobinemia and hemoglobinuria—are present. The passage of reddish urine immediately after exercise and for several hours thereafter is usually the only complaint from affected individuals. Osmotic and mechanical fragility tests are normal. Anemia is uncommon, as less than 1% of the erythrocytes are hemolyzed during an attack. Iron deficiency may occur if exercise and hemolysis are frequent.

CASE STUDY *(continued from page 377)*

The patient's symptoms continued to become worse with frequent seizures, headaches, and dizziness. Her urinalysis results showed a 2+ protein and moderate blood. However, she had normal urinary volume.

5. Based on these results, what is the most likely condition associated with these clinical and laboratory results? Explain.

6. What therapy might be used?

► HEMOLYTIC ANEMIAS CAUSED BY ANTAGONISTS IN THE BLOOD

In addition to the hemolysis caused by abnormal erythrocyte structure or plasma lipid disorders, antagonists such as drugs or venoms and infectious organisms in the environment of the erythrocyte may cause premature destruction (Table 20-1 ✪). This hemolysis is precipitated by either injury to the erythrocyte membrane or to denaturation of hemoglobin.

INFECTIOUS AGENTS

Parasites or bacteria may infect erythrocytes and lead to their destruction. Alternatively, toxins produced by infectious agents may cause hemolysis.

Malarial Parasites

The anemia accompanying malaria is due directly and indirectly to the intracellular malarial parasites that live part of their life cycle in the erythrocyte (Figure 20-4 ■). The anemia resulting from this mechanism is usually mild but can be severe in infection with *Plasmodium falciparum* because of the high levels of parasitemia in this form of malaria. The release of the intraerythrocytic parasite from the cell results in destruction of the cell. On the other hand, the spleen may remove the entire parasitized cell, or splenic macrophages may pit the parasite from the erythrocyte, damaging the cell membrane. Anemia may also result from an immune-mediated process whereby antimalarial antibodies react with malarial antigens on the erythrocyte membrane resulting in removal of the sensitized cell by the splenic macrophages. In some cases, there is a decrease in the concentration of complement regulatory proteins, which may facilitate complement-mediated hemolysis.[35]

Blackwater fever, an uncommon complication of infection with *P. falciparum*, is characterized by massive acute intravascular hemolysis with hemoglobinemia, hemoglobinuria, methemalbuminemia, and hyperbilirubinemia. The mechanism that precipitates this is unclear. One possible mechanism is development of an autoantibody to the infected erythrocyte. Another is a reaction to use of the drug quinine. Use of synthetic quinine drugs has considerably decreased frequency of this complication.

Babesiosis

Babesiosis is a protozoan infection of rodents and cattle that may be transmitted to humans by the bite of a tick or through blood transfusions. On the peripheral blood smear, the parasites appear as intracellular, pleomorphic, ringlike structures resembling ring form trophozoites of *Plasmodium falciparum*. Although infections are often subclinical or mild, moderate anemia and thrombocytopenia may be present. Extravascular hemolysis may occur in a manner similar to that seen with malaria. In a rare fulminating infection, severe anemia, intravascular hemolysis, and hemoglobinuria may be seen. Complications associated with the intravascular hemolysis include renal failure and disseminated intravascular coagulation. Patients who are splenectomized generally have a more severe clinical presentation and parasitemia levels greater than 50%.

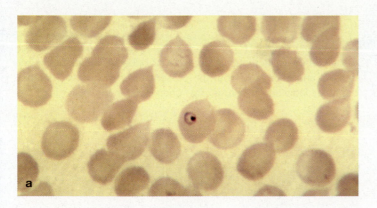
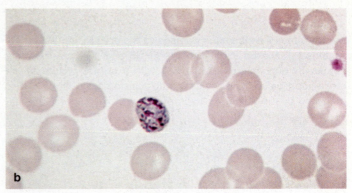

■ **FIGURE 20-4** Peripheral blood smears from patients with malaria. **a.** There is a ring form of malaria in the erythrocyte. **b.** There is an immature schizont form of malaria in the erythrocyte. (Wright stain; 1000× magnification)

✔ **Checkpoint! #7**

Why do malaria and babesiosis result in anemia?

Bartonellosis

One type of bartonellosis—the infection by *Bartonella bacilliformis*—is characterized by an acute, severe febrile hemolytic anemia (Oroya fever). The disease, which is restricted to Columbia, Peru, and Ecuador, is transmitted by sandflies. The rod- or round-shaped (coccobacillary) organisms are readily visualized as single, paired, or chained organisms on or within erythrocytes on Wright- or Giemsa-stained peripheral blood smears during the course of the disease. Several proteins released by the organism are responsible for inducing the pitting or invagination of the erythrocyte membrane. These proteins may help explain the mechanism of cell destruction.[36]

Clostridium perfringens

Rapid hemolysis develops from bacteremia and other infections with *Clostridium perfringens* (as well as with other clostridial species such as *C. septicum*) due to the release of potent hemolysins. The major hemolytic toxin (alpha toxin) is a phospholipase C that hydrolyzes sphingomyelin and lecithin present in the erythrocyte membrane. Hemoglobinuria may be seen; anuria or acute renal failure may develop. The peripheral blood smear shows many microspherocytes and erythrocyte fragments accompanied by thrombocytopenia.

ANIMAL VENOMS

Venoms injected by bees, wasps, spiders, and scorpions may cause hemolysis in some susceptible individuals. The mechanism of damage from the venom from the bite of a brown recluse spider appears to involve the cleavage of glycophorin from the erythrocyte membrane, making it more sensitive to complement-mediated intravascular hemolysis.[37] Although snake bites rarely cause hemolysis directly, they may cause hemolysis secondary to disseminated intravascular coagulation.[38]

Chemicals and Drugs

A variety of chemicals and drugs have been identified that may cause erythrocyte hemolysis; many of these are dose dependent. In addition to causing erythrocyte hemolysis, chemicals and drugs may also produce methemoglobinemia and cyanosis or, in some instances, aplasia of the bone marrow.

Hemoglobinemia and hemoglobinuria may occur as a result of osmotic lysis of erythrocytes. This may occur when water enters the vascular system during transurethral resection or when inappropriate solutions are used during a blood transfusion.

Some drugs known to cause hemolysis in G6PD deficient persons can also cause hemolysis in normal persons if the dose is sufficiently high. The mechanism of hemolysis is similar to that in G6PD deficiency with hemoglobin denaturation and Heinz body formation due to strong oxidants.

The anemia of lead poisoning is usually classified with sideroblastic anemias since the pathophysiologic and hematologic findings are similar. Lead inhibits heme synthesis, causing an accumulation of iron within mitochondria (∞ Chapter 11). However, it is apparent that lead also damages the erythrocyte membrane. This damage is manifested by an increase in osmotic fragility and mechanical fragility.

SUMMARY

Mechanisms of nonimmune damage to the erythrocyte are varied. Of those discussed in this chapter, HUS and TTP are the more commonly encountered, presenting with a classic picture of microangiopathic hemolytic anemia with schistocytes. Classic HUS is mediated by the Shiga-like toxin of *E. coli* O157:H7, while the underlying causes of TTP are varied. Intraerythrocytic parasitic infections with organisms such as malaria or babesiosis can cause hemolysis and anemia without the presence of schistocytes. In susceptible individuals, drugs or chemicals may also lead to hemolysis.

REVIEW QUESTIONS

LEVEL I

1. In which of the following conditions is the formation of schistocytes *not* associated with microthrombi? (Checklist #1, 2)
   a. hemolytic uremic syndrome
   b. hypertension
   c. thrombotic thrombocytopenic purpura
   d. disseminated intravascular coagulation

2. One of the major criteria that distinguishes DIC from other causes of microangiopathic hemolytic anemia is: (Checklist #2)
   a. presence of schistocytes
   b. thrombocytopenia
   c. decreased hemoglobin
   d. abnormal coagulation tests

3. A patient who has anemia with an increased reticulocyte count and increased bilirubin and has many schistocytes on the blood smear may have: (Checklist #2)
   a. MAHA
   b. high cholesterol in the blood
   c. spur cell anemia
   d. immune hemolytic anemia

4. Which of the following organisms *does not* cause damage of the erythrocyte because of an intra-erythrocytic life cycle? (Checklist #4)
   a. *Plasmodium falciparum*
   b. *Babesia* sp
   c. *Bartonella* sp
   d. *Clastridium perfringens*

5. A characteristic finding on a blood smear in MAHA is: (Checklist #3)
   a. target cells
   b. spur cells
   c. schistocytes
   d. echinocytes

6. All of the following are characterized as causes of MAHA *except*: (Checklist #1)
   a. TTP
   b. prosthetic heart valves
   c. HUS
   d. March hemoglobinuria

LEVEL II

1. A 43-year-old woman presents to her physician with a 3 week history of fatigue, constant headache, and low-grade fever. Selected laboratory results include:

   Hemoglobin: 7.5 g/dL   Platelet count: 16×10^9/L
   Hematocrit: 0.23 L/L   Reticulocytes: 11%
   RDW: 15

   Peripheral blood smear showed schistocytes. Which of the following drugs that the patient was taking might cause these symptoms and lab values? (Checklist #2, 4)
   a. ticlopidine
   b. aspirin
   c. estrogens
   d. penicillin

2. A 34-year-old woman is brought into the ER after falling off a ladder while painting her house. Selected lab results include:

   Hemoglobin: 8 g/dL   PT: 36 seconds
   Hematocrit: 0.25 L/L   APTT: >75 seconds
   Platelet count: 20×10^9/L   Fibrinogen: 100 mg/dL

   Peripheral blood smear shows schistocytes. Given these results, what is the most likely diagnosis? (Checklist #2, 4).
   a. HELLP syndrome
   b. TTP
   c. DIC
   d. traumatic hemolytic anemia

3. The following results were obtained on a small child who had easy bruising, tiredness, difficulty breathing, and decreased urinary output. His mother indicated he had an episode of bloody diarrhea about 2 weeks previously but it had not recurred.

   Hemoglobin: 65 g/L; platelets: 41×10^9/L; PT and PTT within normal reference ranges.

   Based on the clinical and limited laboratory findings, what is the most likely condition? (Checklist #2, 4)
   a. TTP
   b. bartonellosis
   c. *Clostridium* sp infection
   d. HUS

REVIEW QUESTIONS (continued)

LEVEL I

7. All of the following are associated with HUS *except:* (Checklist #2)
   a. thrombocytosis
   b. nucleated RBCs
   c. schistocytes
   d. reticulocytosis

8. MAHA is most frequently caused by: (Checklist #1)
   a. physical trauma to the cell
   b. immune destruction
   c. antagonists in the blood
   d. plasma lipid abnormalities

9. Intravascular hemolysis in MAHA would be associated with which of the following parameters? (Checklist #2)

Bilirubin	Haptoglobin
a. decreased	decreased
b. decreased	increased
c. increased	decreased
d. increased	increased

10. MAHA due to HUS is usually seen in which age group? (Checklist #1)
    a. children under 1 year old
    b. females between 20 and 50 years of age
    c. either sex under 50 years of age
    d. males older than 16 years of age

LEVEL II

4. The most likely age group for developing TTP is: (Checklist #2)
   a. female children under 1 year old
   b. females between 20 and 50 years of age
   c. either sex under 5 years of age
   d. males older than 16 years of age

5. Which of the following disorders is *not* characterized by the presence of schistocytes? (Checklist #3)
   a. march hemoglobinuria
   b. insertion of a prosthetic valve
   c. third-degree burns
   d. malignant hypertension

6. A patient with a deficiency in the von Willebrand factor cleaving protein would be at risk to develop what condition? (Checklist #2)
   a. HUS
   b. spur cell anemia
   c. TTP
   d. hereditary acanthocytosis

7. The formation of schistocytes in MAHA is primarily due to: (Checklist #1)
   a. pitting by splenic macrophages
   b. defective cell membranes
   c. increased membrane phospholipids
   d. shearing of erythrocytes by fibrin threads

8. Plasma exchange is used as a primary treatment for which of the following? (Checklist #2)
   a. HUS
   b. TTP
   c. abetalipoproteinemia
   d. DIC

9. The peripheral blood smear from a 6-months-pregnant woman showed the presence of schistocytes. Platelet count was $<60 \times 10^9$/L and her hemoglobin was 75 g/L. She has no history of chronic disease. What laboratory tests might give a clue to the underlying cause? (Checklist #4)
   a. haptoglobin
   b. reticulocyte count
   c. liver enzymes
   d. APTT and PT

10. Hemolytic toxins are the major cause of intravascular hemolysis in diseases or conditions caused by which of the following organisms? (Checklist #5)
    a. *Plasmodium falciparum*
    b. *Babesia* sp.
    c. *Bartonella bacilliformis*
    d. *Clostridium perfringens*

www.prenhall.com/mckenzie
Use the above address to access the free, interactive Companion Web site created for this textbook. Get hints, instant feedback, and textbook references to chapter-related multiple choice questions.

REFERENCES

1. Parsonnet J, Griffin PM. Hemolytic uremic syndrome: Clinical picture and bacterial connection. *Curr Clin Top Infec Dis.* 1993; 13:172–87.

2. Melnyk AM, Solez K, Kjellstrand CM. Adult hemolytic-uremic syndrome: A review of 37 cases. *Arch Intern Med.* 1995; 155:2077–84.

3. Robson WLM, Leung AKC, Kaplan BS. Hemolytic-uremic syndrome. *Curr Prob Pediatr.* 1993; 23:16–33.

4. Gherman RB, Tramont J, Connito DJ. Postpartum hemolytic-uremic syndrome associated with lupus anticoagulant. *J. Reproductive Medicine.* 1999; 44:471–74.

5. Altekruse SF, Cohen M, Swerdlow DL. Emerging foodborne diseases. *Emerging Infect. Dis.* 1997; 3:285–93.

6. Besser RE, Griffin PM, Slutsker L. Escherichia coli O157:H7 gastroenteritis and the hemolytic uremic syndrome: An emerging infectious disease. *Ann. Rev. Med.* 1999; 50:355–67.

7. Sassetti B, Vizcarguenaga MI, Zanaro NL, Silva MV, Kordich L, Florentini L, et al. Hemolytic uremic syndrome in children: Platelet aggregation and membrane glycoproteins. *J Pediatr Hematol Oncol.* 1999; 21:123–28.

8. Cabrera G, Fortenberry J, Warshaw BL, Chambliss CR, Butler JC, Cooperstone BG. Hemolytic uremic syndrome associated with invasive *Streptococcus pneumoniae* infection. *Pediatrics.* 1998; 101: 689–703.

9. VonVigier RO, Seibel K, Bianchetti MG. Positive Coombs' test in Pneumococcus-associated hemolytic uremic syndrome. *Nephron.* 1999; 82:183–84.

10. Wong CS, Jelacic S, Habeeb R, Watkins SL, Tarr PI. The risk of hemolytic-uremic syndrome after antibiotic treatment of Escherichia coli O157:H7 infections. *N Engl J Med,* 2000; 342:1930–36.

11. Tapper D, Tarr P, Avner E, Brandt J, Walddhansen J. Lessons learned in the management of hemolytic uremic syndrome in children. *J Pediatr Surg.* 1995; 30:158–63.

12. Allford SL, Machin SJ. Current understanding of the pathophysiology of thrombotic thrombocytopenic purpura. *J Clin Pathol.* 2000; 53:497–501.

13. Trent K, Neustater BR, Lottenberg R. Chronic relapsing thrombotic thrombocytopenic purpura and antiphospholipid antibodies: A report of two cases. *Am. J. Hematol.* 1997; 54:155–59.

14. Chen D, Kim J, Sutton DMC. Thrombotic throbocytopenic purpura associated with ticlopidine use: A report of 3 cases and review of the literature. *Arch Intern Med.* 1999; 159:311–14.

15. Rose M, Rowe JM, Eldor A. The changing course of thrombotic thrombocytopenic purpura and modern therapy. *Blood Reviews.* 1993; 7:94–103.

16. Moake JL. Thrombotic thrombocytopenic purpura and the hemolytic uremic syndrome. In: *Hematology: Basic Principles and Practice.* Edited by R Hoffman, EJ Benz, SJ Shattil, B Furie, HJ Cohen. New York: Churchill Livingstone; 1991.

17. Moake J. Studies on the pathophysiology of thrombotic thrombocytopenic purpura. *Semin. Hematol.* 1997; 34:83–89.

18. Furlan M, Robles R, Solenthaler M, Wassmer M, Sandoz P, Lammle B. Deficient activity of Von Willebrand factor-cleaving protease in chronic relapsing thrombotic thrombocytopenic purpura. *Blood.* 1997; 89:3097–103.

19. Furlan M, Robles R, Galbusera N, Remozzi G, Kyrle PA, Brenner B, et al. Von Willebrand factor-cleaving protease in thrombotic thrombocytopenic purpura and the hemolytic uremic syndrome. *NEJM.* 1998; 339:1578–84.

20. Tsai HM, Lian ECY. Antibodies to von Willebrand factor-cleaving protease in acute thrombotic thrombocytopenic purpura. *N Engl J Med.* 1998; 339:1585–94.

21. Hymes KB, Karpattkin S. Human immunodeficiency virus infection and thrombotic microangiopathy. *Semin Hematol.* 1997; 34: 117–25.

22. Sutor GC, Schmidt RE, Albrecht, H. Thrombotic microangiopathies and HIV infection: Report of two typical cases, features of HUS and TTP, and review of the literature. *Infection.* 1999; 27:12–15.

23. Lara PN, Coe TL, Zhou H, Fernanco L, Holland PV, Wun T. Improved survival with plasma exchange in patients with thrombotic thrombocytopenic purpura-hemolytic uremic syndrome. *Am J Med.* 1999; 107:573–79.

24. Ellis J, Theodossiou C, Schrwarzenberger P. Treatment of thrombotic thrombocytopenic purpura with the cryosupernatant fraction of plasma: A case report and review of the literature. *Am. J. Med. Sci.* 1999; 318:190–93.

25. Owens MR, Sweeney JD, Tahhan RH, Fortkolt P. Influence of type of exchange fluid on survival in therapeutic apheresis for thrombotic thrombocytopenic purpura. *J. Clin Apheresis.* 1995; 10: 178–82.

26. Rock G, Shumak KH, Sutton DMC, Buskard NA, Nair RC. Cryosupernatant as replacement fluid for plasma exchange in thrombotic thrombocytopenic purpura. *Br J Haematol.* 1996; 94:383–86.

27. Colflesh CR, Agarwal R, Knochel JP. Timing of plasma exchange therapy for thrombotic thrombocytopenia purpura: A brief clinical observation. *Am J Med Sci.* 1996; 31:167–86.

28. Levi M, Ten Cate H. Current concepts: Disseminated intravascular coagulation. *N Engl J Med.* 1999; 341:586–92.

29. Padden MO. HELLP syndrome: Recognition and perinatal management. *Am Fam Physician.* 1999; 60:829–36, 839.

30. Egerman RS, Sibai BM. HELLP syndrome. *Clin Obstet Gynecol.* 1999; 42:381–89.

31. Sibai BM, Ramadan MK, Usta I, Salama M, Mercer BM, Friedman SA. Maternal morbidity and mortality in 442 pregnancies with hemolysis, elevated liver enzymes, and low platelets (HELLP syndrome). *Am J Obstet Gynecol.* 1993; 169:1000–6.

32. Magann EF, Martin JN. Twelve steps to optimal management of HELLP syndrome. *Clin Obstet Gynecol.* 1999; 42:532–50.

33. Maraj R, Jacobs LE, Ioli A, Kotler MN. Evaluation of hemolysis in patients with prosthetic heart valves. *Clinical Cardiology.* 1998; 21:387–92.

34. Schwurman AH, Breederveld RS, Rauwerda JA. Exertional (March) hemoglobinuria. *Neth J Surg.* 1991; 43:39–40.

35. Waitumbi JN, Opollo MO, Muga RO, Misore AO, Stoute JA. Red cell surface changes and erythrophagocytosis in children with severe Plasmodium falciparum anemia. *Blood.* 2000; 95:1481–86.

36. Hendrix LR. Contact-dependent hemolytic activity distinct from deforming activity of Bartonella bacilliformis. *FEMS Microbiology Letters.* 2000; 182:119–24.

37. Tambourgi DV, Morgan BP, deAndrade RM, Magnoli FC, vanDenBerg CW. Loxosceles intermedia spider envenomation induces activation of an endogenous metalloproteinase, resulting in cleavage of glycophorins from the erythrocyte surface and facilitating complement-mediated lysis. *Blood.* 2000; 95:683–91.

38. Boyer LV, Seifert SA, Clark RF, McNally JT, Williams S, Nordt SP, et al. Recurrent and persistent coagulopathy following pit viper envenomation. *Arch Int Med.* 1999; 159:706–10.

SECTION FIVE • NONMALIGNANT DISORDERS OF LEUKOCYTES

21

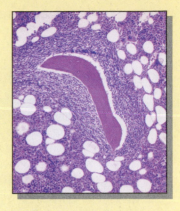

Nonmalignant Granulocyte and Monocyte Disorders

Kathleen M. Mugan, M.Ed.

■ CHECKLIST - LEVEL I

At the end of this unit of study the student should be able to:

1. Recognize neutrophilia from hematologic data and name the common disorders associated with neutrophilia.
2. Explain the quantitative and qualitative neutrophil response to acute bacterial infections.
3. Identify immature granulocytes and morphologic changes (toxic granulation, Döhle bodies, intracellular organisms, and vacuoles) often seen in reactive neutrophilia.
4. Define and recognize *leukemoid reaction, leukoerythroblastosis,* and *pyknotic nuclei.*
5. Distinguish leukemoid reaction from chronic myelogenous leukemia based on laboratory data including the leukocyte alkaline phosphatase.
6. Identify neutropenia from hematologic data and list the common disorders associated with neutropenia.
7. Recognize the conditions associated with spurious, or false, neutropenia.
8. Identify neutrophil nuclear alterations including Pelger-Huët, hypersegmentation, and pyknotic forms.
9. Recognize as abnormal and seek assistance for identification of rare or unusual cytoplasmic abnormalities such as morulae, Alder-Reilly granules, or Chediak-Higashi inclusions.
10. State the common conditions associated with abnormal eosinophil, basophil, and monocyte counts.
11. Define *Gaucher* and *Niemann-Pick diseases.*

■ CHECKLIST - LEVEL II

At the end of this unit of study the student should be able to:

1. Assess the etiology, associated conditions, and peripheral blood findings for immediate, acute, chronic, and reactive neutrophilia.
2. Contrast the hematologic and clinical features for leukemoid reaction and chronic myelogenous leukemia (CML).
3. Organize neutropenia to include etiology and associated conditions, as well as blood and bone marrow findings.
4. Recognize, evaluate, and select appropriate corrective action for spurious or false neutropenia.

■ CHECKLIST - LEVEL II (continued)

5. Appraise the nuclear abnormalities of neutrophils including Pelger-Huët, pseudo-Pelger-Huët, hypersegmentation, and pyknotic nuclei and reconcile them with the appropriate clinical conditions of the patient.

6. Appraise the cytoplasmic abnormalities of neutrophils including toxic granulation, Döhle bodies, vacuoles, intracellular organisms, and morulae and reconcile them with the appropriate clinical conditions of the patient.

7. Recognize, differentiate the cellular abnormalities, and summarize the clinical features of the inherited granulocyte functional disorders (Chediak-Higashi, Alder-Reilly, May-Hegglin, and chronic granulomatous diseases).

8. Evaluate alterations in the relative and/or absolute numbers of eosinophils, basophils, and monocytes and associate them with the clinical condition of the patient.

9. Evaluate the etiology, laboratory findings, and clinical features of the lipid storage disorders.

10. Identify and differentiate the abnormal macrophages seen in Gaucher disease, Niemann-Pick disease, and sea-blue histiocytosis.

11. Construct an efficient and cost-effective reflex testing pathway for follow-up neutrophilia, neutropenia, and qualitative granulocyte abnormalities.

12. Evaluate a case study from a patient with a nonmalignant granulocyte disorder.

KEY TERMS

Agranulocytosis
Basophilia
Döhle bodies
Egress
Eosinophilia
Hypereosinophilic syndrome
Leukemoid reaction
Leukocytosis
Leukoerythroblastic reaction
Leukopenia
Monocytopenia
Monocytosis
Morulae
Myelophthisis
Neutropenia
Neutrophilia
Pelger-Huët anomaly
Pseudoneutrophilia
Reactive neutrophilia
Shift neutrophilia
Shift to the left
Toxic granules

BACKGROUND BASICS

The information in this chapter will build on concepts learned in previous chapters. To maximize your learning experience you should review this material before starting this unit of study.

Level I

▶ Summarize the production, kinetics, distribution, life span, and basic function of neutrophils and monocytes. (Chapter 6)

▶ Describe how leukocytes are counted and differentiated; recognize normal and immature granulocytes. (Chapters 6, 7, 8)

Level II

▶ Describe the role of specific neutrophil granules and enzymes in antimicrobial systems. (Chapter 6)

▶ Identify normal macrophages and discuss their role in the bone marrow and the rest of the reticuloendothelial system. (Chapter 6)

▶ Describe leukocyte maturation and proliferation pools in the bone marrow; describe the role of cytokines in bone marrow release of leukocytes; describe the process of leukocyte egress to tissue. (Chapters 2, 6, 9)

▶ Correlate the function of the reticuloendothelial organs to leukocyte distribution and demise. (Chapter 3)

℮ CASE STUDY

We will address this case throughout the chapter.

Dennis, a 24-year-old male, was taken to emergency surgery to repair several bone fractures sustained in an automobile accident. His previous medical history was unremarkable. He was in excellent health prior to the accident. Consider why this patient's condition could cause abnormal hematologic test results and the possible complications that could occur in this patient during his treatment and recovery. How could this affect hematologic test results?

▶ OVERVIEW

This chapter discusses benign changes in granulocytes and monocytes as a response to various nonmalignant disease states and toxic challenges. These changes include both quantitative and qualitative variations that can be detected by laboratory tests. The chapter is divided into sections covering changes in quantity and morphology of neutrophils, eosinophils, basophils, and monocytes in acquired and inherited states. Emphasis is on recognition of these abnormalities by the laboratory professional and correlation to the clinical condition of the patient.

▶ INTRODUCTION

It is well recognized that changes in leukocyte concentration and morphology are a normal response of the body to various disease processes and toxic challenges. Most often, one type of leukocyte is affected more than the others, providing an important clue to diagnosis. The type of cell affected depends in a large part on the function of that cell (i.e., bacterial infection commonly results in an absolute neutrophilia; viral infections are characterized by an absolute lymphocytosis; and certain parasitic infections cause an eosinophilia). Thus, determination of absolute concentrations of cell types aids in differential diagnosis, especially when the total leukocyte concentration is abnormal.

Leukocytosis refers to a condition in which the total leukocyte count is more than 11.0×10^9/L in an adult. Be aware that reference ranges vary significantly among different sources and laboratories. Refer to Table B on inside cover for leukocyte and differential reference ranges compiled from numerous references.[1-6] Although leukocytosis is usually due to an increase in neutrophils, it may also be related to an increase in lymphocytes or rarely in monocytes or eosinophils.

Quantitative variations of different types of leukocytes are evaluated by performing a total leukocyte count and a differential count. The absolute concentration of each type of leukocyte can be calculated from these two values as described in ∞ Chapter 6.

Absolute cells/L = total leukocyte count/L × percent of cell type from differential

 Checkpoint! #1

A patient's total leukocyte count is 5.0×10^9/L. There are 60% segmented neutrophils, 35% lymphocytes, and 5% monocytes on the differential.

1. Calculate the absolute number of each cell type.

2. Are each of these relative and absolute cell counts normal or abnormal?

Leukopenia refers to a decrease in leukocytes below 4×10^9/L. This condition is usually due to a decrease in neutrophils, but lymphocytes and other cell types may also contribute.

Morphologic or qualitative variations of leukocytes are noted by examination of the stained blood smear. Some qualitative changes affect cell function while others do not. Variations in the appearance of the cell together with its concentration may provide specific clues to the pathologic process.

▶ NEUTROPHIL DISORDERS

Quantitative disorders of neutrophils are usually reflected by changes in the total leukocyte count since neutrophils are the most numerous white blood cells in the peripheral blood. Automated cell counters will flag results outside the reference range. Neutrophilia is more common than neutropenia. On the other hand, qualitative changes in the neutrophils are not detected by automated cell counters. Detection of these changes requires careful microscopic examination of stained blood smears. Qualitative changes may provide important diagnostic information.

QUANTITATIVE DISORDERS

Quantitative abnormalities of neutrophils may occur because of a malignant or benign disorder. The malignant disorders are caused by neoplastic transformation of hematopoietic stem cells and will be discussed in ∞ Chapters 26–31. Benign disorders are usually acquired and may cause an increase (**neutrophilia**) or decrease (**neutropenia**) in neutrophils, but neutrophilia is more common. Table 21-1 ✪ lists three interrelated mechanisms affecting neutrophil concentration in the peripheral blood.

Neutrophilia

The normal neutrophil concentration varies with age and race, so it is important to evaluate the count based on reference ranges for each demographic group. Neutrophilia refers to an increase in the total circulating absolute neutrophil concentration (ANC). In adults, neutrophilia occurs when the concentration of neutrophils exceeds 7.0×10^9/L. (See Table B ✪ on inside cover for age- and race-specific reference ranges.)

✪ **TABLE 21-1**

Factors Affecting Neutrophil Concentration in Peripheral Blood

Bone marrow production and release of neutrophils
Rate of neutrophil egress to tissue or survival time in blood
Ratio of marginating to circulating neutrophils in peripheral blood

Benign neutrophilia occurs most often as a result of a reaction to a physiologic or pathologic process and is called **reactive neutrophilia**. Reactive neutrophilia may be immediate, acute, or chronic and may involve any or all of the three mechanisms listed in Table 21-1 ✪.

Immediate Neutrophilia

Immediate neutrophilia may occur without pathologic stimulus and is probably a simple redistribution of the marginated granulocyte pool (MGP) to the circulating granulocyte pool (CGP). Normally 50% of the neutrophils inside a blood vessel are freely circulating and the other 50% are loosely attached to the vessel endothelial cells (marginated) (∞ Chapter 6). Only cells freely circulating are counted by routine laboratory testing.

The neutrophil increase in immediate neutrophilia is immediate but transient (lasting about 20–30 minutes) and appears to be independent of bone marrow input and tissue **egress**. This type of neutrophilia is also referred to as **pseudoneutrophilia** or **shift neutrophilia** because there is no real change in the number of neutrophils within the vasculature. The increased circulating neutrophils are typically mature, normal cells. This redistribution of neutrophils is responsible for the physiologic neutrophilia that accompanies active exercise, epinephrine administration, anesthesia, and anxiety.

Acute Neutrophilia

Acute neutrophilia occurs within 4–5 hours of a pathologic stimulus (e.g., bacterial infection, toxin). This type of neutrophilia results from an increase in the flow of neutrophils from the bone marrow storage pool to the blood. The neutrophilia is more pronounced than in pseudoneutrophilia, and the proportion of immature neutrophils may increase. More bands appear if the tissue demand for neutrophils creates an acute shortage of segmented neutrophils in the storage pool. Continued demand may result in the release of metamyelocytes and myelocytes. As bone marrow production increases and the storage pool is replenished, the leukocyte differential returns to normal.

Chronic Neutrophilia

Chronic neutrophilia follows acute neutrophilia. If the stimulus for neutrophils continues beyond a few days, the storage pool will become depleted. The mitotic pool will then increase production in an attempt to meet the demand for neutrophils. In this state, the marrow will show increased numbers of early neutrophil precursors including myeloblasts, promyelocytes, and myelocytes. The blood will contain increased numbers of bands, metamyelocytes, myelocytes, and rarely promyelocytes. An increase in the concentration of immature forms of leukocytes in the circulation is termed a **shift to the left**.

Conditions Associated with Reactive Chronic Neutrophilia

Chronic neutrophilia caused by benign or toxic conditions usually is characterized by total leukocytes less than 50×10^9/L and a shift to the left. The immature cells are usually bands and metamyelocytes, but myelocytes and promyelocytes may be seen. Toxic changes including toxic

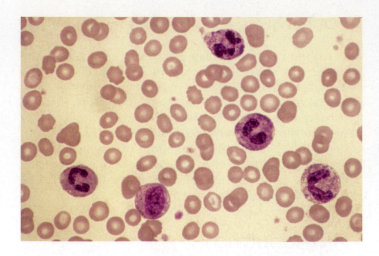

■ **FIGURE 21-1** A leukemoid reaction. There is an increased leukocyte count and a shift to the left. The cells have heavy toxic granulation and Döhle bodies suggesting an infectious or toxic reactive leukocytosis. (Peripheral blood; Wright-Giemsa stain; 1000× magnification)

granulation, **Döhle bodies** (light grayish blue cytoplasmic inclusions), and cytoplasmic vacuoles are often found even if the neutrophil count is normal (Figure 21-1 ■). The leukocyte alkaline phosphatase score may be elevated (∞ Chapter 26). Conditions associated with reactive chronic neutrophilia are listed in Table 21-2 ✪.

Bacterial Infection. The most common cause of neutrophilia is bacterial infection especially with pyrogenic organisms such as staphylococci and streptococci. Depending

✪ TABLE 21-2

Conditions Associated with Neutrophilia

Acute bacterial and fungal infections

Inflammatory processes:
  Tissue damage from burns, trauma, or surgery
  Collagen, vascular, and autoimmune disorders
  Hypersensitivity reactions

Metabolic alterations: uremia, eclampsia, and gout

Neoplasms

Acute hemorrhage or hemolysis

Rebound from bone marrow transplant or treatment with colony-stimulating growth factors

Certain chemicals, toxins, and drugs

Physiologic neutrophilia:
  Strenuous exercise, stress, pain, temperature extremes, childbirth labor, and in newborns

Chronic myeloproliferative disorders*

*In these disorders, increases in neutrophils are not reactive but rather due to a neoplasm of the hematopoietic stem cell.

upon the virulence of the microorganism, the extent of infection, and the response of the host, the neutrophil count may range from $7.0 \times 10^9/L$ to $70 \times 10^9/L$. Usually, the count is in the range of 10–$25 \times 10^9/L$. As the demand for neutrophils at the site of infection increases, the early response of the bone marrow is an increased output of storage neutrophils to the peripheral blood, causing a shift to the left. The inflow of neutrophils from the bone marrow to the blood continues until it exceeds the neutrophil outflow to the tissues, causing an absolute neutrophilia. In very severe infections, the storage pool of neutrophils may become exhausted, the mitotic pool may be unable to keep up with the demand, and a neutropenia develops. Neutropenia in overwhelming infection is a very poor prognostic sign. Chronic bacterial infection may lead to chronic stimulation of the marrow, whereby the production of neutrophils remains high and a new steady state of production develops.

Neutrophilia is neither a unique nor an absolute finding in bacterial infections. Infections with other organisms such as fungi, rickettsia, spirochetes, and parasites may also cause a neutrophilia. Certain bacterial infections are characterized by neutropenia rather than neutrophilia. In a few types of infection such as whooping cough, lymphocytosis, rather than neutrophilia, is typical.[7] Viral infections, although typically accompanied by a lymphocytosis, may present with neutrophilia early in their course.

CASE STUDY (continued from page 384)

Laboratory results on Dennis, the trauma patient, two days after surgery are as follows:

WBC: $14.5 \times 10^9/L$ Segmented neutrophils: 5 %
HGB: 129 g/L Band neutrophils: 50 %
PLT: $180 \times 10^9/L$ Lymphocytes: 40 %
  Monocytes: 5 %

Urine, blood, and wound cultures were ordered.

1. What results, if any, are abnormal?
2. What is the most likely reason for these results?

Tissue Destruction/Injury, Inflammation, Metabolic Disorders. Conditions other than infection that may result in a neutrophilia include tissue necrosis, inflammation, certain metabolic conditions, or drug intoxication. All these conditions produce neutrophilia by increasing neutrophil input from the bone marrow in response to increased egress to the tissue. Examples of these conditions include rheumatoid arthritis, tissue infarctions, burns, neoplasms, trauma, uremia, and gout.

Leukocytes, although defenders of the body, are also responsible for a significant part of the continuing inflammatory process. Damaged tissue releases cytokines that act as chemotactins, causing neutrophils to leave the vessels and move toward the injury site. In gout, for example, depositions of uric acid crystals in joints attract neutrophils to the area. In the process of phagocytosis and death, the leukocytes release toxic intracellular enzymes (granules) and oxygen metabolites. These toxic substances mediate the inflammatory process by injuring other body cells and propagating the formation of chemotactic factors that attract more leukocytes.

Leukemoid Reaction.   Extreme neutrophilic reactions to severe infections or necrotizing tissue may produce a **leukemoid reaction** (Figure 21-1 ■). A leukemoid reaction is a benign leukocyte proliferation characterized by a total leukocyte count usually greater than $25 \times 10^9/L$ with many circulating immature leukocyte precursors. In a neutrophilic–leukemoid reaction, the blood contains many bands and metamyelocytes, increased myelocytes and promyelocytes, and rarely blasts.

Leukemoid reactions may produce a blood picture indistinguishable from that of chronic myelocytic leukemia. If the diagnosis cannot be made by routine hematologic parameters, chromosome studies and leukocyte alkaline phosphatase (LAP) scores may be helpful (Table 21-3 ✪). Contrary to leukemia, a leukemoid reaction is transient, disappearing when the inciting stimulus is removed (e.g., removing tumor, controlling infection). A leukemoid reaction may be seen in chronic infections, malignant tumors, and other inflammatory processes.

✓ Checkpoint! #2

How can CML be distinguished from a leukemoid reaction?

Leukoerythroblastic Reaction.   (Figure 21-2 ■) **Leukoerythroblastic reaction** is characterized by the presence of nucleated erythrocytes and a neutrophilic shift to the left in the peripheral blood. The total neutrophil count may be increased, decreased, or normal. Often, mature erythrocytes in this condition exhibit poikilocytosis with teardrop shapes and anisocytosis. Leukoerythroblastosis is most often associated with chronic neoplastic myeloproliferative conditions, especially myelofibrosis, **myelophthisis** (replacement of normal hematopoietic tissue in the bone marrow by fibrosis, leukemia, or metastatic cancer cells), or in severe hemolytic anemias such as Rh hemolytic disease of the newborn.

Stimulated Bone Marrow States.   When the bone marrow is stimulated to produce erythrocytes in response to hemorrhage or hemolysis, neutrophils may also become caught up in the process, resulting in neutrophilia and a slight shift to the left. Patients whose bone marrow has been stimulated by hematopoietic growth factor hormones such

⊛ TABLE 21-3

Comparison of Laboratory Results in Leukemoid Reactions and Chronic Myelocytic Leukemia (CML)		
	Leukemoid Reaction	**CML**
Leukocyte count	Increased up to 50 × 10⁹/L	Markedly increased (usually >50.0 × 10⁹/L)
Leukocyte differential	Shift to the left with bands, metamyelocytes and myelocytes; neutrophil toxic changes	Shift to the left with immature cells including promyelocytes and blasts; increased eosinophils and basophils
Erythrocyte count	Normal	Often decreased
Platelets	Usually normal	Increased or decreased
LAP	Increased	Decreased
Philadelphia chromosome	Absent	Present
Clinical	Related to primary condition	Systemic (splenomegaly, enlarged nodes, bone pain)

LAP: leukocyte alkaline phosphatase

as granulocyte/monocyte colony stimulating factor (GM-CSF) can demonstrate rapidly increasing total white counts and leukocyte precursors including blasts. Growth cytokines are used to replenish leukocytes after bone marrow transplant, high-dose chemotherapy, or bone marrow failure or prior to autologous blood donation or stem cell apheresis.[10]

Corticosteroid therapy produces a neutrophilia that occurs as a result of increased bone marrow output accompanied by a decreased migration of neutrophils to the tissues. This corticosteroid inhibition of neutrophil migration to the tissues may, in part, explain the increased incidence of bacterial infection in patients on steroid therapy even though the blood neutrophil count is increased. Steroids also inhibit macrophage function.

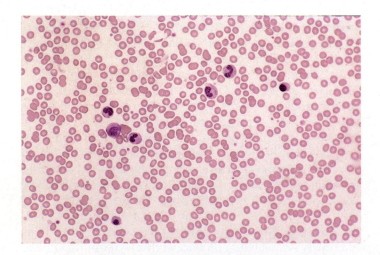

■ **FIGURE 21-2** A leukoerythroblastic reaction. There are nucleated erythrocytes and a shift to the left with band neutrophils and a myelocyte. (Peripheral blood; Wright-Giemsa stain; 500× magnification)

Physiologic Leukocytosis.   Physiologic leukocytosis and neutrophilia are present at birth and for the first few days of life (Table B ⊛ inside cover). The leukocytosis may be accompanied by a slight shift to the left. Physiologic stress including exposure to extreme temperatures, emotional stimuli, exercise, and labor during delivery may cause neutrophilia generally without a shift to the left.

> ✓ ### Checkpoint! #3
>
> *What is the difference between a leukemoid reaction and a leukoerythroblastic reaction?*

Neutropenia

Neutropenia occurs when the neutrophil count falls below 2 × 10⁹/L in whites and below 1.5 × 10⁹/L in blacks. **Agranulocytosis**, a term that refers to a neutrophil count below 0.5 × 10⁹/L, is associated with high probability of infection. Basophils and eosinophils are also commonly depleted in severe neutropenia.

True neutropenia may occur because of the following: (1) decreased bone marrow production, (2) increased cell loss (due to immune destruction or increased neutrophil egress to the tissue), or (3) pseudoneutropenia (increased neutrophilic margination). Spurious, or false, neutropenia can result from neutrophil agglutination or disintegration or from laboratory instrument problems. (See Table 21-4 ⊛ for the most common causes.)

Decreased Bone Marrow Production   Neutropenia may develop as a result of decreased bone marrow production. In this case, the bone marrow shows myeloid hypoplasia, and the M:E ratio is decreased. With defective production, the bone marrow storage pool is decreased, neutrophil egress to tissues is decreased, and both the peripheral blood

✿ TABLE 21-4

Causes of Leukopenia and/or Neutropenia

Infections, especially viral and overwhelming bacterial such as sepsis

Physical agents and chemicals, e.g., radiation and benzene

Drugs: chemotherapy, certain drugs in the classes of sedatives, anti-inflammatory, antibacterial, antithyroid, and antihistamines*

Hematologic disorders:
  Acute leukemia
  Megaloblastic and aplastic anemia
  Splenomegaly

Alloantibodies or autoantibodies, e.g., SLE

Hereditary or congenital disorders

*See *Wintrobe's Clinical Hematology*, 10th ed., Chapter 73, for a more complete list of drugs associated with neutropenia.

circulating pool and the marginal pool decrease. Immature cells may enter the blood in an attempt to alleviate the neutrophil shortage. Cells younger than bands, however, are less efficient in phagocytosis. The end result is a lack of neutrophils at inflammatory sites precipitating overwhelming infections.

Stem Cell Disorders.   Decreased bone marrow production may occur with stem cell failure such as aplastic anemia, radiotherapy, or chemotherapy or with infiltration of hematopoietic tissue by malignant cells (myelophthisis). Forty percent of new leukemia cases present with a low rather than high total white count.[11] This occurs when normal precursor cells in the bone marrow are replaced, but the malignant cells have not had time to egress to the peripheral blood in significant numbers.

Megaloblastic Anemia.   Neutropenia is a characteristic finding in megaloblastic anemia (∞ Chapter 14) and dysmyelopoietic syndromes (∞ Chapter 28). In these cases, however, the marrow is usually hyperplastic. Neutropenia results not from marrow failure but from the abnormal myeloid cells being destroyed before release to the blood (ineffective granulopoiesis).

Chemicals/Drugs.   A wide variety of drugs and chemicals are associated with leukopenia and neutropenia if given in sufficient dosage (Table 21-4 ✿). Chemotherapy and radiation treatment for cancer is a common cause for neutropenia. Pancytopenia from decreased marrow production with its decline in granulocytes predisposes patients with malignancies to frequent and serious infections. Chemotherapy drugs act to cause apoptosis of dividing cells by a variety of mechanisms including direct DNA damage, altering folate receptors, or inhibiting enzymes needed for mitosis. Since blood cell precursors in the bone marrow are also actively dividing, their proliferation is inhibited as well as the tumor

cells'. Prophylactic use of antibiotics and GM-CSF have reduced mortality in chemotherapy patients but infections due to neutropenia remain a serious complication.[10,12]

Congenital and Familial Neutropenia.   Several rare inherited disorders cause neutropenia related to decreased bone marrow production. Periodic or cyclic neutropenia is a curious form of neutropenia that begins in infancy or childhood and occurs in regular 21- to 30-day cycles. The severely neutropenic period lasts for several days and is marked by frequent infections. Between the neutropenic attacks, the patient is asymptomatic. It is believed to be inherited as an autosomal dominant trait with variable expression.[13] Severe congenital neutropenia (SCN), or Kostmann's syndrome, is a rare, often fatal autosomal recessive disorder marked by extreme neutropenia (less than 0.5×10^9/L). The total leukocyte count is often in the normal range. The basic mechanism underlying both of these disorders is unknown, but recent studies have focused on the responsiveness of neutrophil precursors to the hematopoietic growth factor G-CSF.[14,15] Familial neutropenia is a rare benign anomaly characterized by an absolute decrease in neutrophils but usually a normal total leukocyte count. It is transmitted as an autosomal dominant trait and is usually detected by chance.

Increased Cell Loss   Neutropenia may occur as the result of increased neutrophil diapedesis (passage of white cells through blood vessel walls into extravascular tissue). In severe or early infection, the bone marrow may not produce cells as rapidly as they are being utilized, resulting in neutropenia. A wide variety of viral, bacterial, rickettsial, and protozoal infections induce tissue damage, increasing the demand and destruction of neutrophils. Neutropenia resulting from severe infections is often accompanied by marked toxic changes to the granulocytes. These findings predict a dire clinical prognosis, as the organisms appear to be prevailing over the body's immune system.

Immune Neutropenia.   Antibodies may cause a decrease in the number of neutrophils if directed against neutrophil-specific antigens (NA). Leukocytes are destroyed in a manner similar to erythrocytes in immune hemolytic anemia (∞ Chapter 19). In some cases, drugs may precipitate an immunologic response accompanied by the sudden disappearance of cells from the circulation. The immunologic mechanism may include direct cell lysis or sensitization and subsequent sequestration in the spleen.[13] There are two types of immune neutropenia, alloimmune and autoimmune.

Alloimmune neonatal neutropenia occurs when there is transplacental transfer of maternal alloantibodies directed against antigens on the infant's neutrophils. Affected infants may develop infections until the neutropenia is resolved. This immune process is similar to that found in Rh hemolytic disease of the newborn except that the firstborn child is commonly affected in alloimmune neonatal neutropenia.

Two forms of autoimmune neutropenia (AIN) are recognized: primary and secondary. Primary AIN is not associated with other diseases. It develops as antibody-coated neutrophils are sequestered and destroyed by the spleen.[16] This condition of unknown etiology occurs predominantly in young children who subsequently develop fever and recurrent infections. Spontaneous remission usually occurs after a period of 13 to 20 months. Secondary autoimmune neutropenia is generally found in older patients, many of whom have been diagnosed with other autoimmune disorders such as systemic lupus erythrematosus (SLE) or rheumatoid arthritis.

Infections associated with autoimmune neutropenia are not usually life threatening and are treated with routine antibiotic therapy. Intravenous doses of immunoglobulin may be used in severe cases. Laboratory findings are variable. The total leukocyte count may range from normal to decreased, but the neutrophil count is often quite low. Immune neutropenia can be confirmed by testing for antineutrophil antibodies or neutrophil surface antigens by various methods including agglutination tests, immunofluorescense, and enzyme-linked immunosorbent assay (ELISA). The availability of these complex tests varies widely among laboratories.[16–18]

Hypersplenism.   Hypersplenism may result in a selective splenic culling of neutrophils producing mild neutropenia. The bone marrow in this case exhibits neutrophilic hyperplasia. Thrombocytopenia and, occasionally, anemia may also accompany hypersplenism.

Pseudoneutropenia   Pseudoneutropenia is similar to pseudoneutrophilia in that it is produced by alterations in the circulating and marginated pools. Pseudoneutropenia results from the transfer of an increased proportion of circulating neutrophils to the marginal neutrophil pool with no change in the total peripheral blood pool. This temporary shift is characteristic of some infections with endotoxin production and of hypersensitivity. Because of the selective margination of neutrophils, the total leukocyte count drops and a relative lymphocytosis develops.

Spurious, or False, Neutropenia   It is important for the laboratory scientist to recognize when neutropenia is a result of laboratory in vitro manipulations of blood. Table 21-5 ✪ summarizes four in vitro causes of a low neutrophil count:

1. Rarely, neutrophils adhere to erythrocytes when the blood is drawn in EDTA, causing an erroneously low automated white count. If observed on the stained smears, blood can be recollected by fingerstick to make manual dilutions and blood smears without utilizing EDTA.

2. Neutrophils disintegrate over time faster than other leukocytes. If there is a delay in testing the blood, the neutrophil count can be erroneously decreased.

3. In some pathologic conditions, the leukocytes are more fragile than normal and may rupture with the manipulations of preparing blood for testing in the laboratory.

✪ **TABLE 21-5**

Causes of False Low Neutrophil Counts in Clinical Laboratory Testing

EDTA induced neutrophil adherence to erythrocytes

Disintegration of neutrophils over time prior to testing

Disruption of abnormally fragile leukocytes during preparation of the blood for testing

Neutrophil aggregation

4. The neutrophil count may be falsely decreased if the neutrophils clump together, as occurs in the presence of some paraproteins.

✓ **Checkpoint! #4**

How can the correct white cell count be determined when neutrophils clump in the presence of EDTA?

QUALITATIVE OR MORPHOLOGIC ABNORMALITIES OF NEUTROPHILS

Morphologic abnormalities of neutrophils are not detected or flagged by automated cell counters but are identified only by observation of cells on stained blood smears. Cytoplasmic abnormalities are more common than nuclear abnormalities. Most of these cytoplasmic changes (Döhle bodies, toxic granulation, and vacuoles) are reactive transient changes accompanying infectious states. The correct identification of alterations such as intracellular microorganisms can lead to the prompt diagnosis and treatment of life-threatening infections. Recognizing Pelger-Huët or hypersegmented neutrophils can point to the diagnosis of specific conditions that may prove elusive without the morphologic information.

Nuclear Abnormalities

Pelger-Huët   **Pelger-Huët anomaly** (Figure 21-3a) is a benign anomaly, inherited in an autosomal dominant fashion and occurring in about one in 5000 individuals. The neutrophil nucleus does not segment beyond the two-lobed stage. It may also appear round with no segmentation. Nuclear clumping of chromatin is intense, aiding in the differentiation of bilobed cells from true bands. The bilobed nucleus has a characteristic dumbbell shape with the two lobes connected by a thin strand of chromatin. Cells with this appearance are called pince-nez cells. Rod-shaped and peanut-shaped nuclei are also found. The cell is functionally normal. The significance of recognizing this anomaly lies in

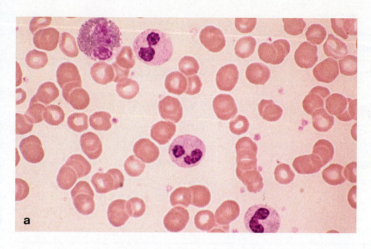

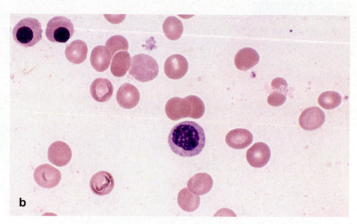

■ **FIGURE 21-3 a.** Pelger-Huët anomaly. Note pince-nez, or eyeglass-shaped, nuclei. These mature cells could easily be confused for bands if not for the highly clumped chromatin. **b.** Pseudo–Pelger-Huët cell with a single round nucleus from a patient with myelodysplastic syndrome. (Peripheral blood; Wright-Giemsa stain; 1000× magnification)

differentiating the benign hereditary defect from a shift to the left occurring with infections.

Acquired, or pseudo, Pelger-Huët anomaly can be seen in myeloproliferative disorders and myelodysplastic states (Figure 21-3b ■). The acquired form is frequently accompanied by hypogranulation because of a lack of secondary granules, and the nuclei acquire a round rather than a dumbbell shape. The chromatin shows intense clumping, aiding in differentiation of these mononuclear cells from myelocytes.

Hypersegmentation Larger-than-normal neutrophils with six or more nuclear segments (hypersegmented neutrophils) are a common and early indicator of megaloblastic anemia. These cells are found together with pancytopenia and macro ovalocytes that typically accompany deficiencies of folate or vitamin B_{12} (∞ Chapter 14). Rarely reported cases of hereditary hypersegmentation of neutrophils are significant only by their need to be distinguished from multilobed nuclei that are associated with disease.[18]

Pyknotic Nucleus Pyknotic, or degenerated, nuclei (Figure 21-4 ■) are found in dying neutrophils in blood or body fluid preparations. The nuclear chromatin breaks down with time, and the lobes become smooth, dark-staining spheres. If the nucleus is round and the cytoplasm not recognized, these necrotic cells can be confused for nucleated erythrocytes by the inexperienced.[19]

Cytoplasmic Abnormalities

Cytoplasmic inclusions are often found in infectious states and, when present, give important diagnostic information to the health care provider (Table 21-6 ✪). These inclusions are Döhle bodies, toxic granules, vacuoles, and intracellular organisms.

Döhle Bodies Döhle bodies are light gray-blue oval inclusions in the cytoplasm of neutrophils and eosinophils (Figure 21-5 ■). Found near the periphery of the cell, these bodies are composed of aggregates of rough endoplasmic reticulum. They are seen in severe bacterial infections, burns, cancer, and other toxic states. Döhle bodies should be looked for whenever toxic granulation or other reactive morphologic changes are present, as they are frequently noted to

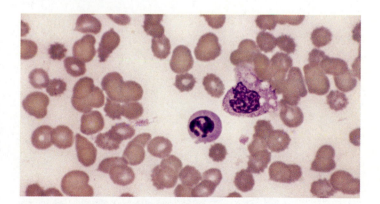

■ **FIGURE 21-4** In the center is a dying cell with a pyknotic nucleus. Note the smooth nuclear material that is breaking up. Above this cell is a band neutrophil with vacuoles and toxic granulation. (Peripheral blood; Wright-Giemsa stain; 1000× magnification)

✔ **Checkpoint! #5**

Describe the difference between hypersegmented and hyposegmented neutrophils and pyknotic nuclei. In what conditions is each seen?

★ TABLE 21-6

Cytoplasmic Inclusions Found in Neutrophils in Infectious Conditions

Inclusion	Morphologic Characteristics	Composition	Associated Conditions
Döhle body	Light gray-blue oval near cell periphery	Rough endoplasmic reticulum (RNA)	Bacterial infections, burns, cancer, toxic, or inflammatory states
Toxic granules	Large blue-black granules	Primary granules	Same as Döhle body
Cytoplasmic vacuole	Clear, unstained circular area	Open spaces from phagocytosis	Same as Döhle body
Bacteria	Small basophilic rods or cocci	Phagocytized organisms	Bacteremia or sepsis
Fungi	Round or oval basophilic inclusions slightly larger than bacteria	Phagocytized fungal organisms	Systemic fungal infections often in immunosuppressed patients
Morulae	Basophilic, granular; irregularly shaped	Clusters of *Ehrlichia* rickettsial organisms	Ehrlichiosis

occur together. Döhle bodies are similar in morphologic appearance to the cytoplasmic inclusions found in May-Hegglin anomaly.

Toxic Granules

Toxic granules are large, deep, blue-black primary granules in the cytoplasm of segmented neutrophils and sometimes in bands and metamyelocytes (Figure 21-6 ■). Primary (nonspecific) granules normally lose their basophilia as the cell matures, so even though about one-third of the granules in the mature neutrophil are primary granules, their presence is obscured. In contrast, toxic primary granules retain their basophilia in the mature neutrophil, perhaps because of a lack of maturation. Also, primary granules may become more apparent as the secondary granules are discharged, fighting bacteria. Toxic granulation is seen in the same conditions as Döhle bodies. Toxic-like granules or inclusions may appear as artifacts with increased staining time or decreased pH of the buffer used in the staining process.

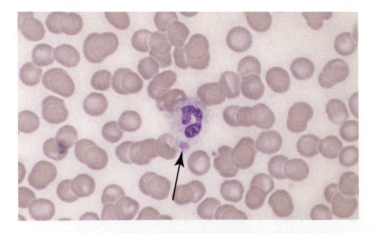

■ **FIGURE 21-5** A band neutrophil with a large bluish inclusion (Döhle body). (Peripheral blood; Wright-Giemsa stain; 1000× magnification)

Cytoplasmic Vacuoles

Cytoplasmic vacuoles appear as clear, unstained areas in the cytoplasm. Vacuoles probably represent the end stage of phagocytosis (Figure 21-6 ■). They are usually seen in the same conditions as toxic granulation and Döhle bodies. Cytoplasmic vacuoles in neutrophils from a fresh specimen are highly correlated to the presence of septicemia.

Vacuoles may also appear as an artifact in blood smears made from blood that has been collected and stored in EDTA. Vacuoles related to storage are more likely to be smaller and more uniformly dispersed than those in toxic states. The artifact can be eliminated by making smears from fresh blood without anticoagulant.

🅔 CASE STUDY *(continued from page 387)*

All cultures were negative for bacteria and fungi.

On further examination of the blood smear, it was noted that there were *no* abnormal cytoplasmic features observed in the neutrophils. However, the nuclei of most of the bands appeared more condensed than normal, and many had two lobes in a dumbbell shape.

3. Given the leukocyte morphology and cultures, what additional condition must now be considered?

4. Explain the clinical significance of the nuclear anomaly described in this patient.

5. Why is the white cell count elevated?

Intracellular Organisms

In most infections, including septicemia, the causative agents are not demonstrable in the peripheral blood. If present, however, microorganisms seen inside of neutrophils should always be considered a significant finding, and the physician should be notified immediately (Figure 21-7 ■)

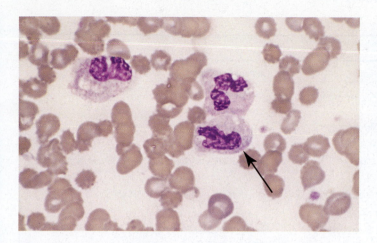

■ **FIGURE 21-6** PMNs and a band neutrophil with vacuoles, toxic granulation. There are also Döhle bodies in the center cell, but they are difficult to see. (Peripheral blood; Wright-Giemsa stain; 1000× magnification)

Bacteria/Fungi. Intracellular histoplasmosis or Candida are sometimes found in the blood of patients with HIV or other severe immunosuppression. Organisms found outside of cells must be interpreted with care. On stained blood smears, it is crucial to distinguish whether the microorganisms came from contaminated equipment or stain or are actually present in the patient's blood. Organisms must also be distinguished from other cytoplasmic material and precipitated stain. All bacteria and yeasts stain basophilic with Wright's stain.

Morulae. *Ehrlichia* sp. has become a significant tick-borne pathogen in humans over the last decade. Ehrlichiosis was first described in a human in the United States in 1986. The disease is characterized by fever, leukopenia, thrombocytopenia, and elevated liver enzymes.[20,21] Most cases of ehrlichiosis occur in April through September, when ticks are

most active. *Ehrlichia* sp. are small, obligate intracellular, coccobacilli bacteria. They infect leukocytes, where they grow within membrane-bound vacuoles (phagosomes). The intracellular organisms are pleomorphic, appearing as basophilic, condensed or loose aggregates of rickettsial organisms. The intracellular microcolonies of *Ehrlichia*, called **morulae**, are observed in leukocytes on stained blood films and may be an important clue to diagnosis (Figure 21-8 ■). The leukocyte eventually ruptures and releases the organisms that then infect other leukocytes. There are at least two species of *Ehrlichia* that infect humans. *E. chaffeensis* infects monocytes and is the causative agent of human monocytic ehrlichiosis (HME). *E. equi* infects granulocytes and is the causative agent of human granulocytic ehlichiosis (HGE). Confirmation of infection is made through serologic determination of antibody titers or by identification of DNA sequences by polymerase-chain-reaction assay. More severe disease and a poorer outcome may occur if diagnosis and therapy are delayed. The pathogenesis of ehrlichiosis may be related to direct cellular injury by the bacteria or a cascade of inflammatory or immune events. Peripheral blood cytopenia is probably the result of sequestration of infected cells in the spleen, liver, and lymph nodes.[22] The bone marrow is usually hypercellular.

Inherited Functional Abnormalities

Functional neutrophil abnormalities are almost always inherited and may or may not be accompanied by morphologic abnormalities. It is suggested that granulocyte functional abnormalities be suspected in patients with recurrent, severe infections, abscesses, or delayed wound healing and in antibiotic resistant sepsis. Table 21-7 ✪ summarizes the functional defects and their clinical features.

Alder-Reilly Anomaly Alder-Reilly anomaly is an inherited condition characterized by the presence of large purplish granules in the cytoplasm of all leukocytes in the

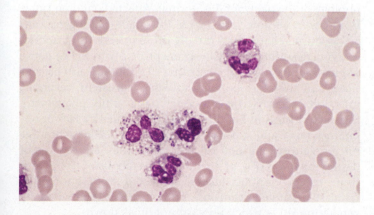

■ **FIGURE 21-7** Intracellular microorganisms. Note the vacuoles and toxic granulation in the cells. (Peripheral blood; Wright-Giemsa stain; 1000× magnification)

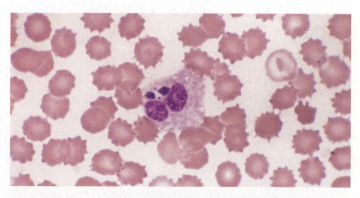

■ **FIGURE 21-8** Morulae in ehrlichiosis. This segmented neutrophil from a patient with human granulocytic ehrlichiosis contains two dense, basophilic inclusions called morulae. (Peripheral blood; Wright-Giemsa stain; 1000× magnification)

⭐ TABLE 21-7

Inherited Qualitative Neutrophil Abnormalities

Condition	Morphologic or Functional Defect	Clinical Features
Alder-Reilly anomaly	Large, dark cytoplasmic granules in all leukocytes; cells function normally	Associated with mucopolysaccharidosis such as Hurler's syndrome
Chediak-Higashi anomaly	Giant fused granules in neutrophils and lymphs; cells engulf but do not kill microorganisms	Serious, often fatal condition with repeated pyrogenic infections
May-Hegglin anomaly	Blue Döhle-like cytoplasmic inclusions in all granulocytes; cells function normally	Bleeding tendency from associated thrombocytopenia
Chronic granulomatous disease (CGD)	Defective respiratory burst; cells engulf but don't kill microorganisms	Recurrent infections especially in childhood
Myeloperoxidase deficiency	Low or absent myeloperoxidase enzyme; cell morphology normal	Usually benign; other bactericidal systems prevent most infections
Leukocyte adhesion deficiency (LAD)	Absence of cell-surface adhesion proteins affecting multiple cell functions; cell morphology normal	Serious condition with recurrent infections and high mortality

inherited group of mucopolysaccharide disorders such as Hurler's syndrome and Hunter's syndrome.[23] (Figure 21-9 ■). The granules can be distinguished from toxic granulation by their staining metachromatically with toluidine blue. The inclusions in lymphocytes tend to occur in clusters in the shape of dots or commas and are surrounded by vacuoles (Gasser's cells). Frequently, the inclusions are seen only in cells of the bone marrow and not in the peripheral blood. The blood cells function normally.

Chediak-Higashi Anomaly
Chediak-Higashi anomaly is a rare autosomal recessive disorder in which death usually occurs in infancy or childhood because of serious pyrogenic (causing fever) infection (Figure 21-10 ■). Giant gray green peroxidase-positive bodies are found in the cytoplasm of leukocytes as well as in most granule-containing cells of all other tissues. The bodies are formed by aggregation and fusion of primary nonspecific and secondary specific neutrophilic granules. This abnormal fusion of cytoplasmic membranes prevents the granules from being delivered into the phagosomes to participate in killing of ingested bacteria.[24] Neutropenia and thrombocytopenia are frequent complications as the disease progresses. The patients have skin hypopigmentation, silvery hair, and photophobia from an abnormality of melanosomes. Lymphadenopathy and hepatosplenomegaly are characteristic.

May-Hegglin Anomaly
May-Hegglin anomaly is a rare, inherited, autosomal dominant trait in which granulocytes contain inclusions similar to Döhle bodies consisting mainly of RNA from rough endoplasmic reticulum[24] (Figure 21-11 ■). Variable thrombocytopenia with giant platelets is characteristic. The only apparent clinical symptom patients may exhibit is abnormal bleeding related to the low platelet count.

Chronic Granulomatous Disease
Chronic granulomatous disease (CGD) is an inherited disorder characterized by defects in the respiratory burst oxidase system. The morphology of the neutrophil is normal. Affected children suffer from recurrent infections with low-grade pathogens (microorganisms that do not usually cause infections in normal individuals). Although CGD occurs primarily in the pediatric population, it is now apparent that CGD should also be considered in the older population when persistent, recurrent infections occur.[25] The abnormal neutrophils phagocytize the microorganisms but do not kill them due to a lack of respiratory burst and superoxide production. Catalase-positive microorganisms are not killed because they are capable of destroying the H_2O_2 of their own metabolism. They continue to grow intracellularly, protected from antibiotics. Catalase-negative organisms, however, kill themselves by generating H_2O_2, which they cannot break down.

The peripheral blood neutrophil count is normal but increases in the presence of infection. Immunoglobulin levels are often increased due to chronic infection.[26] Treatment in-

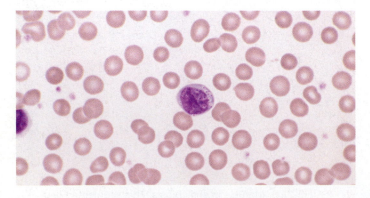

■ **FIGURE 21-9** Lymphocyte from Hurler's disease (mucopolysaccharidoses). Note the halo around the granules. (Peripheral blood; Wright-Giemsa stain; 1000× magnification)

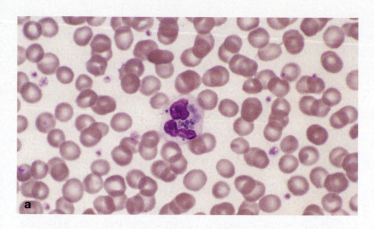
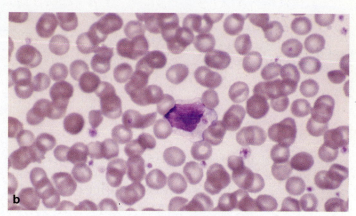

■ **FIGURE 21-10 a.** Neutrophil from Chediak-Higashi syndrome. **b.** Lymphocyte from the same patient as in a. Note the bluish gray inclusion bodies. (Peripheral blood; Wright-Giemsa stain; 1000× magnification)

volves the use of prophylactic antibiotics and early treatment of infections.

The nitroblue tetrazolium dye test (NBT) is useful in detecting the abnormal oxygen metabolism of neutrophils in CGD. Neutrophils are mixed with the yellow dye, nitroblue tetrazolium, and microorganisms. In normal individuals, the leukocytes phagocytize the microorganisms initiating an increase in oxygen uptake. This process leads to an accumulation of oxygen metabolites that reduce the yellow NBT to a blue compound. Neutrophils from individuals with CGD cannot mobilize a respiratory burst, so there is no significant accumulation of metabolites, and the NBT solution retains its yellow color.

Myeloperoxidase Deficiency Myeloperoxidase deficiency is a benign inherited disorder characterized by an absence of myeloperoxidase in neutrophils and monocytes. Although myeloperoxidase is involved in the bacteriocidal process (∞ Chapter 6) by neutrophils, an increase in infec-

tions is not usually a complication of myeloperoxidase deficiency even in homozygous individuals.

The Advia 120 (Technicon H) automated hematology analyzer has very distinct cytograms (graphic depiction of leukocytes produced by automated cell counters) in myeloperoxidase deficiency.[27] This cell-counting system utilizes peroxidase content, nuclear shape, and chromatin to enumerate and classify leukocytes. In myeloperoxidase deficiency the peroxidase cytogram reveals a lack of cells with peroxidase activity, which results in a decreased neutrophil count. The cytogram based on the other cell features, however, reveals a normal distribution of neutrophils. This discrepancy is flagged and can be resolved by reviewing the stained blood smear. The neutrophils are present on the stained smears and appear morphologically normal.

Leukocyte Adhesion Deficiency Leukocyte adhesion deficiency (LAD) is a rare, autosomal recessive disorder characterized by the absence of the leukocyte cell-surface adhesion proteins (integrins), the CD11/CD18 complex (∞ Chapter 6). In LAD there is a deficiency of the CD18 molecules that are important in the cell's ability to kill invading microorganisms. Neutrophils from patients with LAD have multiple defects related to adhesion to endothelial cells, chemotaxis, phagocytosis, respiratory burst activation, and degranulation.[28] Because of defective adhesion proteins, the neutrophils, cannot adhere to endothelial cells of the blood vessel walls and exit the circulation.

Features of LAD include frequent bacterial and fungal infections with persistent leukocytosis and granulocytosis due to increased stimulation of bone marrow.[28] Diagnosis can be made by flow cytometric analysis of neutrophil CD11/CD18 levels using a monoclonal antibody.[15]

Treatment includes prophylactic antibiotics and early, aggressive treatment of infections. Mortality rate in childhood is high, and bone marrow transplantation is recommended in severe cases.

large platelet

■ **FIGURE 21-11** May-Hegglin syndrome. Arrows point to a neutrophil with Döhle-like structures in the cytoplasm and a large platelet. (Peripheral blood; Wright-Giemsa stain; 1000× magnification)

Checkpoint! #6

Explain how you can distinguish if toxic granulation and vacuoles in the PMNs are due to the patient's condition or to artifact.

► EOSINOPHIL DISORDERS

Disorders involving exclusively eosinophils are rare. An increase in the circulating number of these cells is more common and significant than a decrease. Since the lower limit of the reference range is very low, a decrease is difficult to determine and is probably not significant.

REACTIVE EOSINOPHILIA

Eosinophilia refers to an increase in eosinophils above 0.45 × 10⁹/L. Reactive eosinophilia appears to be induced by substances secreted from T lymphocytes. A variety of conditions associated with the cellular immune response (mediated by T lymphocytes) are characterized by eosinophilia including: (1) infection with metazoic parasites, (2) allergic conditions, (3) hypersensitivity reactions, (4) cancer, and (5) chronic inflammatory states. In one study, parasitism and/or inherited allergies explained the eosinophilia in 92% of patients.[29] When the eosinophil concentration is high and there are immature forms present, the blood picture may resemble that seen in chronic eosinophilic leukemia (∞ Chapter 27). The conditions associated with eosinophilia are listed in Table 21-8 ✪.

Tissue invasion by parasites produces an eosinophilia more pronounced than parasitic infestation of the gut or blood. Eosinophils are especially effective in fighting tissue larvae of parasites. Once the larvae become coated with IgG, IgE, and/or complement, the eosinophil becomes aggressive and begins its attack on the parasite. The larva is too large for the eosinophil to phagocytose; instead, the cell molds it-

self around the larva. Intracellular eosinophilic granules fuse with the eosinophil membrane and expel their contents into the space between the cell and the larva. The granular substances attack the larva wall, partially digesting it.[30]

Allergic disorders (asthma, dermatitis, and drug reactions) are frequently characterized by a moderate increase in eosinophils. Large numbers can also be found in nasal discharges and sputum of allergic individuals as well as in the peripheral blood.

Various neoplasms and occult malignant tumors are associated with eosinophilia, which persists until the neoplasm is removed or reduced. Hodgkin lymphoma is occasionally associated with a marked eosinophilia. In some myeloproliferative disorders, especially chronic myelogenous leukemia, eosinophilia is common.

HYPEREOSINOPHILIC SYNDROME

Hypereosinophilic syndrome (HES) is a catchall term used to describe a persistent blood eosinophilia over 1.5 × 10⁹/L with tissue infiltration and no apparent cause (Figure 21-12 ■). If an increased serum IgE is found to accompany the idiopathic eosinophilia, HES may be the result of an immune response. Chronic eosinophilia may cause extensive tissue damage as the granules are released from disintegrating eosinophils. In many cases of HES, the heart is damaged by large numbers of circulating eosinophils. Charcot-Leyden crystals, which are formed from either eosinophil cytoplasm or granules, may be found in exudates and tissues where large numbers of eosinophils migrate and disintegrate. Treatment of HES with corticosteroids, hydroxyurea, and/or α-interferon is sometimes effective in reducing the eosinophil count.

The probability of the patient having eosinophilic leukemia should be considered in HES. In eosinophilic leukemia there are usually increased numbers of myeloblasts and

✪ TABLE 21-8	
Conditions Associated with Quantitative Changes of Eosinophils and Basophils	
Eosinophilia	Parasitic infection
	Allergic conditions, especially asthma, dermatitis, and drug reactions
	Certain hematologic malignancies, Hodgkin lymphoma, CML, and eosinophilic leukemia
	Hypereosinophilic syndrome
Basophilia	Immediate hypersensitivity reactions
	Chronic myeloproliferative disorders especially CML
	Basophilic leukemia
Eosinopenia and basopenia	Both are rare and difficult to determine due to low number of cells normally in circulation

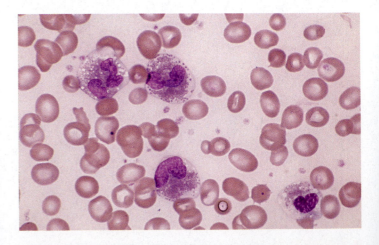

■ **FIGURE 21-12** Hypereosinophilic syndrome. Note the cells are all mature eosinophils. (Peripheral blood; Wright-Giemsa stain; 1000× magnification)

eosinophilic myelocytes, whereas in HES, the eosinophils are mature. In addition, an abnormal chromosome karyotype suggests eosinophilic leukemia rather than HES.

Pulmonary infiltrate with eosinophilia (PIE) syndrome consists of asthma, pulmonary infiltrates, central nervous system involvement, peripheral neuropathy, periateritis nodosa, and local or systemic eosinophilia. This syndrome may be produced by parasitic or bacterial infections, allergic reactions, or collagen disorders. In some cases, no cause can be found.

EOSINOPENIA

Eosinopenia is difficult to establish because of the low normal levels of these cells. Although no eosinophils may be counted in a 100-leukocyte cell differential, a scan of the blood smear under 100–400× magnification should reveal the presence of a few eosinophils. If no eosinophils are noted after scanning the smear, eosinopenia is probably present. Eosinopenia may be seen in acute infections and inflammatory reactions and with the administration of glucocorticosteroids. Glucocorticosteroids and epinephrine inhibit eosinophil release from the bone marrow and increase margination.[31]

▶ BASOPHIL DISORDERS

Basophilia refers to an increase in basophils above $0.15 \times 10^9/L$. Basophilia is associated with immediate hypersensitivity reactions and chronic myeloproliferative disorders (Table 21-8 ✪). Basophils have receptors for IgE, the major immunoglobulin of hypersensitivity states. When the IgE binds to the basophil, the cell degranulates releasing histamine and other inflammatory mediators. Many of these cells can be found in tissues during hypersensitivity reactions.

Basophilia is associated with chronic myeloproliferative disorders including myelofibrosis, polycythemia vera, and especially chronic myelogenous leukemia (CML) (∞ Chapter 27) (Figure 21-13 ■). An absolute basophilia is often helpful in distinguishing CML from a leukemoid reaction or other benign leukocytosis. When the basophil count exceeds 80% of the total leukocyte population and the Philadelphia chromosome is not present, some hematologists prefer to call the disease basophilic leukemia, an extremely rare condition.

A decrease in basophils is even more difficult to establish than eosinopenia. Scanning a blood smear with 100× magnification will reveal a rare basophil in normal individuals. Decreases in basophils are seen in inflammatory states and following immunologic reactions.

✔ Checkpoint! #7

Why are the basophil and eosinophil counts important when assessing the benign or neoplastic nature of a disorder?

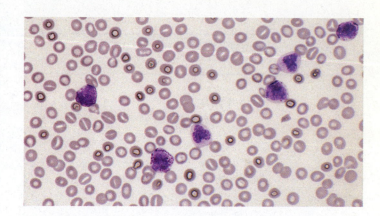

■ **FIGURE 21-13** Peripheral blood from a patient with CML and 30% basophils. (Peripheral blood; Wright-Giemsa stain; 500× magnification)

▶ MONOCYTE/MACROPHAGE DISORDERS

Quantitative disorders are associated with monocytes, whereas the qualitative disorders are associated with macrophages. The qualitative disorders are inherited lipid storage disorders.

QUANTITATIVE DISORDERS

Monocytosis occurs when the absolute monocyte count exceeds $0.8 \times 10^9/L$ (Figure 21-14 ■). It is seen most often in inflammatory conditions and certain malignancies (Table 21-9 ✪). Monocytosis occurring in the recovery stage of acute infections and in agranulocytosis is considered a favorable sign. Monocytes play an important role in the immune cellular response in tuberculosis.

Unexplained monocytosis has been reported to be associated with as many as 62% of all malignancies. Myelodysplas-

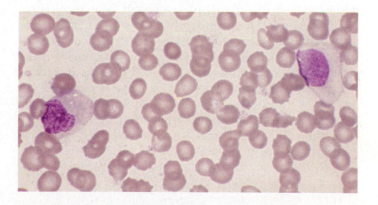

■ **FIGURE 21-14** Peripheral blood from a patient with reactive monocytosis showing two reactive monocytes. (Peripheral blood; Wright-Giemsa stain; 1000× magnification)

⊙ TABLE 21-9

Conditions Associated with Quantitative Changes of Monocytes

Monocytosis	Neoplastic
	Myelodysplastic syndromes
	Myeloproliferative disorders
	Chronic myelogenous leukemia
	Chronic myelomonocytic leukemia
	Acute monocytic, myelomonocytic, and myelocytic leukemias
Reactive	Inflammatory conditions
	Collagen diseases
	Immune disorders
	Certain infections (e.g., TB, syphilis)
Monocytopenia	Stem cell disorders such as aplastic anemia

tic states, acute myelocytic leukemia, and chronic myelocytic leukemia are associated with monocytosis. About 25% of Hodgkin lymphomas are characterized by an increase in monocytes. In these conditions, the monocyte is probably a part of a reactive process to the neoplasm rather than a part of the clonal neoplasm itself. Neoplastic proliferation of monocytes occurs in acute monocytic leukemia and acute and chronic myelomonocytic leukemia (∞ Chapters 27, 29).

Monocytopenia refers to a concentration of monocytes below 0.2×10^9/L and is found in stem cell disorders such as aplastic anemia. A decreased number of circulating monocytes is difficult to establish because of the low normal levels of these cells.

QUALITATIVE DISORDERS

Macrophages are tissue cells developed from monocytes that have egressed from the blood (∞ Chapter 6). The lipid storage disorders are generally categorized as a qualitative disorder of the monocyte/macrophage cell line.

Cells or parts of cells are continually being replaced in the normal process of growth, development, and senescence. The breakdown of cellular debris takes place largely in the phagolysosomes of macrophages as a result of sequential enzymatic degradation. Macrophages are associated with a group of lipid storage disorders in which the cells are unable to completely digest phagocytosed material because of a deficiency of a particular enzyme needed for the degradation process. As a result, the undigested substance accumulates within the cell. The disorders that are diagnosed by abnormal macrophages in hematologic tissue include Gaucher disease, Niemann-Pick disease, and sea-blue histiocytosis.

Gaucher Disease

Gaucher (pronounced gaw-shay) disease is an inherited recessive trait that is characterized by a deficiency of glucocerebrosidase (an enzyme needed to break down the lipid glucocerebroside).[32] In this disease, the macrophage is unable to digest the stroma of ingested cells, and the lipid glucocerebroside accumulates. The clinical findings (splenomegaly and bone pain) of the disease are related to the accumulation of this lipid in macrophages of the lymphoid tissue, spleen, liver, and bone marrow. The macrophages are large (20–80 μm) with small eccentric nuclei. The cytoplasm appears wrinkled or striated, often filled with debris (Figure 21-15 ■). Gaucher cells are present primarily in lymphoid tissue and bone marrow. The spleen and liver become greatly enlarged. Leukopenia, thrombocytopenia, and anemia may occur as the result of their sequestration by an enlarged spleen. A consistent finding useful in the diagnosis of Gaucher disease is an increase in serum acid phosphatase activity.

Cells similar to Gaucher cells may be found in the marrow of individuals with a rapid granulocyte turnover, especially in chronic myelocytic leukemia. The accumulation of lipid in these disorders does not result from a deficiency of an enzyme but rather from the inability of the macrophage to keep up with the flow of fat into the cell from the increased cell turnover. Gaucher disease may be confirmed by demonstrating a decreased leukocyte β-glucosidase activity, whereas the enzyme level is normal or increased in myeloproliferative disorders.

Niemann-Pick Disease

Niemann-Pick disease is a rare autosomal recessive disease, more commonly seen in Ashkenazid Jews. Signs of the disease begin in infancy with poor physical development. The spleen and liver are greatly enlarged. The disease is often fatal by three years of age. The defect is a deficiency of sphingomyelinase (an enzyme needed to break down lipids) resulting in excessive sphingomyelin and ceroid (lipids found in various tissue) storage.[33]

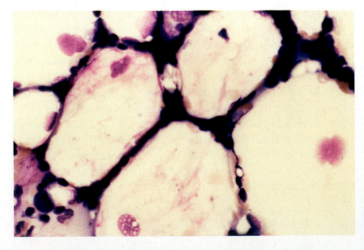

■ **FIGURE 21-15** Gaucher macrophages in bone marrow. (Peripheral blood; Wright-Giemsa stain; 1000× magnification)

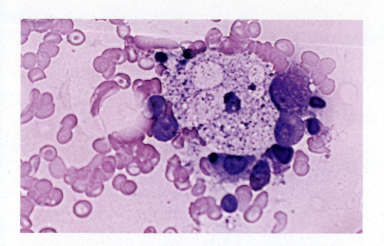

■ **FIGURE 21-16** Macrophage in the bone marrow of a patient with Niemann-Pick disease. Note the foamy cytoplasm with inclusions. (Peripheral blood; Wright-Giemsa stain; 1000× magnification)

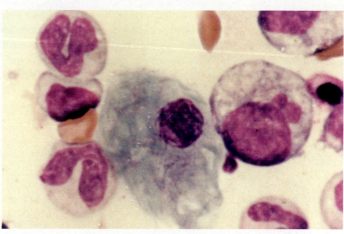

■ **FIGURE 21-17** Sea-blue histiocyte from bone marrow. (Wright stain; 1000× magnification)

Foamy macrophages are found in lymphoid tissue and the bone marrow. (Figure 21-16 ■) The foam cells are large (20–100 μm) with an eccentric nucleus and globular cytoplasmic inclusions. Leukopenia and thrombocytopenia may occur from increased sequestration from the enlarged spleen.

Sea-Blue Histiocytosis Syndrome

Sea-blue histiocytosis syndrome is a primary familial disorder characterized by splenomegaly and thrombocytopenia.[34] Sea-blue staining macrophages are found in the spleen and bone marrow (Figure 21-17 ■). The cell is large (20–60 μm in diameter) with a dense eccentric nucleus and cytoplasm that contains blue or blue-green granules. Considerable variation in clinical manifestations is present, but in most patients the course of the disease is benign.

Miscellaneous Lipid Storage Disorders

Tay-Sachs disease, Sandhoff disease, Fabry disease, Wolman's disease, and Tangier disease are inherited diseases characterized by a deficiency of one or more enzymes that metabolize lipids. As a result of these enzyme deficiencies, abnormal concentrations of lipids accumulate in tissue. These often fatal conditions affect mostly nonhematologic tissue. There are no specific findings in the peripheral blood. Lipid-laden macrophages may be present in the bone marrow.[35]

SUMMARY

Leukocytes respond to toxic, infectious, and inflammatory processes to defend the tissues and limit and/or eliminate the disease process or toxic challenge. This may involve a change in leukocyte concentration, most often increasing one or more leukocyte types. The type of cell affected depends on the cell's function. Thus, a differential count as well as the total leukocyte count aids in diagnosis.

Neutrophilia, an increase in neutrophils, most often occurs as a result of a reaction to a physiologic or pathologic process. The most common cause is bacterial infection. Tissue injury or inflammation may also cause a neutrophilia. Web Figure 21-18 ■ summarizes the laboratory evaluation of neutrophilia.

Neutropenia, a decrease in neutrophils, is less commonly encountered. It may be caused by drugs, immune mechanisms, or decreased bone marrow production. Several inherited conditions are characterized by neutropenia and recurrent infections. Web Figure 21-12 ■ summarizes the laboratory evaluation of neutropenia.

Morphologic abnormalities of neutrophils may be found in infectious states and are important to identify on stained blood smears. These include Döhle bodies, toxic granulation, and cytoplasmic vacuoles. Other morphologic abnormalities include pince-nez cells found in Pelger-Huët anomaly and morulae found in ehrlichiosis.

There are a number of inherited conditions characterized by functional and morphologic abnormalities of the leukocyte. Chronic granulomatous disease and myeloperoxidase deficiency are characterized by defects in the generation of oxidizing radicals after phagocytosing bacteria. The nitroblue tetrazolium dye test is used to detect abnormal oxygen metabolism in CGD. Peroxidase deficient cells can be demonstrated with peroxidase stain. Leukocyte adhesion deficiency (LAD) is identified by the absence of leukocyte cell-surface adhesion proteins. Diagnosis can be made by flow cytometric analysis of neutrophil CD11/CD18 levels using monoclonal antibodies. Other rare leukocyte functional abnormalities include Alder-Reilly anomaly, Chediak-Higashi anomaly, and May-Hegglin anomaly.

Eosinophils are increased in infections with metazoic parasites, allergic conditions, hypersensitivity reactions, cancer, and chronic inflammatory states. Basophilia is seen in hypersensitivity reactions and chronic myeloproliferative disorders, especially chronic myelogenous leukemia. Monocytosis is found in a wide variety of conditions, especially malignancies. Macrophages are associated with a group of lipid storage disorders in which these cells are unable to completely digest phagocytosed material because of a deficiency of a particular enzyme needed for the degradation process.

REVIEW QUESTIONS

LEVEL I

1. Which of the following hematologic values would you expect if the peripheral blood smear revealed toxic granulation of PMNs, Döhle bodies, and vacuoles in PMNs? (Checklist #1, 2)
   a. WBC: 4×10^9/L
   b. differential: 50% neutrophils, 15% bands, 30% lymphs, 5% monocytes
   c. 20% eosinophils
   d. Hb: 10 g/dL; platelets 20×10^9/L

2. An adult white count is 2.0×10^9/L. The differential has 60% segmented neutrophils. Which of the following correctly describes these results? (Checklist #6)
   a. normal
   b. leukocytosis and neutrophilia
   c. leukopenia with normal number of neutrophils
   d. leukopenia and neutropenia

3. Which of the following is the most common cause of neutrophilia? (Checklist #1)
   a. bacterial infection
   b. acute leukemia
   c. following chemotherapy
   d. aplastic anemia

4. Blue-gray oval inclusions composed of RNA near the periphery of neutrophils is a description of: (Checklist #3)
   a. toxic granules
   b. Döhle bodies
   c. vacuoles
   d. primary granules

5. Which of the following is associated with an acute bacterial infection? (Checklist #2)
   a. neutrophilia
   b. neutropenia
   c. eosinophilia
   d. leukocytopenia

6. Which of the following is a common reason for neutropenia in hospitalized patients? (Checklist #6)
   a. chronic myeloproliferative disorders such as CML
   b. chemotherapy and/or radiation treatment for cancer
   c. childbirth
   d. strenuous exercise

LEVEL II

Use the following case study to answer review questions 1–5.

A patient's white count is 30.0×10^9/L. The differential is as follows:

Segmented neutrophils:	54%
Band neutrophils:	10%
Metamyelocytes:	2%
Lymphocytes:	26%
Monocytes:	5%
Eosinophils:	3%

6 Nucleated RBCs/ 100 WBCs

1. Select the additional information most important to assess whether these results are normal or indicate a disease process. (Checklist #1)
   a. platelet count
   b. LAP
   c. patient history
   d. patient age

2. Which of the following correctly describes the absolute neutrophil count (ANC) for the above patient? (Checklist #1, 12)
   a. normal for both an infant and an adult
   b. neutrophilia for both an infant and an adult
   c. normal for an infant and neutrophilia for an adult
   d. normal for an adult and neutrophilia for an infant

3. Which of the following correctly describes the neutrophil concentration if the above patient is an infant? (Checklist #1)
   a. pseudoneutrophilia
   b. leukemoid reaction
   c. leukoerythroblastic reaction
   d. physiologic neutrophilia

4. Which of the following correctly describes the differential if the above patient is an adult? (Checklist #1)
   a. pseudoneutrophila
   b. leukoerythroblastic reaction
   c. agranulocytosis
   d. physiologic neutrophilia

5. If the above patient is an adult, all of the following could probably be considered in the diagnosis *EXCEPT:* (Checklist #1, 2, 12)
   a. myeloproliferative condition
   b. myelophthisis
   c. aplastic anemia
   d. hemolytic anemia

REVIEW QUESTIONS *(continued)*

LEVEL I

7. Which of the following causes a false neutropenia? (Checklist #7)
   a. EDTA induced agglutination
   b. leukemia
   c. splenomegaly
   d. immune neutropenia

8. Which of the following is the most common cause of eosinophilia? (Checklist #10)
   a. parasitic infection
   b. eosinophilic leukemia
   c. CML
   d. asthma and other allergies

9. What substances build up and are ingested by macrophages in the qualitative macrophage disorders such as Gaucher disease? (Checklist #11)
   a. proteins
   b. carbohydrates
   c. lipids
   d. rough endoplasmic reticulum

10. Distinct, large, unidentified inclusions are found in the cytoplasm of many granulocytes. Select the best course of action. (Checklist #9)
    a. ignore them as they probably are not significant
    b. report as intracellular yeast
    c. have a supervisor or pathologist examine the smear for rare or unusual conditions such as Chediak-Higashi
    d. report as toxic granulation

LEVEL II

Qualitative neutrophil abnormalities can sometimes be confused with reactive or toxic conditions. For each set of conditions in questions 6–11, list all lettered features that could help evaluate the patient.
   a. presence of other toxic features (leukocytosis, toxic granulation, Döhle bodies, vacuoles)
   b. abnormal inclusions found in other cells besides neutrophils
   c. other CBC parameters abnormal (RBC, HCT or PLT)
   d. patient symptoms
   e. patient and family history

6. Alder Reilly versus toxic granulation (Checklist #7, 11)

7. May-Hegglin versus toxic Döhle bodies (Checklist #7, 11)

8. Pelger-Huët versus bands (Checklist #5, 11)

9. Chediak-Higashi versus intracellular yeasts or morulae (Checklist #6, 7, 11)

10. Leukemia versus infection (Checklist #2, 11)

11. Toxic vacuoles versus sample with prolonged storage (Checklist #4, 6, 11)

---

www.prenhall.com/mckenzie

Use the above address to access the free, interactive Companion Web site created for this textbook. Get hints, instant feedback, and textbook references to chapter-related multiple choice questions.

REFERENCES

1. Miller DR. Normal blood values from birth through adolescence. Miller D, ed. In: *Blood Diseases of Infancy and Childhood,* 7th ed. St. Louis: Mosby; 1995:30–53.

2. Tonte A, Stevens M. Pediatric and geriatric hematology. Rodak B, ed. In: *Diagnostic Hematology.* Philadelphia: W. B. Saunders; 1995:587–95.

3. Segel GB. Hematology of the newborn. Beutler E, Lichtman MA, Coller B, Kipps TJ, eds. In: *Williams Hematology,* 5th ed. New York, NY: McGraw-Hill; 1995:100–111.

4. Perkins SL. Examination of the blood and bone marrow. Lee GR, Foerster J, Lukens J, Paraskevas F, Greer JP, Rodgers GM, eds. In: *Wintobe's Clinical Hematology,* 10th ed. Baltimore: Williams and Wilkins; 1999:9–35.

5. Reed WW, Diehl LF. Leukopenia, neutropenia and reduced hemoglobin levels in healthy American blacks. *Arch Intern Med.* 1991; 151:501–5.

6. Shoenfeld Y, Modan M, Berliner S, Yair V, Shaklai M, Slusky A, Pinkhas J. The mechanism of benign hereditary neutropenia. *Arch Intern Med.* 1982; 142:797–99.

7. Necheles TF. Quantitative disorders of leukocytes: Differential diagnosis. Seligson D, ed. In: *CRC Handbook Series in Clinical Laboratory Science,* Sect. 1: Hematology. Vol. 2. Boca Raton: CRC Press Inc; 1980:305–8.

8. Stewart, GJ. Neutrophils and deep venous thrombosis. *Haemostasis.* 1993; 23 (suppl. 1):127–40.

9. Dale D.C. Neutrophilia. Beutler E, Lichtman MA, Coller B, Kipps TJ, eds. In: *Williams Hematology,* 5th ed. New York: McGraw-Hill; 1995:824–28.

10. Kallianpur A. Supportive care in hematologic malignancies. Lee GR, Foerster J, Lukens J, Paraskevas F, Greer JP, Rodgers GM, eds. In: *Wintobe's Clinical Hematology,* 10th ed. Baltimore: Williams and Wilkens; 1999:2102–56.

11. Whitlock JA, Gaynon PS. Acute lymphocytic leukemia. Lee GR, Foerster J, Lukens J, Paraskevas F, Greer JP, Rodgers GM, eds. In: *Wintobe's Clinical Hematology,* 10th ed. Baltimore: Williams and Wilkens; 1999:2241–71.

12. Hande KR. Principles and pharmacology of chemotherapy. Lee GR, Foerster J, Lukens J, Paraskevas F, Greer JP, Rodgers GM, eds. In: *Wintobe's Clinical Hematology,* 10th ed. Baltimore: Williams and Wilkens; 1999:2076–101.

13. Athens JW. Neutropenia. Lee GR, Bithell TC, Foerster J, Athens JW, Lukens JN, eds. In: *Wintobe's Clinical Hematology,* 9th ed. Philadelphia: Lea & Febiger; 1993:1589–612.

14. Hestdal K, Welte K, Lie SO, Keller JR, Ruscetti FW, Abrahamsen TG. Severe congenital neutropenia: Abnormal growth and differentiation of myeloid progenitors to granulocyte colony-stimulating factor (G-CSF) but normal response to G-CSF plus stem cell factor. *Blood.* 1993; 82:2991–97.

15. Dinauer M.C. Leukocyte function and nonmalignant leukocyte disorders. *Curr Opin Pediatr.* 1993; 5:80–7.

16. Bux J, Mueller-Eckhardt C. Autoimmune neutropenia. *Sem Hematol.* 1992; 29:45–53.

17. Watts RG. Neutropenia. Lee GR, Foerster J, Lukens J, Paraskevas F, Greer JP, Rodgers GM, eds. In: *Wintobe's Clinical Hematology,* 10th ed. Baltimore: Williams and Wilkens; 1999:1862–88.

18. Jandl JH. Leukocyte anomalies. In: *Blood: Textbook of Hematology,* 2nd ed. Boston: Little, Brown and Company; 1996:785–802.

19. Gall JJ. Laboratory evaluation of body fluids. Stiene-Martin EA, Lotspeich-Steininger CA, Koepke JA. eds. In: *Clinical Hematology,* 2nd ed. Philadelphia: Lipponcott: 1998:400–14.

20. Bakken JS, et al. Human granulocytic ehrlichiosis in the upper midwest United States. *JAMA.* 1994; 272:212–18.

21. Fishbein DB, Dawson JE, Robinson, LE. Human ehrlichiosis in the United States, 1985–1990. *Ann Intern Med.* 1994; 120:736–43.

22. Dumler JS, Bakken JS. Ehrlichial diseases of humans: Emerging tick-borne infections. *Clin Infect Dis.* 1995; 20:1102–10.

23. Reilly WA, Lindsay S. Gargoylism (lipochondrodystrophy): A review of clinical observation in eighteen cases. *Am J Dis Child.* 1948; 75:595–607.

24. Skubitz KM. Qualitative disorders of leukocytes. Lee GR, Foerster J, Lukens J, Paraskevas F, Greer JP, Rodgers GM, eds. In: *Wintobe's Clinical Hematology,* 10th ed. Baltimore: Williams and Wilkens; 1999:1889–1907.

25. Becker CE, Graddick SL, Roy TM. Patterns of chronic granulomatous disease. *J Ky Med Assoc.* 1993; 91:447–50.

26. Athens JW. Qualitative disorders of leukocytes. Lee GR, Bithell TC, Foerster J, Athens JW, Lukens JN, eds. In: *Wintobe's Clinical Hematology,* 9th ed. Philadelphia: Lea & Febiger; 1993:1613–27.

27. McKenzie SB, Metz JA. *Hematology Tech Sample No. H-3* (1991). Chicago: American Society of Clinical Pathology; 1991.

28. Yang KD, Hill HR. Neutrophil function disorders: Pathophysiology, prevention, and therapy. *J Pediatr.* 1991; 119:343–54.

29. Teo CG, et al. Evaluation of the common conditions associated with eosinophilia. *J Clin Pathol.* 1985; 38:305–8.

30. Boggs DR, Winkelstein A. *White Cell Manual,* 4th ed. Philadelphia: F.A. Davis Co; 1983:54–57.

31. Wardlaw AJ, Kay AB. Eosinopenia and eosinophilia. Beutler E, Lichtman MA, Coller B, Kipps TJ, eds. In: *Williams Hematology,* 5th ed. New York: McGraw-Hill; 1995:844–52.

32. Brady RO, Kanfer JN, Bradley RM, Shapiro D. Demonstration of a deficiency of glucocerebroside-cleaving enzyme in Gaucher's disease. *J Clin Invest.* 1966; 45:1112–15.

33. Brady RO, Kanfer JN, Mock MB, Fredrickson DS. The metabolism of sphingomylin: II. Evidence of an enzymatic deficiency in Niemann-Pick disease. *Proc Natl Acad Sci USA.* 1966; 55:366–69.

34. Silverstein MN, Ellefson RD. The syndrome of the sea-blue histiocyte. *Semin Hematol.* 1972; 9:293–307.

35. McGovern MM, Desnick RJ. Abnormalities of the monocyte-macrophage system: The lysosomal storage diseases. Lee GR, Foerster J, Lukens J, Paraskevas F, Greer JP, Rodgers GM, eds. In: *Wintobe's Clinical Hematology,* 10th ed. Baltimore: Williams and Wilkens; 1999:1908–15.

22

Nonmalignant Lymphocyte Disorders

Sue S. Beglinger, M.S.

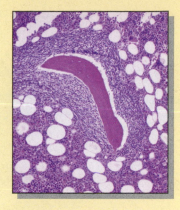

■ CHECKLIST - LEVEL I

At the end of this unit of study, the student should be able to:

1. Identify the infectious agent and describe the clinical symptoms and corresponding leukocyte differential in infectious mononucleosis.
2. Describe and recognize the reactive morphology of lymphocytes found in infectious mononucleosis.
3. Relate the heterophil antibody test to infectious mononucleosis.
4. Calculate an absolute lymphocyte count and differentiate it from a relative lymphocytosis given a differential and leukocyte count.
5. Identify reactive cell morphology associated with viral infections and compare with normal lymphocyte morphology.
6. Describe clinical symptoms of disorders in which a leukocytosis is caused by lymphocytosis.
7. State the complications associated with CMV infections.
8. Identify conditions associated with lymphocytopenia.
9. Explain the pathophysiology of HIV infections and describe how it affects lymphocytes.
10. Describe the abnormal hematological findings associated with AIDS.

■ CHECKLIST - LEVEL II

At the end of this unit of study the student should be able to:

1. Assess and resolve/explain conflicting results between peripheral blood morphology and serologic tests in suspected Epstein-Barr virus (EBV) infection.
2. Describe the pathophysiology of infectious mononucleosis.
3. Assess and correlate antibody titers found in infectious mononucleosis with respect to the various EBV viral antigens.
4. State the pathophysiology of toxoplasmosis infections and explain the resulting lymphocytosis.
5. Differentiate benign lymphocytic leukemoid reactions from neoplastic lymphoproliferative disorders by laboratory results and characteristics of cell morphology.
6. Define the pathophysiology and give clinical findings associated with CMV infection.
7. Propose the cause of lymphocytosis and recognize laboratory features associated with *Bordetella pertussis* infections.

■ **CHECKLIST - LEVEL II** *(continued)*

8. Assess a patient case using the CDC AIDS case surveillance criteria and recommend appropriate laboratory testing.

9. Explain the cytopenia, identify the defect, and recognize the laboratory features in congenital qualitative disorders of lymphocytes.

10. Evaluate a case study from a patient with a lymphoproliferative disorder and conclude from the medical history and laboratory results the most likely diagnosis for the disorder.

KEY TERMS

Acquired immune deficiency syndrome (AIDS)
AIDS-related complex (ARC)
Bordatella pertussis
Cytomegalovirus (CMV)
Epstein-Barr virus (EBV)
Heterophil antibodies
Immunosuppressed
Infectious lymphocytosis
Infectious mononucleosis
Lymphocytic leukemoid reaction
Opportunistic organisms
Severe combined immunodeficiency syndrome (SCIDS)
Toxoplasmosis
Viral load

BACKGROUND BASICS

The information in this chapter will build on the concepts learned in previous chapters. To maximize your learning experience you should review this material before starting this unit of study.

Level I

▶ Describe normal and reactive lymphocyte morphology; identify the distinguishing characteristics of T and B lymphocytes. (Chapter 6)

▶ Calculate absolute cell counts; summarize the relationship between the hematocrit and hemoglobin. (Chapter 7)

▶ Define *antigen* and *antibody* and describe their roles in infectious and noninfectious diseases; summarize the immune response. (Chapter 6)

Level II

▶ Describe the process of T and B lymphocyte differentiation and the function of each subtype; summarize the structure and function of each of the immunoglobulins; describe the immune response. (Chapter 6)

▶ Describe the structure and function of the hematopoietic organs and tissue. (Chapter 3)

▶ Give the principle and application of direct antiglobulin tests in diagnosis of immune mediated anemia. (Chapter 19)

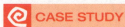 **CASE STUDY**

We will refer to this case study throughout the chapter.
Heidi, a 54-day-old girl, was admitted to the hospital because of recurrent respiratory distress and failure to gain weight. She was born prematurely at 35 weeks gestation by urgent Cesarean section. Her mother was immune to rubella and had negative serologic tests for syphilis. Consider why the lymphatic system should be evaluated in this child and the possible etiology of repeated respiratory problems.

▶ ## OVERVIEW

This chapter discusses benign conditions associated with quantitative and qualitative alterations in lymphocytes. Infectious mononucleosis and other acquired disorders characterized by lymphocytosis are described. This is followed by a discussion of lymphocytopenia and immune deficiency states, both acquired and congenital. Emphasis is on the laboratory features that allow the diseases to be diagnosed and differentiated from neoplastic lymphoproliferative disease.

▶ ## INTRODUCTION

Evidence of disease, especially infectious disease, may be observed by finding abnormal concentrations of lymphocytes and/or reactive lymphocytes on a peripheral blood smear. This finding helps direct the physician's subsequent workup of the patient and aids in the initiation of appropriate therapy. Most disorders affecting lymphocytes are acquired and are characterized by a reactive lymphocytosis. Some acquired disorders result in a lymphocytopenia that may compromise function of the immune system. In the acquired disorders affecting lymphocytes, the change in lymphocyte concentration and morphology is a reactive process. In contrast, in congenital disorders involving lymphocytes, the primary defect is within the lymphocytic system.

► LYMPHOCYTOSIS

Lymphocytosis, an increase in lymphocytes, may be due to a relative or absolute increase in lymphocytes. Absolute lymphocytosis occurs in adults when the lymphocyte count exceeds 4×10^9/L, while relative lymphocytosis is present when the lymphocyte count exceeds 40%. The lymphocyte concentration in children is normally higher than in adults and varies with the child's age (Table B ✪, inside front cover). Lymphocytosis can occur without a leukocytosis.

Lymphocytosis is usually a self-limiting, reactive process that occurs in response to an infection or inflammatory condition. Both T and B lymphocytes commonly are affected but their function remains normal. Occasionally, viral infections may cause functional impairment of the lymphocytes yielding both a qualitative disorder as well as quantitative changes.

Once lymphocytes are stimulated by an infection or inflammatory condition, they enter various states of activation, resulting in a morphologically heterogeneous population of cells on stained blood smears (Figure 22-1 ■). These activated cells may appear large with irregular shapes and cytoplasmic basophilia. Granules may be seen. The nuclear chromatin usually becomes more dispersed (∞ Chapter 6). Occasionally, there is intense proliferation of lymphoid elements in the lymph nodes and spleen, causing lymphadenopathy and splenomegaly, respectively.

Normally, T lymphocytes comprise about 60–80% of peripheral blood lymphocytes. Thus, increases in the concentration of these lymphocytes are more likely to cause changes in the relative lymphocyte count than changes in the B lymphocytes. Absolute lymphocytosis is not usually accompanied by leukocytosis except in infectious mononucleosis, infectious lymphocytosis, *Bordatella pertussis* infection, cytomegalovirus infection, or lymphocytic leukemia. A relative lymphocytosis, secondary to neutropenia, is more commonly found than an absolute lymphocytosis and occurs in a variety of viral infections.

$$\text{Absolute lymphocyte count } (\times 10^9/\text{L}) = \% \text{ lymphocytes} \times \text{WBC count } (\times 10^9/\text{L})$$

It is important to differentiate benign conditions associated with lymphocytosis from neoplastic (malignant) lymphoproliferative disorders (Table 22-1 ✪). The presence of heterogeneous reactive lymphocytes, positive serologic tests for the presence of specific antibodies against infectious organisms, and absence of anemia and thrombocytopenia favor a benign diagnosis. This section will include a discussion of the more common disorders associated with a reactive lymphocytosis.

℮ CASE STUDY (continued from page 404)

Admission CBC on Heidi was: WBC: 7.6×10^9/L; Hct: 0.55 L/L; Plt: 242×10^9/L, and Differential: 84% segs, 2% bands, 4% lymphocytes, 8% monocytes, 2% eosinophils.

1. Does this patient have a leukocytosis or leukopenia?
2. Does this patient have an abnormal lymphocyte count? Explain.

✪ TABLE 22-1

Conditions Associated with Lymphocytosis

Nonmalignant Conditions	Malignant Conditions
Infectious mononucleosis	Acute lymphocytic leukemia
Infectious lymphocytosis	Chronic lymphocytic leukemia
Bordatella pertussis infection	Hairy cell leukemia
Cytomegalovirus infection	Heavy chain disease
Toxoplasmosis	Multiple myeloma
Persistent polyclonal B cell lymphocytosis	Waldenstrom's macroglobulinemia
Viral infection	
Chicken pox	
Measles	
Mumps	
Roseola infantum	
Infectious hepatitis	
Chronic infections	
Tertiary syphilis	
Congenital syphilis	
Brucellosis	
Endocrine disorders	
Thyrotoxicosis	
Addison's disease	
Panhypopituitarism	
Convalescence of acute infections	
Immune reactions	
Inflammatory diseases	

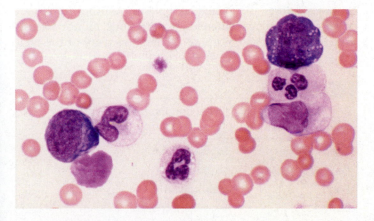

■ **FIGURE 22-1** Two immunoblasts (one o'clock and eight o'clock) and a reactive lymph (three o'clock). These are reactive forms of stimulated lymphocytes and can be found in infectious states, especially viral infections. (Peripheral blood; Wright-Giemsa stain; 1000× magnification)

INFECTIOUS MONONUCLEOSIS

Infectious mononucleosis is a self-limiting lymphoproliferative disease caused by infection with **Epstein-Barr virus (EBV)**. EBV usually affects young adults; the peak age for infection is 14–24 years. In children from lower-income groups, infection usually occurs before 4 years of age, while in more affluent populations, peak infection incidence occurs during adolescence. About 80–90% of adults have had exposure and possess lifelong immunity. The disease, not considered highly contagious, is transmitted through saliva, hence the nickname kissing disease.

Cellular immunity (the function of T lymphocytes) is important in limiting the growth potential of EBV-infected B lymphocytes. Immune compromised individuals are at increased risk of serious infection. EBV-associated B cell tumors and lymphoproliferative syndromes may occur in transplant patients or in patients with acquired immune deficiency syndrome (AIDS).[1] These patients have severe T lymphocyte immunodeficiency. Male children with a rare X-linked lymphoproliferative syndrome, lacking a T lymphocyte response, are unable to limit EBV infection of B lymphocytes. As a result, there is a fatal polyclonal B lymphocyte proliferation.[3]

Pathophysiology

EBV attaches to B lymphocytes by means of a specific receptor, designated CD21, on the B lymphocyte membrane surface.[1] This also is the receptor for the C3d complement component. The virus infects resting B lymphocytes as well as epithelial cells of the oropharynx and cervix. The binding of the virus to the lymphocyte activates the lymphocyte, causing it to express the activation marker CD23.[2] CD23 serves as the receptor for a B lymphocyte growth factor. Once internalized, the virus is incorporated into the B lymphocyte genome, instructing the host's cell to begin production of EBV proteins. These viral proteins are then expressed on the cell membrane. Thus, EBV-infected cells express markers of activated B lymphocytes as well as viral markers. The viral genome is maintained in the lymphocyte nucleus and passed on to the cell's progeny. This results in EBV-immortalized B lymphocytes and possible latent infection.

Acute EBV infection is controlled by a complex, multifaceted cellular immune response. In the first week of illness, there is a polyclonal increase in immunoglobulins. During the second week, however, the number of immunoglobulin secreting B lymphocytes decreases, presumably due to the action of suppressor T lymphocytes. Activated cytotoxic cells that resemble activated killer cells are present early in the course of the disease. These cells are neither EBV-specific nor HLA-restricted (virus nonspecific). Cytotoxic T lymphocytes inhibit the activation and proliferation of EBV-infected B lymphocytes and also participate in the cell-mediated immune response. The majority of the reactive lymphocytes seen in the peripheral blood are the suppressor-cytotoxic T lymphocytes.

Clinical Findings

Prodromal symptoms include lethargy, headache, fever, chills, sore throat, nausea, and anoxia. The classic triad presentation of symptoms are fever, pharyngitis, and lymphadenopathy[3] (Table 22-2 ✪). Children younger than 10 years of age have mild disease and may be asymptomatic.[4,11] The cervical, axillary, and inguinal lymph nodes are commonly enlarged. Splenomegaly occurs in 50–75% of these patients, and hepatomegaly occurs in about 25%. Occasionally, jaundice may develop. Hematologic complications that may occur during or immediately after the disease include autoimmune hemolytic anemia, thrombocytopenia, agranulocytosis, and (very rarely) aplastic anemia. The disease is usually self-limiting, resolving within a few weeks.

Laboratory Findings

Hematologic findings provide important clues to diagnosis in infectious mononucleosis. Serologic tests can confirm diagnosis.

Peripheral Blood   During active viral infection, there is an intense proliferation of lymphocytes within affected lymph nodes. The leukocyte count is usually increased ($12–25 \times 10^9$/L), primarily due to an absolute lymphocytosis. Lymphocytosis begins about 1 week after symptoms appear, peaks at 2–3 weeks, and remains elevated for 2–8 weeks.[5] Lymphocytes usually constitute more than 50% of the leukocytes. Various forms of reactive lymphocytes in the process of immunoblast transformation (>20%) can be found in the peripheral blood. These cells may contain vacuoles (Figure 22-2 ■). Immunoblasts are usually present early in the disease. Plasmacytoid lymphocytes and an occasional plasma cell also may be found. When present, immunoblasts should be distinguished from leukemic lymphoblasts to prevent a misdiagnosis. The chromatin pattern of leukemic lymphoblasts is usually finer than the reticular chromatin of immunoblasts. In addition, immunoblasts generally have a lower N:C ratio with more abundant, sometimes vacuolated, cytoplasm. Another important criterion that helps differentiate infectious mononucleosis from leukemia is the morphologic heterogeneity of the lym-

✪ **TABLE 22-2**

Summary of Typical Clinical and Laboratory Findings in Infectious Mononucleosis

Clinical Findings	Laboratory Findings
Lymphadenopathy	Leukocytosis
Fever	Lymphocytosis
Lethargy	Peripheral blood smear
Sore throat	>20% reactive (atypical) lymphocytes
Splenomegaly	Immunoblasts present
	Heterophil antibodies present
	Positive antigen tests for EBV

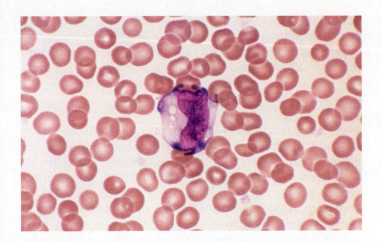

■ **FIGURE 22-2** Reactive (atypical) lymphocyte from a case of infectious mononucleosis. (Peripheral blood; Wright-Giemsa stain; 1000× magnification)

phocyte population characteristic of viral infections, whereas in leukemia there is a homogeneous population. Other diseases associated with a reactive lymphocytosis may be confused with the blood picture of infectious mononucleosis. These include cytomegalovirus infection, viral hepatitis, and toxoplasmosis. The platelet count is often mildly decreased, but concentrations less than 100×10^9/L are rare.

Bone Marrow   Bone marrow aspirations in EBV infection are not indicated, but when performed show hyperplasia of all cellular elements except neutrophils.

Serologic Tests   Serologic tests (tests based on antigen/antibody reactions) are used to differentiate this disease from similar more serious diseases (i.e., diptheria, hepatitis). The blood of patients with infectious mononucleosis contains greatly increased concentrations of antibodies that react with sheep erythrocytes, causing agglutination.[6] These transient antibodies are called **heterophil antibodies**. Other types of heterophil antibodies are found in most individuals and must be differentiated from infectious mononucleosis antibodies. Rapid, specific, and sensitive slide agglutination tests are now available to test for the presence of infectious mononucleosis heterophil antibodies. Other antibodies specific to EBV antigens are also produced by the infected individual at various stages of infection and can be detected by laboratory tests (Table 22-3).

Occasionally, a patient with all the clinical manifestations and peripheral blood findings of infectious mononucleosis will not have a positive heterophil test (heterophil-negative syndrome). In 10–20% of adult cases and in 50% of children younger than 10 years of age, the test is negative in the presence of EBV infection. In other cases, the heterophil-negative syndrome is caused by a non-EBV viral infection. The likely causative agent is cytomegalovirus; however, toxoplasmosis, hepatitis, and drug intoxication also should be considered. Antibody responses may not be detected in **immunosuppressed** individuals (those in whom the immune response is suppressed either naturally, artificially, or pathologically).[7]

Other laboratory tests may be abnormal depending on the presence or absence of complications. Hepatitis of some degree is common and can be a severe complication. An increase in both direct and indirect bilirubin fractions and an increase in serum liver enzymes are common findings. A rare complication of infectious mononucleosis is hemolytic anemia. The anemia appears to be due to cold agglutinins directed against the erythrocyte i-antigen.

Therapy

Since the disease is self-limited, therapy is supportive. Bed rest is recommended if fever and myalgia are present. Strenuous exercise should be avoided for several weeks, especially if splenomegaly is present. Antibiotics are not useful except in the presence of secondary infections.

> ✓ **Checkpoint! #1**
>
> *A patient with lymphocytosis, showing reactive lymphocyte morphology with large, basophilic cells, fine chromatin, and a visible nucleolus has a negative infectious mononucleosis serologic test. What is a possible cause for this altered lymphocyte morphology?*

TOXOPLASMOSIS

Toxoplasmosis is the result of infection with the intracellular protozoan *Toxoplasma gondii*. This obligate parasite can multiply in all body cells except erythrocytes. The infection

✪ TABLE 22-3				
Antibodies to EBV That Are Found in Infectious Mononucleosis				
Stage of Infection	Heterophil Antibodies	VCA-IgM (titer)	VCA-IgG (titer)	EBNA (titer)
Acute (0–3 months)	Present	>1:60	>1:60	Not detected
Recent (3–12 months)	Present	Not detected	>1:160	>1:10
Past (>12 months)	Present	Not detected	>1:40	>1:40

VCA = viralcapsid antigen; EBNA = EBV nuclear antigen.

may be congenital or acquired. Congenital infection, the most serious, results from placental transmission of organisms in the parasitized mother. Congenital infection may cause abortion, jaundice, hepatosplenomegaly, chorioretinitis, hydrocephalus, microcephaly, cerebral calcification, and mental retardation. Acquired infection may be asymptomatic or may cause symptoms resembling infectious mononucleosis. Infection in children and adults is acquired by ingestion of oocysts from cat feces or from inadequately cooked meat. Toxoplasmosis seropositivity is greater in rural children than urban children.[8]

Laboratory findings assist in diagnosis. There is a leukocytosis with a relative lymphocytosis or more rarely an absolute lymphocytosis and an increase in reactive lymphocytes. Most reactive cells are similar to lymphoblasts or lymphoma cells. The heterophil antibody test is negative. Biopsy of lymph nodes shows a reactive follicular hyperplasia and may play an important role in diagnosis. Diagnosis of an active infection is established by confirming a rising titer of toxoplasma antibodies. Immunologically compromised hosts have a more severe infection. The most common hematologic complication is hemolytic anemia, which may be severe.

CYTOMEGALOVIRUS

Infection with the herpes-group virus, **cytomegalovirus (CMV)**, may be the result of congenital or acquired infection. Infection in neonates occurs when organisms from the infected mother cross the placenta and infect the fetus. The newborn demonstrates jaundice, microcephaly, and hepatosplenomegaly. Only about 10% of infected infants exhibit clinical evidence of the disease. The most common hematologic findings in neonates are thrombocytopenia and hemolytic anemia.

Acquired infection is spread by close contact, blood transfusions, and sexual contact. The disease occurs in immunosuppressed individuals, in patients with malignancy, after massive blood transfusions, or in previously healthy adults. It is the most common viral infection complicating tissue transplants and is a significant cause of morbidity and mortality in immunocompromised patients.[9] Infected adults present with symptoms similar to those of infectious mononucleosis, except pharyngitis is absent. Many cytomegalovirus infections are subclinical or cause mild flu-like symptoms.

Laboratory findings include a leukocytosis with an absolute lymphocytosis. Many of the lymphocytes are reactive, but the heterophil agglutinin test is negative. Hepatic enzymes are usually abnormal. Diagnosis is confirmed by demonstrating the virus in the urine or blood or by a rise in the cytomegalovirus antibody titer, except in immunocompromised patients.

CMV is thought to infect neutrophils, which serve as a means of transporting the virus to other body sites. The virus appears to suppress cell-mediated immune function

and induce formation of autoantibodies that have lymphocytotoxic properties.[10,11] There is a decrease in circulating T helper lymphocytes and an increase in T suppressor/cytotoxic lymphocytes.

INFECTIOUS LYMPHOCYTOSIS

Infectious lymphocytosis is an infectious, contagious disease of young children. It may occur in epidemic form. The etiology of the disease is uncertain, but likely viruses are the adenovirus or coxsackie A virus. EBV and CMV are not implicated.[12] The incubation period is from 12 to 21 days. Clinical symptoms, if present, are mild and include diarrhea, gastrointestinal distress, respiratory infection, and fever. Patients also exhibit symptoms of central nervous system involvement, such as headache and vertigo, as well as pain and stiffness of the neck. Pharyngitis and lymphadenopathy are absent.

Laboratory findings help establish the diagnosis. The hemoglobin, erythrocyte count, platelet count, and sedimentation rate are normal. The most striking hematologic abnormality is a leukocytosis of $40\text{--}50 \times 10^9/L$ with 60–97% small, normal-appearing lymphocytes. This is in contrast to the reactive lymphocytes found in most other infectious states that are associated with lymphocytosis.

The lymphocytosis occurs in the first week of illness and falls within the next 3 weeks but may remain elevated for as long as 3 months. The lymphocytosis is primarily due to an increase in T lymphocytes. As the leukocytosis recedes, the eosinophil count may increase to $2\text{--}3 \times 10^9/L$. Within 4–6 weeks, the eosinophil count returns to normal.

BORDETELLA PERTUSSIS

Infection from **Bordetella pertussis** (whooping cough) causes a blood picture very similar to that of infectious lymphocytosis (Figure 22-3 ■). The leukocyte count typically

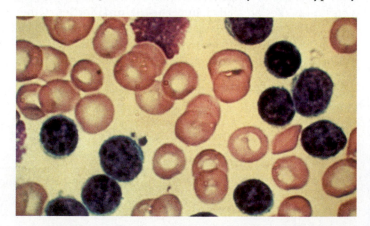

■ **FIGURE 22-3** Lymphoproliferation due to *Bordetella pertussis* (whooping cough). Note the numerous normal-appearing lymphocytes. This self-limiting peripheral blood picture must be distinguished from that of CLL. (Peripheral blood; Wright-Giemsa stain; 1000× magnification)

rises to $15-25 \times 10^9$/L but may reach 50×10^9/L. The rise in leukocytes is caused by a lymphocytosis, although neutrophils also may be increased. Granulocytes may show toxic changes. The lymphocytes are small cells with condensed chromatin and indistinct nucleoli.

A lymphocytosis-promoting factor produced by the bacteria recruits lymphocytes into peripheral circulation and blocks migration back into lymphoid tissue, causing accumulation of lymphocytes in the blood. The lymphocytosis-promoting factor appears to influence T helper cells.[11] Rapid peripheral lymphocytosis is accompanied by decreased cellularity of the lymph nodes.

PERSISTENT LYMPHOCYTOSIS

Persistent lymphocytosis is a rare disorder found in young to middle-aged females who are heavy smokers. It is characterized by a persistent polyclonal B cell lymphocytosis.[13] The disorder is often asymptomatic and found by chance on a routine blood analysis. Symptoms may include fever, fatigue, weight loss, recurrent chest infections, or generalized lymphadenopathy. Hematologic findings are normal except for lymphocytosis and the presence of binucleated lymphocytes. There is a polyclonal increase in serum IgM but low IgG and IgA levels. Bone marrow examination reveals lymphocytic infiltrates. Patients have a benign course.

OTHER DISORDERS ASSOCIATED WITH LYMPHOCYTOSIS

Other disorders accompanied by a reactive lymphocytosis are listed in Table 22-1 ✪. The lymphocytic reactions in these disorders are characterized by an increased relative lymphocyte count with the presence of reactive or immature-appearing lymphocytes (**lymphocytic leukemoid reaction**). Occasionally an absolute lymphocytosis is found. Many of the lymphocytes are large reactive cells with deep blue cytoplasm, fine chromatin, and cytoplasmic vacuoles (Figure 22-4 ■). Reactive cells are usually nonclonal T lymphocytes and large granular lymphocytes. In some viral infections, lymphocytosis is preceded by lymphocytopenia and neutropenia. As the infection subsides, plasmacytoid lymphocytes may be found (Figure 22-5 ■).

In some cases, a lymphocytic leukemoid reaction resembles chronic lymphocytic leukemia. Bone marrow aspiration however, shows minimal, if any, increase in lymphocytes in a lymphocytic leukemoid reaction. Adenopathy and splenomegaly are usually absent. In addition, the patients are usually young, whereas in chronic lymphocytic leukemia, the patients are usually older adults.

PLASMACYTOSIS

Plasma cells are not normally found in the peripheral blood. They may be present, however, with intense stimulation of the immune system, such as occurs in some viral and bacter-

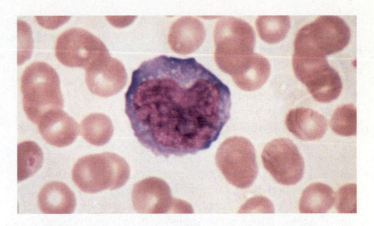

■ **FIGURE 22-4** An immunoblast found in a patient with a viral infection. This cell must be distinguished from a leukemic lymphoblast. (Peripheral blood; Wright-Giemsa stain; 1000× magnification)

ial infections and in disorders associated with elevated serum gamma globulin. They are commonly found in rubeola infections. Circulating plasma cells also may be found in skin diseases, cirrhosis of the liver, collagen disorders, and sarcoidosis. Most often the presence of plasma cells is associated with the neoplastic disorders, plasma cell leukemia, and multiple myeloma.

▶ LYMPHOCYTOPENIA

Some disorders are associated with a lymphocytopenia. Lymphocytopenia occurs in adults when the absolute lymphocyte count is less than 1.0×10^9/L. In children less than 5 years old, the lower normal range varies but it is higher than in adults (Table B ✪, inside front cover). Generally, counts less than 2×10^9/L are abnormal in this population. When the lymphocyte

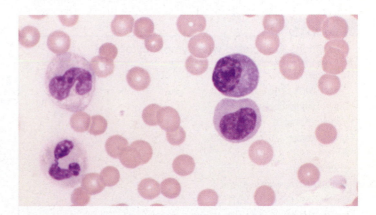

■ **FIGURE 22-5** A reactive lymphocyte (bottom) and a plasmacytoid lymph (top). These cells are associated with infectious states. (Peripheral blood; Wright-Giemsa stain; 1000× magnification)

count is decreased, there may be an impaired ability to mount an immune response, resulting in immunodeficiency.

Lymphocytopenia results from decreased production or increased destruction of lymphocytes, changes in lymphocyte circulation, or other unknown causes (Table 22-4).[14] Corticosteroid therapy causes a sharp drop in circulating lymphocytes within 4 hours. The decrease is caused by sequestration of lymphocytes in the bone marrow. Values return to normal within 12–24 hours after cessation of therapy. Acute inflammatory conditions, including viral and bacterial infections, also may be associated with a transient lymphocytopenia. Carcinoma of the breast and stomach with an associated lymphocytopenia is a poor prognostic sign. Systemic lupus erythematosus is frequently associated with a lymphocytopenia presumably caused by autoantibodies produced against these cells. Chemotherapeutic alkylating drugs for malignancy, such as cyclophosphamide, cause the death of T and B lymphocytes in both interphase and mitosis. Malnutrition is the most common cause of lymphocytopenia. Starvation causes thymic involution and depletion of T lymphocytes. Both congenital and acquired immune deficiencies are associated with lymphocytopenia.

Irradiation causes a prolonged suppression of lymphocyte production. T helper lymphocytes are more sensitive to radiation than T suppressor lymphocytes. It appears that small daily fractions of radiation are more damaging to lymphocytes than periodic large doses. With periodic radiation, the lymphocytes may be able to renew during periods of nonradiation. Aggressive treatment of hematologic malignancies with chemotherapeutics or ionizing radiation can lead to immunodeficiency by depleting short-lived antibody, forming B lymphocytes.

✔ Checkpoint! #2

Why is lymphocytopenia a concern if there is no accompanying leukopenia?

✪ TABLE 22-4

Conditions Associated with Lymphocytopenia

Malnutrition
Disseminated neoplasms
Connective tissue disease (e.g., SLE)
Hodgkin's disease
Chemotherapy
Radiotherapy
Corticosteroids
Acute inflammatory conditions
Chronic infection (e.g., TB)
Congenital immune deficiency diseases
Acquired immune deficiency diseases
Acute and chronic renal disease
Stress

@ **CASE STUDY** *(continued from page 405)*

Heidi weighed 2 pounds 1 ounce at birth. Tests for CMV and toxoplasma infections were negative. At 4 days of age, she was transferred to a special facility for feeding and growth monitoring. She developed a diaper rash that failed to respond to many measures. No thrush was found. At 44 days, she developed pneumonia from coagulase-negative staphylococci that responded to antibiotics. Her WBC count was $12.3 \times 10^9/L$ with a differential of segs 42%, bands 5%, lymphocytes 1%, monocytes 28%, eosinophils 23%, basophils 1%.

3. What is the absolute lymphocyte count?

4. What possible causes exist for these opportunistic infections?

IMMUNE DEFICIENCY DISORDERS

Immune deficiency disorders are characterized by a deficiency of T or B lymphocytes or both. The function of these cells also may be abnormal. This results in an inability to mount a normal immune response. These disorders are characterized clinically by an increase in infections and neoplasms. They may be subgrouped as acquired or congenital.

Acquired immune deficiency syndrome (AIDS) is a common infectious disorder characterized by lymphocytopenia. Due to the frequency with which this disorder is encountered in the clinical hematology laboratory, it will be discussed in more detail next. This is followed by a discussion of the congenital immune deficiency disorders.

Acquired Immune Deficiency Syndrome

Acquired immune deficiency syndrome (AIDS) is a highly lethal immune deficiency disease that was first described in 1981.[15] The disease is caused by infection with a retrovirus, human immunodeficiency virus type I (HIV-1). Recent advances in HIV treatment with combination antiretroviral therapy delay progression to AIDS and death for people infected with HIV.[16]

AIDS is defined by the occurrence of repeated infections with multiple **opportunistic organisms** and an increase in malignancies, especially Kaposi's sarcoma in individuals infected with HIV. Patients infected with HIV progress through three recognized stages: an asymptomatic carrier stage, an **AIDS-related complex (ARC)** stage (mild symptomatic stage), and, finally, symptomatic AIDS with one of the AIDS-defining clinical conditions (discussed later).[17]

Transmission of the virus is through sexual intercourse or contact with blood and blood products. The disease occurs primarily in certain high-risk groups: those who participate in unprotected sexual intercourse with high-risk individuals, homosexual and bisexual men, prostitutes, intravenous drug abusers, Haitians, and hemophiliacs. Although it is most common in men, women who have had sexual relations with someone at high risk of HIV-infection also are at risk, as well as infants born to HIV-infected mothers. Infant infection may be perinatal or occur at birth.

Disease Definition by Clinical Conditions   In 1982, the Centers for Disease Control (CDC) in the United States developed a case definition of AIDS for surveillance purposes. It is revised periodically as more is learned about the disease. It was recently proposed that AIDS case definition should be as comprehensive as possible because many countries will grant social benefits or access to medical care only if HIV infected patients have a diagnosed AIDS-defining illness.[18] The HIV case definition requires[19]:

> The presence of an AIDS defining clinical condition which includes an opportunistic infection or other clinical condition associated with cell-mediated immune defects in a person without a known cause for diminished resistance to disease and laboratory confirmation of HIV infection[20] (Table 22-5 ⊙).

OR

> A CD4 T lymphocyte count less than 200 cells/μL or a CD4 T lymphocyte count that composes less than 14% of the total lymphocytes and laboratory confirmation of HIV infection.

This second definition was added later as it was found that a decrease in CD4 T lymphocytes typically occurs before infection with opportunistic organisms. This second definition may allow preventative treatment in those infected with HIV infection to help delay onset of AIDS defining clinical illnesses.

AIDS case surveillance alone does not reflect accurately the HIV epidemic. To more accurately reflect the trends in HIV infection, the CDC recommends not only AIDS surveillance but also surveillance for HIV infection.[16] This surveillance expansion helps to identify populations with newly diagnosed HIV infection and aids in efforts to prevent HIV transmission.

Laboratory evidence of HIV infection includes positive serologic HIV antibody tests, positive HIV nucleic acid (DNA or RNA), or positive HIV cultures.[16] Almost all children born to HIV-infected mothers have anti-HIV IgG antibodies at birth due to placental transmission of maternal antibodies. However, only 15–30% are infected with HIV. Thus, anti-HIV IgG tests are not reliable until after 18 months in this population. In these cases, HIV nucleic acid detection tests performed after the infant is at least one month of age are almost always positive if the virus is present.[16]

Immune compromised patients without one of the AIDS-defining clinical conditions but with milder symptoms, including weight loss, fever, lymphadenopathy, thrush, chronic rash, or intermittent diarrhea, are included in the ARC category.

Pathophysiology   The etiologic agent of AIDS has been identified as the retrovirus, HIV-1. This virus selectively infects

---

⊙ TABLE 22-5

Clinical Conditions Included in the Centers for Disease Control AIDS Case Definition for Surveillance

Candidiasis of bronchi, trachea, or lungs

Candidiasis, esophageal

Cervical cancer, invasive

Coccidioidomycosis, disseminated or extrapulmonary

Cryptococcosis, extrapulmonary

Cryptosporidiosis, chronic intestinal (>1 month's duration)

Cytomegalovirus disease (other than liver, spleen, or nodes)

Cytomegalovirus retinitis (with loss of vision)

Encephalopathy, HIV related

Herpes simplex: chronic ulcer(s) (>1 month's duration); or bronchitis, pneumonitis, or esophagitis

Histoplasmosis, disseminated or extrapulmonary

Isosporiasis, chronic intestinal (>1 month's duration)

Kaposi's sarcoma

Lymphoma, Burkitt

Lymphoma, immmunoblastic (or equivalent term)

Lymphoma, primary, of brain

Mycobacterium avium complex or *M. kansasii,* (disseminated or extrapulmonary)

Mycobacterium tuberculosis, any site (pulmonary or extrapulmonary)

Mycobacterium, other species or unidentified species, disseminated or extrapulmonary

Pneumocystis carinii pneumonia

Pneumonia, recurrent

Progressive multifocal leukoencephalopathy

Salmonella septicemia, recurrent

Toxoplasmosis of brain

Wasting syndrome due to HIV

(From Appendix B from *MMWR*, 41, No. RR-17, December 1992.)

---

helper T lymphocytes by binding to the CD4 antigen that composes the T lymphocyte receptor (TCR), causing rapid, selective depletion of this lymphocyte subset. Cytolysis of CD4+ lymphocytes results in lymphocytopenia. Once in the cell, HIV sheds its coat and uses reverse transcriptase to make a DNA copy of the viral RNA. The viral DNA is integrated into the host cell DNA. The virus then replicates within the host cell. Monocytes and macrophages also have the CD4 antigen and are infected but are not destroyed by the virus.

Cell-mediated immunity and humoral immunity are abnormal. Cell-mediated immunity declines as CD4 T-lymphocyte-helper function for monocytes, macrophages, and other T lymphocytes declines.[21] Humoral responses are exaggerated with polyclonal B lymphocyte proliferation and increased immunoglobulin production.[22] The B lymphocytes, however, are incapable of responding to signals that trigger resting B lymphocytes.

Laboratory Findings   Multiple hematologic abnormalities are found in AIDS, including leukopenia, lymphocytopenia, anemia, and thrombocytopenia (Table 22-6). Leukopenia is usually related to lymphocytopenia, although neutropenia also may be present.[23] Lymphocytes may include reactive forms. Mild to moderate anemia is present in the majority of HIV-infected individuals and worsens as the disease progresses.[24] Macrocytosis (MCV>110 fL) occurs in up to 70% of patients 2 weeks after receiving zidovudine.[25] Antierythrocyte antibodies may be found in up to 20% of patients with hypergammaglobulinemia. These antibodies react like polyagglutinins and cause a positive direct antiglobulin test (DAT, Coombs' test). Immune thrombocytopenia, indistinguishable from idiopathic thrombocytopenic purpura (ITP), is common (∞ Chapter 36). (ITP is characterized by immune destruction of platelets, causing a thrombocytopenia.)

Disease Monitoring   The severity of CD4 lymphocytopenia and concentration of plasma HIV-1 RNA copies correlate with the severity of disease.[17,26] The normal CD4-to-CD8 ratio in peripheral blood is about 2. In AIDS, this ratio reverses progressively and permanently due to destruction of the CD4 T lymphocytes. The CD4 T lymphocyte count is performed at initial diagnosis and measured periodically to monitor disease progression. In addition, the **viral load** also is monitored. Measuring the number of copies of HIV-1 RNA indicates a patient's viral load.

Therapy   There is no cure for AIDS. Treatment with zidovudine (azodothymidine, AZT) and protease inhibitors appear to lengthen the time between HIV seropositivity and the onset of AIDS.[27] Surveillance studies between 1992 and 1997 determined that careful follow-up and new antiviral treatments decreased the incidence of opportunistic infections in over one-half of the patients on the case definition list.[28]

Health care workers with occupational exposure to HIV (needle-stick injury) should receive immediate antiretroviral therapy.[26] CDC recommends initiation of antiretroviral therapy within 2 hours of a needle-stick injury from a potential HIV source. Combination therapy should consist of two or more antiretroviral drugs and continue for 4 weeks. Laboratory evaluation for adverse effects should be considered after 2 weeks. Health care workers who receive chemoprophylaxis for HIV exposure should enroll in the Centers for Disease Control and Prevention registry (1(888)HIV-4PEP).

✔ **Checkpoint! #3**

Why does infection with HIV result in an increased chance for opportunistic infections?

⊙ **TABLE 22-6**

Common Laboratory Findings in HIV Infections

Leukopenia	Thrombocytopenia
Anemia	Decreased CD4 counts
Macrocytosis	Positive RNA tests for HIV-1

Other Acquired Immune Deficiency Disorders

Some disorders are characterized or accompanied by functional abnormalities of lymphocytes. The lymphocyte count may be normal but in many cases is decreased. Acquired defects of either T or B lymphocytes can result in serious clinical manifestations. Some inflammatory states can transiently impede the response of T lymphocytes to antigen. These include idiopathic granulomatous disorders and malignancy. Sometimes, severe infection by one microorganism impedes the ability of T lymphocytes to react to other infectious organisms. Starvation or severe protein deficiency can severely affect the functional ability of the T lymphocyte.

Congenital Immune Deficiency Disorders

Congenital disorders are usually characterized by a decrease in lymphocytes and impairment in either cell-mediated immunity (T lymphocytes), humoral immunity (B lymphocytes), or both (Table 22-7 ⊙). In contrast to the reactive morphologic heterogeneity of lymphocytes associated with acquired disorders, lymphocytes in congenital disorders are normal in appearance. The functional impairment of the immune response is apparent from birth or a very young age.

Severe Combined Immunodeficiency Syndrome

Severe combined immunodeficiency syndrome (SCIDS) is a heterogeneous group of disorders resulting in major qualitative immune defects. These disorders have a diverse genetic origin with different inheritance patterns and varied severity in clinical manifestation. They are inherited as sex-linked or autosomal-recessive traits. Sporadic forms have been reported. About 75% of individuals with this disease are males.

Both the T and B lymphoid systems are profoundly deficient. The absolute lymphocyte count is usually decreased to less than 0.1×10^9/L, but counts may be normal in infancy. T lymphocytes are absent in peripheral blood, but B lymphocyte numbers may be normal to decreased. Peripheral blood B lymphocytes are unresponsive to mitogens, and immunoglobulin production is decreased. However, these B lymphocytes respond normally when incubated with T lymphocytes in vitro.[22]

Lymph node examination reveals a lack of plasma cells, B lymphocytes, and T lymphocytes. No lymphoid tissue is found in the spleen, tonsils, or intestinal tract. The bone marrow also is deficient in plasma cells and lymphocyte precursors.

Frequent recurrent infections, the presence of skin rashes, diarrhea, and a failure to thrive are characteristic findings in infants with this disorder. Death related to overwhelming sepsis usually occurs within the first 2 years of life. Bone marrow transplantation may be the only hope of survival.

Sex-linked SCIDS.   Sex-linked (X-linked) SCIDS is the most common form of inherited severe combined immunodeficiency, accounting for more than 50% of cases. This form of SCIDS has been mapped to the long arm of the X

⭐ **TABLE 22-7**

Laboratory Findings in Selected Immunodeficiency Disorders

Disorder	Immunoglobulins	B lymphocytes	T lymphocytes	Inheritance
SCIDS (X-linked and autosomal recessive)	↓ IgG, IgM, IgA	↓ or normal	Mature T lymphs absent	Sex-linked (defects at X[q13.1-q21.1]), autosomal recessive, random
Wiskott-Aldrich syndrome	↓ IgM, ↑ IgA, ↑ IgE Normal IgG	Normal	Progressive ↓	Sex-linked (defects at X[p11.3-p11.22])
DiGeorge syndrome	Normal	Normal	↓	Gene deletion (22del[q11])
X-linked agammaglobulinemia	↓ IgG, ↓ IgM, ↓ IgA	↓	Normal	Sex-linked (defects at X[q21.3-q22])
Hereditary ataxia-telangiectasia	Variable, ↑ IgM, ↓ IgG, ↓ IgA, ↓ IgE	Normal	↓	Autosomal recessive (abnormalities of chromosome 7 or 14)

↓ = decreased; ↑ = increased

chromosome (Xql3.1–q21.1). Family history is important in determining the mode of inheritance, although a negative family history of the disease does not rule out an X-linked disease. Up to one-third of the cases show up as a spontaneous mutation.[22,29]

X-linked SCIDS is characterized by absent or severely reduced T lymphocytes. The thymus is hypoplastic. The defect appears to reside in the marrow-derived T precursor cells. T lymphocytes do not mature. B lymphocytes are normal or even increased in number but are functionally abnormal. Immunoglobulin levels are severely depressed. The defect in B lymphocyte function may be partially due to the lack of T lymphocyte help. Additional abnormalities intrinsic to B lymphocytes are probable.

Females who carry the abnormal X-linked SCIDS gene have normal immunity. These carriers can be detected by molecular assays that are used to assess X chromosome inactivation patterns. The mature female cell population is mosaic with one or the other X chromosome inactivated. In female SCIDS carriers, however, only normal X chromosomes are found in the lymphocytes rather than the expected mixture of cells with normal and abnormal X chromosome activation. It has been found that random X chromosome inactivation occurs in these carriers, but the gene product of the X-mutant chromosome does not support lymphocyte maturation. This means that lymphocytes with the mutant X chromosome fail to develop. Thus, the only lymphocytes found in carriers have the active normal X chromosome.

✓ **Checkpoint! #4**

Would you expect female carriers of X-linked SCIDS to be more susceptible to infection than the normal population?

Autosomal SCIDS. The autosomal forms of SCIDS exhibit severe deficiencies of both T and B lymphocytes. The most common form, found in about 50% of autosomal-recessive SCIDS, is due to an adenosine deaminase deficiency.[30,31] The adenosine deaminase gene is located on chromosome 20. Both point mutations and gene deletions have been associated with adenosine deaminase deficiency. Another enzyme deficiency, purine nucleoside phosphorylase, also is a cause of SCIDS. These enzymes degrade purines. Without the enzyme, accumulation of deoxyadenosine triphosphate and deoxyguanosine triphosphate, which are toxic to lymphocytes, occur. Other defects include a deficiency of MHC class II gene expression, interleukin-2 (IL-2) deficiency, and defective assembly of the T lymphocyte receptor/CD3 complex.[22]

@ **CASE STUDY** *(continued from page 410)*

All immunoglobulin levels in the patient were decreased. T and B lymphocyte counts were severely decreased. The peripheral blood smear showed anisocytosis, poikilocytosis (schistocytes), polychromatophilia, and 2 nucleated RBCs/100 WBCs. Her thymus was not detectable on chest films.

5. Is this child more likely to have a congenital or acquired immune deficiency?

6. If she has a congenital immune deficiency, is it more likely she has X-linked or autosomal SCIDS?

7. Are the lymphocytes more likely to be morphologically heterogeneous or homogeneous? Why?

8. What confirmatory test is indicated?

Wiskott-Aldrich Syndrome Wiskott-Aldrich syndrome (WAS) is a sex-linked recessive disease characterized by the triad of eczema, thrombocytopenia, and immunodeficiency. About two-thirds of the children have a family history of the disease, while one-third reflect a spontaneous mutation. Most children die before 10 years of age due to infection or bleeding. Those who survive longer may develop neoplasms of the histiocytic, lymphocytic, or myelocytic systems.

Laboratory findings play an important role in diagnosis of WAS (Table 22-8). There is a progressive decrease in thymic-dependent immunity and depletion of paracortical areas in lymph nodes. Circulating B lymphocyte concentrations are normal, but there is a decrease in T lymphocytes. Antibody production by the B lymphocytes, however, is abnormal.[22] Serum IgM levels are decreased, but IgE and IgA levels are increased. IgG concentrations are usually normal.

One of the most consistent findings is low or absent levels of circulating antibodies to the blood group antigens.[32] This is due to the inability of these children to produce antibodies to polysaccharide antigens. This T-lymphocyte-independent phenomenon suggests that there is an intrinsic B lymphocyte abnormality.

T lymphocyte function is abnormal. The absolute numbers of helper and suppressor T lymphocytes and their ratio is normal to variable. CD43, a highly glycosylated cell marker present on all nonerythroid hematopoietic cells, is abnormal in WAS T lymphocytes. These T lymphocytes are not stimulated by anti-CD43 antibodies or periodate, as are normal T lymphocytes. This highly specific finding is the test of choice when WAS is suspected.[33] Because the gene for CD43 is on chromosome 16 and not the X chromosome, this is probably not the primary defect in WAS.

Abnormal bleeding in the neonatal period is one of the first clinical signs of WAS. The bleeding time is abnormal, but the prothrombin time and activated partial thromboplastin time are normal, indicating the coagulation factor proteins are adequate (∞ Chapter 34). Platelet number and size (volume) are decreased, but megakaryocytes in the bone marrow are normal or increased in number. Splenectomy usually results in correction of platelet concentration and size.

The genetic defect has been localized to the short arm of the X chromosome between Xp11.3 and Xp11.22.[32] Molecular analysis using restriction fragment length polymorphisms reveals that female carriers have selective inactivation of the WAS X chromosome rather than random inactivation of paternal or maternal X chromosomes. This nonrandom inactivation pattern is found in the carrier's T and B lymphocytes, granulocytes, monocytes, and megakaryocytes, indicating all hematopoietic cells in WAS express the defect.

Therapy includes treatment for bleeding and infection. Splenectomy significantly reduces the risk of bleeding complications. Bone marrow transplantation has been used with some success.

✔ Checkpoint! #5

What laboratory findings suggest WAS in a child, and how is the diagnosis confirmed?

DiGeorge Syndrome   DiGeorge syndrome is a congenital immunodeficiency marked by the absence or hypoplasia of the thymus, hypoparathyroidism, heart defects, and dysmorphic facies. Hypocalcemia is typical and the presenting symptom may be seizure due to hypocalcemia. There is usually a decrease in peripheral blood T lymphocytes as well as a decrease in cellularity of the thymic-dependent regions of peripheral lymphoid tissue. The low lymphocyte count is related to a decreased number of CD4 lymphocytes. T lymphocyte function varies. Those children with a hypoplastic thymus may be able to produce enough lymphocytes with normal function to maintain immunocompetence. B lymphocytes are normal in number and function and immunoglobulin levels are normal. Infants exhibit increased susceptibility to viral, fungal, and bacterial infections that are frequently overwhelming. Death occurs in the first year unless thymic grafts are performed.

Cytogenetic studies on these children reveal a deletion within chromosome 22ql1.[34] This defect also is found in a parent of a child with DiGeorge syndrome in 25% of the cases.

Sex-Linked Agammaglobulinemia   Sex-linked (X-linked) agammaglobulinemia (Bruton's disease) is inherited as a sex-linked disease characterized by frequent respiratory and skin infections with extracellular, catalase-negative, pyogenic bacteria. Molecular analysis has revealed that the genetic defect is on the long arm of the X chromosome (q21.3–q22).[22] The genetic mutation results in a block in B lymphocyte maturation at the pre-B-lymphocyte stage. The variable and constant regions of the IgM immunoglobin chain fail to connect. Peripheral blood lymphocyte counts are normal, as are T lymphocytes; there is, however, a decrease in B lymphocytes and an absence of plasma cells in lymph nodes. The serum concentrations of IgG, IgM, and IgA are decreased or absent. Cell-mediated immune function is normal. Monthly injections of gamma globulin are effective in preventing severe infections.

Female carriers of this disease have normal immunity. All their B lymphocytes carry the paternal, normal X chromosome. This suggests the normal X chromosome confers a growth advantage to the normal cells.

Hereditary Ataxia-Telangiectasia   Hereditary ataxia-telangiectasia is inherited as an autosomal-recessive disease. The disease is characterized by progressive neurologic dis-

---

✪ TABLE 22-8

Laboratory Features in Wiskott-Aldrich Syndrome

- Platelets: decreased concentration; small size
- Lymphocytes: decreased or normal concentration; T lymphocytes variable; B lymphocytes usually normal
- Immunoglobulin: IgM decreased; IgE and IgA increased; IgG normal
- Antibodies to blood group antigens absent
- No mitogenic response of lymphocytes to anti-CD43 or periodate

ease, immune dysfunction, and predisposition to malignancy. Affected individuals are ataxic and develop telangiectasias in childhood or adolescence. Telangiectasia is a vascular lesion formed by a dilation of a group of blood vessels that appears as a red line or radiating limbs (spider). Chronic respiratory infection and lymphoid malignancy are the most common causes of death.

These patients have a defect in cell-mediated immunity with hypoplasia or dysplasia of the thymus gland and deple-

tion of thymic-dependent areas in the lymph nodes. B lymphocyte function also is abnormal. There is lymphocytopenia and decreased IgG, IgA, and IgE. IgM levels are increased. Cytogenetic analysis reveals excessive chromosome breakage and rearrangements in cultured cells and clonal abnormalities of chromosome 7 or 14.[35]

SUMMARY

Lymphocytes mount an immune response in inflammatory or infectious states. In these states, the lymphocyte morphology often includes various reactive forms, immunoblasts, and possibly plasmacytoid cells. Quantitative changes in the total lymphocyte concentration occur, which may be either increased or decreased. Although the lymphocyte induces an immune response to eliminate foreign antigens, the cell itself also may serve as the site of infection for some viruses that use lymphocyte membrane receptors to attach to the cell.

Infectious mononucleosis is a common self-limiting lymphoproliferative disorder caused by infection with EBV. Laboratory diagnosis of this disorder includes serologic testing for heterophil antibodies and identification of reactive lymphocytes on Romanowsky-stained blood smears.

AIDS is a disease caused by infection of the CD4 lymphocyte with the retrovirus HIV-1. The virus suppresses the immune response by replicating within and destroying CD4 lymphocytes. CD4 lymphocyte levels and viral loads monitor the progression of the disease. Antiviral treatments in combination with protease inhibitors slow the progression of the disease process. There is no cure for this disease.

Congenital qualitative disorders of lymphocytes include a wide variety of immunodeficiency disorders. Either the T or B lymphocyte or both may be affected. These are usually very serious defects, with most affected individuals succumbing to the disease in childhood. Bone marrow transplant is the only treatment in many cases.

REVIEW QUESTIONS

LEVEL I

1. The infectious agent in infectious mononucleosis is: (Checklist #1)
   a. CMV
   b. HIV
   c. EBV
   d. *Toxoplasmosis gondii*

2. Large reactive (atypical) lymphocytes with dispersed chromatin and irregular cytoplasmic membranes are associated with: (Checklist #2)
   a. infectious lymphocytosis
   b. infectious mononucleosis
   c. cytomegalovirus infection
   d. hepatitis

3. Which of the following best describes the lymphocytes seen in viral infection? (Checklist #5)
   a. large cells with high N:C ratio, immature nucleus, and vacuoles
   b. small cells with high N:C ratio and vacuolated cytoplasm
   c. large cells with deep basophilic cytoplasm and decreased N:C ratio
   d. large cells with immature nuclei and high N:C ratio

LEVEL II

Use this case study for questions 1–3.

A 39-year-old male is seen at the clinic with complaints of nagging cough, weight loss, diarrhea, and low-grade temperature. Results of physical examination show lymphadenopathy, congested lungs, and increased heart rate. Slight splenomegaly and hepatomegaly were noted. A CBC and flow cytometry studies were ordered. Histologic examination of sputum with Gomori's methenamine silver nitrate stain revealed *Pneumocystis carinii*.

Laboratory Data:

Erythrocyte count:	3.86×10^{12}/L
Hb:	13.6 g/dL
Hct:	0.41 L/L
Platelet count:	104×10^9/L
Leukocyte count:	2.8×10^9/L
Differential:	

Segmented neutrophils:	68%	Monocytes:	10%
Lymphocytes:	21%	Eosinophils:	1%

Positive for HIV-1 antibodies

LEVEL I

4. The CD4:CD8 ratio of T lymphocytes in a patient with AIDS is: (Checklist #9, 10)
   a. 2:1
   b. increased
   c. decreased
   d. equal

5. The type of antibodies found in infectious mononucleosis that are used to confirm a diagnosis are: (Checklist #3)
   a. heterophil antibodies
   b. cold agglutinins
   c. PIG antibodies
   d. HIV antibodies

6. The HIV-1 virus infects what type of lymphocytes? (Checklist #9)
   a. B lymphocytes
   b. suppressor T lymphocytes
   c. CD4+ T lymphocytes
   d. CD8+ T lymphocytes

7. A 2-year-old child has a total leukocyte count of 10×10^9/L and 60% lymphocytes. Which of the following best describes the child's blood count? (Checklist #4)
   a. absolute lymphocytosis
   b. relative lymphocytosis
   c. normal lymphocyte count for the age given
   d. absolute lymphocytopenia

Use this case study for questions 8–10.

A 19-year-old female college student went to student health complaining of lethargy and a sore throat over the last two weeks. Physical exam shows pharyngitis, lymphadenopathy, splenomegaly, with a total leukocyte count of 11×10^9/L and 70% lymphocytes (50% of lymphs are reactive).

8. She probably has: (Checklist #1)
   a. HIV
   b. hepatitis
   c. X-linked SCIDS
   d. infectious mononucleosis

9. Her absolute lymphocyte count is: (Checklist #4)
   a. 10×10^9/L
   b. 11×10^9/L
   c. 5.5×10^9/L
   d. 7.7×10^9/L

10. The best description of this patient's leukocyte count is a(n): (Checklist #4)
    a. relative lymphocytopenia
    b. relative neutrophilia
    c. absolute lymphocytosis
    d. absolute neutrophilia

LEVEL II

1. What clinical condition does this patient have? (Checklist #8, 10)
   a. congenital immune deficiency
   b. infectious mononucleosis
   c. ARC
   d. AIDS

2. Which lymphocytes are periodically counted to monitor the disease? (Checklist #8)
   a. infected B lymphocytes
   b. CD4 T lymphocytes
   c. CD8 T lymphocytes
   d. natural killer lymphocytes

3. Which laboratory test is used to follow this patient's disease? (Checklist #8)
   a. HIV-1 viral load
   b. throat swab
   c. serologic test for heterophil antibody
   d. CD43 negative antigen response

4. A clue to differentiating the lymphocytes of infectious mononucleosis from those found in neoplastic lymphocytic disorders is that in neoplastic disorders the lymphocytes are: (Checklist #5)
   a. morphologically similar
   b. heterogeneous morphologically
   c. not increased
   d. reactive

5. A 17-year-old male has a sore throat and lymphadenopathy. He is lethargic and has a temperature of 99.5°F. Laboratory tests reveal a leukocyte count of 13×10^9/L with 65% lymphocytes, most of which are reactive. The heterophil antibody test is positive, the VCA-IgM titer is 1:320, VCA-IgG titer is 1:240, and EBNA is not detectable. What is the most likely explanation for these results? (Checklist #3, 10)
   a. acute EBV infection
   b. EBV infection within the last 3–12 months
   c. EBV infection more than a year ago
   d. no EBV infection present, now, or in the past

6. In female carriers of sex-linked, severe combined immunodeficiency gene, the lymphocytes carry: (Checklist #9)
   a. a normal X chromosome in the T lymphocytes
   b. the mutant X chromosome in T and B lymphocytes
   c. the mutant X chromosome in T lymphocytes
   d. the mutant X chromosome in 50% of T lymphocytes

7. *Bordatella pertussis* infection is characterized by: (Checklist #7)
   a. a positive heterophil antibody test and lymphocytosis
   b. lymphocytopenia and reactive lymphocytes
   c. lymphocytosis with normal appearing lymphocytes
   d. lymphocytosis with reactive lymphocytes

REVIEW QUESTIONS (continued)

LEVEL I

LEVEL II

8. Occasionally, a patient who has been exposed to EBV shows clinical symptoms and reactive lymphocytes but has a negative serologic test. This may be due to: (Checklist #1)
   a. infection with a parasite
   b. infection with *Bordatella pertussis*
   c. infection with syphilis
   d. early infection with no detectable antibody

9. Documentation and surveillance for AIDS in patients includes those who are positive for: (Checklist #8)
   a. HIV viral DNA
   b. EBV viral RNA
   c. heterophil antibodies
   d. any bacterial infection

10. Which of the following nonmalignant conditions is *NOT* associated with a lymphocytosis? (Checklist #5, 7, 9)
    a. whooping cough
    b. Toxoplasmosis gondii
    c. X-linked immunodeficiency syndrome
    d. cytomegalovirus infection

www.prenhall.com/mckenzie

Use the above address to access the free, interactive Companion Web site created for this textbook. Get hints, instant feedback, and textbook references to chapter-related multiple choice questions.

REFERENCES

1. Straus SE, Cohen JI, Tosato G, Meier J. Epstein-Barr virus infections: Biology, pathogenesis, and management. *Ann Intern Med.* 1993; 118:45–58.

2. Foerster J. Infectious mononucleosis. Lee GR, Foerster J, Lukens JN, Paraskevas F, Greer JP, Rodgers GM, eds. In: *Wintrobe's Clinical Hematology,* Vol 2, 10th ed. Baltimore, Md: Williams & Wilken; 1999:1926–55.

3. Bailey RE. Diagnosis and treatment of infectious mononucleosis. *Am Fam Physician.* 1994; 49:879–85.

4. Nathwani D, Wood MJ. Herpes virus infections in childhood:2. *Br J Hosp Med.* 1993; 50:301–8.

5. Peterson L, Hrisinko MA. Benign lymphocytosis and reactive neutrophilia. *Clin Lab Med.* 1993; 13:863–77.

6. Paul JR, et al. The presence of heterophil antibodies in infectious mononucleosis. *Am J Med Sci.* 1932; 83:90–104.

7. Wakiguchi H, Hisakawa H, Kubota H, Kurashiga T. Serodiagnosis of infectious mononucleosis in children. *Acta Paediatr Jpn.* 1998; 40:328–32.

8. Taylor M, Lennon B, Holland C, Caffrey M. Community study of toxoplasma antibodies in urban and rural school children age 4 to 8 years. *Arch Dis Child.* 1997; 77:406–9.

9. Epstein J, Scully C. Cytomegalovirus: A virus of increasing relevance to oral medicine and pathology. *J Oral Pathol Med.* 1993; 22:348–53.

10. Mustafa MM. Cytomegalovirus infection and disease in the immunocompromised host. *Pediatr Infect Dis J.* 1994; 13:249–57.

11. Brown K. Nonmalignant disorders of lymphocytes. *Clin Lab Sci.* 1997; 10:329–35.

12. Gay JC, Athens, JW. Variations of leukocytosis disease. Lee GR, Foerster J, Lukens JN, Paraskevas F, Greer JP, Rodgers GM, eds., In: *Wintrobe's Clinical Hematology,* Vol. 2, 10th ed. Baltimore, Md: Williams & Wilken; 1999:1851.

13. Agrawal S, Matutes E, Voke J, Dyer MJS, Khokhar T, Catovsky D. Persistent polyclonal B-cell lymphocytosis. *Leuk Res.* 1994; 18:791–95.

14. Schoentag RA, Cangiarella J. The nuances of lymphocytopenia. *Clin Lab Med.* 1993; 13:923–36.

15. Gottlieb MS, et al. *Pneumocystis carinii* pneumonia and mucosal candidiasis in previously healthy homosexual men: Evidence of a new acquired cellular immunodeficiency. *N Engl J Med.* 1981; 305: 1425–31.

16. Centers for Disease Control and Prevention. Guidelines for national human immunodeficiency virus case surveillance, including monitoring for human immunodeficiency virus infections and acquired immunodeficiency syndrome. *MMWR.* 1999; 48(RR-13):1–27, 29–31.

17. Centers for Disease Control and Prevention. Prevention and treatment of tuberculosis among patients infected with human immun-

odeficiency virus: Principles of therapy and revised recommendations. *MMWR*. 1998; 47(RR-20):1–51.

18. Albrecht H. Redefining AIDS: Towards a modification of the current AIDS case definition. *Clin Infec Diseases*. 1997; 24(1):64–74.

19. Gold JWM. HIV-1 Infection. *Med Clin North Am*. 1992; 76:1–18.

20. Centers for Disease Control and Prevention. 1993 revised classification system for HIV infection and expanded surveillance case definition for AIDS among adolescents and adults. *MMWR*. 1992; 41(RR-17):1–19.

21. Said JW. Pathogenesis of HIV infection. Nash G, Said JW, eds. In: *Pathology of AIDS and HIV Infection*. Philadelphia: WB Saunders Co.: 1992; 26:15–18. Major Probl Pathol series.

22. Insel RA. Disorders of lymphocyte function. Hoffman R, Benz EJ, Shattil SJ, Furie B, Cohen HJ, Silberstein LE, eds. In: *Hematology: Basic Principles and Practice*. New York, NY: Churchill Livingstone Inc; 1995:819–38.

23. Brynes RK, Gill PS. Clinical characteristics, immunologic abnormalities, and hematopathology of HIV infection. Joshi VV, ed. In: *Pathology of AIDS and Other Manifestations of HIV Infection*. New York: Igaku-Shoin; 1990:21–42.

24. Doukas MA. Human immunodeficiency virus associated anemia. *Med Clin North Am*. 1992; 76:699–709.

25. Aboulafia DM, Mitsuyasu RT. Hematologic abnormalities in AIDS. *Hematol Oncol Clin North Am*. 1991; 5:195–214.

26. Carpenter CCJ, Fischl MA, Hammer SM, et al. Antiretroviral therapy for HIV infection in 1998: Updated recommendations of the International AIDS Society-USA Panel. *JAMA*. 1998; 280:78–86.

27. Ibanez A, Ruiz L, Puig T, Gutierrez C, Sanchez I, Clotet B. Plasma viral load (VL) and CD4 count changes in naive patients at 6 months after initiation of combined therapy with zidovudine (AZT) and zalcitabine (ddC) (abstract). *Interscience Conf. of Antimicrobial Agents*. 1996:208. Abstract I121.

28. Centers for Disease Control and Prevention. Surveillance for AIDS-defining opportunistic illnesses, 1992–1997. *MMWR*. 1999; 47 (SS-2):1–22.

29. Puck JM. Prenatal diagnosis and genetic analysis of X-linked immunodeficiency disorders. *Pediatr Res*. 1993; 33(suppl 1):29–33.

30. Hilman BC, Sorensen RU. Management options: SCIDS with adenosine deaminase deficiency. *Ann Allergy*. 1994; 72:395–403.

31. Rosen FS, Bhan AK. Weekly clinicopathological exercises, case 18-1998: A 54-day-old premature girl with respiratory distress and persistent pulmonary infiltrates. *New Eng J Med*. 1998; 338:1752–58.

32. Peacocke M, Siminovitch KA. Wiskott-Aldrich syndrome: New molecular and biochemical insights. *J Am Acad Dermatol*. 1992; 27:507–19.

33. Peacocke M, Siminovitch KA. The Wiskott-Aldrich syndrome. *Semin Dermatol*. 1993; 12:247–54.

34. Wilson DI, Burn J, Scanbler P, Goodship J. DiGeorge syndrome: Part of CATCH 22. *J Med Genet*. 1993; 30:852–56.

35. Swift M, Heim RA, Lench NJ. Genetic aspects of ataxia telangiectasia. *Adv Neurol*. 1993; 61:115–25.

SECTION SIX • LABORATORY PROCEDURES USED IN DIAGNOSIS OF NEOPLASTIC HEMATOLOGIC DISORDERS

23

Flow Cytometry

Fiona E. Craig, M.D.

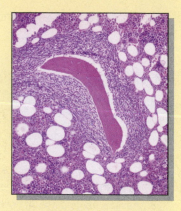

■ CHECKLIST - LEVEL I

At the end of this unit of study the student should be able to:

1. Describe the components of a flow cytometer and the principles of cell analysis.
2. Illustrate by example the clinical applications of flow cytometry.
3. Appraise the use of fluorochrome-labeled antibodies in immunophenotyping by flow cytometry.
4. Give examples of the clinical applications of immunophenotyping by flow cytometry and interpret single dot-plots.
5. Define *clonality* and identify methods for detecting a monoclonal population of cells by immunophenotyping.
6. List the specimens appropriate for immunophenotyping by flow cytometry.
7. Describe how flow cytometry can be used in cell quantitation.
8. Calculate and interpret the absolute CD4 count.
9. Describe reticulocyte counting by flow cytometry and define *immature reticulocyte fraction* (IRF).
10. Explain how flow cytometry can be applied to DNA analysis.
11. List the cells positive for CD34 and explain the purpose of a CD34 count.

■ CHECKLIST - LEVEL II

At the end of this unit of study the student should be able to:

1. Compare and contrast the immunophenotyping results characteristic of chronic lymphocytic leukemia, hairy cell leukemia, and non-Hodgkin lymphoma.
2. Identify the pitfalls that may be encountered in immunophenotyping mature lymphoid malignancies by flow cytometry and generate potential solutions.
3. Compare and contrast the immunophenotyping results characteristic of acute lymphoblastic leukemia and acute myelogenous leukemia.
4. Identify the pitfalls that may be encountered in immunophenotyping acute leukemia and lymphomas by flow cytometry and generate potential solutions.
5. Compare and contrast the usefulness of the sucrose hemolysis test, Ham's test, and flow cytometry immunophenotyping in the diagnosis of paroxysmal nocturnal hemoglobinuria.

■ CHECKLIST - LEVEL II (continued)

6. Select and explain the quality measures that must be enforced in quantitative flow cytometry.

7. Compare and contrast the absolute CD4 count and HIV viral load in the surveillance of HIV infection.

8. Calculate and interpret the S phase-fraction and the DNA index, and give the principle of DNA analysis by flow cytometry.

9. Assess the findings of flow cytometry cell analysis using two or more dot-plots and select the most likely cell represented.

10. Evaluate flow cytometry results to identify problems and generate solutions.

11. Compare reticulocyte counting by flow cytometry with manual methods and assess the advantages of flow cytometry.

12. Interpret the immature reticulocyte fraction (IRF).

13. Summarize the uses of analysis for the CD34 antigen and choose procedures recommended to analyze this antigen.

KEY TERMS

Biphenotypic leukemia
CD designation
Compensation
DNA Index (DI)
Flow chamber
Fluorochromes
Forward light scatter
Gating
Hydrodynamic focusing
Immunophenotyping
Photomultiplier tube
Side light scatter

CASE STUDY

We will address this case study throughout the chapter.

Andrew, a 76-year-old male, had a CBC performed during hospitalization for pneumonia. He was found to have a WBC of 76 × 10^9/L with 80% lymphocytes. Consider the conditions that are associated with these results and the follow-up testing that might be necessary to confirm a diagnosis.

BACKGROUND BASICS

The information in this chapter will build on the concepts learned in previous chapters. To maximize your learning experience you should review these concepts before starting this unit of study.

Level I

▶ Describe the cellular characteristics that differentiate T and B lymphocytes; differentiate the stages of development of granulocytes, lymphocytes, and monocytes. (Chapter 6)

▶ Describe reticulocytes and methods of quantifying them. (Chapters 4, 7, 10)

▶ Summarize the classification of malignant leukocyte disorders. (Chapters 26, 29, 30)

Level II

▶ Summarize the subtypes of malignant disorders and laboratory tests used to help classify them. (Chapters 26, 29, 30, 31)

▶ Describe the abnormality associated with PNH. (Chapter 17)

▶ Outline the cell cycle. (Chapter 2)

▶ Describe the application of IRF. (Chapter 10)

▶ OVERVIEW

The purpose of flow cytometry is to rapidly detect and measure multiple properties of cells so that the cells can be identified and quantitated. This chapter will introduce the principles of flow cytometry and discuss its clinical applications. First, the method of detecting and quantitating particles by flow cytometry is described. This includes specimen requirements and processing and the concept of gating to isolate cells of interest. The remainder of the chapter addresses the uses of flow cytometry in the clinical laboratory. Flow cytometry is currently used to analyze individual cells for the presence of antigens (immunophenotyping) and to quantitate RNA or DNA. Immunophenotyping is one of the tools used for the diagnosis of mature lymphoid malignancies, ALL, AML, HIV, and PNH. This material should be studied together with ∞ Chapters 29, 30, and 31 (neoplastic disorders) to obtain a full understanding of where flow cytometry fits into the diagnostic workup of these disorders. This chapter also introduces the application of flow cytometry in reticulocyte counting and DNA analysis.

▶ INTRODUCTION

A flow cytometer is an instrument capable of detecting molecules on the surface or inside of individual cells or particles. This is achieved by isolating single cells/particles and labeling the molecule of interest with a fluorescent marker. Cells/particles that possess the molecule of interest are recognized by the emission of fluorescent light following excitation. Information is acquired from many thousands of cells/particles and stored on a computer for further analysis. Flow cytometry is currently used in the clinical laboratory for immunophenotyping (identification of antigens using detection antibodies) leukocytes and erythrocytes, enumerating reticulocytes, and analyzing DNA (Table 23-1 ✪).

▶ PRINCIPLES OF FLOW CYTOMETRY

ISOLATION OF SINGLE PARTICLES

Flow cytometry is performed on particles in suspension (e.g., cells or nuclei). The suspension is aspirated and injected into a **flow chamber** (Figure 23-1 ■). The flow chamber is the specimen handling area of a flow cytometer where cells are forced into single file and directed into the path of a laser beam.

The flow chamber contains two columns of fluid. The particles are contained in an inner column of sample fluid that is surrounded by a column of sheath fluid. The sheath and sample fluids are maintained at different pressures and move through the flow chamber at different speeds. This gradient between the sample and sheath fluid keeps the fluids separate (laminar flow) and is used to control the diameter of the column of sample fluid. The central column of sample fluid is narrowed to isolate single cells that pass through a laser beam (**hydrodynamic focusing**) like a string of beads. Laser light is focused on these single cells and can be measured by **photomultiplier tubes** (light detectors) as it is scattered off cells when they pass in front of the beam. If cells have fluorescent molecules attached, the laser light excites the molecules, which then emit light of a specific wavelength. Emitted light is also detected.

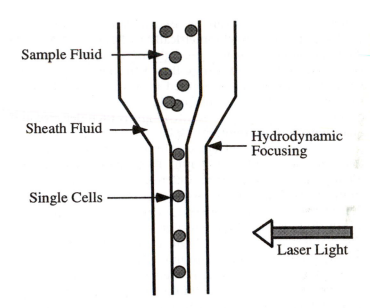

■ **FIGURE 23-1** Flow chamber. The sample fluid, containing a suspension of single cells, is injected into a stream of sheath fluid. The stream is narrowed and directed through the laser beam (hydrodynamic focusing).

LIGHT SCATTERING

When the laser beam interacts with a single particle, light is scattered but its wavelength is not altered. The amount of light scattered in different directions can be used to identify the particle because it is related to the physical properties of the particle (size, granularity, and nuclear complexity). Light scattered at a 90° angle (**side light scatter**) is related to the internal complexity and granularity of the particle. Neutrophils produce a lot of side scatter because of their numerous cytoplasmic granules. Light that proceeds in a forward direction (**forward light scatter**) is related to the size of the particle. Large cells produce more forward scatter than small cells. Therefore, light scattering can be used to distinguish particles and is currently employed by several hematology analyzers to perform differential counting of leukocytes.

✪ TABLE 23-1
Applications of Flow Cytometry

Immunophenotyping
   Lymphoid antigens
   Neutrophilic antigens
   Monocytic antigens
   Terminal deoxynucleotidyl transferase (TdT)
   GPI-linked proteins (CD55 and CD59)
   CD4
   CD34
Reticulocyte counting
DNA analysis

✔ **Checkpoint! #1**

Would a lymphocyte or monocyte have more forward light scatter?

DETECTION OF FLUOROCHROMES

In addition to light scattering, the flow cytometer can be used to detect bound fluorescent markers (**fluorochromes**). These are molecules that are excited by light of one wavelength and emit light of a different wavelength (fluorescent

LEVEL I

    a. bone marrow

    b. lymph node

    c. peripheral blood

    d. skin biopsy

5. Which of the following is a basic criterion of cells that would be processed for chromosome analysis? (Checklist #2)

    a. mitotic activity

    b. protein production

    c. presence of nucleolus

    d. presence of mitochondria

6. In the harvest procedure, how are cells stopped in metaphase? (Checklist #2)

    a. colchicine/colcemid incubation

    b. incubation with hypotonic solution

    c. fixation with Carnoy's fixative

    d. incubation with phytohemagglutinin

7. The ability to identify individual chromosomes depends on which of the following? (Checklist #2)

    a. banding

    b. hypotonic incubation

    c. type of specimen

    d. fixation

8. Which of the following terms would be appropriate for a human cell that has 47 chromosomes? (Checklist #3)

    a. diploid

    b. aneuploid

    c. polyploid

    d. normal

9. Which of the following may result in trisomy? (Checklist #3)

    a. anaphase lag

    b. endomitosis

    c. nondisjunction

    d. chromosome breakage

10. Which of the following would result in an abnormal amount of cellular DNA? (Checklist #3)

    a. balanced translocation

    b. paracentric inversion

    c. pericentric inversion

    d. isochromosome

LEVEL II

2. The breakpoint on chromosome 17 involves which gene? (Checklist #9)

    a. C-ABL

    b. C-MYC

    c. BCR

    d. RARA

3. The identification of this cytogenetic aberration has led to treatment of these patients with which of the following? (Checklist #5, 6)

    a. interferon

    b. interleukin

    c. retinoic acid

    d. vitamin K

Use this case study for questions 4–7.

A 16-year-old girl has fatigue and increased bruising. A CBC shows the following:

Hb: 70g/L

Hct: 0.21L/L

WBC: 35×10^9/L

Platelet count: 60×10^9//L

Differential WBC: 60% blasts with Auer rods

                               10% segmented neutrophils

                               30% lymphocytes

Bone marrow aspirate shows a hypercellular bone marrow with 50% myeloblasts, 10% promyelocytes, 20% myelocytes, 10% metamyelocyte, and 10% RBC precursors

4. Which of the following is most likely to be seen on chromosome analysis of the bone marrow cells? (Checklist #6)

    a. t(8,21)

    b. t(15, 17)

    c. inv(16)

    d. +8

5. Which of the following genes does this translocation involve? (Checklist #9)

    a. BCR/ABL

    b. ETO/AML1

    c. PML/RAR2

    d. 1/AML1

6. What other abnormality might also be expected in this case? (Checklist #6)

    a. −X

    b. −Y

    c. +3

    d. +21

REVIEW QUESTIONS *(continued)*

LEVEL I

LEVEL II

7. Which of the following is the most likely diagnosis? (Checklist #6)
   a. AML-M1
   b. AML-M2
   c. ALL-L3
   d. AML-M3

8. Which of the following is associated with a good prognosis when found in ALL? (Checklist #7)
   a. chromosome count >50
   b. t(9;22)
   c. t(1;19)
   d. chromosome count <46

9. Which of the following is associated with a poor prognosis when found in ALL? (Checklist #7)
   a. chromosome count >50
   b. t(12; 21)
   c. normal karyotype
   d. t(9;22)

10. Which of the following is associated with Burkitt lymphoma/ALL-L3? (Checklist #6)
    a. t(8;21)
    b. t(14;18)
    c. t(12,21)
    d. t(8;14)

REFERENCES

1. Barch M, ed. *The ACT Cytogenetics Laboratory Manual,* 3rd ed. New York: Raven Press; 1997.

2. Caspersson T, Lomakka G, Zach L. The fluorescence patterns of the human metaphase chromosomes-distinguishing characters and variability. *Hereditas.* 1971; 67:89–102.

3. Seabright, M. A rapid banding technique for human chromosomes. *Lancet.* 1971; 2:971–72.

4. Schad C, Kraker W, Tatal S, et al. Use of fluorescent in situ hybridization for marker chromosome identification in congenital and neoplastic disorders. *Am J Clin Path.* 1991; 96:203–10.

5. Mitelman F, ed. *An International System for Human Cytogenetic Nomenclature.* New York: Karger; 1995.

6. Nowell PC, Hungerford DA. A minute chromosome in human, chronic granulocytic leukemia. *Science.* 1960; 132:1497.

7. Rowley JD. A new consistent chromosomal abnormality in chronic granulocytic leukemia. *Nature.* 1973; 243:290–93.

8. Bartram CR, deKlein A, Groffen J, et al. Translocation of C-ABL oncogene correlates with the presence of a Philadelphia chromosome in chronic myelocytic leukemia. *Nature.* 1983; 306:239–42.

9. Faderl S, Talpaz M, Kantarjian HM, et al. The biology of chronic myeloid leukemia. *N Eng J Med.* 1999; 341:164–72.

10. Morric CM, Heisterkamp N, Kennedy MA, Groffen J, et al. Ph-negative chronic myeloid leukemia: Molecular analysis of ABL insertion into M-BCR on chromosome 22. *Blood.* 1990; 76: 1812–18.

11. Lowenberg B, Downing JR, Burnett A. Acute myeloid leukemia. *N Eng J Med.* 1999; 341:1051–62.

12. Willman C. Acute leukemias: A paradigm for the integration of new technologies in diagnosis and classification. *Mod Pathol.* 1999; 12:218–28.

13. de Thé H., Chomienne C, Lanotk M, Deia A, et al. The t(15;17) translocation of acute promyelocytic leukemia fuses the retinoic acid receptor alpha gene to a novel transcribed focus. *Nature.* 1990; 247:SS8–561.

14. Grignani F, Fagioli M, Peticci PG, et al. Acute promyelocytic leukemia: From genetics to treatment. *Blood.* 1994; 1:10–25.

15. Wu X, Wang X, Yao H, et al. Four years experience with the treatment of all-trans-retinoic acid in acute promyelocytic leukemia. *Am J Haematol.* 1993; 43:183–89.

16. Lutterbach B, Westendorf J, Hiebert SW, et al. ETO, a target of t(8;21) in acute leukemia, interacts with the N-COR and mSin3 corepressors. *Mol Cell Biol.* 1998; 18: 7176–84.

17. Westendorf J, Yamamoto C, Hiebert SW, et al. The t(8;21) fusion product, AML-1-ETO, associates with C/EBP-alpha, inhibits C/EBP-alpha-dependent transcription, and blocks granulocytic differentiation. *Mol Cell Biol.* 1998; 18:322–33.

18. Mitterbauer M, Laczika K, Jaeger U, et al. High concordance of karyotype analysis and RT-PCR for CBF beta/MYH11 in unselected patients with acute myeloid leukemia. *Am J Clin Path.* 2000; 113:406–10.

19. Barnard DR, Kalousek DK, Woods WG, et al. Morphologic, immunologic, and cytogenetic classification of acute myeloid leukemia and myelodysplastic syndrome in childhood: A report from the children cancer group. *Leukemia.* 1996; 10:5–12.

20. Morel P, Hebba M, Fenaux P, et al. Cytogenetic analysis has strong independent prognostic value in de novo myelodysplastic syndromes and can be incorporated in a new scoring system: A report on 408 cases. *Leukemia.* 1993; 7:1315–23.

21. Heaney M, Golde DW. Myelodysplasia. *N Eng J Med.* 1999; 340:1649–60.

22. Pederson B. Anatomy of the 5q-deletion: Different sex ratios and deleted 5q bands in MDS and AML. *Leukemia.* 1996; 10:1883–90.

23. Kurtin PJ, DeWald GW, Hanson CA, et al. Hematologic disorders associated with deletions of chromosome 20q: A clinicopathologic study of 107 patients. *Am J Clin Pathol.* 1996; 106:680–88.

24. Carbone P, Santoro A, Giglio MC, Barbara G, et al. Cytogenetic findings in secondary acute nonlymphocytic leukemia. *Cancer Genet. Cytogenet.* 1992; S8:18–23.

25. Pui CH, Evans WE. Acute lymphoblastic leukemia. *N Eng J Med.* 1998; 339:605–15.

26. Pui CH. Acute lymphoblastic leukemia. *Pedi Clin North Am.* 1997; 44:831–44.

27. Khalidi HS, Chang KL, Arber DA, et al. Acute lymphoblastic leukemia: Survey of immunophenotype, French-American-British classification, frequency of myeloid antigen expression, and karyotypic abnormalities in 210 pediatric and adult cases. *Am J Clin Pathol.* 1999; 111:467–76.

28. The Groupe Francais de Cytogenetique Hematologique. Cytogenetic abnormalities in adult acute lymphoblastic leukemia: Correlations with hematologic findings and outcome. *Blood.* 1996; 87:3135–42.

29. Cobaleda C, Gutierrez-Cianca N, Sanchez-Garcia I, et al. A primitive hematopoietic cell is the target for the leukemic transformation in human Philadelphia-positive acute lymphoblastic leukemia. *Blood.* 2000; 95:1007–13.

30. Rubnitz JE, Shuster JJ, Behm FG, et al. Case-control study suggests a favorable impact of TEL rearrangement in patients with B-lineage acute lymphoblastic leukemia treated with antimetabolite-based therapy: A Pediatric Oncology Group study. *Blood.* 1997; 89:1143–46.

31. Raimondi SC, Shurtleff JR, Behm FG, et al. 12p abnormalities and the TEL gene (ETV6) in childhood acute lymphoblastic leukemia. *Blood.* 1997; 90:4559–66.

32. Menolov G, Manolaova Y. Marker band in one chromosome 14 from Burkitt lymphoma. *Nature.* 1972; 237:33.

33. Dalla Favera R, Bregui M, Erickson J, Patterson D, Gallo R, Croce C. Human C-MYC onc gene is located in the region of chromosome 8 that is translocated in Burkitt lymphoma cells. *Proc Natl Acad Sci. USA,* 1982; 79:7824–27.

34. Zutter MM, Hess JL. Guidelines for the diagnosis of leukemia or lymphoma in children. *Am J Clin Pathol.* 1998; 109(Suppl 1):S9–S22.

35. Heim S, Mitleman F. *Cancer Cytogenetics,* 2nd ed. New York: Alan R. Liss, 1996.

36. Knutsen T. Cytogenetic changes in the progression of lymphoma. *Leuk Lymphoma.* 1998; 31:1–19.

37. Frizzera G, Wu D, Inghirami G. The usefulness of immunophenotypic and genotypic studies in the diagnosis and classification of hematopoietic and lymphoid neoplasms. *Am J Clin Pathol.* 1999; 111:S13–S39.

38. Juliusson G, Merup M. Cytogenetics in chronic lymphocytic leukemia. *Sem Onc.* 1998; 25:19–26.

39. Finn WG, Thangavelu M, Peterson LC, et al. Karyotype correlates with peripheral blood morphology and immunophenotype in chronic lymphocytic leukemia. *Am J Clin Pathol.* 1996; 105:458–67.

40. Feinman R, Sawyer J, Tricot G, et al. Cytogenetics and molecular genetics in multiple myeloma. *Hem Onc Clin N Am.* 1997; 11:1–24.

41. Ferrant BA, Labopin M, Gorin NC, et al. Karyotype in acute myeloblastic leukemia: Prognostic significance for bone marrow transplantation in first remission: A European Group for blood and marrow transplantation study. *Blood.* 1997; 90:2931–38.

42. Snyder DS, Nademanee AP, Forman SJ, et al. Long-term follow-up of 23 patients with Philadelphia chromosome-positive acute lymphoblastic leukemia treated with allogeneic bone marrow transplant in first complete remission. *Leukemia.* 1999; 13:2053–58.

43. Van den Berg H, Beverstock G, Westerhof JP, Vossen JM. Chromosomal studies after bone marrow transplantation for leukemia in children. *Bone Marrow Transplant.* 1991; 7:33S–342.

44. Offit K, Burns JP, Cunningham I, Jhawar SC, Black P, Kunan NA, O'Reilly RJ, Chaganti RS. Cytogenetic analysis of chimerism and leukemia relapse in chronic myelogenous leukemia patients after T-cell depleted bone marrow transplantation. *Blood.* 1990; 75:1346–55.

45. Browne PV, Lawler M, Humphries P, McCann SR. Donor-cell leukemia after bone marrow transplantation for severe aplastic anemia. *N Engl J Med.* 1991; 32S:710–13.

46. Bagg A, Kallakury BVS. Molecular pathology of leukemia and lymphoma. *Am J Clin Pathol.* 1999; 112(suppl):S76–S92.

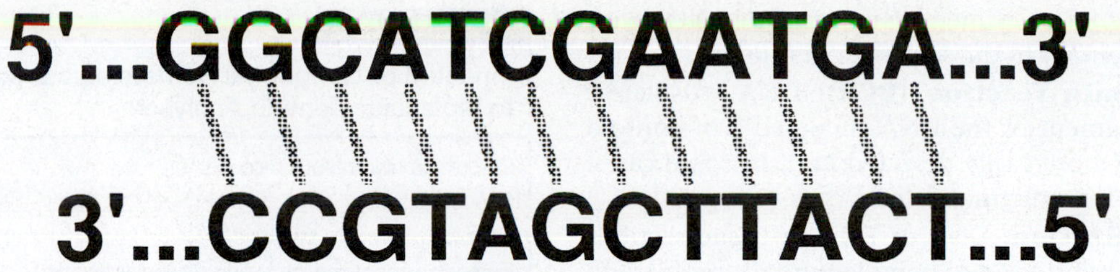

5'...GGCATCGAATGA...3'

3'...CCGTAGCTTACT...5'

■ **FIGURE 25-1** The structure of DNA. DNA is a double-stranded molecule composed of sequences of nucleotides. One strand is bound by hydrogen bonds (shown as diagonal bridges) to its complementary strand. According to the rules of complementary base pairing, the nucleotide adenine (A) is complementary to thymine (T), and guanine (G) is complementary to cytosine (C).

able and are exploited in forensic tests and parentage assays to distinguish one person from another.[2] For example, genes of the human leukocyte antigen (HLA) complex are highly variable among populations, while genes involved in cell division and repair of damaged DNA are virtually identical from person to person.

DNA is composed of two complementary strands of nucleotides (Figure 25-1 ■). In living cells, these complementary strands are bound together by hydrogen bonds except in very short segments that are being actively transcribed or replicated. In the laboratory, however, the two strands of DNA can be fully dissociated by simply heating to 95°C or by placing the DNA in an alkaline solution (high pH). Once the strands are separated, a particular nucleotide sequence of interest can be identified using a DNA **probe**. A probe is simply a single-stranded segment of DNA whose nucleotide sequence is complementary to the target sequence. The

probe binds to the target DNA in a process called **hybridization**. This probe hybridization process forms the basis for all of the laboratory tests that have been developed to analyze specific portions of the human genome (Figure 25-2 ■).

▶ LABORATORY METHODS IN MOLECULAR DIAGNOSTICS

Below are brief descriptions of the most commonly used laboratory tests. These tests are described in greater detail with potential medical applications in the remainder of this chapter.

- **Southern blot analysis:** DNA is isolated, cleaved with restriction endonucleases that cut DNA at specific nucleotide sequences, separated by size using gel electro-

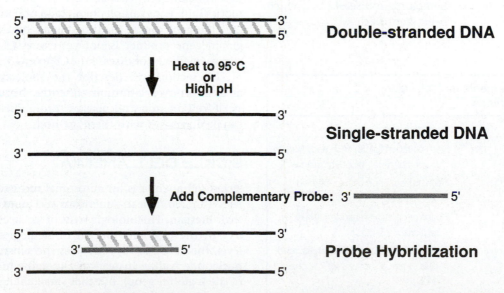

■ **FIGURE 25-2** The two strands of DNA may be dissociated *in vitro* by heating them to 95°C or by treating with a solution of high pH. Once separated, the strands can bind to a DNA probe of complementary nucleotide sequence by a process known as hybridization.

phoresis, transferred to a membrane, and detected with probes complementary to the sequence of interest.

- **Polymerase chain reaction (PCR):** DNA is isolated, and a specific segment of the DNA is copied a billionfold so that it can be more easily detected and, in some cases, further analyzed for structural defects.
- **In situ hybridization:** DNA or RNA in tissue sections on glass slides is hybridized to complementary probes and visualized by microscopy. The architecture and cytology of the tissue are preserved to permit localization of the target sequence to particular cells in the tissue.
- **Fluorescence In Situ Hybridization (FISH):** Whole chromosomes (metaphase or interphase) are hybridized to complementary probes that are labeled with a fluorochrome and visualized by microscopy.
- **DNA sequencing:** The nucleotide sequence is determined in a segment of DNA by replicating one of the DNA strands and monitoring the order in which labeled nucleotides are added to the new strand. DNA sequencing is particularly useful for detecting point mutations located anywhere in the DNA segment.

The specimen requirements for these procedures are listed in Table 25-1 ✪.

▶ INHERITED DISEASES

In the past few years, molecular biologists have identified specific genetic defects underlying various inherited diseases. When a disease-associated genetic defect is identified, the DNA from the defective gene **locus** (specific location on a chromosome) can be used as a probe to study other patient DNA samples for the presence of the defect. Table 25-2 ✪ lists some of the inherited hematologic diseases for which specific genetic defects have been identified.

✪ TABLE 25-1

Specimen Requirements for Molecular Diagnostic Procedures

Procedure	Specimen
Southern blot analysis	Fresh or frozen tissue, fresh body fluid or frozen cell pellet, blood, or marrow
Polymerase chain reaction (PCR)	Fresh, frozen, or paraffin embedded tissue, blood, or body fluid
In situ hybridization	Frozen or paraffin embedded tissue sections
Fluorescence in situ hybridization (FISH)	Fresh cells for metaphase analysis, fixed cells or tissue sections for interphase analysis
DNA sequencing	Fresh, frozen, or paraffin embedded tissue, blood, or body fluid

✪ TABLE 25-2

Inherited or Congenital Hematologic Disorders Amenable to Molecular Genetic Analysis

Chronic granulomatous disease

Gaucher disease

Hereditary hemochromatosis

Hemoglobinopathies, including sickle cell anemia, alpha and beta thalassemias, and hereditary persistence of fetal hemoglobin

Hemolytic anemias such as glucose-6-phosphate dehydrogenase deficiency and McLeod syndrome

Bleeding and thrombotic disorders, including deficiency of coagulation factors V, VII, VIII, IX, XI, XII, and XIII, protein C, protein S, plasmin, plasminogen, and antithrombin, Bernard-Soulier syndrome, platelet storage pool deficiency, von Willebrand disease, factor V Leiden, and prothrombin gene 20210 mutation.

Immunodeficiencies including adenosine deaminase, purine nucleoside phosphorylase, and leukocyte adhesion deficiencies, DiGeorge and Wiskott-Aldrich syndromes, and X-linked lymphoproliferative disorder

Myeloperoxidase deficiency

Porphyrias

Red cell membrane defects including hereditary spherocytosis and elliptocytosis, and paroxysmal nocturnal hemoglobinuria

In inherited diseases, the genetic defect responsible for the illness is present in every nucleated cell of the patient's body, even if gene expression or clinical manifestation is restricted to only one organ or one stage of development. Because the defect is present in all cells, it can be identified in samples that are easily collected such as blood or buccal swabs. Furthermore, the defect can be identified prior to the onset of clinical disease and even in prenatal samples of amniotic fluid. For example, hemoglobinopathies involving the β-globin gene can be identified in a fetus even though the β-globin gene product is not yet expressed nor is there any clinical evidence of disease[3] (∞ Chapter 13).

This section will describe the application of molecular analysis in two common inherited hematologic diseases, sickle cell anemia and venous thrombosis, but many more can be diagnosed with these methods.

SICKLE CELL ANEMIA

Sickle cell anemia is an autosomal recessive disease that affects 1 in 260 African-Americans and almost always shortens their lifespan. The biologic basis of sickle cell anemia is a defect in the β-globin protein of hemoglobin. At the DNA level, the defect always involves the substitution of a single nucleotide (valine instead of glutamine in the sixth **codon** of the β-globin gene), but that small change results in a dramatic alteration of hemoglobin molecules such that they tend to polymerize under conditions of dehydration or low oxygen concentration. Hemoglobin polymerization dimin-

KEY TERMS

- Complementary DNA (cDNA)
- Codon
- DNA sequencing
- Fluorescence in situ hybridization (FISH)
- Gene
- Gene rearrangement
- Genome
- Genotype
- Hybridization
- In situ hybridization
- Linkage analysis
- Locus
- Mutation
- Nucleotide
- Polymerase chain reaction (PCR)
- Probe
- Restriction endonuclease
- Southern blot analysis
- Transcription
- Translation
- Translocation

BACKGROUND BASICS

This chapter builds on concepts learned in other chapters of this textbook. The reader should also have a background of genetic principles. To maximize your learning experience, you should review the following material:

- ▶ Summarize the pathophysiology and etiology of sickle cell anemia. (Chapter 12)
- ▶ Describe the role of oncogenes in the etiology and pathophysiology of cancer. (Chapters 2, 26)
- ▶ Describe the application of cytogenetic analysis in the diagnosis of hematologic disease. (Chapter 24)
- ▶ Summarize the etiology and pathophysiology of leukemia and lymphoma. (Chapters 26, 29, 30, and 31)
- ▶ Describe the congenital aberrations that lead to hypercoagulability and venous thrombosis. (Chapter 38)

CASE STUDY

We will address this case study throughout the chapter.

Ms. Karolton, a 35-year-old female, was seen by her physician with complaints of a 20-pound weight loss in the last 6 months, and fatigue. A CBC revealed a WBC count of 6.5×10^9/L, hemoglobin of 8 g/dL, platelet count of 25×10^9/L. The leukocyte differential showed 71% blasts. The bone marrow revealed 96% blasts. The blasts were negative for myeloperoxidase, Sudan Black B, and combined esterase by cytochemical stains. Cytogenetics revealed t(9;22) (which is characterized by the presence of the Philadelphia chromosome), +8 and +18. Consider the possible disease processes that may be occurring in this patient and laboratory tests that may be helpful in diagnosis and monitoring her disease.

...n determines whether the sickle mutation is present or absent (Figure 25-3 ■).

The Southern blot assay may be adapted to detect many other disease-associated alterations besides the sickle mutation. A key step in the Southern blot procedure is the step in which DNA is cleaved at specific nucleotide sequences by the action of the restriction endonuclease. If a patient's DNA sequence is altered by mutation, translocation, or any other structural defect, then the number and/or size of the resulting restriction fragments is altered accordingly. The restriction fragment(s) containing the gene of interest are identified by probe hybridization. Radiolabeling of the probe permits its subsequent detection by autoradiography. Alternatively, the probe may be labeled with biotin or digoxigenin and detected using colorimetric procedures analogous to what is done in immunoassays of antigen–antibody complexes.

Detection of the Sickle Mutation by Polymerase Chain Reaction

An alternate method of detecting the sickle mutation is by DNA amplification, a procedure in which a particular segment of DNA is copied a billionfold. DNA amplification techniques are revolutionizing our ability to analyze DNA in the clinical laboratory because we now have the capacity to examine an otherwise virtually undetectable sequence of DNA from a small tissue specimen or even a single cell. While several new amplification methods have been recently introduced, the first and most commonly used method is polymerase chain reaction (PCR).[4,5] PCR works by enzymatically replicating one particular segment of DNA (up to about 5000 nucleotides in length) from amidst the entire billion base-pair human genome. This permits rapid, sensitive, and specific identification of a segment of DNA that can then be further tested for a disease-specific genetic defect (Figure 25-4 ■).

Diagnosis of the sickle cell **genotype** (the genetic constitution of a particular person) can be accomplished by PCR amplification of a segment of the β-globin gene harboring the sickle mutation site.[5] The amplified DNA can then be cleaved with the MstII restriction endonuclease and electrophoresed in an agarose gel. Since MstII differentially cleaves normal DNA compared with sickle DNA, a different electrophoretic band pattern is produced depending on whether the sickle mutation is present or not.

Using an alternate amplification strategy called allele-specific PCR, short DNA probes that serve as PCR primers have been designed to preferentially amplify either the normal β-globin sequence or the defective sickle β-globin sequence. This preferential amplification is based on the premise that mutations interfering with primer hybridization result in inhibition of amplification reactions (Figure 25-5 ■).

A major advantage of PCR over Southern blot analysis is that PCR can be performed on much smaller sample volumes since amplification procedures are used to identify rare

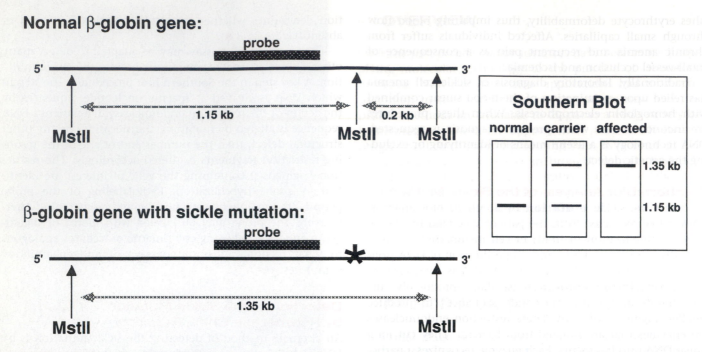

Normal β-globin gene:

probe

5'   3'

1.15 kb   0.2 kb

MstII   MstII   MstII

β-globin gene with sickle mutation:

probe

5'   3'

1.35 kb

MstII   MstII

Southern Blot

normal   carrier   affected

1.35 kb

1.15 kb

■ **FIGURE 25-3** Southern blot analysis of the sickle cell mutation is accomplished by first extracting DNA and then cutting it with MstII restriction endonuclease that cleaves DNA at a specific nucleotide sequence (shown by arrows). Since that specific sequence is present many times in the human genome, MstII cuts genomic DNA into many small fragments. The resultant DNA fragments are separated by size using gel electrophoresis, dissociated into single strands by soaking in an alkaline solution, and then transferred to a nylon membrane by a blotting procedure. To identify the fragment containing the β-globin gene, the membrane is soaked in a radiolabeled DNA probe (shown as a bar) that hybridizes to a complementary segment of the β-globin gene. The pattern of bands recognized by the probe reflects the size of the corresponding restriction fragments, measured in kilobases (kb). A β-globin gene harboring the sickle mutation (shown as a star) fails to cut with MstII at the mutation site, thus altering the band pattern. In this way, a person affected by sickle cell anemia can be distinguished from a carrier (sickle trait) and from a person of normal genotype.

target sequences. PCR is also a more rapid laboratory procedure (1–2 days as compared with >4 days for Southern blot analysis), costs relatively less, and is amenable for use on formalin-fixed paraffin-embedded tissues. However, a drawback of PCR is the meticulous attention required to prevent carryover or contamination of laboratory samples by extraneous DNA.

The sickle cell genotype is relatively easy to diagnose because the specific genetic mutation is identical among all affected individuals. Not all inherited diseases are so straightforward—complex and diverse genetic defects can result in the same clinical syndrome. For example, only about half of all patients with hemophilia A have an identifiable mutation or deletion of the factor VIII gene, while the remaining patients presumably have an occult genetic defect that somehow inhibits expression of the factor VIII protein. In families where the particular genetic defect is known, laboratory tests can be designed to identify the particular defect. Even if the defect is not known, a process called **linkage analysis** can often be used to follow inheritance patterns among family members and predict how likely it is that the disease affects a given individual in the family. In linkage analysis, inheritance patterns are evaluated using the principle that a partic-

ular defective gene of interest is inherited together with adjacent DNA (marker DNA) on the same chromosome.[6] The marker DNA is analyzed since the specific genetic defect is unknown.

INHERITED PREDISPOSITION TO VENOUS THROMBOSIS

There are several inherited mutations that predispose to deep venous thrombosis. The most common is a point mutation at codon 506 in the factor V gene that interferes with catabolism of the encoded coagulation factor. This factor V mutation is quite common, affecting about 5% of the population. Those who inherit it have a sevenfold increased risk of developing thrombosis.

The second most common genetic risk factor for venous thrombosis is a point mutation at position 20210 of the prothrombin gene. This mutation is found in about 2% of the population and is associated with a threefold increased risk of venous thrombosis.

The factor V gene mutation is readily detectable by molecular analysis because it causes loss of an Mnl1 restriction endonuclease cut site. The prothrombin gene mutation is

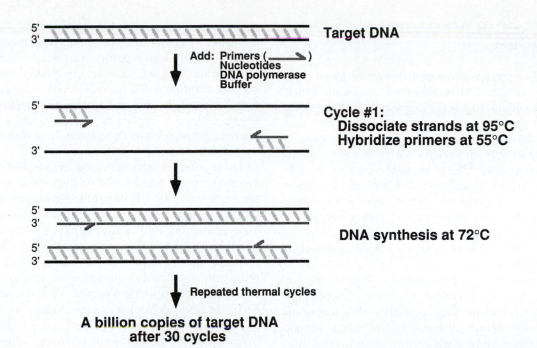

Target DNA

Add: Primers (⟶)
     Nucleotides
     DNA polymerase
     Buffer

Cycle #1:
    Dissociate strands at 95°C
    Hybridize primers at 55°C

DNA synthesis at 72°C

Repeated thermal cycles

**A billion copies of target DNA
after 30 cycles**

■ **FIGURE 25-4** Polymerase chain reaction is a method of enzymatically amplifying a particular segment of DNA through a process of repeated cycles of heating, cooling, and DNA synthesis. First, patient DNA is mixed with the chemicals needed for DNA synthesis. Included are two short DNA probes (called *primers,* shown as half-arrows) that are designed to flank the particular segment of DNA that needs to be amplified. A thermocycler instrument is programmed to sequentially heat and cool the sample. In cycle 1, the sample is heated to 95°C to dissociate complementary strands of DNA, then cooled to 55°C to permit binding of the short DNA probes that serve as primers for subsequent enzymatic DNA replication at 72°C. This replication generates new complementary strands to produce an exact copy of the original target DNA. In subsequent cycles, the products of previous cycles can serve as templates for DNA replication, allowing an exponential accumulation of DNA copies. After 30 cycles, which takes only a couple of hours, approximately a billion copies of the target DNA have been generated.

readily detectable because it adds a HindIII restriction endonuclease site where one was not normally present. The altered restriction enzyme digestion patterns allow for laboratory detection of these mutations using the same strategies described above for sickle cell anemia.

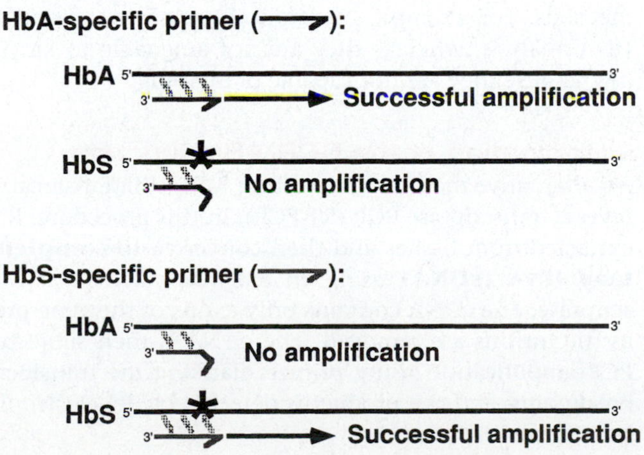

HbA-specific primer (⟶):

HbA 5'⟶3' **Successful amplification**

HbS 5'⟶3' **No amplification**

HbS-specific primer (⟶):

HbA 5'⟶3' **No amplification**

HbS 5'⟶3' **Successful amplification**

✓ Checkpoint! #1

A 40-year-old male is diagnosed with an inherited disease for which a specific point mutation is responsible. His mother died of a similar disease 10 years ago. For purposes of family counseling, the physician wants to know if she had the same mutation. The histology laboratory has archival paraffin-embedded tissue from the mother. What laboratory method(s) are best for detecting the gene mutation?

■ **FIGURE 25-5** One way that polymerase chain reaction can be used to facilitate detection of the sickle mutation is to design primers (shown as half-arrows) that preferentially bind to either normal β-globin or sickle β-globin sequences. If a primer does not match its target sequence perfectly, particularly at the 5' end of the primer where the DNA polymerase initiates replication, then amplification is inhibited. If the primer matches its target, then abundant PCR products are generated. By comparing the yield of the two PCR reactions, it is possible to determine if the sickle mutation is present and whether it is heterozygous or homozygous.

► THE MOLECULAR BASIS OF CANCER

DNA technology provides a powerful new tool to assist in the diagnosis of cancer. Unlike inherited disease in which every nucleated cell in the body contains defective DNA, cancer results when *one* cell acquires genetic defects that stimulate uncontrolled cell division and tumor formation. It is thought that virtually all cancers harbor genetic defects. The specific genes that are altered in tumors and are thereby responsible for tumor formation are called oncogenes (∞ Chapters 2, 26). The unaltered counterpart of an oncogene (proto-oncogene) generally functions to regulate cell growth or differentiation, whereas in tumor cells this function has gone awry as a result of abnormal expression or structural alteration of the gene.

Each time a malignant cell divides, the genetic defect is passed on to its progeny. Therefore, all of the cells within a particular tumor contain the same defective DNA, a concept known as clonality. Because cancers harbor clonal genetic defects, cancer cells may be distinguished from normal cells by DNA probe analysis of the defective gene sequences. Certain oncogene defects are highly characteristic of particular types of cancer and can be used to assist in the diagnosis and classification of those cancers. This section will describe the application of molecular analysis in selected leukemias and lymphomas.

 CASE STUDY *(continued from page 460)*

1. What is the classification of this neoplastic hematologic disorder based on the peripheral blood and bone marrow results?

CHRONIC MYELOGENOUS LEUKEMIA AND THE BCR/ABL TRANSLOCATION

Traditional cytogenetics demonstrates that hematopoietic neoplasms frequently harbor characteristic chromosomal **translocations,** as exemplified by the t(9;22) of chronic myelogenous leukemia (CML) (∞ Chapters 24, 27). A translocation is the breakage of DNA from one chromosome and reciprocal attachment to DNA on another chromosome.

In CML, the characteristic Philadelphia chromosome (Ph[1]) represents a shortened chromosome 22 resulting from a reciprocal translocation between the ABL gene on chromosome 9 and the BCR gene on chromosome 22. This translocation produces a new fusion gene called BCR/ABL that encodes hybrid RNA and hybrid protein. The presence of BCR gene elements enhances the potency of the ABL gene product (a tyrosine kinase enzyme), resulting in uncontrolled cell proliferation. Using a single DNA probe, the molecular

equivalent of the t(9;22) translocation can now be detected in virtually all cases of CML by Southern blot analysis.[7]

About 90% of all patients who have clinical and laboratory features of CML have an identifiable Ph[1] by karyotyping. An additional 5% have an occult translocation that is detectable only by molecular analysis of BCR/ABL. Three different molecular approaches are available—Southern blot analysis, amplification techniques, and fluorescence in situ hybridization.[8]

Those patients with molecular evidence of BCR/ABL share a similar natural history and predisposition to blast crisis. In blast crisis of CML, the BCR/ABL defect is retained, while additional genetic defects account for the more aggressive cytologic appearance and clinical behavior of the tumor. The remaining 5% of tumors suspected of being CML but lacking BCR/ABL do not behave in the same fashion as CML, and these tumors probably represent other myeloproliferative diseases or myelodysplastic syndromes masquerading as CML.

While DNA technology is more sensitive than karyotyping for detecting the CML-associated genetic defect, karyotyping has the advantage of revealing other chromosomal abnormalities besides t(9;22). Therefore, a cost-effective approach to the laboratory workup of suspected CML is to first perform karyotyping and only proceed to molecular testing if the karyotype is nondiagnostic.

Minimal residual disease (MRD) refers to the presence of tumor cells (after therapy) that are not detectable by routine morphologic and radiologic methods but that may result in relapse. Burdens of 10^{10} leukemic cells or more are readily detected by microscopic bone marrow examination. In monitoring tumor burden during therapy, karyotyping is just about as sensitive as Southern blot analysis for detecting low numbers of residual leukemic cells. By either assay, tumors comprising over 5% of sample cellularity are generally detectable. As we will show in the next section of this chapter, amplification strategies (i.e., PCR) are much more sensitive for detecting minimal residual disease (abnormal cells detectable down to 0.01%). Another advantage of molecular technology over karyotyping is the capability to analyze cells that are resistant to entering the cell cycle and are therefore difficult to evaluate by traditional cytogenetic methods. For example, neutrophils are fully amenable to DNA analysis, whereas they are not amenable to karyotyping because they are not capable of dividing.

Amplification of the BCR/ABL Junction

An alternative method of detecting BCR/ABL translocation is reverse transcriptase PCR (RT-PCR). In this procedure, RNA is extracted from tissues and then converted to **complementary DNA (cDNA)** using an enzyme called reverse transcriptase. The cDNA contains only exons of the gene present as the introns are removed. The cDNA is then subjected to PCR amplification using primers flanking the translocation breakpoint, and the product is detected by gel electrophoresis[9] (Figure 25-6 ■).

A recent technologic breakthrough now permits amplification products to be detected without the need for gel electrophoresis. In so-called real-time PCR, products are quantitated as they accumulate in the reaction tube by way of fluorescent probes. This new strategy permits a more accurate assessment of the amount of BCR/ABL in the patient sample, thus allowing tumor burden to be measured at multiple timepoints following initiation of treatment.[10,11]

While RT-PCR is a thousandfold more sensitive than Southern blot analysis or karyotype for detecting low numbers of tumor cells, caution is advised in interpreting test results. It appears that residual BCR/ABL sequences often persist for several months following successful therapy. After this, persistent positive results are predictive of relapse.[12]

A unique benefit of RT-PCR is the ability to distinguish BCR/ABL breakpoints that are characteristic of CML (called p210) from BCR/ABL breakpoints of de novo acute lymphoblastic leukemia (called p190).[13] While these alternate breakpoints appear identical by karyotyping, they are distinct at the molecular level and from a clinical standpoint. They help separate patients with de novo acute leukemia from those presenting in blast crisis of CML. Furthermore, detection of BCR/ABL p190 identifies a subset of acute lymphoblastic leukemia patients who are less responsive to standard chemotherapy regimens.[14]

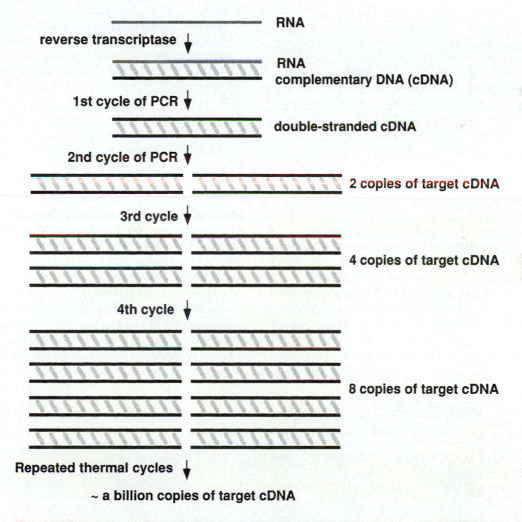

RNA

reverse transcriptase

RNA
complementary DNA (cDNA)

1st cycle of PCR

double-stranded cDNA

2nd cycle of PCR

2 copies of target cDNA

3rd cycle

4 copies of target cDNA

4th cycle

8 copies of target cDNA

Repeated thermal cycles

~ a billion copies of target cDNA

■ **FIGURE 25-6** The rtPCR procedure is a means of determining whether a particular RNA transcript is present in a tissue sample. RNA is extracted from the sample, followed by conversion to complementary DNA (cDNA) using the enzyme reverse transcriptase. This cDNA serves as a template for DNA amplification by the polymerase chain reaction. After 30 cycles, about 1 billion copies of the target cDNA sequence have been generated. These abundant copies can then be readily detected or further analyzed to provide valuable information about the RNA in the patient sample.

Fluorescent in Situ Hybridization (FISH) in CML

A third method of detecting the BCR/ABL translocation uses the FISH procedure. In contrast to the Southern blot and RT-PCR procedures, FISH uses a fluorescent labeled nucleic acid probe that is hybridized directly to cells mounted on glass slides. In this procedure the morphologic information of the cell with the mutation is preserved. However, the cells must be permeabilized and the DNA denatured for hybridization to occur. The molecular probe is allowed to hybidize to the chromosomes in the tissue specimen on the slide. Probe binding can be visualized using a fluorescent microscope. The BCR and ABL probes are each labeled with different color fluorochromes. The BCR/ABL fusion gene causes a colocalization of the two colored probes resulting in a third colored product (Figure 25-7 ■).

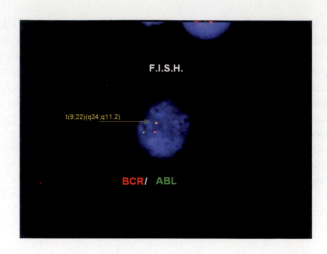

■ **FIGURE 25-7** Identification of the BCR/ABL translocation using FISH. The BCR probe is red and the ABL probe is green. In the cell here, one normal BCR and one normal ABL gene are located on separate chromosomes. However, the other BCR and ABL genes are translocated together on one derivative chromosome, and the juxtaposed probes appear yellowish.

 Checkpoint! #2

A patient with CML was treated with chemotherapy. On subsequent marrow samples the physician ordered molecular testing for residual disease after treatment. The BCR/ABL mutation was not detected 4 months after treatment but was detected at the 8th and 9th months after treatment. Interpret this result.

ACUTE PROMYELOCYTIC LEUKEMIA AND THE PML/RARα TRANSLOCATION

Table 25-4 ✪ displays the characteristic chromosomal defects of myeloid leukemias. One of the most interesting of these cancers is acute promyelocytic leukemia in which t(15;17) juxtaposes the PML gene on chromosome 15 with the retinoic acid receptor alpha (RARα) gene on chromosome 17. Amazingly, leukemias harboring this genetic defect respond to treatment with retinoic acid derivatives, providing one of the first examples where cancer therapy specifically targets a gene product thought to be involved in tu-

morigenesis. Unfortunately, retinoic acid therapy alone is insufficient for cure since the tumor cells eventually become resistant to its effects.[15] Nevertheless, retinoic acid used in combination with other chemotherapeutic agents appears to improve outcomes in affected patients.

Molecular tests are now available to detect the characteristic PML/RARα translocation.[16] These tests are used to assist in the diagnosis and classification of acute leukemia, and to predict response to retinoic acid therapy. In addition, a sensitive test is now available to monitor tumor burden during remission, and the results of this test appear to predict which patients will relapse.[15]

The sensitive molecular assay that is commonly used for detecting PML/RARα is an RT-PCR test. First, RNA purified from the patient sample is converted to cDNA, and then primers flanking the breakpoint between the PML and RARα

✪ TABLE 25-4

Chromosomal Translocations in Myeloid Leukemias

Leukemia	Karyotype	Genes	Clinical Significance
CML	t(9;22)	BCR/ABL	predisposed to blast crisis
CMML	t(5;12)	PDGFRβ/TEL	may progress to acute leukemia
AML-M1 or M2	t(8;21)	ETO/AML1	good response to high-dose ARA-C
AML-M3	t(15;17)	PML/RARα	responds to retinoic acid therapy
AML-M4eo	inv(16)	MYH11/CBFβ	good response to high-dose ARA-C
AML	t(6;9)	DEK/CAN	marrow basophilia is seen

CML = chronic myelogenous leukemia; CMML = chronic myelomonocytic leukemia; t = translocation; inv = inversion; AML = acute myelocytic leukemia

genes are used to specifically amplify the translocation. Amplified products can be seen by gel electrophoresis or by use of labeled internal probes.

Southern blot analysis can also be used to detect PML/RARα, but because the translocation breakpoints vary widely from patient to patient, multiple probes are needed to detect all possible translocations. In contrast, mRNA encoded from the chimeric gene is remarkably homogeneous and therefore more amenable for analysis using RT-PCR. Keep in mind that RNA is much less stable than DNA and must be handled carefully to avoid degradation.

✺ CASE STUDY (continued from page 466)

2. What molecular defect is consistent with the presence of the Philadelphia chromosome?

3. Would molecular analysis assist in diagnosis? Explain.

4. If molecular analysis should be done, which laboratory procedure should be used and what specimen should be obtained?

ONCOGENE TRANSLOCATIONS IN LYMPHOID LEUKEMIAS AND LYMPHOMAS

Lymphomas and lymphoid leukemias commonly contain chromosomal translocations involving the antigen receptor genes, namely the immunoglobulin (Ig) genes expressed by B cells, and the T cell receptor (TCR) genes expressed by T cells. Translocations involving these genes are thought to represent errors occurring during physiologic gene rearrangement (to be described in the next section). Genes located at or near the reciprocal translocation breakpoint are putative oncogenes whose expressions are dysregulated by juxtaposition of the antigen receptor gene.

Table 25-5 ✺ lists the translocations that are most characteristic of lymphoid neoplasms. In most of these tumors, either Ig or TCR genes are juxtaposed with genes that function in regulating cell growth. For example, the myc oncogene of Burkitt lymphoma and the putative bcl1 oncogene (also called PRAD1 or cyclinD1) of mantle cell lymphoma encode proteins that promote cell division.[17–19] In follicular lymphomas, the protein product of the bcl2 oncogene inhibits cell death. Overexpression of these oncogenes appears to be responsible, at least in part, for the development of lymphoid tumors.

Clonal genetic defects often can be detected by Southern blot analysis of the affected oncogene or by amplification of the translocation breakpoint by PCR.[17,20–22] These types of assays, in conjunction with traditional morphologic examination and other laboratory studies, are used to diagnose and classify tumors. While the Southern blot assay is too insensitive to detect minimal residual disease, PCR assays of bcl2/IgH are successful in predicting which patients are likely to relapse with follicular lymphoma.[23]

✺ TABLE 25-5

Chromosomal Translocations in Lymphomas and Lymphoid Leukemias

Lymphoid Neoplasm	Karyotype	Genes*
B cell lymphomas		
Burkitt lymphoma	t(8;14, 2 or 22)	myc/IgH, Igκ, or Igλ
Mantle cell lymphoma	t(11;14)	bcl1/IgH
Follicular lymphoma	t(14;18)	IgH/bcl2
Diffuse large cell lymphoma	t(3;14)	bcl6/IgH
MALT lymphoma	t(11;18)	AP1/MALT1
Lymphoplasmacytoid lymphoma	t(9;14)	PAX5/IgH
B cell leukemias		
Pre-B ALL	t(9;22)	BCR/ABL
Pre-B ALL	t(1;19)	PBX1/E2A
Pre-B ALL	t(17;19)	HLF/E2A
Pre-B ALL	t(12;21)	TEL/AML1
Mixed lineage acute leukemia	t(various;11)	various/MLL
T cell leukemias/lymphomas		
T-ALL	del 1p	TAL1 deletion
Anaplastic large cell lymphoma	t(2;5)	NPM/ALK

*The order of the genes corresponds to the order of the karyotype except for BCR/ABL.

ALL = acutelymphoblastic leukemia; del = deletion

In theory, the best treatment for a tumor would be to eliminate the genetic defect(s) responsible for its uncontrolled growth. Alternatively, if we understood the consequences of a particular genetic defect, it might be possible to wisely intervene in a biochemical pathway to thwart tumor growth or trigger tumor cell death. As further progress is made in tailoring therapy to specific genetic defects, there will be increasing demands on clinical laboratories to detect these genetic defects in patient samples.

Immunoglobulin and T Cell Receptor Gene Rearrangement

All progeny of each B and T lymphocyte have the same gene rearrangement. In addition to any translocation that a lymphoid neoplasm may have, B cell tumors have an additional marker of clonality in their rearranged Ig genes that code for antibody specificity (Figure 25-8 ■). After all, B cell leukemias and lymphomas arise from a single transformed B cell harboring a particular Ig gene rearrangement, and that particular rearrangement is inherited by all tumor cell progeny, resulting in a monoclonal cell population. Therefore, clonal gene rearrangement serves as a marker to distinguish tumor cells from normal cells.[17,21,22] Gene rearrangement can be evaluated by Southern blot analysis using probes targeting the Ig genes (Figure 25-9 ■). Ig gene rearrangement also serves as a marker of commitment to the B cell lineage. Information on clonality and lineage is helpful in

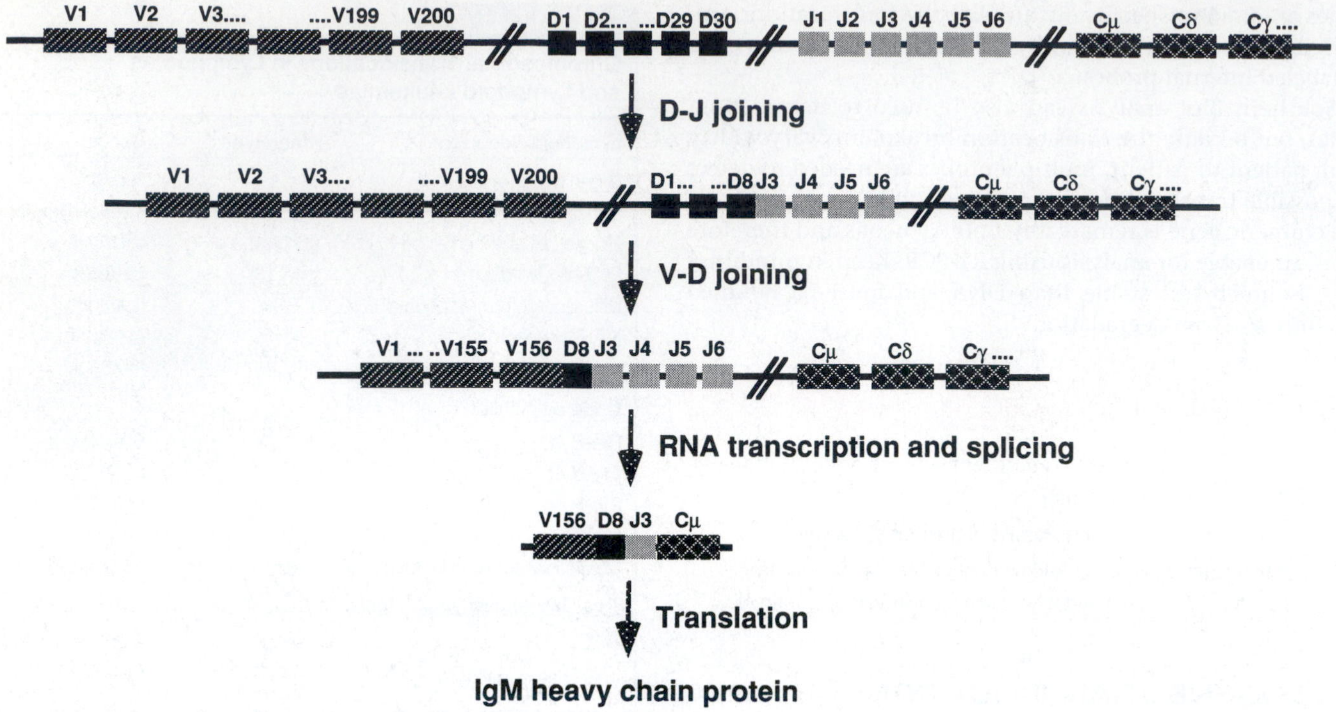

FIGURE 25-8 During B cell differentiation, the immunoglobulin heavy chain gene rearranges to produce a unique coding sequence that determines antibody specificity. This occurs through a process of splicing and deletion whereby one of 30 diversity (D) regions is juxtaposed with one of 6 joining (J) regions, and then with one of 200 variable (V) regions. Finally, constant (C) region splicing determines antibody isotype (IgM, IgD, IgG, IgA, or IgE). In the example depicted here, V, D, J, and $C\mu$ segments are sequentially spliced together to generate a nucleic acid sequence that encodes IgM heavy chain proteins. These heavy chain proteins complex with kappa or lambda light chain proteins (that are also encoded by rearranged genes) to produce a functional antibody molecule. Each developing B cell has different Ig gene rearrangements, so a population of normal B cells is characterized by polyclonal Ig genes. The diversity of these genes and their encoded antibodies permits immune recognition of many different antigens.

distinguishing a B cell neoplasm from benign lymphoid hyperplasia.

Analogous to the process by which B cells rearrange their Ig genes, T cells rearrange their TCR genes to encode a unique antigen receptor expressed on the surface of T lymphocytes. Southern blot analysis of TCR gene rearrangement can serve as a clonal marker for T cell tumors analogous to what was described above for B cell tumors. In the case of T cells, there are four different TCR genes that are capable of rearranging (called TCRα, TCRβ, TCRγ, and TCRδ). Any particular T cell tumor may exhibit rearrangements of one, two, three, or all four of these TCR genes. In clinical laboratories, assays targeting the TCRβ or TCRγ genes are most commonly used to distinguish monoclonal T cell neoplasms from polyclonal reactive processes. The absence of clonal gene rearrangement does not exclude the possibility of a tumor of nonlymphoid origin.

Published guidelines assist with laboratory implementation of gene rearrangement testing by the Southern blot method.[20,22] A typical assay involves DNA extraction, then digestion by two or more separate restriction enzymes, and finally probe hybridization to identify the size of the fragments containing the Ig or TCR genes. Interpretation of Southern blot results involves comparison of band patterns in patient samples with those of normal tissues and weak positive controls that are run in parallel. This technique is sensitive and specific. Lymphoid clones comprising as little as 5% of a sample are reliably detected by Southern blot analysis of the IgH, Ig kappa, and TCRβ genes. As with all clinical laboratory tests, appropriate quality control and proficiency testing are essential.

In recent years, PCR has been implemented as an alternate method of detecting clonal gene rearrangement.[24–26] Current protocols successfully identify clonal IgH gene rearrangement in about 80% of B cell neoplasms. While this is less productive than Southern blot assays, where virtually 100% of B cell neoplasms are identified, amplification techniques still hold promise as laboratory tools because they are fast, less expensive, require a small amount of tissue, and are applicable to paraffin-embedded tissue. Furthermore, the particular rearranged sequences that characterize each lymphoid tumor might be exploited as tumor-specific markers to assist in staging the extent of tumor spread and in monitoring response to therapy.[27]

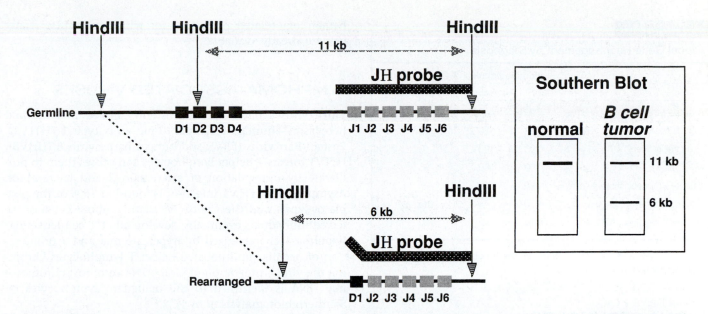

FIGURE 25-9 Rearrangement of the immunoglobulin heavy chain gene involves random splicing of D and J segments to produce a new coding sequence. This process alters the size of DNA fragments produced by the cleaving action of the HindIII restriction endonuclease (shown by arrows). In a B cell tumor, all tumor cells contain exactly the same rearrangement that was present in the original transformed B cell from which the tumor arose. This tumor-related clonal rearrangement is identified as an extra band on a Southern blot hybridized to a JH probe (shown as a bar). In the normal sample, an 11kb band corresponds to the size of the unrearranged (germline) DNA fragment. Although some B cells may be present in the normal sample, their corresponding gene rearrangements are not visible on the Southern blot because the rearrangements are polyclonal and they lie below the threshold of assay sensitivity. In the tumor, an extra band is identified that represents the tumor-specific clonal immunoglobulin gene rearrangement. Residual germline DNA is also present in the tumor, and it is generated from two potential sources: (1) the unrearranged allele of the immunoglobulin gene in tumor cells, or (2) the unrearranged genes present in nontumor cells of the specimen.

Clinical Utility of Gene Rearrangement Testing

The most valuable contribution of gene rearrangement testing is in distinguishing benign from malignant lymphoproliferations. In general, malignant lymphoid tumors exhibit clonal antigen receptor **gene rearrangement** while benign reactive lymphoid hyperplasias do not.

The converse principle is not always true, as exemplified by a few hematopoietic disorders where clonality does not necessarily imply malignancy. These include large granular lymphocytosis and lymphomatoid papulosis, either of which can harbor clonal gene rearrangement even though they often regress without therapy. Because clonality is not always synonymous with malignancy, it is important that DNA probe results be interpreted in the context of clinical information and in correlation with morphologic examination of the tissue to obtain accurate diagnostic and prognostic information.

A second benefit of gene rearrangement testing is in determining the lineage (B versus T) of a lymphoid proliferation. Table 25-6 ✪ reveals that B cell tumors usually have clonal rearrangements of the Ig heavy chain and kappa light chain genes, while T cell tumors usually have clonal rearrangement of the TCRβ and TCRγ genes.[22,26] Sometimes, particularly in acute lymphoblastic leukemias, there are simultaneous Ig and TCR gene rearrangements even though

flow cytometric immunophenotyping suggests no ambiguity with regard to B versus T cell phenotype. Likewise, lymphoid gene rearrangements have been reported in occasional cases of acute myeloid leukemia (but not in nonhematopoietic tumors), implying that gene rearrangement does not necessarily indicate lymphoid origin. We can conclude that immunophenotypic methods are more reliable than gene rearrangement tests for assigning the lineage of hematopoietic neoplasms.

In morphologically equivocal hematopathology specimens, immunophenotyping is generally the first-line ancillary laboratory test, with gene probe studies being reserved as a secondary option.[28] In cases where diagnostic uncertainty remains after morphologic and immunophenotypic examination, gene rearrangement studies were shown to be helpful in 72% of cases (confirmatory in 41%; essential to the diagnosis in 31%).[29]

✔ **Checkpoint! #3**

An enlarged lymph node was biopsied and sent to the laboratory for molecular anlaysis. Lymphoma was suspected. What molecular test(s) could be done on the specimen to determine if the node is malignant and to determine if the cells are of T or B cell origin?

✪ TABLE 25-6

Clonal Gene Rearrangement by Diagnosis

	Immunoglobulin		T Cell Receptors
	IgH	kappa	TCRβ, TCRγ
B-acute lymphoblastic leukemia	100%	40%	30%
CLL, B cell lymphoma	100	100	< 10
Hairy cell leukemia	100	100	0
Myeloma	100	100	30
T-acute lymphoblastic leukemia	20	<1	95
Peripheral T cell lymphoma	<10	<1	80
Mycosis fungioides, ATLL	<10	<1	100

CLL = chronic lymphocytic leukemia (B cell type), ATLL = adult T cell leukemia/lymphoma

▶ DNA TECHNOLOGY IN THE DIAGNOSIS OF INFECTIOUS DISEASE

Molecular technology has provided new methods of detecting microorganisms based on the unique genetic code of each species.[30] Amplification strategies are promising because they are sensitive, specific, and rapid for detecting pathogen-specific nucleic acid sequences. Quantitative amplification assays are useful for monitoring the level of organisms during treatment.

Some organisms exist in the human body as normal flora, and they may or may not eventually cause disease. To investigate this issue, in situ hybridization is helpful for identifying lesion-specific pathogens in biopsy samples.

DNA technology is rapidly becoming a routine method for organism identification in diagnostic laboratories, and it will undoubtedly become the gold standard for detecting those pathogens that are difficult to identify by conventional culture or serology. Table 25-7 ✪ lists numerous

✪ TABLE 25-7

Pathogens of Hematologic Significance Detectable by Molecular Techniques

Cytomegalovirus (CMV)
Epstein-Barr virus (EBV)
Human herpes virus 8 (HHV8)
Human immunodeficiency virus (HIV)
Human T lymphotropic virus type 1 (HTLV1)
Malaria
Mycobacteria
Mycoplasma
Parvovirus B19
Toxoplasma

hematology-related pathogens for which molecular strategies are already available.

LYMPHOMA-ASSOCIATED VIRUSES

Three viruses have been consistently linked to lymphoid neoplasms—human T lymphotropic virus type 1 (HTLV1), Epstein-Barr virus (EBV), and human herpesvirus 8 (HHV8). HTLV1 infects T helper lymphocytes and causes them to proliferate by upregulation of interleukin 2 and its receptor. Asymptomatic HTLV1 infection is found in 15% of the people of Japan and the Caribbean islands. About 0.1% of infected individuals eventually develop adult T cell leukemia/lymphoma characterized by hypercalcemia and a proliferation of peculiar multilobated helper T lymphocytes harboring the virus. Integration of viral cDNA into host chromosomal DNA is identified in the malignant lymphocytes by Southern blot analysis or by PCR.[31]

EBV infects the oropharyngeal mucosa, where it resides in a subset of B lymphocytes. Virtually all persons are infected before adulthood and, once infected, they periodically shed infectious virus in their saliva for the remainder of their lives. EBV is known to cause infectious mononucleosis, and it is suspected of playing a role in the development of some lymphomas. EBV DNA is found in the majority of immunodeficiency-related lymphomas, in 40% of all Hodgkin's disease tissues, in 20% of sporadic Burkitt lymphomas, and in a subset of carcinomas. The best analytic test for confirming tumor-associated EBV is in situ hybridization to EBV encoded RNA (EBER).[32] In this procedure, viral probes are hybridized to viral RNA in paraffin tissue sections on glass slides. Microscopic visualization allows localization of the virus to particular cells in the lesion, such as the Reed-Sternberg cells of Hodgkin's disease (Figure 25-10 ■). EBV viral load measurement by quantitative PCR is a promising new blood test that facilitates diagnosis and monitoring of patients with EBV-related disease.

HHV8 rarely causes disease in healthy individuals, but in AIDS patients it is strongly associated with Kaposi's sarcoma, primary effusion lymphoma, and an atypical lymphoproliferative disorder called multicentric Castleman's disease. The virus can be detected in lesional tissue by in situ hybridization. Affected patients can be monitored using HHV8 viral load assays, which rely on measurement of HHV8 genomic sequences in blood using quantitative PCR.

❷ CASE STUDY *(continued from page 469)*

5. The molecular analysis revealed the BCR/ABL translocation with a p190 breakpoint. What is the diagnosis?

6. Why is this molecular finding helpful in therapy decisions?

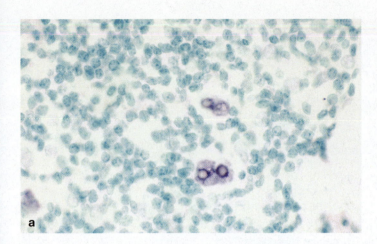
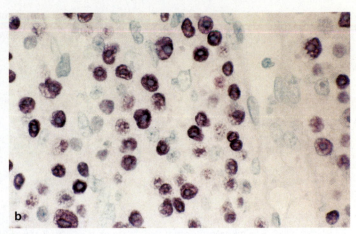

■ **FIGURE 25-10** *In situ* hybridization to Epstein-Barr virus EBER transcripts reveals the localization of the virus to **a.** Reed-Sternberg cells of Hodgkin's disease and **b.** the malignant cells of a diffuse large cell lymphoma, immunoblastic subtype, arising in an immuno-compromised patient. The nuclei of the virus-infected cells are darkly stained as a consequence of a colorimetric reaction occurring at the site of the bound probe.

SUMMARY

In summary, DNA technology provides a powerful new tool for laboratory diagnosis of a wide variety of hematopoietic diseases including inherited diseases, infectious diseases, and malignancies. The laboratory methods that are commonly used include Southern blot analysis, PCR, in situ hybridization, FISH, and DNA sequencing. Inherited hematologic diseases that are amenable to molecular diagnosis include sickle cell anemia and venous thrombosis resulting from factor V or prothrombin gene mutations. Leukemias and lymphomas are quite amenable to molecular diagnosis because these malignancies frequently harbor chromosomal translocations or clonal gene rearrangements. All infectious organisms are suitable targets for molecular detection because each species of organism has a unique genome that hybridizes to a complementary probe. This facilitates molecular diagnosis of infectious diseases and the virus-associated lymphomas.

REVIEW QUESTIONS

LEVEL II

Use this case history for questions 1 and 2.

A 38-year-old woman complained of dizziness, fatigue, and abdominal pain. On physical examination she appeared pale and her spleen was enlarged. Laboratory studies revealed anemia and an elevated leukocyte count of 69×10^9/L. A complete spectrum of granulocytic cells from myeloblasts to neutrophils was present in the blood, and basophils were increased. The neutrophil alkaline phosphatase score was low. The bone marrow was inaspirable, but a biopsy revealed that the marrow was packed with myeloid elements. Cytogenetics could not be performed due to the lack of an adequate marrow aspirate and the inability to induce division of peripheral blood cells. Blood is submitted for molecular diagnostic testing.

1. Which genetic defect is the most appropriate target for molecular testing in order to assist with diagnosis of the patient's hematologic disorder? (Checklist #7)
   a. PML/RARα
   b. bcl2/IgH
   c. BCR/ABL
   d. bcl1/IgH

2. Is there any reason to do molecular testing at a later date on the patient? (Checklist #3, 7)
   a. No, the positive test results are definitive, and nothing more can be accomplished.
   b. Yes, the patient can be monitored to detect residual disease following therapy.
   c. No, but family members should be tested for the same molecular defect.
   d. Yes, the translocation breakpoint must be sequenced to prove which genes are involved.

3. Which of the following reagents is most critical for making a PCR reaction specific for the factor V gene mutation as opposed to the prothrombin gene mutation? (Checklist #2)
   a. primers
   b. nucleotides
   c. DNA polymerase
   d. buffer

REVIEW QUESTIONS *(continued)*

LEVEL II

4. All molecular tests that analyze specific portions of the human genome rely on the principle that: (Checklist #2)
   a. DNA is different in every cell of a particular individual
   b. probes bind to their complementary target sequence through a process called hybridization
   c. restriction endonuclease cut sites remain the same regardless of any mutations
   d. heat or alkaline pH can convert single-stranded DNA to double-stranded DNA.

5. Which of the following assays would be most appropriate for detecting a genetic defect that is present in only 0.1% of the cells in a patient sample? (Checklist #8)
   a. polymerase chain reaction
   b. Southern blot analysis
   c. cytogenetics
   d. immunophenotyping

6. Polymerase chain reaction (PCR) differs from reverse transcriptase PCR (RT-PCR) in the following way(s): (Checklist #8)
   a. ribonucleotides rather than deoxyribonucleotides are added to the reaction mixture of RT-PCR but not PCR.
   b. following amplification, PCR generates a DNA product, whereas RT-PCR generates an RNA product.
   c. RNA rather than DNA serves as the substrate for RT-PCR.
   d. all of the above.

7. Immunoglobulin and T cell receptor gene rearrangement studies can be used to: (Checklist #6)
   a. distinguish B cell leukemia from B cell lymphoma.
   b. determine whether a lymphoid clone is present in a tissue specimen.
   c. prove that a tissue sample is benign.
   d. detect Epstein-Barr virus in a tissue specimen.

8. Which of the following is true about the molecular genetics of cancer? (Checklist #3)
   a. Virtually all cancers are thought to harbor genetic defects.
   b. DNA testing can be helpful in making a diagnosis of cancer.
   c. The genes responsible for tumor formation are called oncogenes.
   d. All of the above.

9. Which of the following is true about the Southern blot procedure? (Checklist #2)
   a. The patient's DNA is cut into fragments using proteinase enzymes.
   b. The electrophoresis step permits the probe to penetrate into the gel.
   c. The probe is labeled so that it can hybridize to its complementary strand.
   d. Interpretation of results relies on visualization of the band pattern.

10. Inherited diseases are characterized by: (Checklist #4)
    a. defective DNA having no effect on gene structure or protein function
    b. acquired mutations that are detected only in diseased organs
    c. the ability to predict inheritance in family members only if the precise genetic defect is known
    d. a genetic defect that is generally present in all tissues of the patient's body

www.prenhall.com/mckenzie

Use the above address to access the free, interactive Companion Web site created for this textbook. Get hints, instant feedback, and textbook references to chapter-related multiple choice questions.

REFERENCES

1. Ross DW. The human genome: Information content and structure. *Hosp Practice*. 1999; 34:49–65.

2. Weedn VW. Forensic DNA tests. *Clin Lab Med*. 1996; 16:187–96.

3. Chui DH, Hardison R, Riemer C, Miller W, Carver MF, Molchanova TP, Efremov GD, Huisman TH. An electronic database of human hemoglobin variants on the World Wide Web. *Blood*. 1998; 91: 2643–44.

4. Lisby G. Application of nucleic acid amplification in clinical microbiology. *Mol Biotechnol*. 1999; 12:75–99.

5. Saiki RK, Scharf S, Faloona F, Mullis KB, Horn GT, Erlich HA, Arnheim N. Enzymatic amplification of beta-globin genomic sequences and restriction site analysis for diagnosis of sickle cell anemia. *Science*. 1985; 230:1350–54.

6. Vnencak-Jones CL. Molecular testing for inherited diseases. *Am J Clin Pathol*. 1999; 112 Suppl:S19–32.

7. Blennerhassett GT, Furth ME, Anderson A, Burns JP, Chaganti RS, Blick M, Talpaz M, Dev VG, Chan LC, Wiedemann LM, et al. Clinical evaluation of a DNA probe assay for the Philadelphia (Ph[1]) translocation in chronic myelogenous leukemia. *Leukemia*. 1988; 2:648–57.

8. Dewald GW, Wyatt WA, Juneau AL, Carlson RO, Zinsmeister AR, Jalal SM, Spurbeck JL, Silver RT. Highly sensitive fluorescence in situ hybridization method to detect double BCR/ABL fusion and monitor response to therapy in chronic myeloid leukemia. *Blood*. 1998; 91:3357–65.

9. Kawasaki ES, Clark SS, Coyne MY, Smith SD, Champlin R, Witte ON, McCormick FP. Diagnosis of chronic myeloid and acute lymphocytic leukemias by detection of leukemia-specific mRNA sequences amplified in vitro. *Proc Natl Acad Sci*. 1988; 85:5698–702.

10. Kreuzer KA, Lass U, Bohn A, Landt O, Schmidt CA. LightCycler technology for the quantitation of BCR/ABL fusion transcripts. *Cancer Res*. 1999; 59:3171–74.

11. Eder M, Battmer K, Kafert S, Stucki A, Ganser A, Hertenstein B. Monitoring of BCR-ABL expression using real-time RT-PCR in CML after bone marrow or peripheral blood stem cell transplantation. *Leukemia*. 1999; 13:1383–83.

12. Radich JP, Gehly G, Gooley T, Bryant E, Clift RA, Collins S, Edmands S, Kirk J, Lee A, Kessler P, et al. Polymerase chain reaction detection of the BCR-ABL fusion transcript after allogeneic marrow transplantation for chronic myeloid leukemia: Results and implications in 346 patients. *Blood*. 1995; 85:2632–38.

13. Melo JV. The diversity of BCR-ABL fusion proteins and their relationship to leukemia phenotype. *Blood*. 1996; 88:2375–84.

14. Westbrook CA, Hooberman AL, Spino C, Dodge RK, Larson RA, Davey F, Wurster-Hill DH, Sobol RE, Schiffer C, Bloomfield CD. Clinical significance of the BCR-ABL fusion gene in adult acute lymphoblastic leukemia: A Cancer and Leukemia Group B Study (8762). *Blood*. 1992; 80:2983–90.

15. Lo Coco F, Diverio D, Falini B, Biondi A, Nervi C, Pelicci PG. Genetic diagnosis and molecular monitoring in the management of acute promyelocytic leukemia. *Blood*. 1999; 94:12–22.

16. Rennert H, Golde T, Wilson RB, Spitalnik SL, Van Deerlin VM, Leonard DG. A novel, non-nested reverse-transcriptase polymerase chain reaction (RT-PCR) test for the detection of the t(15;17) translocation: A comparative study of RT-PCR cytogenetics, and fluorescence in situ hybridization. *Mol Diagn*. 1999; 4:195–209.

17. Medeiros LJ, Carr J. Overview of the role of molecular methods in the diagnosis of malignant lymphomas. *Arch Pathol Lab Med*. 1999; 123:1189–207.

18. Luthra R, Sarris AH, Hai S, Paladugu AV, Romaguera JE, Cabanillas FF, Medeiros LJ. Real-time 5′→3′ exonuclease-based PCR assay for detection of the t(11;14)(q13;q32). *Am J Clin Pathol*. 1999; 112: 524–30.

19. Fan H, Gulley ML, Gascoyne RD, Horsman DE, Adomat SA, Cho CG. Molecular methods for detecting t(11;14) translocations in mantle-cell lymphomas. *Diagnostic Molec Pathol*. 1998; 7:209–14.

20. NCCLS. Immunoglobulin and T-cell receptor gene rearrangement assays. National Committee for Clinical Laboratory Standards; 1995.

21. Gill JI, Gulley ML. Immunoglobulin and T-cell receptor gene rearrangement. *Hematol-Oncol Clin N Amer*. 1994; 8:751–70.

22. Cossman J, Zehnbauer B, Garrett CT, Smith LJ, Williams M, Jaffe ES, Hanson LO, Love J. Gene rearrangements in the diagnosis of lymphoma/leukemia: Guidelines for use based on a multiinstitutional study. *Am J Clin Pathol*. 1991; 95:347–54.

23. Freedman AS, Neuberg D, Mauch P, Soiffer RJ, Anderson KC, Fisher DC, Schlossman R, Alyea EP, Takvorian T, Jallow H, Kuhlman C, Ritz J, Nadler LM, Gribben JG. Long-term follow-up of autologous bone marrow transplantation in patients with relapsed follicular lymphoma. *Blood*. 1999; 94:3325–33.

24. Abdel-Reheim FA, Edwards E, Arber DA. Utility of a rapid polymerase chain reaction panel for the detection of molecular changes in B-cell lymphoma. *Arch Pathol Lab Med*. 1996; 120:357–63.

25. Diaz-Cano S. PCR-based alternative for diagnosis of immunoglobulin heavy chain gene rearrangement: Principles, practice, and polemics. *Diagn Mol Pathol*. 1996; 5:3–9.

26. Krafft AE, Taubenberger JK, Sheng ZM, Bijwaard KE, Abbondanzo SL, Aguilera NS, Lichy JH. Enhanced sensitivity with a novel TCRgamma PCR assay for clonality studies in 569 formalin-fixed, paraffin-embedded (FFPE) cases. *Mol Diagn*. 1999; 4:119–33.

27. Cave H, van der Werff ten Bosch J, Suciu S, Guidal C, Waterkeyn C, Otten J, Bakkus M, Thielemans K, Grandchamp B, Vilmer E. Clinical significance of minimal residual disease in childhood acute lymphoblastic leukemia. European Organization for Research and Treatment of Cancer—Childhood Leukemia Cooperative Group. *New Engl J Med*. 1998; 339:591–98.

28. Kamat D, Laszewski MJ, Kemp JD, Goeken JA, Lutz CT, Platz CE, Dick FR. The diagnostic utility of immunophenotyping and immunogenotyping in the pathologic evaluation of lymphoid proliferations. *Modern Pathol*. 1990; 3:105–12.

29. Davis RE, Warnke RA, Dorfman RF, Cleary ML. Utility of molecular genetic analysis for the diagnosis of neoplasia in morphologically and immunophenotypically equivocal hematolymphoid lesions. *Cancer*. 1991; 67:2890–99.

30. Dumler JS, Valsamakis A. Molecular diagnostics for existing and emerging infections: Complementary tools for a new era of clinical microbiology. *Am J Clin Pathol*. 1999; 112 Suppl:S33–39.

31. Yamaguchi K, Matsuoka M, Takemoto S, Tamiya S, Etoh K, Takatsuki K. DNA diagnosis of HTLV-I. *Intervirology*. 1996; 39:158–64.

32. Gulley ML. Molecular diagnosis of Epstein-Barr virus-related diseases. *J Mol Diagn*. 2001; 3:1–10.

SECTION SEVEN • NEOPLASTIC HEMATOLOGIC DISORDERS

26

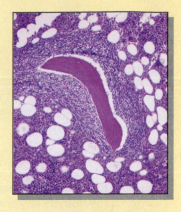

Introduction to Hematopoietic Neoplasms

Jean Sparks, Ph.D., Aamir Ehsan, M.D., Shirlyn B. McKenzie, Ph.D.

■ CHECKLIST - LEVEL I

At the end of this unit of study the student should be able to:

1. Define and differentiate the terms *neoplasm* and *malignant* and identify hematopoietic disorders that may be included in each category.

2. Compare and contrast the general characteristics of the myelodysplastic syndromes (MDS), myeloproliferative disorders (MPD), and acute and chronic leukemias.

3. Name and describe the classification of MDS, MPD, and the leukemias.

4. List the various methods used for categorizing the leukemias.

5. Compare and contrast the laboratory findings of the acute and chronic leukemias.

6. Differentiate proto-oncogenes and oncogenes and summarize their relationship to neoplastic processes.

7. Correlate patient age to the overall incidence of the hematopoietic neoplasms.

8. Explain the usefulness of immunological techniques, chromosome analysis, molecular analysis, and cytochemistry in the diagnosis and prognosis of hematopoietic neoplasms.

9. Predict the prognosis and survival rates of the hematopoietic neoplasms.

■ CHECKLIST - LEVEL II

At the end of this unit of study the student should be able to:

1. Explain how proto-oncogenes are activated and the role oncogenes and tumor suppressor genes and their protein products play in the etiology of hematopoietic neoplasms.

2. Describe the effects of radiation on the incidence of leukemia.

3. Differentiate between the acute and chronic leukemias based on their clinical and hematologic findings.

4. Reconcile the use of chemotherapy for treatment of leukemia.

5. Compare and contrast treatment options for the hematopoietic neoplasms including possible complications.

6. Name the leukomogenic factors of leukemia and propose how each contributes to the development of leukemia.

7. Compare and contrast laboratory features of MDS, MPD, and acute leukemia (AL) and justify a patient diagnosis based on these features.

8. Define the principles, explain the applications, and select appropriate cytochemical stains for bone marrow evaluation.

9. Select laboratory procedures appropriate for confirming cell lineage and diagnosis in hematopoietic neoplasms.

KEY TERMS

Acute lymphocytic leukemia (ALL)
Acute myelocytic leukemia (AML)
Aleukemic leukemia
Auer rods
Benign
Consolidation therapy
Chronic lymphocytic leukemia (CLL)
Chronic myelocytic leukemia (CML)
French-American-British (FAB)
Induction therapy
Leukocyte alkaline phosphatase (LAP)
Leukemia
Leukemic hiatus
Lymphoma
Maintenance chemotherapy
Malignant
Minimum residual disease
Myelodysplastic syndromes (MDS)
Myeloproliferative disorders (MPD)
Neoplasm
Tartrate resistant acid phosphatase (TRAP)

BACKGROUND BASICS

The information in this chapter will serve as a general introduction to the hematopoietic neoplasms (Chapters 27, 28, 29, 30, 31). To maximize your learning experience you should review these concepts before starting this unit of study.

Level I

▶ Summarize the origin and differentiation of the hematopoietic cells. (Chapters 2, 3)
▶ Describe the morphologic characteristics of the hematopoietic cells. (Chapters 4, 6)
▶ Define *oncogenes* and *proto-oncogenes*. (Chapter 2)

Level II

▶ Describe the actions of growth factors and oncogenes. (Chapter 2)
▶ Summarize the cell cycle and identify factors that affect it. (Chapter 2)
▶ Describe the normal structure and function of the bone marrow, spleen, and lymph nodes. (Chapter 3)

CASE STUDY

We will refer to this case study throughout the chapter.
Agnes, a 72-year-old female, was seen by her physician for a persistent cough and fatigue. She had always been in good health and played golf regularly. Upon examination, she was noted to be pale and had slight splenomegaly. A CBC was ordered and the WBC was 83.9×10^9/L. Consider possible explanations for this test result and select reflex tests that should be performed.

▶ OVERVIEW

This chapter provides a general introduction to the neoplastic hematopoietic disorders discussed in detail in Chapters 27–31. It begins with a discussion of oncogenesis including how oncogenes are activated and their association with hematopoietic disease. This is followed by a description of how neoplasms are classified and characterized according to cell lineage, degree of cell differentiation, morphology, cytochemistry, immunophenotype, and genetic abnormalities. The etiology and pathophysiology of the leukemias is examined along with general clinical and laboratory findings. Finally, prognosis and treatment modalities are considered for the disorders.

▶ INTRODUCTION

Neoplasm (tumor) literally means "new growth." Neoplasms arise as a consequence of unregulated proliferation of a single transformed cell. Genetic mutations in the transformed cell reduce or eliminate the cell's dependence on growth factors to regulate proliferation.

Neoplasms may be either malignant or benign. **Benign** neoplasms are formed from highly organized, differentiated cells and do not spread or invade surrounding tissue. *Malignancy* means "deadly," or "having the potential for producing death." A **malignant** neoplasm is a clone of identical, anaplastic (dedifferentiated), proliferating cells. The malignant cells can metastasize. Only malignant tumors are correctly referred to as cancer. Although cancer is actually a malignancy of epithelial tissue, common use of the term includes all malignant neoplasms. A benign neoplasm may be premalignant and progress, with further genetic mutations, to a malignant neoplasm.

Neoplasms of hematopoietic cells in the bone marrow include both benign (premalignant) neoplasms and malignant neoplasms (Figure 26-1 ■). The premalignant neoplasms include the **myeloproliferative disorders (MPD)** and **myelodysplastic syndromes (MDS)**. The malignant bone marrow neoplasms are collectively known as **leukemia**. Malignant cells may or may not circulate in the peripheral blood. The term *leukemia* is used when abnormal cells are seen in both the bone marrow and peripheral circulation. If the abnormal cells are found only in the bone marrow, the term **aleukemic leukemia** is used.

Sometimes, abnormal proliferation of lymphoid cells occurs within the lymphatic tissue, or lymph nodes. These solid tumors are referred to as a **lymphoma**. If the lymphoma affects the bone marrow and the lymphoma cells are found in the peripheral circulation, the leukemic phase of lymphoma is present.

Failure of normal hematopoiesis is the most serious consequence of malignant neoplasms. As the neoplastic cell population increases, the concentration of normal cells decreases

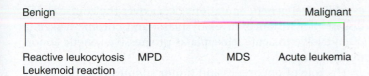

FIGURE 26-1 The spectrum of granulocytic proliferation disorders ranges from benign to malignant processes. Benign granulocyte proliferation is usually a reactive process. Myeloproliferative disorders, myelodysplastic syndromes, and acute myelocytic leukemia (AML) are neoplastic clonal stem cell defects characterized by autonomous proliferation of hematopoietic cells. (Adapted from McKenzie, S.: Chronic Myelocytic Leukemia. *Tech Sample* H-4, 1990. Chicago, ASCP)

resulting in the inevitable cytopenias of normal blood cells (Figure 26-2). If the neoplasm is not treated, the patient usually succumbs to infections secondary to granulocytopenia or bleeding secondary to thrombocytopenia.

▶ ETIOLOGY/PATHOPHYSIOLOGY

Hematopoietic neoplasms occur as the result of a somatic mutation of a single hematopoietic stem cell. Evidence for the clonal evolution of neoplastic cells comes from cytogenetic studies. More than 50% of individuals with leukemia show an acquired abnormal karyotype in hematopoietic cells, whereas other somatic cells are normal. Using these specific cytogenetic markers, normal and malignant cells can be demonstrated to populate the marrow simultaneously. In untreated leukemias and during relapse, the leukemic cells dominate, whereas during remission usually only normal cells can be detected. The MPD, MDS, and lymphomas are also associated with nonrandom genetic abnormalities.

The cell in which a genetic mutation occurs may be a committed lymphoid or myeloid progenitor cell or a more

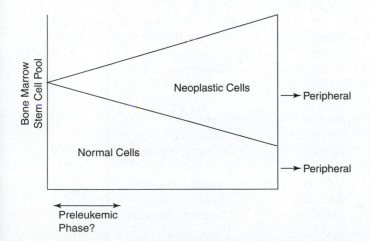

FIGURE 26-2 Clonal expansion of neoplastic cells in the bone marrow in leukemia over a period of time.

primitive progenitor cell that has the potential of differentiating into either lymphoid or myeloid cells, the pluripotential stem cell (multipotential progenitor cell).[1] The mutation can often be identified as a chromosome alteration when cells in mitosis are studied. Occasionally, when chromosome studies are normal, aberrations in DNA at the molecular level can be found. The mutation leads to a neoplastic proliferation of the affected stem cell and its progeny. In acute leukemia, this unregulated proliferation is accompanied by an arrest in maturation at the primitive blast cell stage (dedifferentiation).

✓ Checkpoint! #1

A 62-year-old male presents with an elevated leukocyte count, mild anemia, and a slightly decreased platelet count. His physician suspects leukemia. Explain why the erythrocytes and platelets are affected.

ONCOGENES

Until recently, the actual pathogenic mechanisms of neoplasms have remained obscure. The last several decades have seen enormous progress in our understanding of the pathogenesis of these disorders.

In 1976, J. Michael Bishop and Harold Varmus of the University of California, San Francisco, discovered that normal cells contain genes that can cause cancer/tumors if they become altered or activated.[2] These altered cell genes that cause tumors are referred to as oncogenes (*onco* means "tumor"), while the normal unaltered cellular counterparts of oncogenes are known as proto-oncogenes (∞ Chapter 2). Proto-oncogenes may become activated to oncogenes as a consequence of gene mutation, gene rearrangement, or gene amplification. This alters gene expression or activity/structure of its protein product. In the normal cellular state, proto-oncogenes direct cellular growth, proliferation, and differentiation by encoding proteins that are involved at every level of growth regulation. When altered, these genes are capable of inducing and maintaining cell transformation.

The protein products encoded by proto-oncogenes include:

- Growth factors
- Growth factor receptors
- Proteins involved in signal transduction
- Transcriptional factors (nuclear)

When a proto-oncogene is activated to an oncogene, there is either a qualitative change in the function of the protein product that results in increased activity, a protein that is no longer under normal regulatory control, or a quantitative change that increases the amount of protein produced.

These changes allow cells to proliferate without the normal controls.

Another type of gene recognized as playing a role in neoplastic transformation of cells is the anti-oncogene, or tumor suppressor gene (TSG). The products of the TSGs function by suppressing cellular proliferation and, hence, neoplastic transformation. For example, they trigger apoptosis if DNA can't be repaired, or they block the progression of the cell cycle if DNA is damaged. These genes are recessive, and one copy is sufficient to provide a reasonable amount of normal functioning protein to keep cell growth in check. Mutations to both copies, however, eliminate the block and facilitate tumor growth.

ROLES OF ONCOGENES AND ANTIONCOGENES IN NEOPLASIA

It appears that neoplasia is a multistep process that involves a series of progressive changes. Both oncogenes and tumor suppressor genes play a role in this process. Activation of one oncogene or loss of one tumor suppressor gene is only one step in tumor development. It is probable that multiple oncogenes and tumor suppressor genes acting together may be necessary for development of a malignant neoplasm. This concept of multiple genetic mutations helps explain the high incidence of leukemia in nonhematopoietic disorders associated with hereditary genetic mutations such as Down syndrome. In these conditions, the genetic mutation associated with the nonhematopoietic disorder may be one of the first of multiple steps leading to malignancy. Thus these individuals are at a higher risk of developing a neoplasm. Some neoplasms may progress to more malignant disorders as additional genetic mutations occur over the course of the disease. For instance, myelodysplasia and chronic leukemia often evolve to acute leukemia as progressive genetic abnormalities occur.

The role of oncogenes and tumor suppressor genes in the pathogenesis of neoplasms continues to be investigated. Oncogenes have been identified at the breakpoints of chromosomal aberrations that are commonly present in specific types of leukemias and lymphomas. It appears that chromosome breaks and translocations activate these genes and result in the aberrant expression of the protein product (Table 26-1 ✪). Also, breaks and translocations within a gene sequence may produce a hybrid gene and a new protein product. In chronic myelocytic leukemia (CML), the balanced translocation between chromosmes 9 and 22 results in the formation of a BCR-ABL hybrid gene that acts as an anti-apoptosis gene. Apoptosis is the major form of cell death associated with chemotherapy in tumor cells. The susceptibility of CML cells to treatment may be dependent on the expression of genes that interfere with apoptosis. For more detailed information on oncogenes, refer to Chapter 2.

ACTIVATION OF ONCOGENES

From studies on laboratory animals, several factors have been proposed as playing a role in the activation of oncogenes: (1) genetic susceptibility; (2) somatic mutation; (3) viral infection; and (4) immunologic dysfunction (Table 26-2 ✪).

Genetic Susceptibility

There is strong evidence that hereditary factors and abnormal genetic material have important leukemogenic effects. A

✪ **TABLE 26-1**

Common Genetic Abnormalities in Hematopoietic Neoplasms (for a more complete listing see Table 24-7)

Malignancy	Genetic Abnormality	Involved Genes	Activity
Myeloid leukemia			
CML	t(9;22)	BCR/ABL	Fusion protein
AML-M2	t(8;21)	ETO/AML1	Fusion protein
AML-M3	t(15;17)	PML/RAR-α	Fusion protein
CMMoL	t(5;12)	PDGFRB/TEL	Fusion protein
B cell leukemia			
ALL	t(9;22)	ABL/BCR	Fusion protein
Pre-B ALL	t(1;19)	PBX1/E2A	Fusion protein
CLL	t(14;19)	IGH/BCL3	Deregulated expression
Lymphomas			
Burkitt lymphoma	t(8;14)	MYC/IGH	Transcription regulation
Mantle cell lymphoma	t(11;14)	BCL1/IGH	Transcription deregulation
T cell lymphoma	t(8;14)	MYC/TCR	Transcription regulation
Mixed lineage leukemia	11q23	MLL	Fusion protein

Key: CML = chronic myelocytic leukemia; AML = acute myelocytic leukemia; CMMoL = chronic myelomonocytic leukemia; ALL = acute lymphocytic leukemia; CLL = chronic lymphocytic leukemia.

✪ TABLE 26-2

Factors Proposed to Play a Role in Leukemogenesis

Factor	Example
Hereditary abnormalities	Down syndrome
	Fanconi anemia
	Kleinfelter syndrome
	Bloom syndrome
	Wiskott-Aldrich syndrome
	Blackfan-Diamond syndrome
Somatic mutation	Radiation
	Chemicals
	Drugs
Viral infection	Retroviruses—HTLV-I, II, V, HIV-1
Immunologic disorders	Wiskott-Aldrich syndrome
	Bruton's type X-linked agammaglobulinemia
	Ataxia telangiectasia
	Immunosuppressive therapy

number of individuals who have congenital abnormalities associated with karyotypic abnormalities have a markedly increased risk of developing acute leukemia. Each of these genetic events may potentially activate proto-oncogenes. The best known of the genetic abnormalities associated with leukemia is Down syndrome.[3] Various other congenital disorders also are associated with an increased risk for leukemia, including Fanconi anemia, Kleinfelter syndrome, Bloom syndrome, Wiskott-Aldrich syndrome, and Blackfan-Diamond syndrome.

Further evidence supporting the association of genetic factors with the occurrence of leukemia comes from family studies where increased incidence has been reported in family groups.[4]

Somatic Mutation

Somatic cell mutation is an acquired change in the genetic material of cells other than those involved in reproduction. It is likely that mutations in the chromosome near these proto-oncogenes could play a role in development of neoplasms. More than 50% of patients with leukemia can be demonstrated to have acquired abnormal karyotypes. As the data accumulate from cytogenetic studies, specific, consistent mutations have been found in certain subgroups of hematopoietic neoplasms.

Radiation, some chemicals, and drugs can cause chromosome mutations. Ionizing radiation has long been recognized as capable of inducing leukemia, which is evident from observations of human exposure to radiation from nuclear reactions, therapeutic radiation, and occupational radiation.

An increase in leukemia has been observed after treatment with alkylating agents and other chemotherapeutic drugs used in treatment of many kinds of malignancy. The only specific chemical implicated in causing leukemia, other than those used in medication, is benzene.

Viral Infection

Retroviruses are proven to be responsible for leukemia in laboratory animals, and a few malignancies can be traced to a viral infection of cells in humans.[5] Retroviruses contain a reverse transcriptase that allows them to produce a DNA copy of the viral RNA core. The DNA can then be copied to produce more viral cores, or it can be incorporated into the nuclear DNA of the host cell. The strongest support for the existence of a leukemogenic virus in humans comes from the isolation of several human retroviruses known as human T cell leukemia/lymphoma virus (HTLV-I, II, V) and HIV-1 (human immunodeficiency virus) from cell lines of patients with mature T cell malignancies.[6] Exactly how viruses induce leukemia is unclear, but it is suspected that the incorporation of the viral genome into host DNA may lead to activation of proto-oncogenes.

Immunologic Dysfunction

Increased incidence of lymphocytic leukemia has been observed in both congenital and acquired immunologic disorders. These disorders include the hereditary immunologic diseases Wiskott-Aldrich syndrome, Bruton's type X-linked agammaglobulinemia, and ataxia telangiectasia. An association between long-term treatment of patients with immunosuppressive drugs (e.g., renal transplant) and leukemia also has been observed. Possibly, a breakdown in the cell-mediated immunologic self-surveillance system and/or deficient production of antibodies against foreign antigens leads to the emergence and survival of neoplastic cells.

Other Possibilities

Certain hematologic diseases appear to pose a leukemogenic risk. The leukemia development sometimes appears to be related to the treatment used for the primary disease, whereas in others no such relationship can be found. The highest incidence of acute leukemia is found in individuals with other neoplastic disorders, MPD, and MDS.[7] This has prompted some hematologists to use the term *preleukemia* for these disorders. Perhaps additional genetic mutations as the preleukemic disease progresses result in the frank malignancy, leukemia. Other hematopoietic diseases with an increased incidence of leukemia include paroxysmal nocturnal hemoglobinuria (PNH), aplastic anemia, multiple myeloma, and lymphoma. It is interesting to note that all these hematologic disorders are considered stem cell disorders wherein the primary hematologic defect lies in the myeloid or lymphoid progenitor cells, or pluripotential stem cells.

No single factor is responsible for activation of oncogenes that result in hematopoietic neoplasms, but rather, the disease is produced by a variety of etiologic factors, including genetic factors and environmental exposures. The cause probably varies from patient to patient, and some individuals may be more susceptible than others to oncogene activation.

 Checkpoint! #2

Does a 3-year-old child with Down syndrome have an increased likelihood of developing leukemia? Why or why not?

► HEMATOPOIETIC NEOPLASM CLASSIFICATION

Classifications of hematopoietic neoplasms are considered to be important for three reasons:

1. They allow clinicians and researchers a method of comparison of various therapeutic regimens.

2. They allow a system for identification and comparison of clinical features and laboratory findings.

3. They permit meaningful associations of cytogenetic abnormalities with disease.

The neoplastic disorders of the bone marrow hematopoietic cells can be grouped into three main categories:

• Myeloproliferative disorders (MPD)

• Myelodysplastic syndromes (MDS)

• Acute leukemias (AL)

Each of these three categories can be further subgrouped. In 1976, in an effort to improve and standardize the classification of AL, a group of **French, American, and British (FAB)** physicians proposed a classification and nomenclature system based on the morphologic characteristics of blast cells on Romanowsky-stained smears and the results of cytochemical stains.[8] In the FAB classification, a blast count >30% is diagnostic of leukemia. In 1984, the FAB group proposed a classification for the MDS. This classification uses the blast count and degree of dysplasia in subgrouping the MDS. The MDS are characterized by peripheral blood cytopenias (except chronic myelomonocytic leukemia). The MPDs were recognized by Dameshek in 1951. Myeloproliferative disorders are characterized by neoplastic increases in erythrocytes, leukocytes, and/or platelets.

Both MPD and MDS have a blast count <30%. They may have a chronic or acute course and have the potential of evolving into acute leukemia (Figure 26-1 ■). Of the three groups of neoplastic bone marrow disorders, acute leukemias represent the frank malignant hematopoietic neoplasms with a proliferation of blast cells.

Malignant lymphoproliferative disorders may occur in the hematopoietic system (bone marrow and peripheral blood) or in the lymphoreticular system (lymph nodes and spleen). When the malignant proliferation involves the bone marrow and peripheral blood, the disease is referred to as acute or chronic lymphocytic leukemia. When the malignant proliferation is in the lymphoid tissue, the disease is referred to as a lymphoma (∞ Chapter 31). Lymphomas may eventually spread to the bone marrow and the malignant cells may then be found in the peripheral blood. The acute lymphocytic leukemias are discussed in ∞ Chapter 30. Classification and description of the other malignant lymphoproliferative diseases are discussed in ∞ Chapter 31.

LEUKEMIAS

Leukemias are classified into two broad groups, myeloid and lymphoid, based on the the origin of the leukemic stem cell clone. If myelocytic cells or other cells derived from the CFU-GEMM stem cell predominate, the disease is called *myelogenous leukemia*. If the lymphoid cells predominate, the disease is termed *lymphocytic leukemia*. These two groups are further classified based on the aggressiveness of the illness and differentiation of the leukemic cells: (1) acute, an aggressive disease (**acute myelocytic leukemia, AML; acute lymphocytic leukemia, ALL);** and (2) chronic, a less aggressive form (**chronic myelocytic leukemia, CML; chronic lymphocytic leukemia, CLL**) (Table 26-3 ✪). In acute leukemia there is a gap in the normal maturation pyramid of cells, with many blasts and some mature forms but very few intermediate maturational stages. This gap in maturation is frequently referred to as the **leukemic hiatus**. Eventually, the immature neoplastic cells fill the bone marrow and spill over into the peripheral blood, producing leukocytosis. In the laboratory, the diagnosis of acute leukemia is suggested when examination of the peripheral blood smear reveals the presence of many undifferentiated or minimally differentiated cells. Chronic leukemias are characterized by leukocytosis but <30% blasts with a predominance of more mature cells.

Subtypes of acute leukemia (ALL, AML) can be identified based on morphologic, cytochemical, immunologic, and cytogenetic criteria of the malignant cells (Table 26-4 ✪). Acute leukemias involving the granulocytic, monocytic, erythrocytic, or megakaryocytic cell lines are classified as sub-

✪ TABLE 26-3

Comparison of Acute and Chronic Leukemias

	Acute	Chronic
Age	All ages	Adults
Clinical onset	Sudden	Insidious
Course of disease (untreated)	Weeks to months	Months to years
Predominant cell	Blasts, some mature forms	Mature forms
Anemia	Mild–severe	Mild
Thrombocytopenia	Mild–severe	Mild
WBC	Variable	Increased

✪ TABLE 26-4

Classification of Leukemias

	Myeloid	Lymphoid	Other
Acute leukemia	Myeloblastic	T lymphocytic	Undifferentiated
	Promyelocytic	B lymphocytic	Mixed lineage
	Monocytic	Null cell (unclassified)	Myeloid/natural
	Myelomonocytic		Killer cell
	Erythrocytic		
	Megakaryocytic		
Chronic leukemia	Myelocytic	Lymphocytic	
	Myelomonocytic	Plasmocytic (multiple myeloma)	
		Hairy cell	
		Prolymphocytic	
		Large granular cell lymphocytic leukemia	
		Sézary's syndrome	
		Circulating lymphoma	

types of acute myelocytic leukemia (acute nonlymphocytic leukemia, ANLL) since these cell types develop from the common stem cell, CFU-GEMM (Table 26-5 ✪). The ALL group may be subtyped into L1, L2, and L3 based on morphology and heterogeneity of the bone marrow lymphoblasts (FAB classification) or T, B, and null cell leukemia based on immunophenotype of lymphocytes.

In addition to the above ALs, three other subtypes of acute leukemia are recognized: mixed lineage, undifferentiated, and myeloid/natural killer cell. Mixed lineage leukemia, as its name implies, is characterized by blasts with both lymphoid and myeloid features. Undifferentiated leukemia is characterized by blasts that cannot be identified as lymphoid or myeloid by cytochemical stains and surface markers. The myeloid/natural killer cell acute leukemia coexpresses myeloid (CD33, CD13, CD15) and NK cell-associated antigens (CD56, CD11b), while they lack HLA-DR and T lymph associated antigens, CD3 and CD8. The acute leukemias will be discussed in detail in Chapters 29 and 30.

In the past, chronic leukemias were commonly classified as a distinct group of hematopoietic disorders. More recently, they have been grouped with other chronic neoplastic stem cell disorders, MPD, MDS, and chronic leukemic lymphoid disorders. The bone marrow in chronic leukemias typically exhibits an accumulation of differentiated lymphocytic (CLL) or myelocytic (CML) elements. These cells spill over into the peripheral blood, producing a leukocytosis. The differential count of the bone marrow and peripheral blood are similar with all stages of maturation present but with a predominance of the more mature forms. These chronic leukemias will be discussed in Chapters 27 and 28 with MPD and MDS and in Chapter 31 with lymphoproliferative disorders.

✪ TABLE 26-5

FAB Classification of Acute Leukemia

Acute Nonlymphocytic Leukemias

M0	Acute myeloblastic leukemia without differentiation
M1	Acute myeloblastic leukemia with minimal differentiation
M2	Acute myeloblastic leukemia with maturation
M3	Promyelocytic leukemia, hypergranular
M3m	Promyelocytic leukemia, microgranular variant
M4	Acute myelomonocytic leukemia
M4eo	Acute myelomonocytic leukemia with abnormal eosinophils
M5a	Acute monoblastic leukemia without differentiation
M5b	Acute monoblastic leukemia with differentiation
M6	Acute erythroleukemia
M7	Megakaryocytic leukemia

Acute Lymphocytic Leukemias

L1	Lymphoblastic leukemia with homogeneity
L2	Lymphoblastic leukemia with heterogeneity
L3	Burkitt type lymphoblastic leukemia

ⓔ CASE STUDY *(continued from page 478)*

The CBC results on Agnes were:

WBC:	83.9×10^9/L
RBC:	3.15×10^{12}/L
Hb:	95 g/L
Hct:	0.29 L/L
Platelets:	130×10^9/L
Differential:	segs 12%
	lymphs 88%

1. Given the patient's laboratory results, would this most likely be considered an acute or chronic leukemia? Explain.

MYELOPROLIFERATIVE DISORDERS

The MPDs are characterized by a panhypercellularity of the bone marrow and erythrocytosis, granulocytosis, or thrombocytosis in the peripheral blood. One cell line is usually more prominent than the others, a feature that is used to subgroup these disorders. The neoplastic cell is the pluripotential stem cell. The MPD subgroups are:

- Chronic granulocytic leukemia (CGL)—overproduction of granulocytes
- Polycythemia vera (PV)—overproduction of erythrocytes
- Essential thrombocythemia (ET)—overproduction of platelets
- Agnogenic myeloid metaplasia (AMM)—fibrotic bone marrow (fibrosis is not neoplastic). Also known as myelofibrosis with myeloid metaplasia *(mmm)*.

These disorders will be discussed in Chapter 27.

MYELODYSPLASTIC SYNDROMES

The MDSs are characterized by dysplasia of cells in a hypercellular bone marrow and cytopenia with dysplasia in the peripheral blood. The neoplastic cell is the pluripotential stem cell. The MDSs are divided into five subgroups:

1. Refractory anemia (RA)
2. Refractory anemia with ringed sideroblasts (RARS)
3. Refractory anemia with excess blasts (RAEB)
4. Refractory anemia with excess blasts in transformation (RAEB-T)
5. Chronic myelomonocytic leukemia (CMML)

These disorders will be discussed in Chapter 28.

THE WHO CLASSIFICATION

Recently, genetic features, prior therapy, and a history of myelodysplasia have been shown to have a significant impact on the clinical behavior of the hematopoietic neoplasms. The WHO (World Health Organization) classification was developed by the Society for Hematopathology and the European Association of Hematopologists to better define the hematopoietic neoplasms; first, according to their cell lineage, and second, according to a combination of cell morphology, immunophenotyping, genetic features, and clinical syndrome[9] (Table 26-6 ✪). The classification according to lineage of the neoplastic cells includes four groups: myeloid, lymphoid, mast cell, and histiocytic. There are four major groups of myeloid disease defined by morphology, genetic abnormalities, immunophenotyping, and clinical features:

- Myeloproliferative disorders (MPD)
- Myelodysplasia/myeloproliferative disorders (MD/MPD)
- Myelodysplastic syndromes (MDS)
- Acute myelocytic leukemia (AML)

The MD/MPD group includes diseases that have features of both MDS and MPD such as chronic myelomonocytic leukemia. Each major group is further subgrouped and will be discussed in Chapters 27–30.

A significant change in the WHO classification relates to the blast count used to define and differentiate AML from the other myeloid neoplasms. This classification uses the standard of >20% blasts to define AML. (The FAB standard is that >30% blasts defines AML.) This is based on the observation that patients with 20–30% blasts have a prognosis similar to those with >30% blasts.

In the lymphoid neoplasms, the proposed WHO classification adopts the revised European-American lymphoid neoplasm (REAL) classification. This classification uses morphology, immunophenotype, genetic, and clinical features. There are three groups: B cell, T/NK cell neoplasms, and Hodgkin's disease. The T and B cell neoplasms are grouped into precursor (lymphoblastic) and mature neoplasms. The ALLs are in the

✪ **TABLE 26-6**

WHO Classification of Hematologic Neoplasms

Myeloproliferative Diseases

Chronic myelogenous leukemia, Philadelphia chromosome positive (Ph+)
Chronic neutrophilic leukemia*
Chronic eosinophilic leukemia/hypereosinophilic syndrome*
Chronic idiopathic myelofibrosis
Polycythemia vera
Essential thrombocythemia
Myeloproliferative disease, unclassifiable*

Myelodysplastic/Myeloproliferative Diseases*

- chronic myelomonocytic leukemia
- atypical myelogenous leukemia
- juvenile myelomonocytic leukemia

Myelodysplastic Syndromes

Refractory anemia
- With ringed sideroblasts (RARS)
- Without ringed sideroblasts
Refractory cytopenia with multilineage dysplasia*
Refractory anemia with excess blasts
5q- syndrome*
Myelodysplastic syndrome, unclassifiable*

Acute Myeloid Leukemia[†]

Acute myeloid leukemias with recurrent cytogenetic translocations*
Acute myeloid leukemia with multilineage dysplasia*
Acute myeloid leukemia and myelodysplastic syndrome, therapy related*
Acute myeloid leukemia not otherwise categorized**
Acute biphenotypic leukemia

Acute Lymphoid Leukemias (precursor B- and T-cell neoplasms)

Precursor B cell acute lymphoblastic leukemia* (classified by cytogenetic subgroups)
Precursor T cell acute lymphoblastic leukemia*

B Cell Neoplasms (mature cell neoplasms)[†]

T Cell Neoplasms (mature cell neoplasms)[†]

Hodgkin Lymphoma[†]

[†]subgroups not listed
*not included in FAB classification
**includes subgroups of AML in FAB classification
(The B- and T-cell neoplasms and Hodgkin's disease are discussed in detail in Chapter 31.)

precursor group and include B cell and T cell ALL and Burkitt cell leukemia (L3 in FAB). The mature neoplasms include B cell chronic lymphocytic leukemia (CLL) and hairy cell leukemia.

The REAL classification for lymphoid neoplasms is in general use and is followed in Chapter 31, Malignant Lymphoproliferative Disorders. It remains to be determined if the new WHO proposed myeloid classification will be adopted and used by pathologists, hematologists, and oncologists. In this book, the FAB classification is generally followed for myeloid neoplasms. Comparisons to the WHO classification are made where appropriate.

 Checkpoint! #3

A patient has 50% monoblasts in the bone marrow. Which of the four major types of leukemia does he have, AML, CML, ALL, or CLL?

► EPIDEMIOLOGY

The American Cancer Society predicted that in the year 2002, there would be about 30,800 new cases of leukemia reported in the United States. Of these, about 11,400 would be chronic leukemias. There would be about 10,600 new cases of acute myelogenous leukemia.[10]

Approximately 50% of all leukemias are diagnosed as acute. Although there is some difference in the incidence of the acute leukemias between countries and regions of countries, the differences are not great. However, all leukemias are more prevalent in Jews of Russian, Polish, and Czeck ancestry than in non-Jews. Acute leukemia also is more common in whites than blacks.

Of particular interest is the incidence and morphologic variation of leukemia among age groups (Table 26-7 ✪). Although acute leukemia occurs at all ages, there is a peak incidence in the first decade, particularly from the ages of 2 to 5. This is followed by a decreasing incidence in the second and third decade. Thereafter, the incidence begins to increase, rising steeply after 50 years of age. The cellular type of leukemia, occurring at these peak periods, differs significantly. Most childhood acute leukemias are of the lymphoid type, whereas those occurring in adults are typically myeloid in origin. Chronic leukemias are rare in children. Most chronic myeloid leukemias occur in young to middle-aged adults, while chronic lymphocytic leukemia is found primarily in older adults. MPD and MDS occur most often in adults.

► CLINICAL FINDINGS

Failure of normal hematopoiesis is the most serious consequence of hematopoietic neoplasms. The most frequent symptoms are related to anemia, thrombocytopenia, or neu-

✪ TABLE 26-7

Age Groups Typically Found in Acute and Chronic Leukemias

ALL	children 2–5 years old
CLL:	adults >50 years old
AML:	adults
CML:	adults

tropenia. The major clinical problems are anemia, infection, and bleeding episodes, occurring as frank hemorrhages, petechiae, or ecchymoses. Bone pain due to marrow expansion and weight loss is a common complaint. Physical examination may show hepatosplenomegaly and, occasionally, lymphadenopathy. Organomegaly is more common in chronic leukemias than in the acute forms.

Although the disease originates in the bone marrow, neoplastic cells may infiltrate any tissue of the body, especially the spleen, liver, lymph nodes, central nervous system, and skin. The lesions produced vary from rashes to tumors. Skin infiltration is most commonly found in AML, especially those with a monocytic component. Central nervous system (CNS) involvement is especially common in ALL of childhood. Chloromas, green tumor masses of immature leukocytes, are associated with AML and CML. They are usually found in bone but can be found throughout the body. The green color, which fades to a dirty yellow after exposure to air, is responsible for the descriptive name given to this unique tumor. Presumably, the green color results from the myeloperoxidase content of malignant cells.

► HEMATOLOGIC FINDINGS

Cell counts and morphology are variable in the hematopoietic neoplasms (Table 26-8 ✪). A normocytic (occasionally macrocytic) normochromic anemia is usually present at diagnosis. If not present initially, it invariably develops during progression of the disease.

Thrombocytopenia is usually present at diagnosis in acute leukemia. Thrombocytosis is a common initial finding in MPD. The platelet count in MDS is variable. In both MPD and MDS, however, the platelet count decreases with progression of the disease. Platelet morphology and function also may be abnormal. Especially common are large hypogranular forms, and occasionally, micromegakaryocytes are present.

The leukocyte count may be normal, increased, or decreased. More than 50% of patients with AML do not have a significant leukocytosis at diagnosis. However, if left untreated, leukocytosis eventually develops. On the other hand, in the chronic myeloproliferative and lymphoproliferative neoplasms, leukocytosis at diagnosis is a prominent finding. Normal or decreased leukocyte counts are typical in MDS. Regardless of the leukocyte count, in most cases, an increase in immature precursors is found. Blasts are especially prominent in the acute leukemias. Both absolute and relative monocytosis are common features in the acute myeloid leukemias.

Unique pink-staining granular inclusions called **Auer rods** can be found in the blast cells and promyelocytes of some acute myeloid leukemias. These abnormal granules are believed to be formed from fused primary granules. When AML is suspected, the finding of Auer rods can help establish the diagnosis because these inclusions are not found in ALL.

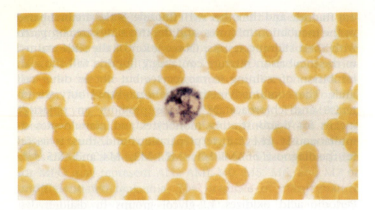

■ **FIGURE 26-8** LAP stain showing neutrophil with a score of 3+. Note strong colored granulation. (Peripheral blood; LAP stain; 500× magnification)

neutrophils contain an increased amount of LAP. Therefore, the LAP score is useful in distinguishing leukemoid reaction/reactive neutrophilia (high LAP) from chronic myelogenous leukemia (low LAP).[18,19]

Freshly prepared peripheral blood smears are obtained from finger-stick capillary blood. Smears should be dried at least one hour before fixation in 10% formalin in methanol. Fixed slides may be stored overnight in a freezer. Improperly stored smears and EDTA anticoagulant may give falsely low LAP scores. The smears are incubated in naphthol AS-BI phosphate at an alkaline pH. The liberated naphthol immediately couples with a diazonium salt (e.g., fast red violet) forming brown to black particles in the cytoplasm of the cells at the enzyme sites (Figure 26-8 ■). After counterstaining, the smears are evaluated microscopically. One hundred segmented neutrophils/bands are counted, and each cell is graded using a scale of 0 to 4+ according to the appearance and intensity of the precipitated dye (Table 26-12 ✪). The number of cells counted in each grade are multiplied by their grades, and the products are summed to obtain a total LAP score (Table 26-13 ✪). LAP is thus a semiquantitative method.

The range of normal scores is 13–130, although there may be slight variation in each laboratory. The range of possible values is 0–400. A score greater than 160 is generally considered increased, and less than 13 is considered decreased. The LAP scores can be increased in leukemoid reaction (infection, inflammation), polycythemia vera, pregnancy, newborns, stress, oral contraceptives, and medications (steroids, estrogen, lithium, growth factors). In secondary erythrocytosis, idiopathic myelofibrosis and essential thrombocytosis, the enzyme activity is usually normal. LAP scores can be decreased in CML, paroxysmal nocturnal hemoglobinuria, idiopathic thrombocytopenic purpura, and sometimes in myelodysplasia. The LAP score may be increased in CML patients in blast crisis or with concurrent infections.

✪ **TABLE 26-13**

Example of a Calculation of a LAP Score

Cell Rating	Number of Cells Counted	LAP Score
0	45	0
1+	30	30
2+	15	30
3+	5	15
4+	5	20
	Total LAP score	95

✔ **Checkpoint! #5**

A pathology resident is evaluating the peripheral blood smear of a 40-year-old male. He suspects a diagnosis of CML. In order to confirm his suspicion, he ordered a LAP score. Do you think that ordering a LAP score will help him in making the right diagnosis?

Acid Phosphatase and Tartrate Resistant Acid Phosphatase (TRAP)

Acid phosphatase is a constituent of lysosomes and is present in most human cells. Acid phosphatase activity is detected by incubating the specimen in naphthol AS-BI phosphoric acid.[20,21] As a result of enzyme activity, naphthol AS-BI is liberated. The liberated naphthol immediately couples with a diazonium salt (e.g., fast garnet) forming an insoluble, visible pigment at the site of enzyme activity. Acid phosphatase activity is present in most normal leukocytes appearing as purplish, dark-red intracellular granules. The acid phosphatase activity in T cell ALL is characteristic, which exhibits focal polarized acid phosphatase activity.

Seven acid phosphatase isoenzymes (0, 1, 2, 3, 3b, 4, and 5) are present in leukocytes. These isoenzymes are cell specific with neutrophils containing isoenzymes 2 and 4, lymphocytes and platelets isoenzyme 3, blasts isoenzyme 3b, and hairy cells isoenzyme 5. All but isoenzyme 5 are sensitive to tartrate inhibition. The hairy cells of hairy cell leukemia exhibit acid phosphatase activity, but may be differentiated from other leukocytes using tartrate inhibition.[22,23] The acid

✪ **TABLE 26-12**

Leukocyte Alkaline Phosphatase: Cell Rating and Staining Characteristics

Cell Rating	Amount	Intensity of Staining
0	None	None
1+	<50%	Faint
2+	50–75%	Moderate
3+	75–100%	Strong
4+	100%	Intense

phosphatase activity within normal leukocytes will be inhibited by tartrate, while enzyme activity within hairy cells is resistant to tartrate inhibition (Figure 26-9 ■). Therefore, hairy cell leukemia is said to be strongly **tartrate resistant acid phosphatase (TRAP)** positive. Weak to moderate TRAP positivity may be seen in activated lymphocytes and Sézary cells, a few cases of chronic lymphocytic leukemia, and prolymphocytic leukemia. Mast cells are also TRAP positive, and the morphology of abnormal mast cells on tissue sections is similar to hairy cell leukemia. Toluidine blue stain is helpful is distinguishing mast cells (positive) from hairy cells (negative).

✓ Checkpoint! #6

A 30-year-old male presented to the emergency room complaining of fatigue, weakness, and gum bleeding. The CBC showed anemia, thrombocytopenia, and a WBC of 30 × 10⁹/L. Evaluation of the peripheral blood smear showed numerous intermediate to large blasts with fine nuclear chromatin and abundant cytoplasm. The bone marrow biopsy contained 60% blasts. No Auer rods were seen after careful evaluation. Several cytochemical stains were then performed. The blasts failed to stain with myeloperoxidase, Sudan black B, and specific esterase; however, the majority of blasts reacted intensely with α-naphthyl esterase. Incubation with sodium fluoride inhibited the staining seen with α-naphthyl esterase. What type of leukemia do you think this patient has?

Terminal Deoxynucleotidyl Transferase

Terminal deoxynucleotidyl transferase (TdT) is a DNA polymerase found in cell nuclei. It is normally present in thymus lymphocytes, in pre-B lymphocytes (hematogones) and in 1–3% of normal bone marrow cells. It is not normally present in peripheral blood lymphocytes or lymph node lymphocytes. TdT is a primitive cell marker and is of value in distinguishing ALL from malignant lymphoma.[24,25] It is also helpful in identifying leukemic cells in body fluid specimens. It is present in 90–95% of ALL (T cell ALL and precursor B cell ALL, but not in B cell ALL). TdT staining may not be beneficial in evaluating acute leukemias as up to 20% of AMLs may show TdT positivity, and over 90% of AML-M0 can be TdT positive. Therefore, when the differential diagnosis is between ALL and AML (i.e., AML-M0), a positive TdT stain is not diagnostically helpful. TdT can be detected by biochemical assays, immunoperoxidase, and enzyme immunoassays and by direct or indirect immunofluorescence using monoclonal antibodies.

✓ Checkpoint! #7

A pathologist is reviewing the slides from the pleural fluid of a 50-year-old male who has hepatosplenomegaly and minimal lymphadenopathy. It is not clear if the mononuclear cells are mature lymphoma cells or leukemic blasts. There is not enough material for flow cytometry to do immunophenotyping, but there is enough to make a few extra cytospin smears. Which stain do you think can be useful in this case?

Toluidine Blue

Toluidine blue is a basic dye that reacts with acid mucopolysaccharides to form red to purple metachromatic granules. A positive reaction is specific for basophils and mast cells. This stain is useful in the diagnosis of mast cell disease and rare cases of AML with basophilic differentiation.[16,26,27] A negative reaction should not rule out neoplasm of these cells because the acid mucopolysaccharides may be scarce or negative in neoplastic disorders.

Reticulin Stain and Masson's Trichrome Stain

Although the presence of fibrosis can be suspected on hematoxylin and eosin (H&E) stained sections, reticulin and trichrome stains are used to evaluate both the presence and extent of fibrosis. Reticulin stain is used to examine the reticulin fibers that form the major framework of the bone marrow. The Gomori methenamine silver staining method for reticulin is more suitable. In hypercellular marrow, the reticulin becomes more prominent, but its structural framework is preserved. In myelofibrosis, reticulin is markedly increased and the structural framework is distorted (Figure 26-10 ■).

Masson's trichrome stain is useful to evaluate the degree of collagenous fibrosis. Normally, collagenous fibrosis is focal and perivascular. Increased staining can be seen in myelofibrosis and indicates severe and dense fibrosis (Figure 26-11 ■).

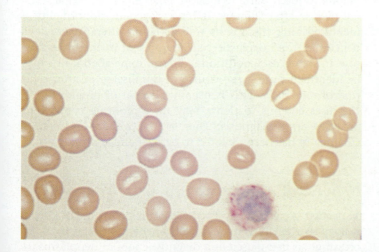

■ **FIGURE 26-9** TRAP stain showing a positive reaction of hairy cell with acid phosphatase that is resistant to tartrate inhibition (reddish granulation). (Peripheral blood; TRAP stain; 500× magnification)

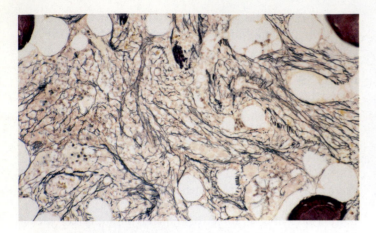

■ **FIGURE 26-10** Bone marrow biopsy stained with reticulin stain showing fibrosis in a patient with myelofibrosis. (Bone marrow; paraffin section, reticulin stain; 200× magnification)

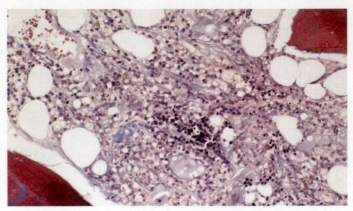

■ **FIGURE 26-11** Bone marrow biopsy stained with Masson's trichrome stain showing collagenous fibrosis (fibers are stained light blue) in a patient with myelofibrosis. (Bone marrow; paraffin section, Masson's Trichrome stain; 400× magnification)

IMMUNOLOGIC ANALYSIS

Immunologic analysis is based on identifying specific membrane antigens (surface markers) that are characteristically found on a particular cell line. Immunologic techniques with monoclonal antibodies are now widely used to identify cell membrane antigens on a variety of cells (∞ Chapter 23). The development of a large number of monoclonal antibodies (produced commercially using hybridomas, cells capable of producing a continuous supply of identical antibodies) to surface antigens on normal and neoplastic cells, together with technical advances in flow cytometry, has greatly enhanced the ability to define leukemic cell lineage, stage of cell development, and clonality. By utilizing a panel of monoclonal antibodies, a more complete picture of the cells' lineage can be determined.

The use of immunologic markers to characterize AML subtypes and myeloid antigenic development has lagged behind the use of these markers in ALL. There are two possible explanations for this lag.[28] The first is that AML, unlike ALL, has two specific cytochemical markers—peroxidase and nonspecific esterase—which help in identifying the myeloid origin of the cells. The second is that to subtype AML, markers for myeloblasts, erythroblasts, monoblasts, and megakaryoblasts need to be identified. Recently, an increasing repertoire of antibodies to myeloid antigens has been developed. These antibodies have helped not only in subtyping the myeloid leukemias but also in identifying the lineage of leukemias that lack specific morphologic and cytochemical characteristics. A more thorough discussion of monoclonal antibodies and their use in the identification of neoplastic hematopoietic disorders can be found in ∞ Chapter 23.

CYTOGENETIC ANALYSIS

Advances in cytogenetics have allowed cytogeneticists to identify characteristic nonrandom karyotypes in the majority of the acute leukemias and in some MPD and MDS.[29,30]

Some specific chromosome changes are consistently associated with a particular neoplastic subgroup and thus are helpful in diagnosis. The t(15;17)(q22;q11) is diagnostic of M3-AML, and the Philadelphia chromosome characterized by t(9;22)(q34;q11.2) confirms a clinical diagnosis of chronic myelocytic leukemia (CML). In the lymphoid leukemias, nonrandom chromosome changes are often associated with either the B or T lymphocyte lineage and provide important prognostic as well as diagnostic information. Chromosomal rearrangements and their accompanying molecular abnormalities can identify distinct clinical groups with a predictable clinical course and response to specific therapy. In addition to helping physicians evaluate their patients, cytogenetic studies help provide new insights into the pathogenesis of neoplastic diseases.

When cytogenetic abnormalities are present they are helpful in identifying remission, relapse, and minimal residual disease after therapy. If the cytogenetic abnormality is identified after therapy as well as before therapy, it is evidence that the neoplastic cells are present in the bone marrow. In some cases, additional chromosome aberrations may be identified during the course of the disease or after a period of remission. This is usually a signal of progression of the disease. Thus, patients may have multiple cytogenetic analyses after diagnosis. Due to the topic's importance, Chapter 24 has been devoted to cytogenetic analysis.

MOLECULAR ANALYSIS

Molecular genetic analysis, the process of using DNA technology to identify genetic defects at the molecular level, increasingly is being used as a diagnostic tool in neoplasms. In some cases the chromosome karyotype is normal but a genetic mutation can be identified at the molecular level. About 5% of patients with CML do not show the typical Philadelphia chromosome on karyotyping, but the BCR-ABL mutation can be identified by molecular techniques. When present, this helps establish or confirm the diagnosis.

Molecular analysis also is helpful in providing clues to the pathogenesis of hematopoietic neoplasms. For example, the specific t(15;17) (q22;q11) mutation found only in acute promyelocytic leukemia (M3 AML) produces an abnormal nuclear hormone receptor, the retinoic acid receptor-alpha (RAR-α). The receptor in its normal form is important in transcription of certain target genes. This specific abnormality is likely involved in the maturation blockage of M3 cells. When patients who have this mutation are treated with retinoic acid derivatives, the cells are induced to differentiate into mature granulocytes.

One of the limitations of molecular genetic analysis is that the specific genetic aberration must be identified first so that probes can be made to detect the gene abnormality. Currently, this technology is helpful in diagnosis of M3-AML, CML, and T and B ALL. Another limitation of molecular techniques is that only a single gene mutation can be identified, so other chromosome mutations are not detected. Thus, it is important for the clinical laboratory scientist to understand the advantages and limitations of each diagnostic procedure and recommend the appropriate combination of testing as well as testing sequence. Chapter 25 discusses molecular genetic techniques and their application in diagnosis of hematopoietic diseases.

 ## Checkpoint! #8

A patient has 35% blasts in the bone marrow. They do not show any specific characteristics that will allow them to be classified according to cell lineage. What are the next steps that the CLS should take with this specimen?

▶ ## PROGNOSIS AND TREATMENT OF NEOPLASTIC DISORDERS

PROGNOSIS

Before the 1960s, a patient diagnosed with acute leukemia could expect to die within a few months. With new treatment modalities, remission rates for both ALL and AML have improved dramatically. Remission is defined as a period of time in which there are no clinical or hematologic signs of the disease.

Approximately 80% of children treated for ALL can be expected to enter a prolonged remission with an indefinite period of survival. The prognosis of ALL in adults is not as good as in children. Two years is the median survival for adults after remission has been achieved. Only 10–25% have achieved a 5-year survival. Poor prognostic factors are listed in Table 26-14 ✪.

✪ TABLE 26-14

Poor Prognostic Indicators in Acute Lymphocytic Leukemia (ALL)

Clinical findings
  Infants
  Patients past puberty
  CNS or mediastinal involvement
Laboratory findings
  High blast counts
  Presence of Philadelphia chromosome

The remission rate in AML is about 55–65%. Approximately 50% of these patients will remain in remission for 3–10 years. Patients who receive bone marrow or stem cell transplants have a better prognosis, especially younger patients. Patients who had a previous myelodysplastic syndrome or chronic myeloproliferative disorder respond poorly to standard chemotherapy.

Survival in the chronic neoplasms is longer. Overall survival in CML appears to be in the range of 1–3 years. After onset of blast crisis, survival is only 1–2 months.[31] Survival in CLL depends on the severity of the disease at diagnosis and ranges from 30 to more than 120 months. Patients with other MDS and MPD diseases usually survive for a year or more, even without treatment. Prognosis for the lymphomas is dependent upon the accurate classification of the cell type and can range from 6 months to 10 years or longer.

 CASE STUDY *(continued from page 486)*

4. Would you expect Agnes to survive more than 3 years or succumb fairly quickly after treatment?

TREATMENT

Chemotherapeutic drug and radiotherapy protocols are developed by cancer and leukemia groups (CALG) and used by cooperative oncology groups (COG) in order to access statistically valid data in a highly efficient fashion.

For treatment purposes, complete remission is defined as the total absence of disease to the limit of testing. Currently standard testing is sensitive to 10^6 cells, so a complete remission is not the same as a cure. More sensitive testing such as PCR or FISH can detect the presence of less than 10^6 tumor cells (∞ Chapter 25). A combination of negative "traditional" tests (peripheral blood and bone marrow blast count and cytogenetics) and positive molecular tests (PCR/FISH) can be called a state of **minimum residual disease** (∞ Chapter 25). A partial remission occurs when there is significant lessening of signs, symptoms, and laboratory values without achieving a total absence of disease. Therapeutic success rates differ by disease and the condition of the patient at time of diagnosis.

Chemotherapy

Chemotherapy is the treatment of choice for leukemia. The goal of this type of therapy is to eradicate all malignant cells within the bone marrow, allowing repopulation with normal hematopoietic precursors. The problem with this type of therapy is that the drugs used in treatment are not specific for leukemic cells. Thus, during treatment, many normal cells also are killed. Complications of traditional therapy are bleeding due to decreased platelet counts, infections due to suppression of granulocyte counts, and anemia due to erythrocyte suppression in the marrow. Supplemental support with recombinant erythropoietin can be used to mitigate the anemia.

Most drugs used to treat leukemia can be included in three groups: antimetabolites, alkylating agents, and antibiotics. The antimetabolites are purine or pyrimidine antagonists, which inhibit the synthesis of DNA. These drugs kill cells in cycle, affecting any rapidly dividing cell. In addition to leukemic cells, the antimetabolites also kill cells lining the gut, germinal epithelium of the hair follicles, and normal hematopoietic cells. This leads to complications of gastrointestinal disturbances, loss of hair, and life-threatening cytopenias.

The alkylating agents (chemical compounds containing alkyl groups) are not specific for cells in cycle but kill both resting and proliferating cells. The drug attaches to DNA molecules, interfering with DNA synthesis. These drugs, as a class, are mutagenic and carcinogenic; they fragment and clump chromosomes, inactivate DNA viruses, and inhibit mitosis but not protein function. The side effects of these compounds include myelosuppression, stomatitis, nausea, and vomiting.

Antibiotics bind to both DNA and RNA molecules, interfering with cell replication. Toxic effects of this therapy are similar to those of alkylating agents.

Since the 1970s, various drug combinations have been found to be more effective than single drug administration. The drugs commonly used and their modes of action are included in Table 26-15 ✪.

Therapy for ALL is divided into several phases. The **induction therapy** phase is designed to reduce the disease into complete remission (i.e., eradicating the leukemic blast population). This is followed by the CNS prophylactic phase. CNS leukemia is the most common form of relapse in young children who have not undergone specific treatment to the brain and spinal column early in remission. The two modes of treatment in the CNS prophylactic phase are cranium irradiation and intrathecal chemotherapy. The third phase is **maintenance chemotherapy,** also called cytoreductive therapy or remission **consolidation therapy.** The need for this type of therapy is controversial. Some studies have shown a slight increase in survival with its use, whereas

✪ TABLE 26-15

Chemotherapeutic Agents Usually Used in Acute Leukemia (AL) Treatment

Drug	Class	Action
Doxorubicin	Anthracycline antibiotic	Inhibits DNA and RNA synthesis
Daunorubicin	Anthracycline antibiotic	Inhibits DNA and RNA synthesis
Idarubicin	Anthracycline antibiotic	Inhibits DNA and RNA synthesis
5-azacytidine	Pyrimidine antimetabolite	Inhibits DNA and RNA synthesis
6-thioguanine	Purine antimetabolite	Inhibits purine synthesis
Methotrexate	Folic acid antimetabolite	Inhibits pyrimidine synthesis
6-mercaptopurine	Purine antimetabolite	Inhibits pyrimidine synthesis
Cytosine arabinoside	Pyrimidine antimetabolite	Inhibits DNA synthesis
Prednisone	Synthetic glucocorticoid	Lyses lymphoblasts
Vincristine	Plant alkaloid	Inhibits RNA synthesis and assembly of mitotic spindles
Asparaginase	*E. coli* enzyme	Depletes endogenous asparagines
Cyclophosphamide	Synthetic alkylating agent	Cross-links DNA strands

others reveal no improvement. Before the institution of CNS prophylactic treatment, there was a high incidence of relapse. The maintenance therapy was designed to prevent this relapse and prolong remission. The purpose of maintenance therapy is to eradicate any remaining leukemic cells. Drug treatment usually continues for 2–3 years. The relapse rate after cessation of all therapy is about 25%.

The treatment regimen for AML is similar to that of ALL. The combination of antileukemic agents is different, but the purpose of chemotherapy is the same—to eradicate the leukemic blasts. CNS involvement is not a common complication of AML; therefore, CNS prophylactic treatment is not a part of the therapy regimen. The induction phase is followed by consolidation (postremission) using drugs at similar doses to those used for induction. Maintenance therapy is controversial but probably not warranted if prior therapy is intense enough.

Permanent remission in CLL is rare. Treatment is conservative and usually reserved for patients with more aggressive forms of the disease. Alkylating agents, chlorambucil and cyclophosphamide, are used. Radiotherapy, bone marrow transplantation, and immunotherapy are also used to treat CLL.

Treatment for the MPD and the MDS is primarily supportive and designed to improve the quality of the patient's life, as few are cured (Table 26-16 ✪).

Bone Marrow Transplant

Bone marrow transplants have provided new hope as a possible cure for hematopoietic disorders; the highest rate of success in transplant patients has occurred with those younger than 40 years of age in a first remission with a closely matched donor. In this procedure, drugs and irradiation are used to bring about remission and eradicate any evidence of leukemic cells. Bone marrow from a suitable donor is then transplanted into the patient to supply a source of normal stem cells.

Autologous transplants have been used when a compatible donor cannot be found. In this procedure, some of the patient's marrow is removed while the patient is in complete remission. The marrow specimen is then treated in vitro with monoclonal antibodies or 4-hydroperoxycyclophosphamide to remove any residual leukemic cells (purged) and cryopreserved. After all traces of leukemia have been removed from the patient by chemotherapy and radiotherapy, the treated marrow is given back to the patient.

Autologous bone marrow transplantation is applied to patients in remission and to those in early relapse. Overall survival appears to be better in those transplanted during the first complete remission. Bone marrow transplantation appears to be successful in many cases; the number of patients who are undergoing this type of therapy is increasing.

Stem Cell Transplants

Peripheral and bone marrow stem cells are being used to reestablish hematopoiesis in the marrow after intensive chemotherapy or radiotherapy in a process called stem cell transplantation. In this procedure, apheresis is used to collect stem cells from the bone marrow or peripheral circulation. These stem cells can come from either the patient or a suitable donor. People who receive a donor's stem cells are given drugs to prevent rejection. Usually 10–21 days following infusion of the stem cells, they begin producing new blood cells. Stem cell transplantation is still a fairly new and complex treatment for leukemia. A more thorough discussion of hematopoietic stem cell transplantation can be found in ∞ Chapter 32.

℮ CASE STUDY (continued from page 493)

5. Is Agnes a suitable candidate for a bone marrow transplant? Why or why not?

Hematopoietic Growth Factors

Recombinant hematopoietic growth factors have been used in the supportive care of AL patients for over a decade. Erythropoietin was introduced in 1989 and has been used in the treatment of chemotherapy-related anemia.[32] Granulocyte colony-stimulating factor (G-CSF) and granulocyte-macrophage colony-stimulating factor (GM-CSF) have been available since 1991 and aid in decreasing the incidence of infection in patients receiving myelosuppressive chemotherapy.[32] Interleukin-11 promotes the maturation of megakaryocytes by stimulating stem cells and megakaryocyte progenitor cells and was introduced for use in 1997.[33] Research continues to be done in the area of cloning additional hematopoietic growth factors in the hopes of accelerating hematopoietic recovery in chemotherapy patients.

Complications of Treatment

Treatment for leukemia can actually aggravate the clinical situation of the patient. Although uric acid levels are commonly elevated in leukemia from an increase in cell turnover, the concentration of this constituent can increase many fold during effective therapy because of the release of nucleic acids by lysed cells. Uric acid is a normal end product of nucleic acid degradation and is excreted mainly by the kidney. In excessive amounts, the uric acid precipitates in renal tubules, leading to renal failure (uric acid nephropathy). Lysed cells also can release procoagulants into the vascular system, precipitating disseminated intravascular coagulation. In this case, the resulting decrease in platelets and coagulation factors can lead to hemorrhage. This complication is especially prevalent in M3 promyelocytic leukemia. The granules of the promyelocytes are potent activators of the coagulation factors.

The chemotherapeutics destroy normal as well as leukemic cells. The cytopenia that develops during aggressive

---

✪ TABLE 26-16

Treatment and Prognosis of Myeloproliferative Disorders (MPD) and Myelodysplastic Syndromes (MDS)

Neoplasm	Treatment	Prognosis
Myeloproliferative disorders		
CML	Chemotherapy, stem cell transplant	3–6 years
PV	Phlebotomy, chemotherapy, no treatment	8–15 years
ET	Chemotherapy, no treatment	>10 years
MMM	Chemotherapy, bone marrow transplant	2–10 years
Myelodysplastic syndromes	Not curable, except with stem cell transplant, chemotherapy	5–50 months, dependent on classification of MDS

lead to death from infection, bleeding, or
anemia. To prevent these life-threatening
episodes, the patient may need supportive treatment, including transfusions with blood components and antimicrobial therapy.

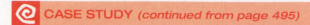

CASE STUDY *(continued from page 495)*

6. What types of treatment are available for our patient Agnes?

SUMMARY

A neoplasm is an unregulated production of cells which can be either malignant or benign. The neoplastic disorders of the bone
marrow hematopoietic cells can be grouped into three main categories:

- Myeloproliferative disorders
- Myelodysplastic syndromes
- Acute leukemias

The myeloproliferative disorders are characterized by an overproduction of erythrocytes, leukocytes, and/or platelets. Myelodysplastic syndromes show peripheral blood cytopenias and dysplasia
of cell maturation. Both MPD and MDS may follow a chronic or
acute course, and both have the potential of evolving into an acute
leukemia. Sometimes, the abnormal proliferation of cells occurs
within the lymphatic tissue or lymph nodes. These solid tumors are
referred to as a lymphoma.

Leukemia is a progressive malignant disease of hematopoietic
stem cells characterized by an inability of these cells to mature into
functional peripheral blood cells. Leukemias may be classified as
acute or chronic based on the aggressiveness of the disease and differentiation of cells. Acute leukemias are characterized by accumulation of immature cells and have a rapid progressive course. Chronic
leukemias are characterized by an accumulation of more differentiated cells and have a slow progressive course. The chronic
leukemias are classified with other chronic neoplastic stem cell disorders—MPD, MDS, and chronic lymphproliferative disorders.

The role of oncogenes in the pathogenesis of hematopoietic
disorders remains under intense investigation. Oncogenes are altered proto-oncogenes that are known to cause tumors. Many
proto-oncogene protein products are involved in cell growth and
include hematopoietic growth factors as well as their cellular receptors, signaling proteins, and transcription factors. Proto-oncogenes

may be mutated to oncogenes by mutagens, viruses, or by chromosome breaks and translocations. Oncogenes may cause production of abnormal growth factors, abnormal amounts of growth
factors, abnormal growth factor receptors, or other abnormalities in
the regulatory mechanisms of cell proliferation and differentiation.

Differentiation and classification of acute leukemias depends on
accurate identification of the blast cell population. Since the lineage of blast cells is difficult to differentiate using only morphologic
characteristics, immunologic phenotyping using monoclonal antibodies and cytochemical analysis are used routinely to help identify
blast phenotypes and stage of cell differentiation. Chromosome
and molecular analyses are helpful since specific mutations are
often associated with specific types of leukemias.

Hematologic findings of hematopoietic neoplasms include anemia, thrombocytopenia (in acute leukemia and MDS), and often
leukocytosis. A shift to the left is consistently found with a combination of blasts and mature cells in acute leukemia. In the chronic
leukemias and other chronic neoplastic stem cell disorders, there is
more of a continuum of cells from immature to mature. Morphologic abnormalities of neoplastic cells is not unusual. Auer rods
may be found in blasts of AML.

Hematopoietic neoplasms are usually treated using a combination of cytotoxic drugs (chemotherapy). The goal is to induce remission by eradicating the leukemic cells. Hematopoietic stem cell
transplants are being used increasingly to restore the marrow after
intense chemotherapy or radiotherapy. Treatment with hematopoietic growth factors is used in some cases to stimulate erythrocyte
production or to stimulate leukemic cells to proliferate, making
these cells more susceptible to cytotoxic drugs. This therapy also
has been used to decrease the neutropenic and thrombocytopenic
period after chemotherapy or radiotherapy.

REVIEW QUESTIONS

LEVEL I

1. A gap in the normal maturation pyramid of cells with many
   blasts and some mature forms is known as: (Checklist #2)
   a. leukemic hiatus
   b. chronic leukemia
   c. mixed cell lineage
   d. lineage restricted

LEVEL II

1. This stain is helpful in distinguishing myeloblasts from lymphoblasts: (Checklist #8)
   a. myeloperoxidase
   b. TRAP
   c. LAP
   d. esterase

REVIEW QUESTIONS (continued)

LEVEL I

2. Auer rods are inclusions found in: (Checklist #5)
   a. myeloblasts
   b. lymphoblasts
   c. erythrocytes
   d. prolymphocytes

3. Chromosome changes in hematologic neoplasms are: (Checklist #8)
   a. present in AL but not MPD or MDS
   b. nonrandom
   c. associated with a poor outcome
   d. not usually present

4. Genes that can cause tumors if activated are: (Checklist #6)
   a. cancer genes
   b. proto-oncogenes
   c. preleukemia genes
   d. tumor-suppressor genes

5. A common characteristic of acute lymphocytic leukemia is: (Checklist #2)
   a. a leukemia of older persons
   b. bone and joint pain
   c. many blast cells with Auer rods
   d. leukocytopenia

6. The FAB classification is used to divide acute leukemias into groups according to: (Checklist #3)
   a. immunology
   b. clinical presentation
   c. cytogenetics
   d. morphology

7. A leukemia that shows a profusion of granulocytes at all stages of development, with the majority of cells being myelocytes and segmented neutrophils, is: (Checklist #2, 5)
   a. AML
   b. CML
   c. ALL
   d. CLL

8. Acute lymphocytic leukemia occurs with greatest frequency in which age group? (Checklist #7)
   a. 1–5 years
   b. 10–15 years
   c. 20–30 years
   d. over 50 years

9. Chronic leukemias primarily affect: (Checklist #2, 7)
   a. all ages, progress rapidly, have immature cells in peripheral circulation
   b. children, progress rapidly, have mature cells in peripheral circulation
   c. young adults, progress slowly, have immature cells in peripheral circulation
   d. adults, progress slowly, have mature cells in circulation

LEVEL II

2. Oncogenes may cause leukemia by: (Checklist #1)
   a. suppressing proliferation of normal cells
   b. activating retroviruses
   c. encoding for an aberrant growth protein
   d. encoding proteins that cause DNA damage

3. The highest levels of serum and urine muramidase are found in this leukemia: (Checklist #3)
   a. M0 AML
   b. M2 AML
   c. CML
   d. M5 AML

4. Which of the following factors has *not* been proposed as playing a role in the causation of leukemia? (Checklist #6)
   a. benzene
   b. therapeutic radiation for Hodgkin's disease
   c. living at high altitudes
   d. chromosome translocations

5. A 3-year-old child with Down syndrome presents with pallor, fatigue, lymphadenopathy, and hepatosplenomegaly. The initial CBC results were: (Checklist #3)

WBC:	18.7×10^9/L	WBC differential:	10 segs
RBC:	2.34×10^{12}/L		27 lymphs
Hb:	5.8 g/dL		63 blasts
Hct:	0.174 L/L		
PLT:	130×10^9/L		

   These findings are suggestive of:
   a. acute lymphocytic leukemia
   b. chronic lymphocytic leukemia
   c. acute myelocytic leukemia
   d. chronic myelocytic leukemia

6. A patient with a hypocellular, dysplastic bone marrow, and anemia and neutropenia in peripheral blood most likely has which of the following neoplasms? (Checklist #7)
   a. MPD
   b. MDS
   c. AML
   d. ALL

7. A 52-year-old female was admitted to the hospital for minor elective surgery. Her pre-op CBC was:

WBC:	49.4×10^9/L
RBC:	4.50×10^{12}/L
Hb:	12.7 g/dL
Hct:	0.38 L/L
PLT:	213×10^9/L
WBC differential:	3% segs
	97% lymphs

LEVEL I

10. A 19-year-old patient's bone marrow is classified by the FAB system as an L3 leukemia. Which of the following best describes this leukemia? (Checklist #2, 3, 5)
    a. CLL
    b. ALL
    c. AML
    d. CML

11. Immunologic phenotyping of the blast cells is important to: (Checklist #8)
    a. help determine cell lineage
    b. identify the etiology of the leukemia
    c. determine if cytogenetic analysis is necessary
    d. replace the need to do multiple cytochemical stains

LEVEL II

What is the best explanation for this patient's leukocytosis and lymphocytosis? (Checklist #3, 7)
    a. ALL
    b. AML
    c. CLL
    d. CML

Case study for questions 8–10:

A 43-year-old male had been working with the Peace Corps in Mexico for the past 10 years. His primary responsibilities were taking x-rays and doing laboratory work at the various clinics. He had been complaining of weakness and fatigue for about a month and had several severe nosebleeds. His CBC upon admission to the hospital was:

WBC: 25.6×10^9/L   WBC differential: 75% blasts with Auer rods

RBC: 3.11×10^{12}/L	20% lymphs
Hb: 8.9 g/dL	3% monos
Hct: 0.267 L/L	2% segs
PLT: 13×10^9/L	

8. Which leukemia is this patient most likely to have acquired? (Checklist #3)
    a. ALL
    b. AML
    c. CLL
    d. CML

9. What would be the most likely causative agent of the leukemia? (Checklist #2)
    a. virus
    b. age
    c. hepatitis
    d. ionizing radiation

10. What treatment would result in the *best* prognosis for this patient if there were no complicating factors? (Checklist #5)
    a. hematopoietic growth factors
    b. stem cell transplantation
    c. radiation therapy
    d. chemotherapy

11. You are doing several cytochemical stains on a bone marrow from a patient who is recently diagnosed with acute leukemia. You are looking at the MPO, and the blasts are negative. However, the reagent is getting close to the expiration date and you are not sure if the stain worked properly. What cells found in the bone marrow normally express myeloperoxidase and could be used to assess the stain's integrity? (Checklist #8, 9)
    a. neutrophils
    b. red cell precursors
    c. megakaryocytes
    d. lymphocytes

REVIEW QUESTIONS (continued)

LEVEL I

LEVEL II

12. A pathologist is looking at the bone marrow aspirate of a 26-year-old male. The marrow is packed with undifferentiated blasts. After careful search, the pathologist could not find any Auer rods. He thinks that the patient most probably has acute lymphoblastic leukemia but by morphology cannot rule out AML. He is thinking of ordering a TdT stain on the slides. Is that going to be useful? (Checklist #8, 9)

a. Yes, TdT is always positive in acute lymphoid leukemia and never in myeloid leukemia.

b. Yes, TdT is always positive in acute myeloid leukemia and never in lymphoid leukemia.

c. No, TdT is positive in the majority of acute lymphoid leukemias and approximately 20% of acute myeloid leukemias can be positive.

d. No, Tdt is positive in the majority of acute myeloid leukemias but approximately 20% of acute lymphoid leukemias can be positive.

www.prenhall.com/mckenzie

Use the above address to access the free, interactive Companion Web site created for this textbook. Get hints, instant feedback, and textbook references to chapter-related multiple choice questions.

REFERENCES

1. Chessells JM, Bailey C, Richards SM. Intensification of treatment and survival in children with lymphoblastic leukaemia: Results of UK Medical Research Council trial UKALL X. Medical Research Council Working Party on Childhood Leukaemia. *Lancet.* 1995; 345(8943):143–48.

2. Bennet JH. Two cases of disease and enlargement of the spleen in which death took place from the presence of purulent matter in the blood. *Edinburgh Med Surg J.* 1845; 64:413.

3. Toll T, Estella J, Illa J, Alcorta I, Mateo M. Acute leukemia in Down syndrome children. *Cytogenet Cell Genet.* 1997; 77(Suppl 1):25–26.

4. Gao Q, et al. Susceptibility gene for familial acute myeloid leukemia associated with loss of 5q and/or 7q is not localized on the commonly deleted portion of 5q. *Genes Chromosomes Cancer.* 2000; 28:164–72.

5. Wyke J. Principles of viral leukemogenesis. *Semin Hematol.* 1986; 23:189–200.

6. Manzari V, et al. HTLV-V: A new human retrovirus in a Tac-negative T cell lymphoma/leukemia. *Science.* 1987; 238(4838):1581–83.

7. Kumar T, Mandla SG, Greer WL. Familial myelodysplastic syndrome with early age of onset. *Am J Hematol.* 2000; 64:53–58.

8. Bennet JM, et al. Proposals for the classification of the acute leukaemias. French-American-British (FAB) Co-operative Group. *Br J Haematol.* 1976; 33:451–58.

9. Harris NL, et al. World Health Organization classification of neoplastic diseases of the hematopoietic and lymphoid tissues: Report of the Clinical Advisory Committee meeting, Airlie House, Virginia, November 1997. *J Clin Oncol.* 1999; 17:3835–49.

10. American Cancer Society. Cancer Facts and Figures 2002. Atlanta: American Cancer Society; 2002.

11. Gabbas AG, Li CY. Acute non-lymphocytic leukemia with eosinophilic differentiation. *Am J Hematol.* 1986; 21:29–38.

12. Stass SA, Pui CH, Melvin S, Rovigatti U, Williams D, Motroni T, et al. Sudan black B positive acute lymphoblastic leukaemia. *Br J Haematol.* 1984; 57:413–21.

13. Sigma Diagnostics. Naphthol AS-D Choloroacetate Esterase and Alpha-Naphthyl Acetate Esterase. St. Louis: Sigma Diagnostics; 1990.

14. Li CY. Leukemia cytochemistry. *Mayo Clin Proc.* 1981; 56:712–13.

15. Shibata A, Bennett JM, Castoldi GL. Recommended methods for cytological procedures in hematology. *Clin Lab Haematol.* 1985; 7:55–74.

16. Yam LT, Li CY, Crosby WH. Cytochemical identification of monocytes and granulocytes. *Am J Clin Pathol.* 1971; 55:283–90.

17. Sigma Diagnostics. *Periodic acid-Schiff staining system: Histochemical demonstration of glycol-containing cellular components in blood or bone marrow films.* St. Louis: Sigma Diagnostics; 1986.

18. National Committee for Clinical Laboratory Standards. Proposed standard: Histochemical method for leukocyte alkaline phosphatase. Villanova, PA: *NCCLS,* 1984; vol.4, no. 14.

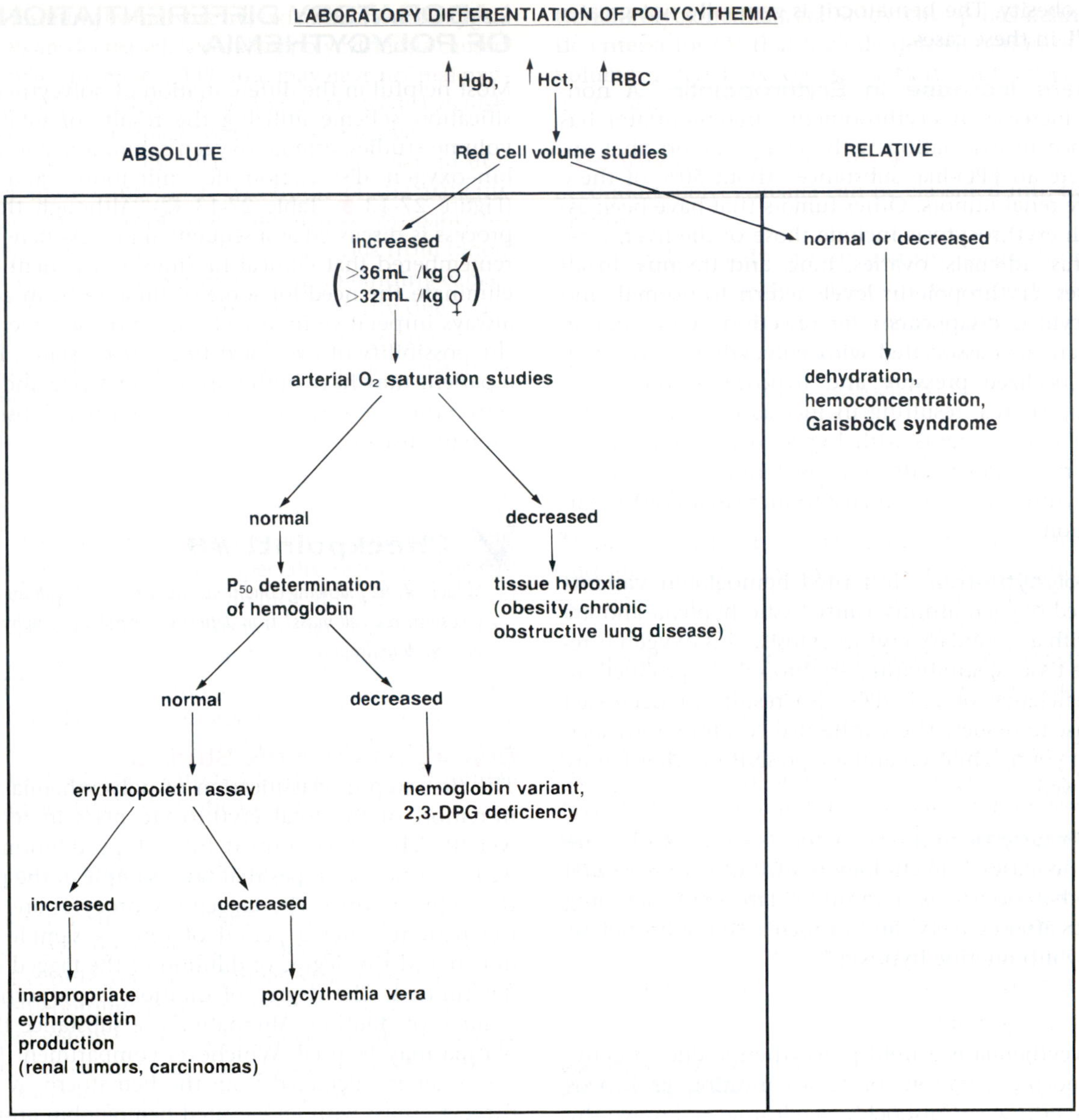

LABORATORY DIFFERENTIATION OF POLYCYTHEMIA

■ FIGURE 27-13 Laboratory differentiation of polycythemia.

smoking. A history and physical exam are essential to establishing an accurate diagnosis.

A normal arterial oxygen saturation demands further investigation. Arterial blood oxygen saturation is a measure of the amount of oxygen brought to the tissues by blood but is no indication of the amount of oxygen actually released. Arterial blood oxygen saturation is normal in the familial high oxygen affinity hemoglobinopathies and in the rare inherited deficiencies of erythrocyte 2,3-DPG, but the hemoglobin releases less than normal amounts of this oxygen to the tissues. The best screening test for a high oxygen affinity hemoglobin variant is a determination of the p50 of blood. p50 is defined as the partial pressure of oxygen at which the

hemoglobin is one-half saturated (∞ Chapter 5). Normal hemoglobin is 50% saturated with oxygen at 26 mm Hg under standard conditions of temperature (37°C) and pH (7.4). Abnormal hemoglobins, with an increased affinity for oxygen, will have a lower p50, meaning that less oxygen is released at an equivalent partial pressure of oxygen. This shifts the oxygen dissociation curve left, resulting in a decrease of oxygen released to tissues, an increase in erythropoietin production, and a concomitant increase in erythrocyte production (∞ Chapters 5, 10). Although hemoglobin electrophoresis should always be performed when an abnormal hemoglobin is suspected, in some cases the hemoglobin variant cannot be diagnosed by electrophoretic patterns as the amino acid

TABLE 27-13

Differential Features of Polycythemia

Feature	PV	Secondary	Relative
Spleen size	↑	N	N
Red cell mass	♂ ≥36 mL/Kg	↑	N
	♀ ≥32 mL/Kg		
Leukocyte count	↑	N	N
Platelet count	↑	N	N
Serum cobalamin	↑	N	N
Arterial O₂ saturation	N	↓	N
Bone marrow	Panhyperplasia	Erythroid hyperplasia	N
Iron stores	↓	N	N
Erythropoietin	↓	N, ↑	N
Chromosome studies	Abnormal (50%)	N	N

N = normal; ↑ = increased; ↓ = decreased

substitutions in globin chains may not change the charge of the molecule.

Erythropoietin Measurement

A normal arterial blood oxygen saturation and normal oxygen dissociation should be followed by urinary erythropoietin assays to distinguish PV from those polycythemias due to an inappropriate increase in EPO. Urinary erythropoietin is low or absent in PV but normal or increased in secondary polycythemias that are associated with tumors and renal carcinomas. In these cases, the increased EPO production is considered inappropriate because tissue hypoxia is not responsible for its synthesis.

✓ Checkpoint! #9

Renal tumors may produce an inappropriate amount of EPO, resulting in what type of polycythemia?

► ESSENTIAL THROMBOCYTHEMIA

Essential thrombocythemia (ET) is a myeloproliferative syndrome affecting primarily the megakaryocytic lineage. There is an extreme thrombocytosis in the peripheral blood together with thrombocytopathy (a qualitative disorder in platelets). There has been considerable controversy over the inclusion of ET as a specific entity in the myeloproliferative disorders since thrombocytosis is often a part of CML, MMM, and PV. In these myeloproliferative disorders, however, the platelet count is usually less than $1,000 \times 10^9$/L,

while in ET the count is almost always greater than $1,000 \times 10^9$/L. In addition, there is a predominant occurrence of hemorrhage and thrombosis, which are a common cause of death in patients with ET. These findings are considered justification to treat ET as a distinct entity of the myeloproliferative disorders.

Synonyms for ET include *primary thrombocythemia, hemorrhagic thrombocythemia,* and *megakaryocytic leukemia.*

PATHOPHYSIOLOGY

Essential thrombocythemia is a clonal disorder of the pluripotential stem cell that affects all three cell lines but chiefly the megakaryocytes. In-vitro culture assay systems have shown that normal megakaryocyte colony formation from CFU-Meg is dependent upon the addition of cytokines. In ET, the normal cell surface receptor for thrombopoietin, c-mpl, is decreased, yet proliferation of progenitor cells ensues autonomously.[42] Serum levels of thrombopoietin are increased.[42] The clonal population of cells appears hypersensitive to cytokines, IL-3 and IL-6, but not to GM-CSF. In addition, TGF-β is decreased, thus minimizing platelet inhibition. These pathologic findings are similar to those found in CML, MMM, and PV making it difficult to diagnose ET. Complicating this distinction is the fact that ET has been found to evolve into PV, MMM, and leukemia.

CLINICAL FINDINGS

Essential thrombocythemia is a rare disorder with peak incidence from 50 to 60 years of age and from 20 to 30 years of age. The younger age of incidence occurs predominantly in women. Bleeding or thrombosis occurs as the most common presenting feature. These problems appear to be more frequent in patients over 59 years of age, with thrombosis occurring more frequently than bleeding at the lower values of thrombocytosis.[43,44]

About half the patients have a palpable spleen but splenomegaly is usually slight. Occasionally, absence of splenomegaly is due to splenic atrophy, resulting from repeated splenic thrombosis and silent infarctions. About 20% of the patients are initially asymptomatic. In these cases the disease is discovered incidentally upon the finding of thrombocytosis and, occasionally, splenomegaly.

LABORATORY FINDINGS

Peripheral Blood

The most striking finding in the peripheral blood is extreme and consistent thrombocytosis (Figure 27-14 ■). Platelet counts are greater than 600×10^9/L and usually range from 1,000 to $5,000 \times 10^9$/L. The peripheral blood smear may show giant bizarre platelets. Platelets may appear in aggregates. Megakaryocytes and megakaryocyte fragments also may be found. However, in many cases, platelet morphology appears normal. Abnormalities in platelet aggregation and adhesiveness suggest defects in platelet function.

Anemia, if present, is proportional to the severity of bleeding and is usually normocytic; however, long standing hemorrhagic episodes may lead to iron deficiency and a microcytic, hypochromic anemia. In about one-third of the patients slight erythrocytosis is present, which may cause confusion with polycythemia vera. Aggregated platelets may lead to an erroneous increase in the erythrocyte count on automated cell counters. Therefore, hemoglobin determinations are a better measurement to assess the anemic status of the patient. Histograms may reveal a high tail on the leukocyte histogram because of platelet clumps. The reticulocyte count may be increased if bleeding is present, and mild polychromatophilia is noted. Peripheral blood abnormalities, secondary to autosplenectomy may occur if the spleen has been infarcted. These abnormalities include Howell-Jolly bodies, nucleated erythrocytes, and poikilocytosis.

A leukocytosis from 27 to 40×10^9/L is almost always present. Occasional metamyelocytes and myelocytes can be found with ET. Mild eosinophilia and basophilia also are observed. The LAP score is normal or increased. Rarely, it may be low. Nucleated erythrocytes are found in 25% of patients.

Bone Marrow

The bone marrow exhibits marked hyperplasia with a striking increase in megakaryocytes, often present in clusters. The background of stained slides shows many platelets. Megakaryocytes are large, with abundant cytoplasm and frequently increased nuclear lobulation. Mitotic forms are increased. Erythroid and myeloid hyperplasia also are evident. Stains for iron reveal normal or increased stores unless chronic hemorrhage has occurred. In some cases reticulin is increased.

Tests of Hemostasis

Laboratory tests alone are unreliable in predicting bleeding or thrombotic complications in ET. The prothrombin time and activated partial thromboplastin time are usually normal, but evidence of low-grade DIC may be present. Although platelet aggregation abnormalities are variable in ET, defective platelet aggregation with epinephrine caused by a loss of platelet α-adrenergic receptors is diagnostic of an MPD and is useful in differentiating ET from secondary thrombocytosis. Spontaneous in vitro platelet aggregation or hyperaggregability is a common finding, and in vivo platelet aggregation is suggested by finding increased levels of β-thromboglobulin (released from platelets). Other platelet abnormalities that have been described in association with ET are included in Table 27-14 ✪.[46] A form of acquired von Willebrand's disease has been described in association with ET. There is a reduction of large multimer forms and reduced levels of ristocetin cofactor activity.

Cytogenetics

The low incidence of clonal abnormalities (about 5%) in ET renders cytogenetic studies less useful than in other MPD.[47] Acquired clonal chromosome aberrations may be identified in the hematopoietic precursors of the bone marrow. There is no diagnostic abnormality reported, but trisomies of Group C chromosomes are commonly seen.

Other Laboratory Findings

Other laboratory tests may be abnormal. Serum cobalamin and the unsaturated cobalamin binding capacity are increased. An increase in cell turnover may cause serum uric acid, LDH, and acid phosphatase to be elevated. Serum potassium may be elevated as a result of in vitro release of potassium from platelets (pseudohyperkalemia). The spurious nature of this hyperkalemia can be verified by performing a simultaneous potassium assay on plasma, which should be normal. Arterial blood gases may reveal a pseudo-

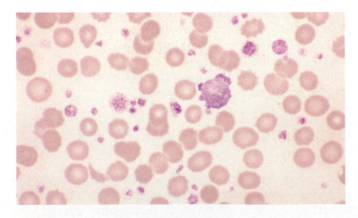

■ FIGURE 27-14 Essential thrombocythemia. Platelets are markedly increased and a giant form is present. (Peripheral blood; 1000× magnification; Wright-Giemsa stain)

✪ TABLE 27-14
Additional Platelet Abnormalities Found in Essential Thrombocytosis
Decreased c-Mpl receptors for thrombopoietin (TPO)
Decreased number of receptors for platelet inhibitor proteins; transforming growth factor-beta (TBF-β), prostaglandin D_2 (PGD^2)
Increased expression of Fc receptors
Reduction of membrane glycoprotein GpIb associated with an increase in GpIIIb and decreased GpIIb
Defective coagulant activity
Impaired serotonin binding and uptake
Changes in the platelet membrane fatty acid composition
Abnormal arachidonic acid metabolism
Increased glyoxalase I activity
Increased lactate production

hypoxia if the sample is not tested promptly. This is due to the in vitro consumption of oxygen by increased numbers of platelets.

PROGNOSIS AND THERAPY

About 50% of the patients with ET survive five years. The prognosis appears to be better in the younger patients. The most common causes of death are thrombosis and bleeding. In some cases, the disease transforms to AML, PV, or MMM.

There is controversy as to which patients with ET require therapy. It is generally agreed that patients with a history of thrombosis or cardiovascular risk factors require therapy to reduce the platelet count. Plateletpheresis is utilized to quickly reduce the platelet count below 1000×10^9/L for control of vascular accidents. Anticoagulants and drugs to inhibit platelet function are sometimes necessary to control thrombosis.

The benefit of specific therapy in asymptomatic patients has not been established. Therapeutic trials with β-interferon show improvement of both hematologic parameters and clinical symptoms on nearly all patients.[48] Withdrawal of interferon, however, leads to recurrence of thrombocytosis. Chronic megakaryocyte suppression is achieved by radiation or chemotherapy. There is concern, however, about the leukemogenic potential of these therapeutic agents.

DIFFERENTIAL DIAGNOSIS

Although the other MPDs have certain diagnostic markers, ET is largely a diagnosis of exclusion. Essential thrombocytosis must be differentiated from a secondary, reactive thrombocytosis (Table 27-15 ✪). Secondary thrombocytosis is associated with many acute and chronic infections, inflammatory diseases, carcinomas, and Hodgkin's disease. The platelet count in ET exceeds $1,000 \times 10^9$/L and is persistent over a period of months or years. Secondary or reactive thrombocytosis rarely reaches $1,000 \times 10^9$/L and is transitory. In addition, in secondary thrombocytosis platelet function is normal, leukocytes and erythrocytes are normal, and splenomegaly is absent.

Differentiation of ET from PV may be difficult. However, marked erythrocytosis together with clinical findings suggestive of hypervolemia is more typical of PV.

The Polycythemia Vera Study Group (PVSG) has proposed a set of diagnostic criteria for ET (Table 27-16 ✪). The first criterion, a platelet count over 600×10^9/L, excludes many cases of secondary thrombocytosis. The second criterion, a hemoglobin less than 13 g/dL, and the third criterion, presence of iron in the bone marrow or failure of response to iron therapy, exclude cases of PV. The fourth criterion, absence of the Ph chromosome, was designed to rule out CML, and the fifth, absence of collagen fibrosis, rules out MMM. The sixth criterion excludes conditions associated with reactive thrombocytosis.

✓ Checkpoint! #10

Is a patient who has a platelet count of 846×10^9/L, splenomegaly, and abnormal platelet function tests of hyperaggregation likely to have reactive or essential thrombocytosis?

✪ TABLE 27-15

Conditions Associated with Thrombocytosis

Essential thrombocythemia (ET)
Polycythemia vera (PV)
Chronic myelocytic leukemia (CML)
Myelofibrosis with myeloid metaplasia (MMM)
Chronic inflammatory disorders
Acute hemorrhage
Hemolytic anemia
Hodgkin's disease
Metastatic carcinoma
Lymphoma
Postsplenectomy
Postoperative
Iron deficiency

✪ TABLE 27-16

Diagnostic Criteria for Essential Thrombocythemia (ET) as Defined by the Polycythemia Vera Study Group

Diagnostic Criteria for ET	Helps Differentiate ET From:
Platelet count >600 × 10⁹/L	Secondary thrombocytosis
Hemoglobin ≤13 g/dL or normal erythrocyte mass	Polycythemia vera
Stainable iron in the marrow or failure of iron therapy to raise the hemoglobin by at least 1 g/dL after one month of iron therapy	Polycythemia vera
Absence of the Philadelphia chromosome	Chronic myelocytic leukemia
Absent collagen fibrosis of marrow or collagen fibrosis in >1/3 biopsied area but no splenomegaly or leukoerythroblastic reaction	Myelofibrosis with myeloid metaplasia
No known cause for reactive thrombocytosis	Reactive thrombocytosis

(Adapted from: Murphy S, Peterson P, Iland H, Lazlo J. Experience of the Polycythemia Vera Study Group with essential thrombocythemia: A final report on diagnostic criteria, survival, and leukemic transition by treatment. *Semin Hematol*, 34: 29-39, 1997)

SUMMARY

The myeloproliferative disorders (MPD) are a group of clonal stem cell disorders characterized by neoplastic production of one or more of the hematopoietic lineages in bone marrow and peripheral blood. There are four MPD subgroups including chronic myeloid leukemia (CML), myelofibrosis with myeloid metaplasia (MMM), polycythemia vera (PV), and essential thrombocythemia (ET).

Although all hematopoietic cell lineages may be involved in the unregulated proliferation in MPD, one cell line is usually involved more than the others. In CML the myeloid cells are primarily affected, in PV the erythrocytes are affected, and in ET the platelets/megakaryocytes are affected. In MMM, the most characteristic finding is a benign proliferation of fibroblasts in the bone marrow. Splenomegaly, bone marrow fibrosis, and megakaryocytic hyperplasia are findings common to all subgroups. The underlying pathophysiology appears to be chromosomal rearrangements that occur in the regions of proto-oncogenes leading to qualitative or quantitative alterations in gene expression and abnormal control of cell growth. Changes in expression of specific hormonal receptors, transcription of DNA, or apoptosis are found.

Abnormal karyotypes in hematopoietic cells may be found in any of the subgroups. The most well-characterized abnormality is the Philadelphia (Ph) chromosome found in up to 95% of individuals with CML. The Ph chromosome is the result of a translocation of genetic material between chromosomes 9 and 22 (9;22) (q34;q11). In CML patients who are Ph chromosome negative, molecular testing reveals a BCR/ABL gene fusion encoding for an abnormal protein, p210. This protein plays a role in the pathogenesis of CML. Trisomies within the Group C chromosomes, trisomy 8 or trisomy 9, are common findings in progressive MPD.

The survival of MPD patients varies with the subgroup. Patients with PV appear to survive longer than patients with CML, MMM, or ET. Any of the subgroups may evolve into acute leukemia, with or without specific therapy. There is currently no cure for any of the MPDs, although bone marrow transplant has a favorable outlook for improving prognosis.

REVIEW QUESTIONS

LEVEL I

1. The most prominent cell line in CML is the: (Checklist #2)
   a. erythroid
   b. myeloid
   c. megakaryocyte
   d. fibroblast

2. The most prominent cell line found in polycythemia vera (PV) is the: (Checklist #2)
   a. erythroid
   b. myeloid
   c. megakaryocyte
   d. fibroblast

3. The Philadelphia chromosome is a gene fusion from a translocation of: (Checklist #4)
   a. chomosomes 8 and 14
   b. chomosomes 9 and 22
   c. chomosomes 12 and 17
   d. chomosomes 15 and 17

4. The peak age for CML is: (Checklist #5)
   a. less than 5 years
   b. 15–30 years
   c. 40–59 years
   d. over 60 years

5. Philadelphia chromosome can be found in patients with: (Checklist #4)
   a. CMML
   b. ALL
   c. ET
   d. polycythemia vera

LEVEL II

Use this case study to answer questions 1–5.

A 45-year-old caucasian woman was admitted to the hospital from the emergency room. She experienced pain in the upper quadrant and bloating for the last several weeks. She had multiple bruises on her legs and arms. She also stated that her gums bled easily when she brushed her teeth. She had been unusually tired and lost about 10 pounds in the last 2 months. Results of physical examination showed a massive spleen. The following laboratory results were noted on blood count admission.

Hb:	7.4 g/dL
Erythrocyte count:	2.9×10^{12}/L
Hct:	.22 L/L
RDW:	18.0
Leukocyte count:	520×10^9/L
Platelet count:	960×10^9/L
Differential:	31% segmented neutrophils
	26% bands
	8% metamyelocytes
	11% myelocytes
	4% promyelocytes
	2% blasts
	4% lymphocytes
	3% monocytes
	5% eosinophils
	6% basophils
	4 nucleated erythrocytes/100 leukocytes
	Occasional micromegakaryocytes

LEVEL I

6. A characteristic peripheral blood finding in patients with myeloid metaplasia is: (Checklist #7)
   a. elliptocytes
   b. dacryocytes
   c. target cells
   d. schistocytes

7. Polycythemia vera (PV) can be distinguished from secondary polycythemia by measuring: (Checklist #9)
   a. hematocrit
   b. plasma volume
   c. hemoglobin concentration
   d. oxygen saturation

8. A 50-year-old man was admitted to the emergency room for chest pain, and a blood count was ordered. The results showed: erythrocyte count 6.5×10^{12}/L; hematocrit 0.60 L/L; leukocyte count 15×10^9/L; platelet count 500×10^9/L. These results indicate: (Checklist #3)
   a. the need for further investigation of a possible diagnosis of MPD
   b. normal findings for an adult male
   c. the patient has experienced a thrombotic episode
   d. a malfunction of the cell counting instrument

9. A patient previously diagnosed with CML now has a platelet count of 540×10^9/L and a leukocyte count of 350×10^9/L with a peripheral blood differential showing: 15% segmented neutrophils, 23% bands, 2% metamyelocytes, 35% blasts, 6% lymphocytes, 4% monocytes, 6% eosinophils, 8% basophils. These results are most consistent with: (Checklist #6)
   a. chronic CML
   b. ET
   c. CML in blast crisis
   d. CMML

10. A patient presenting in ER with a platelet count of over 1000×10^9/L, a leukocyte count of 25×10^9/L, with a normochromic, normocytic anemia should be evaluated for: (Checklist #10)
    a. Philadelphia chromosome
    b. essential thrombocythemia
    c. CMML
    d. primary polycythemia

LEVEL II

There was moderate anisocytosis and poikilocytosis.

A bone marrow aspiration was performed. The marrow was 90% cellular with a myeloid to erythroid ratio of 10:1. The majority of the cells were neutrophilic precursors. There was an increase in eosinophils and basophils. Myeloblasts accounted for 10% of the nucleated cells. Megakaryocytes were increased.

1. What findings suggest that this patient has a defect in the pluripotential stem cell rather than a benign proliferation of hematopoietic cells? (Checklist #4)
   a. the presence of a leukoerythroblastic blood picture
   b. the involvement of several cell lineages in the proliferative process, including neutrophilic cells and platelets
   c. the shift to the left in the neutrophilic cell line
   d. an increase in the RDW

2. Molecular analysis by RT-PCR revealed the presence of a BCR/ABL fusion product. Based on this information, what myeloproliferative disorder is present? (Checklist #1, 3)
   a. CML
   b. PV
   c. ET
   d. MMM

3. What cytochemical stain is used to help differentiate a leukemoid reaction from CML? (Checklist #1, 4)
   a. myeloperoxidase
   b. new methylene blue
   c. leukocyte alkaline phosphatase
   d. Perl's Prussian blue

4. Which of the following terms most accurately describes the peripheral blood picture of this patient? (Checklist #10, 11)
   a. leukemoid reaction
   b. leukoerythroblastic
   c. leukopenia
   d. myelodysplastic

5. What is the best description of the bone marrow? (Checklist #1)
   a. decreased M:E ratio and increased cellularity
   b. increased M:E ratio and decreased cellularity
   c. increased M:E ratio and increased cellularity
   d. decreased M:E ratio and decreased cellularity

6. Extensive bone marrow fibrosis, leukoerythroblastic peripheral blood, and the presence of anisocytosis with dacryocytes are most characteristic of which MPD? (Checklist #6)
   a. CML
   b. PV
   c. ET
   d. MMM

REVIEW QUESTIONS *(continued)*

LEVEL I

LEVEL II

7. A 68-year-old man was seen in the clinic for lethargy, dyspnea, and light-headedness. Results of his blood counts were: erythrocyte count 5.0×10^{12}/L; hematocrit 0.55 L/L; leukocyte count 60×10^9/L; platelet count 70×10^9/L. His differential showed a shift to the left in myeloid elements with 40% eosinophils. The bone marrow revealed 10% blasts. Philadelphia chromosome was negative. He most likely has: (Checklist #10)
   a. polycythemia vera
   b. CML in blast crisis
   c. essential thrombocytosis
   d. chronic eosinophilic leukemia

8. Which of the following is *not* typical of an MPD at the time of diagnosis? (Checklist #1, 2)
   a. hypercellular bone marrow
   b. anemia
   c. leukoerythroblastosis
   d. predominance of blasts in peripheral blood

9. Which of the following does *not* cause secondary polycythemia? (Checklist #7)
   a. chronic obstructive pulmonary disease
   b. smoking
   c. emphysema
   d. dehydration

10. Evidence of clonal proliferation in myeloproliferative disorders can be identified by: (Checklist #8)
   a. G6PD isomers
   b. myeloperoxidase stain
   c. Perl's Prussian blue
   d. trisomy 8

www.prenhall.com/mckenzie
Use the above address to access the free, interactive Companion Web site created for this textbook. Get hints, instant feedback, and textbook references to chapter-related multiple choice questions.

REFERENCES

1. Dameshek W. Some speculations on the myeloproliferative syndromes. *Blood.* 1951; 6:372–75.

2. Douer D, Fabian I, Cline MJ. Circulating pleuripotent haemopoietic cells in patients with myeloproliferative disorders. *Br J Haematol.* 1983; 54:373–81.

3. Gilbert HS, Praloran V, Stanley ER. Increased circulating CSF-1 (M-CSF) in myeloproliferative disease: Association with myeloid metaplasia and peripheral bone marrow extension. *Blood.* 1989; 74:1231–34.

4. Gersuk GM, Carmel R, Pattengale PK. Platelet derived growth factor concentrations in platelet poor plasma and urine from patients with myeloproliferative disorders. *Blood.* 1989; 74:2330–34.

5. Cervantes F, Salgado C, Rozman C. Assessment of iron stores in hospitalized patients. *Am J Clin Pathol.* 1991; 1:105–6.

6. Tefferi A, Ho TC, Ahmann GJ, Katzmann JA, Greipp PR. Plasma interleukin-6 and C-reactive protein levels in reactive versus clonal thrombocytosis. *Am J Med.* 1998; 97:374–78.

7. Landolfi R, De Cristofaro R, Castagnola M, De Candia E, D'Onofrio G, Leone G. Increased platelet-fibrinogen affinity in patients with myeloproliferative disorders. *Blood*. 1988; 71:978–82.

8. Mazzucato M, De Marco L, De Angelis V, De Roia D, Bizzaro N, Casonato A. Platelet membrane abnormalities in myeloproliferative disorders: Decrease in glycoproteins Ib and IIb/IIIa complex is associated with deficient receptor function. *Br J Haematol*. 1989; 73:369–74.

9. Wehmeier A, Tschope D, Esser J, Menzel C, Nieuwenhuis HK, Schneider W. Circulating activated platelets in myeloproliferative disorders. *Thromb Res*. 1991; 61:271–78.

10. Dickstein JI, Vardiman JW. Issues in the pathology and diagnosis of the chronic myeloproliferative disorders and the myelodysplastic syndromes. *Am J Clin Pathol*. 1993; 99:513–25.

11. Epner DE, Roeffler HP. Molecular genetic advances in chronic myelogenous leukemia. *Ann Intern Med*. 1990; 113:3–6.

12. Guo JQ, Wang JY, and Arlinghaus RB. Detection of BCR-ABL proteins in blood cells of benign phase chronic myelogenous leukemia patients. *Cancer Res*. 1991; 51:3048–51.

13. Cortes JE, Talpaz M, Kantarjian H. Chronic myelogenous leukemia: A review. *Am J Med*. 1996; 100:555–70.

14. Rector JT, Veillon DM, Schumacher HR, Cotelingam JD. Chronic leukemias of myeloid origin. *Med Lab Observ*. 1998; 12:28–37,54.

15. Mattson JC, Crisan D, Wilner F, Decker D, Burdakin J. Clinical problem solving using BCL-2 and BCR gene rearrangement analysis. *Lab Med*. 1994; 25:648–53.

16. Hild F, Fonatsch C. Cytogenetic peculiarities in chronic myelogenous leukemia. *Cancer Genet Cytogenet*. 1990; 47:197–217.

17. Tefferi A. The Philadelphia chromosome negative chronic myeloproliferative disorders: A practical overview. *Mayo Cl Proc*. 1998; 73:1177–84.

18. Sawyers C. Chronic myeloid leukemia, *N Engl J Med*. 1999; 340:1330–40.

19. Tien HF, Wang CH, Chen YC, Shen MC, Wu HS, Lee FY, et al. Chromosome and BCR rearrangement in chronic myelogenous leukaemia and their correlation with clinical states and prognosis of the disease. *Br J Haematol*. 1990; 75:469–75.

20. Ahuja H, Bar-Eli M, Arlin Z, Advani S, Allen SL, Goldman J, et al. The spectrum of molecular alterations in the evaluation of chronic myelocytic leukemia. *J Clin Invest*. 1991; 87:2042–47.

21. Imamura J, Miyoshi I, Koeffler HP. p53 in hematologic malignancies. *Blood*. 1994; 84:2412–21.

22. Ponzetto C, Guerrasio A, Rosso C, Avanzi G, Tassinari A, Zaccaria A, et al. ABL proteins in Philadelphia-positive acute leukaemias and chronic myelogenous leukaemia blast crisis. *Br J Haematol*. 1990; 76:39–44.

23. Harris NL, Jaffe ES, Diebold J, Flandrin G, Muller-Hermelink HK, Vardiman J, et al. World Health Organization classification of neoplastic diseases of the hematopoietic and lymphoid tissues: Report of the Clinical Advisory Committee meeting, Airlie House, Virginia, November 1997. *J Clin Oncol*. 1999; 17:3835–49.

24. Galvani DW, Cawley JC. Mechanism of action of alpha interferon in chronic granulocytic leukaemia: Evidence for preferential inhibition of late progenitors. *Br J Haematol*. 1989; 73:475–79.

25. Cornelissen JJ, Ploemacher RE, Wognum BW, Borsboom A, Kluin-Nelemans HC, Hagemeijer A, Lowenberg B. An in vitro model for cytogenetic conversion in CML: Interferon-alpha preferentially inhibits the outgrowth of malignant stem cells preserved in long-term culture. *J Clin Invest*. 1998; 102:976–83.

26. Druker BJ, Sawyers CL, Kantarjian H, et al. Activity of a specific inhibitor of the BCR-ABL tyrosine kinase in the blast crisis of chronic myeloid leukemia and acute lymphoblastic leukemia with the Philadelphia chromosome. *J. Intern Med*. 2001; 250:3–9.

27. Freeburn RW, Gale RE, Watner HM, Linch DC. Analysis of the coding sequence for the GM-CSF receptor alpha and beta chains in patients with juvenile chronic myeloid leukemia. *Exper Hematol*. 1997; 25:306–11.

28. Larson RS, Wolff SN. Chronic myeloid leukemia. Lee GR, Foerster J, Lukens JN, Paraskevas F, Greer JP, Rodgers GM, eds. In: *Wintrobe's Clinical Hematology*, Vol 2, 10th ed. Baltimore: Williams & Wilken; 1999:2342–73.

29. Bain BJ. Eosinophilia-idiopathic or not? *N Engl J Med*. 1999; 341:1141–43.

30. Youman JD, Taddeini L, Cooper T. Histamine excess, symptoms in basophilic chronic granulocytic leukemia. *Arch Intern Med*. 1973; 131:560–62.

31. Zittoun R, Rea D, Ngoc LH, Ramond S. Chronic neutrophilic leukemia. *Ann Hematol*. 1994; 68:55–60.

32. Tefferi A. Medical progress: Myelofibrosis with myeloid metaplasia. *N Engl J Med*. 2000; 342:1255–65.

33. Reilly JT. Pathogenesis of idiopathic myelofibrosis: Role of growth factors. *J Clin Pathol*. 1992; 45:461–64.

34. Paquette RL, Meshkinpour A, Rosen PJ. Autoimmune myelofibrosis. *Medicine*. 1994; 73:145–52.

35. Hoffman R. Agnogenic myeloid metaplasia. Hoffman R, Benz EJ, Shattil SJ, Furie B, Cohen H, Silberstein LE, McGlave P, eds. In: *Hematology: Basic Principles and Practice*, 3rd ed. New York: Churchill Livingstone; 1999:1172–84.

36. Prchal JT, Prchal JF. Evolving understanding of the cellular defect in polycythemia vera: Implications for its clinical diagnosis and molecular pathophysiology. *Blood*. 1994; 83:1–4.

37. Remy I, Wilson IA, Michnick SW. Erythropoietin receptor activation by a ligand-induced conformation change. *Science*. 1999; 283:990–93.

38. Schwartz RS. Polycythemia vera: Chance, death, and mutability. *N Engl J Med*. 1998; 338:613–15.

39. Ellis JT, Peterson P, Geller SA, Rappaport H. Studies of the bone marrow in polycythemia vera and the evolution of myelofibrosis and second hematologic malignancies. *Semin Hematol*. 1986; 23:144–55.

40. Provan D, Weatherall D. Red cells II: Acquired anaemias and polycythaemia. *Lancet*. 2000; 355:1260–68.

41. Danish EH. Neonatal polycythemia. *Prog Hematol*. 1986; 14:55–98.

42. Horikawa Y, Matsumura I, Hashimoto K, Shiraga M, Kosugi S, Tadokoro S, et al. Markedly reduced expression of platelet c-Mpl receptor in essential thrombocythemia. *Blood*. 1997; 90:4031–38.

43. Wang JC, Chen C, Novetsky AD, Lichter SM, Ahmed F, Friedberg NM. Blood thrombopoietin levels in clonal thrombocytosis and reactive thrombocytosis. *Am J Med*. 1998; 104:451–55.

44. van Genderen PJ, Michiels JJ. Primary thrombocythemia: Diagnosis, clinical manifestations and management. *Ann Hematol*. 1993; 67:57–62.

45. Hoffman R. Primary Thrombocythemia. Hoffman R, Benz EJ, Shattil SJ, Furie B, Cohen H, Silberstein LE, McGlave P, eds. In: *Hematology: Basic Principles and Practice*, 3rd ed. New York: Churchill Livingstone; 1999:1188–1201.

46. Schafer AI. Essential thrombocythemia. *Prog Hemost Thromb*. 1991; 10:69–96

47. Tefferi A, Hoagland HC. Issues in the diagnosis and management of essential thrombocythemia. *Mayo Clin Proc*. 1994; 69:651–55.

48. Gisslinger H, Chott A, Scheithauer W, Gilly B, Linkesch W, Ludwig H. Interferon in essential thrombocythaemia. *Br J Haematol*. 1991; 79(Suppl 1):42–47.

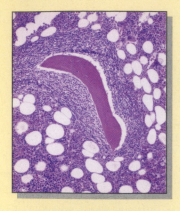

28

Myelodysplastic Syndromes

Louann W. Lawrence, DrP.H.

■ CHECKLIST - LEVEL I

At the end of this unit of study the student should be able to:

1. Define *myelodysplastic syndromes* (MDS) and list general characteristics.
2. List the five subgroups of MDS recognized by the French-American-British (FAB) Cooperative Group and identify key morphological criteria that distinguish each group.
3. Describe laboratory findings and recognize changes in morphology that are characteristic of this group of disorders.

■ CHECKLIST - LEVEL II

At the end of this unit of study the student should be able to:

1. Describe the pathophysiology of MDS.
2. Distinguish among Type I, Type II, and Type III blasts and promyelocytes according to the FAB classification.
3. Summarize treatment and prognosis of MDS.
4. Explain the relationship between MDS and acute leukemia.
5. Assess the results of cytogenetic and molecular tests and correlate with a diagnosis of MDS.
6. List and briefly describe the MDS variants that do not fit into the five subgroups.
7. Differentiate MDS from myeloproliferative disorders, acute leukemia, and other hematologic abnormalities using peripheral blood, bone marrow, and cytogenetic characteristics.
8. Evaluate the laboratory and clinical findings of a patient and propose a diagnostic MDS subgroup.
9. Select laboratory tests that are helpful in diagnosing and differentiating MDSs.

KEY TERMS

Chronic myelomonocytic leukemia (CMML)
Dysplasia
Dyspoiesis
Endomitosis
Micromegakaryocyte
Myelodysplastic syndromes (MDS)
Refractory anemia (RA)
Refractory anemia with excess blasts (RAEB)
Refractory anemia with excess blasts
   in transformation (RAEB-t)
Refractory anemia with ringed sideroblasts (RARS)

BACKGROUND BASICS

The information in this chapter will build on the concepts learned in previous chapters. To maximize your learning experience you should review these concepts before starting this unit of study.

Level I

▶ Create a schematic depicting derivation of different types of blood cells from the pluripotent hematopoietic stem cell. (Chapter 2)

▶ Describe and recognize the cell morphology described by these terms: *ringed sideroblasts* (Chapter 11), *Pelger-Huët anomaly* (Chapter 21), and *megaloblastoid erythropoiesis.* (Chapter 14)

▶ Describe what is meant by ineffective hematopoiesis. (Chapters 10, 27)

▶ Summarize the history and basis of the French-American-British (FAB) classification system to classify malignant leukocyte disorders. (Chapter 26)

▶ Review normal leukocyte development, differentiation, and concentrations in the peripheral blood. (Chapter 6)

Level II

▶ Describe the use of cytochemical and immunological features that distinguish the different types of blasts. (Chapters 23, 26)

▶ Explain how oncogenes and hematopoietic growth factors affect cellular maturation and proliferation. (Chapters 2, 26)

▶ Explain the use of cytogenetics and flow cytometry in diagnosis of malignant disorders. (Chapters 23, 24)

CASE STUDY

We will refer to this case study throughout the chapter.
John Hancock, a 65-year-old white male, was seen in triage with complaints of fatigue, malaise, anorexia, and hemoptysis of recent onset. A CBC was ordered and revealed anemia and a shift to the left in granulocytes. Hematopoietic cells showed dysplastic features. Consider diagnostic probabilities and reflex testing that may provide differential diagnostic information.

▶ OVERVIEW

This chapter describes the neoplastic hematopoietic disorders known as the myelodysplastic syndromes (MDS). It begins with the classification of the disorders into morphologic subgroups according to the FAB classification. The WHO classification is also briefly described and compared to the FAB classification. This is followed by a description of the pathogenesis, incidence, and general clinical and laboratory features including peripheral blood and bone marrow findings. Each subgroup is then described with specific features that allow it to be classified. Variants are also described. Genetic findings common to the MDSs are discussed. The chapter concludes with prognosis and therapy.

▶ INTRODUCTION

The **myelodysplastic syndromes** (MDS) are considered primary, neoplastic, pluripotential stem cell disorders. They are characterized by one or more peripheral blood cytopenias together with prominent maturation abnormalities (**dyspoiesis** or **dysplasia**) in the bone marrow. The peripheral blood cytopenias are the result of ineffective hematopoiesis as evidenced by an accompaning bone marrow hyperplasia. These relatively common entities evolve progressively, leading to aggravation of the cytopenias and, in some cases, transform into a condition indistinguishable from acute leukemia. MDS occurs most commonly in the elderly, although it is being diagnosed with increased frequency in children.

Before the 1980s there was much confusion and disagreement in the literature concerning the criteria for defining, subgrouping, and naming the MDSs. Because of the predisposition of MDS to terminate in leukemia, the term *preleukemia* commonly has been used to describe these disorders. However, the evolution of MDS to acute leukemia is not obligatory, and in fact, many patients die of intercurrent disease or complications of the cytopenia before evolving to leukemia.[1] Whether or not these patients would have developed leukemia had they survived the cytopenic complications is, of course, unknown. In addition, the diagnosis of preleukemia can only be made in retrospect (i.e., after the patient develops leukemia). Thus, the term *myelodysplasia* is more appropriate until the patient actually develops overt leukemia. In the past, MDS has also been described under the terms *refractory anemia with excess blasts, chronic erythremic myelosis, hematopoietic dysplasia, refractory anemia with or without sideroblasts, subacute or chronic myelomonocytic leukemia,* and *smoldering leukemia.* Most hematologists currently consider the terms *dysmyelopoietic syndrome* and *myelodysplastic syndrome* to be more acceptable than *preleukemia* or other synonyms in describing these hematologic disorders. In this book, the term *myelodysplastic syndrome* will be used.

CLASSIFICATION

The French-American-British (FAB) group that earlier proposed criteria for categorizing acute leukemias later proposed a classification scheme for the myelodysplastic syndromes.[2] This classification defines five subgroups based on the blast count and degree of dyspoiesis in the peripheral blood and bone marrow. Hematologists are cautioned that classification in some difficult cases may not always be possible by morphology alone. Overlap between the groups also occurs, delaying definitive characterization. The five subgroups include:

1. Refractory anemia (RA)
2. Refractory anemia with ringed sideroblasts (RARS, RA-S)
3. Refractory anemia with excess blasts (RAEB)
4. Chronic myelomonocytic leukemia (CMML)
5. Refractory anemia with excess blasts in transformation (RAEB-t)

Although the FAB classification system has its limitations, it has been the benchmark for diagnosis of the MDS for the past two decades. Recently, several more comprehensive classification systems have been proposed incorporating information from cytogenetic, immunologic, and molecular diagnostic techniques, as well as clinical and prognostic features of the disease.[3,4] The World Health Organization (WHO) classification system, proposed by a group of American and European pathologists, hematologists, and oncologists, attempts to incorporate morphology, immunophenotype, genetics, and clinical features into classification of all neoplastic diseases of the hematopoietic and lymphoid tissues. This new system makes significant changes in the classification of the MDS.[4] CMML was removed and placed in a newly created category, myelodysplastic/myeloproliferative diseases. RAEB-t was eliminated due to lowering the blast count necessary for a diagnosis of AML from 30% to 20%. Two new categories were added, refractory cytopenia with multilinage dysplasia (RCMD) and 5q–syndrome. (The WHO categories will be addressed briefly later in the chapter.) Because of the newness and proposed status of the WHO system, the FAB classification system will be followed in this chapter.

PATHOGENESIS

The spectrum of clinical and hematological features in MDS is a result of the gradual expansion of abnormal hematopoietic cells and an accompanying increase in premature destruction of these abnormal cells (ineffective hematopoiesis). Cytogenetic, G6PD isoenzyme studies and molecular diagnostic tests support the theory that the abnormal cells in MDS are clones derived from an abnormal stem cell.[5–10]

Chromosome abnormalities are present in over 50% of patients at diagnosis. These abnormalities, detected by standard karyotyping, are present in all hematopoietic cell lines except the lymphoid cell line, which is usually normal, indicating the abnormal clone most probably arises from a myeloid stem cell that can differentiate into granulocyte, monocyte, erythrocyte, or megakaryocyte cell lines.[10–12] Normal clones are found to coexist in the marrow with the abnormal clones. As the disease progresses, the abnormal clone predominates. In those MDS cases that progress to acute leukemia, additional abnormalities in cell cultures and karyotypes can be demonstrated. Therefore, it appears that after the abnormal clone is established, further genetic events may be required for the transformation into acute myelogenous leukemia (AML).[10]

THE ROLE OF ONCOGENES

Control of cellular differentiation, maturation, and proliferation occurs through the interaction of hematopoietic growth factors, with specific cellular receptors (∞ Chapter 2). This interaction causes a complex series of protein and tyrosine kinase phosphorylations and eventually DNA synthesis. The entire process is controlled by cellular proto-oncogenes. When these genes are mutated to oncogenes they can disrupt the process and cause disordered control and neoplasia.[13]

It has been hypothesized that MDS is preceded by a phase in which genetic alterations of hematopoietic cells accumulate before hematologic change or chromosome aberrations occur.[5,14,15] The significance of chromosomal changes in malignant cells is not fully understood, but there is mounting evidence that rearrangements of genetic material may be an important event in the activation of proto-oncogenes to oncogenes.[16,17] Tumor suppressor genes may also play a role in the development of MDS.[9]

"Unbalanced" genetic abnormalities, such as trisomies or whole or partial chromosomal deletions, which are characteristically seen in the MDS, are thought to be responsible for the ineffective hematopoiesis and cytopenias.[18] These chromosomal abnormalities are in contrast to the balanced abnormalities seen in primary AML.

The most frequent chromosome abnormalities in MDS involve chromosomes 5, 7, and 8, all of which carry proto-oncogenes. Chromosome 5 carries the FOS, RAS, and FMS proto-oncogenes; chromosome 7 carries the ERB-D proto-oncogene; and chromosome 8 carries the MYC proto-oncogene. Mutations of the RAS proto-oncogene have been reported in up to 50% of MDS patients[15] and mutations of the FMS in up to 16% of MDS.[14] The RAS, MYC, and FOS proto-oncogenes have been implicated in growth factor mediated signaling mechanisms. If these proto-oncogenes are activated, the abnormal clone in MDS may become immortalized by losing the normal control mechanisms that regulate growth. Some oncogene proteins may be responsible for inhibition of normal hematopoiesis. The role of oncogenes in myelodysplasia needs further exploration.

MATURATION AND PROLIFERATION ABNORMALITIES

Impaired cellular maturation and function due to intrinsic defects in cells of the neoplastic clone is a fundamental pathophysiologic abnormality in MDS as well as in AML. Red cell precursors in MDS patients have been shown to have decreased sensitivity to erythropoietin. Neutrophils in MDS patients may have decreased myeloperoxidase activity leading to increased risk of infection even when cells are quantitatively normal. Platelets may also have functional defects.[12] Progression of MDS to acute leukemia is characterized by a gradual or sudden increase in the blast population with a block in maturation. This is supported by the finding of additional chromosome karyotype abnormalities as progression occurs.[19]

Recent in vitro studies suggest that excessive premature intramedullary cell death of hematologic precursors via *apoptosis* contributes to ineffective hematopoiesis and peripheral blood cytopenias seen in early MDS. The progression to leukemia is associated with a reduction in apoptosis, thereby allowing the expansion of the neoplastic clone.[20] Increased levels of tumor necrosis factor alpha (TNF-α) have been found in the bone marrow of MDS patients, and it is thought to be a mediator of apoptosis. Abnormal levels of other cytokines have also been reported in the serum or marrow of MDS patients, such as IL-1, IL-6, and IL-8.[21]

SECONDARY MDS

Originally, all MDS cases were classified as idiopathic (primary myelodysplasia). Evidence now indicates that a portion of MDS cases, especially those occurring in patients under 50 years of age, are probably secondary to chemotherapy, radiation therapy (therapy-related myelodysplasia, t-MDS), or environmental mutagens.[22,23] In children, MDS may be associated with predisposing conditions such as constitutional chromosome disorders (Down syndrome) and immunodeficiency disorders.[24]

▶ INCIDENCE

MDS occurs primarily in individuals over 50 years of age and has a slight male predominance (approximately 60%).[12] The risk increases sharply with age. Due to the lack of definition and classification of MDS before 1982, the actual incidence of these disorders has not been accurately assessed by large-scale epidemiological studies. Morbidity and mortality statistics are also lacking, partly because MDS is not included as a separate code in the International Classification of Diseases (ICD). The difficulty in making correct diagnoses in the early stages of the disease also contributes to unreliable incidence figures. One source estimated the overall incidence as 3–13 cases per 100,000 per year and the incidence in persons over 70 years as 15–50 cases per 100,000 per year.[10] MDS is more common than AML in patients between 50 and 70 years of age, and the incidence appears to be rising. This rise in incidence may be due to an increased awareness of MDS on the part of physicians and clinical laboratory professionals, an increased application of diagnostic procedures in elderly individuals, and an increase in the number of elderly in the population.[10]

Myelodysplasia is rare in children. Problems in diagnosis may contribute to an underestimation of incidence. The incidence of MDS in children may be approximately the same as the incidence of AML in children. About 15% of acute leukemias in children are AML.[25] One retrospective study indicated that 17% of children with AML had a preleukemic phase (MDS).[26] The median age of children at presentation of MDS is about six years, except for CMML in which the median age is 2.5 years. The male/female ratio is about 1.6:1.

▶ CLINICAL FINDINGS

The most frequent presenting symptoms, fatigue and weakness, are related to an anemia that is refractory to treatment. Less commonly, hemorrhagic symptoms and infection precede diagnosis. These symptoms are related to thrombocytopenia and neutropenia. Many individuals may be asymptomatic, and their disease is discovered upon routine laboratory screening.[11] Infection is a common and life-threatening complication in patients with diagnosed MDS. Neutropenia ($<1 \times 10^9$/L) and the more aggressive subgroups (RAEB, RAEB-t) are associated risk factors for infectious complications.[27] Infection is the most common cause of death. Splenomegaly and/or hepatomegaly is uncommon, except in CMML in which it is present in approximately 30% of cases.

▶ LABORATORY FINDINGS

The MDS present with a range of abnormal morphologic features that can be demonstrated on stained peripheral blood and bone marrow smears. FAB criteria for classification of MDS into subtypes will be presented in a later section of this chapter. Included here are the general hematologic features used to initially define the presence of an MDS (Table 28-1 ✪).

PERIPHERAL BLOOD

The peripheral blood characteristics of MDS are cytopenias and dysplasia. Findings include anemia, neutropenia, and/or thrombocytopenia and occasionally monocytosis. Anemia is the most consistent finding, occurring as an isolated cytopenia in 35% of the cases. Bicytopenia occurs in 30% of the cases and pancytopenia in 19%.[28] Less commonly, an iso-

⊛ TABLE 28-1

Hematologic Abnormalities in Myelodysplastic Syndromes

Findings	Erythroid Series	Myeloid Series	Thrombocyte Series
Peripheral blood	Anemia, macrocytes, oval macrocytes, dimorphism, basophilic stippling, nucleated RBC, Howell-Jolly bodies, sideroblasts, anisocytosis, poikilocytosis, reticulocytopenia	Neutropenia, hypogranulation, abnormal granulation, shift to the left, nuclear abnormalities including pseudo–Pelger-Huët and ring nuclei, monocytosis	Thrombocytopenia, or thrombocytosis, giant forms, hypogranulation, micromegakaryocytes, functional abnormalities
Bone marrow	Megaloblastoid erythropoiesis, nuclear fragmentation and budding, karyorrhexis, multiple nuclei, defective hemoglobinization, vacuolization, ringed sideroblasts	Abnormal granules in promyelocytes, increase in Type I and Type II blasts, absence of secondary granules, nuclear abnormalities, decreased myeloperoxidase, Auer rods in blasts	Micromegakaryocytes, megakaryocytes with multiple, separated nuclei, large mononuclear megakaryocytes, hypogranulation or large abnormal granules in megakaryocytes

lated neutropenia or thrombocytopenia is found. Dysplastic features of one or more cell lines are typical. Functional abnormalities of hematologic cells are also common.[29] Studies show that the higher the degree and number of cytopenias, the worse the prognosis.[30]

Erythrocytes

The degree of anemia is variable but the hemoglobin is generally <10 g/dL. The erythrocytes are usually macrocytic (Figure 28-1 ■), less often normocytic. Oval macrocytes similar to those in megaloblastic anemia are frequently present. A dimorphic anemia with both oval macrocytes and microcytic hypochromic cells is also a common initial finding in the RARS group. Reticulocytes show an absolute decrease but may appear normal if only the uncorrected relative number (percent) is reported. In addition to anemia, qualitative abnormalities indicative of dyserythropoiesis are present. These include anisocytosis, poikilocytosis, basophilic stippling, Howell-Jolly bodies, and nucleated erythrocytes.

Often hemoglobin F is increased (5–6%) and distributed in a heterogeneous pattern. Acquired hemoglobin H has also been found in MDS. Other erythrocyte changes include altered A, B, and I antigens, enzyme changes, and an acquired erythrocyte membrane change similar but not identical to that found in paroxysmal nocturnal hemoglobinuria (PNH).

Leukocytes

Neutropenia is the second most common cytopenia observed in MDS. Neutropenia may be accompanied by the finding of metamyelocytes and myelocytes on the blood smear. Blasts and progranulocytes may also be present. Morphologic abnormalities in granulocytes indicative of dysgranulopoiesis are a hallmark finding in MDS. Dysgranulopoiesis is characterized by agranular or hypogranular

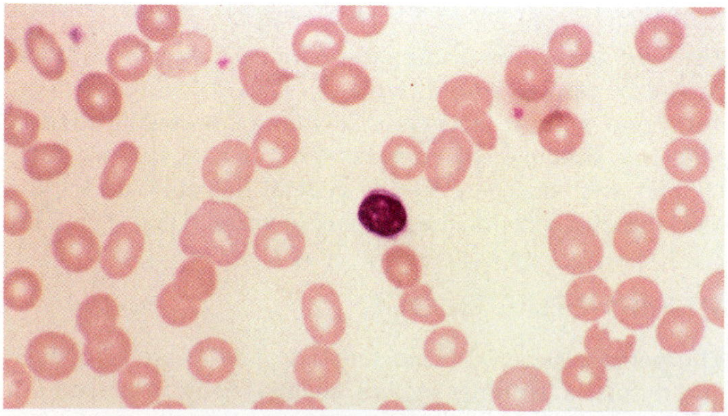

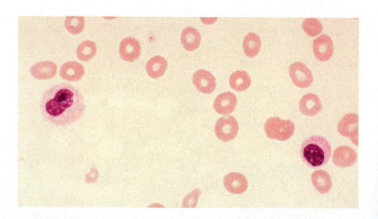

■ **FIGURE 28-2** Peripheral blood film from a patient with MDS showing neutrophils with the pseudo–Pelger-Huët nucleus. One cell's nucleus is peanut shaped and the other is single lobed. The nuclear chromatin is condensed, and the cells contain granules, making identification possible. In many cases, these types of neutrophils are agranular, which makes it difficult to differentiate them from lymphocytes. (Peripheral blood; Wright-Giemsa stain; 1000× magnification)

■ **FIGURE 28-1** A peripheral blood film of a patient with MDS. Note macrocytic cells, and anisocytosis. (Peripheral blood; Wright-Giemsa stain; 1000× magnification)

neutrophils, persistent basophilia of the cytoplasm, abnormal appearing granules, hyposegmentation (pseudo–Pelger-Huët) (Figure 28-2 ■) or hypersegmentation of the nucleus and donut- or ring-shaped nuclei. Care should be taken to distinguish neutrophils with pseudo–Pelger-Huët anomaly and hypogranulation from lymphocytes and to distinguish neutrophilic-band forms with hypogranulation from monocytes. Neutrophils may also demonstrate enzyme defects, such as decreased myeloperoxidase and decreased leukocyte alkaline phosphatase. In some cases, neutrophils exhibit severe functional impairment, including defective bactericidal, phagocytic, or chemotactic properties. Absolute monocytosis is a common finding even in leukopenic conditions.

Platelets

Qualitative and quantitative platelet abnormalities are often present. The platelet count may be normal, increased, or decreased. The lowest platelet counts are associated with CMML and RAEB-t. Giant platelets, hypogranular platelets, and platelets with large fused granules may be seen in the peripheral blood (Figures 28-3 and 28-4 ■). Functional platelet abnormalities include abnormal adhesion and aggregation. As a result, the bleeding time may be prolonged, and other platelet function tests may give abnormal results.

Micromegakaryocytes

Sometimes, circulating **micromegakaryocytes** (small abnormal megakaryocytes), also called dwarf megakaryocytes, can be found in the MDS and myeloproliferative syndromes. Micromegakaryocytes may be difficult to define and are frequently overlooked unless cytoplasmic tags or blebs are present (Figure 28-5 ■). Micromegakaryocytes are believed to represent abnormal megakaryocytes that have lost their ability to undergo endomitosis. (Megakaryocytes undergo a unique maturation process whereby the DNA content duplicates without cell division, resulting in a polyploid nucleus [**endomitosis**]) (∞ Chapter 34). Most of these cells have a

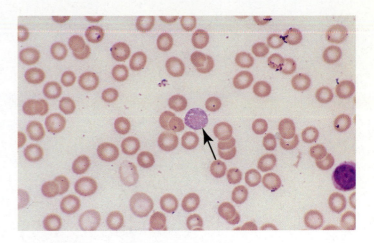

■ FIGURE 28-4 Peripheral blood from a patient with MDS showing large agranular platelet. (Wright-Giemsa stain; 1000× magnification)

single-lobed nucleus and are the size of a lymphocyte. Morphologically they may be confused with lymphocytes but can be distinguished by tags of one or more platelets attached to a nucleus. Some may have pale blue, foamy or vacuolated cytoplasm that resembles a nongranular platelet. The nuclear structure is variable, but many cells have very densely clumped chromatin and stain brown black with Wright-Giemsa stain. Others may have a finer, looser chromatin. These cells are also found in the bone marrow.

✓ **Checkpoint! #1**

How does the typical peripheral blood picture in MDS differ from aplastic anemia?

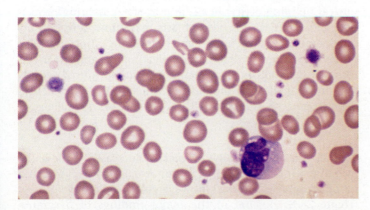

■ FIGURE 28-3 A peripheral blood film from a patient with MDS showing large platelets. (Wright-Giemsa stain; 1000× magnification)

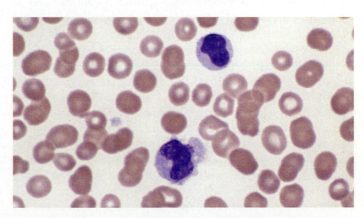

■ FIGURE 28-5 Micromegakaryocyte in peripheral blood film from a patient with MDS. Note the dense chromatin structure and the irregular rim of cytoplasm with cytoplasmic tags. There is an agranular platelet in the field that matches the appearance of the micromegakaryocyte cytoplasm. (Wright-Giemsa stain; 1000× magnification)

Ⓔ **CASE STUDY** *(continued from page 531)*

The results of the CBC on Mr. Hancock were:

RBC:	1.60×10^{12}/L
Hb:	58 g/L
Hct:	0.17 L/L
WBC:	10.5×10^9/L
Platelets:	39×10^9/L
Reticulocyte count:	0.8%
Differential:	44% segmented neutrophils
	7% band neutrophils
	6% lymphocytes
	28% eosinophils
	1% metamyelocytes
	1% myelocytes
	9% promyelocytes
	4% blasts

The neutrophilic cells show marked hyposegmentation and hypogranulation. RBC morphology includes anisocytosis and poikilocytosis, teardrop cells, ovalocytes, and schistocytes.

1. Cytopenia is present in what cell lines?
2. What abnormalities are present in the differential?
3. What evidence of dyspoiesis is seen in the leukocyte morphology?
4. Calculate the MCV. What peripheral blood findings are helpful to rule out megaloblastic anemia?
5. What features of the differential resemble CML? What helps to distinguish this case from CML?

BONE MARROW

Bone marrow examination is necessary to identify the dyshematopoietic element, to determine cellularity, and to establish a diagnosis. In most cases, the bone marrow is hypercellular with erythroid hyperplasia, although normocellular and hypocellular marrows may occur. The hypercellular bone marrow with a peripheral blood picture of cytopenia is the result of premature cell loss in the marrow (ineffective hematopoiesis).[11] The cellularity of the marrow should be interpreted in relation to the patient's age because MDS is commonly found in the elderly. The number of myeloblasts can range from normal to 30% (promonocytes, erythroblasts, promyelocytes, and megakaryoblasts are not included in the blast count). Generally, all cell lines exhibit evidence of dyshematopoiesis.

Bone marrow trephine biopsy may be helpful in establishing the diagnosis of MDS in difficult cases.[31] (Trephine biopsy is the removal of a disc of bone using a cylindrical saw.) Abnormal localization of immature myeloid precursors (ALIP) clustering centrally may be seen in biopsy before an increase in myeloblasts is detected in bone marrow smears.[32] ALIP has been shown to be an indicator of increased risk for

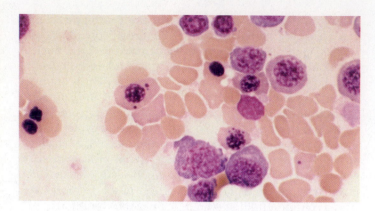

■ **FIGURE 28-6** Meglaoblastoid erythroblasts in the bone marrow of a patient with MDS. (Wright-Giemsa stain; 1000× magnification)

transformation to leukemia and is associated with poor survival. In patients with less than 5% blasts, ALIP may indicate evolution to a more aggressive disease. A biopsy also gives an exact assessment of cellularity and an indication of the amount of reticulin fibers. On the other hand, ringed sideroblasts, nuclear fragmentation and budding, Auer rods, irregular cytoplasmic basophilia, and abnormal staining of primary granules in promyelocytes are more easily identified in bone marrow aspirate smears. Thus, both aspirate smears and biopsy preparations are necessary for accurate diagnosis.

Dyserythropoiesis

The most common bone marrow finding in MDS is nuclear-cytoplasmic asynchrony similar to that seen in megaloblastic anemia (∞ Chapter 14). However, the chromatin is usually thicker and the nuclear chromatin pattern is often described as megaloblastoid (Figure 28-6 ■). The abnormal erythrocytic maturation is not responsive to vitamin B_{12} or folic acid therapy. Giant, multinucleated erythroid precursors can be found (Figure 28-7 ■). Other nuclear abnormalities include nuclear fragmentation, abnormal nuclear shape, nuclear budding, karryohexis, and irregular staining properties. The cytoplasm of normoblasts may show defective hemoglobinization, vacuoles, and basophilic stippling. The presence of ringed sideroblasts, reflecting the abnormal erythrocyte metabolism, is a common finding. *Ringed sideroblasts* are defined as normoblasts in which mitochondrial iron deposits encircle at least one-third or more of the nucleus.

Dysgranulopoiesis

Granulopoiesis is usually normal to increased, unless the overall marrow is hypocellular. Abnormal granulocyte maturation (dysgranulopoiesis), however, is almost always present (Figure 28-8 ■). One of the major findings of dysgranulopoiesis in the bone marrow is abnormal staining of the primary granules in promyelocytes and myelocytes. Sometimes the granules are larger than normal, and other times the

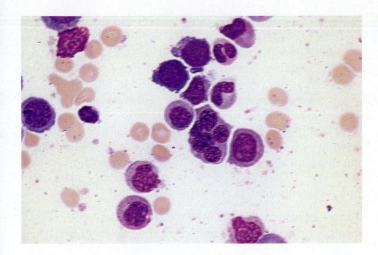

■ FIGURE 28-7 Multinucleated polychromatophilic erythroblast in the bone marrow of a patient with MDS. It is also megaloblastoid. (Wright-Giemsa stain; 1000× magnification)

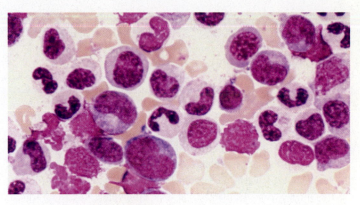

■ FIGURE 28-8 Bone marrow from a patient with MDS. Note the metamyelocytes and bands with a lack of secondary granules. The bands have clear cytoplasm while the metamyelocytes have a bluish cytoplasm. (Wright-Giemsa stain; 1000× magnification)

granules are absent. Secondary granules may be absent in myelocytes and other more mature neutrophils, giving rise to the hypogranular peripheral blood neutrophils. Irregular cytoplasmic basophilia with a dense rim of peripheral basophilia is also characteristic. Nuclear abnormalities similar to those found in the peripheral blood granulocytes may be present in bone marrow granulocytes.

Dysmegakaryopoiesis
Megakaryocytes may be decreased, normal, or increased. Abnormalities in maturation are reflected by the presence of micromegakaryocytes, large mononuclear megakaryocytes, and megakaryocytes with other abnormal nuclear configurations (Figure 28-9 ■). The lack of granules or presence of giant abnormal granules is also characteristic.

OTHER LABORATORY FINDINGS
Serum iron is normal or increased, and the TIBC is normal or decreased. Cobalamin (vitamin B_{12}) and folic acid levels are normal to increased, a feature that helps to differentiate the megaloblastoid features of MDS from the typical megaloblastic features of megaloblastic anemias.

Immunologic analysis has revealed that MDS is associated with a significant decrease in the total number of T lymphocytes together with a decrease in both CD4 and CD8 lymphocyte subsets.[33] The responses of T lymphocytes to mitogens, Ph A, and Con A may be significantly decreased. Although B lymphocytes are quantitatively normal, serum immunologlubulins are often increased, and circulating immune complexes are frequently present. In addition, granulocytic oxidative metabolism as measured by the nitroblue tetrazolium reduction test may be abnormal and chemotaxis impaired.

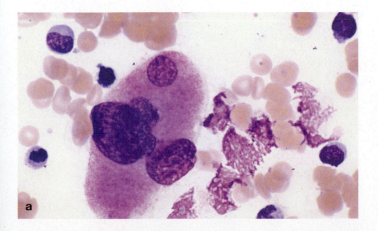

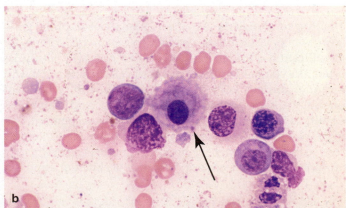

■ FIGURE 28-9 a. Abnormal megakaryocyte from a patient with MDS. b. Micromegakaryocyte in the bone marrow of a patient with MDS. (Both: Bone marrow; Wright-Giemsa stain; 1000× magnification)

Checkpoint! #2

Why is serum vitamin B_{12}, serum folate level, or bone marrow iron stain important in the diagnosis of MDS?

CASE STUDY *(continued from page 536)*

A bone marrow was performed on Mr. Hancock. The marrow showed a cellularity of about 75%. There was myeloid hyperplasia with 12% blasts, 26% promyelocytes, 18% myelocytes, 3% metamyelocytes, 4% bands, and 37% eosinophils. The M:E ratio was 12:1. The myelocytes were hypogranular and some had two nuclei. The erythroid precursors showed megaloblastoid changes. Megakaryocytes were adequate in number but showed abnormal forms with nuclear separation and single nucleated forms.

6. Which of the hematopoietic cell lines exhibit dyshematopoiesis in the bone marrow?

7. How would you classify the bone marrow cellularity?

8. What does the M:E ratio indicate?

9. Identify at least two features of the bone marrow that are compatible with a diagnosis of MDS.

10. What chemistry tests would be helpful to rule out megaloblastic anemia?

▶ ## BLAST CELL CLASSIFICATION

The blast count appears to be the most important prognostic indicator of survival and progression to acute leukemia in MDS. The maximum number of blasts compatible with a diagnosis of MDS is 30% (<20% in the WHO classification). The minimum criteria for a diagnosis of acute leukemia include more than 30% blasts (>20% in the WHO classification).

MORPHOLOGIC IDENTIFICATION OF BLASTS

The dysgranulopoiesis that affects primary azurophilic granules in neoplastic blasts changes the standard criteria for identification and classification of blast cells and promyelocytes. The standard criteria for a blast cell include a cell with a central nucleus with fine nuclear chromatin, prominent nucleoli, a high nuclear:cytoplasmic ratio, and deeply basophilic and agranular cytoplasm. It is now recognized that in MDS and acute leukemia there are some blast-like cells that contain primary azurophilic granules. These early azurophilic granules are not indicative of differentiation but

rather of abnormal neoplastic cells.[34] Consequently, two types of blasts that may be found in the bone marrow and peripheral blood in MDS and AML are recognized: Type I and Type II. More recently, it has been suggested that a third type of blast cell (Type III) be recognized in MDS to improve predictions of progression to acute leukemia and survival.[34] Typical agranular blasts are included in the Type I category. Type II and Type III blasts have typical blast-like features except they contain primary azurophilic granules. The following morphologic criteria have been established for identifying Type I blasts, Type II blasts, Type III blasts, and promyelocytes in MDS and acute leukemia.[34]

Type I Blasts (Figure 28-10 ■). These cells include typical myeloblasts and unclassifiable cells. The nuclear chromatin is

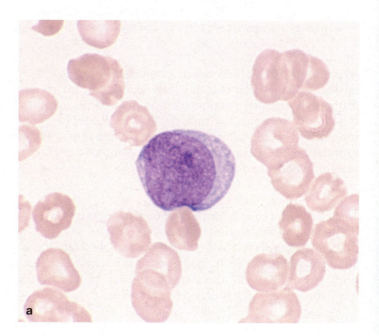

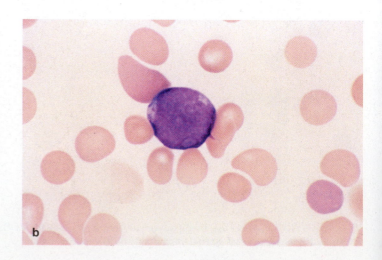

■ **FIGURE 28-10 a.** Type I myeloblast. **b.** Type II myeloblast. (Both: Peripheral blood; Wright-Giemsa stain; 1000× magnification)

finely dispersed with prominent nucleoli. The nuclear cytoplasmic ratio is variable but is higher in the smaller blasts than the larger ones. The cytoplasm contains no granules.

Type II Blasts (Figure 28-10 ■). These cells resemble Type I blasts except that the cytoplasm contains primary granules (fewer than 20) and the nucleus is in a more central position. The nuclear cytoplasmic ratio tends to be lower than that of Type I blasts.

Type III Blasts These cells are similar to Type II blasts except they contain more than 20 granules in the cytoplasm.

Promyelocytes The nucleus is eccentrically placed, and the chromatin pattern is more condensed. The Golgi apparatus is obvious as a clear area adjacent to the nucleus. The nuclear cytoplasmic ratio is low due to the increase in cytoplasm. There are many primary granules present. In some cases of MDS the promyelocyte appears hypogranular or even agranular. In these cases, the abnormal cell can be identified as a promyelocyte by the other nuclear and cytoplasmic criteria. If the azurophilic granules are clumped and heterogeneous in size, the promyelocyte is classified as abnormal.

Using these new criteria for distinguishing blasts and promyelocytes, the minimum criteria for a diagnosis of acute leukemia include more than 30% Type I, Type II, and Type III blasts (exclusive of promyelocytes) in the bone marrow. The maximum proportion of blasts compatible with a diagnosis of MDS is 30% Type I, Type II, and Type III blasts. Often the blast count in the blood is greater than that in the marrow. It has been suggested that when the blast count exceeds 30% in the blood but the bone marrow concentration is less than 30%, the case be regarded as acute leukemia. The blasts in MDS, with the exception of RAEB-t and rarely CMML, usually do not have Auer rods present.

 Checkpoint! #3

Why is it important to correctly identify the number of blasts when evaluating the peripheral blood or bone marrow smear of a patient suspected of having MDS?

CYTOCHEMICAL AND IMMUNOLOGICAL IDENTIFICATION OF BLASTS

Although the blast cells in MDS are derived primarily from myeloid or monocytic precursors, a panel of cytochemical and immunocytochemical reactions should be performed and interpreted to enhance the accuracy of diagnosis[35] (∞ Chapters 23, 26). Peroxidase and Sudan black B identify blasts with a myeloid origin; however, in MDS the blasts may have lower peroxidase activity than normal blasts. Combined esterase stain may be performed on both peripheral blood and bone marrow for a more accurate assessment of monocytic cells. Iron stain may reveal abnormal iron me-

tabolism in erythroblasts with the presence of increased iron stores and ringed sideroblasts. Abnormal carbohydrate metabolism is indicated by the presence of blocks of PAS-positive material in erythrocyte precursors. Abnormal small megakaryoblasts can be difficult to distinguish from lymphoblasts or Type I myeloblasts. They can be readily identified, however, by immunochemistry with antibodies against platelet-specific glycoproteins IIB/IIIA (CD41), or gpIIIA (CD61), or by antibody against factor VIII in histologic sections. Diaminobenzidine can be utilized to identify platelet peroxidase in electron micrographs.[35]

Only a few studies have been reported on the prognostic value of immunophenotyping in MDS. In general, there is no correlation between immunophenotypes and the FAB classification. It has been suggested that increased expression of markers found on immature myeloid cells such as CD13, CD33, CD34, and HLA-DL and decreased expression of NAT-9 (found on mature myeloid cells) may be associated with a worse prognosis and with progression to AML.[36,37] MDS patients with a low percentage of bone marrow cells expressing CD11b had a higher risk of evolution to AML and shorter survival compared to patients with more than 53% of marrow cells expressing CD11b.[37] Standardization of methods to produce comparable results between laboratories must be achieved before surface marker studies can be more fully utilized as diagnostic tools in MDS.[37] Immunological phenotyping using monoclonal antibodies may be useful in identifying the lineage of blasts in those cases of acute leukemia derived from therapy-related MDS. Many of these cases show trilineage dysplasia and are difficult to define according to FAB subgrouping.[38] The specific cellular markers found on different cell lineages in acute leukemia are described in ∞ Chapters 23, 29, 30.

▶ DESCRIPTION OF SUBGROUPS OF MDS

The most widely recognized classification system for MDS is the revised FAB classification proposed in 1982.[2] Some features of the five subgroups of MDS overlap, and some are exclusive to a particular group. The classification criteria are listed in Table 28-2 ✪. They include:

- Percentage of bone marrow blasts
- Percentage of peripheral blood blasts
- Presence or absence of ringed sideroblasts
- Percentage of monocytes present
- Extent of cytopenias
- Degree of dyspoiesis

REFRACTORY ANEMIA

Refractory anemia (RA) occurs with anemia as the primary clinical finding. The anemia is refractory (nonresponsive) to all conventional forms of therapy. Erythrocytes usually

✪ TABLE 28-2

Differentiating Characteristics of FAB Subtypes of Myelodysplastic Syndromes

Characteristic	RA	RARS	CMML	RAEB	RAEB-t
Blasts in PB (%)	<1	<1	<5	<5	≥5
Blasts in BM (%)	<5	<5	≤20	5–20	21–30 and/or Auer rods
Ringed sideroblasts (%)	<15	≥15	variable	variable	variable
Monos in PB	–	–	>1 × 10^9/L	—	—
Monos in BM	–	–	≥20%	—	—

RA = refractory anemia; RARS = refractory anemia with ringed sideroblasts; CMML = chronic myelomonocytic leukemia; RAEB = refractory anemia with excess blasts; RAEB-t = refractory anemia with excess blasts in transformation.

PB = peripheral blood; BM = bone marrow; Monos = monocytes or immature cells of monocytic origin.

(Adapted, with permission, from Lee GR et al. *Wintrobe's Clinical Hematology*, 10th ed., Baltimore: Williams and Wilkins, 1999; p. 2321.)

appear macrocytic, but occasionally they are microcytic or normocytic. The peripheral blood shows reticulocytopenia and signs of dyserythropoiesis, but leukocytes and platelets are usually quantitatively and qualitatively normal. Blast cells are usually absent in the peripheral blood, but if present, they constitute less than 1% of the nucleated cells.

The bone marrow is hypercellular with erythroid hyperplasia and signs of dyserythropoiesis. Megaloblastoid erythropoiesis is present, but it is unresponsive to folic acid or cobalamin. Ringed sideroblasts are absent or present in low numbers. Maturation of neutrophils and megakaryocytes is generally normal. Blast cells compose less than 5% of marrow cells.

For convenience, the rare isolated refractory thrombocytopenias and neutropenias are included in this category even though anemia is absent. Some prefer to call these cases refractory cytopenia.

REFRACTORY ANEMIA WITH RINGED SIDEROBLASTS, OR ACQUIRED IDIOPATHIC SIDEROBLASTIC ANEMIA

Refractory anemia with ringed sideroblasts (RARS), or acquired idiopathic sideroblastic anemia (AISA), is similar to RA, except that ringed sideroblasts account for more than 15% of the nucleated cells in the bone marrow. The anemia is usually macrocytic, less often normocytic. Sometimes there is evidence of a dual population of normochromic and hypochromic cells. The peripheral blood shows reticulocytopenia and often leukopenia. The occurrence of leukopenia in one study was 33% with neutropenia occuring in 7%.[28] Another study found neutropenia in 48% of the cases.[39] Occasionally the platelet count is increased. A few cases exhibit granulocyte and platelet morphologic abnormalities.

The bone marrow is hypercellular with megaloblastoid dyserythropoiesis. If dysgranulopoiesis and dysmegakaryopoiesis are present, it is mild. There are fewer than 5% blast cells in the marrow.

REFRACTORY ANEMIA WITH EXCESS BLASTS

In **refractory anemia with excess blasts (RAEB),** there is cytopenia in at least two cell lines and conspicuous qualitative abnormalities in all three cell lines. The anemia is normocytic or slightly macrocytic with reticulocytopenia. Evidence of dysgranulopoiesis is prominent. There are fewer than 5% blasts in the peripheral blood. Monocytosis without leukocytosis may be present, but the absolute monocyte count does not exceed 1 × 10^9/L, and serum and urinary lysozyme levels are normal. Platelet abnormalities include giant forms, abnormal granularity, and functional aberrations. Sometimes, circulating micromegakaryocytes can be found.

The bone marrow is hypercellular, less often normocellular, with varying degrees of granulocytic and erythrocytic hyperplasia. All three cell lines show signs of dyshematopoiesis. The proportion of blasts varies from 5% to 20%. Abnormal promyelocytes may be present.[40] These abnormal cells have blast-like nuclei with nucleoli and no chromatin condensation, and the cytoplasm contains large bizarre granules. There may be an increase in ringed sideroblasts, but the elevated blast count differentiates RAEB from RARS. In some cases, it is difficult to differentiate RAEB from acute leukemia. Serial examinations are sometimes necessary to make an accurate diagnosis.

It has been shown that there is a difference in survival between patients having 5–10% blasts and those having 11–20% blasts. Those with more than 10% blasts have a worse outcome. The separation of these two groups into RAEB-I (5–10% blasts) and RAEB-II (11–20% blasts) provides a more accurate prognostic classification.[34]

REFRACTORY ANEMIA WITH EXCESS BLASTS IN TRANSFORMATION

Refractory anemia with excess blasts in transformation (RAEB-t) includes those disorders that do not fit into any other MDS category due to an excess of blasts and/or the presence of Auer rods. They are also not typical of acute leukemia because the excess of blasts is insufficient to diagnose AML. This disorder generally has a shorter course than other types of MDS (10-month survival) and has a higher risk of evolving to acute leukemia. Rarely, patients with RAEB-t may have had a previously established form of myelodysplasia.

RAEB-t is similar to RAEB except that any one of the following hematological features may be found: 5% or more blasts in the peripheral blood; 20–30% Type I and Type II blasts in the bone marrow; or the presence of unequivocal Auer rods in granulocyte precursor cells. RAEB-t may resemble AML/M$_2$, which characteristically shows greater than 30% blasts in the bone marrow and Auer rods. Cytogenetic studies may be necessary to differentiate the two. AML/M$_2$ commonly displays t(8;21), while RAEB-t usually shows an unbalanced chromosomal abnormality such as 7q-, 5q–, or del 7.

CHRONIC MYELOMONOCYTIC LEUKEMIA

Chronic myelomonocytic leukemia (CMML) differs from the other subgroups in that it has a myeloproliferative element with a mature granulocytosis in the peripheral blood and many patients have splenomegaly. Since it has features that straddle both myeloproliferative disorders and MDS, it is easily confused with chronic myelocytic leukemia (CML).

Synonyms for this disorder include *subacute myelomonocytic leukemia* and *chronic erythromonocytic leukemia*. Although other subgroups of MDS are not typically associated with organomegaly, 30–54% of patients with CMML have splenomegaly and/or hepatomegaly. Lymphadenopathy is not present. There is usually no skin or gum involvement as is commonly associated with acute myelomonocytic leukemia. The diagnosis is most often made when the patient is seen by a physician for symptoms of anemia, intercurrent infection, or hemorrhagic manifestations. These patients are found to have a predominantly monocytic cellular pattern in the peripheral blood and a myelocytic cellular pattern in the bone marrow. The average time lapse from onset of symptoms until diagnosis is 6–18 months. One study of 41 patients found that 24% had previously been diagnosed with another MDS subgroup or had peripheral cytopenia.[41] Two had agnogenic myeloid metaplasia. None, however, had been treated with cytotoxic drugs.

Although leukocytes are characteristically increased, erythrocytes and platelets are often decreased. Anemia is mild in CMML with an average hemoglobin of 11.7 g/dL. The erythrocytes are normocytic or slightly macrocytic. Thrombocytopenia is present in about 60% of the cases.[42] Giant platelets and hypogranular forms are found. Circulating micromegakaryocytes are sometimes present. The leukocyte count is variable with many in the normal range, some in-creased, and a few decreased. Regardless of the leukocyte count, there is an absolute monocytosis greater than 1×10^9/L and usually greater than 2×10^9/L. Monocytes frequently exhibit morphologic abnormalities. The nuclear pattern varies, but nucleoli are absent and the cells are easily distinguished from blasts. Neutrophils are often increased with or without dysgranulopoiesis. Immature granulocytes, monocytes, and nucleated erythrocytes may be identified on blood smears. Fewer than 5% blasts are found in the peripheral blood.

A constant and significant finding in CMML is the elevation of serum and urinary lysozyme levels. In addition, most patients have an increased uric acid level from increased cell turnover. Vitamin B$_{12}$ and folic acid levels are normal or increased.

Protein electrophoresis reveals hypergammaglobulinemia in over 50% of patients.[33,41] In most cases, it is polyclonal. Although it has been suggested that the abnormal monocytes may be responsible for this phenomenon, no relationship between degree of peripheral monocytosis and presence or absence of gammopathy has been established.

The bone marrow is hypercellular with a proliferation of immature and abnormal myelocytes. Some myelocytes have nuclei with nucleoli and an irregular chromatin pattern somewhere between that of blasts and myelocytes. Some myelocytes appear pyknotic or necrobiotic, whereas others have a monocytoid appearance. Even when myelocytes are increased, there is no apparent leukemic hiatus. Transitional forms in both directions are present. There are frequent reports describing an intermediate or abnormal cell, expressing staining and/or morphological characteristics of both monocytoid and myeloid cells in the bone marrow. Promonocytes may be significantly increased, and up to 20% of the nucleated cells may be blasts. Auer rods may be present in some blasts, especially in progression of the disease. Erythrocyte precursors may be increased, particularly early in the disease. The morphology of erythroblasts is often abnormal with megaloblastoid features and multiple nuclei. Megakaryocytes are usually quantitatively normal, but almost half exhibit some degree of dysmegakaryopoiesis.[41] The presence of a significant peripheral blood and bone marrow monocytosis, trilineage dysplasia, absence of the Philadelphia chromosome, and elevated serum and urine lysozyme help differentiate CMML from CML. Absence of the BCR/ABL fusion gene by molecular analysis is useful to rule out CML (∞ Chapters 25, 27).[11]

CASE STUDY *(continued from page 538)*

Review the peripheral blood and bone marrow features of Mr. Hancock from previous pages.

11. What is the most likely MDS subgroup? Based upon what criteria?

▶ THE WHO CLASSIFICATION

The European Association of Pathologists and the Society for Hematopathology recently proposed the WHO Classification System to better incorporate some of the newer diagnostic techniques along with clinical and prognostic features into a more comprehensive classification system for all hematopoietic malignancies[4] (Table 28-3 ✪). One significant change was to lower the number of bone marrow blasts necessary for diagnosis of AML from 30% to 20%. This eliminated the MDS category of RAEB-t because it was felt that patients in this category (20–30% blasts) have a prognosis similar to that of patients with >30% blasts. Two new categories were added to MDS: refractory cytopenia with multilineage dysplasia (RCMD) and 5q– syndrome. The 5q– syndrome is discussed later in this chapter under Variants of MDS. RCMD was created for cases of MDS with less than 5% blasts that have significant dysplasia involving granulocytic and megakaryocytic cell lines. Recent studies have shown that these cases are more likely to end in death due to bone marrow failure or to progress to acute leukemia than other cases that do not have these distinct features. This category also helps to distinguish these cases from RA and RARS, which typically involve dysplasia in only the erythroid cell line. CMML has features of both the MDS and the myeloproliferative disorders and was placed in a newly created category of diseases, myelodysplastic/myeloproliferative diseases. The clinical acceptance and usefulness of the WHO classification system remains to be determined.

✪ TABLE 28-3

Proposed World Health Organization (WHO) Classification of MDS

- Refractory anemia (RA)
- Refractory anemia with ringed sideroblasts (RARS)
- Refractory cytopenia (myelodysplastic syndrome) with multilineage dysplasia (RCMD)*
- Refractory anemia (myelodysplastic syndrome) with excess blasts (RAEB)
- 5q–syndrome**
- Myelodysplastic syndrome, unclassifiable

*RCMD characteristics: <5% blasts in bone marrow, dysplasia in 2 or more cell lines, poor prognosis
**5q– characteristics: 5q–only chromosomal abnormality present, macrocytic anemia, modest leukopenia, normal to high platelet count, hypolobular megakaryocytes, good prognosis
(Adapted, with permission, from: Harris NL, Jaffe ES, Diebold J, et al. The World Health Organization classification of neoplastic diseases of the haematopoietic and lymphoid tissues: Report of the Clinical Advisory Committee Meeting, Arlie House, Virginia, November 1997. *Histopathology.* 2000; 36:69–87.)

▶ VARIANTS OF MDS

A number of patients have blood and/or marrow findings that cause problems in diagnosis and/or classification. Some of these findings occur often enough to consider them as variants of MDS.

HYPOPLASTIC MDS

Although most cases of MDS are associated with hypercellular or normocellular bone marrows, about 10% have hypocellular marrows. In these cases trephine biopsy is necessary to exclude a diagnosis of aplastic anemia or hypoplastic acute myeloid leukemia (AML). This distinction is important since the diagnosis will have an influence on treatment and prognosis.

Hypocellular MDS should be considered when the bone marrow cellularity is less than 30% or less than 20% in patients over 60 years of age.[43] The criteria for MDS must be met in hypoplastic cases as well as the hypercellular or normocellular cases. Dysplasia can be difficult to identify and dyserythropoiesis has been described in aplastic anemia. Dysmegakaryopoiesis and dysgranulopoiesis, however, are most characteristic of MDS and may be helpful findings. In addition, ALIP (see page 536), indicating an abnormal bone marrow architecture, is typical of MDS. Chromosomal abnormalities, if present, help distinguish MDS from aplastic anemia. The distinction of MDS from AML may be made by the blast count. A count over 30% is indicative of AML.

MDS WITH FIBROSIS

Mild to moderate fibrosis has been described in up to 50% of patients with MDS. The incidence of fibrosis appears to be even greater in therapy-related MDS. If fibrosis is present, other diagnoses should be excluded, including myelofibrosis with myeloid metaplasia (MMM), chronic myelocytic leukemia, and acute megakaryocytic leukemia. Severe myelofibrosis in MDS is not common. In MDS patients with fibrosis there is typically pancytopenia, hypocellular bone marrow with fibrosis, trilineage dysplasia, small megakaryocytes with hypolobulated nuclei, and the absence of hepatomegaly and prominent splenomegaly.[12,44] The increased fibrosis is thought to be produced by liberation of cytokines such as transforming growth factor-β (TGF-β) and platelet derived growth factor from dysplastic megakaryocytes.[11]

UNCLASSIFIABLE MDS

In up to 10% of cases, the MDS does not fit the FAB subgrouping criteria. The most common reason is the presence of overlapping features of trilineage dysplasia and less than 5% blasts. Often the blast count favors the refractory anemia subgroup, but trilineage dysplasia favors the RAEB subgroup. Survival is poor, which favors RAEB. In the WHO classification there is a new subgroup for these MDS cases, refractory cytopenia with multilineage dysplasia (RCMD).

To avoid overlap or contradiction in classifying MDS, a sequential approach has been suggested[45] (Figure 28-11 ■). Classification begins with the blast count, proceeds to the monocyte count and then to the ringed sideroblast count. In this system, the RA subgroup is a classification arrived at by exclusion of the other four.

THERAPY-RELATED MYELODYSPLASIA

Myelodysplasia secondary to alkylating chemotherapy and/or radiotherapy for other malignant or nonmalignant diseases is frequently referred to as therapy-related or treatment-related MDS (t-MDS). It should be kept in mind, however, that

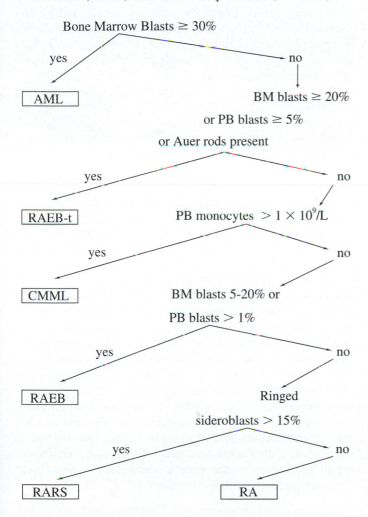

■ **FIGURE 28-11** Sequential approach to classifying MDS according to the FAB criteria. Classification begins with the bone marrow blast count to differentiate MDS from acute leukemia. Key: BM = bone marrow; PB = peripheral blood; AML = acute myeloid leukemia.

MDS may develop as a second primary disorder, unrelated to therapy, especially if MDS develops after a very short or a very long time after therapy. A study of 65 patients with t-MDS or acute leukemia suggests that panmyelosis related to therapy develops in three stages: (1) pancytopenia with myelodysplastic changes and less than 5% blasts; (2) frank MDS which resembles RAEB or RAEB-t; and (3) overt AML.[38] Not all stages are found in all patients, as some present with overt AML while others expire from infection, hemorrhage, or other disease before developing MDS or AML. Development of MDS or acute leukemia appears to be related to the duration, amount, and repetition of the therapy as well as the age of the patient.

Cases of t-MDS tend to have a younger age of onset, an increased frequency and severity of thrombocytopenia, and a greater proportion of patients presenting with RAEB and RAEB-t than cases of primary MDS.[10] The t-MDS are often difficult to classify according to the FAB criteria, and t-MDS has been suggested as a separate category in the WHO classification system.[4] In most cases, the qualitative changes are marked with trilineage involvement, typical of RAEB or RAEB-t. The number of blasts, however, is usually less than 5%, typical of RA. Despite the low percentage of blasts, the clinical course of the disease reflects profound marrow failure, and the outcome is very unfavorable with a median survival of 4–6 months.[38] About 25% of patients have blast counts of 5–20%, which, together with the marked qualitative changes in all cell lines, qualifies for the RAEB classification. The bone marrow is most often hypercellular or normocellular. The finding of increased megakaryocytes is associated with increased fibrosis. Similar to primary MDS, about 30% of t-MDS evolve to acute leukemia.[38]

THE 5q– SYNDROME

MDS patients with an isolated deletion of the long arm of chromosome 5 (del 5q or 5q–) and no other chromosomal abnormalities appear to have a unique disease course characterized by a favorable prognosis and low risk of transformation into AML. There is a marked predominance of cases in women (70%) and the mean age at presentation is 66 years. The main features are macrocytic anemia, moderate leukopenia, normal to increased platelet count, hypolobulated megakaryocytes, and less than 20% blasts in the bone marrow. A number of genes coding for hematopoietic growth factors and their receptors are localized on the long arm of chromosome 5. It has been suggested that loss of these genes and/or tumor supressor genes may be involved in the pathogenesis of disease.[3,12,46] This is a separate MDS subgroup in the WHO classification.

CHILDHOOD MDS

There are few reports of MDS in children. This may be due to lack of a widely accepted classification system and clear diagnostic criteria. In most cases, however, the FAB classification can be applied successfully.[47] Dysplasia in children with MDS is less pronounced; there is a predominance of the more aggressive subtypes (RAEB, RAEB-t); and progression to acute leukemia is faster than in adults.[24,48] Age of two years or less and a hemoglobin F level of 10% or higher are associated with a poor prognosis.[12] Cytogenetic abnormalities are seen in approximately 70% of cases, and monosomy 7 is the most common cytogenetic change. Unlike adults, abnormalities of chromosome 7 do not seem to be associated with a poor prognosis in children. One-third of children with MDS suffer from genetic predisposition syndromes, such as trisomy 21 or trisomy 8.[47] Thus, it is believed that childhood MDS has a different etiology and pathogenesis than the adult form and that genetic predispositon is a factor.[47]

▶ CYTOGENETICS AND MOLECULAR TESTING

Abnormal karyotypes can be demonstrated in up to 50% of individuals with MDS (Table 28-4 ✪). These are acquired clonal aberrations, as are those seen in patients with AML.[36] However, the types of chromosomal abnormalities seen in

✪ TABLE 28-4

Cytogenetic Abnormalities in MDS

Chromosome Abnormality	Frequency (%)
Interstitial or terminal deletion	
del 5q	20
del 7q	10–20*
del 20q	3–5
der or del 11q	2–3
der or del 12p	1–4
Chromosome deletion	
del (7)	10–50*
del (Y)	3–10*
del (17)	3–17*
Chromosome duplication	
trisomy 8	10–15
trisomy 11	3
trisomy 21	2
Translocations	
t(3;3)(q21;q26), or inv 3 (q21;q26)	2–6*
t(1;7)(p11;p11)	1–5*
t(5;17) or t(7;17)(p11;p11)	2–8*
Isochromosome	
Iso (17q)	1–4*
Complex pattern	15–50*

*Higher value denotes frequency in therapy-related MDS.
(Reprinted, with permission, from: List AF, Doll DC. The myelodysplastic syndromes. Lee GR, Foerster J, Lukens J, et al. In: *Wintrobe's Clinical Hematology*, 10th ed. Baltimore: Williams and Wilkins; 1999, p. 2329.)

MDS are usually unbalanced (deletions or extra chromosomes) in contrast to the inversions or translocations seen in AML. The more frequent cytogenetic abnormalities involve structural or numeric abnormalities of chromosomes 5 and 7 and trisomy 8.

The best characterized and most common chromosome defect in MDS is the deletion of the long arm of chromosome 5, known as the 5q–syndrome, discussed previously. Another common abnormality is deletion of the long arm of chromosome 7 (7q–) or deletion of the whole chromosome (–7). The long arm contains the proto-oncogene ERB-B, which is the gene for the receptor of the epidermal growth factor (EGF). This abnormality is most common in pediatric MDS.[49] Trisomy 8 (+8) is found in about 10–15% of the MDS abnormal karyotypes. Chromosome 8 contains the MYC proto-ongogene that codes for a nuclear transcription factor.

Adult MDS patients with chromosome aberrations have a worse prognosis than patients with a normal karyotype and show increased incidence of progression to acute leukemia and complications of marrow failure. The emergence of new abnormal clones is associated with transformation to a more aggressive subgroup of AML.

The t-MDS have more frequent and complex abnormalities than those found in primary MDS. Chromosome changes are almost always present in t-MDS and are usually multiple at diagnosis. The majority of karyotypic abnormalities include abnormalities of chromosomes 5 and/or 7 either singly or in combination with other abnormalities.[50] In Table 28-4 ✪, the higher numbers refer to t-MDS. In contrast to primary MDS, there may be extreme variability in karyotypic aberrations with no two cells exhibiting the same abnormality.

Examination of the bone marrow for cytogenetic abnormalities has become a critical part of the diagnosis and evaluation of the MDS. New techniques such as fluorescence in situ hybridization (FISH) have improved the identification of chromosome abnormalities using specific DNA probes. Molecular diagnostic techniques are also becoming important tools for identification of genetic abnormalities that may aid in more reliable classification and treatment of these diseases. One example is identification of the BCR/ABL fusion gene, which is found in almost all cases of Philadelphia-chromosome-negative chronic myelogenous leukemia (CML) and distinguishes it from CMML. In contrast, another molecular abnormality, the RAS mutation, is uncommon in CML but is present in 40–50% of cases of CMML.[3] In the future, the MDS as well as acute leukemias will be classified according to specific molecular genetic abnormalities along with the corresponding clinical symptoms.

▶ PROGNOSIS

The median survival for all types of MDS is less than two years; however, some patients may survive many years with continuous transfusion therapy. The mortality rate varies

✪ TABLE 28-5

Median Survival and Leukemic Progression in MDS According to FAB Subtype*

FAB Subtype (%)	Median Survival in Months (Range)	% Leukemic Transformation (Range)
RA (25)	37 (19–64)	11 (0–20)
RARS (18)	49 (21–76)	5 (0–15)
CMML (17)	22 (8–60+)	20 (3–55)
RAEB (28)	9 (7–15)	23 (11–50)
RAEB-t (12)	6 (5–12)	48 (11–75)

*Meta-analysis of 1914 patients.
Reprinted from: Sanz GF, Sanz MA. Prognostic factors in myelodysplastic syndromes. *Leukemia Research.* 1992; 16(1):82 with permission from Elsevier Science.

from 58% to 72%. Leukemic transformation ranges in incidence from 10% to 40%.[51] The incidence of transformation appears to be less in RA and RARS. RA and RARS, however, may show progression to RAEB, RAEB-t, and finally, acute leukemia. The most valuable prognostic factor appears to be the percentage of blasts in peripheral blood and bone marrow, with RAEB and RAEB-t having the lowest median survival.[52] (Table 28-5 ✪).

Several scoring systems to be used in conjunction with the FAB criteria have been introduced in the past to aid in predicting survival and acute leukemia risk in the MDS.[53–56] In an attempt to improve on previous systems, recently the International Myelodysplastic Syndrome Risk Analysis Workshop introduced the International Prognostic Scoring System (IPSS)[57,58] (Table 28–6 ✪). This system was developed using data from seven large studies that had previously gen-

erated prognostic systems. The major variables having an impact on disease outcome and risk of evolution to acute leukemia were cytogenetic abnormalities, percentage of blasts in the bone marrow, and number of cytopenias. Other variables that influenced survival were age and gender. Low scores correlate with prolonged survival. The use of scoring is recommended, especially in cases of t-MDS, to determine if those with a more favorable outcome can be identified at initial diagnosis.[35]

ⓔ CASE STUDY *(continued from page 541)*

The karyotype of the patient showed multiple complex abnormalities.

12. Using the International Prognostic Scoring System (IPSS), what is the prognosis for this patient?

► THERAPY

In patients with pancytopenia, morbidity is associated with infection, bleeding, and anemia. The most common causes of death are hemorrhage and infection. Supportive care includes transfusions with leukocyte-depleted erythrocytes and platelets and prophylactic or curative antibiotic therapy. Patients with poor prognosis may be treated more aggressively with AML-type chemotherapeutic regimens. In general MDS patients receiving standard induction therapy as for AML have a lower rate of complete remission, shorter duration of remission, and higher rate of relapse than patients with AML.[12] Differentiation-inducing agents such as cytosine arabinoside (Ara-C) have shown limited success, with

✪ TABLE 28-6

International Prognostic Scoring System (IPSS) for the Myelodysplastic Syndromes

Score Value	Cytopenias	BM Blasts (%)	Karyotype	Total Score	Risk Group	Median Survival (yrs)
0	0–1	<5	Normal, -Y only, del (5q) only del (20q) only	0	Low	5.7
				0.5–1.0	Int. 1	3.5
				1.5–2.0	Int. 2	1.2
0.5	2–3	5–10	Other abns.	>2.5	High	0.4
1.0	—	—	Complex >2 abns. chr 7 abns.			
1.5	—	11–20	—			
2.0	—	21–30	—			

Cytopenias = hemoglobin <10g/dL, platelets <100 × 10⁹/L, or neutrophils <1.8 × 10⁹/L in the peripheral blood; BM = bone marrow; abns. = abnormalities; Int. = Intermediate; yrs. = years; chr. = chromosome
(Adapted, with permission, from: Greenberg PL, Sanz GF, Sanz MA. Prognostic scoring system for risk assessment in myelodysplastic syndromes. *Forum: Trends in Experimental and Clinical Medicine.* 1999; 9(1):17.)

some patients achieving complete remission while others develop myelotoxicity or die from treatment-related causes.[59,60] In the last several years investigators have studied hematopoietic cytokines and growth factors as a possible supportive treatment for MDS. Studies with GM-CSF, G-CSF, and IL-3 show that the growth factors improve the neutrophil count in most cases.[61] Erythropoietin is effective in some patients, leading to decreased requirement for transfusions. Recent studies show that the use of a combination of erythropoietin and G-CSF appears to be effective as support-ive therapy.[12] Stimulation of megakaryopoiesis is least successful.[62] Use of cytokines that stimulate platelet production (IL-11, thrombopoietin) has not been successful due to detrimental side effects. Further studies are needed using combinations of growth factors.

Bone marrow transplant is the only curative treatment available and is the treatment of choice for those under 50 years of age. Allogenic stem-cell transplantation has been the most successful procedure for medically appropriate patients with HLA-matched donors.[12]

SUMMARY

The myelodysplastic syndromes are pluripotential stem cell disorders characterized by one or more peripheral blood cytopenias and prominent cellular maturation abnormalities. The bone marrow is usually normocellular or hypercellular, indicating there is a high degree of ineffective hematopoiesis. Proto-oncogene mutations are commonly found in patients with MDS. Thus, oncogenes probably play a role in the pathogenesis of MDS.

Although anemia is the most common cytopenia, neutropenia and thrombocytopenia also occur. Erythrocytes are macrocytic or less frequently normocytic. Erythropoiesis in the bone marrow is abnormal with megaloblastoid features commonly present. Neutrophils may show hypolobulation of the nucleus and hypogranulation. Megakaryocytes also show megaloblastoid features and hypolobulation of the nucleus. Platelets may be large and agranular.

The FAB group has classified the MDS into five subgroups dependent on the blast count, degree of dyspoiesis and cytopenias, and presence of ringed sideroblasts. These include RA, RARS, RAEB, RAEB-t, and CMML. Those subgroups with higher blast counts and more involvement of cell lines in dyspoiesis are more aggressive disorders. The MDS frequently terminate in acute leukemia. Treatment is primarily supportive unless the patient is a candidate for bone marrow transplant.

REVIEW QUESTIONS

LEVEL I

1. In addition to the number of blasts, what other criterion is essential for a diagnosis of RARS? (Checklist #2)
   a. ≥15% ringed sideroblasts
   b. ≥30% ringed sideroblasts
   c. dyshematopoiesis in all three cell lineages
   d. pancytopenia

2. CMML differs from the other subgroups of MDS because it has: (Checklist #2)
   a. a lymphocytosis in the peripheral blood
   b. a mature granulocytosis in the peripheral blood
   c. a hypocellular bone marrow
   d. a monocytopenia

3. The FAB classification system is based on: (Checklist #2)
   a. immunologic cell markers
   b. cytogenetics
   c. morphology
   d. all of the above

4. The type of anemia usually seen in MDS is: (Checklist #1)
   a. macrocytic, normochromic
   b. normocytic, normochromic
   c. microcytic, hypochromic
   d. normocytic, hypochromic

LEVEL II

1. What is the minimum number of bone marrow blasts needed for a diagnosis of acute leukemia? (Checklist #4)
   a. 29%
   b. 50%
   c. 5%
   d. 30%

2. The t-MDS differ from primary MDS in that t-MDS: (Checklist #6)
   a. is usually the less aggressive subgroup
   b. has more peripheral blood blasts
   c. has fewer and less complex abnormal karyotypes
   d. is more difficult to classify into a subgroup of MDS

3. Progression of MDS to acute leukemia is characterized by: (Checklist #4)
   a. an increase in blast population
   b. decreased bone marrow cellularity
   c. a decreased M:E ratio
   d. splenomegaly

REVIEW QUESTIONS *(continued)*

LEVEL I

5. The most common cytopenia(s) seen in MDS is(are): (Checklist #3)
   a. leukopenia
   b. thrombocytopenia
   c. anemia
   d. a combination of two of the above

6. The typical bone marrow cellularity in MDS is: (Checklist #3)
   a. hypocellular
   b. normocellular
   c. hypercellular
   d. fibrotic

7. The bone marrow in suspected MDS should be stained with the Prussian blue stain to check for: (Checklist #3)
   a. Type II blasts
   b. fibrosis
   c. karyorrhexis
   d. ringed sideroblasts

8. The most common dyserythropoietic finding in the bone marrow in MDS is: (Checklist #3)
   a. megaloblastoid development
   b. impaired hemoglobinization
   c. pseudo–Pelger-Huët cells
   d. agranular cytoplasm

9. The combined esterase stain will be most helpful in establishing a diagnosis in which MDS subgroup? (Checklist #3)
   a. RA
   b. RARS
   c. RAEB
   d. CMML

10. Which of the following are synonyms for myelodysplastic syndrome: (Checklist #1)
    (1) preleukemia
    (2) smoldering leukemia
    (3) dysmyelopoietic syndrome
    (4) myeloproliferative syndrome
    a. 1 and 3
    b. 2 and 4
    c. 1, 2, and 3
    d. 1, 2, 3, 4

LEVEL II

4. A cell resembling a blast that contains 18 primary granules and a centrally located nucleus would be classified as a: (Checklist #2)
   a. Type I blast
   b. Type II blast
   c. Type III blast
   d. promyelocyte

5. The contrast between a hypercellular bone marrow and a cytopenic peripheral blood film seen in MDS is attributed to: (Checklist #1)
   a. premature destruction of abnormal cells in the bone marrow (ineffective hematopoiesis)
   b. production of blood cells outside the bone marrow (extramedullary hematopoiesis)
   c. immune destruction of cells in the peripheral blood
   d. splenic sequestration

6. Which of the following would be most helpful to differentiate CMML from CML? (Checklist #7)
   a. percentage of bone marrow blasts
   b. elevated leukocyte count
   c. presence of nucleated RBCs
   d. karyotype

7. The most effective treatment for MDS is currently considered to be: (Checklist #3)
   a. chemotherapy
   b. immunotherapy
   c. hematopoietic growth factors
   d. bone marrow transplant

Use the following case history to answer questions 8–10.

A patient presents with the following laboratory data:

RBC:	2.30×10^{12}/L
Hgb:	78 g/L
Hct:	0.24 L/L
MCV:	104 fL
RDW:	20
WBC:	8.5×10^9/L
PLT:	140×10^9/L

The differential was normal except for 2% metamyelocytes. Oval macrocytes, a few abnormal NRBC, and a few siderocytes were seen. The bone marrow contained 3% blasts and exhibited hypercellularity with megaloblastoid development in erythroid cells.

8. What is the most probable MDS subgroup? (Checklist #8)
   a. RA
   b. RARS
   c. RAEB
   d. RAEB-t

REVIEW QUESTIONS (continued)

LEVEL I

LEVEL II

9. What other hematologic disorder does this peripheral blood picture resemble? (Checklist #7)
   a. aplastic anemia
   b. megaloblastic anemia
   c. iron deficiency anemia
   d. anemia of chronic disease

10. What laboratory test(s) would be helpful to distinguish the two disorders? (Checklist #7)
    a. serum lysozyme
    b. serum ferritin
    c. serum folate and vitamin B_{12}
    d. combined esterase stain

www.prenhall.com/mckenzie

Use the above address to access the free, interactive Companion Web site created for this textbook. Get hints, instant feedback, and textbook references to chapter-related multiple choice questions.

REFERENCES

1. Coiffier B, Bryon PA, Fiere D, et al. Dysmyelopoietic syndromes: A search for prognostic factors in 193 patients. *Cancer.* 1983; 52:83–90.

2. Bennett JM, Catovsky D, Daniel MT, et al. Proposals for the classification of the myelodysplastic syndromes. *Bri. J Haematol.* 1982; 51:189–99.

3. Mijovic A, Mufti GJ. The myelodysplastic syndromes: Towards a more functional classification. *Blood Reviews.* 1998; 12:73–83.

4. Harris NL, Jaffe ES, Diebold J, et al. The World Health Organization classification of neoplastic diseases of the haematopoietic and lymphoid tissues: Report of the Clinical Advisory Committee Meeting, Airlie House, Virginia, November 1997. *Histopathology.* 2000; 36: 69–87.

5. Raskind WH, Tirumali N, Jacobson R, Singer J, Fialkow PJ, et al. Evidence for a multistep pathogenesis of a myelodysplastic syndrome. *Blood.* 1984; 63:1318–23.

6. Musilova J, Michalova K. Chromosome study of 85 patients with myelodysplastic syndrome. *Cancer Genet. Cytogenet.* 1988; 33:39–50.

7. Okuda T, Yokota S, Maekawa T, et al. Cytogenetic evidence for a clonal involvement of granulocyte-macrophage and erythroid lineages in a patient with refractory anaemia. *Acta Haemat.* 1988; 80:110–5.

8. Prchal JT, Throckmorton DW, Carroll AJ 3rd, Fuson EW, Garns RA, Prchal JF, et al. A common progenitor for human myeloid and lymphoid cells. *Nature.* 1978; 274:590–1.

9. Weimar IS, Bourhis JH, DeGast GC, Gerritsen WR. Clonality in myelodysplastic syndromes. *Leuk Lymph.* 1994; 13:215–21.

10. Aul C, Bowen DT, Yoshida Y. Pathogenesis, etiology, and epidemiology of myelodysplastic syndromes. *Haematologica.* 1998; 83:71–86.

11. List AF, Doll DC. The myelodysplastic syndromes. Lee GR, Foerster J, Lukens J, Paraskevas F, Greer JP, Rodgers GM, editors. In: *Wintrobe's Clinical Hematology,* 10th ed. Baltimore: Williams and Wilkins, 1999; pp. 2320–41.

12. Heaney ML, Golde DW. Myelodysplasia. *New Engl J Med.* 1999; 340 (21):1649–60.

13. Besa EC. Myelodysplastic syndromes (refractory anemia): A perspective of the biologic, clinical, and therapeutic issues. *Med Clin North Am.* 1992; 76:599–617.

14. Bartram CR. Molecular genetic aspects of mylodysplastic syndromes. *Hematol/Oncol Clin North Am.* 1992; 6:557–70.

15. Willemze R, Fibbe WE, Falkenburg JH, Kluin-Nelemans JC, Luin PM, Landegent JE. Biology and treatment of myelodysplastic syndromes: Developments in the past decade. *Ann Hematol.* 1993; 66:107–15.

16. Doll DC, List AF. Myelodysplastic syndromes. *West J. Med.* 1989; 151:161–67.

17. Hirai H, Okada M, Mizoguchi H, et al. Relationship between an activated N-ras oncogene and chromosomal abnormality during leukemic progression from myelodysplastic syndrome. *Blood.* 1988; 71:256–68.

18. Willman CL. Molecular genetic features of myelodysplastic syndromes. *Leukemia.* 1998; 12 (suppl.1):S2–S6.

19. Dormer P, Hershko C, Wilmanns W. Mechanisms and prognostic value of cell kinetics in the myelodysplastic syndromes. *Br. J. Haemat.* 1987; 67:147–52.

20. Mufti GH, Parker JE. Ineffective haemopoiesis and apoptosis in myelodysplastic syndromes. *British J of Haematology.* 1998; 101:220–30.

21. Yoshida Y, Mufti GJ. Apoptosis and its significance in MDS: Controversies revisited. *Leukemia Research.* 1999; 23:777–85.

22. Degnan T, Weiselberg L, Schulman P, Budman DR. Dysmyelopoietic syndrome. *Am J Med.* 1984; 76:122–28.

23. Ciccone G, Mirabelli D, Levis A, et al. Myeloid leukemias and myelodysplastic syndromes: Chemical exposure, histologic subtype, and cytogenetics in a case-control study. *Cancer Genet Cytogenet.* 1993; 68:135–39.

24. Gadner H, Haas OA. Experience in pediatric myelodysplastic syndromes. *Hematol/Oncol Clin North Am.* 1992; 6:655–72.

25. Hasle H. Myelodysplastic syndromes in childhood: Classification, epidemiology, and treatment. *Leuk Lymph.* 1994; 13:11–26.

26. Blank J, Lange B. Preleukemia in children. *J Pediatr.* 1981; 98: 565–68.

27. Pomeroy C, Oken MM, Rydell RE, Felice GA. Infection in the myelodysplastic syndromes. *Am J Med.* 1991; 90:338–44.

28. Juneja SK, Imbert M, Jouault H, Scoazec JY, Sigaux F, Sultan C. Haematological features of primary myelodysplastic syndromes (PMDS) at initial presentation: A study of 118 cases. *J. Clin Pathol.* 1983; 36:1129–35.

29. Noel P, Solberg LA. Myelodysplastic syndromes: Pathogenesis, diagnosis, and treatment. *Crit Rev Oncol/Hematol.* 1992; 12(3):193–215.

30. Sanz GF, Sanz MA. Prognostic factors in myelodysplastic syndromes. *Leuk Res.* 1992; 16:77–86.

31. Rios A, Canizo MC, Sanz MA, et al. Bone marrow biopsy in myelodysplastic syndromes: Morphological characteristics and contribution to the study of prognostic factors. *Br J Haemat.* 1990; 75:26–33.

32. Yoshida Y, Stephenson J, Mufti GJ. Myelodysplastic syndromes: From morphology to molecular biology. Part K. Classification, natural history and cell biology of myelodysplasia. *Int J Hematol.* 1993; 57:87–97.

33. Colombat PH, Renoux M, Lamagnere J, Renous G. Immunologic indices in myelodysplastic syndromes. *Cancer.* 1988; 61:1075–81.

34. Goasguen JE, et al. Prognostic implication and characterization of the blast cell population in the myelodysplastic syndrome. *Leuk Res.* 1991; 15:1159–65.

35. Third MIC Cooperative Study Group Recommendations for a morphologic, immunologic, and cytogenetic (MIC) working classification of the primary and therapy-related myelodysplastic disorders. *Cancer Genet Cytogenet.* 1988; 32:1–10.

36. Kristensen JS. Immunophenotyping in acute leukemia, myelodysplastic syndromes, and hairy cell leukemia. *Dan Med Bulle.* 1994; 41:52–65.

37. Elghetany MT. Surface marker abnormalities in myelodysplastic syndromes. *Haematologica.* 1998; 83:1104–15.

38. Michels SD, McKenna RW, Arthur DC, Brunning RD. Therapy related acute myeloid leukemia and myelodysplastic syndromes: A clinical and morphologic study of 65 cases. *Blood.* 1985; 65: 1364–72.

39. Kushner JP, Lee GR, Wintrobe MM. Idiopathic refractory sideroblastic anemia: Clinical and laboratory investigations of 17 patients and review of the literature. *Medicine.* 1971; 50:139–59.

40. Sultan C, Imbert M, Ricard MF, Marquet M. Myelodysplastic syndromes. Lewis SM, Verwilgen RL. In: *Dyserythropoiesis.* London: Academic Press; 1977.

41. Tefferi A, Hoaglund HC, Therneau TM, Pierre RV. Chronic myelomonocytic leukemia: Natural history and prognostic determinants. *Mayo Clin. Proc.* 1989; 64:1246–54.

42. Miescher PA, Farquet JJ. Chronic myelomonocytic leukemia in adults. *Sem Hematol.* 1974; 11(2):129–39.

43. Dickstein JI, Vardiman JW. Issues in the pathology and diagnosis of the chronic myeloproliferative disorders and the myelodysplastic syndromes. *Am J Clin Pathol.* 1993; 99:513–25.

44. Kampmeier P, Anastasi J, and Vardiman JW. Issues in the pathology of the myelodysplastic syndromes. *Hematol/Oncol Clin North Am.* 1992; 6:501–22.

45. Ho PJ, Gibson J, Vincent P, Joshua D. The myelodysplastic syndromes: Diagnostic criteria and laboratory evaluation. *Path.* 1993; 25:297–304.

46. Boultwood J, Lewis S, Wainscoat JS. The 5q–syndrome. *J of American Society of Hematology.* 1994; 84(10):3253–60.

47. Haas OA, Gadner H. Pathogenesis, biology, and management of myelodysplastic syndromes in children. *Seminars in Hematology.* 1996; 33(3):225–35.

48. Truncer MA, et al. Primary myelodysplastic syndrome in children: The clinical experience in 33 cases. *Br J Haematol.* 1992; 82:347–53.

49. Noel P, Tefferi A, Pierre RV, Jenkins RB, and Dewald GW. Karyotypic analysis in primary myelodysplastic syndromes. *Blood Rev.* 1993; 7:10–18.

50. Iurlo A, Mecucci C, Van Orshoven A, et al. Cytogenetic and clinical investigations in 76 cases with therapy-related leukemia and myelodysplastic syndrome. *Cancer Genet Cytogenet.* 1989; 43:227–41.

51. Ganser A, Hoelzer D. Clinical course of myelodysplastic syndromes. *Hematol/Oncol Clin North Am.* 1992; 6:607–18.

52. Kerkhofs H, Hermans J, Haak HL, Leeksma CHW. Utility of the FAB classification for myelodysplastic syndromes: Investigation of prognostic factors in 237 cases. *Br J Haemat.* 1987; 65:73–81.

53. Mufti GJ, Stevens JR, Oscier DG, Hamblin TJ, Machin D. Myelodysplastic syndromes: A scoring system with prognostic significance. *Br J Haemat.* 1985; 59:425–33.

54. Varela BL, Chuang C, Wall JE, Bennett JM. Modifications in the classification of primary myelodysplastic syndromes: The addition of a scoring system. *Hemat Onc.* 1985; 3:55–63.

55. Aul C, Schneider W. Myelodysplastic syndromes: A prognostic factor analysis of 221 untreated patients. *Blut.* 1988; 57:234.

56. Sanz GF, Sanz MA, Vallespi T, et al. Two regression models and a scoring system for predicting survival and planning treatment in myelodysplastic syndromes: A multivariate analysis of prognostic factors in 370 patients. *Blood.* 1989; 74:395–408.

57. Greenberg P, Cox C, LeBeau MM, et al. International scoring system for evaluating prognosis in myelodysplastic syndromes. *Blood.* 1997; 89(6):2079–88.

58. Greenberg PL, Sanz GF, Sanz MA. Prognostic scoring systems for risk assessment in myeloproliferative syndromes. *Forum.* 1999; 9(1): 17–31.

59. Cheson BD. The myelodysplastic syndromes: Current approaches to therapy. *Ann Intern Med.* 1990; 112:932–41.

60. Willemze R, Fibbe WE, Falkenburg JH, Kluin-Nelemans JC, Kluin PM, Landegent JE. Biology and treatment of myelodysplastic syndromes: Developments in the past decade. *Ann Hematol.* 1993; 66:107–15.

61. Ganser A, Hoelzer D. Treatment of myelodysplastic syndromes with hematopoietic growth factors. *Hematol/Oncol Clin North Am.* 1992; 6:633–53.

62. Arcenas AG, Vadhan-Rah S. Hematopoietic growth factor therapy of myelodysplastic syndromes. *Leuk Lymph.* 1993; 11(suppl 2):65–69.

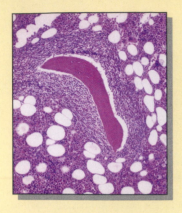

29

Acute Myelogenous Leukemias

Susan J. Leclair, Ph.D.

■ CHECKLIST - LEVEL I

By the end of this unit of study the student should be able to:

1. Define *acute leukemia* and explain the difference between acute myelogenous leukemia (AML) and acute lymphocytic leukemia (ALL).

2. List and define the common variants seen in AML as defined by the FAB classification.

3. Describe and recognize the typical peripheral blood picture (erythrocytes, leukocytes, and thrombocytes) seen in AML.

4. Describe the M:E ratio in bone marrow in acute leukemia (AL).

5. Differentiate Type I, II, and III blasts found in hematopoietic neoplasms.

6. Give the typical results of cytochemical stains in AML.

■ CHECKLIST - LEVEL II

At the end of this unit of study the student should be able to:

1. Compare and contrast the various presentations of AML.

2. Predict the most likely FAB subgroup based on patient history, physical assessment, and laboratory findings.

3. Correlate cellular presentation of AML with prognosis and common complications.

4. Correlate Wright-stain morphology of the AML subgroups with cytochemical stains, flow cytometry, and genetic testing.

5. Evaluate peripheral blood results in relation to oncological therapy (i.e., complete or partial remission, relapse, engraftment).

6. Evaluate patient data from the medical history and laboratory results to determine if a disorder can be classifed, and if not, specify the additional testing to be performed.

7. Compare the WHO and FAB classifications of AML.

KEY TERMS

Acute leukemias (AL)
Auer rods
FAB criteria
Faggot cells
CD33, CD13, CD34
CD19, CD10, CD22
CD7, CD2, CD3, CD5
Phi body
Pseudo–Pelger-Huët cell
Type I myeloblasts
Type II myeloblasts
Type III myeloblasts

BACKGROUND BASICS

The information in this chapter will build upon concepts learned in previous chapters. To maximize your learning experience you should review and have an understanding of these concepts before starting this unit of study.

Level I

▶ Describe the origin and differentiation of hematopoietic cells. (Chapter 2)

▶ Summarize the maturation, differentiation, and function of the leukocyte. (Chapter 6)

▶ Outline the classification and general laboratory findings of the acute leukemias. (Chapter 26)

▶ List and describe the cytochemical stains used to differentiate acute leukemias. (Chapter 26)

Level II

▶ Summarize the role of oncogenes and growth factors in cell proliferation, differentiation, and maturation. (Chapter 2)

▶ Describe the role of molecular analysis in diagnosis and treatment of acute leukemia. (Chapter 25)

▶ Describe the use of immunophenotyping in acute leukemia. (Chapter 23)

▶ Describe the role of cytogenetics in diagnosis and treatment of acute leukemia. (Chapter 24)

ⓔ CASE STUDY

We will refer to this case study throughout the chapter.
Mr. Guerro, a 34-year-old Latin-American male, had been in excellent health until two weeks before admission when he noticed a mild sore throat and was seen at a neighborhood clinic where penicillin was prescribed. He was able to return to work and felt better until four days prior to admission, when he developed a fever and experienced easy bruising. He noticed other bleeding symptoms including gingival bleeding and petechiae. He reported to the emergency room. A CBC revealed a WBC count of 26.2×10^9/L and 6% blasts. He was admitted for further evaluation. Consider what additional laboratory testing may assist in the diagnosis of this patient.

▶ OVERVIEW

This chapter describes the acute myelogenous leukemias (AML), also known as acute nonlymphocytic leukemias (ANLL). It begins with an account of the general laboratory findings in AML. This is followed by a specific description of each subgroup in the FAB classification including clinical and laboratory findings with an emphasis on defining characteristics. The chapter concludes with a look at the current types of therapy used to treat AML.

▶ INTRODUCTION

All **acute leukemias** (AL) are stem cell disorders characterized by malignant neoplastic proliferation and accumulation of immature and nonfunctional hematopoietic cells in the bone marrow. The neoplastic cells apparently escape programmed cell death (apoptosis). The net effect is expansion of the leukemic clone and a decrease in normal cells.[1]

Because leukemia is a clonal expansion of a single transformed stem cell, all acute leukemias begin long before there are any signs and symptoms. It is believed that a tumor burden of 10^{12} cells is sufficient for recognizable signs and symptoms. Lethal levels of tumor burden occur at neoplastic cell numbers of 10^{13-14} or higher. As the tumor burden grows, the normal functional marrow cells decrease. Death from either infection or hemorrhage results in weeks to months unless there is therapeutic intervention.[2]

There are two major categories of acute leukemias classified according to the cellular origin of the primary stem cell defect: AML and ALL. If the defect affects primarily the myeloid stem cells (CFU-GEMM, CFU-GM, CFU-E) the leukemia is classified as AML or acute nonlymphocytic leukemia (ANLL). If the defect affects primarily the lymphoid stem cell, the leukemia is classified as ALL.

The most reliable parameters for defining the neoplastic cells in AML and for classifying into subtypes are combinations of neoplastic cell morphology, cytochemical cellular reactions, immunologic probes to define cell markers, and cytogenetic and molecular genetic abnormalities (∞ Chapter 26).

▶ LABORATORY FINDINGS

PERIPHERAL BLOOD

The peripheral blood picture is quite variable. While it is traditional to describe leukemias as having elevated leukocyte counts, 50% of the cases may have decreased counts or counts within reference range. The leukocyte count ranges from less than 1×10^9/L to more than 100×10^9/L. Regardless of the leukocyte concentration, diagnosis of AL is suggested by the presence of blasts on the blood smear. Blasts usually compose from 15–95% of all leukocytes. Experienced clinical laboratory professionals are able to determine the lineage of the leukemic cells by bright-field microscopy on Romanowsky-stained preparations about 75% of the time. The remainder must be identified through cytochemical, immunologic, and/or genetic methods. Typically, the myeloblast seen in AML is approximately 20 μ in diameter with multiple nucleoli in a nucleus composed of euchromatin (genetically active DNA). Granular structures may be present in the cytoplasm.

The erythrocyte population is typically suppressed, and a hemoglobin value less than 10g/dL is common. Erythrocytes may be slightly macrocytic due to an inability to successfully compete with neoplastic cells for folate or vitamin B_{12}. If bleeding has occurred, there may be a microcytic hypochromic component. The RDW will be elevated. Erythrocyte inclusions such as Howell-Jolly bodies, Pappenheimer bodies, and basophilic stippling reflective of erythrocyte maturation defects may be present. Nucleated erythrocytes may be present in proportion to the anemia or marrow damage.

Platelets are typically also decreased and occasional enlarged forms may be present. As the disease progresses it is possible to visualize more immature platelet forms such as megakaryocytic fragments. The platelet count does not correlate with the potential complication of bleeding. Qualitative platelet defects may also be present.

If AL is suspected by the physician but no blast cells can be detected on the blood smear, or if the leukocyte count is low ($<2 \times 10^9$/L), a buffy-coat smear should be prepared. This preparation will reveal the presence of blast cells when these cells are present in very low concentrations. The finding of blasts with azurophilic granules is helpful in identifying the myeloid nature of the leukemia. When **Auer rods** are present in blasts, they exclude a diagnosis of ALL. Auer rods can be found in myeloblasts, monoblasts, and occasionally in more differentiated monocytic or myelocytic cells.

Other abnormal findings on the blood smear often include monocytosis and neutropenia. The monocytosis frequently precedes overt leukemia. The few mature neutrophils present may demonstrate signs of myelodysplasia: pseudo–Pelger-Huët cells, hypogranulation, and small nuclei with hypercondensed chromatin. Signs of myelodysplasia are especially common in AML-M2.[3,4] Eosinophils and basophils may be mildly to markedly increased. When present, basophilia may help to differentiate leukemia from a leukemoid reaction. Absolute basophilia is not present in a leukemoid reaction.

BONE MARROW

The bone marrow sampling should include both aspirate and biopsy specimens. The quality of marrow specimen is critical for all subsequent analyses. Typically, the bone marrow presentation is hypercellular with decreased fat concentration (based on age), a predominance of blasts, and sometimes an increase in fibrosis. According to the **FAB criteria**

for acute leukemia, blasts must compose more than 30% of the nonerythroid nucleated cells in the marrow (>20% in the WHO classification) to distinguish leukemia from the myelodysplastic syndromes. Frequently, the blast count is close to 100%. Auer rods are present in bone marrow blasts in about half the cases of AML.

Cells can be clumped together, occasionally forming sheets of infiltrate that disturb the usual marrow architecture. In addition to light microscopy evaluation, bone marrow samples should be tested for immunologic markers and genetic mutations.

Checkpoint! #1

What results would you expect to find on the CBC and differential in a suspected case of acute leukemia?

OTHER LABORATORY FINDINGS

Other laboratory findings may reflect the increased proliferation and turnover of cells. Hyperuricemia and an increase in lactate dehydrogenase are common findings resulting from the increase in cell turnover. Hypercalcemia, when present, is thought to be caused by increased bone resorption associated with leukemic proliferation in the bone marrow. Increased serum and urine muramidase are typical findings in those leukemias with a monocytic component.

In the acute promyelocytic leukemia (APL or FAB subtype M3), prolonged prothrombin time and partial thromboplastin time, hypofibrinogenemia, and elevated fibrin degradation products are frequently found in association with ecchymoses and overt bleeding.[5]

CASE STUDY (continued from page 557)

Admission laboratory data on Mr. Guerro are as follows:

RBC:	3.2×10^{12}/L
Hb:	9.7 g/dL
Hct:	30.5%
PLT:	31×10^9/L
WBC:	26.2×10^9/L
Differential	
Blasts:	6%
Promyelocytes:	79%
Myelocytes:	5%
Lymphocytes:	11%

Erythrocyte morphology: Erythrocytes are normochromic and normocytic with rare schistocytes seen.

1. What clues do you have that this patient may have an acute leukemia?

2. Based on the presenting data, what additional testing might be of value?

► CLASSIFICATION

As mentioned in ∞ Chapter 26, investigations have shown that the mutant neoplastic stem cell may arise at multiple points in the differentiation scheme of myeloid cells[6] (Figure 29-1 ■). The original classification was based solely on bright-field microscopy and the patient's signs and symptoms at the time of diagnosis. With the inability to catego-

rize all leukemias by bright-field microscopy, the FAB classification was developed in 1976; it blended morphology and cytochemistry to help identify neoplastic blast lineage.[7] The acute leukemias are gouped into acute myelocytic (AML) and acute lymphocytic (ALL). The AML are further subgrouped into eight subgroups. The M0, M1, M2, M3 subtypes exhibit granulocytic differentiation, differing from each other in the degree of granulocyte maturation.[8] The M4 subtype exhibits both granulocytic and monocytic differentiation, whereas M5 shows predominantly monocytic differentiation; M6 shows erythrocytic differentiation; and M7 megakaryocytic differentiation (Table 26-5).

The FAB approach to diagnosing acute leukemia requires a minimal marrow leukocyte blast count of >30%. [9] Occasionally blasts in the peripheral blood are greater than 30% but blasts in the bone marrow are less than 30%. To permit a diagnosis in this case, it has been proposed that the diagnosis of AML be made if the blast count in either the bone marrow and/or peripheral blood is >30%.[10]

The new proposed World Health Organization (WHO) classification expands the parameters used to classify the neoplastic disorders. The parameters include not only microscopic morphology and cytochemistry but also immunologic probes of cell markers, cytogenetic, and molecular genetic abnormalities and clinical syndrome. In this classification, there are four major AML groups, each with variants or subtypes:

- AML with recurrent cytogenetic translocations. AML with specific cytogenetic abnormalities, distinctive clinical findings, and characteristic hematologic morphology are defined as subgroups.
- AML with severe multilineage dysplasia. There are two variants, those with prior history of MDS and those without prior MDS.
- AML secondary to therapy for another disease. These AMLs are distinctly different from de novo (primary) AML.
- AML not classified. Includes any AML not included in the above subgroups.

The subgroups of the WHO AML classification are included in Table 29-1 ✪. The number of blast cells necessary to support a diagnosis of AL in this classification is >20%.[11]

The WHO classification is the result of a worldwide consensus on classification of the hematopoietic neoplasms. Since proponents of other classifications such as the FAB agreed to adopt the new WHO classification as the standard, this system will most certainly eventually replace the FAB and other less-well-known classification systems.

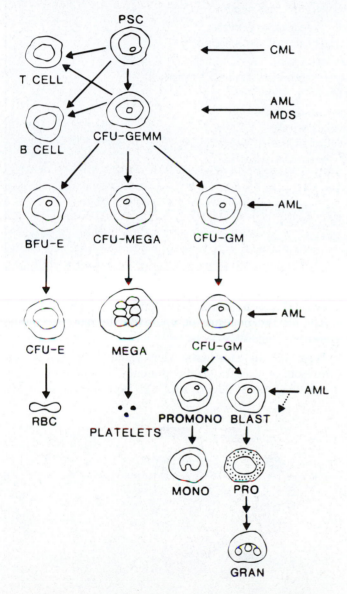

■ **FIGURE 29-1** The possible cells of origin of AML. (PSC—Pluripotential stem cell; CFU—colony-forming unit; GEMM—granulocytic, erythroid, monocytic, megakaryocytic; Mega—megakaryocyte; GM—granulocytic, monocytic; M—monocyte; G—granulocyte; BFU-E—burst-forming unit, erythroid; CFU-E—colony-forming unit, erythroid.) (With permission, from Griffin JD, and Lowenberg B. Clonogenic cells in acute myeloblastic leukemia. *Blood.* 1986;68(6):1305.)

BLAST CLASSIFICATION

Leukemic blasts are abnormal cells and frequently exhibit nuclear/cytoplasmic asynchrony with nuclear maturation lagging. When evaluating cells for the purpose of establishing a diagnosis of AML, the following variations of neoplas-

⊛ **TABLE 29-1**

WHO Classification of AML

Group	Subgroups
Acute myeloid leukemias with recurrent cytogenetic translocations	AML with t(8:21)(q22;q22), AML1(CBFα)/ETO
	Acute promyelocytic leukemia (AML with t[15;17][q22;q11-12] and variants, PML/RARα)
	AML with abnormal bone marrow eosinophils (inv[16][p13q22] or t[16;16][p13;q11], CBFβ/MYH11X)
	AML with 11q23(MLL) abnormalities
Acute myeloid leukemia with multilineage dysplasia	With prior myelodysplastic syndrome
	Without prior myelodysplastic syndrome
Acute myeloid leukemia and myelodysplastic syndrome, therapy related	Alkylating agent related
	Epipodophyllotoxin related (some may be lymphoid)
	Other types
Acute myeloid leukemia (AML) not otherwise categorized	AML minimally differentiated
	AML without maturation
	AML with maturation
	Acute myelomonocytic leukemia
	Acute monocytic leukemia
	Acute erythroid leukemia
	Acute megakaryocytic leukemia
	Acute basophilic leukemia
	Acute panmyelosis with myelofibrosis
Acute biphenotypic leukemia	

tic cells are included in the total blast count when performing a peripheral blood or bone marrow differential:[12]

1. **Type I myeloblasts**: typical myeloblasts with lacy open chromatin and prominent nucleoli, immature deep blue cytoplasm without granules (Figure 29-2 ■).

2. **Type II myeloblasts**: blasts similar to Type I blasts except for the presence of up to 20 discrete azurophilic granules (Figure 29-3 ■).

3. **Type III myeloblasts**: cells resembling the typical myeloblast except for the presence of numerous azurophilic granules (Figure 29-2 ■). (Typically found in M2

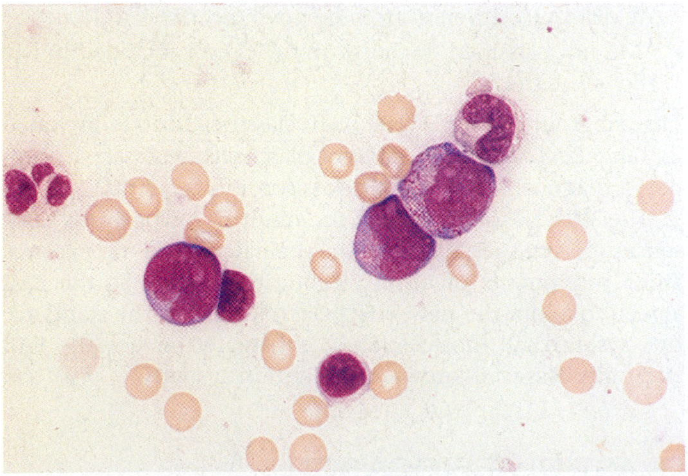

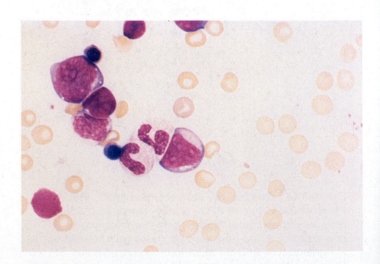

■ **FIGURE 29-2** A Type I blast (left), Type III blast (center), and a promyelocyte (top right). The nuclear chromatin pattern in the two blasts is similar, but the Type III blast has granules. (Bone marrow; Wright-Giemsa stain; 1000× original magnification)

■ **FIGURE 29-3** Type II blast (center) with only a few granules near the periphery of the cell. (Bone marrow; Wright-Giemsa stain; 1000× original magnification)

with a t(8;21) chromosome abnormality, some cases of myelodysplasia and a rare form of M1.)

Other cells recommended to be included in the blast count are: neoplastic promyelocytes associated with M3 AML; monoblasts and promonocytes of M5 AML; and megakaryoblasts of M7 AML.

Since blast cells are undifferentiated cells, they are often difficult to identify by morphology using light microscopy. Cytochemistry and immunophenotyping give additional information that can help define cell lineage (∞ Chapters 23, 26). Also some genetic findings are diagnostic of certain subgroups of leukemia and may be helpful in diagnosis.

✔ Checkpoint! #2

What is the major difference between the FAB and WHO classification systems in differentiating acute leukemia from the other neoplastic hematologic disorders?

CYTOCHEMISTRY

The common cytochemical stains used in the FAB classification include the myeloperoxidase, Sudan black B, naphthol AS-D chloroacetate esterase (specific esterase), and alphanaphthyl esterases (nonspecific esterase). Granulocytic cells stain positive with myelperoxidase and with Sudan black B, while lymphoblasts are negative. Thus these stains help differentiate the acute nonlymphocytic leukemia (ANLL) from ALL. The esterase stains help differentiate precursor granulocytic cells from precursor monocytic cells. Granulocytic cells stain weakly positive with naphthol AS-D chloroacetate esterase. Cells of monocytic lineage stain positive with nonspecific esterase (Table 26-11 ⊙). For a more complete discussion of these stains, refer to ∞ Chapter 26.

CASE STUDY *(continued from page 552)*

3. Based on the peripheral blood examination, what cytochemical stain results would you expect to find on Mr. Guerro's neoplastic cells?

IMMUNOPHENOTYPING

Immunophenotyping is a necessary component of AL classification, especially when the morphological appearance and cytochemistry reactions do not clearly define cell lineage or when it is suspected that more than one neoplastic cell population is present. A specific sequence of testing with monoclonal antibodies should be followed so that if insufficient cells are obtained for complete testing the most useful infor-

mation can be obtained.[13,14] The use of extensive panels is costly and time consuming. In most cases lineage can be determined using a limited, representative panel of monoclonal antibodies.

The first panel of monoclonal antibodies should be those that can differentiate AML from ALL and T-ALL from B-ALL (∞ Chapters 23, 26). About 90–99% of AML can be discriminated from ALL using a panel of antibodies such as that listed in Table 29-2 ⊙.[13–15] Individual facilities will have their own panel of antibodies. Immunophenotyping using monoclonal antibodies for differentiating AML from ALL should include typing for the myeloid antigens **CD33** and **CD13** and the B lymphoid restricted cell antigens, **CD19**, **CD10**, and **CD22**, and the T lymphoid cell antigens **CD2**, **CD3**, **CD5**, and **CD7**. HLA-DR is present on both myeloid and B lymphoid cells. The CD7 antigen is commonly found on neoplastic cells in AML.

Occasionally myeloperoxidase may be identified in blasts at the ultrastructural level when negative by light microscopy. These blasts are considered myeloid in nature if immunophenotyping reveals at least one lineage-specific myeloid antigen.[15]

Immunofluorescence can be used to demonstrate terminal deoxynucleotidyl transferase (TdT) in individual cells. Although originally thought to be lymphoid specific, TdT is now believed to be present on more immature hematopoietic cells including those of myeloid lineage.[13] Therefore TdT should not be used alone in determining lymphoid lineage.

When cytochemistry and immunophenotyping are used together, most cases of AL can be classified into lymphoid or myeloid. Rarely a population of malignant blasts is cytochemically negative by conventional and ultrastructural methods and nonreactive with both lymphoid and myeloid monoclonal antibodies. These leukemias are classified as undifferentiated.

Another uncommon type of acute leukemia is characterized by a blast population with both myeloid and lymphoid markers on the same cell or with two separate populations of malignant blasts, one myeloid and the other lymphoid. This is considered to be a mixed lineage leukemia (biphenotypic). The definition and actual existence of mixed-lineage leukemia is controversial. Some believe that the presence of both myeloid and lymphoid markers on the same cell is an example of lineage infidelity of malignant cells.

The myeloid progenitor cell is capable of differentiation into granulocytes, erythrocytes, monocytes, or platelets. Thus, if the neoplastic clone has myeloid antigens, a second panel of monoclonal antibodies should include antibodies to subtype the AML into granulocytic, monocytic, erythrocytic, and megakaryocytic lineages (Table 29-3 ⊙).

The AML- MO, M6, and M7 can be defined using immunophenotyping. The association of specific immunologic phenotypes with various other FAB subgroups has not been established, although some associations have been made.[16] The monoclonal antibodies that react with most cases of

⊘ TABLE 29-2

Differentiation of ALL from AML Using Immunophenotyping with Selected Monoclonal Antibodies

Leukemia Type	Cell Marker					
	HLA-DR	CD33	CD13	CD19,CD22	CD10	CD2, CD3, CD5, CD7
AML	+	+	+	− (except M2 is CD19+)	−	−
B Lymphocyte	+	−	−	+	+	−
T Lymphocyte	−	−	−	−	+/−	+

AML (subgroups M0-M5) include CD33 and CD13.[16] In addition, the monoclonal antibody that identifies myeloperoxidase, MAI, is helpful, especially when cytochemistry for myeloperoxidase is negative. The **CD34** marker and TdT are present on the least differentiated myeloid cells and are characteristically associated with M0 and M1. The CD34 marker is also found on the neoplastic megakaryoblasts of M7. The AMLs with monocytic differentiation generally have the CD14 and CD11b markers in addition to CD13 and CD33. The promyelocytic cells of M3 are usually negative for the immature myeloid markers HLA-DR and CD34, but positive for CD13 and CD33. Monoclonal antibodies that react with the transferrin receptor (CD71) are helpful in identifying the blasts of M6, as are the lineage specific markers for spectrin and glycophorin A. The blasts of M7 are positive for CD34 and CD33 in early cells. The presence of platelet peroxidase, glycoprotein IIIa (CD61), the glycoprotein IIb and IIb/IIIa complex (CD41) and glycoproteins IX and Ib (CD42a, CD42b) will help identify more mature megakaryoblasts. Cases not defined by these panels should be tested by antibodies that identify subtypes of ALL.

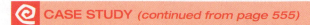

@ CASE STUDY *(continued from page 555)*

4. If the cells from Mr. Guerro's bone marrow were immunophenotyped, which of the following would you expect to be positive? CD 13, CD33, CD34, CD19, CD10, CD7, CD2.

CYTOGENETIC ANALYSES

Two-thirds of patients with AML have detectable cytogenetic abnormalities.[16] Of these, approximately 60% are found to have specific, consistent aberrations. Additional abnormalities may develop in subclones as the disease progresses. A clone is present if two or more cells show identical structural chromosome change or additional chromosomes or if three cells show the same missing chromosome.[17] Therapy-related AML (secondary to alkylating agent therapy) and AML with a history of a previous myelodysplastic disorder have characteristic cytogenetic abnormalities (classified as separate groups of AML in the WHO classification). These aberrations are associated with distinctive clinical findings and out-

⊘ TABLE 29-3

The Pattern of Reactivity with Monoclonal Antibodies Most Commonly Observed in the FAB Subtypes of AML. (TdT is usually used to identify early lymphoid precursors but may also be found in 10–20% of AML, particularly those of M0 and M1 subgroups.)

AML Subgroup	Cell Markers with Monoclonal Antibodies								
	HLA-DR	CD34	CD13	CD33	CD11b	CD14	CD71 Glycophorin A	CD41, CD42, CD61	Other Markers That May Be Present
M0	+	+	+	usually +	usually −	usually −	−	−	−
M1	+	usually +	usually +	+	+ or −	usually −	−	−	−
M2	+	usually −	+	+	+ or −	usually −	−	−	CD19
M3	−	−	+	+	usually −	usually −	−	−	CD2
M4	−	−	+	+	+	+	−	−	CD11c, M4Eo (CD2)
M5	+	usually −	+ or −	+	+	+	−	−	CD11c
M6	+ or −	−	+ or −	+ or −	−	−	+	−	−
M7	usually +	+	−	+ or −	−	−	−	+	−

comes. The nonrandom chromosome abnormalities most commonly associated with the FAB subgroups are listed in ∞ Chapter 24, Table 24-6 ✪, and will be discussed in the sections on FAB subgroups that follow.

In those cases with normal karyotypes, molecular analysis is sometimes helpful. If the expected abnormal karyotype is not found, it may be detected at the molecular level.

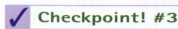

✔ Checkpoint! #3

Explain why molecular analysis is not performed on all suspected cases of acute leukemia.

ASSESSMENT OF BONE MARROW

When a diagnosis of AML or myelodysplastic syndrome is suspected, the first step is an estimation of the bone marrow cellularity, followed by an assessment of the percentage of normoblasts. Further evaluation of the bone marrow depends upon the number of normoblasts present, greater than 50% or less than 50% of all the nucleated marrow cells.

If normoblasts compose more than 50% of all nucleated bone marrow cells, the percentage of nonerythroid blast cells is determined by performing a differential count excluding the erythroid cells. This will help make a differential diagnosis between AML-M6 and myelodysplastic syndrome. If 30% or more of all remaining nonerythroid cells are blasts, the diagnosis is AML-M6, whereas if there are less than 30% blasts in the remaining nonerythroid population, the diagnosis is myelodysplastic syndrome.

If there are fewer than 50% normoblasts in the bone marrow, it is not necessary to exclude the normoblasts from the differential count in order to reach a diagnosis of acute leukemia or myelodysplastic syndrome. The diagnosis of AML-M0–M5 is made when 30% or more of all nucleated bone marrow cells are blasts. This revision in method for counting blast cells when normoblasts exceed 50% of all nucleated marrow cells means that

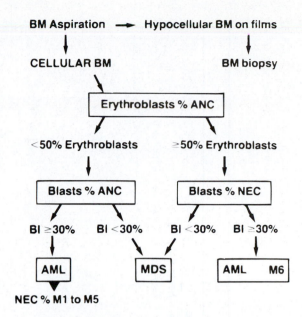

■ **FIGURE 29-4** Suggested steps in the analysis of a bone marrow aspirate to reach a diagnosis. (ANC = all nucleated cells; NEC = nonerythroid cells; AML = acute myeloid leukemia; MDS = myelodysplastic syndrome; M1–M5, M6 = subtypes of AML.) (With permission, from: Bennett JM, et al. Proposed revised criteria for the classification of acute myeloid leukemia. *Ann Intern Med.* 1985; 103:620.)

the criteria for a diagnosis of AML-M6 are different than for other subgroups of AML because M6 can be defined when less than 30% of all marrow cells are leukocyte blasts (Figure 29-4 ■).

For further assessment of the M1–M5 subtypes of AML, only the myeloid cells are evaluated, excluding lymphocytes, plasma cells, mast cells, macrophages, and nucleated erythrocytes. Other criteria designed to distinguish between M1 and M2, between M2 and M4, and between M4 and M5 will be discussed within the description of each subtype in this section (Table 29-4 ✪). For an overall view of the classification scheme, see Table 29-5 ✪.

✪ TABLE 29-4

Bone Marrow Criteria for Classification of AML

Criterion	M1	M2	M3	M4	M5	M6
Blasts (as a % of all nonerythroid cells)	≥90%	30–90%	>30%	>30%	>80% of monocytic cells(5A)	>30%
Erythoblasts (as a % of all nucleated cells)	–	<50%	<50%	<50%	–	>50%
Granulocytic component (as a % of all nonerythroid cells)	<10%	>10%	>10%*	>20%**	<20%	variable
Monocytic component (as a % of all nonerythroid cells)	<10%	<20%	<20%	>20% to <80%†	>80%†	variable

*many promyelocytes with heavy granulation
**includes myeloblasts
†includes monoblasts
Adapted with permission, from Bennett JM, et al. Proposed revised criteria for the classification of acute myeloid leukemia. *Ann. Intern. Med.* 1985; 103:620.

Morphology and Cytochemical Results Used to Classify AML in the FAB Classification

Subtype	Morphologic Features	Cytochemical Features			Leukemia	Other Tests
		Myeloperoxidase or Sudan Black B	Chloroacetate Esterase	Nonspecific Esterase		
M0 Acute myeloblastic leukemia	Myeloblasts without granules	−	−	−	M0	Immunophenotype CD13, CD33, CD34 positive
M1 Acute myeloblastic leukemia with minimal maturation	Myeloblasts, with or without scant granules	+	±	−	M1	−
M2 Acute myeloblastic leukemia with maturation	Myeloblasts with granules, promyelocytes, few myelocytes	+	±	−	M2	−
M3 Acute promyelocytic leukemia	Promyelocytes with prominent granules	+	+	−	M3	Karyotype t(15;17)
M4 Acute myelomonocytic leukemia	Myeloblasts and promyelocytes >20% marrow cells; promonocytes and monoblasts, >20%	+	+	+†	M4	Serum or urinary lysozyme 3 × normal; peripheral monocyte count >5 × 10⁹/L
M5a Acute monoblastic leukemia without differentiation	Large monoblasts with lacy nuclear chromatin and abundant cytoplasm	−	−	+‡	M5	−
M5b Acute monoblastic leukemia with differentiation	Monoblasts, promonocytes, monocytes. Blood monocytosis	−	−	+‡		
M6 Acute erythroleukemia	Megaloblastic erythroid precursors (>50%); myeloblasts (>30%)	+	−	±	M6	PAS—diffuse positivity; immunophenotype CD71 and glycophorin A positive
M7 Megakaryocytic leukemia	Megakaryoblasts, "lymphoid" morphology (L1, L2, M1), cytoplasmic budding	−	±	±‡	M7	plt. peroxidase positive; immunophenotype CD41,CD61 positive

+, usually present; −, usually absent; ±, may or may not be present.
†Incompletely inhibited by sodium fluoride.
‡Inhibited by sodium fluoride.
(From: Lee, GR: *Wintrobe's Clinical Hematology*, 9th ed. Philadelphia, Lea & Febiger, 1993.)

CURRENT FAB CLASSIFICATION

AML-M0

This rather rare leukemia accounts for less than 5% of all AMLs. It is distinguished by the absence of visible granules in the cytoplasm of blasts and negative reactions with cytochemical stains. The blasts, however, may show cytochemical signs of myeloid differentiation at the ultrastructural level or the presence of myeloid lineage markers, CD13 and CD33.[18] (This leukemia may have formerly been classified as undifferentiated AML.) Cells that fulfill these criteria but also have evidence for ultrastructural platelet peroxidase and show the glycoprotein IIb/IIIa (CD41) immunophenotype should be considered to be of the megakaryocytic lineage and the case classified as AML-M7.[12] Since there are no morphologic differentiating features of M0 blasts, immunophenotyping should be used to exclude lymphoid lineage.

AML-M1

This AML variant is most common in adults and in infants less than a year old. Leukocytosis is present in about 50% of patients at the time of initial diagnosis. One identifiable aspect of AML-M1 is its lack of cellular maturation, so it is sometimes referred to as AML-M1 without maturation. Less than 10% of all granulocytic cells show evidence of maturation beyond the blast (Figure 29-5 ■). The predominant cell in the peripheral blood is usually a poorly differentiated myeloblast with fine lacy chromatin and nucleoli. Vacuoles may be present. Occasionally, only a few blast cells are seen in the peripheral blood, but the bone marrow always reveals a sharp increase in blasts. Platelets are generally decreased.

The hypercellular bone marrow reveals that 90% or more of the nonerythroid cells are myeloblasts. The remaining cells are promyelocytes or more mature granulocytes and monocytes. Auer rods are found in the blasts of about 50% of the M1 leukemias. A few blasts may have scant azurophilic granules. If no evidence of granules or Auer rods is present, the blasts may resemble L2 lymphoblasts. Dysmyelopoiesis is almost always present. Dyserythropoiesis and dysthrombopoiesis may also be found.

The myeloperoxidase or Sudan black B stain is positive in more than 3% of the blasts, indicating granulocyte differentiation. Naphthol AS-D chloroacetate S (specific) esterase is strongly positive, but the nonspecific esterases are negative. Auer rods stain similar to reactions in myeloblasts (Table 29-6).

About 50% of patients will have acquired clonal chromosome aberrations in the leukemic cells. If the karyotype is abnormal, the prognosis is significantly worse. Chromosome aberrations associated with this subgroup include trisomy 8(+8), t(9;22), t(6;9). Trisomy 8 is the most frequent chromosome abnormality in AML, and although found most commonly in M1, it may also be found in M3, M4, and M5.

✓ # Checkpoint! #4

What hematologic features help differentiate M0 from M1?

AML-M2

AML-M2 is differentiated from AML-M1 by the presence of more differentiated cells in the bone marrow and is sometimes referred to as AML-M2 with maturation. The M2 variant of AML is most common in adults and accounts for about 30% of AML cases. Together, M1 and M2 account for over 50% of AML cases. As in the M1 variant, leukocytosis is present in about 50% of the patients at initial diagnosis. The remaining 50% have normal counts or are leukopenic. Thrombocytopenia is almost always present. Myeloblasts can usually be found in the blood smears and may be the predominant cell type (Figure 29-6 ■).

The bone marrow is hypercellular and myeloblasts make up from 30 to 89% of the nonerythroid nucleated cells. The myeloblasts are large, with variable amounts of cytoplasm and azurophilic granules. Auer rods are a common finding (Figure 29-5 ■). **Phi bodies** are a variant of Auer rods but they are smaller and not necessarily rod-shaped. All three

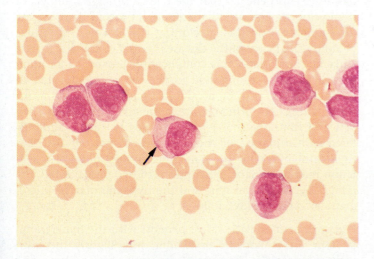

■ **FIGURE 29-5** Peripheral blood film from a patient with AML-M1. The large mononuclear cells are myeloblasts. The cell in the center (arrow) is a myeloblast with an Auer rod. Note the high nuclear-to-cytoplasmic ratio, the fine lacy chromatin, and the prominent nucleoli. (Wright-Giemsa stain; 1000× magnification)

✪ TABLE 29-6

Cytochemical Reactions for Auer Rods

SBB	+
MPO	+
Napthol AS-D chloroacetate esterase	±
PAS	±
Romanowsky	+ or – (occasionally only seen with MPO or SBB)

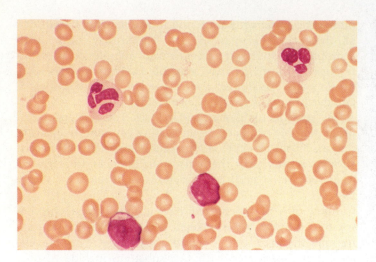

■ **FIGURE 29-6** Peripheral blood film from a patient with AML-M2. Myeloblasts are at the bottom and hypogranulated segmented neutrophils are at the top. (Wright-Giemsa stain; 1000× magnification)

granular inclusions, primary granules, Phi bodies, and Auer rods, will be positive for myeloperoxidase and will also be positive with Sudan black B staining.

The myeloblast nucleus may be round, oval, or reniform, resembling that seen in monocytic cells with fine lacy chromatin and nucleoli. The monocytic component is less than 20%, differentiating M2 from M4. The differentiation characteristic from Ml is that maturation of granulocytes from the promyelocyte stage and beyond is present in more than l0% of the nucleated nonerythroid cells.

Myelocytes and metamyelocytes often show abnormal morphologic characteristics, including nuclear/cytoplasmic maturation asynchrony, hypogranularity, or abnormal granules. Pseudo–Pelger-Huët anomaly in neutrophils and binucleated blasts, promyelocytes, myelocytes, and metamyelocytes can be found.

Eosinophils, basophils, and occasionally plasma cells may be increased. Although in most cases maturation occurs along the line to neutrophils, occasionally bone marrow eosinophilia or basophilia occurs, suggesting the neoplastic cells have entered alternate maturation pathways.[19] These cases are sometimes designated M2E0 or M2 BASO.

Peroxidase, Sudan black B, and naphthol AS-D chloroacetate esterase stains are more strongly positive, and a larger percentage of cells shows reactivity in M2 than in M1. Alpha-naphthyl acetate esterase or alpha-naphthyl butyrate esterase are negative.

Many cases of M2 show a diagnostic chromosome translocation involving chromosomes 8 and 2l, t(8;2l) (q22;q22).[20] The AML1 gene on chromosome 21 and the ETO gene on chromosome 8 are fused in this translocation. The fusion AML1 gene product is a DNA binding subunit that dimerizes with a transcription factor complex, core binding factor (CBF-β). The pathogenesis of this fusion gene

product has not been identified but may be related to the inhibition of normal AML1 gene products. This abnormality has been reported in both M1 and M2 types of AML. When the t(8;21) abnormality is present, additional chromosome changes such as loss of a sex chromosome and 9q– are common. The presence of the t(8;2l) is usually associated with a better prognosis unless additional aberrations are present.

There is a strong association between the t(6;9) chromosome abnormality in M2 and basophilia and/or a previous myelodysplastic syndrome. Basophilia in M2 is also associated with deletion of the short arm of chromosome 12(12p–). The t(9;22) abnormality may also be found but not as frequently as in M1.

✔ **Checkpoint! #5**

A patient with AML has a peripheral blood differential that includes 91% myeloblasts, 3% promyelocytes, 3% granulocytes, and 3% monocytes. Is this an M1 or M2 AML? Explain.

AML-M3, Acute Promyelocyte Leukemia (APL)

The one AML in which female patients outnumber males is AML-M3. Typically seen in young adults and the elderly, this condition is marked by a sudden and severe progression. The presenting signs often include acute disseminated intravascular coagulation.[5] The differential shows a predominance of promyelocytes. The nucleus is very delicate, sometimes showing folding. Auer rods or Phi bodies are commonly found; occasionally multiple rods will be in a single cell.

The most common clinical finding at initial diagnosis is bleeding. It is believed that the release of large numbers of promyelocytic granules that contain a procoagulant initiate disseminated intravascular clotting (DIC). This is a serious complicating factor of the disease.[21] Effective therapy for the leukemia potentiates this complication because large numbers of granules are released from lysed promyelocytes. In addition, there may be a 50-fold increase in tissue factor from dying cells during cytotoxic therapy. There is also evidence of fibrinolysis.[21] Heparin therapy is usually administered with initiation of chemotherapy to prevent DIC, but the treatment is controversial. Other abnormalities of coagulation may be present. Descriptions of two forms of M3, the typical hypergranular type and the hypogranular, or microgranular variant (M3v), follows.[22]

Hypergranular M3

Most patients with the hypergranular type are leukopenic or exhibit only slightly increased leukocyte counts. The count is rarely high. Blasts and promyelocytes with heavy granulation and multiple Auer rods are found (Figure 29-7a).[23] In some cases the typical hypergranularity of promyelocytes is less evident in the peripheral blood than in the bone marrow.[24] Anemia and thrombocytopenia are typical findings.

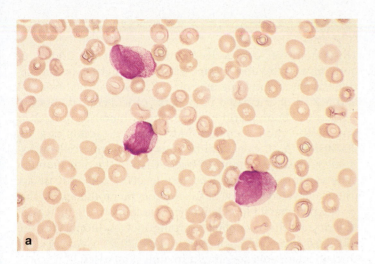
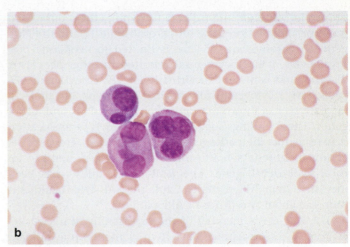

■ **FIGURE 29-7 a.** Peripheral blood film from a patient with AML-M3, hypergranular variant. These promyelocytes have an irregularly shaped nucleus and numerous azurophilic granules. **b.** Peripheral blood film from a patient with AML-M3, microgranular variant. Note the bilobed nuclei and absent or fine granules in these abnormal promyelocytes. (Both: Wright-Giemsa stain; 1000× magnification)

Most cells in the bone marrow are abnormal promyelocytes with heavy azurophilic granulation. Sometimes the granules are so densely packed that they obscure the nucleus. There are also some cells filled with fine, dust-like granules. Cells with multiple Auer rods, sometimes occurring in bundles (**faggot cells**), are characteristic with cytoplasm that is frequently clear and pale blue but may contain a few azurophilic granules or lakes of clear pink material[24] (Figure 29-8 ■). The nucleus varies in shape but is often folded or indented or sometimes bilobed. Often a large number of promyelocytes appear to be disrupted on the blood smear, with azurophilic granules and Auer rods lying over and between intact cells. It is important to distinguish M3 from M2, which may also have a high proportion of promyelocytes. In M2, the granulation is not as heavy and does not pack the cytoplasm as in M3.

Microgranular M3 Variant In contrast to typical hypergranular M3, the leukocyte count in microgranular M3 is usually markedly increased. The predominant cell in the peripheral blood is a promyelocyte with a bilobular, reniform, or multilobed nucleus (resembling that of a monocyte) and cytoplasm devoid of granules or with only a few fine azurophilic granules (Figure 29-7b ■). The nuclear chromatin is fine, with nucleoli often visible. A small abnormal promyelocyte with a bilobed nucleus, deeply basophilic cytoplasm, and sometimes cytoplasmic projections is present as a minor population in most cases but occasionally may be the predominant cell. When cytoplasmic projections are present, the cells resemble megakaryoblasts. Faggot cells are scarce or absent, but single Auer rods may be found. The finding of a few cells with the typical cytoplasmic features of hypergranular M3 will help to distinguish this leukemia from a monocytic leukemia. In contrast to the hypogranular appearance of peripheral blood promyelocytes, the bone marrow promyelocytes are more typical of the cells found in the hypergranular form of M3.

Peroxidase, Sudan black B, and naphthol AS-D chloroacetate esterase are strongly positive. The naphthyl butyrate esterase and alpha-naphthyl acetate esterase for nonspecific esterases are negative. In some cases, cytochemistry results are confusing because the neoplastic cells stain for nonspecific esterase that is fluoride-sensitive or for both specific and fluoride-sensitive nonspecific esterases.

A form of M3 has been described in which some promyelocytes contain metachromatic granules (when stained with toluidine blue).[24] Distinctive features include folded nuclei, hypergranular cytoplasm, and coarse metachromatic granules.

Diagnostic Gene Rearrangement APL is associated with a diagnostic translocation involving chromosomes 15 and 17, t(15;17). This aberration has only been seen in acute

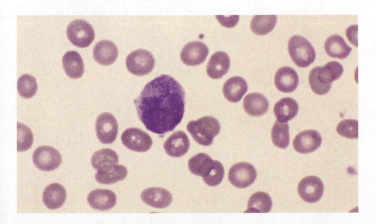

■ **FIGURE 29-8** A faggot cell from promyelocytic leukemia. Notice the bundle of Auer rods. (Peripheral blood; Wright-Giemsa stain; 1000× original magnification)

promyelocytic leukemia (APL).[25] It involves the retinoic acid receptor alpha RAR-α gene on chromosome 17 and the PML gene on chromosome 15 and is limited to neoplastic promyelocytes. It has never been reported in other neoplastic diseases, and is present in virtually all APL cases. Some APL cases have a cytogenetically normal karyotype, but molecular analysis has shown rearrangement of the PML and RAR-α genes. These findings suggest that the t(15;17) translocation is involved in the pathogenesis of the disease. The gene rearrangement results in a fusion RAR-α/PML gene and a reciprocal RAR-α/PML gene. The RAR-α/PML mRNA has been identified in all APL patients, while the RAR-α/PML mRNA is found in about two-thirds of APL patients.[26]

The RAR-α is a member of the superfamily of nuclear receptors. These receptors have two domains, one domain binds DNA and the other domain binds the retinoid hormones. Retinoids are regulators of cell proliferation, differentiation, and embryonal morphogenesis. The RAR-α is activated by binding retinoid. The activated RAR-α then binds to specific sites in DNA where it functions in direct transcriptional control of specific target genes. The role of the fusion gene products in APL has not been determined. It is proposed that the abnormal PML/RAR-α may not act as a normal retinoid receptor, thereby impairing or blocking differentiation.[27] Molecular analysis of the PML/RAR-α gene is important in monitoring therapy and relapse, as the gene disappears with successful treatment but will return as an early marker of relapse.

Retinoic acid has proven to be an effective treatment for inducing complete remission in APL.[28] Molecular analysis has revealed that retinoic acid induces the neoplastic promyelocytes to differentiate to mature granulocytes, thus overcoming the maturation arrest.[29] It is possible that a high concentration of retinoic acid, as is given in induction therapy for APL, somehow overcomes the interference with receptor activation. Cells previously unable to mature and initiate apoptosis are then able to do so. This maturation and apoptosis causes a transitory situation known as hyperleukocytosis, which can produce life-threatening effects. The inordinate amount of endotoxin released as a result of the death and lysis of such a large number of cells can produce a shock-like episode. Hyperleukocytosis will reach its peak 12–14 days after the initiation of therapy.

About 25% of patients given retinoic acid therapy become acutely ill. The mortality rate in these individuals is high. The illness is similar to capillary leak syndrome with fever, respiratory disease, renal impairment, and hemorrhage.[30] The management of the retinoic acid syndrome has not been defined.[31]

✔ Checkpoint! #6

Why is it important to do molecular studies on patients with AML-M3?

AML-M4, Acute Myelomonoblastic Leukemia (Naegeli Type)

This variant of AML derives its name from the finding of both myelocytic and monocytic differentiation in the peripheral blood and bone marrow. It is distinguished from M1 and M2 by an increased proportion of leukemic monocytic cells in the bone marrow or peripheral blood or both. It is one of the most common AML variants, accounting for 20–30% of AML cases. Infiltrations of leukemic cells in extramedullary sites is more frequent than in the pure granulocytic variants. Serum and urinary levels of muramidase are usually elevated because of the monocytic proliferation.

The peripheral blood leukocyte count is usually increased. Monocytic cells (monoblasts, promonocytes, monocytes) are increased to 5×10^9/L or more (Figure 29-9 ■). Anemia and thrombocytopenia are present in almost all cases.

The bone marrow resembles M2, with blasts composing more than 30% of the nonerythroid component. However, the marrow differs from M1, M2, and M3 in that monocytic cells (monoblasts, promonocytes, monocytes) exceed 20% of the nonerythroid nucleated cells. The sum of the myelocytic cells, including myeloblasts, promyelocytes, and later granulocytes, is >20% and <80% of the nonerythroid cells. This bone marrow picture, together with a peripheral blood monocyte count of 5×10^9/L or more (including all stages of monocytic maturation), is compatible with a diagnosis of M4.

The myeloblasts appear as described in M1 and M2. Occasionally myeloblasts and larger blast-like cells containing Auer rods can be seen. Neutrophil precursors contain larger azurophilic granules, although some more mature cells show hypogranularity or **pseudo–Pelger-Huët nuclei.**

Monoblasts are usually large with abundant bluish gray cytoplasm. The nucleus is round or convoluted with delicate chromatin and one or more nucleoli. The bone marrow may reveal erythrophagocytosis by monocytes.

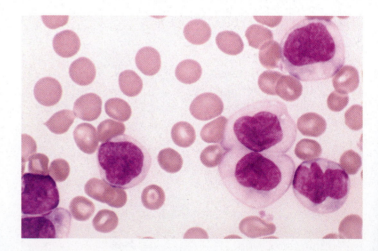

■ **FIGURE 29-9** Peripheral blood film from a case of AML-M4. There are monoblasts and promonocytes present. (Wright-Giemsa stain; 1000× magnification)

TABLE 29-7

FAB Criteria for an M4 Diagnosis

	Bone marrow:	Blasts ≥30% of nonerythroid cells
		Monocytic cells >20% to <80% nonerythroid cells
		Granulocytic component >20% to <80%
AND:	Peripheral blood	≥5 × 10⁹/L monocytic cells
	OR:	
	Peripheral blood	<5 × 10⁹/L monocytic cells and bone marrow monocytic cells ≥20% to <80% of nonerythroid nucleated cells
AND:	Ancillary tests	Serum or urinary lysozyme 3 × normal;
		or: naphthol AS-D chloroacetate esterase and alpha-naphthyl acetate esterase
		or: naphthol AS-D acetate esterase with and without NaFl reveal >20% monocytic cells in bone marrow
	OR:	
	Peripheral blood	≥5 × 10⁹/L monocytic cells
AND:	Bone marrow	Similar to AML-M2 criteria
	Ancillary tests	Serum or urinary lysozyme 3 × normal;
		or: naphthol AS-D chloroacetate esterase and alpha-naphthyl acetate esterase
		or: naphthol AS-D acetate esterase with and without NaFl reveal >20% monocytic cells in bone marrow

Two situations that require additional laboratory testing are when (1) the bone marrow findings are as described above but the peripheral blood monocyte count is less than 5×10^9/L, or (2) when the peripheral blood monocyte count is 5×10^9/L or more but the bone marrow resembles M2 rather than M4. In these cases, ancillary laboratory tests such as lysozyme levels or cytochemical methods are used to confirm the presence of a significant monocytic component and establish a diagnosis of M4 (Table 29-7 ✪).

Cytochemical methods will demonstrate two cell populations in the bone marrow: myeloblasts and promyelocytes; monoblasts and promonocytes. Myeloblasts are positive for peroxidase, Sudan black B, and naphthol AS-D chloroacetate esterase. The nonspecific esterase, alpha-naphthyl acetate esterase, is negative. Monoblasts are negative or only slightly positive for peroxidase and naphthol AS-D chloroacetate esterase and demonstrate a negative or fine granular Sudan black B positivity. The nonspecific esterases are positive and inhibited by sodium fluoride. Some blasts are impossible to distinguish as either myelocytic or monocytic because they have cytochemical reactions of both cell lines.[32] For example, in some cases there is an overlap of blasts with peroxidase and nonspecific esterase positivity.

In some cases of M4 with eosinophilia (M4Eo), abnormal eosinophils account for 5% or more of the nonerythroid nucleated cells in the marrow. There are both eosinophilic and large atypical basophilic granules within the same cell. The nucleus is often monocytoid. These cells stain positive with naphthol AS-D chloroacetate esterase and PAS, whereas normal eosinophils do not. The AML-M2 variant (M2EO) may also have an increase in eosinophils, but these cells have normal granules and stain as typical eosinophils. The eosinophilic variant of M4 (M4Eo) is strongly correlated

with deletion or inversion of the long arm of chromosome 16, inv(16).

Differentiation may also be along the basophilic pathway (M4BASO). Basophilia is associated with t(6;9). Trisomy 4 (+4) and a variety of deletions and translocations involving 11q23 are associated with M4.

AML-M5, Acute Monoblastic Leukemia (Schilling Type)

This subgroup accounts for 5–15% of AML cases. The most common clinical findings in the M5 variant are weakness, bleeding, and a diffuse erythematous skin rash. This disease is usually seen in children or young adults. One of the noticeable aspects of this disease is the degree of gum, CNS, lymph node, and extramedullary infiltrates seen. There are also occasional episodes of DIC. As with M4, there is moderately elevated serum and urine muramidase.

The criterion for a diagnosis of M5 is that 80% or more of all nonerythroid cells in the BM are monocytic (including monoblasts, promonocytes, and monocytes). There are two distinct forms, 5A and 5B, classified according to degree of differentiation (Table 29-8 ✪). It has been suggested that distinction between these particular subtypes is important in prognosis since a smaller degree of maturation (M1 and M5A) is associated with a larger tumor mass and a shorter remission period. The granulocytic component in the bone marrow usually accounts for less than 10% of the nucleated cells but may increase to 20%.

5A Poorly Differentiated This variant is the more frequent AML in children. Monoblasts account for 80% or more of all monocytic cells in the bone marrow (Figure 29-10a ■). The remaining 20% of monocytic cells are mono-

⊘ TABLE 29-8

Criteria for M5 Diagnosis

Variant	Peripheral Blood	Bone Marrow Monocytic Component (Nonerythroid)	Bone Marrow Monoblasts	Maturation Index
M5 A	>5 × 10⁹/L monocytic cells	>80%	>80% of all monocytic components	4%
M5 B	>5 × 10⁹/L monocytic cells	>75%	<80% of all monocytic components	>4%

cytes with only rare promonocytes. Some monoblasts may be found in the peripheral blood (Figure 29-10b ■). The monoblasts are large (up to 40 μ) with voluminous, variably basophilic cytoplasm. Pseudopods with translucent cytoplasm are common. Azurophilic granules may be present. The nucleus is round or oval with delicate chromatin and one or more nucleoli, but Auer rods are not found. Dyshematopoiesis is not conspicuous.

5B Well Differentiated   The well-differentiated form of M5 also reveals more than 80% monocytoid cells in the nonerythroid bone marrow but, in contrast to M5A, monoblasts account for <80% of the monocytic component (Figure 29-11a ■). The remaining cells are promonocytes and monocytes. In some cases, the percentage of blasts is <30%; however, if the total number of monocytes, promonocytes, and monoblasts is >75% in the bone marrow, it still can be called acute leukemia. The promonocytes in the marrow are similar to monoblasts, except that they have a large cerebriform nucleus with delicate chromatin. Nucleoli may be present. The cytoplasm is less basophilic than that of the monoblast, with a ground-glass appearance. Fine azurophilic granules are often present. Monocytes in the peripheral blood are increased and monoblasts are often present (Figure 29-11b ■).

The diagnosis of M5A or M5B is usually confirmed from the results of cytochemical stains. The nonspecific esterase stains, alpha-naphthyl butyrate esterase or alpha-naphthyl acetate esterase, are positive. The specific esterase, naphthol AS-D chloroacetate esterase, is negative. Myeloperoxidase and Sudan black B show absent or weak diffuse activity in the monoblasts.

Abnormalities of the long arm of chromosome 11, with translocations or deletions, are characteristic although not diagnostic for monocytic leukemias. The t(8;16) abnormality is associated with significant phagocytosis. Other chromosome aberrations are similar to those described for M1. The expression of c-fos proto-oncogene on chromosome 14 appears to be enhanced in M4 and M5 leukemia cells.[32] This gene has been linked to normal monocyte-macrophage differentiation.

✓ Checkpoint! #7

How are M5A and M5B differentiated, and what is the significance of making the distinction?

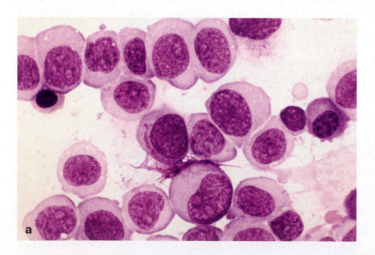
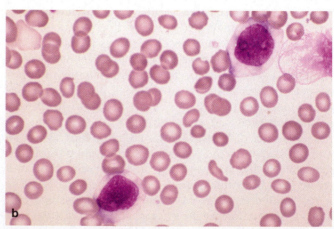

■ **FIGURE 29-10 a.** A smear from a bone marrow aspirate of a patient with M5A AML. The cells are predominately monoblasts and promonocytes **b.** Monoblasts from a case of AML-M5A. (a. Bone marrow; Wright-Giemsa stain; 1000× magnification b. Peripheral blood; 1000× original magnification; Wright-Giemsa stain)

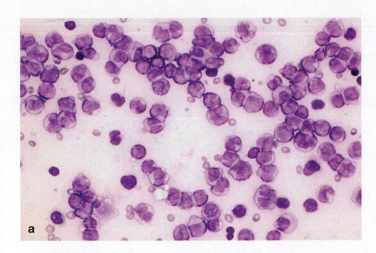
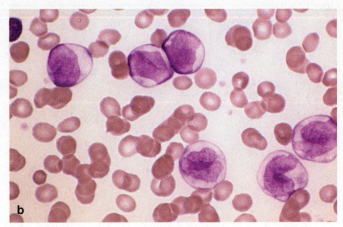

■ **FIGURE 29-11 a.** A smear from a bone marrow aspirate of a patient with AML-M5B. There is a predominance of promonocytes and monoblasts **b.** Monocytic cells, including promonocytes and monoblasts, from acute monocytic leukemia (AML-M5B). (a. Bone marrow; Wright-Giemsa stain; 400× magnification) (b. Peripheral blood; Wright-Giemsa stain 1000× original magnification)

AML-M6, Erythroleukemia (DiGuglielmo's Syndrome)

Erythroleukemia is a rare form of leukemia accounting for less than 5% of AML cases. It is almost nonexistent in children. It primarily affects the erythroid cells. The predominant cell in the bone marrow is the erythroblast, which is why it is referred to as erythroleukemia. Clinical manifestations are similar to those observed in other subtypes of AML. The most frequent presenting symptom is bleeding. As the disease progresses, myelocytic and megakaryocytic involvement in the leukemic process becomes more evident with gradual hyperplasia of these cell lines. Frequently the disease evolves into M1 or M2 acute myeloblastic leukemia. Mean survival is about 11 months.

The most dominant changes in the peripheral blood are anemia with striking poikilocytosis and anisocytosis. Nucleated erythrocytes demonstrate abnormal nuclear configurations similar to those identified in myelodysplasia. The leukocyte alkaline phosphatase score is normal or increased. Leukocytes and platelets are usually decreased. Blasts may be found (Figure 29-12 ■).

The diagnosis of erythroleukemia can be made when more than 50% of all nucleated bone marrow cells are erythroid and 30% or more of all remaining nonerythroid cells are blast cells (Figure 29-13 ■). A rare form called true erythroid leukemia occurs when the bone marrow is replaced by proliferating normoblasts showing no maturation beyond basophilic normoblasts. In this entity, there is no myeloblast proliferation.[33]

The bone marrow normoblasts are distinctly abnormal, with bizarre morphological features. Giant multilobular or multinucleated forms are common (Figure 29-14 ■). Other features include nuclear budding and fragmentation, cytoplasmic vacuoles, Howell-Jolly bodies, ringed sideroblasts, and megaloblastic changes (cobalamin and folic acid levels are normal to increased). Erythrophagocytosis by the abnormal normoblasts is a common finding. Auer rods may be found in the myeloblasts. Dysmegakaryopoiesis is common, with mononuclear forms or micromegakaryoblasts present. Neutrophils may exhibit hypogranularity and pseudo–Pelger-Huët anomaly.

Normoblasts are typically PAS negative; however, in erythroleukemia, some normoblasts, especially pronormoblasts, demonstrate coarse positivity superimposed on diffuse or granular positivity. PAS-positive normoblasts are also found in MDS, other subgroups of AML, iron deficiency anemia, thalassemia, severe hemolytic anemia, and sometimes in megaloblastic anemia. The myeloblastic component of M6 shows reactions similar to those found in M1 both in morphology and in chromosomal aberrations.

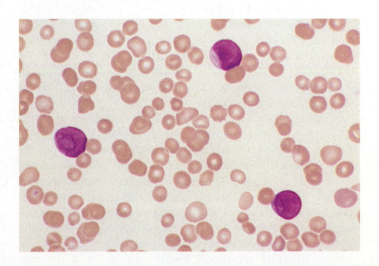

■ **FIGURE 29-12** Myeloblasts in the peripheral blood from a patient with AML-M6. The blast morphology is typical of AML-M1. (Wright-Giemsa stain; 1000× magnification)

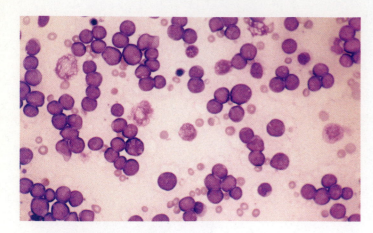

■ **FIGURE 29-13** Smear of a bone marrow aspirate from a patient with erythroleukemia (AML-M6) in blast crisis. Most cells are myeloblasts. (Bone marrow; Wright-Giemsa stain 400× original magnification)

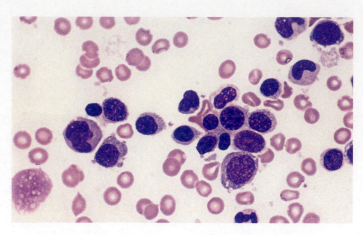

■ **FIGURE 29-14** Erythroblasts with megaloblastoid features in the bone marrow from a case of AML-M6. (Wright-Giemsa stain; 1000× original magnification)

✓ Checkpoint! #8

What is the differentiating hematologic feature of M6 that allows it to be subgrouped?

AML-M7, Acute Megakaryoblastic Leukemia

This acute leukemia has been known by several different names: acute malignant myelosclerosis, acute myelodysplasia with myelofibrosis, and acute myelofibrosis. Because of the similarity of clinical and hematologic findings, all these disorders are believed to represent the same entity, acute megakaryoblastic leukemia. The disease is rare and may occur de novo or as a leukemic transformation of chronic myelogenous leukemia (CML) and myelodysplastic syndromes.[34] Various chemotherapy regimens have been used but remission has not been achieved.

Patients usually present with pallor and weakness because of anemia and bleeding. On physical examination, there is no significant organomegaly.

Peripheral blood pancytopenia is characteristic at initial diagnosis, followed by a high peripheral blood blast count in the later stages of the disease. On careful examination of the blood smear, micromegakaryocytes and undifferentiated blasts may be found. The blasts are pleomorphic without any specific distinguishing characteristics and may resemble lymphoblasts. However, the finding of cytoplasmic blebs is suggestive that these cells are megakaryoblasts. Megakaryocyte fragments may be present.

Bone marrow aspiration usually results in a dry tap. Biopsy reveals increased fibroblasts and/or increased reticulin and greater than 30% blasts. The fibrosis is believed to be secondary to the increase in megakaryocytes. It has been suggested that megakaryocytes secrete a platelet mitogenic factor that stimulates fibroblast proliferation.

Blasts may be identified as megakaryocytic by immunophenotyping, cytochemistry, and electron microscopy.[35] The blasts are highly variable, ranging from small round cells with scant cytoplasm and dense heavy chromatin to cells with moderately abundant cytoplasm with or without granules and nuclei with lacy chromatin and prominent nucleoli. Some blasts may have cytoplasmic blebs. About 20–30% of the blasts are two to three times the size of lymphocytes. Occasionally megakaryocytes with shedding platelets are seen. Dysplasia of all cell lines is a common finding.

Myeloperoxidase, Sudan black B, and chloroacetate esterase staining is negative, distinguishing the megakaryoblasts from myeloblasts. The PAS is positive with distinct localized deposits in more mature cells. Acid phosphatase staining also shows localized positivity. The alpha-naphthyl butyrate esterase is negative, but the alpha-naphthyl acetate esterase is positive, a reaction typical for megakaryoblasts. Undifferentiated blasts may be identified as megakaryoblasts by electron microscopy. The cells exhibit demarcation of the membrane system and a positive platelet peroxidase (PPO) reaction at the ultrastructural level. The PPO activity occurs in the perinuclear space and in the endoplasmic reticulum.

Monoclonal antibodies that react with platelet glycoproteins Ib, IIb/IIIa, and IIIa have been used to identify cells of the megakaryocytic lineage. The antibodies against IIb/IIIa or IIIa recognize both the megakaryoblast and mature megakaryocyte, but the antibody against Ib recognizes only the more mature megakaryocytes.

Abnormalities of chromosome 21 have been described in association with M7. Among patients with Down syndrome who developed acute megakaryoblastic leukemia, all had a translocation of chromosome 21.[36]

CASE STUDY *(continued from page 556)*

A bone marrow aspirate and biopsy was performed on Mr. Guerro to aid in diagnosis. The bone marrow biopsy revealed a hypercellular marrow. The bone marrow aspirate revealed an M:E ratio of 7.8:1. The predominant cell was an abnormal immature cell with an indented or lobulated nuclear configuration. Heavy cytoplasmic granulation was present and multiple Auer rods were seen in several cells. The cells were strongly positive with myeloperoxidase.

5. Based on the morphology and cytochemical staining of these cells, what is the most likely FAB classification?

6. What is the major complication associated with this leukemia?

7. What chromosome abnormality is associated with this leukemia?

▶ **THERAPY**

Traditional chemotherapy is designed to reduce tumor load as rapidly as possible (∞ Chapter 26). Newer treatment modalities include both autologous and allogeneic bone marrow transplants and infusions of donor lymphocyte cells with total body irradiation to increase clonal destruction.

Current research is focusing on the use of monoclonal antibodies, gene therapy, and destruction of the cellular matrix that supports the neoplastic tissue.

Evaluation of therapy by periodic peripheral blood counts is essential for support of patients during chemotherapy. Development of at-risk stages such as pancytopenia, granulocytopenia, and/or thrombocytopenia must be monitored so that early intervention may occur.

One class of medications used in the treatment of AML, the folic acid antagonists, interferes with the synthesis of DNA by inhibiting thymidylate synthetase and by blocking the formation of mature ribosomes. As a consequence, the peripheral blood picture will show a megaloblastoid pancytopenia. Actively proliferating tissues such as malignant cells, bone marrow, fetal cells, dermal epithelium, buccal and intestinal mucosa, and cells of the urinary tract are sensitive to these drugs.

Bone marrow transplantation (∞ Chapter 32), whether allogeneic or autologous, is the only therapeutic choice that currently provides the potential for a prolonged (10+ years) disease-free survival.

CASE STUDY *(continued from page 567)*

8. If this patient were treated with all trans-retinoic acid and two weeks later the blood count was repeated, what would you expect to find?

✓ **Checkpoint! #9**

Predict the peripheral blood picture of a patient on antifolate chemotherapy.

SUMMARY

The acute leukemias (AL) are a heterogeneous group of neoplastic stem cell disorders characterized by unregulated proliferation and blocked maturation. The two major groups of AL are acute myelocytic leukemia (AML) and acute lymphocytic leukemia (ALL). These two major groups are further classified into subtypes based on FAB morphologic criteria, cytochemical stains, immunologic analysis, cytogenetic and molecular abnormalities. The FAB classification describes eight subtypes for AML based on the degree of cellular differentiation and lineage of blasts. The subgroups include, myeloid (M0-M3), monocytic (M4-M5), erythrocytic (M6), and megakaryocytic (M7).

The peroxidase and/or Sudan black B help differentiate AML (peroxidase positive) from ALL (peroxidase negative). Subgrouping the AMLs further requires additional cytochemical stains. Also helpful in differentiating ALs is cytogenetic analysis. The most specific abnormality associated with FAB subgroups is the t(15;17)

found only in M3. This abnormality has been shown at the molecular level to involve the retinoic acid receptor (RAR) gene and the PML gene. Other cytogenetic abnormalities are not specific for a particular subgroup, but some are associated with particular subgroups.

The onset of AL is usually abrupt, and without treatment, the disease progresses. Symptoms are related to anemia, thrombocytopenia, and/or neutropenia. Splenomegaly, hepatomegaly, and lymphadenopathy are common findings.

Hematologic findings include a macrocytic or normocytic, normochromic anemia, thrombocytopenia, and a decreased, normal, or increased leukocyte count. Blasts are almost always found in the peripheral blood. A bone marrow examination is always indicated if leukemia is suspected. The bone marrow reveals more than 30% blasts (FAB) or 20% blasts (WHO).[37]

8. First MIC Cooperative Study Group. Morphologic, immunologic, and cytogenetic (MIC) working classification of acute lymphoblastic leukemias. Report of the workshop held in Leuven, Belgium, April 22–23, 1985. First MIC Cooperative Study Group. *Cancer Genet Cytogenet*. 1986; 23:189–97.

9. Second MIC Cooperative Study Group. Morphologic, immunologic, and cytogenetic (MIC) working classification of the acute myeloid leukaemias. *Br J Haematol*. 1988; 68:487–94.

10. del Canizo MC, et al. Discrepancies between morphologic, cytochemical, and immunologic characteristics in acute myeloblastic leukemia. *Am J Clin Pathol*. 1987; 88:38–42.

11. Harris NL, et al. World Health Organization classification of neoplastic diseases of the hematopoietic and lymphoid tissues: Report of the Clinical Advisory Committee meeting, Airlie House, Virginia, November 1997. *J Clin Oncol*. 1999; 17:3835–49.

12. Cheson BD, et al. Report of the National Cancer Institute-sponsored workshop on definitions of diagnosis and response in acute myeloid leukemia. *J Clin Oncol*. 1990; 8:813–19.

13. Huh YO, Smith TL, Collins P, Bueso-Ramos C, Albitar M, Kantarjian HM, Pierce SA, Freireich EJ. Terminal deoxynucleotidyl transferase expression in acute myelogenous leukemia and myelodysplasia as determined by flow cytometry. *Leuk Lymphoma*. 2000; 37:319–31.

14. Pileri SA, Ascani S, Milani M, Visani G, Piccioli M, Orcioni GF, Poggi S, Sabattini E, Santini D, Falini B. Acute leukaemia immunophenotyping in bone-marrow routine sections. *Br J Haematol*. 1999; 105:394–401.

15. Cascavilla N, Melillo L, D'Arena G, Greco MM, Carella AM, Sajeva MR, Perla G, Matera R, Minervini MM, Carotenuto M. Minimally differentiated acute myeloid leukemia (AML M0): Clinico-biological findings of 29 cases. *Leuk Lymphoma*. 2000; 37:105–13.

16. Tien HF, Wang CH, Lin MT, Lee FY, Liu MC, Chuang SM, Chen YC, Shen MC, Lin KH, Lin DT. Correlation of cytogenetic results with immunophenotype, genotype, clinical features, and ras mutation in acute myeloid leukemia: A study of 235 Chinese patients in Taiwan. *Cancer Genet Cytogenet*. 1995; 84:60–68.

17. An international system for human cytogenetic nomenclature (1978) ISCN (1978). Report of the Standing Committee on Human Cytogenetic Nomenclature. *Cytogenet Cell Genet*. 1978; 21:309–409.

18. Konikova E, Glasova M, Kusenda J, Babusikova O. Intracellular markers in acute myeloid leukemia diagnosis. *Neoplasma*. 1998; 45:282–91.

19. Yamaguchi Y, Nishio H, Kasahara T, Ackerman SJ, Koyanagi H, Suda T. Models of lineage switching in hematopoietic development: A new myeloid-committed eosinophil cell line (YJ) demonstrates tri-lineage potential. *Leukemia*. 1998; 12:1430–39.

20. Sugimoto T, Das H, Imoto S, Murayama T, Gomyo H, Chakraborty S, Taniguchi R, Isobe T, Nakagawa T, Nishimura R, Koizumi T. Quantitation of minimal residual disease in t(8;21)-positive acute myelogenous leukemia patients using real-time quantitative RT-PCR. *Am J Hematol*. 2000; 64:101–6.

21. Meijers JC, Oudijk EJ, Mosnier LO, Bos R, Bouma BN, Nieuwenhuis HK, Fijnheer R. Reduced activity of TAFI (thrombin-activatable fibrinolysis inhibitor) in acute promyelocytic leukaemia. *Br J Haematol*. 2000; 108:518–23.

22. Bennett JM, et al. A variant form of hypergranular promyelocytic leukaemia (M3). *Br J Haematol*. 1980; 44:169–70.

23. Lemez P. A case of acute promyelocytic leukaemia with 'faggot cells' exhibiting strong alpha-naphthylbutyrate esterase activity. *Br J Haematol*. 1988; 68:138–39.

24. Castoldi GL, Liso V, Specchia G, Tomasi P. Acute promyelocytic leukemia: Morphological aspects. *Leukemia*. 1994; 8:1441–46.

25. Iqbal S, Grimwade D, Chase A, Goldstone A, Burnett A, Goldman JM, Swirsky D. Identification of PML/RARalpha rearrangements in suspected acute promyelocytic leukemia using fluorescence in situ hybridization of bone marrow smears: A comparison with cytogenetics and RT-PCR in MRC ATRA trial patients. MRC Adult Leukaemia Working Party. *Leukemia*. 2000; 14:950–53.

26. Gianni M, Ponzanelli I, Mologni L, Reichert U, Rambaldi A, Terao M, Garattini E. Retinoid-dependent growth inhibition, differentiation and apoptosis in acute promyelocytic leukemia cells: Expression and activation of caspases. *Cell Death Differ*. 2000; 7:447–60.

27. Douer D, Ramezani L, Parker J, Levine AM. All-trans-retinoic acid effects the growth, differentiation, and apoptosis of normal human myeloid progenitors derived from purified CD34+ bone marrow cells. *Leukemia*. 2000; 14:874–81.

28. Bruserud O, Gjertsen BT. New strategies for the treatment of acute myelogenous leukemia: Differentiation induction—present use and future possibilities. *Stem Cells*. 2000; 18:157–65.

29. Sun SY, Wan H, Yue P, Hong WK, Lotan R. Evidence that retinoic acid receptor beta induction by retinoids is important for tumor cell growth inhibition. *J Biol Chem*. 2000; 275(22):17149–53.

30. Tallman MS, Andersen JW, Schiffer CA, Appelbaum FR, Feusner JH, Ogden A, Shepherd L, Rowe JM, Francois C, Larson RS, Wiernik PH. Clinical description of 44 patients with acute promyelocytic leukemia who developed the retinoic acid syndrome. *Blood*. 2000; 95:90–95.

31. Cupitt JM. A case for steroids in acute lung injury associated with the retinoic acid syndrome. *Anaesth Intensive Care*. 2000; 28:202–4.

32. Mavilio F, Testa U, Sposi NM, Petrini M, Pelosi E, Bordignon C, Amadori S, Mandelli F, Peschle C. Selective expression of fos proto-oncogene in human acute myelomonocytic and monocytic leukemias: A molecular marker of terminal differentiation. *Blood*. 1987; 69:160–64.

33. Siebert R, Jhanwar S, Brown K, Berman E, Offit K. Familial acute myeloid leukemia and DiGuglielmo syndrome. *Leukemia*. 1995; 9:1091–94.

34. Kinugawa N, Okimoto Y, Hata J. Simultaneous detection of platelet-associated antigen and platelet peroxidase on buffy coat cells from bone marrow in two patients with pediatric acute megakaryocytic leukemia. *J Pediatr Hematol Oncol*. 1999; 21:451–52.

35. Ng KC, Tan AM, Chong YY, Lau LC, Lou J. Congenital acute megakaryoblastic leukemia (M7) with chromosomal t(1;22) (p13;q13) translocation in a set of identical twins. *J Pediatr Hematol Oncol*. 1999; 21:428–30.

36. Malkin D, Brown EJ, Zipursky A. The role of p53 in megakaryocyte differentiation and the megakaryocytic leukemias of Down syndrome. *Cancer Genet Cytogenet*. 2000; 116:1–5.

37. Bennett JM. World Health Organization classification of the acute leukemias and myelodysplastic syndrome. *Int J Hematol*. 2000; 72:131–33.

30

Acute Lymphoblastic Leukemias

Susan J. Leclair, Ph.D.

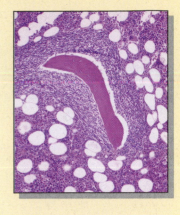

■ CHECKLIST - LEVEL I

At the end of this unit of study the student should be able to:

1. Define *acute lymphoblastic leukemia* (ALL) and differentiate it from acute myeloblastic leukemia (AML).
2. List and define the common variants seen in ALL as defined by the FAB classification.
3. Describe and recognize the typical peripheral blood picture (erythrocytes, leukocytes, and thrombocytes) seen in ALL.
4. Give the typical results of cytochemical stains in ALL.
5. Summarize the clinical signs and symptoms associated with ALL.
6. Define the rare acute leukemias that are not included in AML and ALL groups.

■ CHECKLIST - LEVEL II

At the end of this unit of study the student should be able to:

1. Compare and contrast the various presentations of ALL.
2. Predict the most likely FAB or immunophenotype subgroup based on patient history, physical assessment, and laboratory findings.
3. Correlate cellular presentation with prognosis and common complications in ALL.
4. Correlate Wright stain morphology of the ALL subgroups with cytochemical stains, flow cytometry, and genetic testing results.
5. Evaluate peripheral blood results in relation to oncological therapy (i.e., complete or partial remission, relapse, engraftment).
6. Identify AL from a peripheral blood smear and recommend laboratory tests that may be useful in differentiation of AML and ALL and in classification of subtypes.

CHAPTER OUTLINE

KEY TERMS

Acute undifferentiated leukemia (AUL)
B cell ALL
Bilineage
Biphenotypic
Burkitt cell
Myeloid/natural killer (NK) cell acute leukemia
T cell ALL

BACKGROUND BASICS

The information in this chapter will build upon concepts learned in previous chapters. To maximize your learning experience you should review and have an understanding of these concepts before starting this unit of study.

Level I

▶ Summarize the origin and differentiation of hematopoietic cells. (Chapter 2)
▶ Describe the maturation, differentiation, and function of the lymphocyte. (Chapter 6)
▶ Outline the classification and general laboratory findings of the acute leukemias. (Chapter 26)
▶ Summarize the typical laboratory findings that define acute myeloblastic leukemia. (Chapter 29)

Level II

▶ Summarize the role of oncogenes and growth factors in cell proliferation, differentiation, and maturation. (Chapters 2, 26)
▶ Diagram the maturation scheme for T and B lymphocytes. (Chapter 6)
▶ Describe the role of molecular analysis in diagnosis and treatment of acute leukemia. (Chapter 25)
▶ Describe the use of immunophenotyping in acute leukemia. (Chapters 23, 26)
▶ Describe the role of cytogenetics in diagnosis and treatment of acute leukemia. (Chapters 24, 26)

CASE STUDY

We will refer to this case study throughout this chapter.
John, a 4-year-old white male, is seen by his physician with a complaint of easy fatigue and bruising. His mother states that until one month ago he was a "typical kid." Since then she has noticed increased lassitude, a regression to more baby-like behavior, and loss of appetite. For the past two days, his temperature has been 100°F. Upon physical examination, the child presented as a pale, quiet child of appropriate size for his age. Most systems were unremarkable with the exception of several small shotty lymph nodes felt in the cervical and auxiliary regions. His CBC revealed a WBC count of 40.2 × 10^9/L with 90% blasts. Consider the laboratory testing that may help in the diagnosis of John's illness.

▶ OVERVIEW

This chapter is a study of the acute lymphocytic leukemias (ALL). A summary of clinical signs and symptoms as well as hematologic findings associated with ALL are discussed. A description of the classification systems including the morphologic FAB system, immunologic system, and the WHO system follows. Lastly, the rare acute leukemias that are not grouped into either AML or ALL are briefly reviewed.

▶ INTRODUCTION

Similar to acute myelogenous leukemias, the acute lymphoblastic leukemias are stem cell disorders characterized by malignant neoplastic proliferation and accumulation of immature and nonfunctional hematopoietic cells in the bone marrow. The basic abnormality appears to be a genetic mutation of a single lymphoid stem cell giving rise to a clone of malignant lymphocytes. These lymphoid cells retain the ability to proliferate in an unregulated manner but appear to be frozen in their maturation sequence. As a consequence, they do not develop into mature cells and undergo apoptosis. Thus the leukemic clone expands. The trigger for the original leukemic genetic mutation is unknown but may be a combination of leukemogenic factors. As in AML, the impairment of normal hematopoiesis is the primary cause of concern.

There are two major categories of acute leukemias, classified according to the cellular origin of the primary stem cell defects: AML and ALL. If the defect affects primarily the lymphoid progenitor cell (CFU-L, pre-B or immature T cell), it is classified as acute lymphoblastic leukemia, or ALL. If the defect affects primarily the myeloid progenitor cells, it is classified as AML or ANLL.

As with AML, the most reliable parameters for defining the neoplastic cells and classifying the acute lymphoid leukemias into major categories and subtypes are combinations of the FAB morphologic criteria, cytochemical reactions, immunophenotype, and genetic abnormalities.

▶ CLINICAL FINDINGS

Acute lymphoblastic leukemia (ALL) is primarily a disease of young children, with a peak incidence between the ages of 2 and 5 years. In this population, the signs and symptoms can be insidious and nonspecific. They include: easy fatigue, bruising, low-grade fever, weight loss, and bone/joint pain. Without treatment, survival is short, but with recently developed treatment regimens, most children enter a period of prolonged remission and many appear to be "cured".[1] For an adult with ALL, the onset of signs and symptoms is shorter with more noticeable (or more appreciated) complaints of fatigue, infections, and bruising. Adult onset ALL is not as easily treated as childhood ALL and experiences a lesser quality of remission.

The onset of the disease is usually abrupt and continues in a progressive manner. Symptoms are related to anemia, thrombocytopenia, and neutropenia. Common complaints include fatigue, pallor, fever, weight loss, irritability, and anorexia. Fever is often related to a concomitant infection. Petechiae and ecchymoses are present in over half the patients; actual hemorrhage is less common. Bone pain is noted in about 80% of patients with tenderness, especially over the long bones. Often this complaint is dismissed as "growing pains." When severe, the child refuses to walk or stand. Occasionally children have symptoms related to CNS involvement, including headaches and vomiting. Splenomegaly, hepatomegaly, and lymphadenopathy are common findings. The first evidence of the disease that parents may notice is the presence of small, shotty lymph nodes around the child's hairline during bath time.

✔ Checkpoint! #1

Compare the typical age groups in which AML and ALL are found.

▶ LABORATORY FINDINGS

Study of the peripheral blood and bone marrow is critical to making a diagnosis of ALL.

PERIPHERAL BLOOD

The leukocyte count may be increased, decreased, or normal. About 50% of the patients have leukocytosis due to an abundance of immature lymphoid cells. Neutropenia is often marked, even when the total leukocyte count is increased. Blast cells usually appear in the blood. The blasts are small with scant cytoplasm, indistinct chromatin, and absent or poorly defined nucleoli. The platelet count is usually decreased. Normocytic, normochromic anemia is almost always present and can be severe. Anisocytosis, poikilocytosis, and nucleated erythrocytes, however, are not usually present[2] (Table 30-1).

✪ TABLE 30-1

Laboratory Findings Characteristic of ALL

Peripheral Blood	Leukocyte count usually increased but may be normal or decreased
	Neutropenia
	Lymphoblasts
	Normocytic, normochromic anemia
	Thrombocytopenia
Bone Marrow	Hypercellular
	>30% lymphoblasts (FAB); >20% lymphoblasts (WHO)

℮ CASE STUDY *(continued from page 572)*

The physician ordered a CBC on John. The results are as follows:

WBC:	40.2×10^9/L
RBC:	3.45×10^{12}/L
Hb:	9.7 g/dL
Hct:	0.32 L/L
MCV:	92.7 fL
MCH:	28.1 pg
MCHC:	30.3
RDW:	17.3
PLT:	63×10^9/L

The differential showed 90% lymphoblasts, 8% neutrophils, 1% monocytes, and 1% eosinophils. Rare nucleated erythrocytes are seen on scan. The platelets appear decreased in number.

1. Based upon this data, what would be the initial interpretation of John's presentation?

BONE MARROW

The hypercellular bone marrow reveals replacement of normal hematopoietic cells by lymphoid elements. By traditional FAB definition there are 30% or more lymphoblasts, but in reality most patients have more than 65% blasts present. The morphology of the blasts is variable and will be described with the FAB classification discussed later. Auer rods are not present in lymphoblasts. Intracytoplasmic inclusions have been described in the lymphoblasts of patients with ALL, but the punctate staining and cytochemistry of these inclusions suggest they are probably lysosomal in origin.[3]

In addition to morphology, cytochemistry helps identify the lymphoid nature of these abnormal cells (Table 26-10 ✪). In lymphoblasts, the peroxidase and Sudan black B are negative. The PAS reaction usually demonstrates a coarse granular or block-like positivity. Some myeloid leukemias may also demonstrate this type of reactivity. In AML, however, the granular pattern is superimposed on a diffusely positive background, whereas in lymphoblasts there is no background positivity. Naphthol AS-D chloroacetate, alpha-naphthyl acetate, and alpha-naphthyl butyrate are negative or weakly positive in null cell ALL and B ALL but show localized coarse positivity in T ALL. Acid phosphatase staining shows an intense localized positive reaction in T ALL. In ALL-L3, the vacuoles stain with oil red O indicating the presence of lipid.

℮ CASE STUDY *(continued from page 573)*

2. What is the correct choice of tests that should be used in the initial follow up in this case?

OTHER LABORATORY FINDINGS

As with AML, other laboratory findings are consistent with increased cellular metabolism. Hyperuricemia and an increase in lactate dehydrogenase are common findings resulting from the increase in cell turnover. Hypercalcemia, when present, is thought to be caused by increased bone resorption associated with leukemic proliferation in the bone marrow.

✔ **Checkpoint! #2**

Contrast the malignant neoplastic cells in ALL with those found in AML.

▶ ## CLASSIFICATION

FAB MORPHOLOGIC CLASSIFICATION

The FAB group has defined three subtypes of ALL (L1, L2, L3) based on the morphology and heterogeneity of bone marrow lymphoblasts[4] (Table 30-2). Although these features can vary in each presentation, it is assumed that 90% or greater positivity for a specific cytological feature is significant. The cell features evaluated include:

1. Cell size
2. Nuclear chromatin
3. Nuclear shape
4. Nucleoli
5. Amount of cytoplasm
6. Amount of basophilia in cytoplasm
7. Cytoplasmic vacuolation

Acute Lymphoblastic Leukemia—L1 (ALL-L1)

This is the most common ALL found in children. It appears to have the best prognosis. The key to this subtype is homogeneity of lymphoblasts (Figure 30-1 ■). Most cells within any one case are homogeneous in size, but heterogeneity is compatible with L1 if all other features considered suggest L1. The lymphoblasts are predominantly small, up to twice the size of a small lymphocyte. The chromatin is usually finely dispersed but may appear more condensed in small cells. The chromatin pattern may vary from case to case but is homogeneous within cases. The nuclear shape is regular with occasional clefts or indentations. Nucleoli are not prominent and may be absent. The cytoplasm is scant and only slightly or moderately basophilic.

Acute Lymphoblastic Leukemia—L2 (ALL-L2)

This is the most frequent ALL found in adults. Occasionally, the cells have granular inclusions making it difficult to distinguish L2 from AML-M2, if cytochemical stains are not performed. In contrast to granules in myeloid cells, the granules in lymphoblasts are peroxidase negative and the cells are positive for TdT. In contrast to the blasts of L1, the blasts in L2 demonstrate a marked heterogeneity in any one case and between cases (Figure 30-2 ■). There is a great deal of variability in cell size within each case, but the cells are generally two times the size of small lymphocytes. The nucleus is irregular in shape. The chromatin pattern in any one case is heterogeneous, varying from finely reticular to condensed. Nucleoli are always present but vary in size and number. Often they appear very large. The cytoplasm is abundant with variable basophilia.

Acute Lymphoblastic Leukemia—Burkitt Type (ALL-L3)

This is the rarest form of ALL. It occurs in both adults and children. The lymphoblasts are similar in appearance to those found in Burkitt lymphoma (**Burkitt cell**). The blasts

---

✪ TABLE 30-2

FAB Criteria for the Subtypes of ALL

Morphologic Feature	L1	L2	L3
Cell size	Small	Large, heterogeneous	Large
Nuclear chromatin	Fine or clumped, but homogeneous in cells within a single case	Variable-heterogeneous among cells within a single case	Fine and homogeneous
Nuclear shape	Regular, occasional clefting or indentation common	Irregular, clefting and indentation	Regular, oval to round
Nucleoli	Not visible or small and inconspicuous	One or more, often large and prominent	Prominent, one or more
Cytoplasm			
Amount	Scant	Variable, often moderate to abundant	Moderately abundant
Basophilia	Slight or moderate	Variable, may be deep	Very deep
Vacuolation	Variable	Variable	Often prominent

(Adapted, with permission, from Bennett, JM, et al. Proposals for the classification of the acute leukaemias. *Br J Haematol.* 1976; 33:451.)

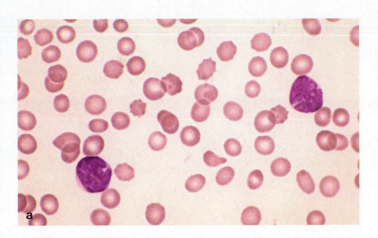

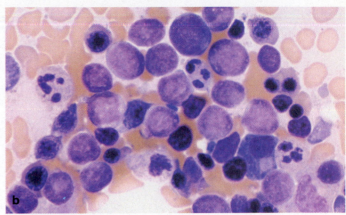

■ FIGURE 30-1 a. Lymphoblasts in peripheral blood from L1 acute lymphocytic leukemia. Notice the nuclear cleavage. b. Lymphoblasts in the bone marrow in a case of L1 ALL. (Both Wright-Giemsa stain; 1000× magnification)

are homogeneous both within and between cases. The cells are large with abundant, intensely basophilic cytoplasm. Surface immunoglobulin is present on L3 cells. There is prominent cytoplasmic vacuolization (Figure 30-3 ■). Vacuoles may also be present in L1 and L2 lymphoblasts but they are much less intense than in L3. The nucleus is oval to round with dense but finely stippled chromatin and one or more vesicular nucleoli.

The rearrangement of the cMYC gene that places it in juxtaposition to the Ig gene is characteristic of ALL-L3. This results in deregulation and overexpression of the cMYC gene. The result is that the cells are perpetually in cycle. The diagnostic cytogenetic aberration is t(8;14)(q24:q32).

It is now generally agreed that ALL-L3 and Burkitt lymphoma are different clinical manifestations of the same disease (∞ Chapter 31).

✓ **Checkpoint! #3**

Contrast the morphology of blasts found in L1, L2, and L3.

IMMUNOLOGIC CLASSIFICATION OF ALL

Immunophenotyping of ALL is essential as it can identify the immunologic subtype (T or B cell) of the neoplastic lymphocyte. This information has important prognostic implications. Immunophenotyping also can distinguish lymphoid from myeloid neoplasms, define mixed cell lineages, and identify minimal residual disease. Research with surface markers and intracellular markers reveals that lymphoblasts in ALL vary considerably in immunologic maturation. In normal lymphoid cells, some antigenic determinants appear

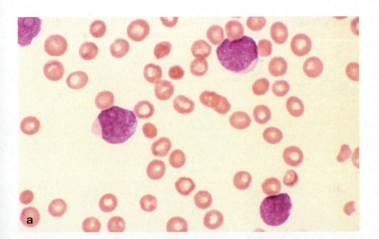

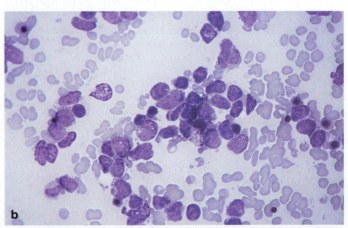

■ FIGURE 30-2 a. Lymphoblasts in peripheral blood from L2 acute lymphocytic leukemia. b. Lymphoblasts in the bone marrow of a patient with ALL-L2. (a. Wright-Giemsa stain; 1000× magnification, b. Wright-Giemsa stain; 500× magnification)

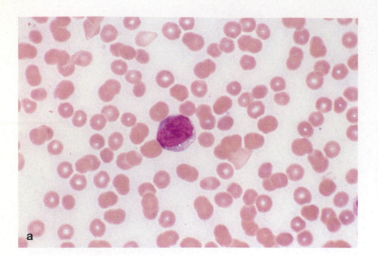
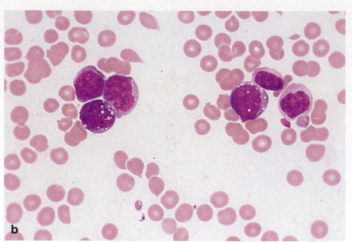

■ FIGURE 30-3 **a.** Lymphoblast in peripheral blood from L3 acute lymphocytic leukemia. Notice the vacuoles. **b.** Lymphoblasts in the bone marrow from the patient in Figure 30-3a. (Both: Wright-Giemsa stain; 1000× magnification)

at a very early developmental stage and disappear with maturity, whereas others appear on more mature cells. Monoclonal antibodies have demonstrated that some leukemic cells may have phenotypes of normal cells while others express an inappropriate combination of antigens (Figures 30-4, 30-5 ■).

The immunologic classification of acute ALL recognizes **T cell ALL** and **B cell ALL**. There are subgroups of B ALL and of T ALL based on cell maturity[5] (Table 30-3 ✪).

B Cell ALL

The B ALL subgroups include early pre-B and pre-B, and mature B cell ALL. The B cell lineage is defined by the presence of the B cell lineage restricted surface antigen CD19 and/or cytoplasmic CD22 (cCD22). The early pre-B lymphoid stage can be determined by the presence of CD34, CD10 (common acute lymphocytic antigen, CALLA), and TdT. Those ALLs with CD10 marker also have been called common ALL.[6] It seems to have the best prognosis of the immunologic subtypes.[7]

The next stage in maturation, the pre-B cell stage, gains the CD20 and surface CD22 (sCD22) antigens as well as cytoplasmic immunoglobulin, but it loses CD34.

The CD19, CD22, CD10, and TdT phenotype is the same as the phenotype of most normal immature B cells in the bone marrow. Therefore, the distinction of normal and neoplastic B cells in the marrow is difficult unless the neoplastic cell also has an abnormal phenotype as a marker of disease. This distinction is important in the detection of minimal residual disease after treatment. In some cases there is a loss of antigen(s) that usually shows synchronous expression with another, or expression of two antigens that are usually not found on the cell together. For example, up to 50% of B ALL express a myeloid antigen, CD13 or CD33. This abnormality makes it easier to differentiate the neoplastic cell from a normal cell. However, the presence of a myeloid antigen may complicate cell identification and make it more difficult to differentiate ALL from AML.

The mature B cell ALL phenotype expresses surface immunoglobulin but lacks CD34 and TdT. CD10 may or may

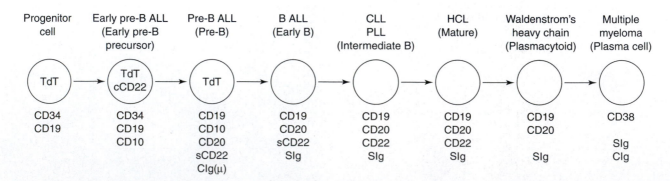

■ FIGURE 30-4 Normal B lymphocyte maturation scheme with leukemic and other lymphoproliferative counterparts. (ALL, acute lymphocytic leukemia; CLL, chronic lymphocytic leukemia; PLL, prolymphocytic leukemia; HCL, hairy cell leukemia; CIg, cytoplasmic immunoglobulin; SIg, surface immunoglobulin)

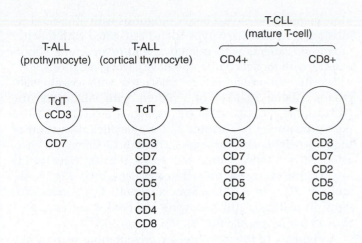

■ **FIGURE 30-5** Normal T lymphocyte maturation scheme with leukemic counterparts. (ALL, acute lymphocytic leukemia; CLL, chronic lymphocytic leukemia)

not be present. Malignancies of later stages of B lymphocyte differentiation are included in the classification of chronic neoplastic lymphoproliferative disorders (∞ Chapter 31).

B cell lineage also is detected by rearrangement of immunoglobulin genes.[8] The assembly of the D-J immunoglobulin genes is the first genetic event that identifies a B cell progenitor. Clonal gene rearrangement helps to differentiate neoplastic B cells from normal B cells. This rearrangement is detected by molecular methods (∞ Chapter 25).

T Cell ALL

Precursor T cell ALL is differentiated using pan T cell markers (markers present on all T cells) CD2, CD3, CD5, and CD7. TdT is present in most and CD10 may also be present (Table 30-3 ✪). The immature T cells differ from more mature T-cells in that they have either both CD4 and CD8 or neither of these antigens. Mature T cells have one or the other. This classification does not recognize the antigenic heterogeneity of T ALL but when utilized with the B ALL markers of CD19, CD10, TdT, CIg, and SIg, 90% of ALL will be classifiable into one of the B ALL or T ALL subgroups[6].

T cell lineage is also detected by rearrangement of the TCR genes using molecular methods. There are four TCR genes capable of rearranging, TCRα, β, γ, and δ. A neoplastic

cell may exhibit rearrangement of one or more of these genes. Detection of a monoclonal TCR gene rearrangement suggests a neoplasm of the T cell (∞ Chapter 25).

T ALL occurs most often in males. A mediastinal mass is a common finding, and the total leukocyte count is usually higher than in other immunologic subtypes.

Although attempts have been made to correlate the FAB subtypes of ALL with the immunologic subtypes, there appear to be no clear distinctions with the exception of L3, which are all B ALL. Most T ALL are L1.

✓ **Checkpoint! #4**

Why is it necessary to immunophenotype the lymphoblasts in ALL if they have been identified as lymphoblasts morphologically?

TERMINAL DEOXYNUCLEOTIDYL TRANSFERASE (TDT)

In addition to identification of lymphocytes by immunophenotyping, certain intracellular enzymes are proving to be helpful in identifying cellular subtypes. The most important of these is terminal deoxynucleotidyl transferase (TdT), a DNA polymerase found in cell nuclei. Its presence can be determined by direct enzyme assay, by indirect immunofluorescence, or with monoclonal antibodies. This enzyme is not present in normal mature lymphocytes but can be found in 65% of the total thymic population of lymphocytes.[9] The TdT positive cells are localized in the cortex. It can also be found in very early B cells and blasts of early myeloid lineage (M0, M1). About 1–3% of normal bone marrow cells are TdT positive. Its value in ALL is to identify primitive lymphoblasts from more mature cells.[10]

@ **CASE STUDY** *(continued from page 573)*

3. If the flow cytometry pattern showed a positive CD10, what would be the classification of this acute leukemia?

4. In this situation, would the therapeutic outcome be considered as favorable or bleak? Why?

✪ **TABLE 30-3**

Cellular Markers Useful in Diagnosis and Classification of ALL

Subgroup	TdT	CD34	CD19	CD22	CD10	CD20	CD2,3,4,5,7	Rearrangement of Ig Genes	cIg	SIg	Rearrangement of TCR Genes
Early pre-B	+	+	+	+(c)	+	−	−	+	−	−	−
Pre-B	+	−	+	+(s)	+	+	−	+	+	−	−
Mature B	−	−	+	+	+/−	+	−	+	−	+	−
Precursor T	+	−	−	−	−	−	+	−	−	−	+

WHO CLASSIFICATION OF ALL

Currently the newer World Health Organization classification of the acute leukemias is attempting to consolidate classification pathways and to include newer methodologies while eliminating subtypes that have been shown to have no current clinical relevance. In this classification, there is considerable movement away from separation based on purely morphologic grounds. For the lymphoblastic leukemias, there is a substitution of precursor B cell ALL morphologic subgroups with cytogenetic subgroups. The other ALL subgroups include precursor T cell ALL and Burkitt cell (B cell) leukemia[11] (Table 30-4).

The WHO classification considers acute lymphoblastic leukemias and lymphoblastic lymphomas to be a single disease with different clinical presentations. Thus, precursor T cell and precursor B cell neoplasms with bone marrow and peripheral blood involvement are acute lymphoblastic leukemias, while precursor T cell and precursor B cell neoplasms presenting as solid tumors are lymphoblastic lymphomas.

✔ **Checkpoint! #5**

A patient has 50% blasts in his bone marrow. Cytochemical stains are negative with peroxidase and Sudan black B. Immunophenotyping is CD19- positive, but CD20-, CD2-, CD10-, and CD7- negative. What additional testing may be helpful to distinguish the immunologic subgroup of this leukemia?

CYTOGENETIC ANALYSES OF ALL

Karyotyping of the ALLs is important for providing prognostic information. Abnormal karyotypes can be demonstrated in 60–75% of the cases of ALL. Abnormalities appear to be more common in B ALL than in T ALL. Both hyperdiploidy and hypodiploidy have been described. Patients who have chromosome counts >50 have a better prognosis with long-term remission. A normal karyotype is also associated with a better prognosis. Patients with numerical and/or structural abnormalities with modal counts <50 have a worse prognosis.

Specific abnormalities are associated with certain subgroups. About 10–15% of children with ALL have the Philadelphia (Ph) chromosome, which is associated with a poor prognosis.[12] (∞ Chapter 27 for a detailed discussion of the Philadelphia chromosome.) The FAB L3 subtype is characterized by a translocation of 8 to 14, t(8;14).[13] The t(4;11) involves the MLL gene (mixed-lineage leukemia), 11q23. Absence of CD10 in B ALL is associated with 11q23 translocations. In particular, the following aberrations are associated with a poor prognosis: t(9;22), t(8;14), t(4;11).[14]

A summary of the morphologic presentations seen in ALL is given in Table 30-1 ✪. A summary of the immunologic, morphologic, cytochemical, and cytogenetic characteristics of ALL subtypes is given in Table 30-5 ✪. The characteristic cytogenetic findings associated with subgroups of ALL can be found in ∞ Chapter 24, Table 24-7.

✔ **Checkpoint! #6**

A 3-year-old patient has 45% lymphoblasts in the bone marrow. The blasts are slightly larger than lymphocytes and appear to be a homogeneous population. The nuclear membrane is regular and nucleoli are not prominent. There is a small amount of moderately basophilic cytoplasm. What is the most likely FAB group of this leukemia? If the cells tested positive for CD19, CD10, and CD34, what is the most likely immunologic subgroup? Why should cytogenetics be done on this patient?

ACUTE LEUKEMIA WITH LINEAGE HETEROGENEITY

The terminology concerning leukemias with lineage heterogeneity is confusing and controversial. The term **bilineage** is generally used to define those leukemias that have two separate populations of leukemic cells, one that phenotypes as lymphoid and the other as myeloid (bilineage). The term **biphenotypic** (mixed lineage leukemia) describes acute leukemias that have myeloid and lymphoid markers on the same population of neoplastic cells. Overall, the incidence of biphenotypic leukemia is quite uncommon. The phenotype combinations can be B lymphoid/myeloid, T lymphoid/myeloid, T/B lymphoid, and one trilineage differentiation.[15] Lack of lineage specificity could be the result of genetic misprogramming, or the leukemic clone could represent a bipotential cell that has retained both lymphoid and myeloid markers during development.[16]

Immunological phenotyping is necessary to define mixed lineage leukemias because there are no definitive morphological and cytochemical features for lymphoid cells. Since

✪ **TABLE 30-4**

The WHO Classification of Acute Lymphoid Leukemias (ALL)

1. Precursor B-cell ALL

   t(9;22)(q34:q11),
   BCR/ABL

   t(v;11q23); MLL rearranged

   t(1;19)(q23:p13),
   E2A/PBX1

   t(12;21)(p12:q22),
   ETV/CBFα

2. Precursor T-cell ALL

⊙ TABLE 30-5

Summary of Laboratory Features Helpful in Classification of ALL

Characteristic	Early Pre-B	Pre-B	Mature B	Precursor T
Gene rearrangement				
Immunoglobulin (Ig)	+	+	+	−
T cell receptor (TCR)	−	−	−	+
Immunologic features				
Cytoplasmic μ	−	+	−	−
Surface Ig	−	−	+	−
Immunophenotype				
CD34	+	−	−	
CD19	+	+	+	−
CD22	+(c)	+(s)	+	−
CD10	+	+	+/−	−
CD20	−	+	+	−
CD2, CD3, CD5, CD7	−	−	−	+
Cytochemistry				
TdT	+	+	−	+
PAS	−	−	−	+

(+ = positive; − = negative; (c) = cytoplasmic; (s) = surface)

lineage markers are generally lineage associated and not lineage specific, a single inappropriate surface marker should not be used as sole evidence for biphenotypic leukemia. Cells should have at least two inappropriate markers to be considered biphenotypic.[17] Biphenotypic leukemia is suspected if the percentage of cells having myeloid markers overlaps with the percentage having lymphoid markers. More specific diagnosis is possible if a double labeling technique utilizing two immunologic markers or a combination of cytochemistry and immunologic markers is used. This procedure distinguishes between mixed lineage (bilineage) and biphenotypic acute leukemias because it can be determined if the same cell has two separate markers.

A more inclusive scheme for identifying mixed-lineage leukemia requires a combination of morphologic, cytochemical, immunologic, and cytogenetic evaluation and subsequent association of these features with one or the other lineage.[18] The importance of an inclusive scheme for classification of leukemia is emphasized by the finding of T cell markers (CD7 and CD2) and a B cell marker (CD19) in a significant number of cases of AML. The blasts in these cases lack any other features of lymphoid lineage, and many express abnormal karyotypes associated with AML rather than ALL. Lineage infidelity may be a characteristic of some malignant cells.[19]

Although mixed-lineage leukemias are uncommon, it is important to identify them in order to determine their actual occurrence, to identify appropriate therapy, and to correlate karyotypic abnormalities.[20]

 Checkpoint! #7

A patient with acute leukemia has two morphologically different types of blasts. One population is positive for CD7 and CD2. The other is positive for CD33 and CD13. What is the most appropriate classification of this leukemia?

UNCLASSIFIED ALL (U-ALL)

Unclassified ALL (also known as null cell ALL, or non-B, non-T ALL) is classified as such because the lymphoblasts lack any of the markers for the other subtypes. Very few ALLs are classified as U-ALL. In some cases, the cells are positive for the HLA-DR and TdT. These two markers are common to less mature T and B lymphocytes, indicating that the common precursor of T and B lymphocytes probably also possesses these markers. Thus, it is possible that the blasts found in U-ALL may represent the committed lymphoid stem cell.

ACUTE UNDIFFERENTIATED LEUKEMIA (AUL)

Occasionally, the blasts of acute leukemia may not stain with the standard cytochemical stains and surface markers. In these cases, the morphology of the blasts is nonspecific. Before a diagnosis of **acute undifferentiated leukemia**

(AUL) is made, electron microscopic studies should be performed to detect ultrastructural evidence of primary granules and/or peroxidase. A positive finding with this technique indicates nonlymphocytic leukemia and is important for treatment decisions. A negative finding with electron microscopy together with the other negative findings indicates a diagnosis of AUL. AUL is predominantly found in adults, and only about one-third of patients respond to the chemotherapy regimens of AML and ALL.

MYELOID/NATURAL KILLER CELL ACUTE LEUKEMIA

A recently recognized acute leukemia, **myeloid/natural killer (NK) cell acute leukemia**, coexpresses myeloid antigens (CD33, CD13, and/or CD15) and NK cell-associated antigens (CD56, CD11b), while lacking HLA-DR and T lymphocyte associated antigens (CD3 and CD8).[21] Most cases morphologically resemble AML-M3v with invaginated nuclear membranes, scant to moderate amounts of cytoplasm, fine to moderately coarse azurophilic granules, and finely granular myeloperoxidase and Sudan black B positivity (weaker than in M3). No faggot cells are present. In contrast to M3 AML, however, the leukemic cells of this group demonstrate cell-mediated cytotoxicity characteristic of NK cells.[22]

The initial leukocyte count is usually high. The percentage of bone marrow blasts is high (47–99%).

In contrast to AML-M3, the leukemic cells of myeloid/NK cell acute leukemia do not show the t(15;17) abnormality or express the PML/RAR-α fusion transcript. Patients do not respond to all trans-retinoic acid (ATRA) therapy. Other cytogenetic abnormalities are sometimes present. It has been suggested that NK cell leukemia may account for some of the mistakenly diagnosed promyelocytic leukemias that do not show a response to ATRA therapy.

Clinical findings overlap with other acute leukemias. Some patients have a bleeding diathesis consisting of petechial and/or mucosal hemorrhage or disseminated intravascular coagulation. Most do not have splenomegaly or hepatomegaly. The median survival is 30 months.

It is suggested that myeloid/NK cell acute leukemia is a distinct disorder and should not be considered a subgroup of AML-M3 or NK large-granular lymphocyte (LGL) leukemia, a lymphoproliferative disorder. Rather, the myeloid/NK cell acute leukemia is thought to be derived from a transformation of a stem cell common to myeloid and NK lineages.[23,24]

 Checkpoint! #8

How can the neoplastic cells in myeloid/NK cell AL be differentiated from the neoplastic cells of AML-M3 if they appear morphologically similar?

▶ THERAPY

A significant number of acute leukemias express inappropriate combinations of antigens making diagnosis challenging. Treatment protocols and prognosis are proving to be more effective and accurate when the leukemic cell is immunologically classified. In addition, therapy response and detection of residual leukemic cells is possible using immunophenotyping, especially when the leukemic cell phenotype deviates from its normal cell counterpart.

The therapy for AL includes chemotherapy, radiotherapy, antibiotics, bone marrow, and stem cell transplants. These are discussed in detail in ∞ Chapters 26 and 34.

SUMMARY

The acute leukemias (AL) are a heterogeneous group of neoplastic stem cell disorders characterized by unregulated proliferation, blocked maturation, or blocked apoptosis. The two major groups of AL are acute myelocytic leukemia (AML) and acute lymphocytic leukemia (ALL). These two major groups are further classified into subtypes based on FAB morphologic criteria, cytochemical stains, immunologic analysis, and cytogenetic and molecular abnormalities. The FAB classification describes three subtypes for ALL. The FAB ALL subgroups are based on morphology of blasts and include L1, L2, and L3. Immunophenotyping in ALL helps subtype the blasts into B or T ALL. There is no clear-cut association between FAB subgroups of ALL and immunologic phenotype except that all L3 ALLs are B ALLs.

The peroxidase and/or Sudan black B help differentiate AML (peroxidase positive) from ALL (peroxidase negative).

Mixed lineage leukemia is used to describe ALs that have two separate cell lines present, myeloid and lymphoid, or two different lymphoid lineages or trilineage cells. *Biphenotypic leukemia* is used to describe ALs that have blasts that possess multicell line markers on the same cell.

Regardless of subtype, the onset of AL is usually abrupt and, without treatment, progresses. Symptoms are related to anemia, thrombocytopenia, and/or neutropenia. Splenomegaly, hepatomegaly, and lymphadenopathy are common findings.

Hematologic findings include a normocytic, normochromic anemia, thrombocytopenia, and a decreased, normal, or increased leukocyte count. Blasts are almost always found in the peripheral blood. A bone marrow examination is always indicated if leukemia is suspected. The bone marrow reveals more than 30% blasts (FAB) or more than 20% blasts in WHO classification.

REVIEW QUESTIONS

LEVEL I

1. Which of the following descriptions is more closely associated with the lymphoblasts seen in ALL-L1? (Checklist #2)
   a. large with a deeply basophilic cytoplasm
   b. homogeneous with moderate basophilia in the cytoplasm
   c. mixed population of large and small cells
   d. medium sized cells with large nucleus and prominent nucleoli

2. Acute lymphoblastic leukemia is most often seen in patients: (Checklist #5)
   a. over the age of 60
   b. age 35–60 years
   c. age 10–35 years
   d. below 5 years

3. The FAB classification of ALL is based on: (Checklist #2)
   a. cytogenetic abnormalities
   b. morphology and cytochemistry of blasts
   c. immunophenotyping of blasts
   d. molecular genetic abnormalities

4. An acute leukemia has morpholocially undifferentiated blasts that are negative with cytochemical stains and immunophenotyping. This should be classified as: (Checklist #6)
   a. acute undifferentiated leukemia
   b. mixed lineage acute leukemia
   c. myeloid/NK cell acute leukemia
   d. null cell acute lymphocytic leukemia

5. Acute leukemia blasts that have myeloid and lymphoid markers on the same cells most likely define what subgroup of leukemia? (Checklist #6)
   a. bilineage
   b. myeloid/NK
   c. biphenotypic
   d. undifferentiated

6. Acute leukemia characterized by morphologically undifferentiated blasts that are negative with conventional cytochemical stains should be: (Checklist #6)
   a. classified as undifferentiated acute leukemia
   b. classified as myeloid/NK leukemia
   c. immunophenotyped before classifying
   d. classified as undifferentiated acute lymphocytic leukemia

7. When Auer rods are found in blasts of a case of acute lymphoblastic leukemia, the leukemia is most probably: (Checklist #2, 6)
   a. undifferentiated leukemia
   b. B lymphocytic leukemia
   c. T lymphocytic leukemia
   d. bilineage leukemia

LEVEL II

1. Cells that are positive for the 8;14 translocation are characteristic of which of the following? (Checklist #4)
   a. T cell ALL
   b. reactive lymphocytosis
   c. mycosis fungoides
   d. Burkitt leukemia

2. Rearrangements of the 11q23 are found in: (Checklist #4)
   a. precursor B cell ALL
   b. Burkitt cell leukemia
   c. precursor T cell ALL
   d. B cell ALL

3. In a case of ALL, the lymphoblasts showed strong localized positivity with acid phosphatase and were positive for CD7 and CD2, negative for CD19, CD24, and CD20. These blasts are most likely: (Checklist #4)
   a. T lymphoblasts
   b. B lymphoblasts
   c. lymphoid stem cells
   d. biphenotypic blasts

4. While performing a differential count on a 2-year-old child, the clinical laboratory scientist identifies 78% blasts and notes the following other data: (Checklist #4, 6)

Hb:	9.5 gm/dL
WBC:	50.3×10^9/L
PLT:	43×10^9/L

   Which of the following cytochemical stains would be expected to be positive?
   a. tartrate-resistant acid phosphatase
   b. periodic acid Schiff
   c. myeloperoxidase
   d. alpha-napthyl butyrate esterase

5. An adult patient with splenomegaly has an increase in mononuclear cells in the peripheral blood. The bone marrow was filled with a heterogeneous collection of blasts with no granulation. The cells in the marrow were negative for myeloperoxidase and Sudan black B. Flow cytometry shows a positive CD20. Which of the following conditions is most likely? (Checklist #4)
   a. early B precursor ALL
   b. common ALL (CALLA)
   c. T cell ALL
   d. B cell ALL

6. BCR/ABL can be seen in: (Checklist #2)
   a. ALL1
   b. Burkitt leukemia
   c. precursor B cell ALL
   d. T cell ALL

REVIEW QUESTIONS *(continued)*

LEVEL I

8. Blasts that are chunky positive with PAS but negative with other cytochemical stains are probably: (Checklist #1, 4)
   a. myeloblasts
   b. monoblasts
   c. megakaryoblasts
   d. lymphoblasts

9. The ALLs are most commonly found in this age group: (Checklist #1, 5)
   a. infants
   b. 2–4 year olds
   c. adults >70 years old
   d. 20–40 year olds

10. Which of the following signs is common in the presentation of childhood ALL? (Checklist #5)
    a. gum infiltration
    b. bone and joint pain
    c. large, painful nodes
    d. eosinophilia

LEVEL II

7. CD10 positive acute lymphoblastic leukemia is most common between the ages of: (Checklist #2)
   a. birth and 1 year
   b. 1 and 4 years
   c. 20 and 30 years
   d. 50 and 70 years

8. What condition is suggested by the following laboratory findings? (Checklist #2, 4)

   WBC: 50.4×10^9/L
   Diff: 75% blasts
            20% segmented cells
            2% lymphs
            3% monos

Peroxidase:	negative
Sudan black B:	negative
Alpha-naphthyl esterase:	negative
Naphthol AS-D chloroacetate esterase:	negative
PAS:	positive

   a. acute lymphoblastic leukemia
   b. acute myelogenous leukemia
   c. chronic granulocytic leukemia
   d. chronic lymphocytic leukemia

9. A 4-year-old male is admitted with the following findings:

WBC:	60×10^9/L
Segs:	15%
Bands:	5%
Blasts:	80%

   The blasts appear to be large with cytoplasmic vacuoles that stain with oil red O. These lymphocytes fluoresce when incubated with a fluorescent labeled anti-immunoglobulin serum and form rosettes when reacted with complement-coated erythrocytes. What type of cell is involved? (Checklist #2, 4)
   a. null cells
   b. T lymphocytes
   c. B lymphocytes
   d. NK cells

10. A 3-year-old male presents with a hemoglobin of 9 gm/dL and a white cell count of 25×10^9/L and a platelet count of 85×10^9/L. A bone marrow reveals a hypercellular marrow with 60% blasts. Choose the cytochemistries that you feel are most in line with the probable diagnosis. (Checklist #1, 2, 4, 6)
    a. myeloperoxidase positive, Sudan black B positive, PAS negative
    b. myeloperoxidase positive, naphthol AS-D chloroacetate esterase positive, alpha-naphthyl acetate esterase negative
    c. myeloperoxidase negative, naphthol AS-D chloroacetate negative, PAS chunky positive
    d. myeloperoxidase negative, Sudan black B positive, naphthol AS-D chloroacetate positive

www.prenhall.com/mckenzie

Use the above address to access the free, interactive Companion Web site created for this textbook. Get hints, instant feedback, and textbook references to chapter-related multiple choice questions.

REFERENCES

1. Shusterman S, Meadows AT. Long-term survivors of childhood leukemia. *Curr Opin Hematol.* 2000; 7:217–22.

2. Ekem I. Childhood acute lymphoblastic leukaemia (ALL) in Ghanaians and Germans: A comparative study. *West Afr J Med.* 2000; 19:50–54.

3. Maitra A, Weinberg AG. Inclusions in lymphoblasts. *Pediatr Dev Pathol.* 1998; 1:573.

4. Bennett JM, Catovsky D, Daniel MT, Flandrin G, Galton DA, Gralnick HR, et al. Proposals for the classification of the acute leukaemias. French-American-British (FAB) Co-Operative Group. *Br J Haematol.* 1976; 33:451–58.

5. First MIC Co-Operative Study Group. Morphologic, immunologic, and cytogenetic (MIC) working classification of acute lymphoblastic leukemias: Report of the workshop held in Leuven, Belgium, April 22–23, 1985. *Cancer Genet Cytogenet.* 1986; 23:189–97.

6. Tiensiwakul P, Lertlum T, Nuchprayoon I, Seksarn P. Immunophenotyping of acute lymphoblastic leukemia in pediatric patients by three-color flow cytometric analysis. *Asian Pac J Allergy Immunol.* 1999; 17:17–21.

7. Cobaleda C, Gutierrez-Cianca N, Perez-Losada J, Flores T, Garcia-Sanz R, Gonzalez M, et al. A primitive hematopoietic cell is the target for the leukemic transformation in human Philadelphia-positive acute lymphoblastic leukemia. *Blood.* 2000; 95:1007–13.

8. De Rossi G, Grossi C, Foa R, Tabilio A, Vegna L, Lo Coco F, et al. Immunophenotype of acute lymphoblastic leukemia cells: The experience of the Italian Cooperative Group (Gimema). *Leuk Lymphoma.* 1993; 9:221–28.

9. Farahat N, Lens D, Morilla R, Matutes E, Catovsky D. Differential TdT expression in acute leukemia by flow cytometry: A quantitative study. *Leukemia.* 1995; 9:583–87.

10. Paietta E, Racevskis J, Bennett JM, Wiernik PH. Differential expression of terminal transferase (TdT) in acute lymphocytic leukaemia expressing myeloid antigens and TdT positive acute myeloid leukaemia as compared to myeloid antigen negative acute lymphocytic leukaemia. *Br J Haematol.* 1993; 84:416–22.

11. Bennett JM. World Health Organization classification of the acute leukemias and myelodysplastic syndrome. *Int J Hematol.* 2000; 72:131–33.

12. Arico M, Valsecchi MG, Camitta B, Schrappe M, Chessells J, Baruchel A, et al. Outcome of treatment in children with Philadelphia chromosome-positive acute lymphoblastic leukemia. *N Engl J Med.* 2000; 342(14):998–1006.

13. Jantunen E, Voranen M, Nousiainen T, Riikonen P. Burkitt leukemia-lymphoma. *Duodecim.* 1995; 111(22):2115–21.

14. Catovsky D, Matutes E, Buccheri V, Shetty V, Hanslip J, Yoshida N, et al. A classification of acute leukaemia for the 1990s. *Ann Hematol.* 1991; 62:16–21.

15. Garcia Vela JA, Monteserin MC, Delgado I, Benito L, Ona F. Aberrant immunophenotypes detected by flow cytometry in acute lymphoblastic leukemia. *Leuk Lymphoma.* 2000; 36:275–84.

16. Killick S, Matutes E, Powles RL, Hamblin M, Swansbury J, Treleaven JG, et al. Outcome of biphenotypic acute leukemia. *Haematologica.* 1999; 84:699–706.

17. Legrand O, Perrot JY, Simonin G, Baudard M, Cadiou M, Blanc C, et al. Adult biphenotypic acute leukaemia: An entity with poor prognosis which is related to unfavourable cytogenetics and P-glycoprotein over-expression. *Br J Haematol.* 1998; 100:147–55.

18. Dunphy CH, Batanian JR. Biphenotypic hematological malignancy with T-lymphoid and myeloid differentiation: Association with t(3;12) (p25;q24.3). Case report and review of the literature. *Cancer Genet Cytogenet.* 1999; 114:51–57.

19. Johansson B, Moorman AV, Haas OA, Watmore AE, Cheung KL, Swanton S, et al. Hematologic malignancies with t(4;11)(q21;q23): A cytogenetic, morphologic, immunophenotypic, and clinical study of 183 cases. European 11q23 Workshop participants. *Leukemia.* 1998; 12:779–87.

20. Lefterova P, Schmidt-Wolf IG. Coexpression of lymphoid and myeloid markers on cell surfaces. *Leuk Lymphoma.* 1997; 26:27–33.

21. Babustkova O, Glasova M, Konikova E, Kusenda J. Leukemia-associated phenotypes: Their characteristics and incidence in acute leukemia. *Neoplasma.* 1996; 43:367–72.

22. Suzuki R, Nakamura S. Malignancies of natural killer (NK) cell precursor: Myeloid/NK cell precursor acute leukemia and blastic NK cell lymphoma/leukemia. *Leuk Res.* 1999; 23:615–24.

23. Paietta E, Gallagher RE, Wiernik PH. Myeloid/natural killer cell acute leukemia: A previously unrecognized form of acute leukemia potentially misdiagnosed as FAB-M3 acute myeloid leukemia. *Blood.* 1994; 84:2824–25.

24. Scott AA, Head DR, Kopecky KJ, Appelbaum FR, Theil KS, Grever MR, et al. HLA-DR–, CD33+, CD56+, CD16– myeloid/natural killer cell acute leukemia: A previously unrecognized form of acute leukemia potentially misdiagnosed as French-American-British acute myeloid leukemia-M3. *Blood.* 1994; 84:244–55.

▶ OVERVIEW

This chapter is a study of the classification of lymphoid malignancies, how the diagnosis is established, and the unique features of selected subtypes. First the etiology and pathogenesis of the disorders are discussed. This is followed by a description of how this broad group of diseases is classified and diagnosed. The remainder of the chapter describes characteristics of the more common types of chronic leukemic lymphoid malignancy, malignant lymphoma, and plasma cell neoplasm.

▶ INTRODUCTION

Lymphoid malignancies are a heterogeneous group of disorders that are composed of cells that resemble one or more stages of normal lymphocyte development. The maturity of the neoplastic cell and the clinical distribution of disease can be used to divide this broad group into four categories: acute lymphoblastic leukemia, chronic leukemic lymphoid malignancies, malignant lymphoma, and plasma cell neoplasms.

Leukemia is a malignant neoplasm that presents with widespread involvement of the bone marrow. Acute lymphoblastic leukemia is a proliferation of blasts belonging to the lymphoid lineage (∞ Chapters 26, 30). The chronic lymphoid leukemic malignancies are composed of mature lymphocytes and usually have an insidious onset and more indolent course than the acute leukemias.

The **lymphomas** are malignant neoplasms that present as tumorous masses that involve the lymphoid organs including lymph nodes, tonsils, spleen, thymus, and lymphoid tissue of the gastrointestinal tract. Although most lymphomas are composed of mature lymphoid cells, blastic malignancies (lymphoblastic lymphoma) do occur. The distinction between leukemia and lymphoma is not always clear-cut. Lymphoblastic lymphoma and acute lymphoblastic leukemia probably represent different clinical manifestations of a single disease entity. Also, patients with leukemia may develop tumors of the lymphoid organs, and lymphoma may spread to involve the bone marrow and peripheral blood.

The **plasma cell neoplasms** are a group of diseases composed of immunoglobulin secreting cells. Unlike the leukemias and lymphomas, this group of diseases contains both benign and malignant neoplasms. Again, the boundary between this group and the malignant lymphomas is not sharp, because lymphoma may contain a subset of cells demonstrating plasma cell differentiation (lymphoplasmacytic lymphoma), and plasma cell neoplasms may demonstrate lymphocytic differentiation (Waldenström's macroglobulinemia). Despite these difficulties in classification, the lymphoid malignancies can be divided into groups that provide information about prognosis and help direct treatment.

▶ ETIOLOGY AND PATHOGENESIS

The genesis of lymphoid malignancy is thought to be a multistep process involving acquired genetic, inherited genetic, and environmental factors.

ACQUIRED GENETIC FACTORS

As described for the leukemias, acquired alterations of proto-oncogenes and tumor suppressor genes have been associated with the development of lymphoid malignancy. Additional targets for genetic damage are the genes involved in programmed cell death (apoptosis) (e.g., *BCL*-2). The **BCL-2 gene** on chromosome 18 is involved in the pathogenesis of follicular lymphoma. Translocation of the BCL-2 gene to the region of the immunoglobulin heavy chain gene, t(14;18), causes an overexpression of the BCL-2 gene. The resulting increase in BCL-2 protein leads to an inhibition of apoptosis. Decreased cell death results in an accumulation of lymphocytes within the lymph node. Therefore, low-grade follicular lymphoma appears to arise from cell persistence rather than uncontrolled cell proliferation.

INHERITED GENETIC FACTORS

The inherited immunodeficiency syndromes, Wiskott Aldrich and ataxia telangiectasia, are associated with a higher incidence of malignant lymphoma.

ENVIRONMENTAL FACTORS

The Epstein-Barr virus (EBV) is associated with the development of several forms of lymphoid malignancy including African Burkitt lymphoma, B cell malignant lymphoma in HIV infected individuals, and Hodgkin lymphoma. Latent infection with EBV is just one of the multiple steps involved in the genesis of these types of lymphoma. EBV infection is acquired orally and is often manifest clinically as infectious mononucleosis. The virus infects B lymphocytes, where it remains latent, under the control of the immune system. The EBV infected cells can proliferate if the host becomes immunocompromised and/or the B lymphocytes acquire additional genetic abnormalities such as the *c-myc* translocation.

Another infectious agent associated with the development of non-Hodgkin lymphoma is *Helicobacter pylori*. Patients with *Helicobacter pylori* induced chronic gastritis have a high incidence of gastric lymphoma of mucosa associated lymphoid tissue (MALT lymphoma). Chronic infection leads to antigen-driven T lymphocyte stimulation and subsequent B lymphocyte activation. Initially the B lymphocytes are polyclonal and entirely dependent on T lymphocyte stimulation. With time the B cell population may become monoclonal and malignant. If the B lymphocyte proliferation is still dependant on T lymphocyte stimulation, the lymphoma may regress following removal of the antigenic stimulus with antimicrobial therapy. Lymphoma that is no longer responsive to antigenic stimulation will probably require more drastic therapy including excision and/or chemotherapy.

 Checkpoint! #1

How does the BCL-2 gene rearrangement differ from most other oncogenes?

▶ DIAGNOSIS OF LYMPHOID MALIGNANCY

Knowledge of the distribution of disease at presentation and the morphologic appearance of the neoplastic cells is essential for the correct diagnosis of lymphoid malignancy. The phenotype and genotype of the malignant cells often assist in diagnosis and classification, determination of prognosis, and detection of residual disease following treatment.

MORPHOLOGIC APPEARANCE

The diagnosis of a lymphoid malignancy is established by examination in the laboratory of a specimen of peripheral blood, bone marrow, and/or other tissue. For most cases of leukemia this involves a CBC and bone marrow sample (aspirate and biopsy). A diagnosis of lymphoma is usually rendered from biopsy or a fine needle aspirate of the mass. In general, normal or reactive proliferations of lymphocytes contain a mixture of cells varying in size, shape, and staining characteristics. The cells present in lymphoid malignancies are usually more homogeneous because of expansion of a single cell type. Less frequently, malignant lymphoid cells can be recognized because of an abnormal or bizarre appearance.

ANCILLARY STUDIES

Sometimes morphology alone is not sufficient to diagnose or subclassify lymphoid malignancies. Several additional studies are available to assist in the diagnosis: immunophenotyping, molecular diagnostics, and cytogenetics. These studies can detect abnormal lymphocytes and/or **clonality** (the presence of identical cells derived from a single progenitor). The cells of malignant lymphoma are thought to derive from a single precursor cell. The progeny from this cell belong to a clone that shares morphologic, immunophenotypic, and genotypic features. In most circumstances clonality is synonymous with malignancy. Clonality can be detected by the identification of only one of the immunoglobulin light chains (kappa or lambda) on B cells or

the presence of a population of cells with an abnormal phenotype such as CD5-positive B lymphocytes (∞ Chapter 23). Clonal rearrangement of immunoglobulin or T cell receptor genes, or the presence of an abnormal translocation can also be used to identify malignant lymphocytes. The presence of characteristic translocations can assist in the diagnosis of a subtype of lymphoid malignancy as in the *bcl-2* rearrangement in follicular lymphoma (∞ Chapters 2, 26).

CLASSIFICATION

Lymphoid malignancies are classified into groups that have a similar clinical course and response to treatment (grading). Although several classification schemes have been proposed, two are currently used in clinical practice: the National Cancer Institute (NCI) working formulation[1] and the World Heath Organization (WHO) classification.[2] The working formulation separates subtypes of malignant lymphoma by their morphologic appearance into three grades (low, intermediate, and high) (Table 31-1 ✪). The histologic features characteristic of low-grade lymphoma include a follicular growth pattern, smaller cells, low mitotic activity, and an absence of apoptosis. In general, low-grade diseases have a long indolent course, and patients often die of disorders other than their lymphoma. High-grade lymphoma usually has a diffuse growth pattern, is composed of larger cells, and displays numerous mitoses and apoptotic bodies. High-grade lymphoma is clinically aggressive and will kill the patient rapidly if not treated. Ironically, current therapeutic regimens are more effective against high-grade than low-grade

✪ TABLE 31-1

Working Formulation of Non-Hodgkin Lymphomas for Clinical Usage[1]

Low-grade	a. Malignant lymphoma, small lymphocytic
	b. Malignant lymphoma, follicular, predominantly small cleaved cell
	c. Malignant lymphoma, follicular, mixed small cleaved and large cell
Intermediate-grade	d. Malignant lymphoma, follicular, predominantly large cell
	e. Malignant lymphoma, diffuse, small cleaved cell
	f. Malignant lymphoma, diffuse, mixed small and large cell
	g. Malignant lymphoma, diffuse, large cell
High-grade	h. Malignant lymphoma, large cell, immunoblastic
	i. Malignant lymphoma, lymphoblastic
	j. Malignant lymphoma, small noncleaved cell
Miscellaneous	Composite, mycosis fungoides, histiocytic, extramedullary plasmacytoma, unclassifiable, other

✪ TABLE 31-2

Proposed WHO Classification of Lymphoid Neoplasms[2]

B cell neoplasms	Precursor B cell neoplasms
	Precursor B lymphoblastic leukemia/lymphoma
	(precursor B cell acute lymphoblastic leukemia)
	Mature B cell neoplasms
	Chronic lymphocytic leukemia/small lympho-
	cytic lymphoma
	B cell prolymphocytic leukemia
	Lymphoplasmacytic lymphoma
	Splenic marginal zone lymphoma
	Hairy cell leukemia
	Plasma cell myeloma
	Extranodal marginal zone B cell lymphoma of
	mucosa associated lymphoid tissue
	Nodal marginal zone B cell lymphoma
	Follicular lymphoma
	Mantle cell lymphoma
	Diffuse large B cell lymphoma
	Mediastinal large B cell lymphoma
	Primary effusion lymphoma
	Burkitt lymphoma leukemia
T cell and NK cell neoplasms	Precursor T cell neoplasm
	Precursor T lymphoblastic leukemia/lymphoma
	(precursor T cell acute lymphoblastic leukemia)
	Mature T cell neoplasms
	T cell prolymphocytic leukemia
	T cell granular lymphocytic leukemia
	Aggressive NK cell leukemia
	Adult T cell lymphoma/leukemia,
	Extranodal NK/T cell lymphoma, nasal type
	Enteropathy-type T cell lymphoma
	Hepatosplenic T cell lymphoma
	Subcutaneous panniculitis-like T cell lymphoma
	Mycosis Fungoides/Sézary syndrome
	Anaplastic large cell lymphoma, T/null, primary
	cutaneous type
	Peripheral T cell lymphoma, not otherwise
	characterized
	Angioimmunoblastic T cell lymphoma
	Anaplastic large cell lymphoma, T/null, primary
	systemic type
Hodgkin lymphoma (disease)	Nodular lymphocyte-predominant Hodgkin lymphoma
	Classical Hodgkin lymphoma
	Nodular sclerosis classical Hodgkin lymphoma
	Mixed cellularity classical Hodgkin lymphoma
	Lymphocyte-rich classical Hodgkin lymphoma
	Lymphocyte depleted Hodgkin lymphoma

lymphoid malignancies. Therefore, many patients with high-grade lymphoma are cured of their disease. Patients with low-grade lymphoma are treated for symptomatic relief, rather than an intention to cure.

The WHO classification is a more complete listing of all lymphoid malignancies (leukemia and lymphoma) (Table 31-2). It combines morphologic findings with the immunophenotype and genotype to separate distinct disease entities such as mantle cell lymphoma and hairy cell leukemia.

STAGING

The prognosis of a patient with a lymphoid malignancy is related to the extent and distribution of disease (**stage**). Determining the stage of disease usually involves radiologic studies, peripheral blood examination, and bone marrow aspiration and biopsy. The Ann Arbor scheme is often used to stage malignant lymphoma (Table 31-3 ✪). Bone marrow involvement indicates disseminated disease, stage IV. Patients with widespread lymphoma usually have a worse prognosis.

The remainder of this chapter describes examples of lymphoid malignancies that illustrate the characteristics of the chronic leukemia lymphoid malignancies, malignant lymphoma, and plasma cell neoplasms.

✓ Checkpoint! #2

How does staging differ from grading in defining and classifying the lymphoid malignancies?

► CHRONIC LEUKEMIC LYMPHOID MALIGNANCIES

The chronic leukemic lymphoid malignancies are a heterogeneous group of disorders displaying a variety of morphologic appearances and immunophenotypes. They are grouped together because they are primarily located in the blood and bone marrow and the malignant cells are mature lymphocytes. Although these malignancies are usually more indolent than

✪ TABLE 31-3

Ann Arbor Staging System for Malignant Lymphoma

I	Single lymph node region or single extralymphatic site (I$_E$)
II	Two or more lymph node regions on same side of diaphragm or with involvement of limited contiguous extralymphatic site (II$_E$)
III	Lymph node regions on both sides of diaphragm, which may include spleen (III$_S$) and/or limited contiguous extralymphatic site (III$_E$)
IV	Multiple or disseminated foci of involvement of one or more extralymphatic organs or tissues with or without lymphatic involvement

the acute leukemias, the prognosis varies with the subtype.[3] The features of the following more common subtypes of chronic leukemic lymphoid malignancy will be discussed further: B cell chronic lymphocytic leukemia, prolymphocytic leukemia, hairy cell leukemia, large granular lymphocyte leukemia, Sézary's syndrome, and circulating lymphoma (Table 31-4 ✪).

✪ TABLE 31-4

Key Features of Subgroups of Chronic Leukemic Lymphoid Malignancies

B cell CLL	Lymphocytosis
	Smudge cells
	Prolymphocytes <10%
	CD19+, CD5+, CD23+
	Surface Ig weak
B cell PLL	Splenomegaly
	Marked lymphocytosis
	Prolymphocytes >55%
	CD19+, CD5−, FMC-7+
	Surface Ig strong
T cell PLL	Splenomegaly
	Skin lesions
	Marked lymphocytosis
	Varied morphologic appearance
	CD3+, CD2+, CD5+, CD4+
	Inv(14)q11q32
Hairy cell leukemia	Pancytopenia
	Circulating hairy cells
	TRAP+
	CD19+, CD5-, CD22+, CD11c+, CD25+
	Surface Ig strong
	Bone marrow dry tap
	Bone marrow "fried egg" appearance
T-cell LGL leukemia	Lymphocytosis
	Anemia
	Neutropenia
	Thrombocytopenia
	Rheumatoid factor present
	CD2+, CD3+, CD8+,
	CD16+, CD56−/+, CD57+/−
	TCR clonally rearranged
	Indolent course
NK LGL leukemia	Lymphocytosis
	Anemia
	CD2+, CD3−, CD8-, CD4-
	CD16+, CD56+/−, CD57−/+
	TCR germ-line
	Rapidly fatal
Sézary's syndrome	Erythroderma (red skin)
	Cutaneous T cell lymphoma
	Circulating malignant cells
	CD2+, CD3+, CD4+, CD7−

B CELL CHRONIC LYMPHOCYTIC LEUKEMIA

Chronic lymphocytic leukemia (CLL) is a disease of adults with a median age of 70 years at diagnosis. Many patients are asymptomatic. The disease is often detected because of a lymphocytosis found on a CBC performed for another reason. Symptoms are often related to anemia, thrombocytopenia, and neutropenia due to replacement of the bone marrow hematopoietic cells by neoplastic lymphocytes. Approximately 10% of patients with CLL develop anemia due to autoimmune mediated hemolysis (∞ Chapter 19). Lymphadenopathy may be present at diagnosis or develop during the course of the disease (*see* small lymphocytic lymphoma).

The diagnosis of CLL is usually established by examination of a peripheral blood specimen. There is an absolute lymphocytosis $>5 \times 10^9$/L. The lymphocytes are small and have scant cytoplasm. The nuclei are usually round, and the chromatin is regularly clumped (block-type chromatin). Nucleoli are inconspicuous (Figure 31-1a ■). A few large, **prolymphocytes** are usually present but represent less than 10% of all lymphocytes. Prolymphocytes have abundant pale-staining cytoplasm and a large central prominent nucleolus.

The neoplastic cells present in CLL appear to be more fragile than normal lymphocytes and often burst open during smear preparation to produce **smudge cells**. Smudge cells can also be found in reactive lymphocytosis and in other neoplasms; therefore, their presence should not be used to diagnose CLL. In fact smudge cells can make the diagnosis of CLL more difficult by preventing visualization of the lymphocytes. The number of these cells can be reduced by mixing a drop of albumin with a drop of blood prior to making the smear.

The differential diagnosis of CLL includes reactive lymphocytosis and the other chronic leukemia lymphoproliferative disorders. Although a provisional diagnosis can usually be made following smear examination, immunophenotyping is often used to establish a definitive diagnosis. B cell CLL is characterized by aberrant expression of the T lymphocyte antigen CD5. Expression of CD23 distinguishes CLL from leukemic mantle cell lymphoma. The cells of CLL usually have weak surface expression of monoclonal immunoglobulin.

CLL may occasionally display plasmacytic differentiation. The neoplastic cells in these cases may have more abundant basophilic cytoplasm and an eccentric nucleus (plasmacytoid lymphocytes), and there may be a monoclonal serum immunoglobulin (M-spike). Plasmacytoid lymphocytes lack the typical immunophenotype of CLL (CD5− and CD23−), and often contain monoclonal cytoplasmic immunoglobulin. CLL with plasmacytic differentiation overlaps morphologically with Waldenström's macroglobulinemia.

CLL is usually an indolent disease. The extent of disease is the most important indicator of prognosis for patients with

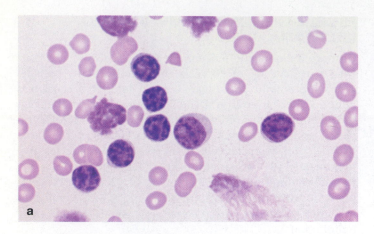
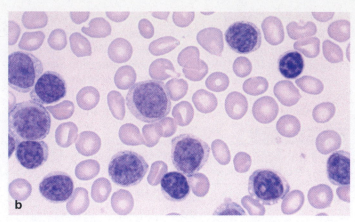

■ **FIGURE 31-1 a.** Chronic lymphocytic leukemia. Small round lymphocytes with clumped chromatin, a larger prolymphocyte with a prominent nucleolus, and numerous smudge cells. **b.** Prolymphocytic leukemia. Numerous large lymphoid cells with prominent nucleoli (prolymphocytes). (Both: Peripheral blood, Wright stain, 1000× magnification)

CLL. Advanced disease is indicated by involvement of many lymph node groups, splenomegaly, hepatomegaly, and/or extensive bone marrow involvement leading to cytopenias. A worse prognosis has also been associated with a karyotype demonstrating multiple cytogenetic abnormalities or the presence of trisomy 12 and a diffuse rather than nodular pattern of bone marrow infiltration. Currently no curative therapy is available. Treatment is reserved for the control of symptoms.

Less than 10% of patients with CLL develop transformation of their disease into one with a worse prognosis. **Richter's transformation** is the development of large cell lymphoma in a patient with CLL. Prolymphocytoid transformation of CLL is associated with an increased number of prolymphocytes.

PROLYMPHOCYTIC LEUKEMIA

Prolymphocytic leukemia (PLL) is an aggressive leukemic disorder of mature B or T lymphoid cells. Approximately 70% of cases are of a B cell lineage.

B Cell PLL

B cell PLL is a disease of adult patients with a male predominance. Although most cases arise de novo, PLL may represent the terminal phase of prolymphocytoid transformation of CLL (see above). The clinical history of CLL is often the only way of identifying the preceding chronic disease. Unlike CLL, patients with PLL usually have marked splenomegaly but minimal lymphadenopathy.

The CBC in patients with PLL reveals marked absolute lymphocytosis, often $>300 \times 10^9$/L, anemia, and thrombocytopenia. The neoplastic cells have a characteristic appearance: large cells with moderate amounts of pale basophilic cytoplasm, mature condensed chromatin, and a single prominent nucleolus (Figure 31-1b ■). Prolymphocytes rep-

resent less than 10% of the lymphocytes seen in CLL and greater than 55% of the lymphocytes present in PLL. Cases with 11–55% prolymphocytes are classified as CLL/PL or CLL mixed cell type. The cell marker phenotype of prolymphocytes often differs from the cells of CLL in demonstrating strong surface immunoglobulin expression, strong CD22, lack of CD11c, expression of FMC-7, and lack of CD5.

B cell PLL is an aggressive disease that usually does not respond to treatment. In contrast, CLL/PL has a variable clinical course.

T Cell PLL

T cell PLL is a rare disorder of adults that also has marked lymphocytosis and splenomegaly. However, patients with T cell PLL have more frequent lymphadenopathy, hepatomegaly, and skin lesions than patients with B cell PLL. The morphologic appearance of T cell PLL is also more variable than that of B cell PLL. The cells of T cell PLL usually have a prominent nucleolus but are medium in size and may have convoluted nuclear outlines. T cell PLL has a mature phenotype with expression of CD3, CD2, and CD5. Most cases are CD4 positive. Although a few cases express both CD4 and CD8, they are negative for TdT. The majority of cases of T cell PLL have cytogenetic abnormalities, most frequently inv(14)q11q32 and trisomy 8q. T cell PLL is an aggressive disorder with a median survival time of only 7.5 months.

HAIRY CELL LEUKEMIA

Hairy cell leukemia (HCL) is a malignant disease presenting in adulthood. There is a higher incidence in males (male: female = 7:1). At presentation, patients usually have massive splenomegaly but lack lymphadenopathy.

Patients with HCL have extensive bone marrow involvement and therefore present with pancytopenia. The white

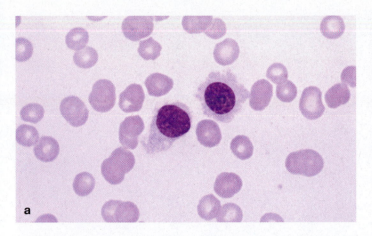
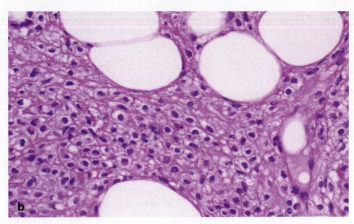

■ **FIGURE 31-2 a.** Hairy cell leukemia. Two abnormal lymphocytes with abundant pale-staining cytoplasm with hair-like projections and relatively finely distributed chromatin. **b.** Hairy cell leukemia. Replacement of hematopoietic precursors by abnormal small lymphocytes with abundant clear cytoplasm ("fried-egg" appearance). (a. Peripheral blood, Wright stain, 1000× magnification; b. Bone marrow, H&E stain, 100× magnification)

blood cell count is low due to both neutropenia and monocytopenia, and therefore patients have an increased susceptibility to infection, especially with mycobacterial organisms.

Although malignant cells are usually present on a peripheral smear, often their number is not sufficient to elevate the WBC. The neoplastic cells (**hairy cells**) have a characteristic abnormal appearance with abundant pale staining cytoplasm, circumferential cytoplasmic projections ("hairs"), oval or reniform nuclei, and relatively fine chromatin (Figure 31-2a ■). The malignant cells show acid phosphatase staining after tartrate incubation (**tartrate resistant acid phosphatase [TRAP]**). Although the morphologic appearance and TRAP staining are characteristic, immunophenotyping is often used to establish a diagnosis. The cells of hairy cell leukemia are B lymphocytes that are strongly positive for CD19, CD20, CD22, CD25, FMC-7, CD103, and CD11c. Although there is usually monoclonal surface immunoglobulin, it may be difficult to demonstrate because of nonspecific binding of the antibodies used to detect surface antigens.

Bone marrow involvement may be diffuse or focal. The neoplastic cells are usually surrounded by fibrosis preventing their aspiration from the bone marrow (dry tap). Bone marrow biopsy sections reveal a monotonous infiltrate of abnormal lymphocytes with small nuclei and abundant pale staining cytoplasm ("fried egg" appearance) (Figure 31-2b ■). Immunohistochemical stains for the B cell antigen CD20 and the marker of hairy cell leukemia DBA may be used to highlight focal disease. Splenectomy specimens reveal marked expansion of the red pulp because of an infiltrate of abnormal cells with the fried egg appearance described in the bone marrow. Lakes of erythrocytes are often formed between the tumor cells (pseudo-sinuses).

Hairy cell leukemia is an indolent disease. Long-lasting remissions are often obtained with the newer chemotherapy agents 2 chlorodeoxyadenosine (2-CDA) and deoxycoformycin.

LARGE GRANULAR LYMPHOCYTE LEUKEMIA

Only 5% of chronic leukemic lymphoproliferative disorders express T cell antigens. These cases were previously referred to as T cell CLL. Subsequent investigation has revealed that the vast majority of these cases represent large granular lymphocyte leukemia (LGL). LGL is characterized by a modest lymphocytosis composed of cells with abundant pale-staining cytoplasm, nuclei with mature clumped chromatin, and azurophilic cytoplasmic granules (Figure 31-3 ■). Large granular lymphocytes (T cell and NK) are a normal component of the peripheral blood. The diagnosis of leukemia is based on the presence of lymphocytosis, an abnormal phenotype, or evidence of clonality using molecular diagnostic or cytogenetic studies.

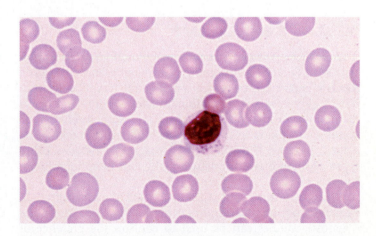

■ **FIGURE 31-3** Large granular lymphocyte leukemia. Lymphocyte with abundant clear-staining cytoplasm and azurophilic cytoplasmic granules. (Peripheral blood, H&E stain, 1000× magnification)

Two categories of LGL are recognized: T lymphocyte and natural-killer cell (NK). Approximately 80% of patients with LGL fall into the T-LGL leukemia category. Their median age at presentation is 55 years. In addition to lymphocytosis, these patients often have anemia, neutropenia, and thrombocytopenia. Anemia may be related to bone marrow infiltration or aplasia of erythroid precursors. Neutropenia and thrombocytopenia may be the result of immune destruction, splenic sequestration, or marrow infiltration. Although splenomegaly is common, lymphadenopathy and hepatomegaly are uncommon. Approximately 25% of patients with T-LGL leukemia have rheumatoid arthritis, and many more are positive for rheumatoid factor. Therefore, many patients with T cell LGL leukemia have the triad defining Felty's syndrome (rheumatoid arthritis, splenomegaly, and neutropenia).

The neoplastic cells are T lymphocytes with the following phenotype: CD2+, CD3+, CD4−, CD5+, CD7+, CD8+, CD16+, CD56−/+, CD57+/−. Molecular diagnostic studies reveal clonal T cell receptor rearrangement.

Patients with T-LGL leukemia usually have an indolent course with greater than 80% actuarial overall survival after 10 years. Death is often due to concurrent infection.

NK-LGL leukemia has a similar morphologic appearance to T-LGL leukemia, but is usually associated with a more acute presentation and aggressive course. The median age at presentation is 39 years. Patients often present with fevers, hepatomegaly, splenomegaly, involvement of the GI tract, and a bleeding disorder. Although anemia is common, neutropenia is rare.

The neoplastic cells have an NK phenotype: CD2+, CD3−, CD4−, CD8−, CD16+, CD56+/−, CD57−/+. Conventional molecular diagnostic studies cannot be used to determine clonality because NK cells do not rearrange the T cell receptor gene.

Unlike T-LGL, NK-LGL is usually an aggressive, rapidly fatal disease with most patients dying of multiorgan failure within 2 months.

SÉZARY'S SYNDROME

A few patients with cutaneous T cell lymphoma (CTCL) present with Sézary's syndrome (erythroderma and circulating **Sézary cells**). Sézary cells are malignant lymphocytes that have a very irregular, convoluted nuclear outline and finely distributed chromatin (Figure 31-4). Abnormal cells can be counted in a blood smear leukocyte differential to determine a Sézary count. The differential diagnosis includes other types of mature and immature malignant lymphoproliferative disorders.

Sézary cells are T cells (CD3+, CD4+) but are usually CD7 negative and may be abnormal in lacking CD5. Molecular diagnostic studies can be used to confirm the presence of malignant cells by demonstrating clonal T cell receptor gene rearrangement. Although the marked nuclear convolutions can also be identified on electron microscopy, this technique is rarely used for diagnosis.

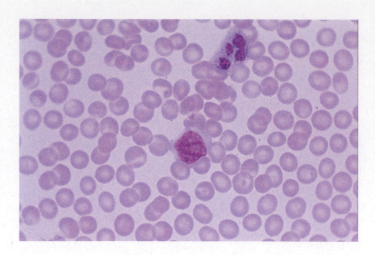

■ **FIGURE 31-4** Sézary syndrome. Abnormal large lymphocyte with relatively finely distributed chromatin and numerous nuclear folds (Sézary cell). (Peripheral blood, H&E stain, 1000× magnification)

CIRCULATING LYMPHOMA CELLS

Patients with non-Hodgkin lymphoma may develop peripheral blood involvement. Circulating lymphoma cells must be distinguished from normal lymphocytes and the cells of chronic leukemic lymphoproliferative disorders. Although the most frequent type of lymphoma to circulate is low-grade follicular lymphoma, other lymphomas may also have a leukemic phase (mantle cell, large cell, Burkitt). The circulating malignant cells of follicular lymphoma often have very irregular nuclear outlines and a deep indentation (cleft) of the nuclear membrane ("buttock" or **"butt" cells**) (see follicular lymphoma). Flow cytometric immunophenotyping can assist in the differential diagnosis by demonstrating monoclonal surface immunoglobulin and a characteristic phenotype (see chronic lymphocytic leukemia, follicular lymphoma, mantle cell lymphoma, Burkitt lymphoma).

✓ **Checkpoint! #3**

The chronic lymphoid leukemic malignancies are a heterogeneous group. What characteristics allow them to be grouped together?

 CASE STUDY *(continued from page 585)*

A CBC revealed a WBC of 20×10^9/L with 60% lymphocytes. Examination of the peripheral blood revealed mature lymphocytes with scant cytoplasm, clumped chromatin, and irregular nuclear outlines.

1. What is the differential diagnosis?
2. What studies could be performed to establish the diagnosis?

► MALIGNANT LYMPHOMA

There are two basic types of lymphoma: Hodgkin and non-Hodgkin lymphoma. They differ in their clinical presentation, morphologic appearance, phenotype, and treatment (Tables 31-5 and 31-6 ✪).

NON-HODGKIN LYMPHOMA

Non-Hodgkin lymphoma of a B cell phenotype has the highest incidence of all the lymphoid malignancies within the United States. It is a heterogeneous group of neoplasms composed of cells that resemble those found in the normal compartments of the lymph node. The following subtypes of non-Hodgkin lymphoma have been selected for further discussion either because they are more common or because they demonstrate important concepts: small lymphocytic lymphoma, follicular lymphoma, mantle cell lymphoma, MALT lymphoma, diffuse large B cell lymphoma, Burkitt lymphoma, lymphoblastic lymphoma, anaplastic large cell lymphoma, and peripheral T/NK lymphoma. (A more complete description of lymphoma subtypes is available in Harris, Jaffe, Stein, et al.[4])

Small Lymphocytic Lymphoma

Small lymphocytic lymphoma (SLL) is the tissue equivalent of chronic lymphocytic leukemia (CLL). The two disorders appear to belong to one disease entity with differing clinical manifestations. Patients with CLL present with peripheral blood lymphocytosis but often develop lymph node involvement. Patients with SLL present with lymphadenopathy but often develop peripheral blood and bone marrow disease.

A lymph node biopsy performed in either CLL or SLL will reveal an essentially diffuse infiltrate of small mature lymphocytes. The small lymphocytes have dense, regularly clumped chromatin and lack nucleoli (Figure 31-5a ■). At low power there is often a vague nodularity due to aggregates of pale large cells (proliferation centers) (Figure 31-5b ■). Although these nodules may be mistaken for follicle germinal centers, they are not composed of follicle center cells. Proliferation centers contain large cells with abundant pale-staining cytoplasm and prominent eosinophilic nucleoli (prolymphocytes). The immunophenotype, cytogenetic findings, and survival are identical to CLL (see previous CLL discussion).

Follicular Lymphoma

Follicular lymphoma is a neoplasm composed of cells originating within the germinal center. It is the most common type of non-Hodgkin lymphoma within the United States. The median age at presentation is 50–60 years. There is no sex predilection. Patients usually present with generalized painless lymphadenopathy, some have peripheral blood involvement (Fig 31-6a), and most have advanced stage disease with bone marrow involvement (Figure 31-6b ■). Involvement of other extranodal sites is unusual.

Lymph node biopsy of follicular lymphoma reveals an infiltrate of lymphoid cells forming poorly circumscribed follicles that resemble germinal centers (Figure 31-6c ■). Although there may be areas with a diffuse growth pattern, there is at least focal follicular growth. Neoplastic follicles differ from reactive follicles in lacking apoptosis of lymphocytes. This is manifest on histology sections as a lack of macrophages engulfing fragments of necrotic cell (**tingible body macrophages**). Tingible body macrophages are found in areas of extensive apoptosis (reactive germinal centers and high-grade lymphoma). The neoplastic infiltrate always contains a mixed population of small cleaved and large cells, but is often more homogeneous than a normal germinal center (Figure 31-6d ■). Follicular lymphoma is graded on the number of large cells per high-power microscopic field (Table 31-7 ✪). The presence of more large cells is often associated with a worse prognosis. Most diagnoses of follicular lymphoma are made using conventional histologic evaluation. Immunophenotyping may be used to confirm the presence of

✪ TABLE 31-5

Differences Between Hodgkin and Non-Hodgkin Lymphoma

Parameter	Hodgkin Lymphoma	Non-Hodgkin Lymphoma
Stage	Usually localized	Usually widespread
Distribution	Usually central nodes	Usually peripheral nodes
Mode of spread	Contiguous	Noncontiguous
Extranodal disease	Uncommon	Common
Peripheral blood	Never involved	May be involved
Cell type	Abnormal bizarre cells	Resembles normal lymphoid cells
Treatment regimen	Often ABVD	Often CHOP

ABVD=doxorubicin, bleomycin, vinblastine, dacarbazine; CHOP=cyclophosphamide, doxorubicin, vincristine and prednisolone

✪ TABLE 31-6

Key Features of Malignant Lymphomas

Follicular lymphoma	nodular growth pattern
	lack of tingible body macrophages
	CD19+, CD5−, CD10+/−
	surface Ig strong
	bcl-2 protein overexpression
	t(14;18)
	bcl-2 gene rearrangement
Mantle cell lymphoma	lack of large cells
	CD19+, CD5+, CD23−, FMC-7+
	surface Ig+
	cyclin-D1 overexpression
	t(11;14)
	bcl-1 rearrangement
MALT lymphoma	accompanied by infectious or autoimmune disease
	localized
	extranodal
	lymphoepithelial lesions
	benign follicles
	heterogeneous neoplastic infiltrate
	phenotype and genotype not specific
Burkitt lymphoma	associated with EBV
	starry sky growth pattern
	CD19+, CD5−, CD10+
	strong surface Ig
	t(8;14)
Anaplastic large cell lymphoma	bizarre, anaplastic cells
	may resemble HD
	T cell or null phenotype
	LCA+/−, CD30+, CD15−
	EMA+/−, EBV−
	t(2;5), Alk-1+/−
Classic Hodgkin lymphoma	Reed-Sternberg cells
	LCA−, CD15+, CD30+, Alk-1−
	often EBV positive
LP Hodgkin lymphoma	growth pattern frequently nodular
	L&H cells
	LCA+, CD20+, CD15−, CD30−
	EBV negative

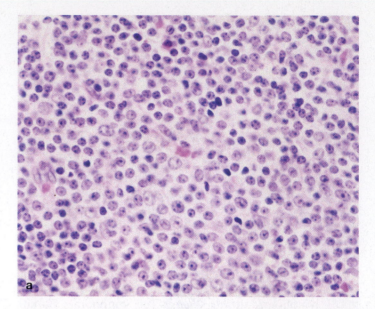

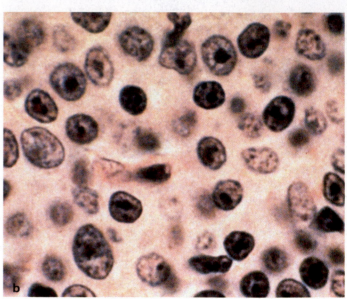

■ **FIGURE 31-5** Small lymphocytic lymphoma. **a.** Small lymphocytes with round nuclei and clumped chromatin. An occasional larger lymphocyte with a prominent nucleolus is present (prolymphocyte). **b.** Proliferation center. Vague nodule containing paler staining larger cells. (a. Lymph node biopsy, H&E stain, 500× magnification, Courtesy of Dr. Steve Swerdlow; b. Lymph node biopsy, H&E stain, 50× magnification)

lymphoma (monoclonal lymphocytes) and confirm the subtype of lymphoma (CD10 positive). Most cases of follicular lymphoma arise because of a chromosome translocation t(14;18) involving the *BCL-2* gene that leads to over-expression of bcl-2 protein in lymphocytes. BCL-2 protein inhibits individual cell necrosis (apoptosis), allowing follicle center cells to accumulate and produce lymphadenopathy. Follicular lymphoma was the first malignant tumor recognized to result

from an inhibition of cell death rather than uncontrolled cell proliferation.

Most patients with follicular lymphoma have an indolent disease with a median survival of 7–9 years. Treatment with chemotherapy and/or radiation therapy is given for relief of symptoms. None of the current therapies for follicular lymphoma are curative. Low-grade follicular lymphoma may progress to a diffuse large cell lymphoma with a median survival of less than 1 year.

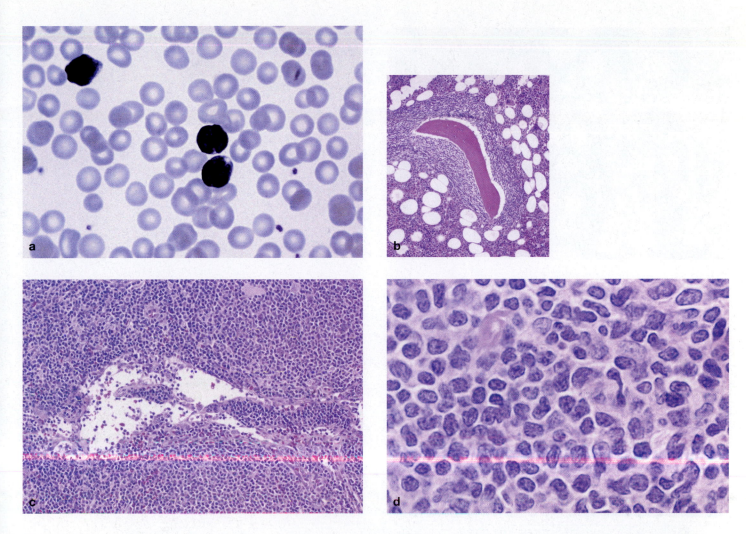

■ FIGURE 31-6 Follicular lymphoma, grade 1. **a.** Circulating lymphoma cells with irregular nuclear outlines. (Peripheral blood, Wright stain, magnification 1000×). **b.** Bone marrow involvement by low grade follicular lymphoma displaying a characteristic paratrabecular growth pattern. (Bone marrow biopsy, H&E stain, magnification 20×). **c.** Loss of the normal lymph node architecture. The abnormal infiltrate forms numerous poorly defined nodules (follicles). (Lymph node biopsy, H&E stain, magnification 20×). **d.** Neoplastic follicle composed of a relatively homogeneous population of small lymphoid cells containing angulated, twisted nuclei. (Lymph node biopsy, H&E stain, magnification 200×)

CASE STUDY *(continued from page 592)*

A cervical lymph node biopsy reveals effacement of the normal architecture by a lymphoid infiltrate with a nodular growth pattern. The nodules contain a relatively homogeneous population of small lymphocytes with irregular nuclear outlines. A few large lymphocytes are present. There is a lack of tingible body macrophages and mitotic figures.

3. What is the cause of the lymphadenopathy?

4. Is this process low grade or high grade?

Mantle Cell Lymphoma

Mantle cell lymphoma (MCL) is a neoplasm derived from the cells of the mantle zone of the lymphoid follicle. The median age at presentation is approximately 60 years, and

there is a male predominance. Most patients present with disseminated disease involving multiple lymph node groups, bone marrow, peripheral blood, spleen, liver, and gastrointestinal tract. Gastrointestinal tract involvement may present as multiple polyps involving the small bowel (lymphomatous polyposis) (Figure 31-7a ■).

✪ TABLE 31-7

Grading of Follicular Lymphoma

Grade	Large Cells/High Power Microscopic Field
1	0–5
2	6–15
3	>15

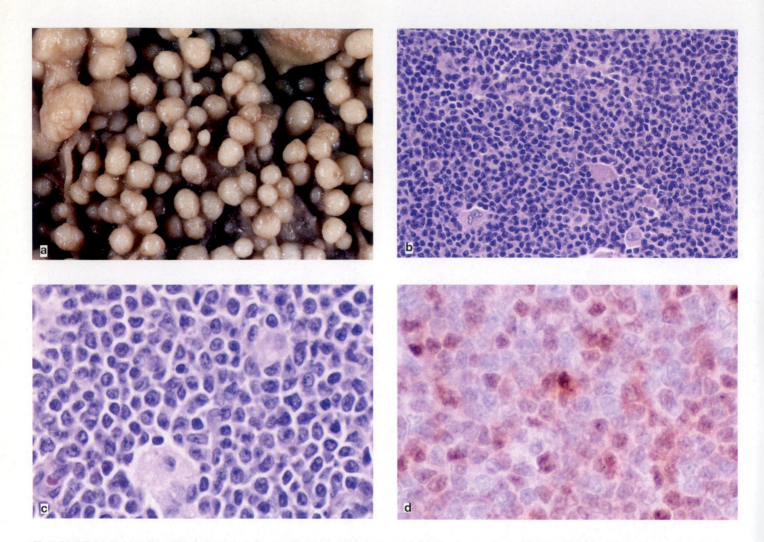

■ **FIGURE 31-7** Mantle cell lymphoma. **a.** Gross photograph of the large intestine in a patient with lymphomatous polyposis of gastrointestinal tract. **b.** Abnormal lymphoid infiltrate in a lymph node displaying a vaguely nodular growth pattern. **c.** Uniform infiltrate of small lymphoid cells with slightly irregular nuclear outlines. **d.** Cyclin D-1 overexpression. (b. Lymph node biopsy, H&E stain, 20× magnification; c. lymph node biopsy, H&E stain, 100× magnification; d. lymph node biopsy, immunohistochemistry stain, 100× magnification)

On histologic sections, mantle cell lymphoma may demonstrate either a diffuse or vaguely nodular growth pattern (Figure 31-7b ■). Occasionally the neoplastic infiltrate surrounds a reactive germinal center (mantle zone pattern). The neoplastic cells are usually small to intermediate in size with round to slightly irregular nuclear outlines (Figure 31-7c ■). Although the morphologic differential diagnosis includes small lymphocytic lymphoma and follicular lymphoma, classical MCL can be distinguished by its absence of large transformed lymphoid cells. Blastic MCL is a morphologic variant that is composed of cells with finely distributed chromatin resembling blasts or large cleaved cells resembling large cell lymphoma.

The correct diagnosis of MCL often requires the use of ancillary studies. Immunophenotyping by flow cytometry reveals the following phenotype: CD19+, CD5+, CD23−, FMC-7+, and sIg+ (strong intensity). Immunohistochemistry reveals nuclear staining for cyclin-D1 protein in approximately 90% of cases of MCL (Figure 31-7d ■). Overexpression of cyclin-D1 is usually the result of a chromosome translocation, t(11;14), that involves the *bcl-1* gene. Although molecular diagnostic studies are available, only approximately 60% of cases of mantle cell lymphoma are routinely identified because of the wide range of breakpoints involved in the t(11;14) translocation. Cyclin D-1 is involved in regulating progression of cells from the G1 to S phase of the cell cycle (∞ Chapter 2). The bcl-1 translocation is thought to lead to neoplastic transformation through loss of cell cycle control.

MCL is a relatively aggressive lymphoma with a poor response to multiagent chemotherapy. The overall median survival is approximately 3–4 years, with the blastic variant having a median survival of only 18 months. Therefore, distinction of MCL from follicular lymphoma and SLL is important. Patients with MCL are often candidates for investigational therapeutic approaches.

Mucosa Associated Lymphoid Tissue (MALT) Lymphoma

MALT lymphoma is a B cell neoplasm derived from mucosa associated lymphoid tissue. Patients with MALT lymphoma usually present with localized extranodal disease (e.g., involving the stomach, salivary gland, lacrimal gland, thyroid, and lung). They often have a preceding chronic inflammatory disorder such as chronic gastritis due to *Helicobacter pylori* infection or autoimmune disease (Sjögren's syndrome or Hashimoto's thyroiditis).

A biopsy of MALT lymphoma often reveals an infiltrate of small to intermediate size lymphocytes intimately associated with epithelial cells (e.g., gastric mucosa, salivary gland ducts). Epithelial structures infiltrated by neoplastic lymphocytes are referred to as **lymphoepithelial lesions** (Figure 31-8a ■). MALT lymphoma is composed of a heterogeneous mixture of small lymphocytes with round or cleaved nuclei and cells with plasma cell differentiation. Often the neoplastic cells have abundant pale-staining cytoplasm and are referred to as monocytoid B cells because of their resemblance to monocytes (Figure 31-8b ■). In addition to the neoplastic cells, the infiltrate often contains benign germinal centers. Infiltration of benign germinal centers by neoplastic cells is referred to as follicular colonization. MALT lymphoma is often difficult to distinguish from reactive lymphoid tissue because of the presence of benign and malignant cells and the varied appearance of the neoplastic cells. The differential diagnosis also includes other lymphomas composed of small lymphocytes, including SLL, MCL, and follicular lymphoma. Ancillary studies can assist in obtaining the correct diagnosis. Monoclonality of immunoglobulin light chains may be demonstrated either by flow cytometry immunophenotyping (surface immunoglobulin on lymphocytes) or by paraffin section immunohistochemistry (cytoplasmic immunoglobulin in cells demonstrating plasma cell differentiation). In contrast to follicular lymphoma and small lymphocytic lymphoma, MALT lymphoma is usually negative for CD10 and CD5.

MALT lymphoma is an indolent disease that was previously considered a reactive condition mimicking lymphoma (pseudolymphoma). MALT lymphoma is now considered malignant because it shares with the non-Hodgkin lymphomas lymphocyte monoclonality and the potential to transform to higher grade, large cell lymphoma. Patients with *Helicobacter pylori* associated gastric MALT lymphoma are often cured with antimicrobial therapy. MALT lymphomas in locations other than the stomach are usually cured using local excision or radiation therapy.

Diffuse Large B Cell Lymphoma

Diffuse large B cell lymphoma is a heterogeneous group of tumors composed of a predominance of large lymphoid cells (Figure 31-9 ■). It represents approximately 20% of all non-Hodgkin lymphoma. Some large cell lymphomas develop as a result of transformation from a lower grade lymphoma (e.g., follicular lymphoma), while others arise *de novo*. Diffuse large B cell lymphoma also forms a subset of lymphomas occurring in HIV infected individuals. Although originally placed in the intermediate grade of the working formulation, many large cell lymphomas behave in an aggressive manner. With intensive chemotherapy complete remission can be achieved in 60–80% of HIV-negative patients. Patients with lymphoma who are HIV-positive usually have a worse prognosis.

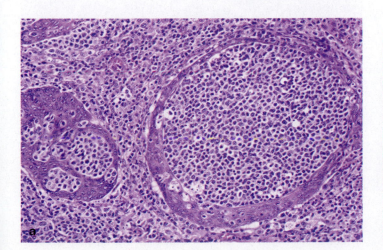
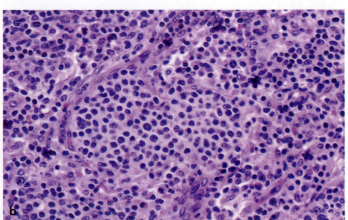

■ **FIGURE 31-8** MALT lymphoma. **a.** Parotid salivary gland involved by low-grade lymphoma of MALT type. Two lymphoepithelial lesions are present demonstrating infiltration of ducts by neoplastic lymphocytes. **b.** Heterogeneous lymphoid infiltrate of MALT lymphoma. Many of the infiltrating cells have abundant clear-staining cytoplasm (i.e., monocytoid B-cells). (a. Parotid gland biopsy, H&E stain, 50× magnification; b. parotid gland biopsy, H&E stain, 100× magnification)

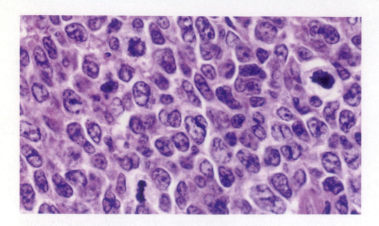

■ **FIGURE 31-9** Diffuse large B-cell lymphoma. Abnormal infiltrate composed of large lymphoid cells with pale-staining, vesicular chromatin, irregular nuclear outlines, and basophilic nucleoli. Several mitotic figures are present. (Lymph node biopsy, H&E stain, 200× magnification)

℮ CASE STUDY *(continued from page 595)*

The previous biopsy established a diagnosis of low-grade non-Hodgkin lymphoma, follicular type. The patient received multiagent chemotherapy for symptomatic relief. Two years following the diagnosis the patient returned with rapidly expanding lymph nodes in her neck. Repeat biopsy revealed effacement of the lymph node architecture by a diffuse infiltrate of large B cells.

5. What is the diagnosis?

6. What is the relationship of this disease to the previous diagnosis?

Burkitt Lymphoma

Burkitt lymphoma is a high-grade non-Hodgkin lymphoma with a high incidence in Africa (endemic subtype). It represents approximately one-third of all pediatric lymphomas occurring outside Africa (sporadic Burkitt lymphoma). Many of the adult cases occur in immunocompromised individuals such as those infected with the HIV virus. Burkitt lymphoma often involves extranodal sites. Endemic Burkitt lymphoma has a predilection for involvement of the facial bones and jaw, while sporadic Burkitt lymphoma often presents with disease involving the intestine, ovaries, or kidney. The Epstein-Barr virus (EBV) is thought to play a role in the pathogenesis of Burkitt lymphoma. EBV DNA is present in most cases of endemic Burkitt lymphoma and approximately one-third of the HIV associated tumors. EBV is found less frequently in the sporadic form. A biopsy of Burkitt lymphoma usually reveals a diffuse infiltrate of tumor cells demonstrating a **"starry sky" appearance** (Figure 31-10a ■). The "sky" represents the blue nuclei of the neoplastic lymphocytes and the "stars" are formed by scattered pale-staining tingible body macrophages. The tumor cells are monomor-

phic, intermediate size cells with nuclei approximately the same size as the nuclei of the tingible body macrophages. There are usually multiple small nucleoli. Mitotic figures and necrotic individual lymphoid cells (apoptotic bodies) are frequent (Figure 31-10b ■). The latter two features are characteristic of high-grade lymphoma.

Burkitt-like lymphoma is a morphologic variant of Burkitt lymphoma that also has features of a high-grade non-Hodgkin lymphoma but differs in its morphologic appearance and genetics. The cells of Burkitt-like lymphoma are more variable in size than those of Burkitt lymphoma and the nucleoli are more prominent and usually single.

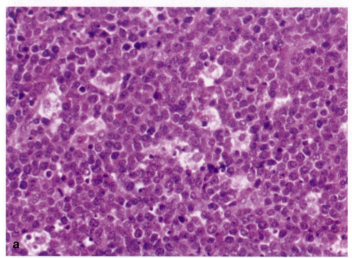

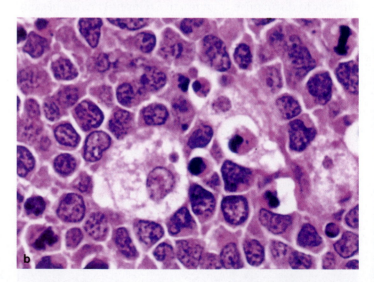

■ **FIGURE 31-10** Small noncleaved lymphoma, Burkitt type. **a.** "Starry-sky" appearance due to pale-staining tingible body macrophages scattered in an infiltrate that appears basophilic due to staining of the tumor cell nuclei. **b.** Intermediate sized lymphocytes with 1–2 nucleoli and scant cytoplasm. Numerous mitotic figures are present. The presence of apoptotic bodies indicates individual cell necrosis. (a. Lymph node biopsy, H&E stain, 100× magnification; b. lymph node biopsy, H&E stain, 500× magnification)

The differential diagnosis for Burkitt lymphoma often includes diffuse large B cell lymphoma and lymphoblastic lymphoma. The immunophenotype of Burkitt lymphoma is not unique and may be shared by diffuse large B cell lymphoma (CD19+, sIg+, CD10+, CD5−). These subtypes of non-Hodgkin lymphoma can be distinguished by cytogenetic and molecular diagnostic studies. Most cases of Burkitt lymphoma have the t(8;14), or less frequently t(2;8) or t(8;22), chromosome translocations that lead to rearrangement of the c-MYC gene.

The presence of surface immunoglobulin allows distinction of Burkitt lymphoma from the L1 and L2 variants of acute lymphoblastic leukemia (ALL). TdT is an enzyme that is present in immature cells and is usually absent in Burkitt lymphoma. Burkitt lymphoma and the L3 variant of ALL are thought to represent different clinical manifestations of the same disease entity.

Burkitt lymphoma is a highly aggressive tumor but is potentially curable with combination chemotherapy.

Lymphoblastic Lymphoma

Lymphoblastic lymphoma is the tissue equivalent of acute lymphoblastic leukemia (ALL). Patients present with a solid tumor involving soft tissue, lymph nodes, or other lymphoid organs such as the thymus. Children are more often affected than adults.

Approximately 20% of lymphoblastic lymphoma are of a B cell lineage and the remaining cases have an immature T cell phenotype. T cell lymphoblastic lymphoma often affects adolescent males who present with a rapidly enlarging mediastinal mass due to involvement of the thymus. Neoplastic blasts may also be seen in the peripheral blood, bone marrow, pleural fluid, and cerebrospinal fluid. A tissue biopsy of lymphoblastic lymphoma usually reveals intermediate to small cells with scant cytoplasm, finely distributed chromatin, and small nuclei (Figure 31-11 ■).

Immunophenotyping is required to distinguish lymphoblastic lymphoma from tissue infiltration by AML (extramedullary myeloid sarcoma) and to identify a T or B cell phenotype. The enzyme TdT is present in the majority of cases of lymphoblastic lymphoma and can be used to help distinguish it from Burkitt lymphoma.

The prognosis of lymphoblastic lymphoma is the same as ALL of the same phenotype.

Anaplastic Large Cell Lymphoma

Anaplastic large cell lymphoma (ALCL) represents less than 10% of all adult lymphomas and 40% of pediatric large cell lymphomas. Two clinical variants have been described: systemic and primary cutaneous.

ALCL is a non-Hodgkin lymphoma that has an appearance and immunophenotype (CD30+) that can be mistaken for Hodgkin lymphoma (HL). Most cases of ALCL are pleomorphic and contain large anaplastic cells resembling Reed-Sternberg cells and Hodgkin variant cells (Figure 31-12 ■).

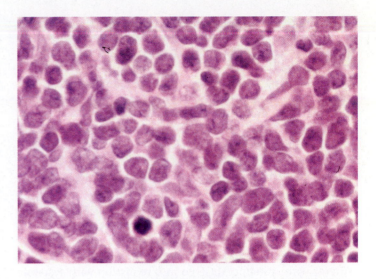

■ **FIGURE 31-11** Lymphoblastic lymphoma. Intermediate size lymphocytes with irregular nuclear outlines, finely distributed chromatin, and very small basophilic nucleoli. A mitotic figure is present. (Lymph node biopsy, H&E stain, 500× magnification)

A few morphologic variants have been described including the monomorphic and small cell variant (SCV). The monomorphic variant is composed of a more monotonous population of intermediate to large CD30+ cells that may be mistaken for diffuse large cell non-Hodgkin lymphoma. The SCV contains only a few CD30 positive large cells and may therefore be mistaken for a reactive process. The tumor cells stain by immunohistochemistry for the CD30 antigen (initially referred to as Ki-1 positive). In contrast to many cases of Hodgkin lymphoma, ALCL usually lacks CD15 expression and evidence of Epstein-Barr virus infection. There is often

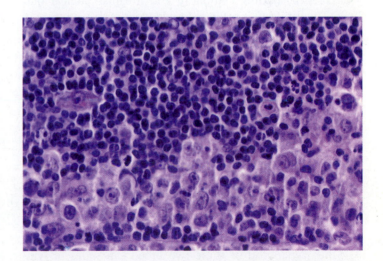

■ **FIGURE 31-12** Anaplastic large cell lymphoma. Abnormal infiltrate of large cells with abundant eosinophilic cytoplasm. The lower third of the picture demonstrates infiltration of the subcapsular sinus. (Lymph node biopsy, H&E stain, 100× magnification)

expression of leukocyte common antigen (LCA) and epithelial membrane antigen. Although cases of B cell ALCL do occur, most are of a T or null (lacking T or B cell antigens) cell phenotype.

Approximately 40% of systemic pleomorphic ALCL and 80% of the monomorphic variant contain the translocation t(2;5) that joins the NPM (nucleophosmin) and ALK (anaplastic large cell kinase) genes. This leads to abnormal expression of ALK protein that can be detected by immunohistochemistry using the ALK-1, ALKc, or p80$^{NPM/ALK}$ antibodies. Immunohistochemistry for the ALK protein can assist in the distinction of ALCL from HL and the separation of primary cutaneous ALCL (ALK negative) from systemic disease. ALK expression is also associated with increased survival.

Primary cutaneous ALCL can be treated successfully by local excision or radiation therapy. Approximately 70% of patients with systemic ALCL go into remission with systemic multiagent chemotherapy, but there is a high rate of relapse.

Peripheral T/NK Cell Lymphoma

Peripheral T/NK cell lymphoma is a group of neoplasms with a mature T lymphocyte or natural killer cell phenotype. They comprise only 15% of lymphomas in the United States. Although several subtypes are described, many of them can only be distinguished on clinical grounds (e.g., nasal T/NK-cell lymphoma). Patients usually present with widespread disease including involvement of extranodal sites such as skin. Although there are a number of morphologic features that can be used to suggest a T cell phenotype, immunophenotyping is essential.

T cell lymphoma usually involves the paracortex of the lymph node, has a diffuse growth pattern, and is rich in vessels. The tumor cells vary in size and may display abundant clear or pale-staining cytoplasm and irregular nuclear outlines. The infiltrate is often heterogeneous with a mixture of histiocytes, plasma cells, eosinophils, and tumor cells (Figure 31-13 ■). Approximately 60% of the cases of T cell lymphoma demonstrate deletion of a T cell antigen (CD5 and/or CD7). An abnormal immunophenotype or the presence of clonal rearrangement of the T cell receptor can assist in the distinction of T cell lymphoma from a reactive process.

Peripheral T/NK cell lymphoma is usually aggressive with frequent relapses. Some patients are cured by combination chemotherapy.

HODGKIN LYMPHOMA

Hodgkin lymphoma differs from non-Hodgkin lymphoma in its clinical presentation and histologic appearance (Table 31-5 ✪). Separation of these two broad categories of lymphoma is important because they are treated with different combinations of chemotherapeutic agents.

Biopsy of Hodgkin lymphoma usually reveals a population of reactive lymphocytes, plasma cells, histiocytes, and eosinophils accompanied by a few tumor cells. The tumor

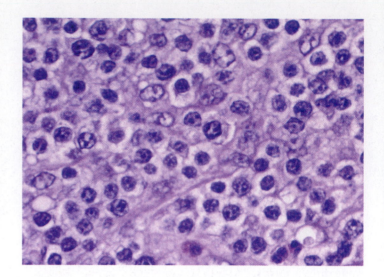

■ **FIGURE 31-13** T cell lymphoma. Diffuse infiltrate of abnormal lymphoid cells with clear cytoplasm. Numerous blood vessels lined by plump eosinophilic endothelial cells are present (high endothelial venules). (Lymph node biopsy, H&E stain, 100× magnification)

cells are large, do not resemble a normal cell counterpart, and demonstrate variations associated with the histologic subtypes of Hodgkin lymphoma. The main histologic types are lymphocyte predominant (LP) and classic Hodgkin lymphoma. Classic Hodgkin lymphoma is further subtyped into nodular sclerosis (NS), mixed cellularity (MC), lymphocyte depletion (LD), and a rare subtype, lymphocyte rich (LR) (Table 31-8 ✪).

The tumor lymphoid cells in classic Hodgkin lymphoma have large, prominent eosinophilic nucleoli and are of uncertain lineage. One variant of tumor cell is characteristically found in all cases of classic Hodgkin lymphoma: the **Reed-Sternberg (R-S) cell**. An R-S cell has two or more nuclear lobes containing inclusion-like nucleoli and an area of perinucleolar clearing (owl's eye appearance) (Figure 31-14a ■).

The three major subtypes of classic Hodgkin lymphoma are distinguished and differentiated by the presence of sclerosis (fibrosis), the presence of specific tumor cell variants, and the proportion of reactive lymphocytes. The NS subtype of Hodgkin lymphoma is characterized by bands of fibrous tissue (Figure 31-14b ■) nodular aggregates of cells and tumor cells with cytoplasmic clearing and delicate, multilobated nuclei (**lacunar cells**) (Figure 31-14c ■).

LD Hodgkin lymphoma has very few reactive lymphocytes and many tumor cells. The diagnosis of MC Hodgkin lymphoma is made after excluding the other classic subtypes: NS, LD, and lymphocyte rich.

LP Hodgkin lymphoma is composed of numerous reactive lymphocytes and rare tumor cells. The tumor cells in LP Hodgkin lymphoma include the lymphocytic and histiocytic variant (**L&H**, or **popcorn cell**), which is characterized by a multilobated nucleus with delicate nuclear membranes, finely

⭐ TABLE 31-8

Classification of Classic Hodgkin Lymphoma

Type	Sclerosis	Lymphocytes	Tumor Cells	Variants	Cell Type
NS	present	++	++	lacunar	?
MC	−	++	++	−	?
LD	−	+	++++	−	?
LR	−	++++	+	−	?
LP	−	++++	+	L&H	B cell

NS = nodular sclerosis classic subtype, MC = mixed cellularity classic subtype, LD = lymphocyte depletion classic subtype, LR = lymphocyte rich classic subtype, LP = lymphocyte predominance subtype; ? = uncertain cell of origin, + = few, ++++ = many

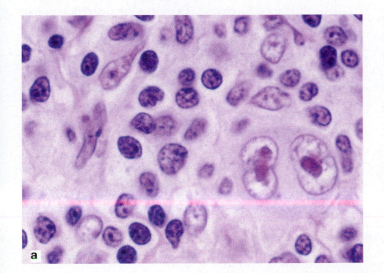

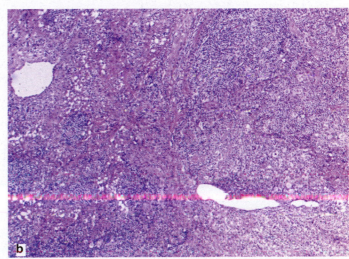

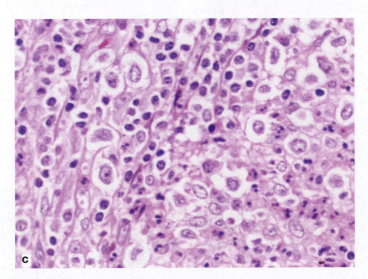

■ **FIGURE 31-14** Hodgkin lymphoma, classic type, nodular sclerosis subtype. a. Reed-Sternberg cell with two nuclear lobes and prominent, eosinophilic nucleoli giving an owl's eye appearance. The background contains many small lymphocytes and a few pale eosinophilic histiocytes. b. Bands of fibrous tissue isolate nodules containing an abnormal cellular infiltrate (nodular sclerosing pattern). c. Lacunar cells with abundant clear staining cytoplasm, delicate nuclear membranes, and small basophilic nucleoli. (a. Lymph node biopsy, H&E stain, 200× magnification; b. lymph node biopsy, H&E stain, 20× magnification; c. lymph node biopsy, H&E stain, 100× magnification)

granular chromatin, and indistinct nucleoli (Figure 31-15 ■). The L&H cell has a B cell phenotype (LCA+ [Leukocyte Common Antigen], CD20+, CD15–) (Table 31-8 ✪).

The morphologic differential diagnosis of Hodgkin lymphoma includes reactive lymphadenopathy, carcinoma, and non-Hodgkin lymphoma (e.g., anaplastic large cell lymphoma). Immunohistochemistry may assist in the diagnosis. The tumor cells of classic Hodgkin lymphoma are negative for LCA (leukocyte common antigen) and ALK, and positive for the CD30 antigen. They may also be positive for CD15 and/or EBV.

Currently the 5-year survival for patients with stage I or IIA Hodgkin lymphoma is approximately 90%, and for stage IV 60–70%.

> ✓ **Checkpoint! #4**
>
> *What cell characteristically distinguishes Hodgkin lymphoma from non-Hodgkin lymphoma? Describe this cell.*

▶ PLASMA CELL NEOPLASMS

Plasma cell neoplasms are a diverse group of disorders that rarely involve lymph nodes and usually secrete monoclonal immunoglobulin into the serum and or urine. They can be divided into disease entities by the distribution of disease (solitary versus multiple lesions and bone versus extramedullary), the characteristics of the immunosecretory protein produced (IgM, immunoglobulin heavy or light chain only) and the appearance of the malignant cell (plasma cells, lymphoplasmacytoid lymphocytes) (Table 31-9 ✪).[3] The following more common plasma cell neoplasms will be discussed in more detail: multiple myeloma, plasmacytoma, monoclonal gam-

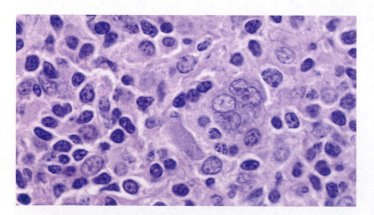

■ **FIGURE 31-15** Hodgkin lymphoma, lymphocyte predominant subtype. Large L&H ("popcorn") cell with multilobated nucleus, delicate nuclear membranes, and small basophilic nucleoli. The background contains many small lymphocytes and histiocytes with pale-staining, eosinophilic cytoplasm. (Lymph node biopsy, H&E stain, 200× magnification)

✪ **TABLE 31-9**

Plasma Cell Disorders

Monoclonal gammopathy of undetermined significance (MGUS)

Plasmacytoma

Multiple myeloma

Waldenström's macroglobulinemia

Primary amyloidosis

Heavy chain disease

mopathy of undetermined significance, and Waldenström's macroglobulinemia. Their key features are outlined in Table 31-10 ✪. Primary amyloidosis is a monoclonal proliferation of plasma cells producing an abnormal immunoglobulin that is deposited in tissues (amyloid). Heavy chain disease is characterized by the production of immunoglobulin heavy chain fragments only. The clinical presentation and morphologic features vary with the class of heavy chain produced.

MULTIPLE MYELOMA

Multiple myeloma is the most frequent of the plasma cell neoplasms. It is a malignant disorder that forms multiple tumors throughout the skeletal system (lytic bone lesions) (Figure 31-16a ■). The median age at diagnosis is 65 years, and there is a male predominance. Patients often present with bone pain and/or pathologic fractures due to tumor infiltration. Approximately 20% of patients are asymptomatic, and the diagnosis is made following the incidental finding of a monoclonal serum protein.

✪ **TABLE 31-10**

Key Features of Plasma Cell Neoplasms

Neoplasm	Features
Multiple myeloma	Lytic bone lesions
	"M"-spike on serum/urine electrophoresis
	Rouleaux on blood smear
	>30% plasma cells in bone marrow
Plasmacytoma	Localized mass
	Monoclonal plasma cells
Monoclonal gammopathy of undetermined significance	Monoclonal serum protein
	Monoclonal protein <3 gm/dL
	Bence-Jones proteins absent
	Lytic bone lesions absent
	Bone marrow plasma cells <10%
Waldenström's macroglobulinemia	Lymphadenopathy
	Hyperviscosity syndrome
	IgM monoclonal protein
	Plasmacytoid lymphocytes

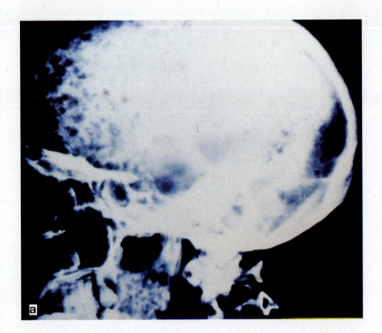

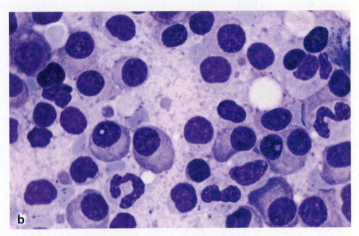

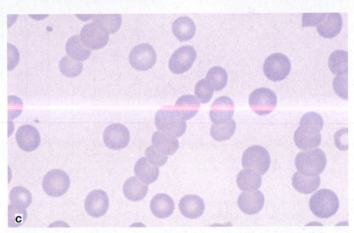

■ **FIGURE 31-16** Multiple myeloma. **a.** Skull x-ray demonstrating multiple lytic bone lesions giving a "moth-eaten" appearance. **b.** Replacement of hematopoietic precursors by an infiltrate of plasma cells. Plasma cells appear normal, but represent >30% of the cells present. **c.** Stacking of the erythrocytes due to the presence of increased globulin (Rouleaux). (b. Bone marrow aspirate, Wright stain, 1000× magnification; c. peripheral blood, Wright stain, 1000× magnification)

Examination of the bone marrow from a lytic lesion or from the posterior iliac crest will reveal an abnormal infiltrate of plasma cells replacing the normal hematopoietic cells. In multiple myeloma, plasma cells usually form greater than 30% of all bone marrow cells (Figure 31-16b ■). Although neoplastic plasma cells may appear normal, abnormal forms with more finely distributed chromatin, nucleoli or intranuclear inclusions that contain immunoglobulin (**Dutcher bodies**) are often present. Neoplastic plasma cells rarely circulate in the blood, but the peripheral smear is often abnormal due to stacking of the erythrocytes (**rouleaux** formation) (Figure 31-16c ■). The stained blood smear has a blue background due to the increased serum protein.

Serum protein electrophoresis (SPEP) reveals increased protein with a narrow range of electrophoretic mobility (M spike) (Figure 31-17 ■). An M spike can be characterized by immunofixation electrophoresis (IFE) to confirm the presence of a monoclonal protein and determine the immunoglobulin class (Figure 31-17c ■). The monoclonal protein usually contains one immunoglobulin light chain (kappa or lambda) and one heavy chain with the following incidence: IgG > IgA > IgM > IgD > IgE. Normal immunoglobulin production is usually decreased leading to functional hypogammaglobulinemia. Plasma cell neoplasms may produce monoclonal immunoglobulin with an excess of light chains, light chains only, heavy chains only, or non-

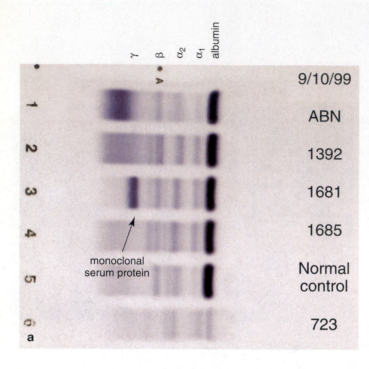

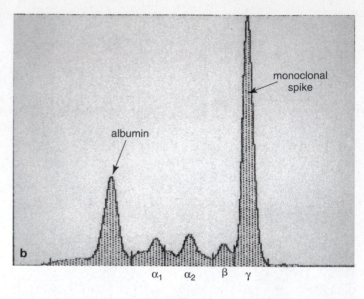

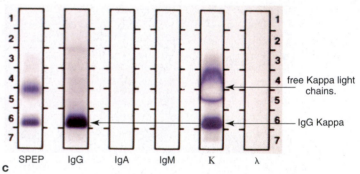

■ **FIGURE 31-17** Monoclonal gammopathy. a. Serum protein electrophoresis. Sample 1681 displays a band in the early gamma region. b. Densitometry scan reveals a "spike" in the gamma region. A similar spike was found in the urine. c. Immunofixation electrophoresis performed on a urine sample reveals two monoclonal bands composed of IgG kappa and free kappa light chains (Bence-Jones proteins).

secretory plasma cells. Patients with light chain only disease may have a normal SPEP because the protein is excreted into the urine. Free light chains in the urine are referred to as **Bence-Jones proteinuria**.

The prognosis of multiple myeloma is poor, with a median survival of only 6 months without therapy. The median survival can be increased to 3 years with chemotherapy, and an increased survival has been reported with autologous bone marrow and peripheral blood stem cell transplants. Infection is a major cause of death.

PLASMACYTOMA

A plasmacytoma is a localized, tumorous collection of monoclonal plasma cells that may lead to a monoclonal spike on SPEP. The prognosis is related to the location. Many patients with plasmacytoma of bone develop additional lesions and ultimately develop multiple myeloma. Plasmacytoma of the upper respiratory tract has a good prognosis with only rare recurrence after excision and a low incidence of dissemination.

MONOCLONAL GAMMOPATHY OF UNDETERMINED SIGNIFICANCE (MGUS)

Identification of a monoclonal spike is not diagnostic of multiple myeloma. The prevalence of an M spike increases with age and is present in 3% of asymptomatic patients over 70 years of age. The significance of finding an M spike depends on the presence of features indicating another overt plasma cell disorder such as multiple lytic lesions in multiple myeloma. Therefore, MGUS is a diagnosis of exclusion. There is no treatment for MGUS. Although most patients have stable disease and die of other causes, an overt plasma cell dyscrasia such as multiple myeloma develops in approximately 25% of patients.

WALDENSTRÖM'S MACROGLOBULINEMIA

Waldenström's macroglobulinemia is a malignant plasma cell neoplasm that has a different clinical presentation and morphologic appearance from multiple myeloma. Patients present with lymphadenopathy, hepatomegaly, splenomegaly, and/or hyperviscosity syndrome (visual impairment, headache, dizziness, deafness). Unlike patients with multiple myeloma, those with Waldenström's do not have lytic bone lesions. The malignant cells are a mixed population of lymphocytes, plasma cells, and plasmacytoid lymphocytes and may resemble those seen in small lymphocytic lymphoma. The serum protein contains monoclonal immunoglobulin light chain (kappa or lambda) combined with IgM heavy chain. IgM is a large molecule that leads to increased serum viscosity and the hyperviscosity syndrome.

The median survival for patients with Waldenström's macroglobulinemia is 4 years. Plasmapheresis can alleviate many of the symptoms related to increased viscosity.

 Checkpoint! #5

What clinical finding differentiates multiple myeloma from other plasma cell neoplasms?

SUMMARY

The lymphoid malignancies are a diverse group of diseases that vary in their clinical presentation, morphologic appearance, immunophenotype, and genotype. The malignant cells resemble one or more of the stages of normal lymphocyte development. The lymphoid malignancies can be classified as acute lymphoblastic leukemia, chronic leukemic lymphoid malignancy, and lymphoma. The leukemic entities are characterized by peripheral blood and bone marrow involvement while lymphomas have tumorous masses involving the lymph nodes and other lymphoid tissue. The diagnosis often requires a combination of conventional morphology and ancillary studies. The ancillary studies include immunophenotyping, molecular dianostics, and cytogenetics. Although the classification of lymphoid malignancies is complicated, it is important to separate distinct disease entities that have a predictable outcome and response to specific therapy.

REVIEW QUESTIONS

LEVEL I

1. Which of the following is the most likely distribution of disease in a patient with leukemia? (Checklist #3)
   a. a lytic bone lesion
   b. a tumorous mass involving lymph nodes
   c. a tumorous mass involving the tonsil
   d. widespread involvement of the bone marrow

2. A 60-year-old male being evaluated for insurance purposes was found to have lymphocytosis. Peripheral smear revealed a uniform population of small mature lymphocytes. Which of the following is the most likely diagnosis? (Checklist #3, 7)
   a. acute lymphoblastic leukemia
   b. chronic lymphocytic leukemia
   c. infectious mononucleosis
   d. malignant lymphoma

3. Which of the following findings indicate(s) the presence of a lymphoid malignancy? (Checklist #2)
   a. clonal immunoglobulin gene rearrangement
   b. population of lymphocytes expressing only one immunoglobulin light chain
   c. population of lymphocytes expressing an abnormal phenotype
   d. all of the above

LEVEL II

1. Which of the following is involved in the pathogenesis of low-grade follicular lymphoma? (Checklist #8)
   a. genes involved in apoptosis
   b. inherited immunodeficiency
   c. proto-oncogenes
   d. tumor suppressor genes

2. Which type of lymphoma can be cured by antimicrobial therapy? (Checklist #8)
   a. Burkitt lymphoma
   b. Hodgkin lymphoma
   c. MALT lymphoma
   d. HIV-associated non-Hodgkin lymphoma

3. A lymph node biopsy is performed in a patient with lymphadenopathy. Which of the following findings would support a diagnosis of a reactive proliferation rather than malignant lymphoma? (Checklist #9)
   a. a mixed population of cells varying in size, shape, and color
   b. clonality
   c. presence of large, bizarre cells
   d. mitotic activity

LEVEL I

4. Which of the following is used in the working formulation to group cases of malignant lymphoma? (Checklist #9)
   a. karyotype
   b. genotype
   c. morphology
   d. phenotype

5. A lymph node biopsy reveals a nodular infiltrate of small, mature lymphoid cells with an absence of mitoses and apoptosis. Which of the following is the correct classification of this lymphoma? (Checklist #9)
   a. high-grade
   b. high-stage
   c. low-grade
   d. low-stage

6. Which of the following lymphoid malignancies is most likely to have circulating neoplastic cells? (Checklist #3, 6)
   a. chronic lymphocytic leukemia
   b. high-grade lymphoma
   c. low-grade lymphoma
   d. Hodgkin lymphoma

7. Which of the following studies is (are) used in the WHO classification of lymphoid malignancies? (Checklist #9)
   a. genotype
   b. morphology
   c. phenotype
   d. all of the above

8. A bone marrow performed for staging purposes revealed involvement by non-Hodgkin lymphoma. This finding indicates that the disease is: (Checklist #9)
   a. high-grade
   b. high-stage
   c. low-grade
   d. low-stage

9. A peripheral smear performed on a 35-year-old male with lymphocytosis reveals numerous smudge cells. Which of the following does this finding indicate? (Checklist #3, 8)
   a. chronic lymphocytic leukemia
   b. infectious mononucleosis
   c. acute lymphoblastic leukemia
   d. the finding is not diagnostic

10. Peripheral smear examination of a patient with chronic lymphocytic leukemia reveals 8% prolymphocytes. This finding is consistent with which of the following diagnoses? (Checklist #8)
    a. chronic lymphocytic leukemia
    b. prolymphocytic leukemia
    c. prolymphocytoid transformation
    d. Richter's transformation

LEVEL II

4. A CBC performed on a 65-year-old female reveals lymphocytosis. A bone marrow reveals replacement of the hematopoietic precursors by an infiltrate of mature lymphocytes. Which of the following is the most likely course of the disease? (Checklist #5)
   a. cure following therapy
   b. rapid progression
   c. slow progression
   d. spontaneous remission

5. Which of the following phenotypes is characteristic of chronic lymphocytic leukemia? (Checklist #1)
   a. CD19+, CD5+, CD23+
   b. CD19+, CD5–, CD23+
   c. CD19+, CD5+, CD23–
   d. CD19+, CD5–, CD23–

6. A CBC performed on an 80-year-old female reveals an absolute lymphocyte count of 8×10^9/L. Examination of the peripheral blood smear reveals a uniform population of small lymphocytes. Which of the following procedures would be most likely to establish a diagnosis? (Checklist #1, 5)
   a. cytogenetics
   b. flow cytometry immunophenotyping
   c. immunoglobulin gene rearrangement
   d. lymph node biopsy

7. A patient presents with a lymphocyte count of 350×10^9/L. Peripheral blood examination reveals large cells with moderate amounts of pale basophilic cytoplasm, mature condensed chromatin, and prominent nucleoli. Which of the following is the most likely clinical finding? (Checklist #5)
   a. massive splenomegaly
   b. lymphadenopathy
   c. lytic bone lesions
   d. lymphomatous polyposis

8. A CBC performed on a 60-year-old male with a history of rheumatoid arthritis revealed neutropenia and an absolute lymphocytosis. Examination of the peripheral smear revealed many lymphocytes with abundant pale staining cytoplasm and cytoplasmic granules. Which of the following is the most likely phenotype? (Checklist #1, 5)
   a. CD3+, CD2+, CD57+
   b. CD19+, CD5+, CD57–
   c. CD2+, CD3–, CD56+
   d. CD19+, CD10+, CD34+

REVIEW QUESTIONS *(continued)*

LEVEL I

LEVEL II

9. A patient with a previous diagnosis of small lymphocytic lymphoma (SLL) is found to have peripheral blood lymphocytosis. The lymphocytes are small and have round nuclei with clumped chromatin. Which of the following is the most appropriate interpretation? (Checklist #3)
   a. This represents the same disease process (SLL).
   b. The patient has a new lymphoid malignancy: chronic lymphocytic leukemia.
   c. The lymphoma has transformed.
   d. The patient has developed a therapy-related malignancy.

10. A lymph node biopsy revealed an infiltrate of small lymphoid cells with a vaguely nodular growth pattern. Flow cytometry revealed a monoclonal population of B cells expressing CD5. Immunohistochemistry revealed nuclear staining for cyclin-D1 protein. Which of the following is the most likely diagnosis? (Checklist #3)
   a. mantle cell lymphoma
   b. small lymphocytic lymphoma
   c. chronic lymphocytic leukemia
   d. follicular lymphoma

REFERENCES

1. National Cancer Institute sponsored study of classifications of non-Hodgkin lymphomas: Summary and description of a working formulation for clinical usage. The Non-Hodgkin Lymphoma Pathologic Classification Project. *Cancer.* 1992; 49:2112–35.

2. Harris NL, Jaffe ES, Diebold J, et al. World Health Organization classification of neoplastic diseases of the hematopoietic and lymphoid tissues: Report of the Clinical Advisory Committee Meeting, Airlie House, Virginia, November 1997. *J Clin Oncol.* 1999; 17:3835–49.

3. Brunning R, McKenna RW. Tumors of the bone marrow. In: *Atlas of Tumor Pathology.* AFIP Third Series, Fasc 9; 1993:1–491.

4. Harris NL, Jaffe ES, Stein HS, et al. A revised European-American classification of lymphoid neoplasms: A proposal from the International Lymphoma Study Group. *Blood.* 1994; 84:1361–92.

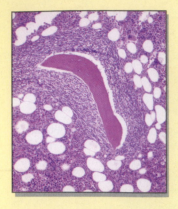

CHAPTER OUTLINE

32

Hematopoietic Stem Cell Transplantation

Aamir Ehsan, M.D.

CHECKLIST - LEVEL I

At the end of this unit of study, the student should be able to:

1. Describe the sources of hematopoietic stem cells and characteristics of each.
2. Identify the diseases that can be treated with different sources of hematopoietic stem cells.
3. List characteristics of stem cells.
4. Describe the significance of ABO and HLA antigens for stem cell transplant.
5. Identify the infections that are serious complications during the peritransplant period.
6. Describe the significance and effects of graft-versus-host disease (GVHD) and compare to graft-versus-leukemia (GVL) process.

CHECKLIST - LEVEL II

At the end of this unit of study, the student should be able to:

1. Summarize the collection and processing of hematopoietic stem cells and assess the success of these procedures.
2. Explain the role of the clinical laboratory professional in stem cell transplantation.
3. Select and outline methods to enumerate hematopoietic stem cells.
4. Explain the complications of stem cell transplant, assess the patient's risk of developing them, and select the most appropriate form of transplant to treat them.
5. Formulate the sequence of events for a patient who will receive a stem cell transplant.
6. Select laboratory tests used to determine engraftment and assess engraftment given results of these tests.

KEY TERMS

Allogeneic
Apheresis
Autologous
Chimerism
Clonogenic
Conditioning regimen
Cryopreserved
Engraftment
Graft-versus-host disease (GVHD)
Graft-versus-leukemia (GVL)
In situ hybridization
Polymorphic
Purging
Syngeneic transplantation
Variable number tandem repeats (VNTR)

BACKGROUND BASICS

This chapter will build on concepts learned in previous chapters. To maximize your learning experience you should review the following material before starting this unit of study.

Level I

▶ Describe the origin and differentiation of hematopoietic cells. (Chapter 2)

▶ Outline the classification and explain the etiology and pathophysiology of neoplastic hematologic disorders. (Chapter 26)

▶ Explain the role of chemotherapy and radiotherapy in treatment of neoplastic hematologic disorders. (Chapters 26, 27, 29, 30, 31)

Level II

▶ Describe the role of cytokines and bone marrow microenvironment in maturation and differentiation of hematopoietic stem cells; explain the role of oncogenes in cancer development. (Chapter 2)

▶ Explain the use of molecular genetic technology and cytogenetics in diagnosis and prognosis of neoplastic hematopoietic disorders. (Chapters 24, 25)

▶ Correlate subgroups of neoplastic hematologic disorders with laboratory findings and prognosis. (Chapter 26)

CASE STUDY

We will refer to this case study throughout the chapter.
Brandon, a 35-year-old male (weight 80 kg), was recently diagnosed with AML-M2 and received induction chemotherapy. Day 21 bone marrow reveals no evidence of residual leukemia. Two weeks later, circulating blasts were seen in the peripheral blood. Brandon is being evaluated for a stem cell transplant. Consider the laboratory's role in evaluation for the transplant, the collection and processing of the stem cells, and determination of engraftment.

▶ OVERVIEW

The use of stem cells in the therapy of neoplastic hematopoietic disorders is becoming commonplace. The laboratory's role in this therapy is critical and requires that the clinical laboratory professional not only know the associated laboratory tests but also know why the tests are necessary and how they relate to the overall process of stem cell transplantation. This chapter reviews the sources of hematopoietic stem cells (HSCs); the use of allogeneic, autologous, and umbilical cord stem cells in treating a variety of malignant and nonmalignant disorders; the mobilization, collection, enumeration of mononuclear cells (MNCs) and CD34 positive cells; the procedures used to assess transplant success (**engraftment**), and the role of the clinical laboratory professional during this process.

▶ INTRODUCTION

Hematopoietic stem cell transplantation (HSCT) is a recognized therapeutic modality for leukemias, lymphomas, solid organ tumors, and a variety of metabolic and immunologic disorders (Table 32-1 ✪). The concept of stem cell transplantation (SCT) came from experiments done five decades ago when it was observed that mice given intravenous marrow infusions could overcome lethal doses of radiation.[1,2] Later, in the 1960s, the first successful bone marrow transplant was performed on a leukemia patient using marrow donated by the leukemic patient's brother.

After the early successful **allogeneic** bone marrow SCTs (transplantation of stem cells between genetically dissimilar but human-leukocyte-antigen-matched[HLA-matched]-individuals) using fresh anticoagulated bone marrow from HLA-matched siblings or family members, clinical practice has expanded to include the use of **autologous** bone marrow stem cells (transplantation or infusion of a person's own stem cells), autologous and allogeneic peripheral blood stem cells (PBSCs), and umbilical cord stem cells. The ability of the body to mount an immune response is controlled by the HLA genes. These genes code for histocompatible antigens found on the surface of essentially all nucleated cells (∞ Chapter 6).

▶ ORIGIN AND DIFFERENTIATION OF HEMATOPOIETIC STEM CELLS

HSCs are rare cells that can be found in the bone marrow and occasionally in the peripheral blood of healthy individuals. Self-renewal and multilineage differentiation are the two distinct biologic properties that make HSCs remarkable. Pluripotent stem cells differentiate into myeloid and lymphoid stem cells (Figure 2-11 ■). Myeloid stem cells produce three types of committed/progenitor cells that differentiate

⚙ TABLE 32-1

Diseases That Can Be Treated with Stem Cell Transplantation

Hematologic		Nonhematologic
Neoplastic	**Non-neoplastic**	
Acute lymphoblastic leukemia	Aplastic anemia	Solid organ malignancies (breast, ovarian, neuroblastoma, Wilm's tumor, germ cell)
Acute myelogenous leukemia	Paroxysmal nocturnal hemoglobinuria	
Chronic myelogenous leukemia	Thalassemia	Inborn error of metabolism (e.g., Hurler's syndrome)
Idiopathic myelofibrosis	Sickle cell disease	Severe combined immunodeficiency disease
Chronic lymphocytic leukemia	Fanconi's anemia	Wiskott-Aldrich syndrome
Myelodysplastic syndrome	Congenital pure red cell aplasia	Congenital leukocyte dysfunction syndromes
Non-Hodgkin lymphoma		Malignant osteopetrosis
Hodgkin lymphoma		
Multiple myeloma		

into erythroid, granulocyte-macrophage, and megakaryocytic cell pathways. The lymphoid stem cells differentiate into T cells, B cells, and possibly natural killer cells. The committed progenitor cells have been called colony-forming units (CFUs) because they give rise to colonies of differentiated progeny in vitro (∞ Chapter 2). From these CFUs arise morphologically recognizable precursors of differentiated cells (pronormoblast, myeloblast, monoblast, megakaryoblast) that further differentiate into mature cells. In summary, pluripotent stem cells have the capacity to self-renew and differentiate. With additional divisions, their progeny, the committed progenitor cells, become progressively restricted to proliferation and differentiation into a single cell line. The committed cell lacks the property of self-renewal.

▶ ## SOURCES OF HEMATOPOIETIC STEM CELLS AND TYPES OF STEM CELL TRANSPLANTS

HSCs for clinical use[3] can be harvested from the bone marrow, peripheral blood, and umbilical cord blood (UCB). Fetal bone marrow and liver are also rich in stem cells, but because of ethical issues their use is limited. HSCs, unlike other tissues and organs destined for transplant, are not routinely taken from cadavers. One reason for this is because in most situations the stem cell donor receives hematopoietic cytokines for a few days before the stem cells are harvested to maximize stem cell yield.

ALLOGENEIC STEM CELL TRANSPLANTATION

Allogeneic transplantation is the infusion of HSCs from another individual (donor) into the patient (recipient). In the past, the usual source of stem cells has been the bone marrow, but now allogeneic transplants using PBSCs are more common. Allogeneic transplants are often indicated when the disease process involves the patient's own stem cells, making them potentially unsuitable for transplant (Table 32-2 ⚙). Allogeneic transplant is usually performed for therapy of acute leukemias, chronic myelogenous leukemia (CML), aplastic anemia, hemoglobinopathies, immune deficiencies, and metabolic genetic disorders.[4,5]

There are three important factors to consider for successful allogeneic stem cell transplantation. Adequate numbers

⚙ TABLE 32-2

Type of Transplant, Sources of Stem Cells, and Diseases in Which These Stem Cells Are Used

Type of Transplant	Source of Stem Cells	Diseases
Allogeneic	Bone marrow Peripheral blood Cord blood	Acute leukemias, CML, nonmalignant hematologic conditions (see Table 32-1), immunologic and inherited diseases
Autologous	Peripheral blood Bone marrow	Hodgkin lymphoma, NHL, solid organ tumors, MM
Syngeneic	Peripheral blood Bone marrow	Any disorder treated by allogeneic/autologous transplant except a genetic disease

CML = chronic myelogenous leukemia; NHL = non-Hodgkin lymphoma; MM = multiple myeloma

of HSCs should be present in the graft, so that when infused into the recipient's circulation, engraftment in the marrow microenvironment will occur. Donor stem cells should be tolerated by the recipient's immune system so that rejection of the graft does not occur, and immune cells of the donor should tolerate host tissue so that severe **graft-versus-host disease (GVHD)** does not occur. Graft-versus-host disease occurs when immunocompetent donor T lymphocytes recognize non-self HLA antigens on the host cells and initiate cell injury.

Highly incompatible tissues are almost certain to be rejected. Compatibility is based on the recognition of certain cell markers as "self" by the immune system. The most critical of these appear to be the HLA, also known as the major histocompatibility complex (MHC). The HLA system is a highly **polymorphic** (occurring in several forms) system.

Genes present on the short arm of chromosome 6 encode HLA antigens. HLA class I antigens are encoded by three loci: HLA-A, HLA-B, and HLA-C. HLA class II antigens are encoded by another three loci: HLA-DR, HLA-DP, and HLA-DQ. Serological and molecular testing methods are available to HLA-type individuals.[6,7] Although the candidate donors and recipients are tested for HLA-A, -B, -C, -DR, and -DQ antigens, an HLA match requires only that the donor and recipient have compatible HLA-A, HLA-B, and usually HLA-DR antigens. An optimum clinical result occurs when the donor and recipient are matched at the HLA-A, HLA-B, and HLA-DR loci. Even with a complete match, graft rejection and GVHD can occur, indicating the possibility of incompatible, unrecognized antigens by the current testing methods or other antigens not encoded by MHC. On the other hand, successful transplant may occur even with some degree of HLA-mismatch.[8,9]

Approximately 30% of patients requiring allogeneic transplant will have a matched sibling donor and another 2 to 5% will have a partially matched related donor.[10] If family members do not match or are not available, the search for an unrelated HLA-matched donor is made through the National Marrow Donor Program (NMDP).[11] This type of transplant is called a matched unrelated donor (MUD) transplant. The NMDP was established in 1987 and currently has over 3 million registered donors. Even with such a large donor pool in the NMDP, there are certain limitations for the MUD transplant. First, because of HLA polymorphisms there are difficulties in locating HLA-matched donors. Second, the length of time to find a compatible allograft is about 4–6 months. Third, the cost of a donor search/procurement is high. Fourth, the racial distribution in the NMDP is unbalanced, limiting its usefulness for patients of minority origins, particularly those of African and Asian heritage. However, considerable efforts are being made to recruit minority donors. Finally, with MUD transplant there is an increased chance of graft failure, GVHD, and opportunistic infections.

The initial donor selection for an allogeneic transplant is based on HLA compatibility with the recipient. The ABO blood group antigens do not need to be matched between donor and recipient for successful transplantation because these antigens are not expressed on HSCs. Stem cell donors are tested for the same infectious diseases as are required by the Food and Drug Administration (FDA) for volunteer blood donors. Most transplant centers will absolutely exclude donors only if they are found to have serologic evidence of HIV infection. Before receiving the allogeneic HSC infusion, the recipient is treated with conditioning chemotherapy and/or total body irradiation.[12] Depending upon the underlying disease, this regimen may serve two purposes. First, it provides an antitumor effect, and second, it is immunosuppressive so that the recipient better tolerates the donor cells. The goal of giving high-dose chemotherapy/radiotherapy is to destroy all the malignant cells. This therapy is also toxic to normal bone marrow cells. The patient's marrow is then rescued with normal cells by infusing the donor stem cells. As in solid organ transplantation, recipients must also be given additional immunosuppressive therapy such as cyclosporine or tacrolimus to minimize graft rejection and GVHD.

Syngeneic transplantation is the use of bone marrow or PBSCs from an identical twin. This type of transplant is rare, but could be used for any disorder treated by allogeneic or autologous transplant except genetic diseases that affect both twins. In this uncommon situation, there should be no risk of rejection or GVHD, and no special immunosuppressive drugs need be given.

ⓔ CASE STUDY *(continued from page 609)*

Brandon had a bone marrow examination, and there were 6% blasts present. He has four siblings.

1. Is Brandon a candidate for a stem cell transplant?
2. If yes, what form of transplant is required for him?
3. What testing should be done on Brandon to proceed with the transplant?

AUTOLOGOUS STEM CELL TRANSPLANTATION

Autologous stem cell transplantation involves the infusion of the patient's own bone marrow or PBSCs. These stem cells are collected prior to intensive or myeloablative chemotherapy and/or radiotherapy, which are aimed at eliminating the malignant cells. After therapy, the collected stem cells are infused into the patient to reestablish hematopoiesis. Autologous transplantation is usually indicated when (1) the patient's stem cells are not affected by the disease, and (2) the underlying disease is potentially responsive to high-dose chemotherapy and/or radiotherapy. This type of transplant is commonly utilized for Hodgkin lymphoma, non-Hodgkin lymphoma; multiple myeloma; solid organ tumors including breast, ovarian, and testicular cancers; and pediatric neoplasms such as neuroblastoma and Wilm's tumor (Table 32-2 ✪).

Autologous PBSC transplant also can be performed if the disease involves the patient's marrow. However, in this case a number of other factors should be evaluated (age, underlying disease, degree of marrow involvement, response to previous chemotherapy, and donor availability). The use of autologous stem cells for transplant in a subset of acute leukemias, myeloproliferative disorders, and myelodysplastic syndrome (MDS) is currently being assessed.[13–15]

There are advantages as well as disadvantages to autologous stem cell transplantation. One important advantage is that it is not necessary to identify HLA-matched donors. Immunosuppression is not used, and thus graft rejection and GVHD are not an issue. Peritransplant mortality is low, and the procedure is relatively well tolerated by older patients. Some disadvantages of autologous transplant include the possibility of neoplastic cells in the stem cell product that could cause disease recurrence; difficulty in obtaining adequate stem cells if the patient has received extensive prior therapy; and the **graft-versus-leukemia (GVL)** effect sometimes seen with allogeneic transplant is not possible. (GVL effect is a favorable effect seen when immunocompetent donor T cells present in the allograft destroy the recipient's leukemic cells. The significance of GVL is described later in the chapter.)

✓ Checkpoint! #1

A physician is evaluating a 28-year-old patient with a history of acute lymphoblastic leukemia for PBSC transplantation. The laboratory professional found circulating leukemic blasts in the peripheral blood. Is this patient a candidate for an autologous PBSC transplant?

UMBILICAL CORD STEM CELL TRANSPLANTATION

Umbilical cord blood contains sufficient numbers of HSCs to provide short-term and long-term engraftment in related and unrelated recipients.[16–18] The first cord blood transplantation was performed in 1988, in a 5-year-old boy with Fanconi's anemia.[19] Clinical data indicate that cord blood from siblings and unrelated donors can be used to reconstitute hematopoiesis in patients with malignant and nonmalignant disorders.[16–18,20] As a result of the early successes with cord blood transplantation from sibling donors, pilot programs for the banking of unrelated donor cord blood were initiated in various countries around the world. Cord blood contains sufficient numbers of HSCs for engraftment in

✪ TABLE 32-3	
Advantages and Disadvantages of Using Cord Blood Stem Cells vs Marrow Stem Cell Donors	
Advantages	**Disadvantages**
Cord blood is abundantly available.	The total number of stem cells is generally inadequate for most adult transplant patients.
Cord blood stem cells can be collected without risk to the mother or infant.	May have reduced GVL effect.
Cord blood can be frozen and readily available on demand.	Only one unit is available for each transplant procedure.
The ethnic balance of a given population of donors can be maintained.	
The risk of latent viral contamination (CMV, EBV) is low.	
Cord blood does not contain mature T cells, and therefore is likely less immunogenic and will reduce the incidence of GVHD.	

most recipients weighing less than 40 kg. However, cord blood transplants have been attempted with some success in patients weighing more than 40 kg. The advantages and disadvantages of cord blood over marrow are given in Table 32-3 ✪.

✓ Checkpoint! #2

A patient with CML needs a stem cell transplant. What would be the best form of transplant for him, and what antigen type needs to be matched?

► COLLECTION AND PROCESSING OF HEMATOPOIETIC STEM CELLS

The collection and processing of hematopoietic stem cells requires a team of clinical laboratory professionals as well as physicians.

BONE MARROW

Collection of bone marrow stem cells (allogeneic or autologous) is a surgical procedure that is performed in the operating room under general or local anesthesia. The marrow is taken from the posterior iliac crest with harvest needles and syringes. Approximately 1 liter of marrow is harvested, in order to provide an adequate number of mononuclear cells (MNCs). When the marrow is harvested, it contains a mixture of red blood cells, white blood cells, MNCs, platelets, plasma, and fat particles. If a marrow recipient is ABO compatible with the donor, the marrow can be infused immediately after filtering the fat and small bone particles. Otherwise the marrow can be further processed to remove a mononuclear cell layer that can be frozen and stored.

PERIPHERAL BLOOD

Because stem cells are rare in the peripheral blood (less than 0.01%) various regimens have been tried to mobilize stem cells in the marrow to enter the peripheral blood and increase the number of circulating MNCs. Transplanting more stem cells means more rapid hematopoietic recovery.[21] For autologous PBSC collection, patients may receive cytotoxic chemotherapy (e.g., Cytoxan), hematopoietic cytokines (e.g., granulocyte colony stimulating factor [G-CSF]; granulocyte-macrophage colony stimulating factor [GM-CSF]); or a combination of chemotherapy and cytokines to mobilize stem cells.

After cytotoxic and cytokine therapy, the stem cells in the marrow rebound and are mobilized to the peripheral blood where they can be collected by **apheresis.** Apheresis is a procedure whereby whole blood is separated into various components. One of the components is retained and the remaining constituents are recombined and returned to the individual.

The optimum timing for collection of PBSCs after cytotoxic and growth factor therapy is sometimes unpredictable, and the time of harvest varies depending upon the mobilization protocol. Some centers determine timing of PBSC collection based on a preapheresis peripheral blood CD34 count.[22]

For allogeneic PBSC collection, hematopoietic cytokines (G-CSF or GM-CSF) are given to normal, healthy donors to mobilize stem cells, and then the MNCs are collected by apheresis.

 CASE STUDY *(continued from page 611)*

There is an HLA-matched sibling who has agreed to be a donor for Brandon.

    4. Should the source of stem cells be peripheral blood or bone marrow? Why?

UMBILICAL CORD BLOOD

If UCB is collected as a source for stem cells, the mother must sign an informed consent. A complete medical history of the parents is obtained. Cord blood is usually collected from a delivered placenta or sometimes from an undelivered placenta (after the baby is delivered and the cord is being clamped). A large-bore needle is inserted into the umbilical vein, and blood is collected into a sterile collection bag containing anticoagulant. Several methods are used to separate MNCs from the whole cord blood including Ficoll-Hypaque, modified Ficoll-Hypaque gradient method, and addition of hydroxyethyl starch (HES).[23,24] Table 32-3 ✪ shows the advantages and disadvantages of cord blood stem cells versus marrow stem cell donors. The cord blood is not usually processed if certain conditions are present, as shown in Table 32-4 ✪.

PURGING

Purging is a technique by which undesirable cells that are present in the product are removed. Purging is performed on the stem cell product that has been collected by apheresis. Depending upon the source of stem cells and clinical conditions in which these HSCs are used, a variety of purging techniques (mechanical, immunological, and pharmacological) are available.[25]

When a patient with a history of solid tumor is undergoing an autologous transplant, the bone marrow and, to a lesser extent, PBSCs may be contaminated with occult tumor cells. Therefore removal of tumor cells, if present, is theoretically highly desirable.

In an allogeneic transplantation, GVHD is a potential complication. GVHD is an immunologic response that results from the presence of donor origin CD8-positive T suppressor cells that may interact with the host's CD4-positive T helper cells. If the donor T lymphocytes are removed from the allograft by purging, then GVHD can be prevented or its severity can be reduced. However, some of these T cells seem to be necessary for marrow engraftment and for achievement of the GVL effect. GVL is a favorable response, usually seen because the T cells present in the graft may have an active role in destroying the residual leukemic cells of the recipient. In support of this possibility, patients receiving T cell depleted grafts are known to be at higher risk for disease relapse than patients receiving unmanipulated grafts for the same disease.

✪ **TABLE 32-4**

Conditions in Which Stem Cells Are Not Usually Collected/and or Processed from the Cord Blood

Inadequate volume collected from an individual placenta (less than 40 mL)

Preterm delivery (less than 36 weeks)

Fever of greater than 100°F (38°C) in mother

Premature rupture of membranes

Meconium staining of the fluid

Family history of inherited diseases

Congenital anomalies in the infant

CRYOPRESERVATION AND STORAGE

HSCs from bone marrow, PBSCs, or cord blood can be effectively **cryopreserved** (maintaining of the viability of cells by storing at very low temperatures) for months or years before transplantation. When the stem cells are frozen or thawed, cell injury or loss of viability of stem cells results from intracellular crystal formation and cellular dehydration.

To achieve the optimum cryopreservation without compromising the cell viability, a cryoprotectant agent is used.[25] The most common cryoprotectant used is either 10% DMSO (dimethylsulfoxide) or 5% DMSO and 6% HES. The DMSO diffuses rapidly into the cells and increases intracellular solute concentration, thus decreasing intracellular ice crystal formation and preventing cell lysis.

After optimizing the concentration of the stem cells in the presence of cryoprotectant, tissue culture media and autologous plasma are frozen in many small plastic bags. The freezing rate seems to be an important factor for viable cell recovery. The freezing is usually performed in the chamber of a programmable device into which liquid nitrogen is pumped to maintain the desired rate. After completion of the freezing program, the bags are removed from the chamber and placed in a liquid nitrogen refrigerator, in either liquid or vapor phase at −196°C.

INFUSION

The patient is premedicated with antihistamine and antiemetic (sometimes diuretics and/or steroids). The frozen bags are immediately thawed in a 37°C water bath just before the infusion. The infusion is carried out as quickly as possible to dilute the cell suspension with the patient's blood volume because DMSO in liquid phase can be toxic to stem cells. The most common adverse reactions associated with cryopreserved stem cells are chills, nausea, vomiting, fever, allergic reactions, transient cough, and shortness of breath. Adverse events from infusion can be related to DMSO-induced histamine release, therefore, some centers thaw and dilute or wash the cell suspension to remove the DMSO. Cell loss and clumping may be a problem with this approach.

▶ QUANTITATION OF HEMATOPOIETIC STEM CELLS

The quantity of stem cells or CD34+ cells that can be obtained varies greatly from donor to donor. For PBSCs, one or more apheresis procedures are needed to get the appropriate dose for engraftment and hematopoietic recovery. Because the outcome of engraftment depends upon the number of stem cells present in the product, the HSCs (from bone marrow, PBSCs, or cord blood) are quantitated by one of the three methods described next.

DETERMINATION OF MONONUCLEAR CELL COUNT

It is known that stem cells are mononuclear cells. In addition, other cells are also mononuclear (like immature myeloid cells, lymphocytes, and monocytes), thus, counting MNCs provides a very indirect estimate of the number of stem cells present in the sample (Figure 32-1 ■). The volume of cells necessary to achieve a satisfactory dose for successful engraftment may be determined from the MNC count. The dose is usually specified as the number of MNCs per kilogram of the recipient's body weight. Laboratories quantify the MNCs by automated cell counters or by hemacytometers.

CD34 ENUMERATION BY FLOW CYTOMETRY

Stem cells express CD34 antigen, and enumeration of these cells by immunophenotyping has become a routine practice. When bound to fluorescent dyes, anti-CD34 antibodies offer a rapid method of enumerating stem cells using a flow cytometer. Flow cytometric enumeration of CD34+ cells has been shown to be the most useful indicator of the hematopoietic reconstitutive capacity of SCT.

The major difficulty with the analysis of CD34+ cells is the low number of cells present in the specimen. The sensitivity of the method is 1 in 10,000. Procedures to measure CD34+ cells vary widely. Optimally 100 CD34+ cells and 75,000 CD45+

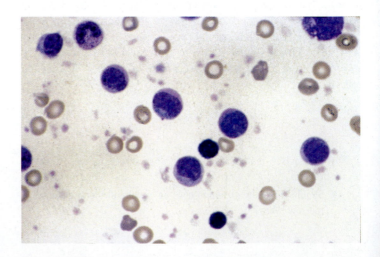

■ **FIGURE 32-1** Wright's stain slide prepared for the manual differential count from the stem cell product showing myeloid precursors and mononuclear cells.

(leukocytes) events should be acquired in order to optimize the accuracy of analysis.[26,27] The CD34 count is calculated in conjunction with the total leukocyte counts.[27,28] These results should be reported as soon as possible because the clinical decision to collect more stem cells depends upon CD34 yield. CD34 counts can be performed on peripheral blood and stem cell product. Some centers determine timing of PBSC collection based on a peripheral blood CD34 count.[22] If the CD34+ cells are lower than required, the decision may be made to perform more (or postpone) apheresis or "prime" the patient in a different manner.

CELL CULTURE FOR COLONY FORMING UNITS (CFUS)

Flow cytometry analysis identifies cells only by their antigenic markers and thus cannot identify cells that are **clonogenic;** only culture techniques can demonstrate clonogenecity. An in vitro clonogenic assay is a culture system containing stem cells and various growth factors. The culture is incubated for 14–15 days on a semisolid medium (agar or methylcellulose). The colonies generated from committed myeloid and erythroid hematopoietic progenitors can be differentiated and counted (Figure 32-2).

The advantage of the clonogenic assay is that this system tests the capacity of progenitor cells to divide and may predict the engraftment potential of the stem cell product.[29,30] The two-week incubation period needed in this method is a distinct disadvantage when data are needed for immediate clinical decisions. There is great variability in the results of clonogenic assay systems from different institutions due to variance in reagent lots and the level of staff expertise. Commercial kits are now available that may aid in the standardization of clonogenic assays.

✔ **Checkpoint! #3**

You receive a peripheral blood specimen in the hematology laboratory with a request for a mononuclear cell count and analysis of CD34+ cells. Without any further information, why should you consider this a STAT request?

► COLLECTION TARGET FOR STEM CELLS

The recipient's body weight will determine the adequate dose of stem cells. The exact number of stem cells needed to ensure engraftment is not known, but cell doses of $2.5–5.0 \times 10^6$ CD34+ cells per kilogram recipient weight are desirable; earlier engraftment will be observed with even higher doses.[31,32] For a transplant using umbilical cord blood, greater than 3.0×10^7 of total nucleated cells per kilogram recipient weight are desirable.

CASE STUDY *(continued from page 613)*

PBSCs were collected by apheresis from the sibling. Enumeration of CD34 count indicates that the total CD34+ cells collected are 6×10^6/kg.

5. Is this an adequate dose for SCT?

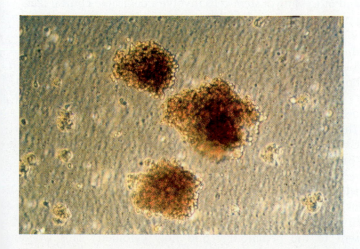
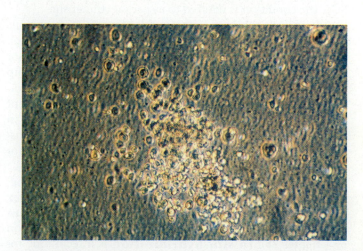

■ **FIGURE 32-2** Cell culture colonies: a. erythroid colonies; b. myeloid colonies (on semisolid medium).

► HEMATOPOIETIC ENGRAFTMENT

The **conditioning regimen** given to patients for stem cell transplantation causes severe myelosuppression in recipients and also may affect T and B cell immunity (usually in an allogeneic setting). After the conditioning regimen, the HSCs are usually given to restore the marrow function. Typically a period of pancytopenia follows, during which the patient is prone to develop infections and bleeding complications. To reduce the period of pancytopenia, growth factors such as G-CSF or GM-CSF may be given.[32,33]

EVIDENCE OF SHORT-TERM ENGRAFTMENT

After transplant, the time for engraftment depends on the number of CD34+ cells in the graft. The period of pancytopenia may last from a few days to 2–4 weeks. Myeloid recovery is followed by platelet and red cell recovery. Short-term evidence of hematopoietic engraftment exists when the absolute neutrophil count is over 500 μL and platelet count is over 20,000/μL with no need for platelet transfusion. The period of pancytopenia after PBSC transplant when compared to bone marrow transplant is somewhat shorter. After cord blood transplants, neutrophil recovery may take 5–6 weeks and the platelets usually engraft late (median time 80 days).[20]

EVIDENCE OF LONG-TERM ENGRAFTMENT

In an SCT recipient, when testing reveals that all hematopoietic cells are derived from an allogeneic donor, the condition is referred to as full **chimerism** (the presence of donor hematopoietic cells in a recipient). When a recipient's hematopoietic cells persist together with donor cells after SCT, the condition is referred to as partial chimerism.

To evaluate the long-term engraftment of HSCs, various laboratory methods have evolved.[34] Detection of red cell antigens was among the first tests used to evaluate donor cell engraftment. For example, if the recipient's blood group is O and the donor's blood group is A, then after hematopoietic engraftment with complete chimerism, the recipient may type as group A. However, because of the long life span of red cells and multiple blood transfusions during transplantation, the red cell antigens are no longer used for chimerism studies.

Currently, the most widely used tests for evaluating long-term engraftment are in situ hybridization (ISH) with sex chromosomes and typing of **variable number tandem repeat** (VNTR) polymorphism by DNA amplification (∞ Chapter 25). **In situ hybridization** is a technique for detection of specific DNA or RNA sequences in tissue sections or cell preparations using a labeled complementary nucleic acid sequence probe. The ISH is applicable only when the donor and recipient are of the opposite sex. Variable number tandem repeats are DNA sequences that are tandemly repeated in a genome and can vary among different individuals. This test for chimerism is applicable in allogeneic transplant settings where testing a person's VNTRs can distinguish donor and recipient cells.

In summary, the clinical applications of chimerism tests in marrow transplantation are to document donor cell engraftment, evaluate persistence of donor cells, and to assess recurrence of disease.

 ✓ **Checkpoint! #4**

A physician wants to evaluate the engraftment on a male patient who received SCT from his brother four months ago. What laboratory tests should be performed to make this assessment?

 CASE STUDY *(continued from page 615)*

Stem cells were collected and frozen for Brandon.

6. Does Brandon need to undergo any form of therapy before the transplant?

► ROLE OF THE CLINICAL LABORATORY PROFESSIONAL IN STEM CELL TRANSPLANTATION

Once the decision to undertake an SCT is made, the collection and processing of stem cells involve a dedicated clinical laboratory staff that works as a team (Figure 32-3 ■). The process of SCT involves the clinical laboratory professionals working in the department of hematology, apheresis, blood bank, microbiology, flow cytometry, molecular/HLA, cytogenetics, and bone marrow transplant laboratories (Figure 32-4 ■).

Let's take an example of a patient for whom the clinical decision for autologous stem cell transplant has been made. This patient will receive cytotoxic chemotherapy, G-CSF, or both. For PBSC collection, the patient undergoes apheresis. (In an allogeneic transplant setting, both the donor and recipient cells are typed for HLA antigens in the molecular/HLA laboratory before stem cells are collected.) The apheresis staff spends 4–6 hours with the patient to get a good yield of MNCs. After the product has been collected, the sample is sent to the hematology and flow cytometry labs where WBC/MNCs and CD34 counts are performed on a sample collected by apheresis.

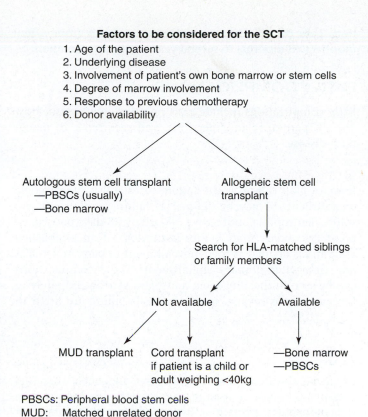

Factors to be considered for the SCT
1. Age of the patient
2. Underlying disease
3. Involvement of patient's own bone marrow or stem cells
4. Degree of marrow involvement
5. Response to previous chemotherapy
6. Donor availability

PBSCs: Peripheral blood stem cells
MUD: Matched unrelated donor

■ **FIGURE 32-3** Decision making process in the stem cell transplantation. The evaluation of the patient for SCT is usually done at the time of primary diagnosis. For allogeneic SCT, a donor is selected based on HLA compatibility. If family members do not match or are not available, the search for an unrelated HLA-matched donor is made through the NMDP. If the patient is a child or small adult (less than 40 kg), then the cord blood registry/banks may also be an option. In general, if the disease involves the patient's own stem cells, allogeneic transplant is a valid option. Autologous transplant is planned when the disease has not affected the patient's own stem cells. On the other hand, autologous PBSC transplant may be performed even if the disease involves the patient's marrow, but a number of other factors should be evaluated, as shown in this algorithm.

The bone marrow transplant laboratory staff will process and cryopreserve the stem cells for future use. The cells' viability is checked, samples for bacterial cultures are taken, and the cell culture may be set up for enumeration of CFUs. On the day of transplant, the clinical laboratory staff (usually of the bone marrow lab) thaws the units for the infusion.

After the transplant, short-term engraftment is evaluated with a complete blood count in hematology. For evaluation of long-term engraftment, the sample is sent to the cytogenetic and molecular/HLA laboratories to perform chimerism studies. Throughout the course of the transplant, the blood bank personnel provide special blood components that are required during the process of transplantation.

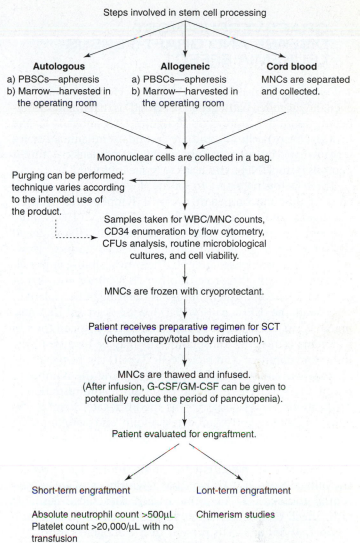

■ **FIGURE 32-4** Steps involved from the time the patient is diagnosed with the disease to the final infusion of stem cell product. For autologous transplant, the stem cells are usually collected from peripheral blood or sometimes harvested from the bone marrow. If the stem cells are collected from the peripheral blood, then the patient may receive cytotoxic chemotherapy, growth factors, or both to mobilize stem cells into the blood, which are then collected by apheresis. For an allogeneic transplant, an HLA-matched family member donor or an HLA-matched donor from the NMDP is considered. The stem cells are collected from the iliac crests in a surgical procedure. In an allogeneic setting, stem cells can also be collected by apheresis from peripheral blood after mobilizing the donor with growth factors. Whatever the method of collection, after collecting the required number of stem cells from peripheral blood, bone marrow, or cord blood, samples are taken for appropriate tests and stem cells are cryopreserved for later infusion. Before the transplant, the patient receives a high dose of chemotherapy and/or radiotherapy to destroy the tumor cells. This therapy can be toxic to normal organs including bone marrow. The marrow is rescued by transplanting frozen stem cells that have been reserved for a particular patient.

▶ GRAFT-VERSUS-HOST DISEASE AND GRAFT-VERSUS-LEUKEMIA EFFECT

The exact mechanism for GVHD is not yet clearly known. However, the suggested pathogenesis of GVHD is that immunocompetent donor T lymphocytes recognize HLA antigens on the host (recipient) cells and initiate secondary inflammatory injury mediated by inflammatory cytokines (interleukin-1, tumor necrosis factor [TNF]). This leads to tissue injury.[35,36]

Three factors necessary to set the stage for GVHD are presence of immunocompetent donor T lymphocytes, HLA alloantigens, and an immunosuppressed host. GVHD is more frequent and severe in recipients of partially HLA-matched sibling allografts or in grafts from unrelated donors.[8] However, GVHD also occurs after HLA-identical sibling donor allografts, indicating the role of other HLA minor antigens or factors that are not usually tested at the time of transplant.

Overall, the risk of acute GVHD for the degree of HLA mismatch is less in recipients of cord stem cell transplant than in recipients of marrow transplant. This may be because of the immature nature of cord blood cells. GVHD can be prevented or its severity may be reduced by decreasing the number of donor T lymphocytes from the graft and/or administration of medications like cyclosporine A, methotrexate, steroids, cyclophosphamide, antithymocyte globulin, and tacrolimus.[37,38]

Recipients of T cell depleted marrow experience less GVHD, but have a higher incidence of relapse and higher graft failure than patients with unmanipulated marrow for the same disease. It is known that T lymphocytes are also essential for marrow engraftment and to achieve desirable GVL effect. GVL is the favorable effect seen when immunocompetent donor T cells present in the allograft destroy the recipient's leukemic cells.[39] For example, in patients with CML who relapse after allogeneic SCT, donor lymphocyte infusion (DLI) can induce a potent GVL effect and reestablish complete remission in most of the patients. DLI is the infusion of small numbers of lymphocytes collected by apheresis from the original graft donor to the allograft recipient who is at high risk of relapse of disease or who has relapsed.[40]

The critical question is how many T lymphocytes need to be removed from the allograft to avoid GVHD and yet allow marrow engraftment and GVL effect. This issue is controversial. Any number should be interpreted with caution because the T cell concentration required to achieve long-term engraftment, control of GVHD, and beneficial GVL effect also depends on the disease and the degree of HLA disparity.

▶ COMPLICATIONS ASSOCIATED WITH STEM CELL TRANSPLANTATION

Complications of stem cell transplants can be divided into early and late complications. Early complications usually are those that occur during the first 100 days after transplanta-tion. Late complications are those that occur from a few months (>3 months) to several years posttransplantation.

EARLY COMPLICATIONS

Early complications include graft rejection, graft-versus-host disease, peritransplant infections, and recurrence of malignant disease.

Graft Rejection

Primary graft failure is the failure to establish hematologic engraftment. It may be defined as failure to attain an absolute neutrophil count above 500 μL by 28 days post-transplant. Secondary graft failure is the loss of an established graft and is defined as the redevelopment of pancytopenia at any time after primary engraftment. These complications can be seen in the allogeneic transplant setting and rarely in the autologous setting. Causes of graft failure are listed in Table 32-5 ✪.

Graft-versus-Host Disease

GVHD can be either acute or chronic. Acute GVHD generally occurs in the first three months after allogeneic stem cell transplantation and usually involves the recipient's skin (maculopapular dermatitis), liver (elevation of bilirubin, abnormal liver function tests), and gastrointestinal tract (nausea, vomiting, diarrhea). Chronic GVHD is defined as symptoms appearing 80–100 days posttransplantation.

Peritransplant Infections

In the peritransplant period, when the patient has been immunosuppressed and has a low neutrophil count, the risk of opportunistic infection is very high. Infections can be bacterial, protozoal, fungal, and/or viral. These infections during the first 3 months posttransplant may be serious and, rarely, life threatening. Reactivation of cytomegalovirus (CMV, a group of the herpes virus family) and herpes simplex are the most common. In the United States, CMV prevalence in the population ranges from 50 to 85%. SCT patients are particularly vulnerable to CMV infection. Infections may be primary, but superinfection with a second strain or a reactivation of latent disease also occur. The complications include pneumonitis, gastroenteritis, and retinitis. Fatal CMV pneumonia occurs in 10–15% of patients.

The relative risk for CMV infection among SCT patients depends upon the serostatus of the donor and recipient.[41] A

✪ TABLE 32-5

Causes of Graft Failure

Inadequate quantity of stem cells
HLA disparity between donor and recipient
Significant T cell depletion of the allograft
Decreased degree of immunosuppression

REFERENCES

1. Jacobson LO, Marks
   spleen protection or
   Med. 1949; 34:1538–

2. Lorenz E, Uphoff D, I
   injury in mice and g
   Cancer Inst. 1951; 12:

3. O'Reilly RJ. Allogenic
   and future directions.

4. Speck B, Bortin MN
   McGlave PB, et al.
   chronic myelogenous

5. Deeg HJ, Klingeman
   Transplantation, 2nd e

6. Begovich AB, Erlich H
   tion: New polymerase
   273:586–91.

7. Beatty PG. The immu
   Transfus Med Rev. 1994

8. Beatty PG, Clift RA,
   Martin PJ, et al. Marre
   than HLA-identical sik

seronegative recipient of seropositive transplant is at significant risk of primary transfusion-transmitted CMV infection. Seropositive recipients of seropositive transplants may develop reactivation or superinfection of CMV.

In selecting donors for a CMV negative patient, preference is given to an HLA-compatible donor who is seronegative for CMV. SCT patients who are at significant risk of acquiring transfusion-transmitted CMV also should receive cellular components that carry a reduced risk of CMV. It has been shown that CMV resides in leukocytes, and studies have indicated that leukocyte-reduced cellular blood components can prevent CMV infection. However, equivalent efficacy of leukocyte-reduced and CMV-seronegative cellular components in preventing transfusion associated (TA)-CMV is not yet completely resolved. Most transplant physicians believe that a CMV-seronegative recipient also should receive CMV-seronegative cellular blood components if the stem cell donor is CMV-seronegative. If the CMV-negative blood component is not available, transfusing a leukocyte reduced filtered component may effectively prevent the transmission of CMV disease.

Recurrence of Malignant Disease

Patients who undergo autologous transplantation are more at risk of dying from disease recurrence than from transplant-related complications. After autologous transplant, recurrence of the original disease can occur because of incomplete eradication of malignant cells or the presence of residual neoplastic cells in the autograft that have not been adequately eliminated by purging techniques. Patients who receive an allogeneic transplant rather than an autologous transplant for hematologic malignancies have a lower relapse rate; however, the risk of leukemic relapse varies from 5 to 70%. This variability depends upon the diagnosis and stage of the disease, the degree of immunosuppression, whether the allograft is matched or mismatched, and the presence or absence of GVHD.

Other Complications

Other complications after SCT include symptoms and clinical signs of toxicity related to chemotherapy and radiotherapy. These include mucositis, myocarditis, pericarditis, pneumonitis, hemorrhagic cystitis, and adverse drug reactions. A condition called veno-occlusive disease is a serious liver disorder complicating up to 50% of marrow transplants. Veno-occlusive disease is diagnosed clinically and is characterized by right upper quadrant pain, weight gain, and jaundice. Other features include ascites, hepatomegaly, hyperbilirubinemia, encephalopathy, and renal failure or multiorgan failure.

LATE COMPLICATIONS

Late complications can be secondary to pretransplantation chemotherapy/radiotherapy, continued effects of acute complications, and/or immunosuppressive states leading to delayed infections. These complications include hypothyroidism, hypogonadism, cataracts, growth retardation in pediatric patients, neuropathies, and sometimes development of second malignancies (non-Hodgkin lymphoma, myelodysplastic syndrome, and leukemia).

 Checkpoint! #5

A CMV-seronegative patient requires SCT. Two HLA-matched donors are available. Is it important to know the CMV status of the stem cell donor? If the stem cell donor is CMV-seronegative and the patient requires red cell transfusion during the peritransplant period, what blood components (in terms of CMV status) would you select for this patient?

 CASE STUDY *(continued from page 616)*

(continued from page 616)

Brandon received stem cells from his HLA-matched sibling and successfully engrafted. Three months later he developed diarrhea, skin rash, and jaundice.

7. What could be the possible cause for this?

SUMMARY

HSCT is a recognized therapeutic modality for leukemias, lymphomas, solid organ tumors, and a variety of metabolic/immunologic disorders. Sources of HSCs can be bone marrow, peripheral blood, and umbilical cord blood. For an autologous transplant, the patient's own stem cells are collected, frozen, and used later for hematopoietic reconstitution. For allogeneic transplant, the donor is selected based on the best HLA match from either family members or an unrelated donor.

Quantitation of stem cells can be performed by counting the MNCs, CD34+ cells, and CFUs. Before transplant the patient undergoes conditioning chemotherapy/radiotherapy and then the stem cells are infused. Routine blood counts and chimerism studies (in allogeneic SCT only) can be performed to assess the engraftment. Complications of stem cell transplant include graft rejection, GVHD, opportunistic infections, recurrence of malignant disease, and others.

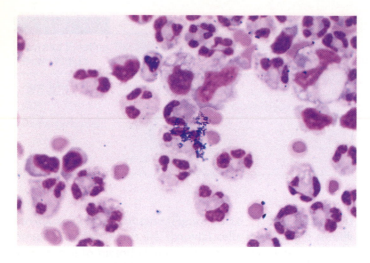

■ **FIGURE 33-21** Stain precipitate on top of the cell, with precipitate in focus and cells slightly out of focus.

lial cells and is dependent on four factors: capillary hydrostatic pressure, plasma oncotic pressure, lymphatic resorption, and capillary permeability.[2] Any pathologic state affecting one or several of these four factors may result in abnormal fluid collection, or **effusion**, in the pleural, pericardial, and peritoneal spaces. In the pleural spaces, accumulation of at least 300 mL is necessary to be detected on chest x-ray, and in the peritoneal cavity accumulation of at least 500 mL is necessary to be detected by abdominal x-ray.[2]

An effusion may accumulate due to a systemic disease state (**transudate**) or as a result of a primary pathologic state of the area (**exudate**). Transudates are frequently a result of increased capillary hydrostatic pressure, such as seen with congestive heart failure, or decreased plasma oncotic pressure, such as seen with hypoproteinemia due to nephrotic syndrome or liver failure. A transudate will most often

have a specific gravity of 1.015 or less, a total protein of 3.0 g/dL or lower, a ratio of effusion total protein to serum total protein of less than 0.5, a ratio of effusion lactate dehydrogenase (LD) to serum LD of less than 0.6, and usually a total leukocyte count $<1000/\mu L$.[1,2]

An exudate is formed by increased capillary permeability and/or decreased lymphatic resorption. An exudative effusion can be caused by many different pathologic processes, such as bacterial infections, viral infections, neoplasms, and collagen vascular diseases. An exudate will have a specific gravity >1.015, a total protein >3.0 g/dL, a ratio of total fluid protein to serum protein >0.5, a ratio of fluid LD to serum $LD>0.6$, and usually a total leukocyte count $>1000/\mu L$.[1,2]

A **chylous** effusion has a characteristic milky, opaque appearance that remains in the supernatant after centrifugation. Chylous effusions result from leakage of lymphatic vessels. In the pleural cavity (chylothorax), this is due to leakage of the major thoracic duct. In the peritoneal cavity, chylous effusions result from blockage of the lymphatic vessels. In both the pleural and peritoneal cavities, this most often results from malignancy such as lymphoma or carcinoma or from trauma. This type of fluid is rich in chylomicrons, has elevated triglycerides (>110 mg/dL), and the predominant cells are lymphocytes.[2,4] A **pseudochylous** effusion is also milky and results from a chronic, long-standing effusion due to such conditions as tuberculosis and rheumatoid pleuritis.[2] Pseudochylous effusions do not contain chylomicrons and usually have triglycerides <50 mg/dL. There will be a mixed reactive cell population with many inflammatory and necrotic cells.

@ **CASE STUDY** *(continued from page 624)*

Radiologic studies show a large effusion in the right pleural cavity. A thoracentesis is performed and 1 liter of thick, yellow fluid is aspirated. Laboratory studies show a total protein of 4.5 g/dL (serum = 6 g/dL), lactate dehydrogenase 40 U/L (serum = 50 U/L), and total leukocyte count of 20,000/µL with 90% segmented neutrophils, 10% histiocytes, and many degenerating cells.

1. Is this a transudate or exudate?
2. Is this a chylous fluid?

NONSPECIFIC REACTIVE CHANGES

The term *nonspecific reactive changes* refers to effusions that have an inflammatory cell response that is not diagnostic for any specific disorder. In various pathologic states, certain types of white blood cells may be present in increased numbers. Bacterial infections will have a predominance of segmented neutrophils while viral, fungal, and mycobacterial infections may have a predominance of lymphocytes or

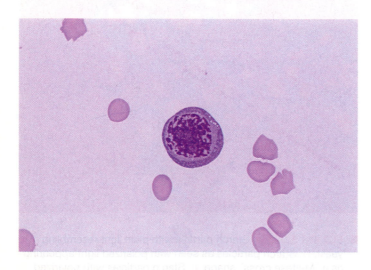

■ **FIGURE 33-22** Early cell degeneration.

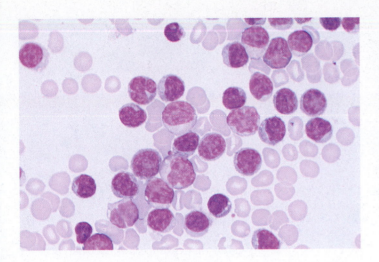

■ **FIGURE 33-23** Reactive lymphocytes in pleural fluid.

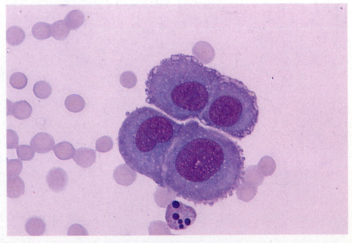

■ **FIGURE 33-25** Spontaneous LE cell formation in pleural fluid.

show a mixed inflammatory response. As in peripheral blood, neutrophils may have toxic granulation, Döhle bodies, and cytoplasmic vacuoles.

Lymphocytes are frequently reactive and transformed, simulating lymphoma cells. The most helpful feature in distinguishing reactive lymphocytes from lymphoma cells is that reactive lymphocytes consist of a heterogeneous population of cells with varying nuclear shape, amount of cytoplasm, and degree of cytoplasmic basophilia (Figures 33-23 and 33-24 ■). Lymphoma cells will be homogeneous, with the same nuclear and cytoplasmic features. The morphology of the lymphoma cells will depend on the particular type of lymphoma.

In rare cases, spontaneous formation of lupus erythematosus (LE) cells is apparent. An LE cell is a macrophage, either neutrophil or monocyte, that has phagocytosed a nucleus showing a homogeneous, smooth chromatin pattern

(Figure 33-25 ■). The finding of these cells is suspicious but not diagnostic for systemic lupus erythematosus (SLE). Other autoimmune type disorders may also show the LE cell phenomenon. Nevertheless, identification of these cells can be extremely helpful in arriving at a difficult diagnosis. The LE cell should not be mistaken for simple phagocytosis of cells by macrophages, which is frequently seen. The chromatin of the usual phagocytosed cell is not smooth or homogeneous.

Mesothelial cells may show nonspecific reactive changes, which include multinuclearity, presence of nucleoli, mitotic activity, and sometimes an increase in cell size (Figures 33-26 and 33-27 ■). Occasionally, there also may be an increased nuclear-cytoplasmic ratio and nuclear folding simulating carcinoma. Reactive mesothelial cells also may tend to cluster and appear cohesive; however, nuclear molding is not seen (Figure 33-28 ■). In cases where it is very difficult to distinguish reactive mesothelial cells from malignant cells,

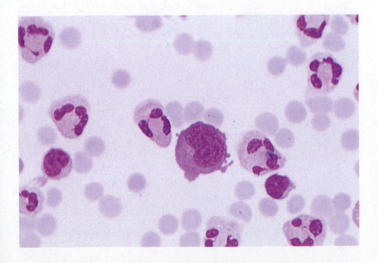

■ **FIGURE 33-24** Reactive lymphocytes in pleural fluid.

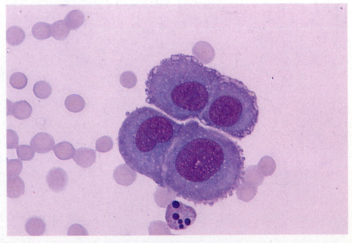

■ **FIGURE 33-26** Reactive mesothelial cells in pleural fluid.

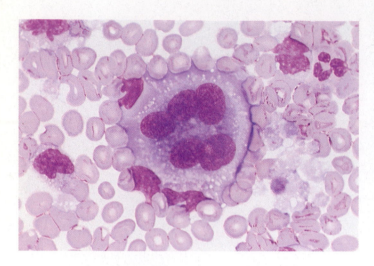

■ FIGURE 33-27 Multinucleated reactive mesothelial cells in pleural fluid.

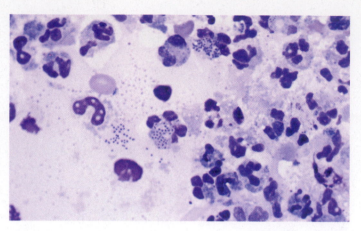

■ FIGURE 33-29 Intracellular and extracellular bacterial cocci, joint fluid.

cytology preparations will usually be definitive as alcohol fixation and Papanicolaou stain yield better nuclear detail.

✓ **Checkpoint! #2**

A 32-year-old woman has right-sided chest pain and shortness of breath that has worsened over a two-week period. Chest radiologic studies reveal a right pleural effusion, and a thoracentesis is performed. The pleural fluid specimen on a cytocentrifuged, Wright-stained slide reveals cells similar to that seen in Figure 33-7. What is the best interpretation of this finding? If there is a strong concern that this may represent a low-grade lymphoma, what would be the best way to determine whether these are benign on malignant lymphocytes?

MICROORGANISMS

Most types of pathogenic bacterial and fungal organisms will stain with Wright's stain and are detectable on a routine cytocentrifuge preparation. Bacteria will stain blue regardless of the gram-stain features. It is important to demonstrate the organisms intracellularly as this is an indication of true pathogenicity rather than in vitro contamination (Figures 33-29 and 33-30 ■). Once bacteria are recognized with Wright's stain, it is helpful to prepare a second cytocentrifuge slide for a gram stain to confirm the presence of bacteria and to be able to give additional information to the physician while cultures are pending.

Most pathogenic yeasts are found in CSF, as opposed to pleural, pericardial, or peritoneal fluids. These organisms may or may not be found intracellularly. The different types of pathogenic yeast show some distinguishing features on Wright's stain. This morphologic variance can be used as a

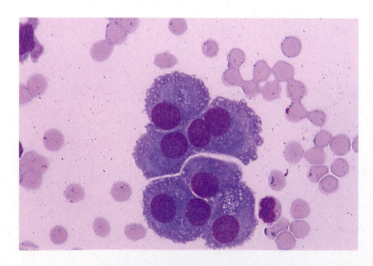

■ FIGURE 33-28 Reactive mesothelial cells in pleural fluid.

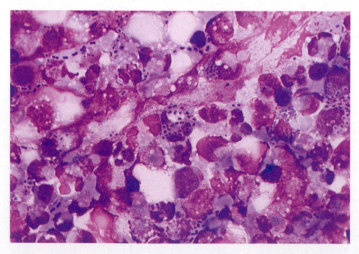

■ FIGURE 33-30 Intracellular and extracellular bacteria, bacilli, peritoneal fluid.

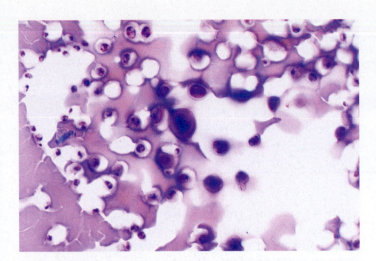

■ **FIGURE 33-31** *Cryptococcus neoformans*, CSF.

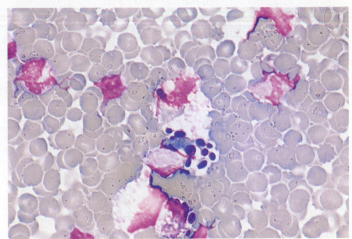

■ **FIGURE 33-33** *Candida albicans*, CSF.

clue for an initial impression of the specific type of yeast, but cultures must be obtained for definitive identification. The most frequently seen fungal organisms in fluids are *Cryptococcus*, *Histoplasma*, *Candida albicans*, and *Candida tropicalis* (Figures 33-31, 33-32, 33-33, and 33-34 ■). Refer to Table 33-4 ✪ for a comparison of morphology.

@ **CASE STUDY** *(continued from page 632)*

A cytocentrifuged, Wright-stained slide is prepared and a photomicrograph is taken (Fig. 33-35).

3. What would be an appropriate next step to determine whether the material seen is debris or true organisms?

Some of the large tissue cells showed features of degeneration and features suspicious for malignancy.

4. How should this be interpreted?

MALIGNANT CELLS IN FLUIDS

The pleural, pericardial, or peritoneal fluids may contain malignant cells, and their identification is critical for accurate diagnosis.[5,6,7] In some patients, a diagnosis of malignancy may already have been established by other tissue sampling (biopsy or excision), and finding the malignant cells in fluid establishes a condition of tumor metastasis. For other patients, the finding of malignant cells in fluid may be the initial diagnosis of a malignancy, and if a sample is not sent to cytology, the recognition of malignancy on the hematology laboratory preparation is critical in establishing an early diagnosis. Malignant cells in fluids can usually be distinguished as hematopoietic in origin (leukemia, lymphoma) versus nonhematopoietic (carcinoma, sarcoma), and in some cases further specification of cell type is also possible. It is important to look at the entire cellular area of the slide with

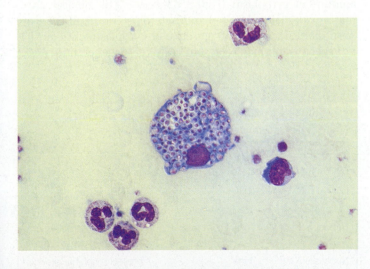

■ **FIGURE 33-32** *Histoplasma capsulatum*, multiple organisms in histiocyte; buffy coat, peripheral blood.

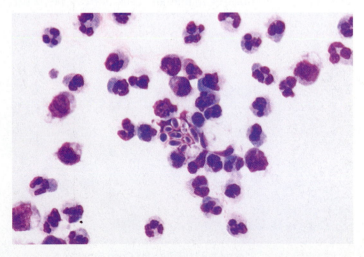

■ **FIGURE 33-34** *Candida tropicalis*, peritoneal fluid.

✪ TABLE 33-4

Comparison of Morphology of Pathologic Yeast as Seen with Wright Stain

Histoplasma	Cryptococcus	Candida albicans	Candida tropicalis
Usually small, often intracellular, distinct non-staining cell wall, partially staining interior	Wide variation in size, usually extra-cellular, capsule not visible on air dried preparations, either solidly stained with "wrinkled" appearance, or partial internal staining	Can be extracellular and intracellular, moderate size, stains solid; rarely may see pseudohyphae formation	Can be extracellular and intracellular, moderate size, dark blue with red internal staining

a low power objective (10×) to detect suspicious clusters of cells. In any one sample, there may be only a few malignant cells present that are difficult to find.

General features that can be seen in almost any type of malignant cell include an irregular nuclear membrane, unevenly distributed chromatin, and nucleoli that also have an irregular membrane (Table 33-5 ✪).[6] The nuclear-cytoplasmic ratio will vary, with small cell carcinoma cells having minimal cytoplasm and adenocarcinoma cells having as much or more cytoplasm as a benign mesothelial cell. The nuclear membrane irregularity may be jagged or may show multiple folds. When nucleoli are present they are frequently prominent and irregular in shape (Figure 33-36 ■). Mitotic activity by itself is not a reliable sign of malignancy as reactive mesothelial cells may undergo mitosis. Cytoplasmic vacuoles are also not a reliable finding for malignancy as this may be seen as a part of early degeneration in many cells. None of the features described can be used alone to diagnose malignancy. All of the features must be looked for and evaluated together. For example, one type of malignancy may show smooth nuclear membranes but with unevenly distributed chromatin and irregular nucleoli (Table 33-6 ✪).

The most common nonhematopoietic malignancies seen in body fluids are small cell carcinoma (oat cell) and adenocarcinoma. Small cell carcinoma cells have the same general morphologic findings of malignant cells but can be distinguished from other types of carcinoma cells because of the characteristic high nuclear-cytoplasmic ratio, blast-like chromatin, absence of nucleoli or nonprominent nucleoli, and frequent nuclear molding (Figure 33-37 ■). Nuclear molding is the process of the nucleus of one cell molding around the shape of an adjacent cell. Nuclear molding occurs with cohesive growth of cells requiring the presence of tight junctions between the cytoplasmic membranes of the cells. Therefore, this may be seen in any type of carcinoma but is most often seen with small cell carcinoma. Some cells also may have a paranuclear "blue body," which is an inclusion that has not yet been characterized and may represent early cell degeneration or phagocytosed material. Depending on the orientation of the cell, the blue body may appear to be intranuclear. The blue body has been described only in small cell carcinoma and rarely in sarcoma.[8] The blue body is seen only with air dried, Wright-stained preparations (Figure 33-38 ■). If the malignant cells are noncohesive, small cell carcinoma could be mistaken for a hematopoietic malignancy, and the finding of a blue body would be a good clue for the diagnosis of small cell carcinoma.

Adenocarcinoma differs from small cell carcinoma in that the overall size of an adenocarcinoma cell is larger than a small cell carcinoma cell with a moderate to abundant amount of cytoplasm (Figure 33-39 ■). The nuclear chromatin is partially clumped and heterogeneous, and there are prominent nucleoli. The presence of cytoplasmic vacuoles is not specific and may represent early cell degeneration.

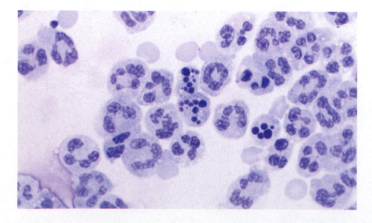

■ **FIGURE 33-35** Pleural fluid. (Figure for Case Study questions number 3 and 4.)

✪ TABLE 33-5

Comparison of Morphologic Features of Reactive Mesothelial Cells versus Malignant Cells

Cell Features	Reactive Mesothelial Cells	Malignant Cells
Nuclear membrane	smooth	irregular, jagged
Chromatin	evenly distributed	unevenly distributed
Nucleoli	absent or present with smooth membrane	prominent, frequently multiple, irregular membrane
Nuclear molding	none	present in non-hematopoietic malignancies

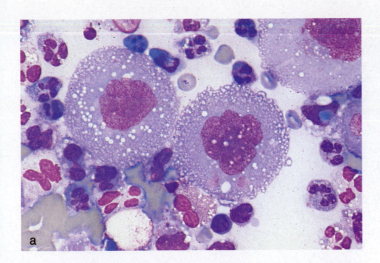

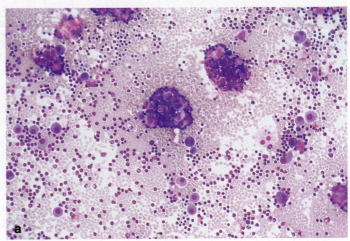

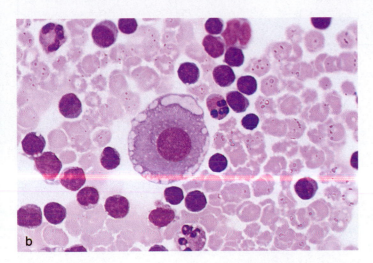

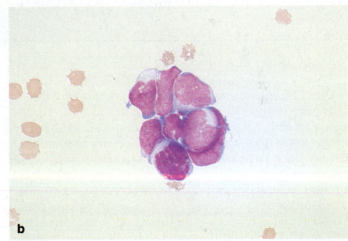

■ **FIGURE 33-37** **a.** Small cell carcinoma, pleural fluid, showing tight cell clusters (original magnification, 25x). **b.** Small cell carcinoma.

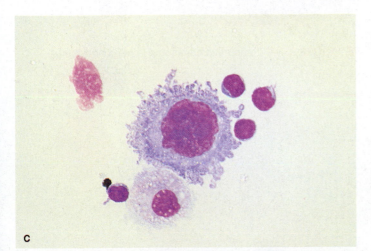

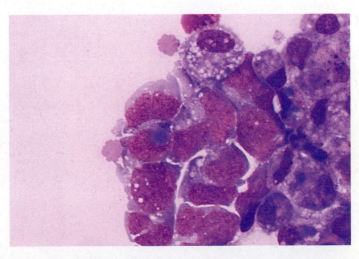

■ **FIGURE 33-36** **a.** Malignant cells (adenocarcinoma), pleural fluid. **b.** Benign mesothelial cell to contrast with features of malignant cell. **c.** Single malignant cell (adenocarcinoma), pleural fluid.

■ **FIGURE 33-38** Small cell carcinoma, paranuclear "blue body" in malignant cell.

⭐ **TABLE 33-6**

General Morphologic Findings of Benign Mesothelial Cells and Malignant Cells. Any given cell may show variable features so that all must be evaluated before deciding if a body fluid sample is benign or malignant. No single feature can be used to diagnose malignancy.

	Mesothelial Cell	Adenocarcinoma	Small Cell Carcinoma	Large Cell Lymphoma	Leukemic Blasts
Cell size	large—15–30 μ	large to giant	moderate to large	moderate to large	small to moderate
Chromatin	loose, homogeneous	partially clumped heterogeneous	slightly course, homogeneous	partially clumped, heterogeneous	smooth, lace-like homogeneous
Nucleoli	none to small and regular	prominent, multiple, irregular	none to small and not prominent	small to prominent, irregular	variable
Nuclear membrane	smooth	irregular, jagged	irregular, jagged, folded	irregular, jagged, folded	smooth or irregular, folded
N:C ratio	low, 1:3–5	low, 1:3 or less	high, 1:1.25	high to moderate 1:1.25–1:2	high to moderate 1:1.25–1:1.75
Intercell relationship	individual or clumped, no nuclear molding	usually clumped, ± nuclear molding	clumped with nuclear molding; occasionally individual	individual, no clumping, no nuclear molding	individual, no clumping, no nuclear molding

Other types of carcinoma and sarcoma can be found in body fluids (Figures 33-40, 33-41, 33-42, and 33-43 ■). The features seen with Wright's stain are not as specific as from a cytology preparation, and the latter is necessary to specifically identify the type of malignancy. For example, squamous cell carcinoma can look like adenocarcinoma with Wright's stain; however, in most cases these are readily distinguishable on cytology preparations (Figure 33-44 ■). Certain types of malignant cells may contain clues for the cellular origin. Melanoma cells may have melanin pigment that will be demonstrable with Wright's stain, and hepatocellular carcinoma may have bile pigment (Figures 33-45 and 33-46 ■). The presence of these pigments can be suspected with Wright's stain but must be confirmed with more specific staining techniques.

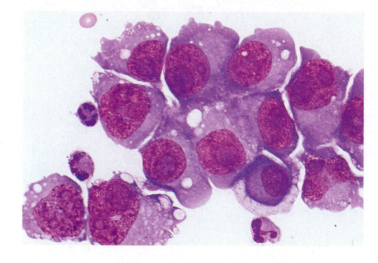

■ **FIGURE 33-40** Pancreatic carcinoma in peritoneal fluid.

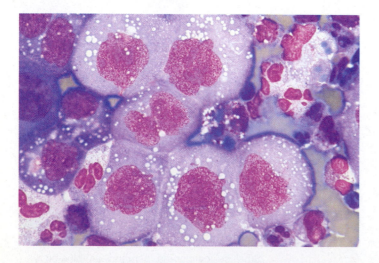

■ **FIGURE 33-39** Adenocarcinoma in pleural fluid.

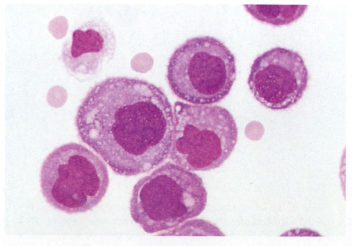

■ **FIGURE 33-41** Gastric adenocarcinoma in pleural fluid.

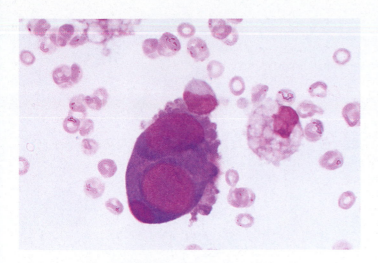

■ FIGURE 33-42 Liposarcoma in pleural fluid.

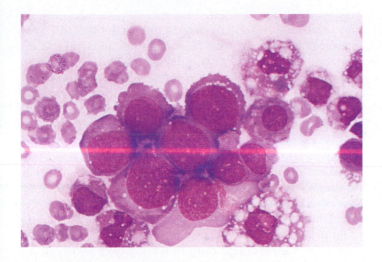

■ FIGURE 33-43 Germ cell tumor (spermatocytic seminoma) in pleural fluid.

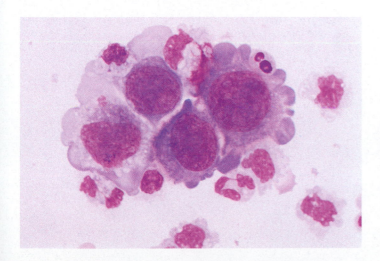

■ FIGURE 33-44 Squamous cell carcinoma in pleural fluid.

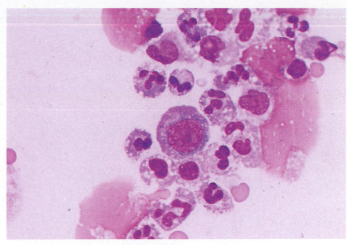

■ FIGURE 33-45 Malignant melanoma in pleural fluid with melanin pigment in malignant cells.

> ✓ **Checkpoint! #3**
>
> *When examining a cytocentrifuged, Wright-stained slide of a body fluid specimen, what are the best features to use in determining if tissue cells are benign or malignant?*

Practically any type of hematopoietic malignancy can be found in body fluids, including lymphocytic and nonlymphocytic leukemias, lymphomas, Hodgkin disease, and plasma cell[9] neoplasms. Generally, the abnormal cells found in the body fluids in these disorders will have the same morphologic features as are seen in peripheral blood and bone marrow. The acute leukemias will only occasionally involve the pleural, pericardial, or peritoneal cavities and more often will be seen in the CSF. Blasts appear larger on cytocentrifuge

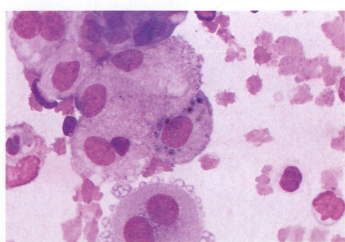

■ FIGURE 33-46 Bile pigment in macrophage in peritoneal fluid due to cholangiocarcinoma.

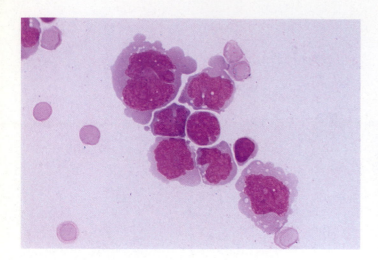

■ FIGURE 33-47 Large cell lymphoma in pleural fluid.

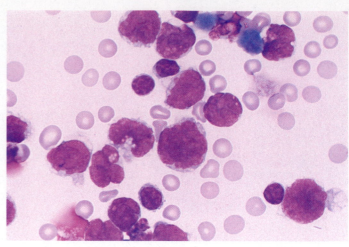

■ FIGURE 33-49 Lymphoblastic lymphoma, T cell type, in pleural fluid.

preparations than on peripheral blood smears, and the nuclear membrane may be surprisingly irregular. Auer rods can be seen, and if necessary, unstained slides can be prepared for cytochemistry stains and terminal deoxynucleotidyl transferase (TdT) to differentiate the blasts (∞ Chapter 26). Lymphoblasts will have a very high nuclear-cytoplasmic ratio, and the nucleus may be folded or convoluted.

The morphology of non-Hodgkin lymphoma in the body fluids will depend on the particular type of lymphoma. Again, the nuclear membrane may be surprisingly irregular. Large cell lymphoma will have cells that are moderate in size to large with irregular nuclei, partially clumped chromatin, and sometimes prominent nucleoli (Figure 33-47 ■). The cytoplasm is low to moderate in amount and basophilic. The cells are discohesive, but if the fluid is very cellular, the cells may be thrown together and have the appearance of carcinoma cell clusters; nuclear molding will not be seen. Small

noncleaved cell lymphoma (Burkitt or non-Burkitt) will have intermediate size cells with more than one nucleoli and an immature blast-like chromatin (Figure 33-48 ■). Frequently, prominent cytoplasmic vacuoles are apparent. Small cell lymphoma is the most difficult to diagnose and may look like a benign lymphocytic infiltrate. In these cases, flow cytometry is valuable in demonstrating a clonal population of cells (∞ Chapter 23). T cell lymphoma may show markedly irregular, convoluted nuclei; however, marker studies are necessary to confirm T or B cell origin of the neoplastic cells (Figures 33-49, and 33-50 ■). This may be accomplished by flow cytometry or by immunoperoxidase techniques on cytocentrifuge prepared slides.

Primary effusion (body cavity) lymphoma is a high-grade lymphoma that is found only in a body cavity without an associated solid tumor mass. This unique malignancy has been reported in patients who are immunocompromised,

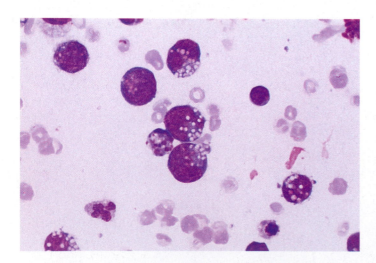

■ FIGURE 33-48 Small noncleaved cell (Burkitt) lymphoma in pleural fluid.

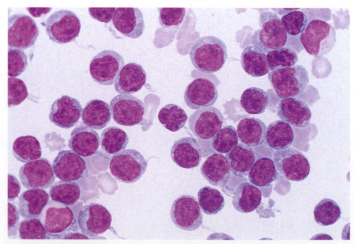

■ FIGURE 33-50 Small lymphocytic lymphoma.

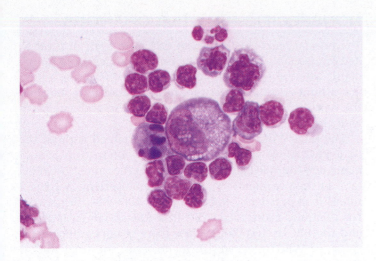

■ **FIGURE 33-51** Hodgkin disease, pleural fluid.

usually HIV-positive, and is associated with HHV-8 (human Herpes virus 8, also known as Kaposi sarcoma associated Herpes virus, KSHV).[10,11] The morphology of the cells is similar to either anaplastic large cell lymphoma, immunoblastic lymphoma, or small noncleaved cell lymphoma. These malignant cells are usually B cell derived, but lack surface associated antigens for T or B cell lineage.

Hodgkin lymphoma can occasionally be seen to involve pleural fluid (Figures 33-51 and 33-52 ■). The malignant Hodgkin cell is large with a moderate to abundant amount of cytoplasm, large nuclei, and prominent nucleoli. If the nucleus is bilobated or if the cell has two nuclei, it may be a Reed-Sternberg cell. The other cells present consist of varying numbers of small lymphocytes, eosinophils, histiocytes, and plasma cells. If a patient has a diagnosis of Hodgkin disease already established by other tissue biopsy, the malig-

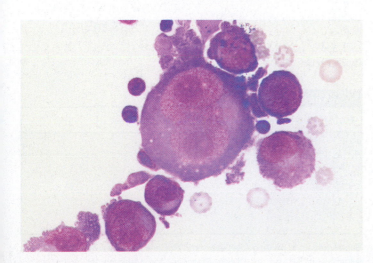

■ **FIGURE 33-52** Hodgkin disease with Reed-Sternberg cell, pleural fluid.

nant cells (either Hodgkin cell, Reed-Sternberg cell, or multinucleated variants) must still be identified in the effusion sample to diagnose involvement of the fluid.

CASE STUDY *(continued from page 635)*

After 3 weeks, the patient improves significantly, but the chest pain and effusion does not resolve. A repeat thoracentesis is performed. Laboratory studies show protein 4.7 g/dL (serum = 6 g/dL), lactate dehydrogenase 50 U/L (serum = 60 U/L), and total nucleated cell count 3,000/μL. A cytocentrifuged, Wright-stained slide is examined, and the differential count shows 30% segmented neutrophils, 20% lymphocytes, 10% histiocytes, and 40% tissue cells. A photomicrograph of the tissue cells is seen in Figure 33-53.

5. Is this an exudate or transudate?

6. What is the most appropriate interpretation of these findings?

► CEREBROSPINAL FLUID

Cerebrospinal fluid (CSF) is different from the pleural, pericardial, and peritoneal fluids in that it exists in the normal state. However, CSF is normally acellular so that the presence of any cells even at a low count is suggestive of a pathologic state. A common problem when evaluating CSF is to distinguish a true CNS hemorrhage versus a spinal tap procedure that causes hemorrhage (traumatic tap). Both of these will present as grossly bloody fluids. If the total erythrocyte count (red blood cell [RBC] count) in the first tube collected is significantly higher than in the last tube collected, it is in favor of a traumatic tap. Xanthochromia is a pink to orange fluid supernatant produced by the breakdown products of hemoglobin and is usually thought to indicate true CNS hemorrhage. Xanthochromia will occur, however, if a grossly bloody fluid from a traumatic tap sits for some time before it is centrifuged. A definitive sign of CNS hemorrhage is phagocytosis of erythrocytes by histiocytes (erythrophagocytosis) (Figure 33-54 ■). It takes approximately 18 hours for histiocytes to mobilize and phagocytose erythrocytes after a hemorrhage. If the hemorrhage is older, hematoidin crystals may be seen intracellularly or extracellarly (Figure 33-55 ■). Hematoidin is a product of hemoglobin catabolism.

✓ **Checkpoint! #4**

A 47-year-old man is found comatose at home by his wife. During examination in the emergency room, a spinal tap is performed and grossly bloody spinal fluid is obtained. The total red blood cell count in the first tube is the same as that in the third tube. A cytocentrifuged, Wright-stained slide shows findings similar to that seen in Figure 33-54. What is the most appropriate interpretation?

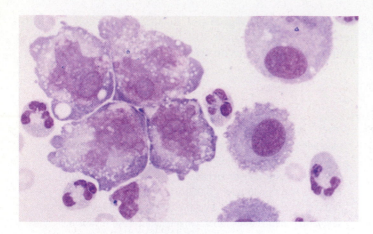

■ **FIGURE 33-53** Pleural fluid. (Figure for Case Study question number 6.)

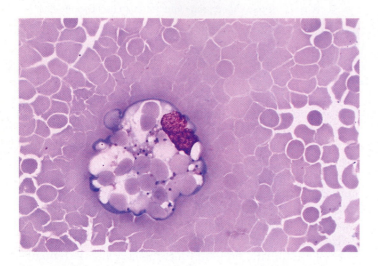

■ **FIGURE 33-54** Erythrophagocytosis.

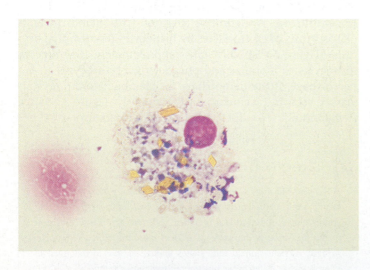

■ **FIGURE 33-55** Hematoidin crystals in macrophage in CSF.

NONSPECIFIC REACTIVE CHANGES

The normal leukocyte counts of CSF have been difficult to determine (Table 33-7 ✪).[1,2] The normal ranges listed for pediatric ages are somewhat controversial as they have a high upper limit. Most important for interpretation is to consider the types of white blood cells present and to correlate them with clinical findings.

The total WBC count cannot be interpreted without the total RBC count. When a specimen is obtained as a traumatic tap, the WBC and RBC will reflect the same WBC/RBC ratio as the peripheral blood of the same patient. A general rule is to expect 1 to 2 WBC for every 1000 RBC in the CSF. For example, if the total WBC in a CSF specimen is $10/\mu L$ and the RBC is $10,000/\mu L$, then there is no significant increase of WBC (pleocytosis). If, however, the total RBC is $100/\mu L$ with a WBC of $10/\mu L$, then there is a significant increase of WBC indicative of a pathologic state.[12] When a patient has an elevated or decreased peripheral blood WBC or RBC, then it is best to use the following calculation to determine if the CSF WBC is significant:[1,2]

$$\text{Corrected CSF WBC} = \text{total WBC of fluid} - \frac{\text{WBC of blood} \times \text{RBC of fluid}}{\text{RBC of blood}}$$

For example, a 21-year-old man has fever, headache, and a stiff neck. A spinal tap is performed. Laboratory studies reveal the following:

	Total RBC	**Total WBC**
CSF	$50,000/\mu L$	$250/\mu L$
Peripheral blood	$3.5 \times 10^{12}/L$	$3 \times 10^{9}/L$

The physician asks if the CSF WBC count represents peripheral blood contamination or a true increase indicative of meningitis. Since the patient has peripheral leukopenia and anemia, the formula should be used to answer this question.

$$\text{Corrected CSF WBC} = 250/\mu L - \frac{(3.0 \times 10^{9}/L) \times (50,000/\mu L)}{3.5 \times 10^{12}/L}$$

$$\text{Corrected CSF WBC} = 250/\mu L - 50/\mu L$$

$$\text{Corrected CSF WBC} = 200/\mu L$$

✪ TABLE 33-7

Reference Range for Leukocytes in CSF per μL

Age	Reference Range
Adults	0–5
5–puberty	0–10
1–4	0–20
<1	0–30

Based on data from Kreig AF, Kieldsberg CR: Cerebrospinal fluid and other body fluids. Henry SB, ed. In: *Clinical Diagnosis and Management by Laboratory Methods.* Philadelphia: W.B. Saunders; 1996, and from Kieldsberg C, Knight J: *Body Fluids,* 3rd ed. Chicago: ASCP Press; 1993.

Hence there is a significant increase in the CSF WBC.

In general, the type of predominant white blood cell present has the same diagnostic indication as seen in the peripheral blood. For example, a predominance of neutrophils most often indicates a bacterial meningitis, a predominance of lymphocytes correlates with viral and fungal meningitis, and an increase of eosinophils may indicate a parasitic infection or allergic and drug reactions. More detailed correlations of possible diagnosis and type of cell increase is available in other sources.[1,2,13]

As with the pleural, pericardial, and peritoneal fluids, reactive lymphocytes must be distinguished from lymphoma cells (Figure 33-56 ■). Hematopoietic precursors including megakaryocytes are present if the spinal tap needle penetrated the vertebral bone, drawing back a portion of bone marrow. This is most often seen in infants, but may occur in adults with osteoarthritis.[14]

Mesothelial cells are not present in CSF, but other tissue cells such as arachnoid cells and choroid plexus cells can be seen. These are most often present in CSF from infants or from adults who have had some type of manipulation such as surgery, shunt, or reservoir. It is very unusual to see these cells from a simple spinal tap procedure in an adult.

MICROORGANISMS

The same types of microorganisms described in pleural, pericardial, and peritoneal fluids may be present in CSF samples. As mentioned earlier, it is critical to distinguish intracellular bacteria from stain precipitate. A Gram stain is most helpful in this situation. The most common yeast organism seen in CSF is cryptococcus (Figure 33-31 ■). Once cryptococcus is suspected from the cytocentrifuge prepared slide, an India ink preparation should be performed by the microbiology laboratory to confirm the presence of the characteristic large capsule of cryptococcus. If only very few organisms are pre-

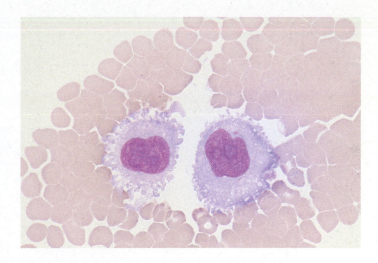

■ FIGURE 33-57 Adenocarcinoma, CSF.

sent, however, the India ink preparation may be negative as unconcentrated CSF is used for the India ink. Cultures must be obtained to confirm the type of organism present.

MALIGNANT CELLS

Much of the description of malignant cells in pleural, pericardial, and peritoneal fluids holds true for spinal fluid examination as well.[15] Carcinoma cells tend to be less cohesive in spinal fluid than in other fluids and may simulate hematopoietic malignancies. Since mesothelial cells do not exist in the CSF, the presence of any large tissue cells should be considered suspicious for malignancy (Figures 33-57, 33-58, and 33-59 ■). Malignant cells, however, must be differentiated from the benign choroid plexus cells, ependymal cells, and arachnoid cells. This is done by evaluating the cells for standard features of malignancy as described earlier.

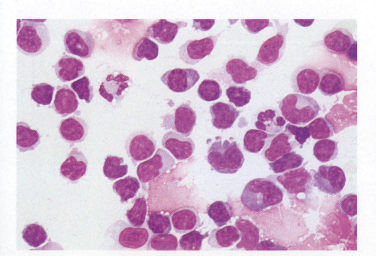

■ FIGURE 33-56 Reactive lymphocytes, CSF.

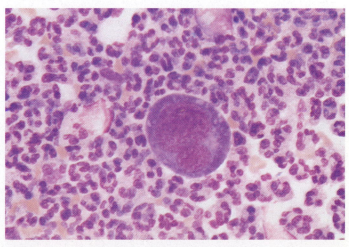

■ FIGURE 33-58 Large cell undifferentiated carcinoma with intense chemical acute meningitis, CSF.

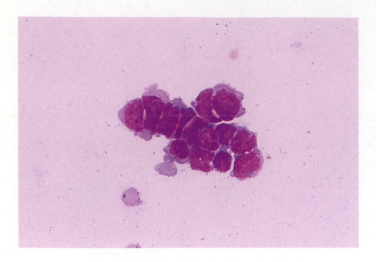

■ FIGURE 33-59 Small cell carcinoma, CSF.

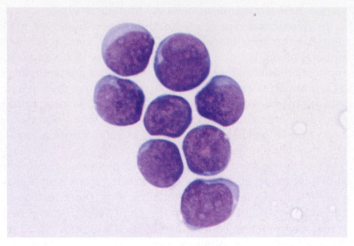

■ FIGURE 33-61 Acute lymphocytic leukemia, CSF.

Cytology preparations will usually be definitive. Benign tissue cells usually are seen only in CSF from infants or from adults who have recent neurosurgery or a shunt or reservoir in place.

Rarely, cells from primary CNS neoplasms may be found in the CSF. Medulloblastoma is a malignant tumor usually occurring in the cerebellum of pediatric patients and has a morphologic appearance similar to small cell carcinoma (Figure 33-60 ■). Patient history from the physician would be necessary to distinguish the origin of the tumor.

Acute lymphocytic leukemia more often involves the CNS than acute nonlymphocytic leukemia (Figures 33-61, 33-62, and 33-63 ■). When erythrocytes are present, care must be taken not to overinterpret the presence of blasts that simply represent peripheral blood contamination. If no erythrocytes are present, even a low number of blasts (1% to 2%) may be indicative of CNS involvement.[16] Special studies

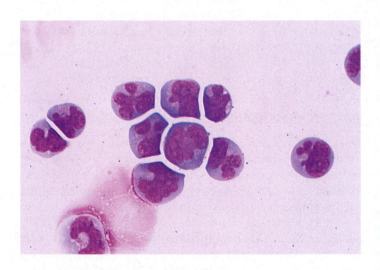

■ FIGURE 33-62 Acute myelomonocytic leukemia, CSF.

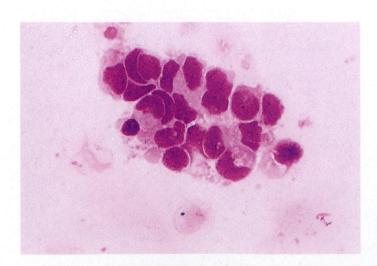

■ FIGURE 33-60 Medulloblastoma, CSF.

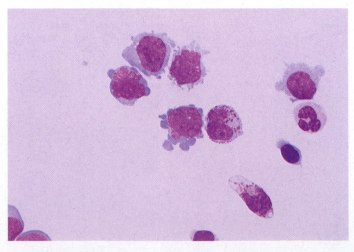

■ FIGURE 33-63 Blast crisis of chronic myelocytic leukemia with myeloblasts in CSF.

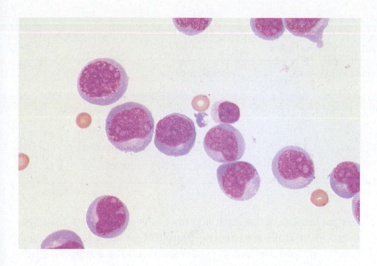

■ **FIGURE 33-64** High-grade lymphoma, small noncleaved cell type, CSF.

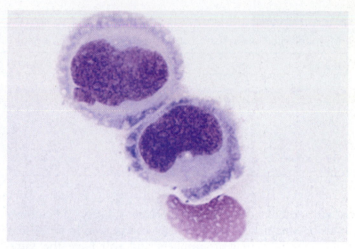

■ **FIGURE 33-65** Cerebral spinal fluid. (Figure for Case Study question number 7)

such as cytochemistry stains, TdT, and surface markers by immunoperoxidase stains or flow cytometry may be helpful[17] (∞ Chapters 23, 26).

Any type of lymphoma may involve the CNS, but more often seen are the high-grade lymphomas such as lymphoblastic, immunoblastic, and small noncleaved cell. Primary CNS lymphoma is seen more often in recent years because of the relatively high incidence of this malignancy in patients who are HIV-positive. The lymphomas in HIV-positive patients are high-grade and frequently correspond to small noncleaved cell, pleomorphic type, or B immunoblastic (Figure 33-64 ■).

pseudogout) from septic processes. Other disease states can induce an inflammatory response; however, it is usually not possible to diagnose these by joint-fluid examination alone. Certain diagnoses can be suspected when comparing the total WBC count with percent segmented neutrophils present; however, there is great overlap, and morphologic examination by cytocentrifuge preparations can be extremely helpful (Table 33-8 ✪).[18,19]

Joint fluids that have a total WBC of 50,000 to 200,000/μL are suggestive of an infectious or crystal-induced etiology. If the differential count shows 90% or more segmented neu-

✐ CASE STUDY *(continued from page 641)*

After an extensive work up, the patient is found to have a primary adenocarcinoma of the right upper lung lobe. A surgical resection is performed. Six months later, the patient has severe headaches. A spinal tap is performed and a photomicrograph of the cells is seen in Figure 33-65.

7. What is the most appropriate interpretation of these cells?

▶ JOINT FLUID

Synovial fluids tend to be thick and viscous due to the presence of hyaluronic acid, a mucopolysaccharide substance secreted by the lining synovial cells. If the fluid is too thick to proceed with cell counts, the use of hyaluronidase can be very helpful to loosen the fluid. Joint fluid is most often aspirated to distinguish crystal-inducing diseases (gout,

✪ TABLE 33-8

General Grouping of Diagnosis by Total WBC and Percent Neutrophils in Synovial Fluid Analysis. There is some overlap of diagnostic groups and other studies are necessary to reach an accurate diagnosis.

Total WBC	0–5,000/μL <30% neutrophils osteoarthritis, traumatic arthritis, neuropathic arthropathy, pigmented villonodular synovitis
Total WBC	2,000–200,000/μL >50% neutrophils rheumatoid arthritis, Lupus erythematosus, Reiter's syndrome, rheumatic fever, ankylosing spondylitis
Total WBC	50,000–200,000/μL >90% neutrophils Infectious—bacterial, mycobacterial, fungal
Total WBC	500–200,000/μL <90% neutrophils Crystal induced—gout, pseudogout, apatite arthropathy
Total WBC	50–10,000/μL <50% neutrophils RBC present Hemorrhagic—trauma, hemophilia, anticoagulant, pigmented villonodular synovitis, neuropathic arthropathy, hemangioma

⊛ **TABLE 33-9**

Morphologic Comparisons of Commonly Seen Birefringent Crystals and Particles

Crystal	Birefringence	Color Parallel to Quartz Compensator	Morphology
Monosodium urate	strong	yellow	long, thin, needle-like, intra- and extracellular
Calcium pyrophosphate	weak	blue	short, rectangular, intra- and extracellular
Cholesterol	strong	variable	large plate-like, notched, extracellular
Steroids	strong	variable	amorphous, intra- and extracellular
Talc particles	strong	yellow and blue	maltese cross shape, extracellular

trophils, then an infectious agent is most likely and cultures must be obtained. Microorganisms can be seen in joint fluid if present in sufficient numbers and will have the same morphology as previously described. Bacterial organisms are more common and pathogenic yeasts are only rarely seen.

When the total WBC is in the range of 2,000 to 200,000/ μL with greater than 50% neutrophils in the differential count, entities such as rheumatoid arthritis (RA), systemic lupus erythematosus (SLE), Reiter's syndrome, and so forth should be considered. Rarely, spontaneous LE cell formation may occur. The LE cell is suggestive of SLE; however, it is not diagnostic and also may be seen in RA. The so-called RA cell is a neutrophil containing granules of immune complexes. These cells are not specific for a diagnosis of RA. The Reiter's cell is a macrophage with vacuoles containing debris of phagocytosed neutrophils. The debris may also be unrecognizable blue material. These cells are also nonspecific and not diagnostic for Reiter's disease.

Synovial cells can become proliferative in a reactive setting similar to mesothelial cells. Reactive synovial cells may also be multinucleated and may occur in clusters, and their nuclei may have small, regular nucleoli. Theoretically, malignant cells may be seen in synovial fluid; however, this is extremely rare.[20]

EXAMINATION FOR CRYSTALS

The three most common types of crystals present in joint fluid are monosodium urate crystals seen in gout, calcium pyrophosphate crystals seen in pseudogout, and cholesterol crystals present in different types of chronic arthritides such as RA. Examination for crystals on a cytocentrifuge-prepared slide is superior to a standard wet preparation as the cytocentrifuge concentrates the specimen. Samples that may be negative with wet preparation may actually show crystals on the concentrated cytocentrifuge slide. Using cytocentrifuge prepared slides also decreases the biologic hazard when handling wet preparations. If sufficient numbers of crystals are present, they can be seen with plain light microscopy on a Wright-stained cytocentrifuge slide. However, polarized light must be used to confirm birefringence[21] (described later). If fewer crys-

tals are present, polarization is necessary to see them initially. Every joint fluid sent to the hematology laboratory for cell counts should have a crystal examination. Some Wright's stain techniques result in dissolution of the monosodium urate crystals. Therefore, it is best to prepare two cytocentrifuge slides, one for Wright's stain and one left unstained. Both slides should be examined for crystals on multiple specimens to determine if a particular stain technique dissolves the monosodium urate crystals (Table 33-9 ⊛).

Birefringence refers to the ability of a particular material to refract light rays. This is determined by using a polarizing microscope. A fixed light filter (analyzer) is placed above the specimen and a rotating filter (polarizer) is placed below the specimen. Both filters allow light to pass in only one direction. When the polarizer is rotated 90 degrees to the analyzer, no light can pass, yielding a "dark field." If the specimen contains birefringent material, it will change the direction (refract) of the light rays allowing them to pass through the analyzer, and the birefringent material will be seen as a bright particle or crystal.[21] A quartz compensator is used to further identify a crystal by determining the velocity of the light rays passing through the grain (axis) of the crystal.

Monosodium urate (MSU) crystals should be reported as intracellular and/or extracellular. MSU crystals are typically long, thin, and needle-like with pointed ends (Figure 33-66a ■). They may be seen singly or in bundles. MSU crystals are strongly birefringent and are brilliant with polarized light (Figure 33-66b ■). A quartz compensator must be used to determine positive or negative birefringence. MSU are negatively birefringent and when aligned parallel to the axis of the compensator will show a yellow color; when turned perpendicular to the axis of the compensator, the color changes to blue (Figure 33-66c ■).[1,2,21]

Calcium pyrophosphate crystals (CPP) may also be seen intracellularly and/or extracellularly. CPP crystals are typically short, rectangular, and weakly birefringent so that they may be difficult to see with polarized light (Figures 33-67a and 33-67b ■). When aligned parallel to the axis of a quartz compensator, the CPP crystals are blue, and the color changes to yellow when crystals are perpendicular to the axis of the compensator (Figure 33-67c ■).[1,2,21] Occasionally, a joint fluid may have both MSU and CPP crystals; the presence of one does not exclude the other.

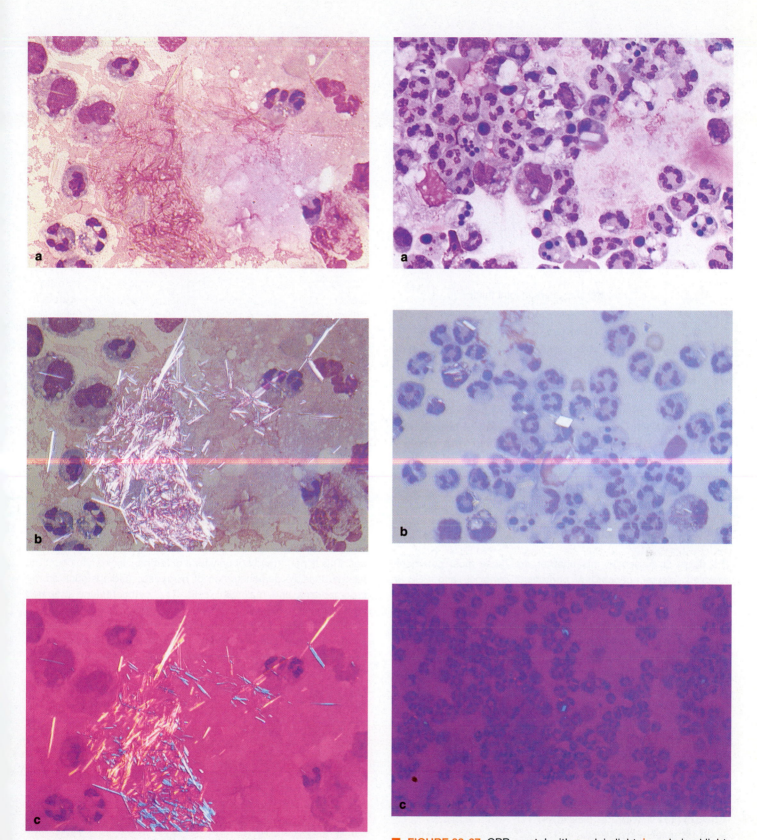

■ FIGURE 33-66 MSU crystal with a. plain light, b. polarized light, and c. quartz compensator with crystal showing yellow parallel to quartz line and crystal with blue perpendicular to quartz line.

■ FIGURE 33-67 CPP crystal with a. plain light, b. polarized light, c. quartz compensator with yellow crystal perpendicular to quartz line and blue crystal parallel to quartz line.

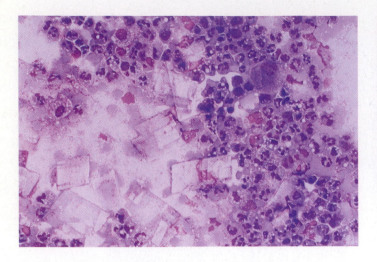

■ **FIGURE 33-68** Cholesterol crystals in joint fluid.

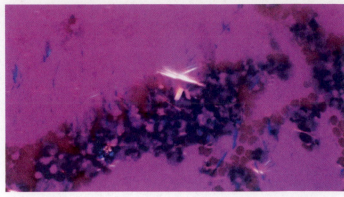

■ **FIGURE 33-69** Synovial fluid. (Figure for Checkpoint #5.)

Cholesterol crystals have a characteristic notched-plate shape and are birefringent (Figure 33-68 ■). These crystals are present in chronically inflamed joints such as seen in rheumatoid arthritis.

Starch particles are distinguished from pathogenic crystals by a characteristic Maltese-cross shape with polarized light (Figure 33-20 ■). If a joint has been injected with steroids, the steroid particles can be seen intracellularly and extracellulary. Steroid particles do not have a crystal shape and are amorphous but birefringent.

> ✓ **Checkpoint! #5**
>
> *A 57-year-old man has an acutely swollen, painful, reddened joint in his left great toe. Joint fluid is aspirated, and a photomicrograph is taken (Figure 33-69). This picture is taken with polarized light using a quartz compensator. What is the most appropriate interpretation of this finding?*

SUMMARY

The fluids discussed in this chapter are those most commonly sampled: pleural, pericardial, peritoneal, synovial, and CSF. In pathologic conditions the amount of fluid can increase (effusion). An effusion can be a transudate or an exudate. Chylous effusions are milky and result from leakage of lymphatic vessels. Common cell types seen in these fluids include white blood cells, tissue cells, and malignant cells. Examination of cellular morphology in body fluids is a critically important procedure for hematology laborato-ries. This is performed not only for a differential leukocyte count but for the possible demonstration of diagnostic findings such as microorganisms and malignant cells. The cytocentrifuge prepared Wright-stained slide yields excellent morphology of cells and can significantly aid in timely diagnosis of patients with effusions of unknown etiology. The hematology laboratory must take an active role in correlating morphologic findings with additional studies that may be necessary such as cultures, special stains, and cytology.

REVIEW QUESTIONS

LEVEL I

1. The types of body fluids other than peripheral blood that are frequently sent to the hematology laboratory include which of the following? (Checklist #1)
   a. cerebrospinal fluid
   b. pleural fluid
   c. pericardial fluid
   d. all of the above

LEVEL II

1. A specimen is sent to the laboratory labeled "ascites." What type of procedure was used to obtain this fluid? (Checklist #1)
   a. thoracentesis
   b. lumbar puncture
   c. pericardial aspiration
   d. paracentesis

REVIEW QUESTIONS (continued)

LEVEL I

2. The pleura, pericardium, and peritoneum are composed of what type of cell? (Checklist #2)
   a. white blood cell
   b. epithelial cell
   c. mesothelial cell
   d. squamous cell

3. Anatomically, where is the visceral pleura located? (Checklist #1)
   a. innermost aspect of the abdominal wall
   b. outermost portion of the heart
   c. innermost aspect of the chest wall
   d. outermost portion of the lung

4. Which of the following cell type(s) when seen in cerebrospinal fluid may be considered normal and not a sign of pathologic disease? (Checklist #2)
   a. arachnoid cells
   b. choroid plexus cells
   c. ependymal cells
   d. all of the above

5. The finding of possible bacterial organisms on a cytocentrifuged, Wright-stained slide would be easiest to confirm by which of the following? (Checklist #5)
   a. gram stain
   b. silver stain
   c. culture
   d. electrophoresis

6. Which of the following may be seen as artifact on a cytocentrifuged, Wright-stained slide? (Checklist #8)
   a. hypersegmentation of neutrophils
   b. stain precipitate
   c. cytoplasmic projections of lymphocytes
   d. all of the above

7. Which of the following best characterizes a chylous fluid? (Checklist #4)
   a. transparent, yellow, low nucleated cell count
   b. opaque, bloody, many neutrophils
   c. cloudy, yellowish-green, many histiocytes
   d. opaque, white, many lymphocytes and chylomicrons

8. A 45-year-old man has pleural effusions on the right and left side. A right-sided thoracentesis is performed and a sample is sent to the laboratory. The fluid-serum protein ratio is 0.3, the fluid-serum LD ratio is 0.4, and the total nucleated cell count is low. Which of the following best describes this fluid? (Checklist #4)
   a. chylous
   b. exudate
   c. pseudochylous
   d. transudate

LEVEL II

2. Which of the following cell types is responsible for the production of cerebrospinal fluid? (Checklist #2)
   a. choroid plexus
   b. arachnoid
   c. neutrophils
   d. mesothelial

3. A 25-year-old woman develops a left-sided pleural effusion while recovering from bacterial pneumonia. A thoracentesis is performed and the following laboratory results are reported:

	Serum	Fluid
Protein	6.5 g/dL	5 g/dL
LD	75 U/L	60 U/L

   These results would be best interpreted as which of the following? (Checklist #3)
   a. chylous
   b. exudate
   c. pseudochylous
   d. transudate

4. A 56-year-old woman has a three-week history of abdominal pain. A peritoneal effusion is found. After paracentesis, a sample is sent to the laboratory. Examination of the cytocentrifuged, Wright-stained slide shows clusters of large cells that have abundant cytoplasm, smooth nuclear membranes, evenly distributed chromatin, and no nucleoli. An occasional multinucleated cell is found with the same features. These cells most likely represent: (Checklist #5)
   a. reactive mesothelial cells
   b. adenocarcinoma cells
   c. small cell carcinoma
   d. ependymal cells

5. A 60-year-old man who has smoked cigarettes since the age of 16 years has left-sided chest pain. A thoracentesis sample is sent to the laboratory. The cytocentrifuged, Wright-stained slide is examined and there are clusters of large cells that have irregular, jagged nuclear membranes, prominent and irregular nucleoli, and unevenly distributed chromatin. These cells most likely represent: (Checklist #5)
   a. reactive mesothelial cells
   b. adenocarcinoma cells
   c. large cell lymphoma
   d. reactive histiocytes

6. Referring to the case in question 5, the protein, LD, and other studies would most likely reveal that this is a(n): (Checklist #3)
   a. exudate
   b. chylous fluid
   c. transudate
   d. pseudochylous fluid

LEVEL I

9. Which of the following is (are) a morphologic feature characteristic of malignant tissue cells? (Checklist #6)
   a. irregular nuclear membrane
   b. evenly distributed chromatin
   c. prominent, irregular nucleoli
   d. a and c only

10. The finding of which of the following in joint fluid is most helpful to establish a diagnosis of gout? (Checklist #7)
   a. monosodium urate
   b. cholesterol
   c. starch particles
   d. neutrophils

LEVEL II

7. A 65-year-old man has a painful, swollen elbow. A joint aspiration is performed and a sample is sent to the laboratory. A cytocentrifuged slide is examined with polarized light and a quartz compensator. Birefringent crystals are seen intracellular and extracellular; they are needle-like in appearance and are yellow when oriented parallel to the quartz compensator. These crystals would be best identified as which of the following? (Checklist #8)
   a. calcium pyrophosphate
   b. cholesterol
   c. monosodium urate
   d. steroids

8. Referring to the case in question 7, which of the following is the most likely diagnosis? (Checklist #8)
   a. gout arthritis
   b. pseudogout arthritis
   c. rheumatoid arthritis
   d. systemic lupus erythematosus

9. A 55-year-old man is brought to the emergency room in a comatose state. He was found at home by his son and appears to have fallen from a ladder. A spinal tap is performed and reveals the following:

Color:	red
Appearance:	bloody
RBC:	100×10^9/L
WBC:	0.10×10^9/L
Differential WBC:	80% segmented neutrophils
	15% lymphocytes
	5% monocytes

Which of the following would be the most specific finding for a true CNS hemorrhage vs traumatic spinal tap in this patient? (Checklist #6)
   a. crenated red blood cells
   b. xanthochromia of the supernatant
   c. erythrophagocytosis by histiocytes
   d. WBC of 0.1×10^9/L

10. Referring to the patient in question 9, what is the significance of the white cell count of 0.1×10^9/L? (Checklist #9)
   a. This is diagnostic for bacterial meningitis.
   b. This is diagnostic for early viral meningitis.
   c. This is expected for the amount of hemorrhage.
   d. This is diagnostic for fungal meningitis.

REFERENCES

1. Kreig AF, Kieldsberg CR. Cerebrospinal fluid and other body fluids. Henry SB, ed. In: Clinical Diagnosis and Management by Laboratory Methods. Philadelphia: W. B. Saunders; 1996.

2. Kieldsberg C, Knight J. *Body Fluids,* 3rd ed. Chicago: ASCP Press; 1993.

3. Lau MS, Pien FD. Eosinophilic pleural effusions. *Hawaii Med J.* 1990; 49:206–7.

4. Horn KD, Penchansky L. Chylous pleural effusions simulating leukemic infiltrate associated with thoracoabdominal disease and surgery in infants. *Am J Clin Path.* 1999; 111:99–104.

5. Ultmann J. Malignant effusions. *CA-Cancer,* 1991; 41:166–79.

6. Clare N, Rone R. Detection of malignancy in body fluids. *Lab Med.* 1986; 17:147–50.

7. Kendall B, Dunn C, Solanki P. A comparison of the effectiveness of malignancy detection in body fluid examination by the cytopathology and hematology laboratories. *Arch Pathol Lab Med.* 1997; 121:976–79.

8. Wittchow R, Laszewski M, Walker W, Dick F. Paranuclear blue inclusions in metastatic undifferentiated small cell carcinoma in the bone marrow. *Mod Pathol.* 1992; 5:555–58.

9. Mitchell MA, Horneffer MD, Standiford TJ. Multiple myeloma complicated by restrictive cardiomyopathy and cardiac tamponade. *Chest.* 1993; 103:946–47.

10. Nador RG, Cesarman E, Chadburn A, et al. Primary effusion lymphoma: A distinct clinicopathologic entity associated with the Kaposi's sarcoma-associated herpes virus. *Blood.* 1996; 88:645–56.

11. Knowles D, Chadburn A. Lymphadenopathy and the lymphoid neoplasms associated with the acquired immune deficiency syndrome. *Neoplastic Hematopathology,* Knowles D, ed. In: 2nd ed. Philadelphia: Lippincott Williams and Wilkins, 2001.

12. Bonadio WA, Smith DS, Goddard S, Burroughs J, Khaja G. Distinguishing cerebrospinal fluid abnormalities in children with bacterial meningitis and traumatic lumbar puncture. *J Infect Dis.* 1990; 162:251–54.

13. Greenlee JE. Approach to diagnosis of meningitis: Cerebrospinal fluid evaluation. *Infect Dis Clin North Am.* 1990; 4:583–98.

14. Craver RD, Carson TH. Hematopoietic elements in cerebrospinal fluid in children. *Am J Clin Pathol.* 1991; 95:532–35.

15. Bigner SH. Cerebrospinal fluid (CSF) cytology: Current status and diagnostic applications. *J Neuropathol Exp Neurol.* 1992; 51:235–45.

16. Odom L, Wilson H, Jamieson B, et al. Significance of blasts in low cell count cerebrospinal fluid specimens from children with acute lymphoblastic leukemia. *Cancer.* 1990; 66:1748–54.

17. Homans AC, Barker BE, Forman EN, Cornell CJ Jr, Dickerman JD, Truman JT. Immunophenotypic characteristics of cerebrospinal fluid cells in children with acute lymphoblastic leukemia at diagnosis. *Blood.* 1990; 76:1807–11.

18. Shmerling RH, Delbanco TL, Tosteson A, Trentham D. Synovial fluid tests: What should be ordered? *JAMA.* 1990; 264:1009–14.

19. Freemont AJ, Denton J, Chuck A, Holt PJ, Davies M. Diagnostic value of synovial fluid microscopy: A reassessment and rationalisation. *Ann Rheum Dis.* 1991; 50:101–7.

20. Li CY, Yam LT. Blast transformation in chronic myeloid leukemia with synovial involvement. *Acta Cytol.* 1991; 35:543–45.

21. Judkins S, Cornbleet PJ. Synovial fluid crystal analysis. *Lab Med.* 1997; 28:774–79.

SECTION NINE • HEMOSTASIS

34

Primary Hemostasis

Linda Larson, M.S.

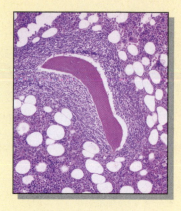

■ CHECKLIST - LEVEL I

At the end of this unit of study the student should be able to:

1. Define *hemostasis, blood coagulation,* and *thrombosis.*
2. Explain the general interaction of the systems involved in maintaining hemostasis.
3. Distinguish the events that occur in primary hemostasis from those that occur in secondary hemostasis.
4. Differentiate the primary hemostatic plug from the secondary hemostatic plug.
5. Name the three types of blood vessels and explain the general role of the vasculature and of normal endothelial cells in aiding and preventing activation of the hemostatic system.
6. Describe the normal morphology and number of platelets on a peripheral blood smear and state the normal concentration in the blood.
7. Name and describe the cell that is the precursor of platelets in the bone marrow.
8. Identify and define the steps in the normal sequence of events of platelet activation following injury to the endothelium.
9. Describe the role of the primary hemostatic plug in the cessation of bleeding.

■ CHECKLIST - LEVEL II

At the end of this unit of study the student should be able to:

1. Identify key histologic features of each type of blood vessel and explain the metabolic functions of endothelial cells in hemostasis.
2. Describe the development of megakaryocytes and platelets in the bone marrow to include the action of humoral factors, the stem cells and progenitor cell compartment, the recognizable features of the morphologic stages, and the mechanism of release from the marrow to peripheral blood.
3. Define *endomitosis* and *polyploidy.*
4. Identify three key substances that are stored in the platelet dense bodies and five key substances stored in the platelet alpha granules and explain the role of each in hemostasis.
5. Outline steps the platelets undergo in forming the primary hemostatic plug, including the biochemical mediators necessary for platelet adhesion, platelet aggregation, and platelet secretion.
6. Correlate various platelet functions with platelet ultrastructure features responsible for them.
7. Identify platelet agonists and predict their effect on platelet function.
8. Describe the biochemical roles of the secreted contents of the platelet granules in hemostasis.

■ **CHECKLIST - LEVEL II** *(continued)*

9. Correlate activation with changes in the platelet ultrastructure and biochemistry.

10. Describe the roles of the platelet in secondary hemostasis.

11. State the life span of platelets in the peripheral blood.

KEY TERMS

Agonist
Alpha granules
Arachidonic acid (AA)
Clot retraction
Demarcation membrane system (DMS)
Dense bodies
Dense tubular system (DTS)
Endomitosis
Glycocalyx
Glycoprotein Ib (GPIb)
Glycoprotein IIb/IIIa (GPIIb/IIIa)
Hemostasis
Open canalicular system (OCS)
Platelet activation
Platelet adhesion
Platelet aggregation
Platelet procoagulant activity
Platelet secretion
Polyploidy
Primary hemostatic plug
Secondary hemostatic plug
Thrombogenic/nonthrombogenic
Thrombopoietin (TPO)
Thrombosis

The information in this chapter will build on the concepts learned in previous chapters. To maximize your learning experience you should review these concepts before starting this unit of study.

Level I

▶ Hematopoiesis: Describe the bone marrow production of blood cells. (Chapters 2, 3)

Level II

▶ Stem cells and growth factors: Summarize the hierarchy of stem and progenitor cells in the bone marrow and the growth factors that direct the proliferation and maturation of blood cells. (Chapter 2)

▶ Adhesion molecules: Describe the general biology of integrins and other adhesion molecules. (Chapter 6)

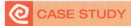
CASE STUDY

We will refer to this case study throughout the chapter.
John, a 20-year-old male, has acute lymphocytic leukemia (ALL). He is receiving chemotherapy. Two weeks after his second treatment he noted small reddish-purple spots on his lower legs and ankles. A CBC revealed: Hb 9 g/dL; WBC 2 × 10⁹/L; platelets 19 × 10⁹/L. Consider what may be responsible for the pancytopenia and the potential consequences of this condition.

▶ OVERVIEW

This chapter is the first of a section in this text that describes the processes involved when blood clots in response to an injury. Actions of the blood vessels and platelets in hemostasis are collectively called primary hemostasis, while actions of the protein coagulation factors are called secondary hemostasis. This chapter discusses primary hemostasis. The physical structure and functions of the blood vessels in hemostasis are described first. Platelets are discussed next under the major topics of production, structure, and functions.

▶ INTRODUCTION

Blood normally circulates within a closed system of vessels. A traumatic injury, such as a cut to the finger, severs blood vessels and results in bleeding. To minimize blood loss, normally inert platelets and dissolved proteins in the plasma mobilize to form an insoluble mass, or structural barrier, that occludes the injured vessels. The barrier is limited to the injury site so that normal circulation is maintained in vessels elsewhere in the body. In other words, the hemostatic system is activated when it is needed and where it is needed. The same elements provide a continuous surveillance system that prevents leakage of plasma and cells into the tissues in normal circumstances.

The process of forming the barrier to blood loss and limiting it to the injured site is **hemostasis**. Hemostasis is from the Greek words *heme,* meaning blood, and *stasis,* meaning to halt. The barrier mass is known as the hemostatic plug, blood clot, or thrombus. It is formed by the process of blood coagulation.

Hemostasis occurs in stages called primary hemostasis, secondary hemostasis, and fibrinolysis. During primary hemostasis, the platelets interact with the injured vessels and with each other. This interaction results in a clump of platelets that is known as the **primary hemostatic plug.** The primary hemostatic plug temporarily arrests bleeding, but it is fragile and easily dislodged from the vessel wall.

Subsequently, insoluble strands of fibrin become deposited on the primary platelet plug to reinforce and stabilize it and to allow healing of the wound without further blood loss. Generation of fibrin constitutes the stage of secondary hemostasis. Fibrin is formed by a series of complex biochemical reactions from soluble plasma proteins (coagulation factors) as they associate with the injured blood vessels and with the platelet plug (∞ Chapter 35). The plug, or clot, is then called the **secondary hemostatic plug** (Figure 34-1 ■). The blood has changed from a liquid to a solid at the site of injury.

✪ TABLE 34-1
Components of Hemostasis
Vasculature
Platelets
Proteins
• Fibrin-forming proteins
• Fibrinolytic proteins
• Inhibitors

After the wound has healed, additional components of the hemostatic system break down and remove the clot in the fibrinolysis stage. All of the phases and components of the hemostatic system are controlled by physiologic and biochemical inhibitors.

Injury also can occur to intact, unsevered blood vessels. In this case, blood clot formation occurs on an interior surface of the damaged vessel wall and results in an abnormal condition called **thrombosis.**

In summary, hemostasis occurs because of the interaction of the blood vessels, the platelets, and certain plasma proteins (Table 34-1 ✪). Proteins of hemostasis include those that form fibrin, those that are involved with fibrinolysis, and those that inhibit all stages of the process. This chapter will focus on primary hemostasis. The structure and functions of the blood vessels (vascular system or vasculature) and the platelets as they form the primary hemostatic plug will be described. Secondary hemostasis (fibrin formation) and fibrinolysis will be described in Chapter 35. Disorders of hemostasis that result in bleeding symptoms will be discussed in Chapters 36 and 37, and disorders that result in thrombosis symptoms will be discussed in Chapter 38.

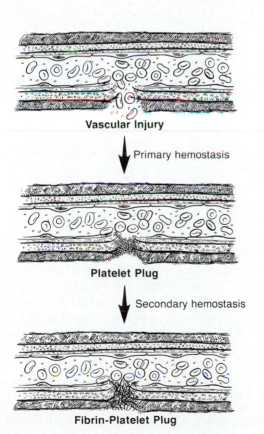

Vascular Injury

↓ Primary hemostasis

Platelet Plug

↓ Secondary hemostasis

Fibrin-Platelet Plug

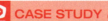

CASE STUDY *(continued from page 654)*

1. Does John have a defect in primary or secondary hemostasis?

■ **FIGURE 34-1** Stages of hemostasis after vascular injury. Bleeding occurs after an injury to a blood vessel. The hemostatic system is activated to prevent excessive blood loss. Hemostasis occurs in two stages: (1) during primary hemostasis the platelets aggregate at the site of the injury and form the platelet plug (primary hemostatic plug); (2) during secondary hemostasis fibrin develops to strengthen the platelet plug forming the fibrin-platelet plug (secondary hemostatic plug).

► **ROLE OF THE VASCULAR SYSTEM**

The vascular system consists of three types of blood vessels: arteries, veins, and capillaries (Table 34-2 ✪). The arteries carry blood from the heart to the capillaries. The veins return blood from the capillaries to the heart. The vessels in which hemostasis occurs are primarily the smallest veins (*venules*) and, to a lesser degree, the smallest arteries (*arterioles*). Venules and arterioles are 20–200 μm in diameter.

✪ TABLE 34-2

Structure and Functions of Blood Vessels of the Microcirculation

Blood Vessel	Structural Characteristics	Functions
Arterioles	20–200 μm in diameter Basement membrane Primary component is smooth muscle Fibroblasts Thicker wall of collagen and extracellular matrix	Site of hemostatic activity following injury Regulate blood pressure by change in diameter Endothelial cell hemostatic functions
Venules	20–200 μm diameter Basement membrane Few smooth muscle cells Few fibroblasts Primary component is thin layer of collagen and extracellular matrix No elastic fibers	Major site of hemostatic activity following traumatic injury Exchange nutrients, oxygen, and waste products Regulate vascular permeability Endothelial cell hemostatic functions
Capillaries	5–10 μm diameter Single endothelial cell lumen Basement membrane No smooth muscle cells No collagen fibers No elastic fibers	No hemostatic function except those of endothelial cells Exchange nutrients, oxygen, and waste products

STRUCTURE OF BLOOD VESSELS

The structure of all blood vessels is similar (Figure 34-2 ■). It consists of a central cavity, the lumen, through which the blood flows. The lumen is lined with a continuous, single layer of flattened cells called endothelial cells. Endothelial cells separate the blood from the underlying tissues. They provide a protective environment for the cellular elements of the plasma. Overlapping portions of their cytoplasm interconnect the individual endothelial cells.

The luminal surface of the endothelial cells (surface on the inside of the vessel) has a thin coating of complex protein and carbohydrate substances (mucopolysaccharides) called the **glycocalyx**. The abluminal surface (the surface on the tissue side) is attached to a basement membrane that consists of a unique form of collagen, type IV, embedded in a matrix of adhesive proteins.

Three layers of tissue in the vessel wall vary in thickness and composition depending on the size and type of vessel. Histologically on cross section, the layers of the walls of veins and arteries appear distinct (Figure 34-2a ■). The innermost layer, tunica intima, consists of the endothelial cell monolayer, the basement membrane, subendothelial connective tissue that holds them together, and in arteries, an organized internal elastic membrane.

The middle layer, tunica media, is thicker in arteries than in veins. In arteries, smooth muscle cells predominate and are surrounded by loose connective tissue primarily consisting of elastin fibers, collagen fibers, reticular fibers, and proteoglycans. The tunica media of veins contains only a few smooth muscle cells, less elastin fibers, and a similar matrix

of connective tissue. In response to a variety of physiologic stimuli, the smooth muscle cells of the tunica media contract and expand, which constricts or dilates the lumen.

The tunica adventitia, the outer coat, is thicker in veins than in arteries. In this layer there are a few fibroblasts embedded in the collagen and other connective tissues. The fibroblasts synthesize and secrete the fibers and other components of the matrix. Mast cells are present in some layers of veins (∞ Chapter 6).

The third type of blood vessel, the capillary (Figure 34–2b ■), connects the arterioles and venules. Capillaries collectively compose, by far, the largest surface area of all types of blood vessels, although they are individually the smallest. They are approximately 5–10 μm in diameter, just large enough for single blood cells to traverse. Single endothelial cells form the lumen of a capillary with their cytoplasm wrapped around in circular form. Tissue beneath the basement membrane of a capillary is sparse and contains no smooth muscle cells.

FUNCTIONS OF BLOOD VESSELS

After injury, the damaged vessels initiate hemostasis. The first response of the vessels to the injury is constriction or narrowing of the lumen of the arterioles to minimize the flow of blood to the wounded area and the escape of blood from the wound site. Vasoconstriction occurs immediately and lasts a short time.

The mechanism of vasoconstriction is complex. It is caused in part by neurogenic factors and in part by several regulatory substances that interact with receptors on the sur-

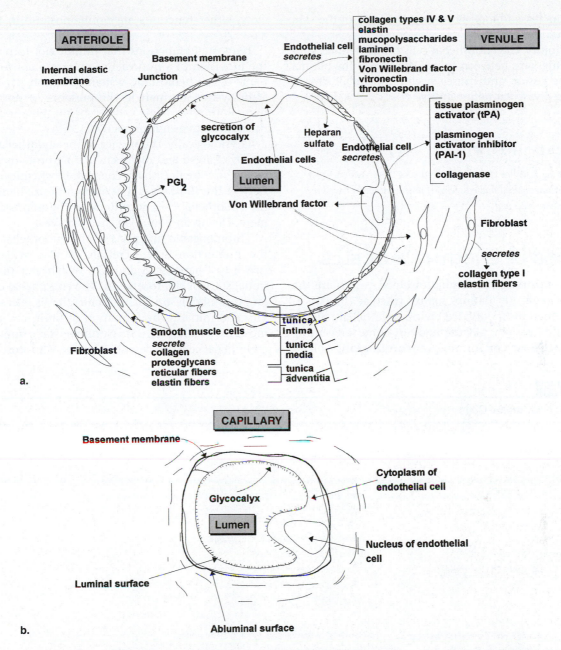

ARTERIOLE

Internal elastic membrane

Basement membrane

Junction

Endothelial cell *secretes*

collagen types IV & V
elastin
mucopolysaccharides
laminen
fibronectin
Von Willebrand factor
vitronectin
thrombospondin

VENULE

secretion of glycocalyx

Heparan sulfate

Endothelial cell *secretes*

tissue plasminogen activator (tPA)

plasminogen activator inhibitor (PAI-1)

collagenase

Endothelial cells

PGI_2

Lumen

Von Willebrand factor

Fibroblast

secretes

collagen type I
elastin fibers

Fibroblast

Smooth muscle cells
secrete
collagen
proteoglycans
reticular fibers
elastin fibers

tunica intima
tunica media
tunica adventitia

a.

CAPILLARY

Basement membrane

Glycocalyx

Lumen

Cytoplasm of endothelial cell

Nucleus of endothelial cell

Luminal surface

Abluminal surface

b.

■ **FIGURE 34-2** Structure and function of the blood vessel wall, comparing and contrasting arterioles, venules, and capillaries. a. Arterioles and venules. Endothelial cells, smooth muscle cells, and fibroblasts synthesize and secrete the components of the subendothelial matrix of connective tissue and the basement membrane proteins. The wall of arterioles is primarily smooth muscle cells and contains elastin in contrast to the venule, which has only sparse smooth muscle cells. The media of arterioles is the most prominent layer, while the adventitia layer is the largest in venules. b. A capillary consists primarily of endothelial cells and basement membrane with very little connective tissue.

face of cells of the blood vessel wall. The regulating substances include serotonin and thromboxane A_2 (both products of platelet activation) and endothelin-1 (which is produced by damaged endothelial cells). These substances may aid in prolonging vasoconstriction.[1]

In contrast, the endothelial cells synthesize and secrete a prostaglandin, PGI_2, also called prostacyclin. PGI_2 counteracts constriction by causing vasodilation of the arterioles.[2] Vasodilation increases the blood flow to the injured area to bring fresh supplies of blood clotting substances in the plasma. The increased blood flow causes redness of the skin at the wound site.

Also after injury, the endothelial cells of the venules contract, producing gaps between them. Fluid from the plasma leaks into the tissues and causes swelling (edema). This is called increased vascular permeability.

✓ **Checkpoint! #1**

Think about the last time that you injured your finger with a paper cut. Did your finger bleed immediately? If not, what might have prevented immediate bleeding?

FUNCTIONS OF ENDOTHELIAL CELLS

Endothelial cells lining the lumina of blood vessels are the principle elements regulating many vascular functions. Some of the functions modulated by the endothelial cells are hemostatic and, as such, aid the body in either preventing (**nonthrombogenic**) or forming (**thrombogenic**) blood clots. Other functions are nonhemostatic in nature (Table 34-3 ✪).

Hemostatic functions that inhibit clot formation include the provision of a nonreactive environment for the components of the hemostatic system. Components of the hemostatic system are inert in the presence of normal endothelium. Both physiologic and biochemical interactions provide the nonreactive environment.[3]

Physiologically, the surface of the endothelial cells is negatively charged and repels circulating proteins and platelets, which also are negatively charged. Biochemically, a wide variety of the substances that are synthesized and secreted by the endothelial cells contribute to the nonreactive environment. Details are found on the Web site.

Thrombogenic functions of the endothelial cells include the production and secretion of von Willebrand factor (vWF) (∞ Chapters 35 and 37), which aids platelets in the initial stage of clot formation. The endothelial cells also contain thromboplastin (tissue factor) that is released during injury and initiates the formation of fibrin for secondary hemostasis (∞ Chapter 35). Nonhemostatic functions of the endothelial cells are described on the Web site.

TABLE 34-3

Functions of Endothelial Cells

Function	Consequence
Hemostatic functions	
Nonthrombogenic	
Negatively charged surface	Repels platelets and hemostatic proteins
Heparan sulfate	Inhibits fibrin formation
Thrombomodulin	Inhibits fibrin formation
PGI$_2$ (Prostacyclin)	Vasodilation; inhibits platelet aggregation
Tissue plasminogen activator (tPA)	Activates fibrinolytic system
Plasminogen activator inhibitor (PAI-1)	Inhibits activation of fibrinolytic system
Endothelin	Vasoconstriction
Nitric oxide	Vasodilation
Thrombogenic	
Produce and process von Willebrand factor	Carrier of factor VIII in plasma; platelet adhesion
Tissue thromboplastin	Initiates fibrin formation
Nonhemostatic functions	
Selective blood/tissue barrier	Keeps cells and macromolecules in vessels; allows nutrient and gas exchange
Process blood-borne antigens	Cellular immunity
Synthesize and secrete connective tissue:	
Basement membrane collagen	Backup protection for endothelial cells
Collagen of the matrix	Platelet adhesion
Elastin	Vasodilation and vasoconstriction
Fibronectin	Bind cells to one another
Laminin	Platelet adhesion after injury
Vitronectin	Bind cells to one another; ? Platelet adhesion
Thrombospondin	Bind cells to one another; ? Platelet adhesion

(Key: ? = possibly)

When endothelial injury occurs and bleeding starts, platelets and coagulation proteins in the plasma physically contact subendothelial tissues. Interactions then occur among the vessel wall, platelets, and hemostatic proteins in the plasma so that a blood clot forms to stop the bleeding.

The amount of blood lost from a vessel depends on its size and type as well as on the efficiency of the hemostatic mechanism. Hemostasis is most effective in arterioles and venules. Capillaries lack a vessel wall and are not contributors to hemostasis. When larger vessels are severed, hemostatic plug formation takes longer and may not be sufficient to stop bleeding. The pressure is much higher in arteries, and the flow may be so rapid that clots cannot form.

✓ **Checkpoint! #2**

What actions of the endothelial cells prevent clotting from occurring within the blood vessels?

▶ **PLATELETS IN HEMOSTASIS**

The second major component of the hemostatic system is the blood platelets. The role of platelets in hemostasis was first established by Bizzozero in 1882.[4] He noted that they were clumped together as part of thrombi in the mesenteric vessels of rabbits and guinea pigs.

Platelets are seen on a Romanowsky-stained peripheral blood smear as small, anuclear cells with prominent reddish purple granules (Figure 34-3). They circulate as discoid-shaped structures, approximately 2–3 μm in diameter. The normal concentration of platelets in the blood is 150–440 × 10^9/L. ∞ Chapter 7 describes methods of counting platelets.

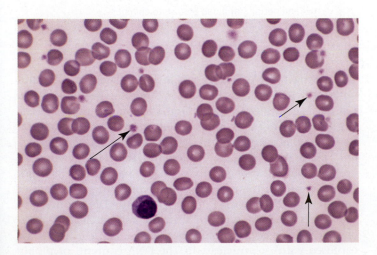

■ **FIGURE 34-3** Peripheral blood smear. The arrows point to platelets. (Wright-Giemsa stain; 1000 × magnification)

The following sections of this chapter will discuss the production of platelets in the bone marrow, their ultrastructure, and their various roles in hemostasis.

PLATELET PRODUCTION

Platelets are produced in the bone marrow from the same progenitor cell as the erythroid and myeloid series (CFU-GEMM) (Figure 34-4 ■). The platelet precursor cell is a megakaryocyte. Platelets are fragments of the cytoplasm of megakaryocytes. The cells of the megakaryocyte lineage include actively proliferating progenitor cells as well as postmitotic megakaryocytes undergoing maturational development.

Megakaryocyte Progenitor Cell Compartment

Megakaryocyte progenitor cells are responsible for the expansion of megakaryocyte numbers and proliferate in response to a number of mitotic cytokines. The CFU-GEMM differentiates into a committed megakaryocyte progenitor cell (∞ Chapter 2). Using cell culture techniques to grow human adult bone marrow progenitor cells, researchers have defined a hierarchy of megakaryocyte progenitor cells that develops through stages identified as BFU-Mk and CFU-Mk. Surface antigens and growth characteristics differentiate the two stages. The BFU-Mk is CD34$^+$, HLA-DR$^-$, c-kit$^+$ while the CFU-Mk is positive for all three antigens. In culture, BFU-Mk produce multifocal colonies (bursts) of 100–500 megakaryocytes, while the CFU-Mk produce single colonies of 4–32 megakaryocytes. A progenitor cell that is more primitive than the BFU-Mk has been grown in cultures of fetal bone marrow and is called the high proliferative potential cell-megakaryocyte (HPPC-Mk).[5] Morphologically, progenitor cells appear as small indistinguishable lymphoid-like cells.[6]

Regulation of Platelet Production

A regulatory process maintains an adequate concentration of platelets in the peripheral blood. Production of platelets by the bone marrow can be increased or decreased according to need. The stimulus for production is the platelet mass in circulating blood plus the megakaryocyte mass in the bone marrow.[7]

Cytokines and growth factors, such as interleukin-3 (IL-3), GM-CSF, and stem cell factor, influence the progenitor stages of megakaryocytes to proliferate, similar to their action on other myeloid cell lines.[7,8] Interleukins-6 and -11 also affect megakaryocyte development, particularly the maturation phases, but only when they work in synergy with each other and with other cytokines.[9]

The major humoral factor regulating platelet development is **thrombopoietin** (TPO). TPO influences all stages of megakaryocyte production from the HPPC-Mk level to the release of mature platelets from the bone marrow.[10,11] Megakaryocytes grown in culture undergo apoptosis in the absence of TPO.[12]

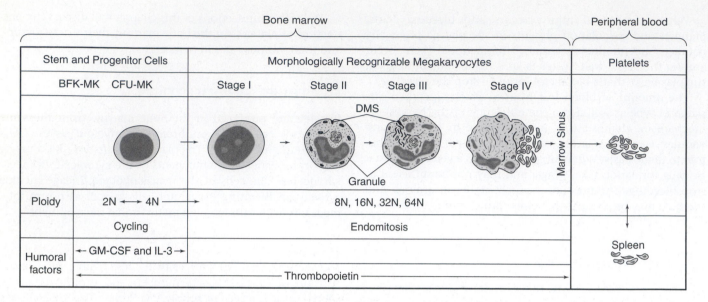

■ **FIGURE 34-4** Production of platelets. Progenitor cells become committed to the megakaryocyte lineage. Committed progenitor stages are BFU-Mk and CFU-Mk. Megakaryoblasts undergo a series of endomitoses until nuclear maturation is complete at 8N to 64N ploidy levels. Cytoplasmic maturation occurs at ploidy levels of 8N or higher. Morphologic features of each stage of cytoplasmic maturation are described in the text. Growth factors GM-CSF and IL-3 influence proliferation of the stem and progenitor cells. Thrombopoietin influences all stages of megakaryocyte production. Platelets are first released through the endothelial cells of the marrow sinuses as proplatelets. Proplatelets break into mature platelets and are released into the peripheral blood.

The presence of TPO had been suspected since the 1950s. It was not until 1994, however, that several research groups first isolated it. The gene for TPO was cloned shortly after its discovery. By 1997, TPO was made by recombinant DNA techniques, and its effects have been studied in vitro and in clinical trials to treat patients with certain platelet disorders. TPO is produced in the liver, the kidney, and the spleen, and possibly in the bone marrow in patients who have low platelet counts.[7,10] Thrombopoietin is structurally related to the erythrocyte growth factor, erythropoietin.[7]

TPO maintains a constant number of platelets in the peripheral blood by binding to its receptor, Mpl (CD110), on circulating platelets and bone marrow megakaryocytes and progenitors.[7] More information on the Mpl receptor can be found at *<www.ncbi.nlm.nih.gov/prow/guide/11586825_g.htm>*. Bound TPO is not available to stimulate proliferation of bone marrow progenitor cells. Therefore, the higher the peripheral platelet count, the more TPO is bound and stimulation of bone marrow production is reduced. When the platelet count decreases, more TPO is free to bind to megakaryocyte progenitor cells in the bone marrow.[10] TPO appears to work both independently and in synergy with the other growth factors mentioned above. The effects of TPO in patients with low numbers of platelets are to increase the number of megakaryocytes in the bone marrow, increase the size and DNA content (ploidy level) of megakaryocytes, and increase the rate of maturation of the megakaryocytes.[11] The number of circulating platelets can be increased from 3 to 10 times by administration of TPO.[10]

✓ **Checkpoint! #3**

What would be the effect on the platelet count if a patient had a mutation in the gene for thrombopoietin that resulted in inability of the gene to code for functional mRNA?

CASE STUDY *(continued from page 655)*

2. If John were given TPO, how would you expect his bone marrow and peripheral blood picture to change?

Stages of Megakaryocyte Development

When progenitor cell receptors are stimulated by TPO and other growth factors, megakaryocyte differentiation results. The blast cell undergoes a maturation sequence that is different from that of other marrow cells in that nuclear maturation takes place first and is largely complete before cytoplasmic maturation begins. Following an initial series of proliferative (mitotic) cell divisions, the precursor cells begin a unique nuclear maturation process consisting of a series of endomitoses. With each **endomitosis,** the DNA content of the cell is doubled but cell division and nuclear division does not take place.[9] The cells become **polyploid** (not to be confused with polynucleated). The DNA content, or ploidy level of the cells (normally 2N) may range from 4N to 64N (within the same nuclear envelope) or potentially larger. The

8N stage is the first recognizable stage on a bone marrow smear because it is at this stage that megakaryocytes begin to be significantly larger than other cells in the bone marrow. The 16N stage is the most common ploidy class in adult humans.

Cytoplasmic maturation may begin at nuclear ploidy levels of 8N or greater, but the stage at which maturation occurs varies from cell to cell. In general, nuclear maturation ceases when cytoplasmic maturation begins. The reason for variability in cytoplasmic maturation at different ploidy levels is not known. Clinical conditions associated with the presence of large platelets on the peripheral blood smear are noted to have more megakaryocytes with lower ploidy (shifted left). Increased ploidy of the nucleus of an individual megakaryocyte might result in more cytoplasm and, thus, more platelets from that megakaryocyte.

Four arbitrary stages of megakaryocyte development are described according to their morphologic appearance on Romanowsky-stained bone marrow smears. Differentiating characteristics defining these stages are the nuclear morphology, cytoplasmic appearance, and relative size of the cell as determined by the ploidy class. The four stages are described in Table 34-4 ✪. Figure 34-5 ■ shows an early megakaryocyte and a mature megakaryocyte. In general, as the megakary-

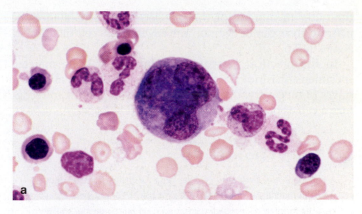
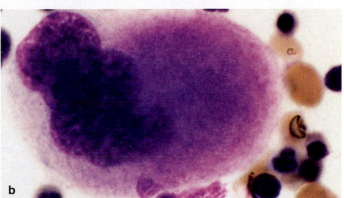

■ **FIGURE 34-5 a.** Early megakaryocyte. **b.** Mature megakaryocyte. (Bone marrow; Wright-Giemsa stain; 1000× magnification)

ocyte matures, the cytoplasm changes from blue, nongranular, and scant in the blast stage to completely granular, with a pinkish hue in the mature stage. The nucleus changes from a single lobe with fine chromatin and visible nucleoli to lobulated with coarse chromatin and no visible nucleoli. Comparing the photographs of the two megakaryocytes, the volume of cytoplasm in a maturing megakaryocyte increases from the early stage to the final stage. The early stage may have a few granules in the cytoplasm, but the cytoplasm of the mature cell appears completely filled with azurophilic granules. The granules first appear in the Golgi region and eventually spread throughout the cytoplasm.

In addition to granules, the cytoplasm of a maturing megakaryocyte develops an internal membrane called the **demarcation membrane system (DMS).** The demarcation membrane is not visible in the light microscope and is first seen in electron micrographs at the promegakaryocyte stage. The origin of this membrane is unknown, but it is speculated that it is derived by invagination of the original outer membrane of the megakaryocyte since the receptors in the two membranes are identical. Alternatively, the Golgi may synthesize it. As the DMS forms, small areas of the megakaryocyte cytoplasm are separated. These areas will eventually become the platelets, and the DMS will become

✪ TABLE 34-4

Developmental Stages of Megakaryocytes

	Name	Characteristics
Stage I	Megakaryoblast	6–24 μm diameter Scant basophilic cytoplasm No visible granules Round nucleus Visible nucleoli
Stage II	Promegakaryocyte	14–30 μm diameter More cytoplasm, primarily blue Few visible cytoplasmic granules Nucleus lobulated or indented Beginning demarcation membrane with electron microscopy
Stage III	Granular megakaryocyte	16–56 μm diameter More cytoplasmic granules Abundant cytoplasm, beginning pink color Multilobulated nucleus No visible nucleoli

Stage IV	Mature megakarocyte	20–60 μm diameter
		Abundant pinkish, very granular
		    cytoplasm
		Demarcation zones indistinctly
		    present
		Multilobulated nucleus
		No visible nucleoli

the outer membrane of the platelets.[8] The separated cytoplasmic areas can be seen on the edges of the cell pictured in Figure 34-5b ■.

In the practical day-to-day evaluation of bone marrow specimens, it is not necessary to distinguish the maturation stages of megakaryocytes. It is, however, important to recognize a cell as being of the megakaryocyte lineage.

 Checkpoint! #4

If a patient has a mutation in the gene for thrombopoietin that resulted in inability of the gene to code for mRNA, how would you expect the number of megakaryocytes seen on bone marrow smears to be affected?

Release of Platelets

The primary site of megakaryocyte development and platelet production is in the bone marrow. Mature megakaryocytes, situated less than 1 μm from a bone marrow sinus, shed platelets directly into the sinuses. Platelets appear to be released from megakaryocytes in groups called proplatelets, which are protrusions of megakaryocyte cytoplasm or pseudopods. Seven to eight proplatelets from each megakaryocyte are extruded through the cytoplasm of endothelial cells and into the marrow sinuses. It is thought that the proplatelets then break up into individual platelets. Alternatively, the megakaryocyte cytoplasm could randomly break up into platelets within the marrow space. The nucleus of the megakaryocyte remains in the marrow and is thought to degenerate and to be removed by the macrophage system.

Whole intact megakaryocytes are occasionally released from the marrow, circulate in the peripheral blood, and be-come trapped in capillary beds in the spleen and lungs. These cells also may release platelets to the peripheral blood.[13]

Approximately 5 days are required for a megakaryoblast to develop to the platelet-producing stage. Two-thirds of the platelets that are released into the peripheral blood circulate in the bloodstream. The other third is sequestered in the spleen and is in equilibrium with those platelets in the circulation. The average life span of platelets in the peripheral blood is approximately 9.5 days.

PLATELET STRUCTURE

Circulating inert platelets are disc-shaped cells with smooth surfaces. Unlike the exterior surfaces of erythrocytes and leukocytes, platelets have several openings resembling holes in a sponge. The openings are membranous channels that extend deep into the interior of the cells.

Circulating platelets repel one another and the surfaces of the endothelial cells that line the interior cavity of blood vessels. After an injury, many changes affecting the platelet morphology and biochemistry take place. The changes cause the platelets to become "activated," after which they interact to form the primary hemostatic plug. To understand the activation process, the normal platelet ultrastructure must be considered.

The platelet ultrastructure is divided into four arbitrary regions or zones: the peripheral zone, the structural zone, the organelle zone, and the membrane systems[11] (Figure 34-6 ■ and Table 34-5 ✪). The components of each region have specific functions in activated platelets and are discussed in the following sections.

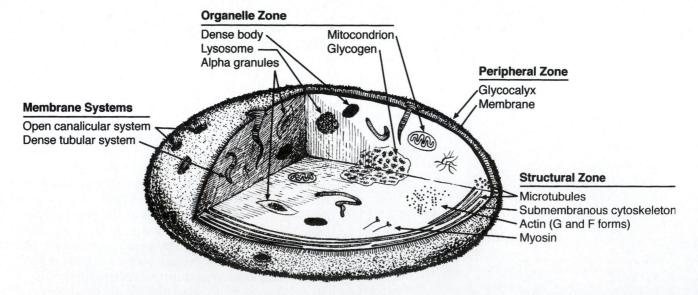

Organelle Zone
Dense body
Lysosome
Alpha granules
Mitocondrion
Glycogen

Peripheral Zone
Glycocalyx
Membrane

Membrane Systems
Open canalicular system
Dense tubular system

Structural Zone
Microtubules
Submembranous cytoskeleton
Actin (G and F forms)
Myosin

■ **FIGURE 34-6** Diagram of platelet ultrastructure. (Modified, with permission, from Thompson AR, Harker LA. *Manual of Hemostasis and Thrombosis*, 3rd ed. Philadelphia: F.A. Davis; 1982.)

⊛ TABLE 34-5

Platelet Ultrastructure and Functions

Zone and Component	Function
Peripheral zone	Adhesion and aggregation
Glycocalyx	
Proteins, glycoproteins, mucopolysaccharides	
Phospholipid bilayer	
Phospholipids	Asymmetric arrangement; Source of arachidonic acid
Integral proteins	
Glycoproteins Ib/IX, IIb/IIIa	Adhesion and aggregation
Enzymes	Activation
Structural zone	Structure and support
Microtubules	
Cytoskeletal network	
Actin	
Actin-binding protein	
Cytoplasmic meshwork	
Actin	
Myosin	
Organelle zone	Secretion and storage
Granules	
Dense bodies	Nonprotein mediators (ADP)
Alpha granules	Protein mediators
Lysosomes	Enzymes
Microperoxisomes	Unknown
Mitochondria	
Glycogen	
Membrane systems	Secretion and storage
Open canalicular system	Secretion of granule contents
Dense tubular system	Calcium storage site

Peripheral Zone

The peripheral zone of the platelet consists of a phospholipid membrane covered on the exterior by a fluffy surface coat and on the interior by a thin submembranous region between the cytoplasmic membrane and the next layer. Microfilaments are present in the submembranous region, the nature of which is described later.

The surface coat, or **glycocalyx,** is thicker on platelets than on other cells. It consists of several glycoproteins, proteins, and mucopolysaccharides that are probably adsorbed from the plasma, including coagulation factor V, von Willebrand factor, and fibrinogen (∞ Chapters 35 and 36). The glycocalyx also is found on the surface membrane of the interior channels. Some of the surface proteins are receptors for substances that cause **platelet activation.**

The cytoplasmic membrane has a typical trilaminar structure of a bilayer of phospholipid and embedded integral proteins. The membrane is the former demarcation membrane of the parent megakaryocyte. An asymmetric arrangement of the phospholipids is an important factor in the function of activated platelets. Phosphatidylcholine and sphingomyelin, which are neutral in charge, are concentrated on the outer half, while negatively charged phospholipids (phosphatidylserine, phosphatidylinositol, and phosphatidylethanolamine) predominate on the inner half of the bilayer.[1] The phospholipid asymmetry is maintained in resting platelets by an ATP-dependent amino phospholipid translocase that actively pumps phosphatidylethanolamine and phosphatidylserine from the outer to the inner leaflet.

The integral proteins are receptors for stimuli involved in platelet function. Approximately 30 have been identified as glycoproteins, and a nomenclature system has been developed. They may be abbreviated GP and are numbered with Roman numerals from I to IX according to electrophoretic migration by decreasing molecular weight. Glycoproteins Ib, IIb, and IIIa are most significantly associated with abnormal platelet function.

Glycoprotein Ib (GPIb) is a receptor for von Willebrand factor (Figure 34-7a ■). It is noncovalently associated with GPV and GPIX in the membrane. The function of GPV is not known, and no clinical bleeding problems are associated with its absence. Rare bleeding disorders are associated with abnormalities of GPIb and with GPIX. The complex will be referred to in this text as GPIb/IX.

Glycoprotein Ib has two chains, α and β. The GPIbα chain is larger and contains the binding sites for vWF, thrombin, ristocetin (used in the platelet aggregation test described in ∞ Chapter 39). The binding sites are located on the major portion of GPIb called glycocalicin. The glycocalicin portion extends from the surface of the platelet and can be removed by proteolytic enzymes. The remainder of GPIbα is associated with the GPIbβ chain and spans the phospholipid bilayer. On the cytoplasmic side both the α and the β portions are associated with actin-binding protein. Each platelet contains approximately 25,000 GPIb molecules.[14] GPIb/IX functions in the platelet adhesion process described later. GPIb/IX is recognized by monoclonal antibodies as CD42. The alpha chain is CD42b and the beta chain is CD42c.

Glycoproteins IIb and IIIa together form a complex (GPIIb/IIIa) and become the receptor for fibrinogen (Figure 34-7b ■). The **GPIIb/IIIa** complex also binds other circulating adhesive proteins such as von Willebrand factor, thrombospondin, vitronectin, and fibronectin. There are approximately 80,000 copies per platelet externally and another 30,000 copies on the internal membranes.[15]

Glycoprotein IIb, the larger of the two subunits, is a two-chain protein. The α chain is embedded in the phospholipid bilayer, and the β chain protrudes from the platelet surface. Part of the β chain is the HPA-3 (formerly Bak[a]) platelet alloantigen. Glycoprotein IIIa is a single chain polypeptide and is associated with the GPIIb portion that lies within the phospholipid bilayer. The small surface portion of GPIIIa contains the HPA-1 (formerly Pl[A1]) antigen. The cytoplasmic

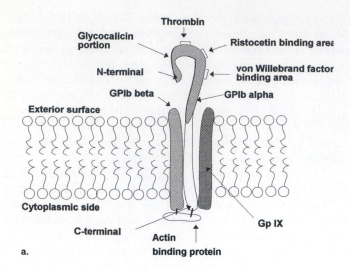

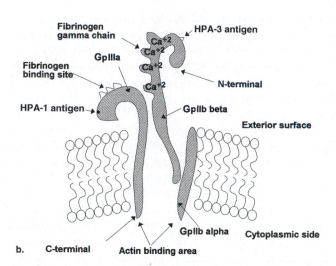

FIGURE 34-7 Structure of platelet membrane glycoproteins. **a.** Glycoprotein Ib is composed of an alpha and a beta chain. Both span the phospholipid bilayer. The alpha chain is larger and contains the binding sites for thrombin, ristocetin, and vWF. Actin-binding protein is attached to the cytoplasmic side. Glycoprotein IX associates with glycoprotein Ib. **b.** Glycoproteins IIb and IIIa associate in a complex after platelet activation. Binding sites for fibrinogen as well as platelet-specific antigens are present. Cytoplasmic portions of each component have binding areas for actin.

sides of the two proteins are associated with actin in the platelet cytoskeleton. The GPIIb/IIIa complex is a latent receptor "hidden" in resting platelets and "appears" (i.e., is induced to a state in which it can bind fibrinogen) when platelets are activated. It is required for platelet aggregation as described later. GPIIb/IIIa is an integrin of the $\alpha_{IIb}\beta_3$ type. Monoclonal antibodies recognize these proteins as CD41/CD61.

Arachidonic acid, an unsaturated fatty acid, is a major component of the phospholipid portion of the membrane. It is a precursor of very potent stimulators that cause platelet aggregation and vessel constriction. The region beneath the membrane consists of actin filaments similar to those in the structural layer described next.

✔ Checkpoint! #5

If a patient inherited a mutation of the gene for glycoprotein IIIa that resulted in its absence, what two platelet antigens would be decreased or absent?

Structural Zone

The structural zone consists of *microtubules* and a network of proteins. The functions of the structural zone are to support the plasma membrane, maintain the resting discoid shape of the platelet, and provide a means of change in shape when the platelet is activated.

Microtubules are composed of the protein tubulin. They are a bundle of from 8 to 24 tubules, which are located beneath the submembranous region of microfilaments and completely surround the circumference of the platelet.

The protein network consists of actin, actin-binding protein, and several other structural proteins, and it forms a cytoskeleton that supports the plasma membrane (Web Figure 34-1 ■). Actin is the most abundant protein in platelets, accounting for 15–20% of the total protein. It has two forms, G (globular) and F (filamentous). The F form consists of several polymerized G molecules. Approximately 30–40% of the actin in a resting platelet is in the F form, with the remainder in the G form. Actin-binding protein is attached to the cytoplasmic side of the GPIb/IX complex and anchors actin to the membrane.[13]

Actin also is part of a network of structural support throughout the cytoplasm. In the cytoplasm it is associated with myosin, along with several other contractile proteins similar to those of smooth muscle. Unlike smooth muscle, in which the ratio of actin to myosin is about 7:1, the platelet ratio is 100:1. This network also supports the resting discoid shape. Significant changes in actin structure and location occur when platelets become activated.

Organelle Zone

The organelle zone is beneath the microtubule layer and consists of mitochondria, glycogen particles (which support the platelet's metabolic activities), and four types of granules dispersed within the cytoplasm. The granules are *dense bodies, alpha granules, lysosomal granules,* and *microperoxisomes.* The granules serve as storage sites for proteins and other substances essential for platelet function. Generally, mature platelets do not have ribosomes or rough endoplasmic reticulum.

The **dense bodies** are so named because they appear more dense in electron microscope preparations than the

✪ TABLE 34-6

Composition and Functions of Platelet Dense Body Contents

Component	Function
ADP (nonmetabolic)	Agonist for platelets
ATP (nonmetabolic)	Agonist for cells other than platelets
Other nucleotides	Unknown
Inorganic phosphates	Unknown
Calcium	Source of adequate extracellular calcium
Serotonin	Vasoconstriction; platelet agonist

✪ TABLE 34-7

Composition and Functions of Platelet Alpha Granule Proteins

Protein	Functions
Group I—hemostatic proteins	
Fibrinogen	Platelet aggregation
	Conversion to fibrin
Factor V	Fibrin formation
von Willebrand factor	Platelet adhesion
	Carries factor VIII for fibrin formation
Plasminogen	Converted to plasmin that lyses fibrin
Plasminogen activator inhibitor	
(PAI-1)	Inhibits activation of fibrinolysis
α_2-antiplasmin	Inhibits plasmin
Group II—nonhemostatic proteins	
Platelet-specific	
β-thromboglobulin	Chemotactic for neutrophils
	Inactivates heparin
Platelet factor 4	Inactivates heparin
Platelet-derived growth factor (PDGF)	Promotes regrowth of smooth muscle cells
Not platelet-specific	
Albumin	Unknown
Thrombospondin	Interacts with several adhesive proteins and stabilizes platelet aggregates
Fibronectin	Unknown but may help bind platelets to various proteins at the wound site

other types of granules. These bodies contain mediators of platelet function and hemostasis that are not proteins: ADP, ATP, and other nucleotides as well as phosphate compounds, calcium ions, and serotonin (Table 34-6 ✪). The ADP in the dense bodies is known as the nonmetabolic, or storage, pool of ADP to distinguish it from metabolic ADP found in the cytoplasm. The metabolic pool provides energy for normal platelet metabolism, whereas the storage pool is important in the platelet aggregation reactions.

Alpha granules are the most numerous of the four types of granules. Alpha granules contain two major groups of proteins (Table 34-7 ✪). One group consists of proteins that are similar to hemostatic proteins found in the plasma. Some, such as von Willebrand factor and factor V, are synthesized in the megakaryocyte as the platelets develop.[16] Others, such as fibrinogen, immunoglobulins, and albumin, are absorbed from the plasma by megakaryocytes and packaged in the alpha granules during thrombopoiesis.[9] The second group includes proteins with a variety of functions. Some are found exclusively in platelets (e.g., platelet factor 4 and β-thromboglobulin). Some proteins are growth factors that affect the growth and gene expression of smooth muscle cells in the blood vessel wall (e.g., platelet derived growth factor). Plasminogen activator inhibitor is present in platelet alpha granules in addition to being synthesized by endothelial cells. Platelet alpha granules also contain a number of adhesive proteins including fibronectin, vWf, vitronectin, and thrombospondin.

Lysosomal granules contain several hydrolytic enzymes and are similar to the lysosomes found in other cells. The function of the microperoxisomes is unknown.

Platelets contain all the necessary enzymes for the glycolytic and tricarboxylic acid cycles and for glycogen synthesis and degradation. About 50% of the platelet's energy (ATP) is derived from the glycolytic pathway and about 50% is derived from the tricarboxylic acid cycle.

Membrane Systems

The fourth structural zone of the platelet is a system of membranes. One type of membrane, the surface-connected **open canalicular system (OCS),** is the membrane that surrounds the twisted channels leading from the platelet surface to the interior of the platelet. This membrane is derived from the demarcation membrane system of the parent megakaryocyte and functions in platelet storage and secretion.

A second type of membrane is the **dense tubular system (DTS),** which originates from the smooth endoplasmic reticulum of the megakaryocyte. It is one of the storage sites for calcium ions within platelets. The channels of the DTS do not connect with the surface of the platelet.

The two membrane systems, OCS and DTS, fuse in various areas of the platelet cytoplasm to form membrane complexes that appear to be important regulators of the intracellular calcium concentration. The concentration of calcium ions within the platelet cytoplasm is important in regulating platelet metabolism and activation.

PLATELET FUNCTION

Platelet Roles in Hemostasis

Platelets are involved in several aspects of hemostasis (Table 34-8 ✪). One role appears to be that of passive surveillance of the blood vessel endothelial lining for gaps and breaks. Although the exact nature of this role is somewhat controversial, it has been shown that platelets maintain the

⊙ TABLE 34-8

Platelet Roles in Hemostasis

Surveillance of blood vessel continuity
Formation of primary hemostatic plug
Surface for coagulation factors to make secondary hemostatic plug
Aid in healing of injured tissue

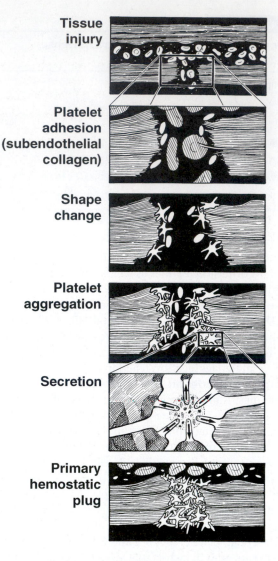

■ **FIGURE 34-8** Diagram of platelets forming the primary hemostatic plug. Tissue injury causes platelets to adhere to subendothelial collagen. Shape change, aggregation, and secretion of granule contents follow. Additional platelets become activated by the secreted substances and clump together, eventually forming a mechanical barrier that halts the flow of blood from the wound.

continuity or integrity of the vessels by filling in the small gaps caused by the separation of endothelial cells. They attach to the underlying exposed collagen fibers of the subendothelium and prevent blood from escaping. A decrease in the number of platelets in the peripheral blood results in leaking of blood through these gaps into the tissues.

When injury occurs and there is an actual break in the continuity of the lining of the vessels, the platelets react by forming the primary hemostatic plug. By sticking first to exposed collagen and then to each other, the platelets form a mass that mechanically fills openings in the vessels and limits the loss of blood from the injury site.

Following plug formation, membrane phospholipids of the aggregated platelets provide a reaction surface for the proteins that make fibrin. Fibrin stabilizes the initial platelet plug, and the entire mass of fibrin and platelets constitutes the secondary hemostatic plug.

As a fourth role, platelet derived growth factor stimulates smooth muscle cells and possibly fibroblasts to multiply and replace the cells that were damaged, allowing the injured tissues to heal.

The steps and mechanisms that result in primary and secondary hemostatic plug formation are described below.

Formation of the Primary Hemostatic Plug

Platelets circulating in blood vessels do not interact with other platelets or other cell types. Circulating platelets are disc-shaped and inert in the environment of normal endothelium. Injury to the blood vessels causes a change in the normal environment, and in response the platelets become activated. The primary hemostatic plug is the result of the transformation of the platelets from an inactive (nonadhesive) to an active (adhesive) state. The plug forms in a specific sequence of steps that are called adhesion, aggregation, and secretion (Figure 34-8 ■).

Platelet Adhesion
Platelet adhesion, the first step in primary hemostatic plug formation, is the attachment of platelets to collagen fibers in the subendothelium. When endothelium is injured and bleeding occurs, platelets escape from the blood vessel and flow into the tissues. Since surfaces in the tissues are components to which platelets are not normally exposed, they immediately bind to collagen fibers present in these tissues. Platelet adhesion to collagen requires the presence of von Willebrand factor (vWf) and the GPIb/IX receptor of the platelet membrane.

vWf, which is synthesized by endothelial cells, is both stored within the cells (in Weible Palade bodies) and secreted into the plasma and into the subendothelium, where it is bound to collagen (Web Figure 34-2 ■ and ∞ Chapter 36). vWf molecules consist of a series of from 2 to 50 identical subunits. Each subunit has receptor sites for GPIb/IX on the platelet surface in addition to its collagen binding sites. As platelets leave the lumen of the vessel, they adhere to the immobilized vWf by attachment of GPIb/IX to the receptor sites on vWf; thus, vWf becomes a "bridge" connecting the platelet to the collagen fibers (Web Figure 34-2 ■). While there are numerous other adhesion molecules in the tissues and many other receptors on the platelet surface, platelets are preferentially attracted to collagen via vWf under the physical forces (shear forces) that occur in the microcirculation. Because of the rapid flow of blood in the smaller vessels, the shear force is high. Most cells are carried quickly through the wound to the surface of the skin. Platelets, however, adhere to vWf in the subendothelium under the conditions of high shear.

Over time each platelet "zippers" along the collagen fiber by attachment to several of the other adhesive proteins of the connective tissue matrix. In this way the platelet eventually spreads itself over the surface of the collagen.[17] Many platelets spread in a similar manner until a monolayer of platelets covers the surface of the subendothelium.

Much of what is known about this phase of platelet function has been learned from studying patients with two diseases in which platelets fail to adhere properly: Bernard-Soulier disease and von Willebrand disease. Patients with Bernard-Soulier disease have mutations in one of the genes of the GPIb/IX complex that cause either decreased amounts of the complex on the platelet surface or abnormal function of the complex (∞ Chapter 36). Patients with von Willebrand disease have mutations in the gene for von Willebrand factor (∞ Chapter 37).

Adhesion of platelets to collagen fibers via vWf triggers a series of morphologic and functional changes known as platelet activation. Activation is a complex process that is not totally understood. The process includes changes in metabolic biochemistry, shape, surface receptors, and membrane phospholipid orientation. Key outcomes of activation are the activation of GPIIb/IIIa receptors for fibrinogen and the ability of the platelets to secrete the contents of their granules into the surrounding tissue. Only activated platelets are able to proceed with the subsequent steps in the formation of the primary hemostatic plug. Once activated, the platelet response becomes self-perpetuating and, through strict control mechanisms, remains localized to the injured area.

Changes in platelet biochemistry will be described first. A number of substances have been shown to stimulate platelets and to activate them. Some substances are generated by the platelets themselves, and some by other cells in the injured tissue. Some are normally present within cells but are released when the cells are injured. Some have been tested experimentally in in vitro tests, but their in vivo significance is unknown.

An agent that induces platelet activation is called an **agonist.** Each agonist binds to the platelet surface at its specific platelet receptor. A signal is transmitted (transduced) internally by the receptor, and then a series of reactions in the interior of the platelet leads to subsequent platelet responses. The signal transduction mechanisms in the platelet are similar to those of other cells.

Actions of the most familiar agonists—collagen, ADP, thrombin, epinephrine, thromboxane A_2, and arachidonic acid—and their receptors are linked with guanine nucleotide-binding (G) proteins on the inner leaflet of the phospholipid membrane. When the platelet adheres to collagen, G proteins are activated and, in turn, activate enzymes in the platelet membrane. The activated enzymes cleave specific membrane phospholipids. The resulting lipid products are "second messengers" that transmit the signal to interior parts of the cells.

The pathways and second messenger products of two membrane enzymes, phospholipase C and phospholipase A_2, are important in platelet activation. Products of both enzymes mobilize calcium ions from storage sites in the DTS and influx from outside of the cell into the cytoplasm. Resting platelets have very low levels of ionic calcium in the cytoplasm. Subsequently, many cellular systems that are idle in resting platelets become activated by the increase in calcium ions. There is a direct relationship between the amount of cytoplasmic-free calcium and the extent of stimulation. Details describing the pathways of phospholipase C activation can be found on this text's companion Web site as well as Web Figure 34-3 ∎.

Phospholipase A_2 is stimulated by the increase in cytoplasmic calcium and hydrolyzes arachidonic acid from the second carbon of the glycerol backbone of membrane phospholipids. **Arachidonic acid (AA)** is an unsaturated fatty acid and a precursor of a variety of regulatory substances. In the platelet, thromboxane A_2(TXA_2) is synthesized from AA by the enzymes cyclo-oxygenase and thromboxane synthase (Figure 34-9 ∎).

Within the platelet, thromboxane A_2 stimulates secretion from the platelet granules. Normal secretion will not occur if TXA_2 synthesis is blocked, and subsequent steps in platelet function will be seriously impaired. Ingestion of aspirin inhibits cyclo-oxygenase and prevents affected platelets from synthesizing TXA_2 (∞ Chapter 36). TXA_2 also diffuses out of the cell to enhance vasoconstriction and to function as a platelet agonist to perpetuate the activation process. TXA_2 is a labile compound and is spontaneously converted into an inert form, TXB_2, a short time after its synthesis.

Of the agonists listed above some, such as ADP and epinephrine, are classified as weak because they require platelet aggregation for secretion to occur; presumably TXA_2 must be generated before they can be effective as agonists. Collagen and thrombin are strong agonists. They cause all of the platelet responses without the presence of TXA_2 or platelet aggregation. Thrombin is probably the most potent activator of platelets in vivo.[13]

Another platelet membrane enzyme, adenyl cyclase, is activated when prostaglandin mediators generated as a response to the injury contact platelet membrane G-protein receptors. Activated adenyl cyclase produces cyclic AMP (cAMP) within the platelet cytoplasm. cAMP activates protein kinase enzymes that, in turn, phosphorylate proteins and inhibit platelet aggregation. This is one means of limiting and localizing the formation of the hemostatic plug.[18]

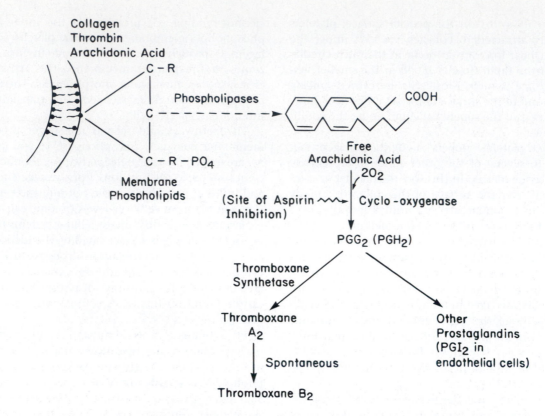

■ **FIGURE 34-9** Biochemical pathways of thromboxane A_2 formation in the platelet. Stimulation of platelet membranes (both intracellular granule and cytoplasmic membranes) by agonists (e.g., collagen, thrombin, arachidonic acid) results in liberation of arachidonic acid from membrane phospholipids. Cyclo-oxygenase incorporates two molecules of oxygen forming prostaglandin PGG_2 (PGH_2 in the reduced form). Thromboxane synthetase converts PGG_2 to thromboxane A_2. Thromboxane A_2 is spontaneously converted to inactive thromboxane B_2. Alternatively, PGG_2 can be converted to other prostaglandins and in endothelial cells to PGI_2, a powerful platelet inhibitor.

Activation continues with a change in shape of the platelet when the internal calcium level reaches a threshold. Shape change is the transformation from disc-shaped cells to spheres with spiny projections from the surface called pseudopods. It involves proteins in the structural zone including the membrane cytoskeletal proteins, actin and myosin of the cytoplasmic lattice, and the microtubules.

The result of the shape change is that each platelet has a larger membrane surface area for biochemical reactions and a greater chance of contact with other platelets. As platelets

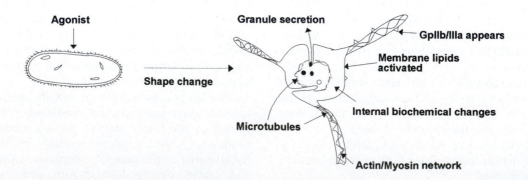

■ **FIGURE 34-10** Platelet shape change after stimulation by an agonist. Pseudopods develop on the platelet surface and contain a network of actin and myosin; membrane phospholipids are activated; glycoprotein IIb/IIIa receptors appear; internal biochemical changes occur; and granule secretion follows.

spread over the collagen surface they fill in spaces between the pseudopods over time and fit together in a jigsaw puzzle effect. Shape change will lead to succeeding responses if the stimulus from the agonists is strong enough and the intracellular calcium level becomes high enough. In the absence of these events, the platelet will return to its original discoid shape.

The third element of activation results in the appearance of the active GPIIb/IIIa receptor to which soluble fibrinogen binds. GPIIb/IIIa appears soon after platelet activation with any agonist. The mechanism by which the fibrinogen receptor appears is not known. Resting platelets do not express functional GPIIb/IIIa complex or, at least, are unable to bind fibrinogen. This prevents unactivated platelets from aggregating as they circulate in the plasma. Some authors describe the appearance of the active GPIIb/IIIa receptor as a merging of the two proteins or as a change in their conformation after stimulation by an agonist.

The fourth aspect of platelet activation is the changes in the platelet membrane that allow platelets to function in secondary hemostasis. Fibrin-forming proteins (coagulation factors) must bind to the surface of the activated platelets. This function is known as the platelet procoagulant activity and is discussed later. Activation of platelets is summarized schematically in Figure 34-10 ■ and in Web Table 34-1 ✪.

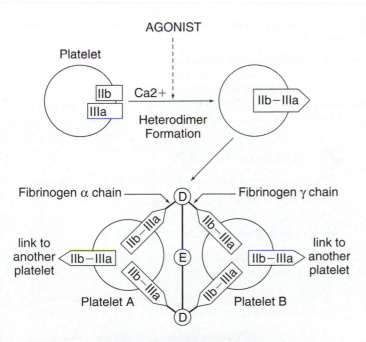

■ **FIGURE 34-11** Platelet aggregation. Agonist stimulation causes fibrinogen receptors, glycoprotein IIb/IIIa, to appear on the platelet surface. Fibrinogen binds horizontally to two platelets by peptide sequences at the terminal end of its gamma and alpha chains in the D domains, one gamma chain to GPIIb/IIIa receptors on each platelet. Fibrinogen thus becomes a bridge between the two platelets.

✔ **Checkpoint! #6**

If a patient with Bernard-Soulier disease or von Willebrand disease cut a finger, would you expect bleeding to stop as fast as the bleeding stops when you cut your own finger? Why?

Platelet Aggregation   After adherent platelets (platelets adhered to collagen via vWF) are activated, primary hemostatic plug formation continues with a phase known as aggregation. **Platelet aggregation** is the attachment of platelets to one another and is a stimulated event. Newly arriving platelets flowing into the bleeding tissue become activated by contact with agonists such as ADP and TXA_2 (released by activated platelets), products from the damaged tissue and endothelial cells, and thrombin (a procoagulant enzyme generated by tissue factor/factor VIIa) (∞ Chapter 35). With activation, the new platelets undergo shape change and exposure of their GPIIb/IIIa sites (receptors for fibrinogen). The fibrinogen bound to activated platelets serves as a bridge, linking GPIIb/IIIa molecules on two adjacent platelets. Additional platelets arriving in the area then stick to those that were already adhering to collagen.

Fibrinogen is able to link two platelets because of its molecular structure (∞ Chapter 35). Briefly, fibrinogen is composed of two pairs of three polypeptide chains: alpha, beta, and gamma. The C terminal ends of each set of three peptide chains forms a D domain on each end of the molecule. The N-terminal ends of all six chains meet in the center of the molecule in the E domain. One fibrinogen molecule attaches to the GPIIb/IIIa receptors on two different platelets via binding sites at the carboxy terminal end of the γ chains of its D domains.[18] (Figure 34-11 ■). The α chains also contain sequences for platelet binding. Approximately 40,000 to 50,000 molecules of fibrinogen are bound to each activated platelet. Fibrinogen binding is reversible for a time, but after about 10 to 30 minutes it becomes irreversible. Calcium is needed for platelet aggregation to occur, whereas platelet adhesion does not require calcium.

Sources of fibrinogen and calcium are both the plasma and internal platelet storage granules, which provide high concentrations of both constituents in the injured area. The role of calcium in platelet aggregation is not fully known, but the need for calcium can be inferred by observations of platelets on a blood smear. Platelets are found in clumps of various sizes on smears prepared from a needle tip or capillary blood sample. On smears prepared from blood that has been anticoagulated by a calcium-sequestering agent such as EDTA, platelets are singly dispersed, and platelet clumps are seen only rarely.

The importance of GPIIb/IIIa receptors in platelet aggregation was demonstrated by studying patients with Glanzmann thrombasthenia (∞ Chapter 36). Persons with this rare disease lack functional GPIIb/IIIa receptors, and their platelets do not aggregate in response to various agonists in platelet aggregation tests (∞ Chapter 39). Patients who have

Figure 34-11 labels:

AGONIST

Platelet

IIb / IIIa   Ca2+ ↑   IIb—IIIa

Heterodimer Formation

Fibrinogen α chain — D — Fibrinogen γ chain

link to another platelet   IIb—IIIa   E   IIb—IIIa   link to another platelet

Platelet A   IIb—IIIa   IIb—IIIa   Platelet B

D

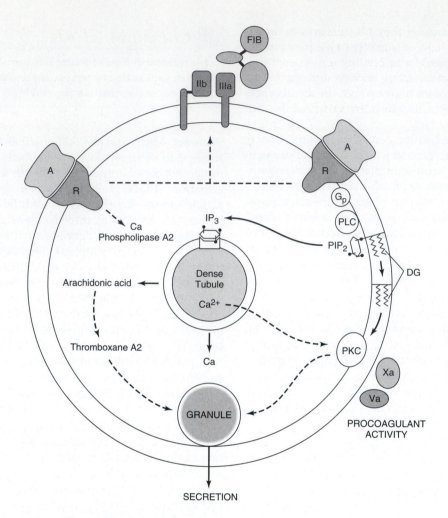

■ **FIGURE 34-12** Schematic diagram showing platelet biochemical changes after activation. See text and Web site for explanation. (Key: IIb, IIIa = GPIIb/IIa receptor; FIB = fibrinogin; DG = diacylglycerol; G = guanine nucleotide binding protein; IP₃ = inositol-3-phosphate; PLC = phospholipase C; PKC = protein kinase C; PIPₐ = phosphatidylinositol phosphate; A = agonist; R = receptor

decreased levels of fibrinogen also have abnormal platelet aggregation (∞ Chapter 36). Other adhesive proteins such as vWf, thrombospondin, and fibronectin also bind to the GPIIb/IIIa receptor, but their roles in platelet aggregation are not clear.

In in vitro test systems, aggregation occurs in two phases called primary and secondary aggregation. During primary aggregation, platelets adhere loosely to one another. If the stimulus by agonists is weak, primary aggregation is reversible. Secondary aggregation takes longer and results in irreversible platelet aggregation. It begins as the platelets start to release their own ADP and other granule contents and to synthesize TXA₂ as described later. The released substances act as agonists, which continue the platelet stimulation. If platelets are unable to release ADP and/or to synthesize TXA₂, secondary aggregation will not occur, and the platelets will disaggregate. The in vivo result might be that bleeding from a wound will take longer to stop.

✓ Checkpoint! #7

Your finger is still bleeding at this point, but the platelets are aggregating to form the primary hemostatic plug. Let's review the key events:

a. To what do platelets first adhere?

b. What bridge and what platelet membrane receptor are needed for platelet adhesion?

c. What bridge and what platelet membrane receptor are needed for platelets to attach to one another?

d. What is the attachment of platelets to one another called?

Platelet Secretion (Release) Following adhesion and shape change, platelets begin to discharge granule contents into the surrounding area. This process is known as **platelet**

secretion, or release. Secretion is an energy-dependent process and requires ATP. It occurs gradually, before or concurrently with secondary aggregation.

Secretion has been speculated to occur in two ways. In one mechanism, the open canalicular system fuses with membranes of granules that have been centralized deep within the interior of the platelet. The contents are then extruded through the OCS to the outside. Alternatively, the membranes of some granules fuse with each other and then subsequently with the plasma membrane. The contents are, again, emptied to the outside of the platelet.

Secretion is self-supporting. Some of the released substances function as agonists that stimulate membrane receptors on additional platelets. Stimulation of the receptors causes the internal calcium level to rise, and then more release occurs. The platelets eventually become degranulated.

Roles of the Granule Contents. The dense bodies release their contents into the surrounding tissue (Table 34-6). The release of ADP from dense bodies is considered to be of primary importance as ADP functions as an agonist, producing a positive feedback mechanism in the continued stimulation and recruitment of new platelets to the aggregate. The receptor for ADP has recently been identified. Stimulation by ADP results in the typical response of increased cytoplasmic calcium, more release, and appearance of active fibrinogen receptors (GPIIb/IIIa).[14]

Calcium is released extracellularly with the ADP from the dense bodies. This calcium is nonmetabolic and is not involved in the internal stimulation processes. The extruded calcium is believed to provide a high concentration outside the platelets necessary for fibrinogen attachment and for other enzymatic reactions that take place on the platelet exterior surface. Other components and their functions are listed in Table 34-6 ✪.

The alpha granules contain a wide variety of proteins. Some are specific for the platelet, and others, such as fibrinogen, are similar to hemostatic proteins found in the plasma. A partial list of the substances released from the alpha granules is found in Table 34-7 ✪.

The platelet-specific proteins are platelet factor 4 (PF4) and β-thromboglobulin (βTG). PF4 is called the heparin neutralizing factor. Heparin is an anticoagulant used in the treatment of patients who clot excessively (thrombosis) (∞ Chapter 38). Endothelial cells synthesize heparin-like molecules and express them on their surface. PF4 binds to the heparin-like substances on the endothelial cell surface. Heparin administered for therapeutic purposes can capture and complex with the bound PF4. The activity of the therapeutic heparin is thus neutralized. PF4 also has many other actions including chemotactic activity for neutrophils, monocytes, and fibroblasts. The role of βTG, which is actually a family of proteins, is uncertain, but it is believed to attract fibroblasts chemotactically and may, therefore, promote healing of the wound. βTG also binds heparin, but not as well as PF4.

Thrombospondin constitutes about 20% of the protein released from the platelet alpha granules. It is also synthesized by other cells, including endothelial cells, and is found in the extracellular connective tissue. It may function to stabilize the aggregated platelets.[14]

Platelet-derived growth factor (PDGF) is a mitogen for smooth muscle cells and also may contribute to healing of the wounded tissue, but it can contribute to thrombus formation in abnormal situations.

vWf, factor V, and fibrinogen are proteins in the alpha granules that are similar to hemostatic proteins of the plasma. Factor V may function as a receptor on the platelet surface for hemostatic proteins (factor Xa and prothrombin, ∞ Chapter 35) and is a cofactor in the process of fibrin formation. The functions of vWf and fibrinogen have been discussed previously. Plasminogen activator inhibitor (PAI-1), when released from activated platelets, appears to protect newly formed clots from lysis. Protein S and α_2-antiplasmin are among other inhibitors of clot lysis found in the alpha granules. The presence of these hemostatic proteins in the platelet granules may serve as an additional source of these components to ensure an adequate supply at the time of injury.

Platelet activation and biochemical reactions leading to aggregation are summarized in Figure 34-12.

Primary Hemostatic Plug Eventually the platelets form a barrier that seals the injury and prevents further loss of blood. The barrier is called the primary hemostatic plug. When the primary hemostatic plug is formed, the bleeding stops. The time for bleeding to cease depends on the depth of the injury and the size of the blood vessel involved. Superficial wounds, in which only capillaries and small vessels are affected, usually stop bleeding within 10 minutes.

✔ **Checkpoint! #8**

Your finger has now stopped bleeding. Outline the steps of primary hemostasis that have occurred.

ⓔ CASE STUDY *(continued from page 660)*

3. The physician explained to John that the reddish purple spots on his legs and ankles were tiny pinpoint hemorrhages into the skin. Explain the relationship of these hemorrhages to the platelet count.

Platelets and Secondary Hemostasis

The primary platelet plug is relatively unstable and is easily dislodged. As an illustration, you can probably recall accidentally causing trauma to a fresh cut and having the bleeding begin again. The primary platelet plug is stabilized and anchored firmly to the vessel wall by the process of secondary hemostasis.

During secondary hemostasis, fibrin forms amid and around the aggregated platelets. Platelets enhance the fibrin forming processes by mechanisms that are fully explained in ∞ Chapter 35. The proteins that interact enzymatically to form fibrin must be assembled on a lipid surface, where the reactions take place. The membrane phospholipids of activated platelets are the primary source of this lipid surface.

Fibrin-forming proteins do not bind to resting platelet surfaces in the normal circulation. However, during activation of platelets after injury, membrane phospholipids flip-flop, and negatively charged phospholipids that are normally more concentrated on the inner leaf of the bilayer move to the outer leaflet.[11] This allows coagulation factors to bind to the platelet surface, become activated, and initiate fibrin formation. The capacity of stimulated platelet surfaces to catalyze the fibrin-forming processes is called **platelet procoagulant activity.** Platelet factor 3 activity is another (older) name for platelet procoagulant activity. The fibrin-platelet plug is the secondary hemostatic plug.

The entire platelet-fibrin mass then contracts to a firmer, more cohesive clot. This contraction is called **clot retraction.** An adequate number of intact platelets are needed for clot retraction to occur. The process of clot retraction can be observed in a test tube of blood when no anticoagulant is added. A few minutes after unanticoagulated blood is placed into the test tube, it begins to gel. The gel is due to the formation of fibrin, with the blood cells caught in it. The mass of fibrin and trapped cells shrinks over a period of 2 to 24 hours as the serum is extruded from the fibrin mass.

Clot retraction is believed to occur by the association of adjacent platelet pseudopods with each other and with the fibrin strands. Actin and other contractile proteins within the pseudopods cause the platelets to contract. In vivo, the result of clot retraction is a cohesive mass of platelets and fibrin that seals the wounded vessel and prevents further blood loss. Contraction also permits the return of a more normal blood flow through the vessel. The stabilized platelet-fibrin mass will remain in place until fibroblast repair of the wound results in permanent healing.

ⓔ CASE STUDY *(continued from page 671)*

4. What is the most likely cause of John's pancytopenia?

5. Why would the administration of growth factors such as EPO and TPO be considered in this case?

SUMMARY

Blood clots after an injury by a series of complex biochemical reactions called hemostasis. The purpose of hemostasis is to temporarily reconstruct continuity of injured vessels so that external loss of blood is minimized. The components of hemostasis are found in the plasma and in the tissues that comprise the blood vessel walls. All of the components are inert until activated by the injury.

Hemostasis occurs in phases called primary hemostasis, secondary hemostasis, and fibrinolysis. This chapter discussed the primary hemostasis phase. During primary hemostasis, the blood vessels and the platelets cooperatively form an aggregate of platelets that mechanically fills the openings in the injured blood vessels and stops bleeding from the wound site. The injured blood vessels contribute by constricting and secreting a variety of biochemical mediators that affect all of the subsequent steps of hemostasis.

The roles of the platelets are to adhere to the injured areas of the blood vessel walls, and to aggregate by attaching to one another and by secreting substances that are stored in their granules. The secreted substances help to attract and activate new platelets that are added to the aggregate and that help the growth of new tissue to permanently heal the wound. The surface of the aggregated platelets is required for the reactions of secondary hemostasis.

REVIEW QUESTIONS

LEVEL I

1. Hemostasis is: (Checklist #1)
   a. the process of maintaining the body temperature
   b. termination of bleeding following a traumatic injury
   c. the process of forming a hematoma
   d. regulation of kidney function

LEVEL II

1. The cells that line the central cavity of all blood vessels and related tissues are called: (Checklist #1)
   a. epithelial cells
   b. endothelial cells
   c. capillaries
   d. smooth muscle cells

REVIEW QUESTIONS (continued)

LEVEL I

2. Which of the following is the primary element that prevents blood from clotting inside blood vessels? (Checklist #5)
   a. fibrinogen
   b. arteriole
   c. endothelial cells
   d. platelets

3. The bone marrow cell that is the precursor of platelets is called: (Checklist #7)
   a. neutrophil
   b. erythrocyte
   c. endothelial cell
   d. megakaryocyte

4. Immediately after an injury the action of the blood vessels in hemostasis is: (Checklist #5)
   a. thrombosis
   b. aggregation
   c. vasoconstriction
   d. vasodilation

5. Which of the following has happened when a cut finger initially stops bleeding? (Checklist #8, 9)
   a. vasoconstriction of vessels proximal to the cut
   b. vasodilation of vessels distal to the cut
   c. aggregated platelets have formed the primary hemostatic plug
   d. fibrin formation has been completed and the secondary hemostatic plug has formed

6. A reasonable reference range for platelets in the peripheral blood is: (Checklist #6)
   a. $1.5–4.0 \times 10^9$/L
   b. $150–400 \times 10^9$/L
   c. $4.0–11.0 \times 10^{12}$/L
   d. $4.0–11.0 \times 10^9$/L

7. The first step in platelet function after an injury is: (Checklist #8)
   a. fibrin formation
   b. release of ADP
   c. platelet aggregation
   d. platelet adhesion to collagen

8. When platelets bind to one another the process is called: (Checklist #8)
   a. platelet secretion
   b. fibrin formation
   c. platelet adhesion
   d. platelet aggregation

9. Which of the following best describes the normal morphology of platelets on a peripheral blood smear? (Checklist #6)
   a. They are larger than erythrocytes
   b. They are filled with azurophilic granules
   c. They are light blue in color without granules
   d. They have large nuclei

LEVEL II

2. The normal life span of platelets in the peripheral blood is: (Checklist #11)
   a. 8 hours
   b. 1 day
   c. 10 days
   d. 100 days

3. Platelet dense bodies are storage organelles for _____, which are released after activation. (Checklist #4)
   a. calcium, ADP, and serotonin
   b. fibrinogen, glycoprotein Ib, and von Willebrand factor
   c. ADP, thromboxane A_2, and factor V
   d. lysosomal granules, ATP, and factor VIII

4. Which of the following is the platelet receptor needed for platelet adhesion? (Checklist #5)
   a. thrombin
   b. actin
   c. von Willebrand factor
   d. glycoprotein Ib/IX

5. Platelet glycoprotein IIb/IIIa complex is: (Checklist #5)
   a. a membrane receptor for fibrinogen
   b. secreted from the dense bodies
   c. secreted by endothelial cells
   d. also called actin

6. The formation of thromboxane A2 in the activated platelet: (Checklist #8)
   a. is needed for platelets to adhere to collagen
   b. is caused by the alpha granule proteins
   c. requires the enzyme cyclooxygenase
   d. occurs via a pathway involving von Willebrand factor

7. What effect does thrombopoietin have on the megakaryocyte? (Checklist #2)
   a. decreases the number of platelets formed
   b. speeds maturation in the bone marrow
   c. induces release of the cell to the peripheral blood
   d. decreases rate of endomitosis and ploidy

8. The function of microtubules in the resting platelet is to: (Checklist #6)
   a. keep a high level of calcium in the cytoplasm
   b. store and sequester calcium
   c. provide a negative charge on the platelet surface
   d. maintain the disc shape

9. Contents of the platelet granules may be released from the platelet: (Checklist #5)
   a. through the open membrane system after fusion with the granules
   b. through the microtubules after fusion with the granules
   c. by disintegration of the platelet plasma membrane
   d. by the mitochondria

REVIEW QUESTIONS (continued)

LEVEL I

10. All of the following are involved in hemostasis *except:* (Checklist #2)
    a. vasoconstriction by the blood vessels
    b. adhesion and aggregation by the platelets
    c. fibrin formation by proteins in the plasma and platelets
    d. regulation of blood pressure

LEVEL II

10. Which of the following is true about the relationship between ADP and platelets? (Checklist #7)
    a. ADP is necessary for platelet adhesion.
    b. ADP released from the dense bodies is required for adequate platelet aggregation.
    c. ADP is synthesized in the platelet from arachidonic acid.
    d. ADP is released from the alpha granules of the platelets.

REFERENCES

1. Jandl JH. *Textbook of Hematology,* 2nd ed. Boston: Little, Brown and Company; 1996.

2. Hajjar KA, Esmon NL, Marcus AJ, Muller WA. Vascular function in hemostasis. Beutler E, Lichtman MA, Coller BS, Kipps TJ, Seligsohn U, eds. In: *William's Hematology,* 6th ed. New York: McGraw-Hill; 2001:1451–69.

3. Rodgers GM. Endothelium and the regulation of hemostasis. Lee GR, Foerster J, Lukens J, Paraskevas F, Greer JP, Rodgers GM, eds. In: *Wintrobe's Clinical Hematology,* 10th ed. Baltimore: Williams & Wilkins; 1999:765–73.

4. Bizzozero J. Ueber einen neuen Formbestandtheil des Blutes und dessen Rolle bei der Thrombose und der Blutgerinnung. *Virchows Arch Pathol Anat.* 1882; 90:261–332.

5. Bruno E, Hoffman R. Human megakaryocyte progenitor cells. *Semin Hematol.* 1998; 35:182–91.

6. Gerwirtz AM. Human megakaryocytopoiesis. *Semin Hematol.* 1986; 23:27–42.

7. Wendling F. Thrombopoietin: Its role from early hematopoiesis to platelet production. *Haematologica.* 1999; 84:158–66.

8. Zucker-Franklin D. Megakaryocyte and platelet structure. Hoffman R, Benz EJ Jr, Shattil SJ, Furie B, Cohen HJ, Silberstein, McGlave P, eds. In: *Hematology: Basic Principles and Practice,* 3rd ed. New York: Churchill Livingstone; 2000:1730–40.

9. Cramer EM. Megakaryocyte structure and function. *Curr Opin Hematol.* 1999; 6:354–61.

10. Long MW. Thrombopoietin stimulation of hematopoietic stem/progenitor cells. *Curr Opin Hematol.* 1999; 6:159–63.

11. Stenberg PE, Hill RJ. Platelets and megakaryocytes. Lee GR, Foerster J, Lukens J, Paraskevas F, Greer JP, Rodgers GM, eds. In: *Wintrobe's Clinical Hematology,* 10th ed. Baltimore: Williams & Wilkins; 1999:615–60.

12. Osada M, Komeno Y, Todokoro K, et al. Immature megakaryocytes undergo apoptosis in the absence of thrombopoietin. *Exp Hematol.* 1999; 27:131–38.

13. Brass LF. Molecular basis for platelet activation. Hoffman R, Benz EJ Jr, Shattil SJ, Furie B, Cohen HJ, Silberstein LE, McGlave P, eds. In: *Hematology: Basic Principles and Practice,* 3rd ed. New York: Churchill Livingstone; 2000:1753–70.

14. Parise LV, Boudignon-Proudhon C, Keely PJ, Naik UP. Platelets in hemostasis and thrombosis. Lee GR, Foerster J, Lukens J, Paraskevas F, Green JP, Rodgers GM, ed. In: *Wintrobe's Clinical Hematology,* 10th ed. Baltimore: Williams & Wilkins; 1999:661–83.

15. Parise LV, Smyth SS, Coller BS. Platelet morphology, biochemistry, and function. Beutler E, Lichtman MA, Coller BS, Kipps TJ, Seligsohn U, ed. In: *Williams Hematology,* 6th ed. New York: McGraw-Hill; 2001:1357–1408.

16. Plow EF, Ginsberg MH. Molecular basis for platelet function. Hoffman R, Benz EJ Jr, Shattil SJ, Furie B, Cohen HJ, Silberstein LE, McGlave P, eds. In: *Hematology: Basic Principles and Practice,* 3rd ed. New York: Churchill Livingstone; 2000:1741–52.

17. Sixma JJ, van Zanten GH, Banga J-D, Nieuwenhuls HK, de Groot PG. Platelet adhesion. *Semin Hematol.* 1995; 32:89–98.

19. Hawiger J. Adhesive ends of fibrinogen and its antiadhesive peptides: The end of a saga? *Semin Hematol.* 1995; 32:99–109.

35

Secondary Hemostasis and Fibrinolysis

Mary Ann Weller, Ph.D.

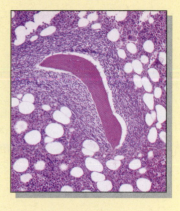

■ CHECKLIST - LEVEL I

At the end of this unit of study the student should be able to:

1. Define *hemostasis*. Identify the three systems involved in the hemostatic mechanism.
2. Differentiate primary and secondary hemostasis.
3. List the coagulation factors using Roman numerals and common names and determine how each is evaluated in lab testing.
4. Classify the coagulation factors into groups and discuss their characteristics.
5. Describe the mechanism of action of the coagulation proteins.
6. Diagram the sequence of reactions in the coagulation cascade according to the historic concepts of intrinsic, extrinsic, and common pathways.
7. Identify the factors involved in contact activation.
8. Define *fibrinolysis;* identify the major components of the fibrinolytic system; explain why fibrinolysis is a necessary component of hemostasis.
9. List the fragments resulting from fibrinolytic degradation; compare and contrast the fragments resulting from degradation of fibrinogen and fibrin.
10. List the major biochemical inhibitors that regulate secondary hemostasis.

■ CHECKLIST - LEVEL II

At the end of this unit of study the student should be able to:

1. Explain the interactions of the three systems involved in hemostasis.
2. Describe the domain structure of the coagulation factors; determine how this structure affects the action of the serine proteases; explain the significance of the noncatalytic regions.
3. Summarize the formation of complexes on a phospholipid surface and explain the significance of these complexes to hemostasis.
4. Integrate the role of contact factors with other systems (complement activation, fibrinolysis, inflammation).
5. Diagram the physiologic pathway of blood coagulation.
6. Evaluate the importance of vitamin K in hemostasis.
7. Describe the roles of thrombin in hemostasis.
8. Compare and contrast physiologic and systemic fibrinolysis.

■ **CHECKLIST - LEVEL II** *(continued)*

9. Describe the physiologic controls of hemostasis, including: blood flow, feedback inhibition, liver clearance, and inhibitors (antithrombin, tissue factor pathway inhibitor, protein C, and protein S).

10. Evaluate a case study from a patient with a defect in hemostasis; using the medical history and laboratory results, determine the diagnosis.

KEY TERMS

γ Carboxylation
Coagulation factors
Common pathway
Contact group
Extrinsic pathway
Extrinsic Xase
Fibrin degradation (split) products (FDP or FSP)
Fibrinogen group
Fibrinolysis
Intrinsic pathway
Intrinsic Xase
PIVKA
Plasminogen activator inhibitors (PAI)
Plasminogen activators
Prothrombinase complex
Prothrombin group
Serine protease
Serpin
Thrombomodulin
Tissue-type plasminogen activator (t-PA)
Transglutaminase
Urokinase-type plasminogen activator (u-PA)
Vitamin K-dependent
Zymogen

BACKGROUND BASICS

The information in this chapter will build on the concepts learned in previous chapters. To maximize your learning experience you should review these concepts before starting this unit of study.

Level I

▶ Define and summarize *primary hemostasis.* (Chapter 34)
▶ Discuss the role of platelets in primary hemostasis. (Chapter 34)

Level II

▶ Describe the structure of the platelet phospholipid membrane. (Chapter 34)
▶ Review protein structure and properties of enzymes. (previous chemistry and biology courses)

 CASE STUDY

We will address this case throughout the chapter.

Shawn, a 10-year-old boy, was seen by his physician for recurrent nosebleeds and anemia. History revealed that the epistaxis began when he was about 18 months old. The nosebleeds occurred one or two times a month and began spontaneously. The mother reported that Shawn seemed to bruise easily. No lesion was found in the nose. No history of drugs was noted. The family history indicated that the boy's grandparents were cousins. The patient had a brother who died at 10 years of age of intracranial hemorrhage. Parents and all other relatives showed no bleeding problems. As you read this chapter consider which of the three physiologic compartments involved in hemostasis could be responsible for Shawn's bleeding history and how this diagnosis could be established.

▶ ## OVERVIEW

Hemostasis requires interaction of platelets, blood vessels (primary hemostasis), and coagulation proteins (secondary hemostasis). The previous chapter described primary hemostasis. This chapter serves as an introduction to the plasma protein systems contributing to hemostasis (secondary hemostasis). It begins with an overview of hemostasis and defines the distinctions between primary and secondary hemostasis. The coagulation proteins are presented in related groups for initial discussion of general properties, mechanisms of action, and protein structure. The functional interactions of these procoagulant proteins are described from the classical perspective of intrinsic, extrinsic, and common pathways. The fibrinolytic system (components, activators, and inhibitors) is presented, and the products of fibrinolytic degradation are defined. The various components contributing to the control of hemostasis are discussed, including physiologic processes (blood flow, liver clearance), positive and negative feedback mechanisms, and natural inhibitors. The chapter concludes with an updated perspective of the hemostatic system, referred to as the physiologic pathway.

► INTRODUCTION

Hemostasis is the process by which the body prevents loss of blood from the vascular system and maintains it in a fluid state. Although often thought of as clot formation, it also includes clot dissolution and vessel repair. The process involves a series of complex and highly regulated events linking platelets, vascular endothelial cells, and coagulation proteins (referred to as **coagulation factors**). The interaction of these three elements at the cell and molecular level determines if equilibrium between excessive bleeding (hemorrhage) and clotting (thrombosis) is maintained (Figure 35-1 ■).

As discussed in Chapter 34, hemostasis can be viewed as consisting of two stages: primary and secondary hemostasis. Primary hemostasis (∞ Chapter 34), the formation of the unstable platelet plug, is the first response to vascular injury. Secondary hemostasis, the rapid reinforcement of the unstable platelet plug with a chemically stable fibrin clot, follows immediately and includes a series of interdependent, enzyme-mediated reactions. The endpoint of these reactions is the generation of thrombin that transforms the soluble protein fibrinogen to insoluble fibrin to stabilize the platelet plug.

The process of fibrin formation is well balanced and controlled, limiting clot formation to the ruptured vessel. Localization of the response to the site of injury prevents widespread coagulation activation. The reactions are amplified to the appropriate degree, while natural inhibitors limit the proteolytic activity of the activated clotting factors. Fibrin formation is also controlled by negative feedback: large quantities of thrombin, the last enzyme formed, destroy coagulation cofactors in the rate-limiting steps of its own production. Once the fibrin clot has served its purpose of plugging the injured vessel and the vessel begins to repair itself, the fibrin is digested by plasmin, an enzyme of the fibrinolytic system.

The study of hemostasis is complicated and involves many interrelating parts and control mechanisms. No part of the system acts alone. Our approach will be to study each part individually and then integrate the concepts.

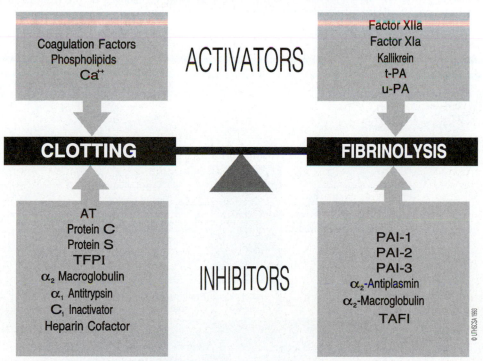

■ FIGURE 35-1 The coagulation system is kept in balance by activators and inhibitors of clotting and fibrinolysis. Clotting occurs when blood vessels are damaged and activators of coagulation factors are released. Clotting is kept in control because fibrinolysis is initiated in response to clotting activation. Inhibitors of both clotting and fibrinolysis serve to bring the system back into balance. An upset in the activation or inhibition of either clotting or fibrinolysis will cause thrombosis or bleeding.

► THE HEMOSTATIC MECHANISM

The reactions involved in hemostasis were originally described as occurring in a cascade[1] or waterfall-like[2] fashion in which circulating, inactive coagulation factors, called **zymogens**, are sequentially activated to their active enzyme forms. Each zymogen serves first as a substrate and then as an enzyme. A simplified diagram of the cascade is shown in Figure 35-2 ■. In vitro, initiation of the cascade occurs via two pathways. The **intrinsic pathway** requires enzymes and protein cofactors originally present in plasma. The **extrinsic pathway** requires enzymes and protein cofactors present in plasma as well as an activator, tissue factor, not found in blood under normal conditions. Both converge in a third path called the **common pathway** to generate the fibrin clot. The traditional analysis of the coagulation process assigns each of the coagulation factors to the intrinsic, extrinsic, or common pathway as indicated in Table 35-1 .

The conceptualization of intrinsic, extrinsic, and common pathways evolved from observations of reactions occurring in vitro (in test tubes) and has contributed to our knowledge of how coagulation occurs in vivo. For clinical laboratory professionals, understanding hemostasis from an in vitro diagnostic perspective is important. The concept of the three pathways, combined with available tests for in vitro evaluation of the intrinsic system (partial thromboplastin time [PTT]) and the extrinsic system (prothrombin time [PT]) are invaluable in diagnosing clinical bleeding disorders.

We continue to use the model of intrinsic, extrinsic, and common pathways as the basis of our understanding of this complicated system. We also realize that in vivo the system functions quite differently, and is not so compartmentalized. The current concept of hemostasis is of one pathway, explained later in this chapter as the physiologic pathway.

✓ **Checkpoint! #1**

What is the major distinction between the so-called extrinsic and intrinsic pathways?

@ **CASE STUDY** *(continued from page 676)*

Screening tests for evaluating hemostasis were done on Shawn. The child was found to have a platelet count of 242 × 10⁹/L. Bleeding time was 8 seconds. The prothrombin time (PT) was 29.5 seconds with a control of 12.0 seconds. The activated partial thromboplastin time (APTT) was 51.0 seconds with a control of 55.4 seconds. Liver function tests were normal.

1. What do the results of the screening tests (platelet count, bleeding time, prothrombin time (PT), and activated partial thromboplastin time (aPTT) indicate?

2. What component of the hemostatic mechanism is most likely affected?

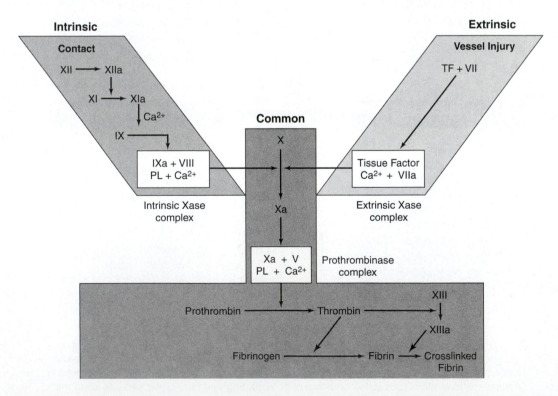

■ FIGURE 35-2 A simplified version of the coagulation cascade showing the cascade or waterfall-like sequence of reactions. Boxes indicate complex formation. (PL=platelet phospholipid)

✪ TABLE 35-1

Coagulation Factors in Intrinsic, Extrinsic, and Common Pathway

Intrinsic Pathway	Extrinsic Pathway	Common Pathway
Prekallikrien	VII	X
HMWK	Tissue factor (TF; III)	V
XII		II
XI		I
IX		
VIII		

▶ THE COAGULATION FACTORS

The coagulation factors are the proteins involved in hemostasis. Some have been assigned Roman numerals I through XIII by the International Committee on Nomenclature of Blood Coagulation Factors.[3] Each Roman numeral was assigned according to the order of discovery of the respective factor, not its place in the reaction sequence. Each factor has one or more common names or synonyms in addition to the Roman numeral designation (Table 35-2 ✪). The letter *a* following the Roman numeral indicates that the factor has been activated. It is no longer a zymogen but has enzymatic activity. There are, however, several exceptions to this terminology. Factor II (prothrombin), in its activated form, is preferentially known as thrombin rather than factor IIa. When fibrinogen (factor I) is cleaved by thrombin, it is preferentially called fibrin. Tissue factor was assigned factor III and calcium was assigned factor IV, but the Roman numeral designations are no longer used. Factor VI is no longer included in the coagulation sequence as it was found to be activated factor V. High molecular weight kininogen and prekallikrein were never assigned Roman numerals.

The coagulation factors were discovered when physicians saw patients with a life-long history of bleeding problems. Studies of the affected patient's blood revealed that certain proteins were functionally deficient. These proteins have now been isolated and characterized as to their composition and biochemical functions (Table 35-2 ✪). In addition, the coagulation proteins have been sequenced and the chromosomal location of their genes identified, providing useful information for understanding hereditary problems (Table 35-2 ✪).

℮ CASE STUDY *(continued from page 678)*

3. What evidence exists to indicate that Shawn has a hereditary bleeding disorder?

4. Are the nosebleeds significant in considering a diagnosis?

PROPERTIES OF THE BLOOD COAGULATION FACTORS

Similarities among the structural and functional properties of the coagulation factors permit division into three groups: the **prothrombin group**, the **fibrinogen group**, and the **contact group** (Table 35-3 ✪).

Prothrombin Group

The prothrombin group of proteins includes prothrombin (factor II), factors VII, IX, and X. These factors have a molecular mass ranging from 50,000 to 100,000 Daltons. The factors in the prothrombin group are produced in the liver, and all contain the γ-carboxyglutamic acid rich region called the GLA-domain that is critical for the calcium binding properties of these proteins. The prothrombin group is also referred to as **vitamin K-dependent** because its members require vitamin K (see later section) to be functional.

Fibrinogen Group

The fibrinogen group includes fibrinogen (factor I) and factors V, VIII, and XIII. All are acted upon by thrombin during coagulation. They have the highest molecular weights of all the factors, ranging from 300,000 to 350,000 Daltons. These factors are not found in serum because they are consumed during clotting.

Contact Group

The contact group includes factors XI and XII, prekallikrein (PK), and high molecular weight kininogen (HK). The proteins have molecular weights ranging from 80,000 to 173,000 Daltons. The contact group is involved in the initial activation of the intrinsic pathway and requires contact with a negatively charged surface for activation. With the exception of factor XI, the contact factors do not appear to play an essential role in hemostasis in vivo.[4] However, this group of factors is integrally related to other physiologic systems. The activated forms of the contact group can activate the fibrinolytic, kinin, and complement systems, as well as the coagulation system. These factors are found in serum after clotting has taken place.

MECHANISM OF ACTION OF THE COAGULATION FACTORS

The coagulation proteins may function as a cofactor, substrate, or enzyme. Enzymes act as either a serine protease or a transglutaminase.

Cofactors

Factors V and VIII function as *cofactors*. They are required for the conversion of specific zymogens to the active enzyme form. Factors Va and VIIIa have no enzymatic activity of their own. HK functions as a cofactor for the contact activation phase of coagulation, and protein S is a cofactor for

⊙ TABLE 35-2

Summary of the Properties of Coagulation Factors

Factor	Common Name(s)	Description	t1/2 (hours)	Function	Plasma Concentration	Chromosome
I	Fibrinogen	6-chain glycoprotein MW 340,000	72–120	Substrate; fibrin precursor	250–350 mg/dL	4
II	Prothrombin	Single-chain glycoprotein MW 72,000	67–106	Serine protease Thrombin precursor	100 μg/mL	11
III	Tissue factor	Single-chain, transmembrane lipoprotein MW 45,000	NA	Cofactor in extrinsic Xase complex; not found in circulation	NA	1
IV	Calcium	Element	NA	Cofactor in some Coagulation reactions	8.8–10.5 mg/dL	—
V	Proaccelerin	Single-chain glycoprotein MW 330,000	12–36	Cofactor in prothrombinase complex	4–14 μg/mL	1
VII	Proconvertin (Stable factor)	Single-chain glycoprotein MW 50,000	5–8	Serine protease; constituent of extrinsic Xase complex	0.5 μg/mL	13
VIIIc	Antihemophiliac factor	Heterodimer glycoprotein MW 80,000 (light chain) 90–200,000 (heavy chain)	8–12	Cofactor; complexed with vWf; constituent of intrinsic Xase complex	0.15 μg/mL	X
vWf	von Willebrand factor	Multimeric glycoprotein MW 250,000 (subunit)	22–40	Platelet adhesion	8–10 μg/mL	12
IX	Plasma thromboplastin component (PTC)	Single-chain glycoprotein MW 57,000	48–72	Serine protease; constituent of intrinsic Xase complex	4 μg/mL	X
X	Stuart factor	Two-chain glycoprotein MW 56,000	48–60	Serine protease; constituent of prothrombinase complex	4–6 μg/mL	13
XI	Plasma thromboplastin antecedent, (PTA)	Two-chain glycoprotein MW 160,000	48–84	Serine protease; contact factor	2–7 μg/mL	4
XII	Hageman factor	Single-chain glycoprotein MW 80,000	48–60	Serine protease; contact factor	23–39 μg/mL	5
XIII	Fibrin stabilizing factor	Multimeric glycoprotein MW 320,000	72–120	Transglutaminase; stabilizes fibrin	10–20 μg/mL	6
HMWK	Fitzgerald factor (Flaujeac factor)	Monomeric α-globulin MW 120,000	156	Cofactor; complexed with prekallikrein and Factor XI; contact factor	70–90 μg/mL	3
Prekallikrein	Fletcher factor	Monomeric γ-globulin MW 100,000	35	Serine protease complexed with HMWK; contact factor	35–45 μg/mL	4

Key to abbreviations: t1/2 = biologic half-life; MW = molecular weight in Daltons; HMWK = high molecular weight kininogen.

TABLE 35-3

Coagulation Factor Groups Based on Physical Characteristics

Contact Group	Prothrombin Group	Fibrinogen Group
Characteristic: Requires contact with a surface for activation	Characteristics: Require vitamin K for synthesis; need Ca^{++} to bind to a phospholipid surface; adsorbed from plasma by BaSO$_4$.	Characteristics: Large molecules; absent from serum (consumable).
XII	II	I
XI	VII	V
Prekallikrein	IX	VIII
HMWK	X	XIII

activated protein C (see later section). Tissue factor may be considered a cofactor for factor VIIa.

Substrate

Fibrinogen is classified as a *substrate* because it is acted upon by the enzyme, thrombin. It is the only coagulation protein that, as a substrate, does not become an activated enzyme.

Enzymes

The coagulation proteins that have enzymatic activity are secreted as zymogens. Zymogens are proenzymes or inactive precursors that must be modified to become active. Activation may involve either: (1) a conformational change (twist, turn, or bend) in the molecule, or (2) hydrolytic cleavage of a specific zymogen peptide bond. The coagulation zymogens are rapidly activated in a cascade sequence. Initially, a small number of zymogens are activated, and each sequentially activates the next one in the cascade, resulting in amplification of the initial stimulus.

The family of **serine proteases,** which includes thrombin, factors VIIa, IXa, Xa, XIa, XIIa, and the digestive enzymes chymotrypsin and trypsin, have a functional serine in their active sites and a common catalytic mechanism. They selectively hydrolyze arginine- or lysine-containing peptide bonds of other zymogens converting them to serine proteases. In contrast to digestive enzymes, which cleave peptide bonds indiscriminately, each serine protease involved in the coagulation cascade is highly specific for its substrate.

Factor XIIIa is the only coagulation protein with **transglutaminase** activity. It catalyzes the formation of isopeptide bonds between glutamine and lysine residues on fibrin, forming stable covalent crosslinks.

VITAMIN K-DEPENDENT COAGULATION PROTEINS

Six of the blood coagulation proteins, including prothrombin, factors VII, IX, and X, and proteins C and S, require vitamin K to become functional. Vitamin K is a fat-soluble vitamin found in green leafy vegetables, fish, and liver. Some gram-negative intestinal bacteria also synthesize it. Vitamin K is necessary for the **γ-carboxylation** of glutamic acid residues in the GLA domains of these proteins. The addition of an extra COOH (carboxyl) group to the γ-carbon of the glutamic acid residues (γ-carboxylation) is a postribosomal modification. It is essential for binding the factor to negatively charged phospholipid surfaces via Ca^{2+} bridges.[5] In the absence of vitamin K, the factors are synthesized by the liver and can be found in the plasma. However, they are nonfunctional because they lack the COOH groups necessary for binding to Ca^{2+} on phospholipid membranes (Figure 35-3 ■).

The vitamin K-dependent factors lacking the COOH modification have previously been referred to as **PIVKA** (**P**rotein **I**nduced by **V**itamin **K** **A**bsence or Antagonists). The Inter-

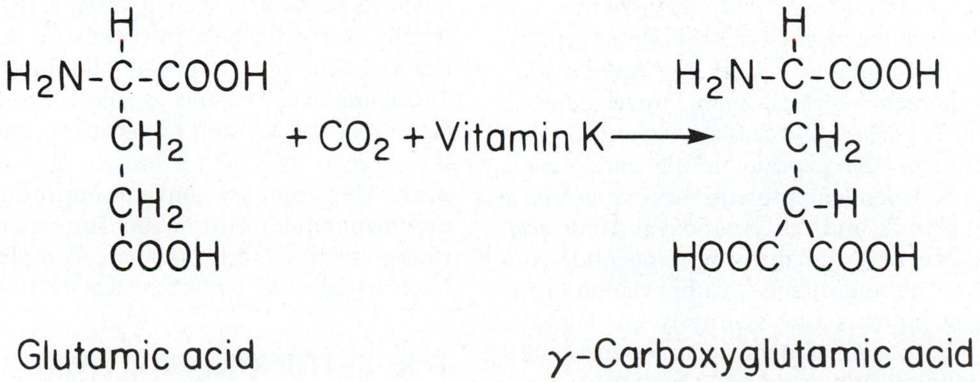

$$H_2N-\overset{\overset{\displaystyle H}{|}}{\underset{\underset{\displaystyle COOH}{|}}{\underset{\displaystyle CH_2}{|}}}{C}-COOH \quad + CO_2 + \text{Vitamin K} \longrightarrow \quad H_2N-\overset{\overset{\displaystyle H}{|}}{\underset{\underset{\displaystyle HOOC \quad COOH}{|}}{\underset{\displaystyle CH_2}{|}}}{C}-COOH$$

Glutamic acid   γ-Carboxyglutamic acid

■ **FIGURE 35-3** The vitamin K-dependent γ-carboxylation of glutamic acid. The coagulation factors in the prothrombin group must undergo this postribosomal carboxylation of glutamine residues in order to become functional. In factor activation, calcium binds to the carboxyl groups of the protein and to the phospholipid surface of the platelet.

national Committee on Thrombosis and Haemostasis has suggested using the term *acarboxy* instead. Vitamin K antagonistic drugs like warfarin/coumadin result in the production of inactive proteins by the liver by inhibiting the g-carboxylation process. The nonfunctional and functional forms of the factors are identical with respect to antigenic determinants and amino acid composition.

✓ Checkpoint! #2

Will a patient who is vitamin K-deficient produce any of the vitamin K-dependent factors? Why is vitamin K so vital to the formation of coagulation complexes?

STRUCTURE OF THE BLOOD COAGULATION PROTEINS

The blood coagulation proteins are made up of multiple functional units called domains that are derived from common ancestral genes.[6] Domains can be classified as catalytic or noncatalytic depending on their function. Catalytic domains contain the active site of the enzyme and are involved in activating other proteins. Noncatalytic domains contain regulatory elements. Similarities are noted among proteins involved in the hemostatic mechanism (Web Figure 35-1 ■).

The *catalytic domain* that is common to all serine proteases involved in blood clotting is highly homologous to trypsin. Conversion of an inactive proenzyme to an active enzyme by cleavage of a peptide bond, also known as zymogen activation by limited proteolysis, is the function of this domain.

The noncatalytic domains give each coagulation factor its own unique identity, making each highly specific in its activity and activation. They are regulatory elements serving to bind calcium and promoting interaction with phospholipids, cofactors, receptors, and substrates. Some of the most common noncatalytic domains include: the signal peptide, the propeptide/γ-carboxyglutamic acid rich domain, epidermal growth factor domain, apple domain, finger domain, and kringle domain. The *signal peptide* is a short domain that permits translocation of the peptide to the endoplasmic reticulum. Vitamin K-dependent proteins have a *propeptide* between the signal peptide and the γ-carboxyglutamic *acid-rich domain* (called the GLA-domain). The propeptide contains the recognition site that directs γ-carboxylation of the vitamin K-dependent proteins after synthesis. The GLA domain contains 10–12 γ-carboxyglutamic acid residues and is essential for Ca^{2+} binding. When bound, Ca^{2+} mediates the interaction between a factor and a phospholipid surface by forming a bridge.

The *epidermal growth factor domain* (EGF), *finger domain*, and *apple domains* are thought to be involved in binding to cofactors, activators, or substrates. The *kringle domain* is a lysine-binding site and is responsible for the affinity of proteins (plasminogen, plasmin, tissue plasminogen activator) for fibrin. There are other domains whose functions are as yet unknown (Web Figure 35-2 ■).

✓ Checkpoint! #3

Why are the domains of the serine proteases involved in blood clotting so important in the hemostatic mechanism?

► THE COAGULATION CASCADE

The coagulation cascade is composed of four interacting sets of reactions: complex formation on phospholipid membranes; intrinsic pathway; extrinsic pathway; and common pathway.

COMPLEX FORMATION ON PHOSPHOLIPID MEMBRANES

The coagulation cascade occurs on cell surface membranes. Clotting factors bind to the phospholipid membrane surface and rearrange until a complex including enzyme, substrate, and cofactor is formed.[7] Subendothelial tissue, exposed when blood vessel injury occurs, and the platelet surface provide the critical membranes for coagulation in vivo. The membrane serves to decrease the Km of the reaction between enzyme and substrate and to localize the reaction to the site of injury.[8]

Three procoagulant complexes including **extrinsic Xase, intrinsic Xase,** and prothrombinase assemble on the phospholipid membrane (Figure 35-4 ■). Extrinsic Xase is formed when tissue factor (TF), an integral membrane lipoprotein, is exposed to blood when vessel injury occurs. TF binds factor VII or VIIa in the presence of Ca^{2+}, giving rise to the factor VIIa/TF complex that activates factor X. The intrinsic Xase assembles on membrane surfaces when factors IXa and VIIIa bind to phospholipid in the presence of Ca^{2+}. This complex also activates factor X to Xa. In a similar way, factors Xa and Va bind to negatively charged membranes in the presence of Ca^{2+} to form the **prothrombinase complex**. This complex converts prothrombin, also bound to the membrane, to thrombin. The rate of prothrombin activation by the prothrombinase complex is about 300,000 times higher than by factor Xa activation alone.[9]

THE INTRINSIC PATHWAY

Contact Factors

The four contact factors include factor XII, factor XI, prekallikrein (PK), and high molecular weight kininogen (HK). The contact factors are activated when exposed to and

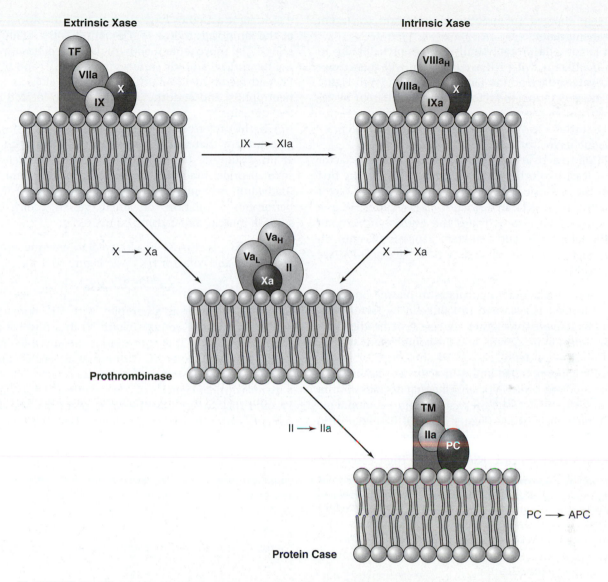

■ **FIGURE 35-4** Schematic illustration of the coagulation complexes forming on a phospholipid surface. The vitamin K-dependent proteases (factors VIIa, IXa, and Xa and thrombin are shown associated with their cofactors (TF, factors VIIIa, Va, and trombomodulin (TM), respectively) and substrates (factors IX and X, prothrombin, and protein C (PC), respectively) on the membrane surface. (APC= activated protein C)

adsorbed to negatively charged surfaces such as glass, kaolin, celite, and ellagic acid. Activation of these factors does not require Ca^{2+}; thus, in vitro activation (or "pre-activation") may occur in citrated patient samples stored in glass tubes for prolonged periods before testing. Patients deficient in factor XII, PK, and HK do not bleed abnormally despite a prolonged APTT; thus it is unlikely that these factors play a significant role in hemostasis in vivo. They do, however, contribute to fibrinolysis, inflammation, complement activation, angiogenesis, and kinin formation. At least 50% of patients with factor XI deficiency have bleeding abnormalities, suggesting that factor XI is an important accessory to blood coagulation but it is probably not essential.

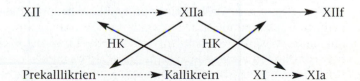

Factor XII Factor XII (Hageman factor) is produced by the liver. It is activated by contact with negatively charged surfaces in a phenomenon called autoactivation. Many nonphysiologic substances (glass, kaolin, ellagic acid)[10] have been associated with in vitro factor XII autoactivation. The nature of the physiologic surfaces responsible for autoactivation is still in question but is most likely cellular membranes or negatively charged subendothelial structures (collagen, basement membrane).

Bound factor XIIa proteolytically cleaves prekallikrein to kallikrein. Kallikrein, with HK as a cofactor, will then reciprocally activate surface bound factor XII to XIIa (Web Figure 35-3 ■). The generation of factor XIIa and kallikrein by reciprocal activation serves to amplify the reactions. Factor XIIa can be further cleaved by kallikrein yielding smaller factor XII fragments (factor XIIf).

In addition to activating prekallikrein to kallikrein, factor XIIa has at least two other enzymatic functions. As the first enzyme in the intrinsic pathway, factor XIIa converts factor XI to its active form, XIa, in a reaction that requires HK as a cofactor. Factor XIIa also activates the fibrinolytic system. Factor XIIa, factor XIa, and kallikrein generate plasmin directly, although much less efficiently than t-PA or u-PA (see later section)(Figure 35-5 ■).

Prekallikrein   Prekallikrein circulates in plasma bound to HK. In this form it is activated to kallikrein by factor XIIa. Kallikrein can activate three other biologic systems, the kinin system, the fibrinolytic system, and the complement system. Kallikrein, a serine protease, cleaves HK into smaller biologically active fragments called kinins. It activates plasminogen to plasmin, a potent proteolytic enzyme that degrades fibrin. Plasmin, in turn, can activate the first and third components of the complement cascade (Figure 35-5 ■). Kallikrein also serves as a chemoattractant for neutrophils and monocytes.

High Molecular Weight Kininogen   High molecular weight kininogen serves as a cofactor in activation of contact factors and is the source of kinins. The two forms of kininogen found in plasma are high molecular weight kininogen (HK) and low molecular weight kininogen (LK). Both forms are produced by the liver. HK accelerates the rate of surface-dependent activation of factor XII and the rate of PK activation by factor XIIa.

Different activities have been located to various domains of the kininogen molecule. Domain 4 is the bradykinin region.[11] The procoagulant activity of HK depends on its binding to artificial anionic surfaces (domain 5)[12] and binding to PK and factor XI (domain 6).[13] Binding sites for platelets, neutrophils, and endothelial cells are also located on these two domains.[14]

HK, the preferred substrate for kallikrein, is a single-chain glycoprotein that can be cleaved by kallikrein into a two-chain disulphide-bonded molecule with the release of a small peptide, bradykinin, composed of nine amino acids. Bradykinin has many actions including increasing vessel permeability, dilation of small vessels, contraction of smooth muscle, and causing pain.

Factor XI   Factor XI is activated to a serine protease by factor XIIa and cofactor HK (Web Figure 35-4 ■).

$$XI \xrightarrow{\text{XIIa, HK}} XIa$$

Factor XI circulates as a complex with HK. Both thrombin and factor XIa can activate factor XI in a positive feedback reaction. It may be that thrombin is the physiologically relevant activator of factor XI, with minimal need for factor XIIa activation. The substrate for factor XIa is factor IX. Although patients with deficiencies of other contact factors (factor XII, PK, and HK) do not have bleeding problems, about 50% of patients with a factor XI deficiency (Hemophilia C) experience abnormal bleeding after surgery or injury. Whether bleeding occurs is not determined exclusively by factor XI levels, since levels are similar in patients who have bleeding problems and those who do not.

Other Factors in the Intrinsic Pathway
Factor IX

Factor IX is activated by factor XIa in the presence of Ca^{2+} (Web Figure 35-5 ■).

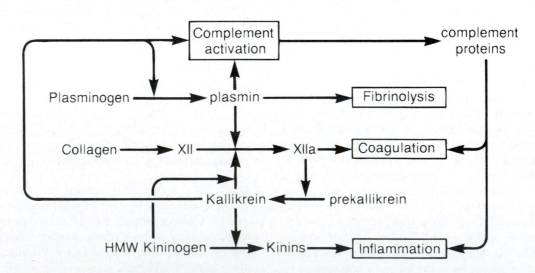

■ FIGURE 35-5 Role of contact factors in physiologic systems.

$$XIa$$
$$\downarrow$$
$$IX \xrightarrow{} IXa$$
$$Ca^{2+}$$

When activated, factor IXa forms a complex (intrinsic Xase) with cofactor VIIIa and Ca^{2+} on the surface of activated platelets to activate factor X (Figure 35-6 ■).

$$IXa + VIIIa$$
$$\textbf{activated platelet surface}$$
$$Ca^{2+}$$
$$\downarrow$$
$$X \xrightarrow{} Xa$$

The extrinsic pathway complex, factor VIIa/TF also activates factor IX (see later section). This extrinsic pathway for factor IX activation bypasses the contact activation system.

Factor IX is a single-chain glycoprotein produced by the liver. Factor IXa (but not factor IX) binds to phospholipid surfaces in the presence of calcium. It binds to activated platelets but not to resting platelets. It is one of two coagulation proteins (factors VIII and IX) that are encoded on the X chromosome. The severe bleeding that results from a deficiency of factor IX (Hemophilia B) indicates that it has a critical role in blood coagulation.

Factor VIII   In plasma, factor VIII circulates in association with von Willebrand factor (vWf) (Figure 37-2 ■). The circulating complex is composed of two distinct, noncovalently bonded subunits: factor VIII with procoagulant activity (previously referred to as VIII:C) and the portion that carries the von Willebrand factor activity (previously referred to as VIII:vWf). Each portion has distinct functions and biologic and immuno-

logic properties (∞ Chapter 37). Binding to vWf stabilizes factor VIII and protects it from inhibition or degradation.

Factor VIII is a heterodimer composed of light- and heavy-chain polypeptides. Factor VIII is synthesized at several sites in the body, but the liver appears to be the most important. Factor VIII is heat labile; its activity is lost at room temperature. The cofactor function of factor VIII can be markedly enhanced by small amounts of thrombin. Thrombin activates factor VIII to VIIIa by proteolytic cleavage, which dissociates factor VIIIa from the vWf molecule. Factor VIII complexed to vWf is blocked from binding to phospholipids and activated platelets. After proteolytic activation of factor VIII by thrombin, vWf is released, permitting factor VIIIa interaction with the platelet surface. Factor VIIIa has no enzymatic activity of its own; as part of the intrinsic Xase complex, it functions as a cofactor for factor IXa. However, large amounts of thrombin destroy the procoagulant function of factor VIIIa. Like factor IX, the gene for factor VIII is located on the X chromosome, and the factor is critical to normal blood coagulation. A deficiency of factor VIII results in Hemophilia A.

von Willebrand Factor (vWf)   von Willebrand factor is a glycoprotein synthesized by endothelial cells and megakaryocytes. vWf is synthesized as a large monomer of 250,000 Daltons, but undergoes posttranslational modification involving the formation of dimers and subsequently higher multimers. vWf circulates in the plasma as a family of molecules (multimers) of a wide range of sizes (0.5–>20 million Daltons) with the largest forms having the highest degree of hemostatic activity. However, most vWf molecules bind only one factor VIII molecule (resulting in a molar ratio of 1:1). Mature vWf multimers are stored within α-granules of platelets and in Weibel-Palade bodies of endothelial cells. They are released from these intracellular stores following injury or stimulation by thrombin, histamine, or fibrin. Platelet and endothelial cell vWf generally consists of larger multimers than are found in plasma and are not complexed with factor VIII.

vWf has two roles, contributing to both primary and secondary hemostasis. First, it mediates adhesion of platelets to the vessel wall by the simultaneous binding of vWf to GPIb on platelet surfaces and to collagen on the subendothelium. High molecular weight multimers of vWf contain the highest number of platelet and other cell surface binding sites. These molecules can serve as *intercellular bridges* between platelets, between platelets and subendothelium, or between platelets and endothelial cells. Second, vWf carries factor VIII in plasma. vWf binds to and stabilizes factor VIII by a noncovalent interaction, and the two proteins circulate as a vWf/VIII complex.

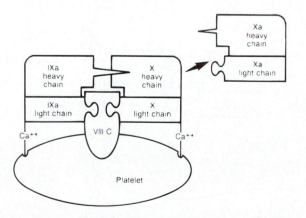

■ **FIGURE 35-6** The complex formed by the sequential activation of the intrinsic pathway (factors IXa, VIII, Ca^{2+}) activates factor X. The cofactor, factor VIII, binds to the platelet phospholipids (PF3) and serves to orient factors IXa and X to enhance activation of factor X. Factors IX and X are bound to the platelet surface via Ca^{2+} bridges.

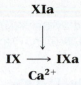 **Checkpoint! #4**

Which components of the intrinsic pathway are believed to be essential for in vivo hemostasis?

THE EXTRINSIC PATHWAY

Factor X can also be activated by the extrinsic pathway. The extrinsic activation involves factor VII and a cofactor, tissue factor (TF or tissue thromboplastin). When vessel injury occurs, nonvascular cells with TF on their surface are exposed to the blood. TF binds factor VII and factor VIIa in the presence of calcium, forming the VIIa/TF complex. Once formed, this complex initiates the extrinsic pathway of blood coagulation. The VIIa/TF complex (extrinsic Xase) converts factor X to factor Xa, as does the intrinsic Xase complex. The VIIa/TF complex can also activate factor IX of the intrinsic pathway, bypassing the need for contact activation. Factor Xa can feed back to activate more VII to VIIa.

$$\begin{array}{cc} \textbf{VIIa/TF} & \textbf{VIIa/TF} \\ \downarrow \textbf{Ca}^{2+} & \downarrow \textbf{Ca}^{2+} \\ \textbf{X} \longrightarrow \textbf{Xa} & \textbf{IX} \longrightarrow \textbf{IXa} \end{array}$$

Tissue Factor

Tissue factor is a transmembrane lipoprotein. It was originally named factor III and has also been called tissue thromboplastin. TF is found on the plasma membrane of most nonvascular cells. It is widely distributed in many tissues, but is especially rich in the brain, lungs, and placenta. Monocytes and endothelial cells can be stimulated to produce TF by endotoxin, complement component 5a, immune complexes, interleukin-1, or tumor necrosis factor.[15] TF and the platelet phospholipid surface have similar functions in coagulation. Both attract calcium ions to facilitate the formation of the enzyme complexes at the site of injury.

Factor VII

Factor VII is one of the vitamin K-dependent proteins produced by the liver. In the blood, factor VII circulates in two forms: the inactive zymogen, factor VII, and low levels of the active enzyme, factor VIIa.[16]

As with intrinsic activation of coagulation, there is positive feedback in activating the extrinsic pathway as well. When TF and factor VII are bound in a complex, factor VIIa can autocatalyze more factor VII to factor VIIa. Additionally, factor Xa associated with a phospholipid surface can feedback to activate factor VII, increasing the amount of VIIa formed.[17]

 ### Checkpoint! #5

Historically, the major importance for initiating coagulation was assigned to either the intrinsic or the extrinsic pathway. What are some observations that suggest that the classic concepts were not accurate?

THE COMMON PATHWAY

The common pathway converges with the intrinsic and extrinsic pathways, which both activate factor X.

Factor X Activation

Factor X can be activated by the VIIa/TF/Ca^{2+} complex (extrinsic Xase) or the FIXa/FVIIIa/Ca^{2+}/phospholipid complex (intrinsic Xase).

$$\begin{array}{c} \textbf{VIIa/TF/Ca}^{2+} \\ \downarrow \\ \textbf{X} \longrightarrow \textbf{Xa} \\ \uparrow \\ \textbf{IXa/VIIIa} \\ \textbf{Ca}^{2+}\textbf{/PL} \end{array}$$

Thrombin Generation

Factor Xa then forms a complex with cofactor V, phospholipid, and Ca^{2+}. This prothrombinase complex acts to optimally activate prothrombin to thrombin.

$$\begin{array}{c} \textbf{Xa/Va/Ca}^{2+}\textbf{/PL} \\ \downarrow \\ \textbf{Prothrombin} \longrightarrow \textbf{Thrombin} \end{array}$$

Factor X Factor X is another vitamin K-dependent protein produced by the liver. It binds to phospholipid membranes in the presence of calcium.

Factor V Factor V, produced by the liver, is also called labile factor because its activity deteriorates quickly at room temperature. About 25% of factor V in the blood is found in the α-granules of platelets, from which it is secreted during platelet activation.[18]

Thrombin or factor Xa can convert factor V to its activated form, factor Va. Both factors V and Va are membrane-binding proteins that do not require Ca^{2+} for binding. Factor Va binds to specific sites on the activated platelet surface, delineating the formation of the prothrombinase complex (Fig-

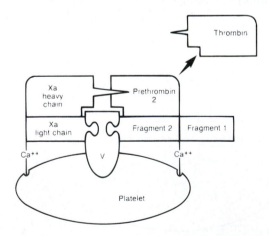

■ **FIGURE 35-7** The prothrombinase complex (factors Xa, Va, Ca^{2+}, PL) activates prothrombin to thrombin. Factor V binds to the platelet phospholipid surface (PF3) and serves to orient factor Xa and prothrombin to enhance the formation of thrombin. Factor X and prothrombin are bound to the platelet surface via Ca^{2+} bridges. This complex is very similar to the complex formed by the intrinsic pathway (factors IXa, VIIIa, Ca^{2+}, PL).

ure 35-7 ■). It appears that membrane-bound factor Va is the attachment site for factor Xa on platelets.

Prothrombin   Prothrombin is a vitamin K-dependent protein, produced by the liver. Like the other vitamin K-dependent proteins, it contains GLA residues. Alpha-thrombin is derived from the carboxy-terminal half of the molecule, and is composed of an α- and β-chain linked by a disulfide bond. It does not contain the GLA domain of prothrombin and thus does not bind to negatively charged phospholipids. It does contain the catalytic domain (Figure 35-8 ■).

Roles of Thrombin

Thrombin generation is critical for normal hemostasis. This protein functions as a procoagulant by cleaving fibrinopeptides A and B from fibrinogen to create fibrin monomer; activating factors V, VIII, and XIII to greatly amplify its own formation; stimulating endothelial cells to release vWf, PAI-1, and to express TF[19]; and stimulating platelet aggregation. Thrombin can suppress fibrinolysis by activating the thrombin activatable fibrinolysis inhibitor, TAFI. Conversely, thrombin also has antithrombotic functions that serve to dampen its own formation. Thrombin binds to thrombomodulin and activates protein C, and it stimulates endothelial cells to release tissue plasminogen activator and endothelium derived relaxing factor (EDRF [nitric oxide]).

CASE STUDY *(continued from page 679)*

5. What coagulation factors are included in the extrinsic pathway?
6. What factors are included in the intrinsic pathway?
7. What factors are included in the common pathway?
8. An abnormal PT and a normal APTT would indicate a problem with which factor?

Formation of Fibrin

The insoluble fibrin clot is formed from fibrinogen in three distinct steps:

1. Hydrolytic *cleavage* of arginine-glycine bonds by thrombin, releasing A and B fibrinopeptides from the α and β chains, forming fibrin monomer
2. Spontaneous *polymerization* of fibrin monomers to form fibrin polymers
3. *Stabilization* of the fibrin polymers by factor XIIIa

Fibrinogen   The fibrinogen molecule is a large (350,000 Dalton), trinodular glycoprotein found in plasma and platelet α-granules. Platelets do not synthesize the protein

Prothrombin Conversion to Thrombin

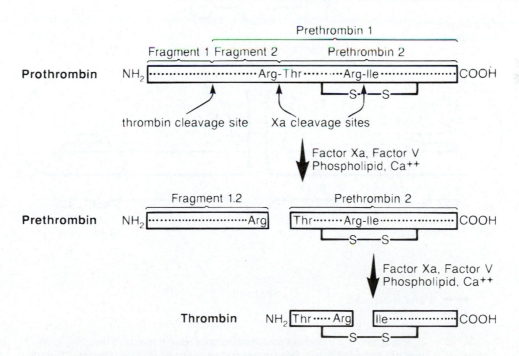

■ **FIGURE 35-8** The prothrombin molecule is a single-chain glycoprotein that can be divided into the "pro" portion (fragment 1 and fragment 2 or fragment 1.2) and the thrombin portion (prethrombin 2). Factor Xa proteolytically cleaves the molecule between the "pro" and thrombin portions releasing fragment 1.2 and prethrombin. Prethrombin is further cleaved into two disulfide bonded chains forming the potent enzyme thrombin.

but absorb it from plasma. Fibrinogen is the most abundant coagulation protein, with a plasma concentration of 2–3 mg/mL (representing about 2% of the total plasma protein concentration). Fibrinogen is encoded by three separate genes located on chromosome 4.

Fibrinogen is composed of three pairs of nonidentical polypeptide chains referred to as Aα, Bβ, and γ chains[20] (Figure 35-9 ■). Three disulfide bonds join the three pairs of chains. Electron microscopy has demonstrated the folding of the molecule into a trinodular structure.[21] The central nodule, called the E-domain, is referred to as the N-terminal disulfide knot (N-DSK) because the amino terminal ends of all six polypeptide chains join to form this region. The two outer nodules, called the D-domains, are made up of the carboxyterminal ends of the β and γ chains and a short sequence of the α chain. The Aα chain has a long polar appendage at the carboxy-terminal end that folds back toward the N-DSK. The D- and E-domains are separated from each other by 111–112 amino acids forming a triple-stranded α-helical structure called the coiled-coil domain.

Release of FBPs A and B. Thrombin binds to the central E domain of fibrinogen and cleaves arginine-glycine bonds. It releases a short peptide containing 16 amino acids from the Aα chain (fibrinopeptide A) as well as a 14 amino acid peptide from the Bβ chain (fibrinopeptide B). The resulting molecule is called fibrin monomer. Only the release of fibrinopeptide A is required for clot formation.

Assembly of Fibrin Polymers. The cleavage of fibrinopeptides A and B exposes binding sites in the central E-domain. These binding sites interact with complementary sites on the γ-chain of the D-domain of other fibrin monomers creating a D-E contact. The aggregation continues by the addition of a third monomer forming a D-D contact as well as another D-E contact. The use of x-ray crystallography to study fibrinogen has provided insights into the mechanism by which fibrin self-assembles. The crystal structures show a mechanism for electrostatic steering to guide the alignment of fibrin polymers during polymerization.[22] The noncovalent interaction of the nodules leads to the initial formation of two-stranded protofibrils. The protofibrils aggregate in an overlapping pattern called half-staggered array. The protofibrils then aggregate into thick fibers through lateral associations held together by weak interactions.

Fibrinogen Structure

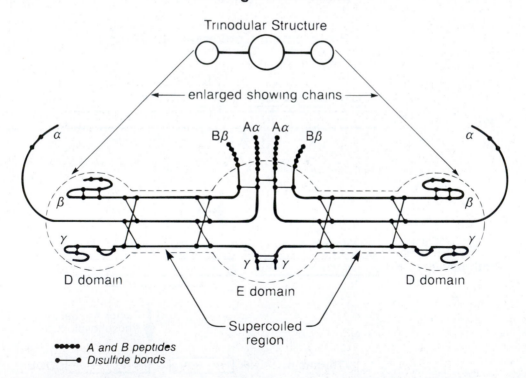

- ●●●● *A and B peptides*
- ●—● *Disulfide bonds*

■ FIGURE 35-9 Fibrinogen is a trinodular structure composed of three pairs (Aα, Bβ, γ) of disulfide binded polypeptide chains. The central nodule is known as the E domain. Thrombin cleaves small peptides, A and B, from the α and β chains in this region to form fibrin. The central nodule is joined by supercoiled α-helices to the terminal nodules also known as the D domains.

Fibrin Stabilization. Spontaneously polymerized fibrin strands are unstable, but the α and γ chains of adjacent fibrin strands are subsequently covalently crosslinked by factor XIIIa. The crosslinking strengthens the clot and provides resistance to chemical and enzymatic digestion compared to the uncrosslinked polymer (Figure 35-10 ■).

Factor XIII The final reaction in fibrin formation is the stabilization of the fibrin polymer catalyzed by factor XIIIa. Factor XIII circulates as a heterotetramer (A_2B_2) and is activated to factor XIIIa by thrombin cleavage. The expression of factor XIIIa activity requires its interaction with calcium ions, causing a conformational change that exposes its active center. Factor XIII is found evenly distributed between plasma and platelets. There is strong evidence that plasma factor XIII is synthesized by the megakaryocyte and is stored in the soluble (nongranular) fraction of the platelet.

Factor XIIIa is a calcium-dependent transglutaminase that is responsible for catalyzing the formation of covalent bonds between glutamine and lysine residues of the fibrin polymer.

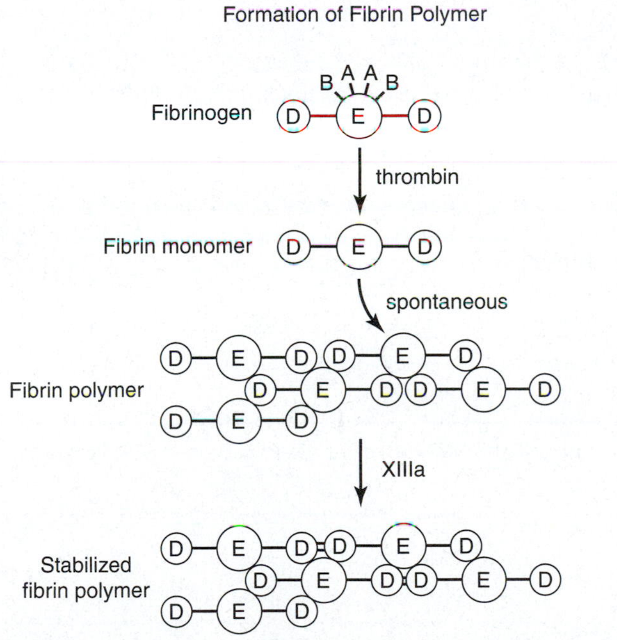

These bonds are formed between the terminal domains of γ chains and between polar appendages of α chains of neighboring monomers. The covalently cross-linked fibrin network produces a fibrin clot with increased mechanical strength and increased resistance to proteolytic digestion by plasmin. The presence of these unique bonds is responsible for the liberation of specific fibrin degradation products when plasmin digests the clot. In contrast to the hydrogen-bonded monomers, the factor XIIIa-stabilized fibrin polymer is not soluble in 5M urea or monochloroacetic acid (∞ Chapter 39).

✓ Checkpoint! #6

What are the three steps in the formation of an insoluble fibrin clot?

► THE FIBRINOLYTIC SYSTEM

The fibrinolytic system is activated in response to activation of the coagulation cascade. This system digests the fibrin clot through proteolysis.

INTRODUCTION

Fibrin formation occurs as a consequence of coagulation, inflammation, and tissue repair. When no longer needed, fibrin must be removed so that normal vessel structure and function can be restored. The process of removal of fibrin is called **fibrinolysis.** The fibrinolytic system is responsible for dissolving clots and maintaining a patent vascular system. The key components in this system are: (1) the inactive proenzyme, plasminogen, (2) plasminogen activators, (3) plasmin, (4) fibrin, (5) fibrin/fibrinogen degradation (split) products, and (6) inhibitors of plasminogen activators and plasmin (Table 35-4 ✪). With close regulation and control, the fibrinolytic system acts locally at sites of fibrin accumulation without causing systemic effects. If the activity of the fibrinolytic system is increased (e.g., deficiencies of inhibitors α_2-antiplasmin, PAI-1) there is an increased bleeding tendency. Conversely, activity of the system may decrease (e.g., deficiency of plasminogen, plasminogen activators, or elevated inhibitors), resulting in thromboembolic tendencies.

Fibrin formation essentially initiates fibrinolysis. When clotting begins, the zymogen plasminogen binds to fibrin throughout the clot. Tissue plasminogen activator (t-PA) also binds to fibrin, which increases its enzymatic activity so it can efficiently convert plasminogen to plasmin. Plasmin then digests fibrin to soluble degradation products, producing several well-characterized fragments. The system is in-

Formation of Fibrin Polymer

■ **FIGURE 35-10** Thrombin cleaves the A and B fibrinopeptides from the E domain of fibrinogen to form fibrin monomer. The cleavage apparently changes the negative charge of the E domain to a positive charge. This permits the spontaneous growth of fibrin polymers as the positively charged E domain assembles with the negatively charged D domains of other fibrin monomers. The polymer is initially joined by hydrogen bonds. FXIIIa in the presence of Ca^{2+} is responsible for catalyzing the formation of covalent bonds between glutamine and lysine residues of adjacent monomers (D domains), thus stabilizing the lattice formation.

⊙ TABLE 35-4

Summary of Properties of the Components of the Fibrinolytic System

Component	Description	Function	t1/2	Concentration	Chromosome
I. Fibrinolytic component					
Plasminogen	Single-chain glycoprotein MW 80,000	Zymogen; precursor of plasmin	2.2 days	0.2 mg/mL	6
Plasmin	Dimeric glycoprotein MW 92,000	Serine protease; cleaves fibrin	0.1 sec	—	—
II. Activators of plasminogen					
t-PA	Glycoprotein MW 70,000	Serine protease; complexed with inhibitor PAI-1; activates plasminogen	4 min	5 ng/mL	8
u-PA	Single-chain glycoprotein (scu-PA) MW 54,000	Serine protease; low enzymatic activity until cleaved to tcu-PA by plasmin; activates plasminogen	7 min	4 ng/mL	10
III. Inhibitors					
Plasminogen activator Inhibitor-1 (PAI-1)	Single-chain glycoprotein MW 52,000	Proteinase inhibitor (SERPIN): Inhibits plasminogen activators (t-PA and u-PA)	3 days	0.02 μg/mL	7
Plasminogen activator inhibitor-2 (PAI-2)	Glycoprotein Two forms: MW 60,000 (secreted); 47,000 (intracellular)	Proteinase inhibitor (SERPIN): Inhibits plasminogen activators (t-PA, u-PA)	—	trace	18
α_2-antiplasmin	Single-chain glycoprotein MW 70,000	Complexes with plasmin and inhibits kallikrein, thrombin, t-PA	3 days	1 μM	17
Thrombin activated fibrinolysis inhibitor (TAFI)	Single-chain protein MW 60,000	Carboxypeptidase B: inhibits plasminogen activation	10 min	73 nM	13

Key to abbreviations: t-PA = tissue plasminogen activator; u-PA = urinary-type plasminogen activator; MW = molecular weight in Daltons; SERPIN = serine protease inhibitor.

hibited by the action of plasminogen activator inhibitors (PAIs) and by the plasmin inhibitor, α_2-antiplasmin.

The plasminogen activators, tissue-type plasminogen activator (t-PA) and single-chain urokinase-type plasminogen activator (scu-PA), preferentially activate plasminogen on the surface of fibrin. When associated with the fibrin surface, plasmin is protected from rapid inhibition by α_2-antiplasmin so that efficient degradation of a fibrin clot may occur (Figure 35-11 .) If free plasmin leaks into the circulation, these plasmin molecules are rapidly inactivated by α_2-antiplasmin. Thus the activity of this potentially dangerous proteolytic enzyme is localized to the fibrin clot.

✓ Checkpoint! #7

Why is the process of fibrinolysis a vital part of the hemostatic mechanism? Why must it be closely regulated and controlled?

PLASMINOGEN AND PLASMIN

Plasminogen is synthesized by the liver. It has five kringle domains, which are critical in the regulation of fibrinolysis. The kringles contain lysine binding sites that are responsible for the affinity of plasminogen and plasmin for fibrin, plas-

The Fibrinolytic System

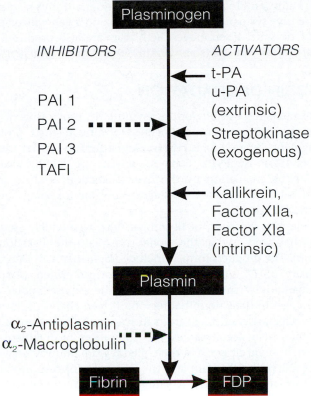

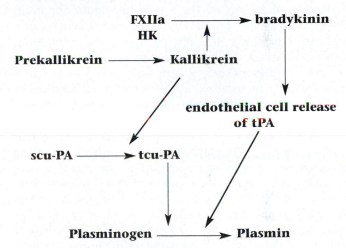

■ **FIGURE 35-11** The fibrinolytic system can be activated by the extrinsic activators, tissue plasminogen activator (t-PA) derived from endothelial cells, and urokinase-type plasminogen activator (u-PA), or the intrinsic activator, kallikrein. Exogenous activator, streptokinase, may also activate the system. Plasmin, the product of activation, controls coagulation by digesting fibrin to fibrin degradation products (FDP) and by degrading factors V, VIII, and XII. The inhibitors of plasminogen activation, plasminogen activator inhibitor-1 (PAI-1), plasminogen activator inhibitor-2 (PAI-2), plasminogen activator inhibitor-3 (PAI-3), and the inhibitors of plasmin (α_2-antiplasmin and α_2-macroglobulin) serve to control the fibrinolytic system. Activated protein C (PCa) inhibits PAI-1 and may enhance release of t-PA, thus enhancing fibrinolysis. The fibrinolytic system, like the clotting system, is intricately regulated by these activators and inhibitors.

min activation, and the interaction of plasmin with α_2-antiplasmin. Plasminogen activators convert plasminogen into its active two-chain form, the serine protease plasmin, by hydrolysis of a single peptide bond.

The proteolytic enzyme plasmin has the potential capacity to degrade and destroy most proteins. However, the formation and inactivation of plasmin is highly regulated in vivo, thus the enzyme is active only temporarily and locally. Activation occurs much more efficiently at the fibrin surface, as the proenzyme as well as its activators have affinity for fibrin.

ACTIVATORS OF FIBRINOLYSIS

Activators of plasminogen can be found in blood (intrinsic) and in most tissues (extrinsic). Some substances not normally present in blood during the coagulation and fibrinolytic processes (exogenous) can gain access to the circulation in pathologic states and activate plasminogen as well. The exogenous activators include commercially available therapeutic agents used in treatment of thrombotic disorders.

Intrinsic Activators

Plasminogen activators involved in the contact phase of the intrinsic pathway are referred to as intrinsic activators. Factor XIIa, factor XIa, and kallikrein all have the ability to activate plasminogen to plasmin. Kallikrein can affect fibrinolysis by converting single-chain urokinase (scu-PA, an extrinsic activator) to its more active two-chain form (tcu-PA), and by liberating bradykinin from HK. Bradykinin then stimulates release of t-PA (another extrinsic activator) from endothelial cells.

In vitro activation of factor XII results in plasmin formation. The process is amplified when plasmin further activates more factor XIIa. In vivo, the importance of intrinsic activators may be mediated via kallikrein conversion of scu-PA to tcu-PA, which has increased ability to activate plasminogen.

Extrinsic Activators

There are two physiologic extrinsic plasminogen activators: **tissue-type plasminogen activator (t-PA)** and **urokinase-type plasminogen activator (u-PA)**. Both are serine proteases having a high degree of specificity for converting plasminogen to plasmin by cleaving a single bond. Each has different structural, functional, and immunologic properties.

Tissue-type plasminogen activator (t-PA) is produced mainly by vascular endothelial cells and seems to be the predominant activity in the circulatory system. In vivo, t-PA is released from the endothelial cells by stimuli such as thrombin, bradykinin, exercise, venous stasis, and desmopressin (DDAVP) administration.[23] t-PA includes a finger domain, an epidermal growth factor domain, and two kringle domains. The domains are involved in binding to fibrin, fibrin-specific plasminogen activation, rapid clearance in vivo, and binding to endothelial receptors.[24]

Plasminogen activation by t-PA in plasma is relatively inefficient. However, because of the high affinity of t-PA for fibrin-bound plasminogen, activation of plasminogen by t-PA (which is slow in the absence of fibrin) is markedly increased when both proteins are bound to fibrin. Single-chain t-PA can be activated to a two-chain form; however, t-PA is unique among the serine proteases in that it is fully active toward its substrate plasminogen in its single-chain form, especially in the presence of fibrin.

Urokinase-type plasminogen activator (u-PA) is found in plasma and urine. However, it functions mainly in the tissues, where it plays an important role in digesting the extracellular matrix, enabling cells to migrate.[25] This process is important in wound healing, embryogenesis, inflammation, and cancer metastasis. u-PA is secreted as a single-chain molecule (scu-PA) that is converted to a two-chain form (tcu-PA) by plasmin or kallikrein. The scu-PA has significant fibrin affinity, but has little proteolytic or activator activity until it is cleaved to tcu-PA.[26] Although tcu-PA can activate both fibrin-bound plasminogen and circulating plasminogen, tcu-PA activation of plasminogen is increased tenfold in the presence of fibrin. The localized generation of small amounts of fibrin-bound plasmin converts scu-PA to tcu-PA, bringing about the reciprocal activation of plasminogen and scu-PA.

A specific receptor for u-PA, urokinase plasminogen activator receptor (u-PAR), plays an important role in localizing u-PA-catalyzed plasminogen activation. The receptor confines u-PA to the cell surface and facilitates activation of u-PA to tcu-PA. Binding of u-PA to u-PAR increases the activation of plasminogen sixfold. The u-PAR is a glycosyl phosphotidylinositol (GPI) anchored protein. This protein is deficient in paroxysmal nocturnal hemoglobinuria (∞ Chapter 17).

Lipoprotein(a) (Lp[a]), an LDL-like particle similar in structure to plasminogen, has been shown to inhibit the activation of plasminogen by t-PA and u-PA[27] because it competes with plasmin for fibrin binding. This displaces plasmin into the blood, where it is rapidly inactivated by α_2-antiplasmin, making the effects of Lp(a) antifibrinolytic. Lp(a) also blocks inhibition of t-PA by PAI-1 in the presence of fibrinogen or heparin, resulting in a profibrinolytic effect. The overall effect of Lp(a) on fibrinolysis depends largely on the concentrations of PAI-1, t-PA, and Lp(a).

Exogenous Activators

In addition to these physiologically important plasminogen activators, different bacterial species produce efficient plasminogen activators of their own. Streptokinase, derived from β-hemolytic streptococci, is not a serine protease but assumes enzyme activity when complexed with plasminogen. Streptokinase is used as a therapeutic agent to dissolve clots. However, streptokinase has no preferential action toward plasminogen bound to fibrin. It acts equally well on plasminogen molecules in the circulation and thus results in extensive systemic plasmin activation and a generalized proteolytic state. Plasminogen activators are also produced by *Staphyloccus aureus* (staphylokinase) and by *Yersinia pestis*.

FIBRIN DEGRADATION

Plasmin is responsible for the asymmetric, progressive degradation of fibrin (or fibrinogen), forming distinct protein fragments referred to as **fibrin degradation (split) products (FDP or FSP)**. These fragments are rapidly cleared from the circulation by the liver. Detection of these fragments in the plasma is of diagnostic value for some hemostatic disorders.

Plasmin digestion of fibrinogen has been widely studied and has been used as the model to explain the digestion of fibrin. The products formed include fragments X, Y, D, and E (Figure 35-12 ■). Fragment X is formed when plasmin cleaves a few small peptides from the exposed polar appendages in the C-terminal region of the α-chains of fibrinogen. Liberation of β1-42 from the N-terminal portion of the β-chain also accompanies the formation of fragment X. Next, a single cleavage in the coiled region, midway between one D-terminal domain and the E-central domain, produces a uninodular fragment D and a binodular fragment E-D (fragment Y). Plasmin then cleaves fragment Y in the coiled

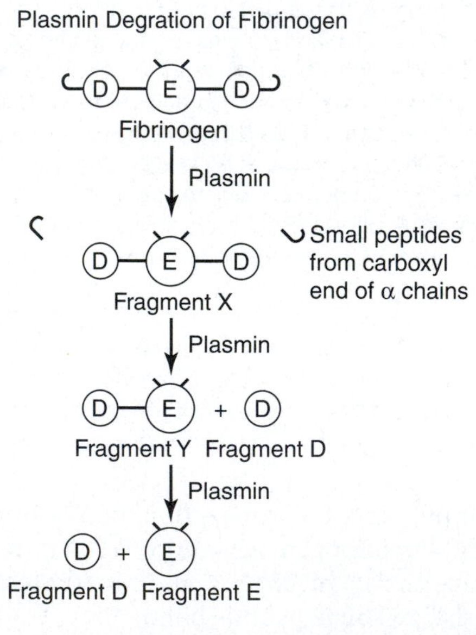

Plasmin Degration of Fibrinogen

■ **FIGURE 35-12** The degradation of fibrinogen by plasmin occurs in well-defined sequential steps. First, small peptides are cleaved from the carboxyl ends of α-chains producing fragment X. The E domain retains the A and B peptides. The fragment X is still capable of reacting with thrombin to form fibrin. Next, one of the D domains is cleaved from the fragment X, producing fragment Y (DE) and a fragment D. Further cleavage of the fragment Y produces D and E fragments.

region between the remaining E and D domains, producing fragment E and another fragment D. Ultimately each fibrinogen molecule is degraded into two D fragments, one E fragment, and a few small peptides.

Plasmin degradation of fibrin monomer and non-crosslinked fibrin polymer is essentially identical to that of fibrinogen. Plasmin degradation of crosslinked fibrin, however, is slower and produces different degradation products because of the intermolecular bonds induced by factor XIIIa. The potential sites of proteolytic attack are the same, but because of the crosslinking of the fibrin polymer the sites may be inaccessible to plasmin. Some of the crosslinked fibrin degradation products are combinations of X, Y, D, and E fragment complexes from two or more crosslinked fibrin monomers (e.g., DD/E, YD/DY, YY/DXD) (Figure 35-13 ■). The smallest unique degradation product is called D-dimer and is made up of two fragment D pieces crosslinked together. The D-dimer test is a specific marker for plasmin degradation of fibrin.

The fibrin fragments, if present in sufficient concentration, can exert an anticoagulant effect on the clotting system. Fragment X can still react with thrombin, but very slowly. Fragment X thus competes with fibrinogen for thrombin, so that less fibrin is formed. Fragments Y and D inhibit the polymerization of fibrin monomers, and fragment E inhibits thrombin. The fragments can also interfere with primary hemostasis by inhibiting platelet aggregation.

If free in plasma, plasmin can cause proteolytic degradation of factors V, VIII, and XII as well as components of the kinin and complement systems. The rapid formation of complexes between free plasmin and its inhibitor, α_2-antiplasmin, controls this potentially dangerous proteolytic process. If inactivation of plasmin is not sufficiently controlled, a systemic fibrinolytic state results. This is characterized by plasminogen activation, depletion of α_2-antiplasmin,

and fibrinogen breakdown. Physiologic fibrinolysis, which occurs when plasmin is attached to fibrin, is highly fibrin specific and not associated with a systemic fibrinolytic state.

 Checkpoint! #8

Why are the plasmin degradation products of fibrinogen and fibrin different?

INHIBITORS OF FIBRINOLYSIS

The fibrinolytic proteins are held in check by fibrinolytic inhibitors.

Plasminogen Activator Inhibitors (PAI)

Several inhibitors control and modulate the fibrinolytic system to prevent systemic fibrinolysis (Table 35-4 ✿). Most belong to a family of serine-protease inhibitors called **serpins** that inhibit target molecules by formation of a 1:1 stoichiometric complex. The primary regulators are the **plasminogen activator inhibitors (PAIs)**. Four proteins with PAI activity have been identified (PAI-1, PAI-2, PAI-3, and protease nexin-1).

Plasminogen activator inhibitor-1 (PAI-1) appears to be the primary physiological inhibitor of t-PA. PAI-1 is produced by endothelial cells, hepatocytes, smooth muscle cells, and adipocytes. PAI-1 reacts with t-PA, tcu-PA, but not scu-PA. In plasma, PAI-1 acts as an acute phase reactant and behaves in a similar fashion as C-reactive protein. Elevated PAI-1 levels result in a decrease in t-PA activation of plasminogen and a shift in the hemostatic balance toward hypercoagulability (∞ Chapter 38). Deficiency of PAI-1 results in a serious bleeding disorder due to unregulated and excessive fibrinolysis.

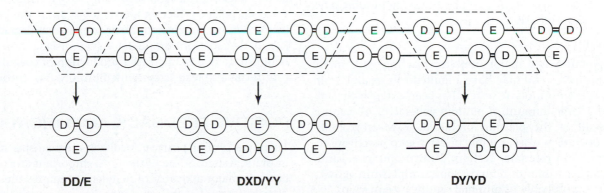

DD/E   DXD/YY   DY/YD

■ **FIGURE 35-13** Fibrin digestion by plasmin occurs at cleavage sites identical to those of fibrinogen. However, because of the covalent bonds of the factor XIIIa stabilized polymer, digestion is slower. Derivatives also are different as some sites are not accessible in the lattice formation. In this schematic drawing, some of the derivatives of plasmin digestion of fibrin are depicted. (Adapted, with permission, from: Beutler E, et al, eds. *Williams Hematology.* New York: McGraw Hill; 1995.

PAI-2 is the second plasminogen activator inhibitor. PAI-2 is found in placenta and in macrophages. Levels are very low except in pregnancy, when it is drastically elevated. Its precise role remains to be determined, but PAI-2 preferentially inhibits u-PA.

PAI-3 is probably the protein C inhibitor. These two molecules are immunologically and functionally identical.

Thrombin Activatable Fibrinolysis Inhibitor (TAFI)

Thrombin-activatable fibrinolysis inhibitor (TAFI) is a recently discovered plasma protein that inhibits fibrinolysis.

TAFI is a procarboxypeptidase B, activated by the thrombin/thrombomodulin complex.[28] The mechanism of action involves formation of a ternary complex involving TAFI-thrombin-thrombomodulin. Recent evidence suggests that TAFI suppresses fibrinolysis by removing carboxy-terminal lysine and arginine residues from fibrin, thereby eliminating the fibrin binding sites for plasminogen.[29] The active form, TAFIa, protects the fibrin clot from degradation by inhibiting the binding and activation of plasminogen. Thus, thrombin generation can, in principle, result in the suppression of fibrinolysis. Thrombomodulin has a role in down-regulating both fibrinolysis and coagulation by activating TAFI as well as protein C (see later section).

α_2-Antiplasmin

α_2-Antiplasmin (AP) is produced and secreted by the liver. It is the principle physiologic inhibitor of plasmin. AP rapidly inhibits plasmin, and interferes with the absorption of plasminogen to fibrin. Some AP molecules are crosslinked to fibrin by factor XIIIa during clotting, thus increasing the initial resistance of fibrin to the action of plasmin. This allows repair processes to start before clot lysis is initiated. In the circulation, AP reacts quickly with free plasmin, first binding reversibly to plasmin, then forming a stable complex with the enzyme and irreversibly inhibiting it. Circulating AP thus makes an important contribution to limiting systemic fibrinolysis. Plasmin bound to fibrin is protected from inactivation by AP because fibrin occupies the same binding sites on plasmin as would AP.

α_2-Macroglobulin

α_2-Macroglobulin is a major inhibitor reacting with many different proteases and may have a limited role as a plasmin inhibitor. If the fibrinolytic system has been extensively activated and a large amount of plasmin generated, AP cannot neutralize all of the plasmin produced. α_2-Macroglobulin will then operate as a second line of defense to inactivate remaining plasmin (see later section). Antithrombin, α_1-antitrypsin, and C1 inhibitor all have some antiplasmin activity *in vitro* but are probably of minimal significance in vivo.

> ℮ **CASE STUDY** *(continued from page 687)*
>
> 9. Does any evidence exist to indicate a problem with Shawn's fibrinolytic system?

► PHYSIOLOGIC CONTROL OF HEMOSTASIS

The dynamic process of fibrin formation is normally limited to the site of vascular injury. However, the fact that blood flows presents an extraordinary problem to the regulation of hemostasis. Activated factors and/or platelets must be kept at the site of injury. They must be controlled so they are inactive when distant from a site of vessel damage, so that even with intense activation of the hemostatic mechanism such as occurs in massive trauma, blood remains fluid in uninvolved vessels. The physiologic mechanisms responsible for controlling hemostasis include: control of blood flow, liver clearance, negative and positive feedback of activated clotting factors, and biochemical inhibitors (naturally occurring anticoagulants).

BLOOD FLOW

Vasoconstriction and activation of clotting factors are necessary for clot formation to begin. Initially, vessel constriction enhances clot formation by slowing blood flow through the injured vessel. As blood pools, creating an area of stasis, platelets and coagulation factors are brought in close proximity, promoting the initiation of primary and secondary hemostasis. Neither stasis alone nor the activation of coagulation factors in flowing blood will result in clot formation. The slowing down of blood flow by vasoconstriction of the injured vessel is an important initial step for adequate fibrin formation. Return to normal blood flow through an area of injury then serves to limit coagulation by continually diluting the concentration of activated factors.

LIVER CLEARANCE

The liver is the site of production of many of the clotting factors, making it a vital organ for normal hemostasis. Activated coagulation factors are removed from the circulation by the liver, as are plasmin and complexes of degraded fibrin (fibrin degradation products). Liver disease can result in hemorrhage due to decreased production of coagulation factors. It can also lead to systemic fibrinolysis or thrombosis.

POSITIVE FEEDBACK AMPLIFICATION

There are several positive feedback mechanisms in the hemostatic system. Some of the most important are: (1) thrombin, as a major activator of platelets, promotes the release of platelet factor Va and the exposure of negatively charged phospholipid surfaces used for assembly of protein coagulation complexes; (2) thrombin activates factors V and VIII; (3) factor Xa feeds back to activate factor VII; (4) factor Xa has limited ability to activate factor VIII in a reaction that may be important before significant quantities of thrombin are produced (Figure 35-14 ■).

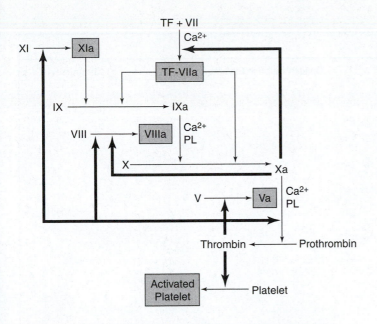

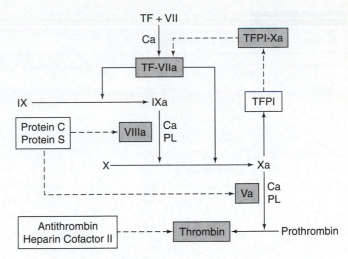

■ **FIGURE 35-14** Positive feedbacks in coagulation. Positive feedbacks are indicated by heavy arrows. Shaded boxes indicate targets. (Adapted, with permission, from: Beutler E, et al: *William's Hematology*. New York: McGraw-Hill; 1995)

■ **FIGURE 35-15** Major naturally occurring inhibitors of coagulation. Open boxes indicate inhibitors. Dashed lines show direction of inhibition. Shaded boxes indicate targets.

NEGATIVE FEEDBACK INHIBITION

Some of the activated factors have the potential to destroy other factors in the coagulation cascade. This process of feedback inhibition limits the production of the enzymes. Thrombin has the ability to activate factors V and VIII, but at higher concentrations it inactivates them. Factor Xa first enhances the activity of factor VII and then, through the action of tissue factor pathway inhibitor, is itself inactivated in a reaction that requires factor VIIa/TF. Clotting is also controlled indirectly by fibrin, the end product of the cascade. Fibrin has a strong affinity for thrombin. Once adsorbed onto the fibrin complex, thrombin is very slowly released, limiting the amount of thrombin available to cleave more fibrinogen to fibrin. In addition, fibrin degradation products produced by plasmin digestion function as inhibitors of fibrin formation by interfering with the conversion of fibrinogen to fibrin and the polymerization of fibrin monomers.

BIOCHEMICAL INHIBITORS

Naturally occurring inhibitors are soluble plasma proteins that regulate the enzymatic reactions of serine proteases. They prevent the initiation or amplification of the coagulation cascade (Table 35-5 ✿) (Figure 35-15 ■). The natural inhibitors include:

1. Antithrombin
2. Heparin cofactor II
3. Protein C
4. Protein S
5. Tissue factor pathway inhibitor
6. α_2-macroglobulin
7. α_1-antitrypsin
8. C1-inhibitor
9. Thrombin activatable fibrinolysis inhibitor (see under fibrinolysis)
10. α_2-antiplasmin (see under fibrinolysis)

Antithrombin, α_1-antitrypsin, heparin cofactor II, C1-inhibitor, and α_2-antiplasmin are all members of the serpin family of serine protease inhibitors. **Serpins** inhibit their target enzymes by formation of a covalent complex between the active site serine of the enzyme and the reactive center of the serpin. Conformational changes are induced in both molecules, trapping the enzyme within the serpin.

Antithrombin

Antithrombin (AT), (formerly called antithrombin III), is a member of the serpin family of serine protease inhibitors and can neutralize all the serine proteases including thrombin, XIIa, XIa, IXa, Xa, and kallikrein. It also inhibits plasmin. AT forms a 1:1 complex with each target protease, but the reaction is slow without heparin. Inhibition of its target proteases is accelerated three to four orders of magnitude by the cofactor heparin. Likewise, AT must be present for heparin to function as an anticoagulant.

Antithrombin is produced by endothelial cells, the liver, and possibly megakaryocytes. In vivo, heparin is located in the granules of mast cells and basophils, though under normal circumstances heparin is not released from mast cells into the circulation and cannot be detected in plasma. While only small amounts of naturally occurring heparin are found in the blood, vascular endothelium is rich in heparin-like molecules called heparan sulfate proteoglycans (HSPGs).

⊕ **TABLE 35-5**

Summary of Naturally Occurring Inhibitors

Component	Description	Function	Concentration in Plasma	t1/2	Chromosome
Protein C	Two-chain glycoprotein; MW 62,000	Serine protease: inactivates factors Va and VIIIa	2–6 μg/mL	8–10 hr	2
Protein S	Single-chain glycoprotein; MW 75,000	Cofactor for APC inhibition of factors Va & VIIIa	20–25 μg/mL	42 hr	3
Thrombomodulin	Transmembrane protein; MW 450,000	Cofactor/modulator: Endothelial cell receptor for thrombin; activates protein C when bound to thrombin; stimulates endothelial cells to release t-PA and EDRF	NA	–	–
Antithrombin	Single-chain glycoprotein MW 58,000	Proteinase inhibitor (SERPIN): inhibits thrombin, factors Xa, IXa XIa, XIIa, kallikrein plasmin, t-PA	125–290 μg/mL	61–72 hr	1
Heparin cofactor II	Glycoprotein MW 66,000	Proteinase inhibitor (SERPIN): inhibits thrombin	31–67 μg/mL	–	22
C1 esterase inhibitor	Single-chain glycoprotein MW 105,000	Proteinase inhibitor (SERPIN): inhibits kallikrein, plasmin, C1, factors XIIa, XIa	18 mg/dL	–	–
Protein C inhibitor (PAI-3)	Single-chain protein MW 57,000	Proteinase inhibitor (SERPIN): inhibits APC	5.3 μg/mL	23 days	–
α_1-antitrypsin (α_1-proteinase inhibitor)	Protein MW 55,000	Proteinase inhibitor (SERPIN): inhibits factor XIa, thrombin, kallikrein, plasmin, t-PA	1300 μg/mL	144 hr	–
Tissue factor pathway Inhibitor (TFPI)	MW 40,000	Proteinase inhibitor: inhibits factor VIIa and factor Xa	0.05–0.15 μg/mL	1–2 min	–
α_2-macroglobulin	Dimeric protein MW 725,000	Proteinase inhibitor: inhibits kallikrein, plasmin, thrombin, t-PA	2–5 μM	–	12

Key to abbreviations: SERPIN = serine protease inhibitor; t-PA = tissue plasminogen activator; MW = molecular weight in Daltons; APC = activated protein C; PAI = plasminogen activator inhibitor.

These endothelial-cell-associated proteins have heparan side chains with the correct carbohydrate sequences needed for AT recognition. Both thrombin and AT bind here and are brought close together. AT undergoes a conformational change, making its reactive site more accessible to the serine site of thrombin. The thrombin/AT complex then dissociates from the proteoglycan and the heparan sites are free to bind with other thrombin/AT molecules. Dermatan sulfate, another glycosaminoglycan located in the vessel wall, has little catalytic effect on AT but is a potent catalyst for heparin cofactor II (HC II).

As an anticoagulant, heparin molecules are structurally and functionally heterogeneous. In commercial preparations of heparin, less than one-third of the molecules have catalytic activity. Among naturally occurring heparin-like proteoglycans, less than 10% are active. The low-molecular-weight heparins (therapeutic antithrombotic agents) can inactivate factor Xa, but are less effective in inactivating thrombin. When the size of the heparin fraction decreases, the ratio of inactivation of factor Xa versus thrombin increases. This property serves to increase the half-life of thrombin in relation to factor Xa. When AT levels fall below

60% of normal, patients are unresponsive to antithrombotic therapy with heparin.

Heparin Cofactor II

Heparin cofactor II (HC II) inhibits thrombin but is inactive with other coagulation proteases. HC II bound to heparin potentiates the inhibition of thrombin by 1000×. Because the affinity of HC II for heparin is less than that of AT, a higher concentration of heparin is needed to accelerate its thrombin inhibition. It has been suggested that HC II may function as a second-line inhibitor of thrombin and that it may be involved in the inhibition of thrombin in extravascular locations. HC II may also play a role in protection from thrombosis during pregnancy.[30]

Protein C and Protein S

The protein C pathway is a major inhibitory mechanism involved in control of blood coagulation. Unlike the other inhibitory mechanisms directed at the proteases of the coagulation cascade, activated protein C inhibits two of the nonproteolytic regulatory cofactors of coagulation: cofactors Va and VIIIa.

Protein C and its cofactor, protein S, are vitamin K-dependent proteins synthesized in the liver. The protein C pathway is illustrated in Figure 35-16 ■.

As depicted in this scheme, thrombin is generated at the site of injury. Excess thrombin is carried downstream and binds to thrombomodulin on the EC surface. **Thrombo-** modulin is an integral membrane protein named for its ability to change the specificity of thrombin from a procoagulant to an anticoagulant. Thrombomodulin-bound thrombin has less ability to clot fibrinogen, to activate factor V, or to stimulate platelets.[31, 32] Binding appears to cause a conformational change in the thrombin molecule that allows it instead to rapidly activate protein C in the presence of Ca^{2+}. Activated protein C (APC) is released from the thrombin/thrombomodulin complex (T:TM) and inactivates factors Va and VIIIa. The zymogens, factors V and VIII, are resistant to the action of APC.

To function effectively, APC must interact with protein S, forming a 1:1 stoichiometric complex in the presence of Ca^{2+} and a phospholipid surface. Two forms of protein S circulate in the blood: (1) free protein and (2) protein that is noncovalently associated with C4b-binding protein (C4b-BP). The free form of protein S is the only effective cofactor for APC. When bound to a cell surface, the complex of protein C–protein S is capable of inactivating factors Va and VIIIa. The complex may also promote fibrinolysis by neutralizing plasminogen activator inhibitor.

An endothelial protein C receptor (EPCR) is found on the endothelial cells of larger vessels.[33] When EPCR binds protein C, it augments protein C activation by increasing the affinity of the T:TM complex for protein C.[34] When activated by the T:TM in the microcirculation, APC rapidly dissociates from the endothelial cells. It dissociates more slowly from the endothelium of larger vessels because of binding to EPCR. When bound to EPCR, APC is not capable of inactivating factor Va (and probably factor VIIIa) but can be inhibited by various proteinase inhibitors. When the APC dissociates from the EPCR, it can bind protein S and then inactivate FVa. It has been suggested that the EPCR/APC complex catalyzes cleavage of plasma or cellular substrates yet to be identified.[35]

APC is slowly neutralized by protein C inhibitor (PAI-3), α_1-antitrypsin, and α_2-macroglobulin. Protein C inhibitor is a serpin that has a procoagulant effect. Deficiency of either protein C or S results in severe thromboembolic disease. Patients have been described with normal amounts of protein C and S in their plasma, yet activation of protein C fails to prolong their clotting time. This abnormality (factor V Leiden), referred to as APC resistance, is due to a mutation in one of the cleavage sites of factor Va.[36] As a result, factor Va is not destroyed by APC, accounting for the inability of APC to prolong the clotting time in vitro, as well as the patient's thromboembolic tendency in vivo.

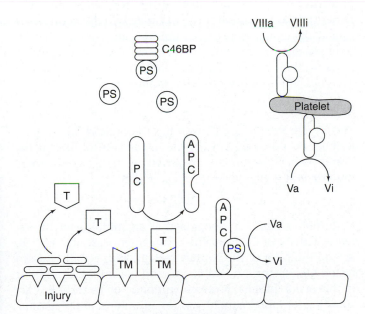

Vascular Endothelium

■ **FIGURE 35-16** Protein C pathway. Thrombin forms on the vessel wall at the site of injury. Thrombomodulin on the endothelial cell forms a complex with thrombin. This complex activates protein C, which then inactivates factors Va and VIIIa. (key: PC=protein C; PS=protein S; T=thrombin; TM=thrombomodulin; APC=activated protein C; C4bBP=complement binding protein)

Tissue Factor Pathway Inhibitor

Tissue factor pathway inhibitor, or TFPI (formerly called extrinsic pathway inhibitor, lipoprotein associated coagulation inhibitor, and antithromboplastin), inhibits the factor VIIa-tissue factor complex, suppressing the activity of the extrinsic pathway.

The endothelium is thought to be the major source of TFPI in vivo, although it has also been detected in megakaryocytes, macrophages, and the microglia of the brain. TFPI carried by platelets is released following stimulation with thrombin or other agonists.[37] The range of TFPI concentrations is broad among normal individuals. Plasma concentration of TFPI correlates with LDL levels because much of the circulating TFPI is bound to lipoproteins.[38]

TFPI is a potent inhibitor of factor Xa and the factor VIIa/TF complex and a modest inhibitor of plasmin. The inhibitor inactivates factor Xa by binding to the serine active site in 1:1 stoichiometry. This binding is not calcium dependent. The inhibition of factor VIIa/TF by TFPI involves the formation of a complex of VIIa-TF-Xa-TFPI after a small quantity of factor Xa has been formed (Figure 35-17 ■). This quaternary complex forms as the result of several binding steps. First, TFPI binds to factor Xa; second, this TFPI/Xa complex then binds to the membrane-bound factor VIIa/TF complex in a calcium-dependent reaction.[39]

TFPI has a novel mechanism of action. It acts as a Kunitz-type inhibitor, feigning to be a good substrate for the enzyme, but actually inducing slowing or cessation of enzyme activity after binding. Analysis of the structure of TFPI reveals the molecular basis for the capacity of the inhibitor to neutralize two proteases simultaneously. TFPI has three inhibitor domains: the first domain inhibits the factor VIIa/TF complex and the second directly inhibits factor Xa. The target of the third inhibitory domain is unknown.[40]

TFPI–induced feedback inhibition of the extrinsic pathway explains the need for both the extrinsic and intrinsic coagulation pathways. An advantage of this mechanism is that inhibition of factor VIIa is delayed until factor Xa is formed upon exposure of tissue factor to blood. Once factor Xa is produced, TFPI prevents continued activation of factor X by the factor VIIa/TF complex (as well as activation of fac-

tor IX by the factor VIIa/TF complex). This implies that further activation of factor X must occur through the intrinsic pathway by the factor IXa-VIIIa complex. While initial activation of factor Xa occurs via the extrinsic pathway, sustained activation requires activation of factor IXa via the intrinsic pathway.[41] This explains the bleeding associated with factor deficiencies of the intrinsic pathway. Even in the event of tissue damage and tissue factor generation, deficiencies of factors VIII or IX will not permit enough activation of factor X to maintain normal hemostasis.

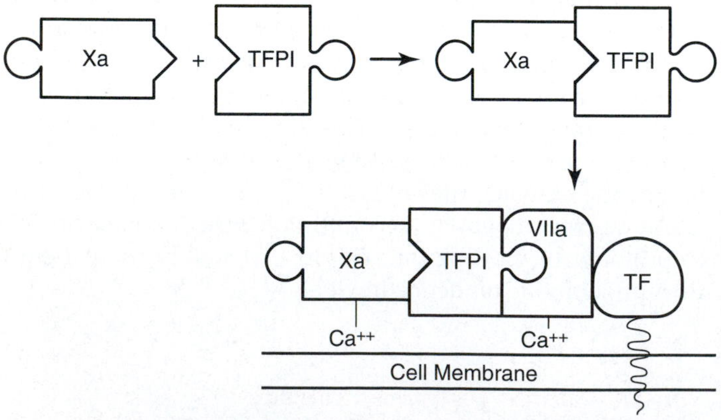

α_2-Macroglobulin

α_2-Macroglobulin is capable of inhibiting several serine proteases, including thrombin, factor Xa, plasmin, and kallikrein. The rate of inhibition is relatively slow when compared to other inhibitors, and enzymatic activity is not completely neutralized.

The glycoprotein α_2-macroglobulin is widely distributed in the body. Its concentration changes with age, with highest levels in infants and children. It also may appear elevated in pregnancy, in women using oral contraceptives, and in a number of other disorders. Following initial binding to the target enzyme, α_2-macroglobulin undergoes a conformational change essentially trapping the enzyme, preventing binding to its substrate. However, the catalytic site of the protease is left intact. For example, thrombin bound to α_2-macroglobulin can continue to slowly cleave fibrinogen to fibrin. This suggests that α_2-macroglobulin may function primarily as a clearance mechanism for serine proteases rather than as an inhibitor of enzymatic activity because the α_2-macroglobulin/protease complexes are rapidly cleared from plasma. On the other hand, α_2-macroglobulin is an important inhibitor of kallikrein, accounting for about 50% of the kallikrein inhibitory activity in plasma.

α_1-Antitrypsin

The glycoprotein α_1-antitrypsin has the capacity to inhibit a number of proteases, but its role in the control of coagulation is probably secondary. Its activity is thought to be more important at the tissue level.

C1-Inhibitor

C1-inhibitor was first recognized as an inhibitor of the esterase activity of C1 from the complement cascade. As well, it is an inhibitor of the contact system, with activity toward factor XIIa, factor IXa, kallikrein, and plasmin. C1-inhibitor is the major plasma protease inhibitor of factor XIIa, accounting for more than 90% of the inhibition in the plasma. C1-inhibitor binds to factor XIIa with 1:1 stoichiometry and irreversibly inactivates the enzyme.

■ **FIGURE 35-17** The inhibition of factor VIIa/TF by tissue factor pathway inhibitor (TFPI) occurs as the result of a multistep process. First, TFPI binds to factor Xa. This results in a conformational change of TFPI that promotes binding of the Xa/TFPI complex with the factor VIIa/TF complex in a calcium dependent reaction.

✔ **Checkpoint! #9**

Why are naturally occurring inhibitors important in the hemostatic mechanism?

CASE STUDY *(continued from page 694)*

10. Why were liver function tests done on Shawn?
11. What is the significance of normal results in a patient with hemostatic disease?

▶ THE PHYSIOLOGIC PATHWAY

While it has been traditional to divide the hemostatic mechanism into intrinsic and extrinsic pathways, it is now accepted that such a discrete division does not occur in vivo. Current thought is that tissue factor is the key initiator of coagulation in vivo (Figure 35-18 ■).

Tissue factor is not normally expressed on cells in contact with blood. It is found on the surface of a variety of cell types outside of the vasculature, so that upon injury, cells expressing tissue factor are exposed to the blood. TF then captures factor VII or factor VIIa with high affinity. Because TF is an integral membrane protein, the complex is anchored to the site of injury. Factor VIIa/TF then activates factor X to Xa and the common pathway continues. The extrinsic activation of factor X would seem to make the activation of factor X by the intrinsic Xase complex (factor IXa, factor VIIIa, PL, and Ca^{2+}) unnecessary, but clinical observations have demonstrated the absolute necessity of these factors for normal hemostasis. Patients with deficiencies of factor VIII and factor IX have major bleeding problems (hemophilia A and hemophilia B, respectively). Likewise patients with deficiencies of factors II, V, VII, and X have bleeding tendencies. It is obvious that the factors II, V, VII, VIII, IX, and X are all essential for hemostasis. The observation that factor VIIa/TF also activates factor IX to IXa has led to a revision of our concept of the clotting mechanism because it showed that extrinsic pathway activation could activate factor X through both pathways (Figure 35-18 ■).

The significance of the apparent duplication of activity was unclear until it was shown that the efficiency of activation of factor X by the factor IXa/factor VIIIa complex is significantly greater than the efficiency of the factor VIIa/TF complex alone. Likewise, the dependence on factor IXa/factor VIIIa is even stronger in the presence of TFPI, which inhibits the factor VIIa:TF complex. This unique enzyme (TFPI) requires that the system become activated (i.e., generation of factor Xa) be-

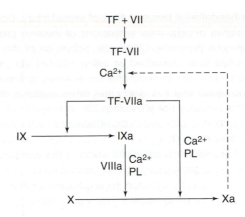

■ **FIGURE 35-18** Tissue factor initiation of the physiologic pathway by activation of factors IX and X. Dotted line indicates positive-feedback activation of TF-VII by Xa.

fore the inhibitor can work. This mechanism appears to allow soluble factor VIIa to survive in plasma in the absence of factor Xa/TFPI. Activation of factor X by factor VIIa/TF is insufficient to support hemostasis without the reinforcement of factor IXa/factor VIIIa activation of factor X.

These facts explain the observation that patients with hereditary deficiencies of factor XII, PK, and HK have a markedly prolonged PTT (which suggests an abnormality in the intrinsic pathway), but they do not have abnormal bleeding in vivo. Also, the fact that the factor VIIa/TF complex activates factor X *and* factor IX suggests a central role for factors VIII and IX in clotting initiated by the TF/extrinsic pathway and explains why a deficiency of either factor results in severe bleeding. Because a deficiency of factor XI is not always linked to a bleeding problem, the in vivo role of factor XI in hemostasis is uncertain.

CASE STUDY *(continued from page 699)*

A specific assay for factor VII activity was done on Shawn and both of his parents. The patient's factor VII activity was found to be 3% of that in normal plasma. Prothrombin and factor X activities were normal. The factor VII activity of the child's father and mother was 50% and 47%, respectively. (The normal range of factor VII activity is 70–120%.)

12. Do these findings explain the patient's bleeding history?

SUMMARY

The hemostatic mechanism functions to keep blood fluid within the vasculature and to prevent excessive blood loss upon vascular injury. Platelets, vascular endothelial cells, and numerous coagulation proteins interact to maintain a balance between bleeding and clotting in vivo. Primary hemostasis occurs through activation of platelets and results in the formation of an unstable platelet plug. This is subsequently reinforced by the formation of fibrin (coagula-tion), resulting in stabilization of the platelet plug, or secondary hemostasis.

The process of fibrin formation is a carefully controlled process, limited to areas of damage within the vascular network. Localization of the response to the site of injury prevents widespread coagulation activation. Activation of the coagulation system occurs on phospholipid membrane surfaces (activated platelets) or on

■ **CHECKLIST - LEVEL II** *(continued)*

8. Explain the biochemical mechanism of the effect of aspirin on platelet function and recommend a time frame for patients to refrain from taking aspirin and related anti-inflammatory drugs prior to platelet function testing.

9. Summarize the effect of aspirin, alcohol, and antibiotics on platelet function.

KEY TERMS

Bernard-Soulier disease
δ-storage pool disease
Ecchymoses
Epistaxis
Glanzmann's thrombasthenia
Gray platelet syndrome
Hematoma
Heparin induced thrombocytopenia (HIT)
Idiopathic (immune) thrombocytopenic purpura (ITP)
Ischemia
Necrosis
Neonatal alloimmune thrombocytopenia (NAIT)
Nonthrombocytopenic purpura
Petechiae
Primary thrombocytosis
Purpura
Secondary (reactive) thrombocytosis
Thrombotic thrombocytopenic purpura (TTP)
Vasculitis

BACKGROUND BASICS

The information in this chapter will build on the concepts learned in previous chapters. To maximize your learning experience you should review these concepts before starting this unit of study.

Level I

▶ Hemostasis: Describe how a blood clot forms after an injury, especially the role of platelets in cessation of bleeding. (Chapter 34).

▶ Immunology: Define/describe: antigen/antibody reactions, classes of immunoglobulins, the process of immune complex formation. (Chapter 6)

▶ Immune hemolytic anemia: Summarize the pathophysiology of the immune hemolytic anemias. (Chapter 19)

▶ Laboratory methods: Correlate the automated platelet count with the platelet count estimate on a peripheral blood smear. (Chapters 8 and 42)

▶ Laboratory methods: Identify artifacts that can cause spuriously increased or decreased automated platelet counts. (Chapters 8 and 42)

Level II

▶ Hemostasis: Correlate the functions of the blood vessels, platelets, and coagulation factors in forming a blood clot. (Chapters 34 and 35)

▶ Neoplastic leukocyte disorders: Summarize the consequences of malignant diseases of the bone marrow, particularly as they relate to the production of platelets. (Chapters 26–31)

▶ Cytokines: Describe how the bone marrow utilizes cytokines and growth factors to produce blood cells. (Chapter 2)

▶ Flow cytometry: Recognize and correctly utilize the CD nomenclature of cellular antigens. (Chapter 23)

CASE STUDY

We will address this case study throughout the chapter.
Mohammed, a 15-year-old male from Saudi Arabia, was admitted to the emergency room after an automobile accident with several superficial cuts and bruises to the head and arms. He was bleeding profusely but seemed to have more severe bleeding than would be expected from the nature of his wounds. Consider possible causes of this abnormal bleeding and the laboratory tests that might be used to differentiate and diagnose the cause.

▶ OVERVIEW

This chapter is the first of two that will describe abnormalities of the hemostatic system that result primarily in bleeding. It begins with a discussion of general clinical and laboratory aspects of hemostatic disorders. Following the general topics, defects in primary hemostasis, including the vascular system and platelets will be discussed. For each defect, the pathophysiologic basis and the clinical manifestations will be presented, but the major emphasis will be on the laboratory involvement in the diagnosis and/or treatment of the conditions. It is important to identify the cause so that appropriate treatment or prevention practices can be implemented.

▶ INTRODUCTION

As you have seen in ∞ Chapters 34 and 35, hemostasis functions to minimize the amount of blood lost from a disruptive injury to the blood vessels and to prevent blood from leaking out of intact vessels. The hemostatic system includes vasoconstriction of the blood vessels, primary hemostatic plug formation by the platelets, fibrin formation by soluble plasma proteins, and inhibitors that prevent inappropriate clot formation and allow the system to become active only when and where it is needed. Adequate hemostasis is dependent on a large number of intricately balanced mechanisms. Abnormalities of one or more components in the process of clot formation (i.e., the blood vessels, the platelets, or the clotting factors) can lead to excessive bleeding. Failure in the regulation of excessive clot formation leads to thrombosis.

▶ DIAGNOSIS OF BLEEDING DISORDERS

CLINICAL MANIFESTATIONS OF BLEEDING DISORDERS

A patient with a clinically significant bleeding disorder will present to the physician with hemorrhagic symptoms. Bleeding symptoms range from the presence of more bruises than usual to hemorrhaging that is life threatening. The severity of the bleed is generally in proportion to the severity and to the type of defect.

The type of bleeding may indicate which aspect of the hemostatic mechanism is defective. A defect in a component of primary hemostasis usually results in bleeding from the skin or mucous membranes such as the nose. Bleeding symptoms in patients with coagulation factor abnormalities, on the other hand, are usually internal, into deeper tissues and joints.

Bleeding from subcutaneous blood vessels (capillaries) into intact skin may be visualized as petechiae, ecchmyoses, or hematomas (Figure 36-1 ■). **Petechiae** are small red to purple spots in the skin, less than 3 mm in diameter. They result from blood leaking through the intact endothelial lining of capillaries. Petechiae usually occur on the extremities because of the high venous pressure. When they arise spontaneously without trauma, they are painless. Several petechiae in one area may merge into a larger bruised area. Petechial lesions are characteristic of abnormalities of platelets and blood vessels and usually are not seen in coagulation factor disorders.

Ecchymoses are bruises that are larger than 3 mm in diameter and also are caused by blood escaping through endothelium and into intact subcutaneous tissue, perhaps from a vessel larger than a capillary. They are red or purple when first formed and become yellowish green as they heal. Ecchymoses may appear spontaneously or with trauma, and may be painful and tender. They may occur when there are abnormalities of blood vessels, platelets, or coagulation factors.

A bruise is called a **hematoma** when blood leaks from an opening in a vessel and collects beneath intact skin. It is blue or purple and slightly raised. Hematomas can occur in any organ or tissue and may be in the form of a clot.

The word **purpura,** meaning purple, is used ambiguously but generally refers to both petechiae and ecchymoses. Purpura is also used as part of the name of diseases in which these typical symptoms occur.

When ecchymoses and petechiae are found in greater than normal numbers and with less than usual trauma, the condition is termed *easy bruisability.* Another term used often in describing clinical manifestations of bleeding disorders is *excess bleeding.* Excess bleeding from superficial cuts and scratches occurs when platelets fail to form an effective primary hemostatic plug. Excess bleeding means that the bleeding occurs for a longer time and is more profuse than normal for the patient or compared with a normal person. Blood may escape from visceral organs into any body cavity or from mucous membranes into any body orifice. Frank bleeding is characteristic of both platelet and coagulation abnormalities.

PHYSICIAN'S EVALUATION OF A PATIENT WITH ABNORMAL BLEEDING

Excessive bleeding may be caused by a local disruption of the vasculature such as a bleeding ulcer or by a generalized failure of the hemostatic mechanism. In some cases both may be present, and then the local problem is compounded. It is the physician's responsibility to determine the cause of the bleeding and to prescribe proper treatment. This is done by obtaining an accurate medical history, performing a thorough physical examination, and ordering and interpreting the results of appropriate laboratory tests.

Questions in several categories are included in the patient's history:

- Age of onset
- Type of symptoms
- Family history

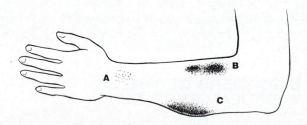

■ **FIGURE 36-1** Schematic drawing of bleeding manifestations in intact skin. a. petechiae; b. ecchymosis; c. hematoma.

- Other diseases
- Drug history
- Exposure to toxins

The answers should enable the physician to decide if a bleeding disorder exists and help define the affected portion of the hemostatic system. The first category concerns the age at which symptoms first began. Occurrence at or shortly after birth indicates an inherited disorder, although onset later in life does not rule this out. Bleeding from the umbilical cord and circumcision suggest coagulation factor defects.

A second category concerns the persistence and severity of the symptoms, which may be revealed by inquiring if the symptoms have continued throughout life, have occurred as a single event, or have been intermittent. Bleeding in excess of that expected from a tonsillectomy, tooth extraction, trauma, injury, surgery, or childbirth may provide clues.

The family history is helpful to determine if other family members have similar symptoms. A pedigree analysis may determine the type of inheritance. Patients with inherited abnormalities do not always have a positive family history, however, because spontaneous mutations occur in several of the hemostatic disorders.

The presence of associated disease such as malignancy, aplastic anemia, leukemia, uremia, liver disease, or infections must be excluded. These conditions may be associated with secondary platelet disorders and/or coagulation defects.

A history of drug therapy is important to consider. Many drugs are known to affect the hemostatic mechanism and different drugs affect different portions of the system. Aspirin, chemotherapeutic drugs for malignancies, and coumarin anticoagulants are examples, but there are many others. The reader is referred to other texts that provide extensive lists of specific drugs that have been implicated in acquired hemostatic defects.[1,2]

Finally, past or present exposure to toxic chemicals such as benzene, insect sprays, or hair dyes should be investigated.

On physical examination, the type and sites of bleeding will be noted, as well as whether the bleeding is from single or multiple sites and whether it is spontaneous or the result of trauma. Using the information from the history and physical examination, the physician will order appropriate laboratory tests to confirm and classify the presence of abnormal hemostasis.

LABORATORY EVALUATION OF ABNORMAL BLEEDING

No individual laboratory test can fully evaluate defective hemostasis, so initially a battery or group of screening tests is usually ordered. Based on the results of these tests, the physician can determine if a detectable abnormality of hemostasis does exist and order the confirmatory tests necessary to define the disorder. Minimal screening tests include:

- Platelet count
- Prothrombin time (PT)
- Activated partial thromboplastin time (APTT).

The results of one or more of these tests will be abnormal in most patients with hemostatic disorders, and they will usually be within the reference ranges if the patient does not have a defect in the hemostatic system. In patients with disorders of primary hemostasis, the PT and APTT are usually normal and the platelet count may or may not be abnormal.

When the history warrants and results of these screening tests are normal, a vascular disorder or functional platelet defect is likely. Confirmatory tests of platelet function may then be ordered. These include the bleeding time, the closure time, platelet aggregation tests, and flow cytometry for platelet function. In the absence of abnormal results of platelet function testing, the physician may investigate the possibility of a vascular disorder.

If the PT and/or the APTT are abnormal, a coagulation factor disorder is indicated (∞ Chapter 37). A wide range of confirmatory testing is available to specify the diagnosis (∞ Chapter 39).

In some patients with mild disease, the screening tests will not be sensitive enough to detect an abnormality. Other patients may have conditions that do not affect the screening tests. In such cases, a knowledgeable physician in the field of bleeding disorders may direct the clinical investigation using the information of the clinical history and physical examination.

Remembering that laboratory testing for the hemostatic system consists of a number of tests, each of which tells the story of a specific part of the hemostatic system, it is important for a clinical laboratorian to correlate and understand the significance of the results of all hemostasis tests and to correlate the results with the patient's condition. In this way you can be watchful for results that might be in error, justify your results if they are questioned, or recommend additional testing procedures to a physician.

 Checkpoint! #1

Assume that you are the clinical laboratory scientist collecting a blood specimen from a patient with a suspected bleeding disorder. You noticed petechiae and several bruises on the patient's arm. What screening tests would the physician likely have ordered? What results of these tests would you expect (normal or abnormal) in this patient?

▶ DISORDERS OF THE VASCULAR SYSTEM

Since the blood vessels are actively involved in hemostasis in a variety of ways (∞ Chapter 34), a structural abnormality or damage to either the endothelial lining of blood vessels or to

✪ TABLE 36-1

Characteristics of Inherited Disorders of the Vascular System

Disorder	Gene	Effect	Chromosome	Laboratory Findings
Hereditary hemorrhagic telangiectasia	Endoglin	Abnormal transforming growth factor-β	9q and 12q	Normal
Ehlers-Danlos syndromes	Multiple collagen genes	Fragility of blood vessels	Multiple	BT* Increased
Marfan syndrome	Fibrillin-1	Decreased strength and elasticity of blood vessels	15	BT* Increased
Osteogenesis imperfecta	Type I procollagen (COLA1 & 2)	Patchy, defective bone matrix	2	Not significant
Pseudoxanthoma elasticum	Unknown	Calcification of vessels	Unknown	Not significant

* BT=Bleeding time

subendothelial structures may result from, or lead to, a variety of clinical manifestations and disease conditions. These disorders can be either inherited or acquired secondary to another condition. The hereditary vascular diseases are caused by abnormal synthesis of subendothelial connective tissue components[3–8] (Table 36-1 ✪). Acquired vascular disorders are caused either by abnormal subendothelium or by altered endothelial cells (Table 36-2 ✪).

Symptoms seen in vascular disorders are, for the most part, of the superficial type, such as easy bruising, petechiae, or lesions that mimic them but are actually not caused by bleeding. Bleeding in the congenital vascular diseases is usually external, resulting from tears in the skin. Bleeding in the acquired disorders is usually from breaks in the blood vessels into intact skin, resulting in easy bruising and petechiae.

✪ TABLE 36-2

Classification of Acquired Disorders of the Vascular System

Purpura due to decreased connective tissue
    Senile purpura
    Cushing syndrome and corticosteroid therapy
    Scurvy
Purpura associated with paraprotein disorders
    Paraproteins
    Amyloidosis
Purpura due to vasculitis
    Henoch-Schönlein purpura
    Infections
    Drugs
Miscellaneous causes of purpura
    Mechanical purpura
    Artificially induced purpura
    Easy bruising syndrome
    Purpura fulminans

The diagnosis of blood vessel disorders is most often made by exclusion. That is, by finding no positive evidence for a disorder of platelets, coagulation factors, or fibrinolysis in a patient who has bleeding symptoms. The platelet count and screening tests for coagulation factors are usually normal in blood vessel disorders. A template bleeding time and other platelet function testing are also usually normal, but may be prolonged in some vascular disease states.

When platelets are normal in number, purpura are considered to be caused by damage to the blood vessels and the condition is called **nonthrombocytopenic purpura.**

HEREDITARY DISORDERS OF THE VASCULAR SYSTEM

The hereditary disorders of the vascular system are summarized in Table 36-1 ✪. They are very rare, and while bleeding is a common symptom, hemostasis tests are not necessary for diagnosis. A more complete description of these disorders is available on this text's companion Web site.

ACQUIRED DISORDERS OF THE VASCULAR SYSTEM

Acquired disorders of the vascular system are seen quite often and are characterized by bruising and petechiae. Defects of either the vessel wall or the endothelial cells may be caused by conditions that decrease the supportive connective tissue in blood vessel walls, infections or allergic conditions, the presence of abnormal proteins in the vascular tissues, or mechanical stress. The acquired disorders of the vasculature are shown in Table 36-2 ✪.

Purpura Due to Decreased Connective Tissue

The diseases in this category are due to a decreased amount of supportive connective tissue in the blood vessel walls.

Rodgers GM, eds. In: *Wintrobe's Clinical Hematology,* 10th ed. Baltimore: Williams & Wilkins; 1999:1579–1613.

12. Bussel JB, Schreiber AD. Immunothrombocytopenic purpura, neonatal alloimmune thrombocytopenia, and post transfusion purpura. Hoffman R, Benz EJ Jr, Shattil SJ, Furie HJ, Cohen HJ, eds. In: *Hematology: Basic Principles and Practice,* New York: Churchill Livingstone; 1991:1485–94.

13. George JN, Woolf SH, Raskob GE, et al. Idiopathic thrombocyotopenic purpura: A practice guideline developed by explicit methods for the American Society of Hematology. *Blood.* 1996; 88:3–40.

14. Davis, GL. Quantitative and qualitative disorders of platelets. Steine-Martin EA, Lotspeich-Steininger CA, Koepke JA, eds. In: *Clinical Hematology: Principles, Procedures, Correlations,* 2nd ed., Philadelphia: Lippincott; 1998:717–34.

15. Ware RE and Zimmerman SA. Anti-D: Mechanisms of action. *Semin Hemat.* 1998; 35:14–22.

16. Tarantino MD, Goldsmith G. Treatment of immune thrombocytopenia. *Semin Hemat.* 1998; 35:28–35.

17. George JN and Raskob GE. Idiopathic thrombocytopenic purpura: A concise summary of pathophysiology and diagnosis in children and adults. *Semin Hemat.* 1998; 35:5–8.

18. McCrae KR, Samuels P, Schreiber AD. Pregnancy associated thrombocytopenia: Pathogenesis and management. *Blood.* 1992; 80:2697–2714.

19. Kelton JG. The serological investigation of patients with autoimmune thrombocytopenia. *Thromb Haemost.* 1995; 74:228–33.

20. Warkentin TE. Heparin-induced thrombocytopenia: A ten-year retrospective. *Annu Rev Med.* 1999; 50:129–47.

21. Levine SP. Miscellaneous causes of thrombocytopenia. Lee GR, Foerster J, Lukens J, Paraskevas F, Greer JP, Rodgers GM, eds. In: *Win-trobe's Clinical Hematology,* 10th ed. Baltimore: Williams & Wilkins; 1999:1623–32.

22. Woodman RC, Harker LA. Bleeding complications associated with cardiopulmonary bypass. *Blood.* 1990; 76:1680–97.

23. Hoffman R, Silberstein MN, Hromas R. Primary thrombocythemia. Hoffman R, Benz EJ Jr, Shattil SJ, Furie B, Cohen HJ, Silberstein LE. In: *Hematology: Basic Principles and Practice,* 2nd ed. New York: Churchill Livingstone; 1995:1174–84.

24. Levine SP. Thrombocytosis. Lee GR, Foerster J, Lukens J, Paraskevas F, Greer JP, Rodgers GM, eds. In: *Wintrobe's Clinical Hematology,* 10th ed. Baltimore: Williams & Wilkins; 1999:1648–60.

25. Evans VJ. Platelet morphology and the blood smear. *J Med Tech.* 1984; 1:689–95.

26. Lopez JA, Andrew RK, Afshar-Karghan V, Berndt MC. Bernard-Soulier syndrome. *Blood.* 1998; 91:4397–418.

27. Fausett B, Silver RM. Congenital disorders of platelet dysfunction. *Clin Obstet Gynecol.* 1999; 42:390–405.

28. Coller BS. Hereditary qualitative platelet defects. Beutler E, Lichtman MA, Coller BS, Kipps TJ, eds. In: *William's Hematology,* 5th ed. New York: McGraw-Hill; 1995:1364–85.

29. Bennett JS. Hereditary disorders of platelet function. Hoffman R, Benz EJ Jr, Shattil SJ, Furie B, Cohen HJ, Silberstein LE. In: *Hematology: Basic Principles and Practice,* 2nd ed. New York: Churchill Livingstone; 1995:1909–25.

30. Weiss HJ. Scott syndrome: A disorder of platelet coagulant activity. *Semin Hemat.* 1994; 31:312–19.

31. Nurden, AT. Inherited abnormalities of platelets. *Thromb Haemost.* 1999; 82:468–80.

32. Rinder HM. Platelet function testing by flow cytometry. *Clin Lab Sci.* 1998; 11:365–72.

■ CHECKLIST - LEVEL II (continued)

5. Select laboratory tests and identify clinical symptoms t ease, deficiencies of factors VIII and IX, Bernard-Souli basthenia.

6. Select and interpret the results of the laboratory tests f tors VIII and IX.

7. Describe the pathophysiology of the conditions that re hemostatic system and select confirmatory laboratory p

8. Select and describe the laboratory screening methods cies and inhibitors of hemostatic proteins.

9. Describe the significance and clinical implications of th agulants and select laboratory procedures that confirm factor inhibitors and nonspecific factor inhibitors.

10. Compare and contrast the clinical and laboratory findir cular coagulation with those found in thrombotic throm uremic syndrome.

11. Choose laboratory methods that would differentiate be ondary fibrinolysis and support your selection.

KEY TERMS:

Acquired inhibitors (circulating anticoagulants)
Afibrinogenemia
Anticardiolipin antibodies (ACA)
Consumption coagulopathy
CRM+
CRM−
Disseminated intravascular coagulation (DIC)
Dysfibrinogenemia
Hemophilia A
Hemophilia B
Hemorrhagic disease of the newborn
Hypofibrinogenemia
Lupus anticoagulant (LA)
Platelet-type-pseudo-VWD
Primary fibrinogenolysis
Ristocetin induced platelet agglutination (RIPA)
vWf multimers
vWf: ristocetin cofactor activity (vWf:RCoF)
von Willebrand disease (VWD)
von Willebrand factor antigen (vWf:Ag)

▶ OVERVIEW

This chapter will discuss disorders of clotting factors tha sult in excess bleeding. Deficiencies of most of the fi forming proteins are included in this category, as wel

✪ TABLE 37-1

Bleeding Characteristics in Disorders of Secondary Hemostasis

Symptoms typical of secondary hemostatic disorders
- Delayed bleeding
- Deep muscular bleeding
- Spontaneous joint bleeding

Symptoms common to primary and secondary hemostatic disorders

Ecchymoses	Gingival (gums) bleeding
Gastrointestinal bleeding	Increased bleeding after tooth extraction
Hematuria	Intracranial bleeding
Hypermenorrhea	Epistaxis

on how the clot-forming proteins function, and they do not differentiate qualitative from quantitative defects. A functionally defective coagulation factor will prolong the clotting screening test but may still be recognized by immunologically based procedures in the laboratory. Individuals who have these functionally defective factors that can be detected immunologically are said to be positive for cross-reacting material **(CRM+)**. Patients in whom the clotting factor is decreased both functionally and immunologically are negative for cross-reacting material **(CRM−)** (Web Figure 37-1 ■).

Clinical bleeding symptoms in patients with coagulation factor deficiencies differ from those seen in platelet defects (Table 37-1 ✪). These patients bleed from the rupture of small arterioles rather than from capillaries. The sites of bleeds are into deep muscular tissues and joints rather than the superficial areas seen in platelet disorders. Hematomas are common and can be massive. Patients also experience delayed bleeding from cuts. Patients with coagulation factor defects usually have normal platelets. Therefore, a typical primary hemostatic plug is formed after a superficial cut, which initially arrests the blood flow, and the cut stops bleeding. Delayed bleeding occurs because, in the absence of stabilization with fibrin formation, the plug dislodges and the cut begins to bleed again at a later time. The second bleed will usually continue for a longer time, with the loss of a greater quantity of blood.

Patients with coagulation factor deficiencies may experience ecchymoses, excess bleeding from traumatic injuries, or bleeding from the body sites listed in Table 37-1 ✪. Some of these symptoms are also seen in patients with platelet disorders. Retroperitoneal bleeding and hematuria also are common, while petechiae are not usually seen in disorders of secondary hemostasis.

The physician's evaluation and laboratory investigation of a bleeding patient proceeds as described in ∞ Chapter 36. The battery of screening tests will usually show a normal platelet count, but the PT, the APTT, or both will be prolonged (Table 37-2 ✪). The thrombin clotting time may be abnormal in disorders of fibrinogen. When the history and results of the screening tests indicate, additional testing to

tory tests described previously.[10] In this scheme there are three major categories: types 1, 2, and 3. The three major categories depend on whether the patient has a quantitative or a qualitative defect and, in the case of quantitative defects, the extent of the quantitative deficiency. Types 1 and 3 VWD are both quantitative deficiencies of vWf. Type 1, the most common type, is a mild form of VWD in which patients have a partial deficiency of vWf. This is known as the classic type. Type 3 patients have an absolute absence of vWf in platelets and plasma (a severe form of the disease). Type 2 patients have qualitatively abnormal vWf of various kinds.[11] The structure of a vWf protein with sites of mutations is depicted in Figure 37-2. Some characteristics of the vWf types are shown in Table 37-4 . These subtypes are discussed in more detail on the text's companion Web site. Table 37-5 ✪ summarizes laboratory test results in all types and subtypes of VWD.

✓ Checkpoint! #1

A. Why do patients with type 1 VWD have 25–50% of vWf in their plasma?

B. Why do they have a corresponding decrease in factor VIII in their plasma?

Two additional forms of VWD are **platelet-type-pseudo-VWD** and acquired von Willebrand syndrome. These conditions are not VWD because, while clinical bleeding symptoms and laboratory test results are similar to those in VWD, they are not caused by mutations in the vWf gene.

Pseudo-VWD is a platelet disorder that results in increased affinity of the platelet GPIb/IX receptor for vWf. It is similar to VWD type 2B, but in pseudo-VWD, the defect is in the platelet receptor for vWf, usually resulting in increased binding of the larger multimers of plasma vWf to platelet GPIb. This results

in a decrease of large vWf multimers and factor VIII in the plasma. In addition, GPIIb/IIIa receptors are exposed and platelets aggregate, resulting in thrombocytopenia.

Acquired VWD syndrome is called a syndrome rather than a disease because it is not caused by vWf mutations. Acquired VWD is very rare and has been reported in fewer than 100 patients. It is associated primarily with lymphoproliferative diseases such as multiple myeloma, lymphoma, or chronic lymphocytic leukemia. The pathogenic mechanism of acquired VWD varies from patient to patient. Acquired VWD is diagnosed with the same laboratory tests used for inherited VWD: factor VIII coagulant activity, vWf:Ag, and vWf:RCoF. There is, however, no way to distinguish inherited from acquired VWD by laboratory tests. The diagnosis is based on a clinical history of no prior bleeding problems in the patient or family and the presence of a disease that is associated with acquired VWD.[12]

Prenatal Diagnosis.   Prenatal diagnosis of VWD is available but is usually reserved for patients with severe types of the disease. Type 2 is easily identified prenatally by PCR techniques, while diagnosis of type 3 is more difficult.[3]

Therapy.   Patients with mild VWD who are not experiencing clinical bleeding do not require therapy. For patients who are actively bleeding, several preparations are available to raise the level of vWf in the plasma of VWD patients. The classic treatment for VWD is to inject cryoprecipitate preparations that contain all molecular forms of vWf including the large multimer forms. The precipitate contains factor VIII and fibrinogen in addition to vWf. A drawback is that cryoprecipitate cannot be treated to inactivate blood borne viruses and, therefore, carries a risk of transmission of blood borne disease.

The current preferred method of treatment is a modified antidiuretic hormone, deamino-D-vasopressin (DDAVP), which was found to induce endothelial cells to release vWf

---

✪ TABLE 37-4

Description of von Willebrand Disease (VWD) Subtypes

Type	Description	% of VWD	Mutation Sites
1	Partial quantitative deficiency with normal structure and function of the multimers	70–80	Multiple
2	Qualitative disorder with functionally abnormal vWf		
2A	Decreased platelet adhesion because of absence of largest multimers	10–15	A2—either defective synthesis of largest (qualitative deficiency) multimers or increased loss A1, D2
2B	Increased affinity for platelet GPIb and absence of largest multimers	<5	A1
2M	Decreased platelet adhesion via GPIb/IX but not because of absence of largest multimers	Rare	A1
2N	Decreased affinity for factor VIII (autosomal recessive)	Rare	D', part of D3
3	Absence of vWf in platelets and plasma	0.5–5 per million	Varied 64% characterized

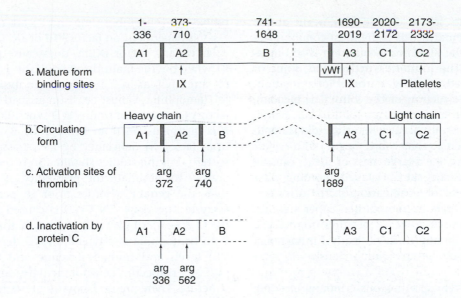

■ **FIGURE 37-3** Schematic diagram depicting factor VIII. **a.** The mature protein with domains A1, A2, B, A3, C1, and C2. Grayed areas are regions containing acidic amino acids. **b.** The circulating form of factor VIII with variable portions of the B domain removed and attached to vWf at the acidic region preceeding domain A3. **c.** Sites of activation by thrombin at Arg residues 372, 740, and 1689. The heavy chain is split, forming a 3-chain structure, and factor VIII is removed from vWf. **d.** Sites of proteolytic inactivation of factor VIII by activated protein C (APC) at Arg 336 and Arg 562. (Key: Arg = arginine)

mutation occurs in all members of a family, resulting in a similar clinical expression of disease in affected members of the family.

Factor IX Mutations Factor IX deficiency, or hemophilia B, is also known as Christmas disease (*Christmas* was the surname of an affected family first reported). Heterogeneous mutations in the factor IX gene or its regulatory components result in hemophilia B. A database of mutations worldwide is available at **<www.umds.ac.uk/molgen>**, and includes over 600 mutations in 1918 patients.[18,19] Point mutations (mis-sense and nonsense) account for 95% of the abnormalities. Other abnormalities include deletions of various portions of the gene and insertions. The clinical severity depends on the type of mutation and the region of the gene affected. Some factor IX deficient patients are CRM–, approximately one-third are CRM+, and some have reduced levels of antigen (CRMR). CRM+ hemophilia B patients have a mutation in the structural gene resulting in production of an abnormal molecule. These patients have normal levels of factor IX antigen and variably reduced levels of factor IX activity. Patients who are CRM– may have large deletions of the gene and are at risk for developing inhibitors and anaphylactic reactions to replacement therapy.

Clinical Aspects of the Hemophilias Clinical manifestations of hemophilia vary with the amount of factor present and are classified as severe, moderate, or mild disease

(Table 37-7 ✪). The variation in clinical symptoms is largely the result of the type and site of the mutation (e.g., factor VIII deficient patients who have mutations at the thrombin-cleavage sites of factor VIII are unable to activate it, or patients with the inversion mutation have no factor VIII activity and severe bleeding symptoms).

✪ **TABLE 37-7**

Clinical Findings in Deficiencies of Factors VIII and IX

Factor VIII or IX Level, U/dL	Severity	Symptoms
0–1	Severe	Frequent spontaneous hemarthrosis with crippling
		Frequent severe, spontaneous hemorrhage (intracranial, intramuscular)
2–5	Moderate	Bleeding at circumcision
		Infrequent spontaneous joint and tissue bleeds
		Profuse bleeding after surgery or trauma
		Serious bleeding from minor injuries
6–30	Mild	Rare spontaneous bleeds
		Profuse bleeding after surgery or trauma
		May not be discovered until bleeding episode occurs

Clinical symptoms in severe disease may begin at the time of circumcision. Hemarthrosis is the most common feature of severe hemophilia. Bleeding into a joint is accompanied by intense pain. The joint fills with blood, some of which is not reabsorbed, causing chronic inflammation, pain, and eventually destruction of the joint. The bleeding may be triggered by even minor trauma. Joint bleeds, particularly into the knee, generally occur when the child starts to walk. Subcutaneous hematomas may begin with slight trauma and spread to involve a large mass of tissue, causing purple discoloration of the skin. Delayed bleeding after minor cuts, characteristic of coagulation factor disorders, may be seen. Epistaxis is rare in hemophilia. Other manifestations include hematuria and excess bleeding from dental extractions. The most common cause of death is intracranial hemorrhage, which may occur spontaneously or after trauma.

Hemarthrosis and severe spontaneous crippling bleeding into muscles are usually found in severe disease. These symptoms are not seen in those with moderate or mild severity. More characteristic of moderate hemophilia is excessive bleeding after traumatic injury. Mild deficiencies of factor VIII or IX may be symptomless and unsuspected until a surgical procedure or major traumatic injury results in severe bleeding. While the site of bleeding varies from individual to individual, the clinical severity of deficiencies of both factors remains similar within families.

Laboratory Evaluation of the Hemophilias Laboratory tests are required to screen for abnormalities of coagulation factors and then to confirm and quantitate the specific factor that is deficient (∞ Chapter 39). Screening tests (APTT) are expressed as time, usually in seconds. Confirmatory assays are expressed in units of activity. Normal plasma is considered to have 1 unit (U) per mL of activity, or 100 units (U) per dL.

Table 37-2 ✪ shows the results of screening tests in a variety of hemostatic disorders. The APTT is prolonged in both factor VIII and IX deficiencies. The APTT is lengthened inversely to the level of factor present in the patient's plasma, when the level is below the sensitivity of the testing methodology. Levels of 20 U/dL or less of factor IX and 30 U/dL of factor VIII will consistently prolong the APTT.

Definitive diagnosis is made on the basis of the results of specific factor assays. Precautions to be used in interpreting results include: (1) factor VIII levels are lower in persons with blood group O than other blood groups (corresponding to the level of vWf) so the blood type must be considered when diagnosing factor VIII deficiency; (2) screening test systems may not be sensitive enough to detect mild deficiencies at levels between 20 and 50 U/dL. In these cases, the physician may order a factor assay on the basis of the patient's history.

The results of additional laboratory tests are shown in Table 37-3 ✪ and are compared with the results in type 1 VWD. All platelet testing results are normal in the hemophilias. The thrombin time and PT are normal since neither assay is dependent on factor VIII or IX. One abnormal molecular variant, factor IXBm, does cause prolongation of the PT when bovine brain thromboplastin is used instead of rabbit thromboplastin.[20] Tests for fibrinolysis also are normal.

Hemophilia A must be distinguished from deficiencies of factors IX or XI and from VWD types 2N and 3. Hemophilia A is distinguished from hemophilia B by factor assays and from factor XI deficiency by factor assays and inheritance pattern. Mixing studies should also be performed in the laboratory to eliminate the possibility of an inhibitor rather than the genetic disorder prior to performing the factor assay testing. Type 2N VWD is caused by abnormalities of the D' domain of vWf that prevent factor VIII from binding.[3] Both hemophilia and type 2N VWD demonstrate low factor VIII levels and normal structure and functional tests for vWf:Ag, ristocetin cofactor activity, and vWf multimeric structure. There are no laboratory tests to distinguish hemophilia A from VWD type 2N, but patients with type 2N VWD would not respond well to factor VIII replacement therapy. Patients with type 2N VWD exhibit autosomal recessive inheritance. Type 3 VWD could be differentiated on the basis of a homozygous or double heterozygous inheritance pattern and by a decrease of vWf:Ag in both platelets and plasma.

✔ Checkpoint! #4

Referring to Table 37-3 *, explain why the platelet function tests are abnormal in VWD and not in factor VIII or IX deficiencies.*

Carrier Detection and Prenatal Diagnosis Daughters of hemophilic males and women who have hemophilic sons are obligate carriers of the disease. Obligate carriers generally do not require further testing. Daughters of obligate carriers may inherit either X chromosome from their mother, and thus may be either carriers or normal. Female carriers of X-linked disorders are usually asymptomatic because they have one functional allele. As described by Mary Lyons, inactivation of one of the X chromosomes occurs randomly in each somatic cell of a female. Theoretically, in a carrier of an X-linked disorder, random inactivation would result in approximately 50% of the cells having a functional X chromosome active, while the remaining 50% would have the X chromosome bearing the mutant allele. A female carrier of factor VIII or factor IX deficiency is expected to have approximately 50% of the normal plasma level of the factor in question. Detection of the carrier state cannot, however, be based on merely finding half of the normal activity in a factor assay. Approximately 6% to 20% of women studied may be erroneously classified either as normal or as carriers for two reasons. First, inactivation of the X chromosomes is not always randomly distributed. A carrier may have func-

tional factor
than 50% of h
may be in the
of the norma
show clinical
the case of fac
and is physiol
and several oth
rise of factor V
factor IX coag
contraceptives.

Detection o
the plasma for
deficiency, the
vWf:Ag levels i
activity levels.[2]
tected in this w
testing with pro
in intron 22 m
DNA testing me
available for scre
carriers of factor
factor IX activity
cult to detect tha

Prenatal diagr
vantages over ph
by X chromosom
els, and testing c
methods are avai
the type of muta
can be done at 1
studies such as res
of the enormous
the considerable s
agnosis is not ava
limited by the fact
cases arise from ne
is not known, it is

Direct sampling
possible in some i
formed on the bloc
multaneous use of
sound analysis for
available. Patients
sis (even when preg
ered) so that physic
vent bleeding if the

Therapy. The key
is replacement of clo
cally, hemostasis fo
plasma factor levels
bleeding requires at
tients who are activ

hemophilia A, and when factor IX is deficient, the dis
is hemophilia B.

X-linked disorders are usually inherited by sons
their carrier (heterozygous) mothers who have an abno
allele on one X-chromosome and a normal allele on
other. Fifty percent of the sons will be expected to in
the abnormal gene. Males have only one X-chromoso
thus if they inherit an abnormal allele on that chromoso
they are affected with hemophilia. In the case of factor
or IX deficiency, they are able to synthesize little or nor
the clotting factor, depending on the particular mutation

Hemophilia A is a deficiency of the factor VIII portio
the factor VIII/vWf complex, as opposed to VWD in wh
the vWf portion of the complex is abnormal (discussed
viously). Patients with hemophilia A have normal circu
ing levels of normal functional vWf. Thus, their platelets
here properly to collagen and the formation of a nor
primary hemostatic plug is not disrupted. Patients with
mophilia B have an intact VIII/vWf complex and, likew
have normal primary hemostatic plug formation. The ab
mal bleeding in both diseases is caused by delayed and i
equate fibrin formation.

Clinical symptoms are identical in both deficiencies. T
can only be distinguished by laboratory testing. The c
mon clinical and laboratory aspects of the hemophilias
be discussed later after a discussion of the genetic mutati
specific for factor VIII or factor IX.

Hemophilia has been known for several centuries. It
contributed to world history by its presence in the r
families of Europe, particularly Great Britain, Russia,
Spain, through Queen Victoria, who was a carrier for he
philia A. Originally, all patients with X-linked bleeding
orders were believed to have the same disease. This idea
challenged when, in 1947, Pavlovsky observed that
longed recalcification times (the test available then) on
patients with hemophilia were corrected when the test
performed on mixtures of the two plasmas.[13] In 1952, th
groups of investigators reported patients who were missi
new factor that became known as factor IX.

The overall prevalence of the hemophilias is appr
mately 1 in 5,000–10,000 male births. Approximately 8
of the patients have factor VIII deficiency, and the rema
ing 20% are deficient in factor IX. Hemophilia A is secon
VWD in the overall frequency of inherited bleeding di
ders. In approximately 30% of the affected individuals, th
is no positive family history of the disease, indicating t
new genetic mutations occur often.

Factor VIII Nomenclature   In 1985 the Internatio
Committee on Thrombosis and Hemostasis published
ommendations that defined nomenclature for functio
and immunologic properties of the factor VIII/vWf c
plex.[14] Prior to these recommendations, the literature re
ring to factor VIII and vWf was quite confusing. By the
1980s the genes for both factor VIII and vWf had been id

vel of factor VIII or factor IX in the
37-8).

ies are treated with cryoprecipitate
VIII concentrates as described for
actor VIII concentrate is prepared by
e activity of factor VIII is slightly re-
e, and the large vWf multimers are
ed by hemophiliacs at home as pro-
event extensive bleeding and have
ling, enabling these individuals to

been realized with the use of con-
ecause the plasma of up to 20,000
e one lot of the product. Most pa-
therapy before 1984 were exposed
c, and the HIV viruses. Since 1984,
treatments have been used to inac-
titis viruses, and concentrates are
wever, for a time, 90% of patients
eficiency had HIV antibodies and
surface antigen. Since 1987 no new
ttributed to the administration of
es in North America, and transmis-
rarely been documented.
ission, factor VIII products free of
d by using monoclonal antibodies
III (rfactor VIII). Rfactor VIII is also
an albumin must be added to the
nd this has been reported to cause
rvovirus. The most recently devel-
eplacement therapy is a recombi-
he B domain is deleted. This type
uire the albumin additive.
herapy in patients capable of pro-
mildly affected hemophilia A and
DDAVP, which stimulates storage
to the plasma.
eated with whole plasma or with
tain factors II, VII, and X (pro-

Disseminated Intravascular Coagulation

Disseminated intravascular coagulation (DIC) is a condition in which the normal balance of hemostasis is altered, allowing the uncontrolled inappropriate formation and lysis of fibrin within the blood vessels. Fibrin is deposited diffusely in the capillaries as well as in the arterioles and venules. As fibrin is formed, several clotting proteins as well as naturally occurring inhibitors and platelets are consumed faster than they are synthesized (**consumption coagulopathy**). The result is an acquired deficiency of multiple hemostatic components. Fibrinolysis follows fibrin formation as a natural sequence of the hemostatic process. These events are the same processes that occur in normal hemostasis, except they are happening at the wrong time and in the wrong place. As a result of consumption of coagulation factors and platelets and the formation of FDP, the patient begins to bleed at the same time that disseminated clotting is occurring.

Incidence   DIC occurs in approximately 1 in 1000 hospital patients. About 20% of the cases are asymptomatic and suspected only on the basis of laboratory data. It can occur at any age, although it is most often seen in the very young and in the elderly.

Etiology   DIC is a syndrome, not a disease. It is a secondary group of symptoms that is always triggered by a primary condition that does not necessarily involve coagulation. Any disease state, singly or in combination with others, can trigger the DIC syndrome. Events that trigger DIC often involve the introduction of TF into the blood stream. TF may enter the blood from mechanical injury to tissues or from injury to the endothelial cells. Once in the blood TF initiates fibrin formation.

Conditions most often associated with developing DIC are summarized in Table 37-10 ✪. Infections, particularly those that are septic, are the most common trigger. The trigger mechanism of infections is likely cytokines (IL-1, IL-6, and/or TNF) released into the tissues by the inflammatory response, which activate endothelial cells. Resting endothelium does not express TF, but endothelial cells activated by cytokines or injured by endotoxin express TF activity. The full DIC response is seen in 30% to 50% of patients with Gram-negative or Gram-positive septicemia.[33]

Complications of pregnancy likely cause DIC because amniotic fluid acts as a thromboplastin to activate fibrin formation pathways. With massive tissue or blood cell injury it is thought that TF-like substances, such as fat and phospholipids, enter the circulation and activate coagulation. In one study, most patients with head trauma had laboratory evidence of DIC caused by procoagulants entering the circulation from the injured brain tissue.[34] The trigger mechanism of malignant cells is a variation of tissue injury. Some malignant cells express a TF-like substance, while others have been shown to produce a cysteine protease capable of directly activating factor X.[33,35] Figure 37-4 ■ summarizes the potential activation sites in the hemostatic system.

✪ **TABLE 37-10**

Clinical Conditions Associated with the Development of DIC

Infections	Bacterial (endotoxins)
	Viral
	Fungal
	Rickettsial
	Protozoal
Complications of pregnancy	Abruptio placentae
	Amniotic fluid embolism
	Retained placenta
	Toxemia
	Intrauterine fetal death
	Septic abortion
Neoplasms (malignant)	Solid tumors
	Leukemia, particularly AML-M3
Massive tissue injury	Burns
	Trauma
	Head injury
	Extensive surgery
	Extracorporeal circulation
Vascular injury	Shock
	Hypotension
	Hypoxia
	Acidosis
Miscellaneous	Snake bite
	Heat stroke
	Any disease

Pathophysiology   Once the initiating event has occurred, thrombin is formed within the circulation. Unlike the physiologic formation of the hemostatic plug in which thrombin generation remains limited and localized at the site of vessel injury, DIC results in generalized or systemic activation of coagulation. The circulating thrombin acts on its substrates as they circulate in the same manner as it does after an injury-induced localized formation of fibrin (∞ Chapter 35). This unregulated overexpression of thrombin results in the consumption of fibrinogen, factors V, VIII, and XIII (the natural substrates of thrombin), as well as a depletion of prothrombin (the precursor zymogen). Thrombin is a potent agonist of platelets, inducing platelet activation and aggregation. Thrombin also binds to receptors on endothelial cells, inducing endothelial release of t-PA, which in the presence of the newly formed fibrin, activates plasminogen to plasmin and triggers an aggressive secondary fibrinolysis. As plasmin is generated, plasminogen becomes depleted. DIC results from a failure of the mechanisms that limit blood clotting and thrombin generation (the normal inhibitory pathways to prevent the systemic effects of thrombin).

The coagulation inhibitors AT, HC II, and thrombomodulin (TM), normally effective in regulating the localized gen-

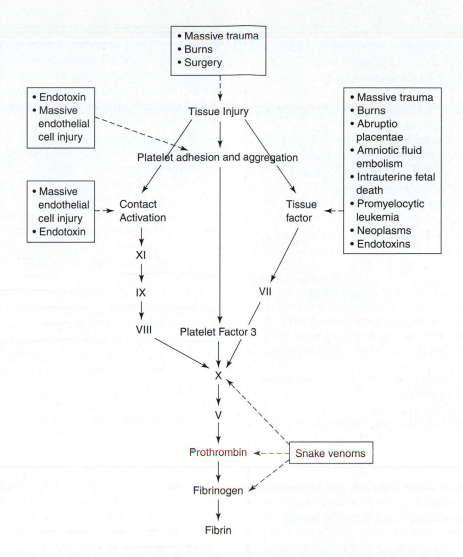

■ FIGURE 37-4 Conditions that initiate DIC activate the hemostatic pathways in a variety of ways. Normal hemostasis is shown by solid arrows. Processes that trigger DIC are shown in the boxes, and broken arrows indicate proposed sites of activation. (Adapted with permission from: Grosset AMB, Rodgers GM. Acquired coagulation disorders. Lee GR, Foerster J, Lukens J, Paraskevas F, Greer JP, Rodgers GM, eds. In: *Wintrobe's Clinical Hematology*, 10th ed. Baltimore: Williams & Wilkins; 1999:1733–80.)

eration of thrombin, are overwhelmed in DIC. Deficiencies of AT, protein C, and protein S are induced as they are utilized in removing their activated substrates from the circulation. Also, IL-1 and TNF (elevated in sepsis) decrease TM expression on endothelium, resulting in decreased activity of the PC/PS inhibitory mechanism (∞ Chapter 35).

Plasma levels of fibrinopeptides A and B (FPA and FPB) and D-dimer are elevated because of the actions of thrombin on fibrinogen and of plasmin on fibrin. FDPs interfere with fibrin formation and platelet function, contributing to the bleeding tendency.

All of these events may result in bleeding as the clotting mechanism is activated and procoagulant components become depleted. The pathogenesis of DIC is summarized in Figure 37-5 ■.

Clinical Aspects The symptoms seen in patients with DIC result from the presence and activation of thrombin, plasmin, platelets, endothelium, and proteolytic inhibitors within the bloodstream and vary from patient to patient because of the complex interactions between these components. Because clotting factors and platelets are consumed, bleeding symptoms are favored in some patients. Thrombosis is the dominant process in other patients. In addition, the intensity and duration can result in either an acute or chronic clinical course. Patients with acute disease tend to manifest hemorrhagic symptoms, whereas in those with chronic disease thrombosis is more likely to predominate.[35] The more commonly recognized acute form begins with sudden onset of severe bleeding and is seen in 80%–90% of patients with DIC. In the chronic form (10%–20% of patients)

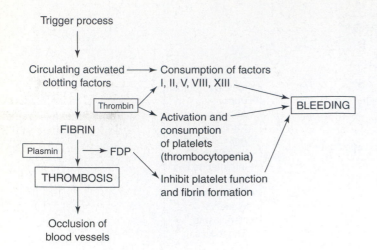

■ **FIGURE 37-5** Pathogenesis of DIC. Activation of hemostasis by triggering processes leads to clotting and bleeding simultaneously. Intravascular fibrin formation results in occlusion of vessels. During clotting several coagulation factors and platelets are consumed, leading to bleeding. (Adapted from: Grosset AMB, Rodgers GM. Acquired coagulation disorders. Lee GR, Foerster J, Lukens J, Paraskevas F, Greer JP, Rodgers GM, eds. In: *Wintrobe's Clinical Hematology*, 10th ed. Baltimore: Williams & Wilkins; 1999:1733–1780.)

the stimulus that triggers clotting is weaker, and the natural homeostatic mechanisms are sufficient to replace depleted hemostatic components.

Hemorrhages and thrombosis occur predominantly in the microvasculature and are responsible for the clinical manifestations. In patients with acute DIC whose disease course is hemorrhagic, bleeding begins abruptly and generally occurs from three or more sites simultaneously.[29] Sites of bleeding tend to correspond to the tissues involved in the triggering event. Possible bleeding manifestations include hematuria, gastrointestinal and respiratory tract bleeding, intracranial bleeding, epistaxis, oozing from needle puncture sites, surgical drains or sutures, spontaneous bruising, and petechiae. Bleeding may be profuse, leading to death.

At the same time, small strands of fibrin (microclots) form inside blood vessels and obstruct the microvasculature. Because blood vessels are occluded, tissue anoxia and microinfarcts in various organs occur. Manifestations are renal failure, coma, liver failure, respiratory failure, skin necrosis, gangrene, and venous thromboembolism.

Shock is a common feature and may be either a cause or an effect of DIC. The association of shock with DIC is complex and not well understood. Shock is likely induced because cytokine generation and products of the kinin and complement systems cause increased vascular permeability and hypotension. The mortality rate of DIC is 50% to 60%.

Laboratory Evaluation The diagnosis of DIC is primarily made by the physician based on the patient's clinical symptoms. There is no single laboratory test that will estab-

lish a diagnosis of DIC, nor any combination of tests that are specific for DIC. Laboratory tests are ordered to confirm a suspected clinical diagnosis. Screening tests that are usually ordered by the physician include a platelet count, blood smear, PT, APTT, fibrinogen determination, and D-dimer test. Some laboratories include a test for AT. These tests demonstrate the generation of both thrombin and plasmin and may also reflect the severity of the consumption of hemostatic elements. Table 37-11 ✪ shows the typical laboratory results in patients with DIC.

The platelet count, the most useful parameter, may fall to levels of $40–75 \times 10^9$/L. The platelet count is decreased in 97% of patients. A decrease in the platelet count may be difficult to identify in patients whose usual platelet count is in the upper normal range, and serial platelet counts clearly demonstrating decreasing values are more useful than a single determination.

The PT and APTT may be prolonged because of the decrease in factors II, V, and VIII and fibrinogen, although their alteration is not as consistent as the platelet count. One or more of these tests are prolonged in 60–75% of patients with DIC.[29] Occasionally, early in the disease process, these tests may be shorter than normal, perhaps due to the presence of factors that are already activated, and which would require less time for clot formation in vitro.[29]

In severe disease, the fibrinogen level may drop to 10–50 mg/dL but is decreased in only 23% to 71% of patients.[33] Fibrinogen is an acute phase reactant, and the protein increases in inflammatory conditions. Since many patients with DIC have underlying disease, their fibrinogen levels may have been initially elevated because of the acute phase response.

The D-dimer test to demonstrate the presence of FDPs and, therefore, generation of plasmin, is elevated in 93% of patients and provides good evidence in favor of DIC.[29] D-dimers are present only after factor XIII stabilization of fibrin. D-dimers confirm that activation of coagulation has taken place, but they are not specific for DIC. The D-dimer test may be positive in several other clinical conditions such as after surgery and in patients with renal disease or pulmonary emboli. In most laboratories the D-dimer test has replaced a similar latex test for fibrin degradation products that fails to distinguish between plasmin degradation products of fibrinogen and fibrin.

A test to demonstrate a decrease in AT has been recommended by some clinicians. AT decreases in concentration early in the disease process as it combines with and inactivates thrombin and other serine proteases. It is decreased in 89% of patients. Examination of the blood smear reveals the presence of schistocytes in 50% of patients. Schistocytes are produced as blood cells are forced through the fibrin webs that clog the blood vessels. However, fragmented RBC rarely constitute >10% of the red cells on the peripheral smear.

Other laboratory tests that may be abnormal in DIC but generally are not necessary for a diagnosis in most cases are the thrombin time and serial specific factor assays for factors

⊙ TABLE 37-11

Typical Laboratory Findings in Acquired Disorders of Hemostasis Associated with Bleeding

Test	DIC	Primary Fibrinogenolysis	Severe Liver Disease	Vitamin K Deficiency	Specific Factor Inhibitor	Lupus Anticoagulant
Screening tests						
Platelet count	Dec	N	Dec	N	N	N
PT	Inc	Inc	Inc	Inc	N (inc with factor VII)	N
APTT	Inc	Inc	Inc	Inc	Inc (except factor VII)	Inc
						Inc
TT	Inc	Inc	Inc	N	N	N
Definitive tests						
Fibrinogen	Dec	Dec	Dec	N	N	N
D-dimer	Inc	N	N	N	N	N
Latex FSP test	Inc	Inc	N/inc	N	N	N
Plasminogen	Dec	Dec	N/dec	N	N	N
Fibrinopeptide A	Inc	N	N	N	N	N
Natural inhibitors						
Antithrombin	Dec	N	Dec	N	N	N
Protein C	Varies	N	Dec	Dec	N	N
Protein S	Varies	N	Dec	Dec	N	Varies
Miscellaneous						
Blood smear	Schistocytes	N	Macrocytes, target cells, acanthocytes	N	N	N

Key to abbreviations: Inc = increased; Dec = decreased; N = normal; PT = prothrombin time; APTT = activated partial thromboplastin time; TT = thrombin time; FSP = fibrin split products

V and VIII or prothrombin (to demonstrate decreased factor levels/increased consumption). The TT is increased because of the presence of FDPs as well as the decreased fibrinogen level and is abnormal in 58% of patients. Additional tests of thrombin generation include tests for fibrin monomers, FP-A and -B, thrombin-AT complexes, and prothrombin fragment 1.2 (∞ Chapter 39). They are all potentially useful parameters, but at present are mainly research tools.

Therapy   Treatment for DIC is to first eliminate the underlying cause, if possible. After that it is controversial. The acute form is often self-limited and will disappear when the fibrin is completely lysed. Replacement therapy using platelets, red cells, cryoprecipitate, or fresh frozen plasma are used when indicated (patients with clear laboratory evidence of DIC and bleeding).[36] Low molecular weight heparins have been found helpful in those patients with strong clinical and laboratory evidence of DIC and predominant thromboembolic manifestations, or in patients in whom replacement therapy fails to alleviate excessive bleeding and increase the level of clotting factors. Newer approaches to therapy are to replace the depleted physiologic inhibitors: AT, PC, and TFPI with concentrates. Clinical trials are being conducted on

some of these products. Under most circumstances, patients with DIC should not be treated with fibrinolytic inhibitors.

The chronic form of DIC is usually seen secondary to disseminated carcinoma, in which case elimination of the precipitating event is difficult. Heparin therapy sometimes may be helpful if thrombosis is life threatening because it will stop intravascular fibrin formation. It is administered with caution, however, because fatal bleeding has occurred with its use.

 Checkpoint! #8

A. *Why is thrombocytopenia usually present in a patient with DIC?*

B. *Which hemostasis laboratory screening tests (PT and APTT), if any, will the following affect:*

Decreased factor V?

Decreased factor VIII?

Decreased fibrinogen?

Decreased antithrombin?

C. *Which laboratory test results would distinguish DIC from hemophilia A?*

Primary Fibrinogenolysis

Primary fibrinogenolysis is a condition similar to DIC, but it requires differentiation so that proper treatment can be instituted. In primary fibrinogenolysis plasminogen becomes inappropriately activated to plasmin without concomitant thrombin generation. Plasmin then circulates and, if it overwhelms the antiplasmin inhibitors, will degrade fibrinogen, factors V, VIII, and XIII, plus other coagulation factors (and other proteins). Eventually an acquired deficiency of the proteins develops and leads to bleeding symptoms that resemble DIC.

Similar pathologies can cause the two conditions, but liver disease is one of the most common triggers of primary fibrinogenolysis. Differentiating the two conditions with laboratory tests is sometimes difficult. Patients with primary fibrinogenolysis may have an abnormal PT, APTT, thrombin time, fibrinogen assay, and increased fibrin(ogen) degradation products but normal D-dimer and fibrin monomer tests because stabilized fibrin is not formed. The level of fibrinopeptide A is normal in primary fibrinogenolysis but elevated in DIC.[37] Table 37-11 ✪ compares laboratory test results in these two conditions with other acquired hemostatic disorders.

Therapy for primary fibrinogenolysis is with epsilon aminocaproic acid (EACA), a specific inhibitor of plasmin. EACA is dangerous if administered to patients with DIC; therefore, the diagnosis of DIC needs to be excluded before the drug is given.[37]

Liver Disease

Liver disease affects all hemostatic functions. Most hemostatic proteins (those involved in fibrin formation, in fibrinolysis, as well as hemostatic inhibitors) are synthesized in the liver (∞ Chapter 35; Web Table 37-1 ✪). The liver macrophages play a major role in removal of activated factors and products of activation, such as the fibrinopeptides, fibrin degradation products, and plasminogen activators. When the liver is diseased, these functions are diminished.[37]

Laboratory tests in liver disease may resemble DIC, and in fact, an element of DIC may also be present. Differentiating the two conditions is a difficult task for the physician. Table 37-11 ✪ compares the results of laboratory testing. The decreased production of proteins involved in fibrin formation may cause all screening coagulation tests to be prolonged, including the PT, APTT, and thrombin time. The fibrinogen concentration is usually normal but may stabilize in the low normal range. An abnormal fibrinogen molecule may be synthesized that has an increased content of sialic acid and may cause defective clot formation.

The platelet count may be decreased for several reasons including hypersplenism (from backing up of the portal blood supply when it is unable to enter the liver), alcohol toxicity of the bone marrow, or utilization of the platelets if DIC is present.

FDPs are increased because the liver cells are unable to remove them from the circulation. Incomplete removal of plasminogen activators may result in systemic formation of plasmin and subsequent proteolysis of fibrinogen, resulting in a slight increase of FDPs. Excess fibrin or fibrinogen degradation products may impair blood coagulation and result in platelet dysfunction. The D-dimer test may be normal and may be one way of differentiating DIC from liver disease.

Clinical bleeding is minimal except in severe liver disease, when ecchymoses and epistaxis may occur. Bleeding from local lesions in the GI tract is common. Therapy involves the use of replacement products as needed.

Vitamin K Deficiency

Vitamin K is needed by hepatic cells to complete the post-translational alteration of factors II, VII, IX, and X and proteins C and S (∞ Chapter 35). In the absence of vitamin K, precursor proteins are synthesized by the hepatic cells, but because γ-carboxyglutamic acid residues are absent, the calcium-binding sites are nonfunctional. Deficiency of vitamin K results in induced functional deficiencies of all of these proteins. If the level of functional proteins falls below 30 U/dL, bleeding symptoms may result, and the PT and/or the APTT will be prolonged.

Sources of vitamin K are green, leafy vegetables in the diet and synthesis by bacteria in the GI tract. Symptomatic vitamin K deficiency is most often seen in newborns in the first days of life, called **hemorrhagic disease of the newborn**. Because their livers are still immature, synthesis of the vitamin K-dependent factors in newborns is 30% to 50% of adult levels. Almost all neonates are vitamin K deficient, presumably as a result of deficient vitamin K in the mother, and/or the lack of colonization of the colon by vitamin K producing bacteria in the neonate. This deficiency is more prevalent in breast-fed babies, since human milk contains less vitamin K than cow's milk. It is critical to determine whether a prolonged PT or APTT in a newborn is due to vitamin K deficiency or to a decreased synthetic capacity of the liver. In some infants, particularly those born prematurely, the levels of the clotting factors are low enough to cause bleeding symptoms.

Manifestations of hemorrhagic disease of the newborn are bleeding in the skin or from mucosal surfaces, from circumcision, generalized ecchymoses, large intramuscular hemorrhages, and (rarely) intracranial bleeds. In the laboratory, the PT and possibly the APTT are more prolonged than expected at this age. Specific factor assays for factors II, VII, IX, and X are markedly decreased. The BT and the platelet count are within normal limits (Table 37-11 ✪).

Hemorrhagic disease of the newborn is prevented in the United States by administration of vitamin K to all newborns. In countries where this practice has recently been stopped, the disease occurs occasionally.

Causes of vitamin K deficiency in adults include malabsorptive syndromes such as sprue, obstruction of the biliary tract (because bile salts are necessary for absorption), and prolonged broad-spectrum antibiotic therapy that abolishes normal flora of the intestine. Vitamin K administration corrects the deficiency within 24 hours.

Acquired Pathologic Inhibitors

Acquired inhibitors of blood coagulation, also called **circulating anticoagulants**, develop pathologically in patients with certain disease states, as well as in some who have no apparent underlying condition. Almost all are immunoglobulins, either IgG or IgM, and can be either alloantibodies or autoantibodies. Two types of inhibitors are described: those directed toward a single coagulation factor and the lupus anticoagulant (LA).

Inhibitors of Single Factors

Pathologic inhibitors against most coagulation factors have been reported. They are usually seen in patients with inherited factor deficiencies who have received replacement treatment for bleeding complications, but they are also associated with other conditions such as diseases or drugs and are sometimes seen in patients who are otherwise healthy. With the exception of antibodies to factors VIII and IX, they are extremely rare. These inhibitors are recognized because of their interference with or neutralization of clotting factor activity. The following discussion will concentrate on the factor VIII and IX inhibitors.

Clinical Aspects. Inhibitors to factors VIII and IX are observed most often in association with the hemophilias. Approximately 15% to 20% of patients with hemophilia A and 1% to 3% of patients with hemophilia B develop alloantibodies to the respective deficient factor. Thirty-five percent of hemophilia A patients with the inversion mutation described earlier develop factor VIII inhibitors. Most patients with inhibitors have severe disease with very low coagulant levels of the affected factor. Most patients also have received replacement therapy for their factor deficiency, although there is no correlation between the amount of treatment received and the development of inhibitors. In hemophilia A patients, the antibody specificity is directed toward the coagulant antigen (VIII:Ag) only and not the vWf portion of the VIII/vWf complex. Although most inhibitors develop in severe or moderate forms of hemophilia, they may also be found in some patients with mild forms of hemophilia A.

Factor VIII inhibitors (autoantibodies) may also be found in nonhemophilic patients. Occasionally they develop in otherwise healthy individuals who most often are older patients or females during or following a pregnancy. Disease states associated with factor VIII inhibitors include autoimmune and lymphoproliferative diseases or multiple myeloma. Autoantibodies to other clotting factors may appear in similar circumstances as the factor VIII inhibitors.

The clinical course of patients with inhibitors is variable but can resemble that of patients with severe hemophilia and result in fatal consequences in 10% to 20% of cases. In hemophilic patients, bleeding may begin while the patient is receiving therapy. In patients who have not received therapy

for 1 to 2 years the antibody level often decreases, but an anamnestic response may be seen within 2 to 4 days after reexposure. The antibody may also disappear spontaneously.

Laboratory Evaluation. Laboratory test results in patients with factor VIII or IX inhibitors resemble those in patients with severe factor deficiencies. The APTT will be markedly prolonged and other screening tests will be normal (Table 37-11 ✪). Mixing studies can be done as a screening procedure to distinguish between a true factor deficiency and an inhibitor (∞ Chapter 39). If an inhibitor is present, the test on the mixture will remain prolonged. Assays for specific inhibitors can then be performed (∞ Chapter 39).

Therapy. The type of therapy used for patients with factor VIII inhibitors depends on whether the patient is a low or high responder and on the titer of the inhibitor. Low responders (25% of hemophiliacs with inhibitors) are patients with low titer inhibitors that do not rise after further exposure to factor VIII. Patients with inhibitors that rise markedly with further exposure to factor VIII (anamnestic response) are known as high responders (~75% of hemophiliacs with inhibitors). For those who are low responders experiencing life-threatening symptoms, large amounts of factor VIII may be administered in hopes of overcoming the antibody. If human factor VIII cannot be used because the inhibitor level is too high, factor IX complex products or porcine factor VIII may be used in an attempt to bypass the need for factor VIII. Factor IX complex concentrates contain prothrombin and factors VII, IX, and X. While the substance(s) responsible for factor VIII bypassing activity remain(s) unknown, evidence suggests that it is activated factor IX. Recombinant factor VIIa is a new product being evaluated for effectiveness and safety and appears to be promising.[37] Recombinant factor VIIa works by activating factor X and bypassing the need for factors VIII or IX in the formation of fibrin and thus is equally effective in both hemophilia A and B patients with inhibitors.

Lupus Anticoagulant

The second type of inhibitor of major clinical importance is the **lupus anticoagulant (LA)**, so called because it was first discovered in patients with systemic lupus erythematosus (SLE). Approximately 6% to 16% of patients with SLE develop LA. The term *LA* is a misnomer because LA is more frequently encountered in patients without lupus and has been associated with a variety of other autoimmune diseases, neoplasias, certain infections, and the administration of drugs such as chlorpromazine or procainamide, as well as in apparently normal individuals. Even though it has now been associated with many diseases, it is still called the lupus anticoagulant. It is usually discovered by finding an unexpectedly prolonged APTT, and sometimes PT, while performing routine coagulation studies.

LAs are a family of autoantibodies that were originally thought to be directed toward phospholipid (antiphospholipid antibodies).[38] Another group of antibodies in the antiphospholipid family are **anticardiolipin antibodies (ACA).** They behave in a similar manner to LA, and 73% of patients with LA also have ACA.[39] Immunologically, both LA and ACA are usually IgG but may be IgM or a mixture of both. The antibody combines with the phospholipid surfaces of test reagents used in the APTT, and occasionally the PT, prolonging the test results. Both LA and ACA were originally thought to react only with phospholipid. Further studies of antibody specificity revealed that ACA require the presence of a protein, β_2-glycoprotein I (β_2-GPI), to be associated with the phospholipid on the surface of the cells to which they bind,[39] and LA were directed against epitopes on prothrombin. These ACA and LA antibodies react with β_2-GPI and prothrombin in solution, and then the antigen–antibody complex binds to anionic phospholipids in the test systems. Recent theories of the origin of LA suggest that it is formed in vivo after damage to endothelial cells exposes anionic phospholipids that bind prothrombin and trigger antibody formation.[38,40] A comparison between LA and the pathogenesis of heparin-induced thrombocytopenia (∞ Chapter 36) is made because both antibodies bind with the aid of proteins to phospholipid surfaces, activate cells, and result in thrombosis.[40] Because of the variability of clinical findings, it is likely that there is a wide variety of LA antibodies in different patients.

Clinical Aspects.   The lupus anticoagulant is a laboratory phenomenon and is not associated with clinical bleeding symptoms. Patients have undergone major surgery with no complications. An occasional patient with LA may have clinically significant bleeding, but this is usually attributable to a coexistant abnormality in addition to the LA (e.g., thrombocytopenia, prothrombin deficiency, etc.). While bleeding symptoms generally are not seen in the presence of LA, 30–40% of affected patients demonstrate thrombosis (∞ Chapter 38).

Laboratory Evaluation.   LA is difficult to identify in the laboratory. There is no single assay that detects all LAs in all patients; instead, a combination of tests must be performed. Table 37-11 ✪ shows typical laboratory test results and comparisons to other acquired conditions. (The sensitivity of the APTT reagent for LA detection varies with different commercial reagents used for the test. Some commercial APTT reagents have been created to be very sensitive to the presence of LA.)

A sequence of suggested tests for evaluating a patient's plasma for the presence of LA, recommended by the Subcommittee on Lupus Anticoagulant/Antiphospholipid Antibody of the Scientific and Standardization Committee of the International Society of Thrombosis and Haemostasis is outlined in Table 37-12 ✪.[41]

The diagnosis of LA requires that the specimen and any normal plasma used for mixing studies be collected carefully and centrifuged at high speeds to remove platelets because procoagulant phospholipids from platelet activation in plasma samples reduce the sensitivity of the screening test

✪ **TABLE 37-12**

Recommended Approach for Identification of the Lupus Anticoagulant (LA)[41]

Screening procedures—two or more using single concentration of phospholipid

1. Demonstrate at least one prolonged phospholipid-based clotting test (e.g., APTT)
2. Demonstrate at least one additional prolonged LA screening test (e.g., dilute Russell's viper venom time [dRVVT], Plasma clot time [PCT], Kaolin clotting time [KCT])

Confirmatory procedures—modification of abnormal screening procedure by altering phospholipid content of the test procedure, which demonstrates that the LA is dependent on phospholipid

1. Reducing phospholipid concentration in test reagent to accentuate prolonged test (e.g., diluting the test reagent)
2. Neutralizing the effect of the LA by increasing the phospholipid in the test system (e.g., frozen-thawed platelets [platelet neutralization procedure] platelet vesicles hexagonal phase phospholipid)

Additional requirements for documenting LA

1. Mixing studies with normal platelet free plasma not corrected
2. Exclusion of presence of heparin in the sample (e.g., normal thrombin time/reptilase time)
3. Proof that another coagulopathy is not present or concurrent; Specific factor assays to rule out a factor deficiency; Detailed clinical history

reagents. Some laboratories use a 0.2 μm cellulose filter to remove platelets. The platelet count of the plasmas must be less than 10×10^9/L.[39]

The first criterion in identifying LA is that at least one laboratory test that uses phospholipid in the reagent (e.g., the APTT) must be prolonged. This prolonged test must then be repeated on a mixture of patient's plasma and normal plasma to distinguish between an inhibitor and a single factor deficiency (see mixing studies, ∞ Chapter 39). In the presence of an inhibitor, no correction will be noted. A specific factor deficiency may also be ruled out by factor assays and by the clinical history of the patients. The possibility of the presence of heparin causing the prolonged APTT must also be eliminated. Heparin can be identified by observing a prolonged thrombin time and a normal reptilase time (∞ Chapter 39). At least one additional abnormal screening test for the LA must be demonstrated.

A confirmatory test is then performed to prove that the antibody is directed toward phospholipids. Confirmatory tests are modifications of the screening tests (that were originally abnormal) that alter the amount of phospholipid in the test system. The modifications are to alter the amount of phospholipid by either reducing the amount of phospholipid in the reagent or by adding an excess of phospholipid to the test system. The most sensitive tests for detecting the inhibitor contain only limited amounts of procoagulant

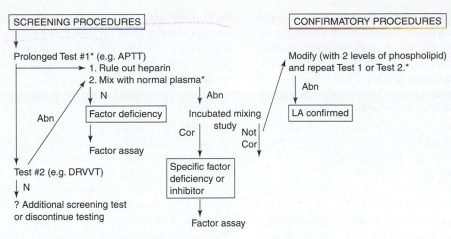

| SCREENING PROCEDURES | CONFIRMATORY PROCEDURES |

Prolonged Test #1* (e.g. APTT)
→ 1. Rule out heparin
→ 2. Mix with normal plasma*

Modify (with 2 levels of phospholipid) and repeat Test 1 or Test 2.*

Factor deficiency

Factor assay

Test #2 (e.g. DRVVT)

? Additional screening test or discontinue testing

Incubated mixing study

Specific factor deficiency or inhibitor

Factor assay

LA confirmed

* Plasma samples must be platelet free.

■ **FIGURE 37-6** A flow chart for an approach to the diagnosis of the lupus anticoagulant (LA). At least two screening phospholipid-based screening tests (tests using one concentration of phospholipid) must be prolonged. Mixing studies must be uncorrected with normal plasma. The presence of heparin must be ruled out. Confirmatory tests are performed by modifying the abnormal screening tests with two levels of phospholipid. (Adapted from: Brandt JT, Triplett DA, Alving B, Scharrer I. Criteria for the diagnosis of lupus anticoagulants: An update. *Thromb Haemost.* 1995; 74:1185–90.) (Key: Cor = corrected; N = normal; Abn = abnormal; LA = lupus anticoagulant; APTT = activated partial thromboplastin time; dRVVT = dilute Russell's viper venom time)

phospholipids (dilute Russell's viper venom time, dilute PTT, or the PT performed with very dilute tissue factor—the tissue thromboplastin inhibition [TTI] test) and remain prolonged. When excess phospholipid is added to the test system, there is an overabundance of phospholipid, the antibody is overwhelmed, and the original prolonged test time is shortened to the normal range. The platelet neutralization procedure (∞ Chapter 39) is a popular confirmatory test. In this test, washed, frozen, and thawed platelets, an abundant source of phospholipid, are added to the patient's plasma and correct the prolonged screening test. Figure 37-6 ■ outlines a flow chart for an approach to the laboratory testing for LA.

CASE STUDY *(continued from page 745)*

A thrombin time was performed on Scott and the results were within the laboratory's reference range.

The laboratory then performed mixing studies. Scott's plasma was mixed with normal plasma, and the APTT was repeated on the mixture. The result of the APTT on the mixture was 36 sec.

8. What do the results of the APTT on the mixture of Scott's plasma with normal plasma indicate?

9. What test should be performed next?

10. If a factor VIII assay was done with results of <1 U/dL, what molecular studies should be done?

11. What therapy is indicated for this patient?

12. What complications from the therapy are possible?

▶ FLOW CHARTS

Flow charts that outline reflex testing procedures that the laboratory can follow to investigate abnormal hemostatic screening tests are included on this text's companion Web site.

▶ HEMOSTASIS IN THE NEWBORN

Blood coagulation studies in the newborn present special challenges to the laboratory. At birth, liver synthesis of several of the clotting proteins is at a lower level than in normal adults. Some proteins do not reach adult levels until 6–12 months of age. Laboratory screening tests are prolonged and also are dependent on the age of the child and the presence of accompanying diseases. These factors influence the interpretation of the laboratory tests.

Obtaining an adequate blood sample is of utmost importance but technically extremely difficult. Even with maximum attention to quality control, there is the possibility of spuriously altered results. A venous sample is preferred to capillary or arterial blood. Obtaining the sample from an indwelling catheter should be avoided because of the danger of heparin contamination.

Adding anticoagulant to the syringe allows one to draw blood more slowly while minimizing the risk of clotting. The amount of anticoagulant must be reduced when the infant's hematocrit is above 65% because of the reduced plasma volume.

Because the total volume of blood in newborns is only 250–350 mL, efforts must be made to minimize the amount of sample drawn. Some suggestions for minimizing the amount of plasma needed for testing are to eliminate duplicate testing when performing the PT or APTT and to run several factor assays using diluted plasma rather than the screening tests.[42] Micro adaptations of several routine procedures, using 5–40 μL of plasma, have been developed.[43]

NORMAL HEMOSTASIS IN THE NEWBORN

Platelets and the proteins of the coagulation and fibrinolytic systems are first detected in fetuses at 10 to 11 weeks of gestation. Table 37-13 ✪ shows expected values for various laboratory tests for preterm and term infants at birth compared with results in older children and adults, as well as the ages when adult levels of the proteins are reached.

Platelet counts reach adult levels by 27 weeks of gestation and, therefore, should be in the normal adult range at birth. As with adults, platelet counts of less than 100×10^9/L should be considered abnormal. Counts of $100–150 \times 10^9$/L are borderline and should be repeated. Decreased platelet aggregation with low levels of ADP and with collagen, epinephrine, and thrombin are found at birth but normalize within several weeks. Platelet agglutination with ristocetin, on the other hand, is increased in newborns, which must be considered when diagnosing VWD. Drugs that affect platelet function, such as aspirin, when taken by the mother, will also influence hemostasis in the fetus.

Concentrations of the coagulation proteins for term and preterm infants, older children, and adults are shown in Table 37-14 ✪. The fibrinogen group of factors is at normal adult levels at birth. The concentrations of the proteins of the prothrombin and contact factor groups are decreased at birth, due to newborn liver immaturity. They reach adult levels at varying times (Table 37-14 ✪). Usually the levels of these clotting factors are not low enough to affect hemostasis, unless a stressful situation is present. vWf, on the other hand, is increased at birth and gradually decreases over the first 6 months of life.[44]

Natural inhibitors that are synthesized by the liver are also decreased in newborns (Table 37-14 ✪). Adults with levels of AT equivalent to infants are considered at risk for thrombosis. Infants do not have this problem because the procoagulant proteins that are inactivated by AT are also decreased. Levels of PC and PS are decreased to 10% to 50% of adult levels in term infants, but are not balanced by a corresponding decrease in the proteins that they inhibit.[42] PC levels are still low at 6 months.[43] Plasminogen levels are also decreased, and FDPs are similar to adult values.

The decrease in hemostatic factors in term and preterm infants affects coagulation tests (Table 37-13 ✪). The PT is prolonged ~3 seconds compared to adults, because of the low levels of factors II, VII, and X. However, a PT of greater than 17 seconds should be considered abnormal in the newborn.[45] Values in the normal adult range are usually achieved in 3 to 4 days.

The APTT is also prolonged ~2–3 seconds in term infants and may be significantly prolonged in preterm infants. This test is dependent on the factors of the intrinsic system and is particularly sensitive to the contact factors. Results of this test are also highly dependent upon the reagent used.[42,44] Adult levels may be reached in 4 to 6 months.[45] The thrombin clotting time is abnormal even though the fibrinogen level is normal, and may be explained by the presence of a distinct fetal fibrinogen molecule with altered function. The thrombin time becomes normal within a few days after birth.

In general, hemostatic values in preterm infants differ from adults as discussed above. They also differ from term infants, but erratically so, and by 6 months of age their values are comparable to those of term infants.[46]

✪ TABLE 37-13

Laboratory Tests in Preterm and Term Infants as Compared to Adults and Older Children

Test	Preterm Infant (32–36 Weeks) (Day 1)	Term Infant (37–41 Weeks) (Day 1)	Adults and Older Children	Age Adult Level Reached
Platelet count, $\times 10^9$/L	150–430	174–456	150–450	Before birth
Platelet aggregation	Abnormal	Abnormal	Normal	One month
PT, sec	10.6–16.2*	13–20	11–13	Comparable at birth
APTT, sec	27.5–79.4*	42.9 ± 5.80**	11–13	By 6 months
TT, sec	19.0–30.4*	23.5 ± 2.38**	19.7–30.3*	At birth
FDP	Normal	Normal	Normal	Before birth

*from: Andrew M, Paes B, Milner R, et al. Development of the human coagulation system in the healthy premature infant. *Blood.* 1988; 72:1651–57.
**from: Andrew M, Paes B, Milner R, et al. Development of the human coagulation system in the full-term infant. *Blood.* 1987; 70:165–72.
Key to abbreviations: PT = prothrombin time; APTT = activated partial thromboplastin time; TT = thrombin time; FDP = fibrin degradation products

⊛ TABLE 37-14

Levels of Hemostatic Proteins in Preterm and Term Infants as Compared to Adults and Older Children*

Protein	Preterm Infants* (27–31 Weeks) (U/dL)(Day 1)	Term Infants** (38–41 Weeks) (U/dL)(Day 1)	Adults and Older Children (U/dL)	Age Adult Level Reached
Coagulant proteins—fibrinogen group				
Fibrinogen, mg/dL	256 ± 70	215 ± 35	200–400	Before birth
Factor V	91 ± 33	56–200	64–162	Before birth
Factor VIII	82–224	134 ± 54	50–200	Before birth
Factor XIII				
A subunit	32–108	79 ± 26	105 ± 25	Before birth
B subunit	35–127	76 ± 23	97 ± 20	Before birth
Coagulant proteins—prothrombin group				
Factor II (Prothrombin)	20–77	48 ± 11	108 ± 19	6 months
Factor VII	21–113	66 ± 19	105 ± 19	5 days
Factor IX	19–65	53 ± 19	109 ± 27	6 months
Factor X	11–71	40 ± 14	106 ± 23	6 months
Coagulant proteins—contact group				
Factor XI	8–52	38 ± 14	97 ± 15	After 6 months
Factor XII	10–66	53 ± 20	108 ± 28	After 6 months
Prekallikrein	9–57	37 ± 16	112 ± 25	After 6 months
HMWK	9–89	54 ± 24	92 ± 22	1 month
Fibrinolytic protein				
Plasminogen	112–248	195 ± 35	336 ± 34	6 months
Naturally occurring inhibitors				
Antithrombin	14–62	63 ± 12	105 ± 13	3 months
Protein C	12–44	35 ± 9	96 ± 16	After 6 months
Protein S	14–38	36 ± 12	92 ± 16	3 months
Heparin cofactor II	0–60	43 ± 25	96 ± 15	6 months

*Compiled from: Andrew M, Paes B, Milner R, et al. Development of the human coagulation system in the healthy premature infant. *Blood.* 1988; 72:1651–57.
**Compiled from: Andrew M, Paes B, Milner R, et al. Development of the human coagulation system in the full-term infant. *Blood.* 1987; 70:165–72.

COMMON BLEEDING DISORDERS IN THE NEONATE

Although the coagulation systems of the well term and preterm infants show low levels of many procoagulant, anticoagulant, and fibrinolytic proteins, hemostasis is usually functionally balanced, and neither thromboses nor hemorrhages occur. However, abnormalities of hemostasis may be present in ~1% of newborns. The classification of the most common problems is dependent on whether the child is considered sick or well. Sick infants include those with prematurity, perinatal infection, respiratory distress syndrome, metabolic derangements, and/or birth asphyxia. Babies considered sick usually have either DIC, isolated platelet consumption independent of a decrease in clotting factors, or liver failure.

In well babies, the most common abnormalities of hemostasis are immune thrombocytopenia, vitamin K deficiency, hemophilia, or bleeding from a localized vascular lesion. It is difficult to diagnose some hereditary bleeding disorders in the neonatal period, particularly mild or moderate deficiencies of factor IX and VWD. Severe forms of factor VIII or IX deficiencies are easier to diagnose. Early onset vitamin K deficiency bleeding (within the first 24 hours of life) is usually due to placental transfer of maternal drugs that inhibit vitamin K activity in the baby, including dilantin or other anticonvulsants, antibiotics, and oral anticoagulants.

Bleeding manifestations in babies with DIC are similar to other patients with the syndrome and include bleeding from puncture sites, the GI tract, or other locations. The PT and APTT are markedly prolonged, and thrombocytopenia is present in symptomatic babies.

One of the most common causes of death in premature infants is intracranial hemorrhage. Many of these are patients who have severe respiratory distress syndrome or a familial bleeding diathesis (hemophilia or other hereditary coagulation deficiency).

Thrombosis may also occur in infants, particularly those with indwelling catheters, those born to diabetic mothers, or those with predisposing medical conditions (e.g., asphyxia, infection, respiratory distress syndrome). Neonatal hypercoagulability may also be seen in infants with a hereditary thrombophilia (∞ Chapter 38).

SUMMARY

This chapter includes a discussion of the conditions associated with abnormal secondary hemostasis. These conditions encompass those in which fibrin is formed too slowly or is lysed too rapidly so that excessive bleeding results. Also included is a discussion of the unique hemostatic status of newborns.

Abnormal fibrin formation occurs in patients with mutations of the genes that code for the circulating hemostatic proteins and result either in decreased synthesis or abnormal function of the protein. The most common of these disorders are X-linked deficiencies of factors VIII and IX, called the hemophilias. von Willebrand factor is complexed with factor VIII in the circulation, and when deficient may result in a bleeding diathesis. Rarer deficiencies of the remaining coagulation factors and of components of fibrinolysis may result in excessive bleeding. However, in the case of factor XII, prekallikrein, and high molecular weight kininogen, no clinical bleeding symptoms are present in spite of abnormal in vitro laboratory test results. Some patients with deficiencies of these three components may have an increased risk for thrombosis. Laboratory screening tests and specific factor assays establish the diagnosis in disorders associated with coagulant protein deficiencies.

Newborns are at higher risk for bleeding and may have prolonged PTs and APTTs until the vitamin K-producing intestinal bacteria and liver production of the various coagulation factors are established.

REVIEW QUESTIONS

LEVEL I

1. A patient who has a deficiency of a clotting factor may have: (Checklist #1)
   a. inherited an abnormal gene from a parent
   b. acquired the deficiency because of another disease
   c. a decrease in amount of the particular factor in the blood
   d. all of the above

2. Patients who have deficiencies of clotting factors usually have abnormal bleeding because: (Checklist #1, 2)
   a. fibrin formation is slower and less effective than normal
   b. platelets do not aggregate normally
   c. fibrin is formed too fast and in too large a quantity
   d. fibrin is broken down as fast as it is formed

3. The clotting factor that is deficient in a patient with hemophilia A is: (Checklist #4)
   a. factor VII
   b. factor VIII
   c. factor IX
   d. factor XIII

Use the following case study to answer questions 4–6.

An 18-year-old female bled profusely following extraction of a tooth. She had a history of sporadically increased menstrual bleeding and nosebleeds. She had an appendectomy at age 10 with no unusual bleeding. A workup in the coagulation laboratory showed the following:

LEVEL II

1. Referring to the case study for Level I questions 4–6, the results of the platelet aggregation studies indicate that the patient has a defect in: (Checklist # 4)
   a. factor VIII
   b. platelet adhesion
   c. fibrinolysis
   d. the intrinsic system of fibrin formation

2. The inheritance pattern of von Willebrand disease is usually: (Checklist #3)
   a. autosomal dominant
   b. autosomal recessive
   c. X-linked recessive
   d. not inherited, usually acquired

3. Type I von Willebrand disease is characterized by: (Checklist #4)
   a. decreased amounts of large multimers of von Willebrand factor
   b. increased amounts of large multimers of von Willebrand factor
   c. decreased amounts of all von Willebrand factor multimers
   d. decreased amounts of small von Willebrand factor multimers only

REVIEW QUESTIONS (continued)

LEVEL I

Laboratory test	Patient results	Laboratory reference range
Platelet count	312×10^9/L	150–440×10^9/L
Bleeding time	9.5 minutes	2–9 minutes
Closure time	Increased	
Prothrombin time	11.5 sec	10–12 sec
Activated partial thromboplastin time	38.0 sec	23–36 sec
Factor VIII assay	20 U/dL	50–150 U/dL
Factor IX assay	102 U/dL	50–150 U/dL
Platelet aggregation studies	Normal: ADP, collagen, epinephrine Abnormal: ristocetin	

4. Which laboratory tests are outside of their reference range? (Checklist #2)
   a. all tests shown
   b. platelet aggregation with ristocetin, activated partial thromboplastin time, factor VIII assay
   c. platelet count, prothrombin time, factor IX assay
   d. prothrombin time, activated partial thromboplastin time, factor IX assay

5. The most probable cause of this patient's bleeding is: (Checklist #3, 10)
   a. a vascular disorder
   b. factor IX deficiency
   c. von Willebrand disease
   d. disseminated intravascular coagulation

6. One of the laboratory tests that is abnormal in this patient that is different from that of a patient with hemophilia A is: (Checklist #5, 6)
   a. factor VIII assay
   b. factor IX assay
   c. platelet aggregation studies with ADP
   d. platelet aggregation studies with ristocetin

7. What result of the platelet count would you expect in a patient with hemophilia A? (Checklist #5)
   a. normal
   b. increased
   c. decreased
   d. unpredictable

8. A patient with DIC most likely would have: (Checklist # 8)
   a. a prolonged PT
   b. a prolonged APTT
   c. a decreased platelet count
   d. all of the above

LEVEL II

4. Which laboratory procedure analyzes von Willebrand factor qualitatively for abnormalities of the molecular structure? (Checklist #4)
   a. ristocetin-induced platelet aggregation
   b. factor VIII assay
   c. SDS-page gel electrophoresis
   d. activated partial thromboplastin time

5. Von Willebrand disease is caused by: (Checklist #3)
   a. genetic mutations in the factor VIII gene
   b. genetic mutations in the von Willebrand factor gene
   c. genetic mutations in the glycoprotein Ib gene
   d. exposure to dyes and chemicals

6. In which of the following conditions would the presence of delayed bleeding and deep muscular hematomas be most likely? (Checklist #1, 5)
   a. factor VIII deficiency
   b. factor XII deficiency
   c. a patient who is heterozygous for factor V deficiency
   d. a patient with dysfibrinogenemia

7. In which of the following diseases would you most likely find an abnormal prothrombin time? (Checklist #4, 7)
   a. factor VIII deficiency
   b. factor IX deficiency
   c. disseminated intravascular coagulation
   d. prekallikrein deficiency

8. Which of the following is true concerning acquired circulating pathologic inhibitors to single coagulation factors: (Checklist #9)
   a. They do not cause bleeding symptoms.
   b. They cause the same symptoms in the patient as an inherited deficiency of the same factor.
   c. They are often found in patients with von Willebrand disease.
   d. They are antibodies to the phospholipid in the coagulation reagents.

9. In the condition known as disseminated intravascular coagulation (DIC): (Checklist #7)
   a. factors V and VIII become increased in activity
   b. fibrinolytic activity is absent
   c. the patient has a single coagulation factor deficiency
   d. fibrinogen and platelets become depleted

10. One laboratory test that is helpful in diagnosing the lupus anticoagulant is: (Checklist #9)
    a. D-dimer test
    b. dilute Russell's viper venom test
    c. factor XI assay
    d. platelet count

REVIEW QUESTIONS (continued)

LEVEL I

9. The cause of DIC is: (Checklist # 8)
   a. inherited deficiency of factor X
   b. a reaction to another disease that causes the hemostatic system to become activated
   c. a deficiency of vitamin K
   d. an antibody to factor VIII

10. In a newborn infant one would expect: (Checklist #9)
    a. the APTT test to be shorter than that in an adult
    b. the APTT test to be longer than that in an adult
    c. the platelet count to be lower than that in an adult
    d. the platelet count to be higher than that in an adult

LEVEL II

REFERENCES

1. Sadler JE. Biochemistry and genetics of von Willebrand factor. *Ann Rev Biochem*. 1998; 67:395–424.

2. Mazurier C, Ribba AS, Gaucher C, Meyer D. Molecular genetics of von Willebrand disease. *Ann de Genet*. 1997; 41:34–43.

3. Wagner DD, Ginsburg D. Structure, biology, and genetics of von Willebrand factor. Hoffman R, Benz EJ Jr, Shatill SJ, Furie B, Cohen HJ, Silberstein LE, eds. In: *Hematology: Basic Principles and Practice*, 2nd ed. New York: Churchill Livingstone; 1995:1717–25.

4. Sadler JE, Gralnick HR. Commentary: A new classification for von Willebrand disease. *Blood*. 1994; 84:676–79.

5. Federici AB. Diagnosis of von Willebrand disease. *Hemophilia*. 1998; 4:654–60.

6. Vischer UM, de Moerloose P. Von Willebrand factor: From cell biology to the clinical management of von Willebrand's disease. *Crit Rev Oncol/Hematol*. 1999; 30:93–109.

7. Ginsburg D, Bowie EJW. Molecular genetics of von Willebrand disease. *Blood*. 1992; 79:2507–19.

8. Veyradier A, Fressinaud E, Meyer D. Laboratory diagnosis of von Willebrand disease. *Int J Clin Lab Res*. 1998; 28:201–10.

9. Favaloro EJ, Facey D, Henniker A. Use of a novel platelet function analyzer (PFA-100) with high sensitivity to disturbances in von Willebrand factor to screen for von Willebrand's disease and other disorders. *Am J Hematol*. 1999; 62:165–74.

10. Sadler JE. A revised classification of von Willebrand disease. *Thrombo Haemost*. 1994; 71:520–25.

11. Ginsburg D. Molecular genetics of von Willebrand disease. *Thromb Haemost*. 1999; 82:585–91.

12. Tefferi A, Nichols WL. Acquired von Willebrand disease: Concise review of occurrence, diagnosis, pathogenesis, and treatment. *Amer J Med*. 1997; 103:536–40.

13. Pavlovsky A. Contribution to the pathogenesis of hemophilia. *Blood*. 1947; 2:185–91.

14. Marder VJ, Mannucci PM, Firkin BG, Hoyer LW, Meyer D. Standard nomenclature for factor VIII and von Willebrand factor: A recommendation by the International Committee on Thrombosis and Haemostasis. *Thromb Haemost*. 1985; 54:871–72.

15. Greenberg CS, Orthner CL. Blood coagulation and fibrinolysis. Lee GR, Foerster J, Lukens J, Paraskevas F, Greer JP, Rodgers GM, eds. In: *Wintrobe's Clinical Hematology*, 10th ed. Baltimore: Williams & Wilkins; 1999:684–764.

16. Lillicrap D. Molecular diagnosis of inherited bleeding disorders and thrombophilia. *Sem Hematol*. 1999; 36:340–451.

17. Kaufman RJ, Antonarakis SE. Structure, biology, and genetics of factor VIII. Hoffman R, Benz EJ Jr, Shatill SJ, Furie B, Cohen HJ, Silberstein LE, eds. In: *Hematology: Basic Principles and Practice*, 2nd ed. New York: Churchill Livingstone; 1995:1633–48.

18. Attali O, Vinciguerra C, Treciak MC, et al. Factor IX gene analysis in 70 unrelated patients with haemophilia B: Description of 13 new mutations. *Thromb Haemost*. 1999; 82:1437–42.

19. Giannelli F, Green PM, Sommer, SS, et al. Haemophilia B: Database of point mutations and short additions and deletions—eighth edition. *Nucleic Acids Res*. 1998; 26:265–68.

20. Roberts HR, Gray TF III. Clinical aspects of and therapy for hemophilia B. Hoffman R, Benz EJ Jr, Shatill SJ, Furie B, Cohen HJ, Silberstein LE, eds. In: *Hematology: Basic Principles and Practice*, 2nd ed. New York: Churchill Livingstone; 1995:1678–85.

21. Bretter DB, Kraus EM, Levine PH. Clinical aspects of and therapy for hemophilia A. Hoffman R, Benz EJ Jr, Shatill SJ, Furie B, Cohen HJ, Silberstein LE, eds. In: *Hematology: Basic Principles and Practice*. 2nd ed. New York: Churchill Livingstone; 1995:1648–63.

22. Giangrande PLF. Pregnancy in carriers of haemophilia. 1997: *http://www.medicine.ac.uk/ohc/carrier.htm*.

23. Peyvandi F, Mannucci PM. Rare coagulation disorders. *Thromb Haemost*. 1999; 82:1207–14.

24. Galanakis DK. Fibrinogen anomalies and disease. *Hematol/Oncol Clin NA*. 1992; 6:1171–87.

25. Mosesson, MW. Hereditary abnormalities of fibrinogen. Beutler E, Lichtman MA, Coller BS, Kipps TJ, Seliqsohn U, eds. In: *William's Hematology*, 6th ed. New York: McGraw-Hill; 2001:1659–71.

26. Owren CA, Bowie EJW, Thompson JH. *The Diagnosis of Bleeding Disorders*, 2nd ed. Boston, MA: Little Brown & Co; 1975.

27. Cooper DN, Millar DS, Wacey A, Pemberton S, Tuddenham EGD. Inherited factor X deficiency: Molecular genetics and pathophysiology. *Thromb Haemost*. 1997;78:161–72.

28. Roberts HR, Hoffman M. Hemophilia and related conditions: Inherited deficiencies of prothrombin (factor II), factor V, and factors

VII to XII. Beutler E, Lichtman MA, Coller BS, Kipps TJ, eds. In: *William's Hematology,* 5th ed. New York: McGraw-Hill; 1995: 1413–39.

29. Bick RL. *Disorders of Thrombosis and Hemostasis: Clinical and Laboratory Practice.* Chicago: ASCP Press; 1992.

30. Katona E, Haramura G, Karpati L, Fachet J, Muszbek L. A simple, quick one-step ELISA assay for the determination of complex plasma factor XIII (A_2B_2). *Thromb Haemost.* 2000; 83:268–73.

31. Kaufman RJ, Antonarakis SE, Fay PJ. Factor VIII and hemophilia A. Colman RW, Hirsh J, Marder VJ, Clowes AW, George JN, eds. In: *Hemostasis and Thrombosis: Basic Principles and Clinical Practice,* 4th ed. Philadelphia: Lippincott Williams & Wilkens; 2000:135–56.

32. Rodgers GM, Greenberg CS. Inherited coagulation disorders. Lee GR, Foerster J, Lukens J, Paraskevas F, Greer JP, Rodgers GM, eds. In: *Wintrobe's Clinical Hematology,* 10th ed. Baltimore: Williams & Wilkins; 1999:1682–1732.

33. Levi M, de Jonge E, van der Poll T, ten Cate H. Disseminated intravascular coagulation. *Thromb Haemost.* 1999; 82:695–705.

34. Scherer RU, Spangenberg P. Procoagulant activity in patients with isolated severe head trauma. *Crit Care Med.* 1998; 26:149–56.

35. Feinstein DI, Marder VJ, Colman RW. Consumptive thrombohemorrhagic disorders. Colman RW, Hirsh J, Marder VJ, Clowes AW, George JN, eds. In: *Hemostasis and Thrombosis, Basic Principles and Clinical Practice,* 4th ed. Philadelphia: Lippincott Williams & Wilkens; 2000: 1197–1234.

36. Baglin T. Disseminated intravascular coagulation: Diagnosis and treatment. *BMJ.* 1996; 312:683–87.

37. Grosset AMB, Rodgers GM. Acquired coagulation disorders. Lee GR, Foerster J, Lukens J, Paraskevas F, Greer JP, Rodgers GM, eds. In: *Wintrobe's Clinical Hematology,* 10th ed. Baltimore: Williams & Wilkins; 1999:1733–1780.

38. Thiagarajan P, Shapiro SS. Lupus anticoagulants and antiphospholipid antibodies. *Hemat/Oncol Clin NA.* 1998; 12:1167–92.

39. Court EL. Lupus anticoagulants: Pathogenesis and laboratory diagnosis. *Brit J Biomed Sci.* 1997; 54:287–98.

40. Arnout J. The pathogenesis of the antiphospholipid syndrome: A hypothesis based on parallelisms with heparin-induced thrombocytopenia. *Thromb Haemost.* 1996; 75:536–41.

41. Brandt JT, Triplett DA, Alving B, Scharrer I. Criteria for the diagnosis of lupus anticoagulants: An update. *Thromb Haemost.* 1995; 74: 1185–90.

42. Montgomery RR, Marlar RA, Gill JC. Newborn hemostasis. *Clin Haematol.* 1985; 14:443–60.

43. Johnston M, Zipursky A. Microtechnology for the study of blood coagulation system in newborn infants. *Can J Med Tech.* 1980; 42:159–64.

44. Andrew M, Paes B, Milner R, et al. Development of the human coagulation system in the full-term infant. *Blood.* 1987; 70:165–72.

45. Hathaway W, Corrigan J, for the Subcommittee. Normal coagulation data for fetuses and newborn infants. *Thromb Haemost.* 1991; 65:323–25.

46. Andrew M, Paes B, Milner R, et al. Development of the human coagulation system in the healthy premature infant. *Blood.* 1988; 72:1651–57.

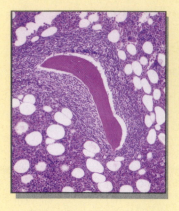

38

Thrombophilia

Lynne Williams, Ph.D.
Cheryl Swinehart, M.S.

CHAPTER OUTLINE

■ CHECKLIST - LEVEL I

At the end of this unit of study the student should be able to:

1. Define *hypercoagulability, thrombophilia, thrombus,* and *thrombosis.*

2. Describe the physiological processes involved in hypercoagulability.

3. Explain how a thrombus becomes a thromboembolus.

4. List two differences between a white thrombus and a red thrombus and the risk factors predisposing to the formation of each.

5. Define *deep vein thrombosis* (DVT); explain how it is diagnosed and what clinical conditions can result.

6. Describe the role of heparin in the neutralization of activated coagulation factors by antithrombin.

7. Diagram the relationship of protein C and protein S to the coagulation pathway and explain why a deficiency of either might lead to a thrombotic tendency.

8. Explain why both molecular (antigenic) and functional assays should be performed for diagnosing antithrombin, protein C, or protein S abnormalities in a patient.

9. Describe activated protein C resistance (APCR) and explain its contribution to thrombophilia.

10. List two side effects of heparin therapy and what hematology procedures should be monitored to prevent these complications.

11. Identify the difference between unfractionated and low molecular weight heparin (LMWH).

12. Discuss how oral anticoagulants like coumadin decrease a person's risk for thrombosis and the best way to monitor oral anticoagulation.

■ CHECKLIST - LEVEL II

At the end of this unit of study the student should be able to:

1. Evaluate the utility of laboratory tests in differential diagnosis of arterial and venous thrombotic disease.

2. List four clinical manifestations suggestive of an inherited thrombophilia and explain why many patients are not diagnosed.

3. Explain the differences between Type I and Type II deficiencies of protein C, protein S, and antithrombin; given values for antithrombin or protein C and S assays, determine the type of deficiency in a patient.

rin. The activ
thrombus that
tually obstruct
off and lodges
ing myocardia
ment for arteri
drugs (e.g., asp
Traditional
creased predis
of arterial thrc
sion, smoking
However, since
coronary thro
risk factors, th
laboratory test
botic event. Hi
have been con
novel risk fac
While the clini
sistent, some c
thrombotic ter
New approa
arterial disease
vated lipoprot
elevated PAI-1
tein (CRP). No
bosis. Tests sug
(elevated fibri
fibrinolytic act
tendency but r
is the recent re
role in the initi
inflammation
markers of infl
clinical athero
tant, with elev
acute injury, ir
the introductic
its potential as
being evaluate
and serum amy
teins) strongly
esis. Evidence c
in advance of
and women, ir
early and prece

VENOUS T

Thrombi forme
termed **red th**
blood cells trap
platelets and le
gions of slow c
ments that hav

■ **CHECKLIST - LEVEL II *(continued)***

4. List two deficiencies that can cause warfarin- (coumadin-) induced skin necrosis and give potential treatment options.
5. Defend the use of both a clotting and molecular assay for diagnosis of APCR.
6. Describe the two most common mutations leading to hyperhomocysteinemia.
7. Explain how increased levels of prothrombin or fibrinogen might predispose to thrombosis.
8. Describe how deficiencies of plasminogen or plasminogen activator or increased levels of plasminogen activator inhibitor could lead to thrombosis.
9. Identify secondary disorders leading to thrombosis.
10. Describe and explain the treatment of a thrombotic episode.
11. Explain how the INR has standardized prothrombin times.
12. Evaluate the use and monitoring of thrombolytic therapy in treatment of thrombosis.
13. Given a patient history and appropriate laboratory results, interpret the data to determine a probable diagnosis.

KEY TERMS

Activated protein C resistance (APCR)
Antiphospholipid antibody syndrome (APLS)
Deep vein thrombosis (DVT)
Dysfibrinogenemia
Embolus
Factor V Leiden (FVL)
Hypercoagulable
Hyperhomocysteinemia
Low molecular weight heparin (LMWH)
Pulmonary embolism (PE)
Red thrombi
Thromboembolism (TE)
Thrombolytic therapy
Thrombophilia
Thrombophlebitis
Thrombosis
Thrombus
White thrombi

BACKGROUND BASICS

Information in this chapter will build on concepts learned in previous chapters. To maximize your learning experience you should review these concepts before starting this unit of study.

Level I

- Primary hemostasis: Describe the mechanisms of platelet activation and the functions of platelets in both primary and secondary hemostasis. (Chapter 34)
- Secondary hemostasis: Outline the coagulation cascade and the components contributing to fibrin formation. List the components and the function of the fibrinolytic system and the products of fibrinolytic activation (FDPs). List the mechanisms that maintain normal physiologic control of hemostasis, particularly the inhibitors of both coagulation and fibrinolysis. (Chapter 35)

Level II

- Secondary hemostasis: Describe the mechanism of activation of serine proteases (complex formation on a phospholipid surface). (Chapter 35)
- Secondary hemostasis: Summarize the physiologic controls that limit activation of coagulation and fibrinolysis to the sites of vessel injury. (Chapter 35)
- Secondary hemostasis: Describe the method of activation and physiologic function of the inhibitors of coagulation and fibrinolysis. (Chapter 35)

CASE STUDY

We will address this case study throughout the chapter.

A. C. is a 37-year-old woman recently diagnosed with deep vein thrombosis (DVT) of the right leg. She is dehydrated and on oral contraceptives. She is also on coumadin.

Consider possible factors contributing to the thrombosis in this patient and the laboratory tests that might be used to differentiate and diagnose the cause.

▶ OVERVIEW

This chapter describes imbalances between procoagulant and anticoagulant processes in the hemostatic system that result in an increased tendency to form thrombi (thrombophilia). The chapter begins with a summary of the factors

that influe
nous blood
that form
bophilia is
that contr
thrombopl
manifestat
phasis is o
torial disea
tioned in
chapter en
pies for the

► INTF

The humar
procoagula
fibrinolytic
systems are
clotting oc
more proce
activity), th
bosis is th
a vessel kn
ditions can

The thre
stasis are a
vascular en
teins (Table
tithrombog
agulation f
cause releas
or loss of n
thrombom
tithrombin
circulating
subendoth
vated by ti
vessels. Ina
from decre
inadequate
blood flow
flow serves
from their s

Thrombi
tem, includ
lation. Thr
trapped cel
hemodynar
thrombi. T
clot; howe
(either in v
cavities). T
logic event

BACKGROUND BASICS

The information in this chapter will build on the concepts learned in previous chapters. To maximize your learning experience you should review these concepts before starting this unit of study.

Level I

► Role of blood vessels in hemostasis: Describe the vascular contributions to hemostasis. (Chapter 34)

► Formation of the primary platelet plug: Summarize the steps involved in the formation of the primary platelet plug. (Chapter 34)

► Coagulation cascade: List the coagulation factors and the sequence of events involved in the coagulation cascade. (Chapter 35)

► Biochemical inhibitors: Describe the biochemical inhibitors that regulate the coagulation cascade. (Chapter 35)

► Fibrinolytic system: List the factors and the sequence of events involved in fibrinolysis. (Chapter 35)

Level II

► Qualitative and quantitative platelet disorders: Define the defect and identify the cause of impaired hemostasis in the following disorders of primary hemostasis: Bernard-Soulier syndrome, Glanzmann's thrombasthenia, drug-induced platelet disorders, and immune thrombocytopenic purpura. (Chapter 36)

► Inherited disorders of secondary hemostasis: Define the defect and identify the cause of impaired hemostasis in the following disorders of secondary hemostasis: von Willebrand disease, hemophilia A, and hemophilia B. (Chapter 37)

► Acquired disorders of secondary hemostasis: Summarize the etiology and the pathophysiology of the acquired disorders of hemostasis, including disseminated intravascular coagulation,

vitamin K deficiency, lupus-like anticoagulant, and factor VIII inhibitor. (Chapter 37)

► Inherited and acquired hypercoagulable states: Summarize the effect on the hemostatic system of factor V Leiden, protein C deficiency, antithrombin III deficiency, and protein S deficiency. (Chapter 38)

► OVERVIEW

This chapter describes tests performed in the coagulation laboratory that are used to investigate a hemostatic disorder as indicated by either patient history or physical examination. Screening tests are used to place the defect in one of several broad categories with definitive diagnosis subsequently established using more specialized testing. Screening tests for defects of primary hemostasis include a platelet count and/or bleeding time, while screening tests for defects of secondary hemostasis are generally the prothrombin time (PT) and the activated partial thromboplastin time (APTT). In some cases, screening tests are performed to assess the patient's hemostatic status before surgery.

Coagulation test results are highly dependent on the appropriateness and integrity of the blood specimen. Thus, the chapter begins with a discussion on specimen collection and processing. The tests are grouped according to the part of the coagulation system that they assess: primary hemostasis, secondary hemostasis, and fibrinolysis. The last section of this chapter deals with laboratory tests used to assess hypercoagulable states and monitor anticoagulant therapy. A general description of each test includes the theory of the test, a summary of the procedure, and expected results. A detailed procedure for selected tests can be found on the text's companion Web site.

► SPECIMEN COLLECTION AND PROCESSING

The accuracy of coagulation tests relies on proper collection, processing, and storage, if the testing cannot be performed immediately.

SPECIMEN COLLECTION

Whole blood should be collected aseptically by venipuncture using an evacuated tube system or a syringe (∞ Chapter 7). When using the evacuated tube system, the first, second, or third tube collected may be used as the coagulation specimen.[1-3] However, two factors are important considerations in selection of the tube sequence: (1) the venipuncture must be trouble-free (i.e., without trauma), and (2) if the second or third tube is used for the coagulation specimen, the tubes collected prior should not contain an anticoagulant or clot-promoting substance. In the case of a difficult phlebotomy or when certain coagulation studies are requested, the two-syringe technique may be appropriate to minimize chance contamination of the specimen due to release of tissue factor. When using the two-syringe technique, the blood from the second syringe should be used for the coagulation specimen. The possibility of heparin contamination must be considered when blood is collected from an indwelling catheter. To prevent this, the line should be flushed with saline and the first 5 mL of blood discarded.

The anticoagulant of choice for coagulation studies is 3.2% sodium citrate.[1-4] The proper ratio of anticoagulant to whole blood is 1:9. Studies have shown that high hematocrits have less effect on the overall anticoagulation of the specimen when using 3.2% sodium citrate compared to 3.8% sodium citrate.[5] However, the NCCLS guideline continues to recommend adjusting the amount of anticoagulant used when the patient's hematocrit exceeds 55%[4] (see Web Figure 39-1 ■ for the correction formulas). The use of a collection tube containing the standard amount of anticoagulant when a patient's hematocrit exceeds 55% will result in a relative increase in anticoagulant causing the sample to be over-anticoagulated.

SPECIMEN PROCESSING

Citrate anticoagulated whole blood is centrifuged to obtain plasma for coagulation testing. Depending on the test, either platelet-poor or platelet-rich plasma may be required.

Platelet-Poor Plasma

Proper processing of the specimen is required in order to obtain reliable results. To obtain platelet-poor plasma (PPP), the specimen is centrifuged for 15 minutes at 2500 × g. Platelet-poor plasma should contain <10 × 10^9/L platelets. The separated plasma may either be left on top of the erythrocytes or be removed from the packed cells using a plastic pipet and placed in a capped plastic tube. The separated plasma may be stored at 18–24°C or 2–4°C for up to 4 hours before testing. If testing cannot be performed within this time period, platelet-poor plasma should be separated from the cells and stored at –20°C for no longer than 2 weeks or –70°C for no longer than 6 months. Frozen samples should be thawed rapidly at 37°C and tested immediately. Samples for coagulation testing should never be stored in self-defrosting freezers, as the freeze–thaw cycles will compromise sample integrity.

Platelet-Rich Plasma

Several coagulation procedures require the use of platelet-rich plasma (PRP), rather than platelet-poor plasma (e.g., platelet aggregation studies). To obtain platelet-rich plasma, the specimen is centrifuged for 10 minutes at 200 × g as soon as possible after collection. Platelet-rich plasma will contain 200–300 × 10^9/L platelets. Platelet-rich plasma should be separated from the packed cells using a plastic pipet and placed in a covered plastic tube. If testing is not performed immediately, platelet-rich plasma may be stored at room temperature (18–24°C) for up to 3 hours.

> ### Checkpoint! #1
>
> *Why have most clinical laboratories switched from 3.8% to 3.2% sodium citrate for specimen collection in coagulation studies?*

► LABORATORY INVESTIGATION OF PRIMARY HEMOSTASIS

Laboratory testing to evaluate primary hemostasis includes tests for platelet concentration and function. The platelet count was described in Chapter 7. The bleeding time and platelet aggregation tests for platelet function will be discussed here.

BLEEDING TIME

Screening for defects of primary hemostasis is evaluated using the bleeding time (BT).[6,7] It is an in vivo measurement of platelet function. Several factors affect the bleeding time including platelet numbers, platelet function, and vascular integrity (∞ Chapter 34). The test is not significantly prolonged in most disorders that result in prolongation of the PT or APTT. The BT measures the time required for bleeding to cease from a superficial cut of the skin. In addition to platelet number and function, the BT is influenced by the depth, location, and direction of the incision, skin thickness, and skill of the clinical laboratory professional.

Several methods have been used to perform the bleeding time. The oldest method, the Duke bleeding time, utilized a lancet to make a puncture in the ear lobe. In 1941, Ivy improved the bleeding time technique by creating a constant venous pressure with a blood pressure cuff (40 mmHg) and performing the test on the forearm with a lancet. The template bleeding time, which is utilized today, is a modification of the Ivy bleeding time. By using a template, the incision made is a consistent length and depth. Disposable bleeding time devices are used to perform the template bleeding time. The template bleeding time procedure is provided on the companion Web site. The BT is the length of time required for bleeding to cease. The general **reference interval** for the BT is 1–9 minutes.

In order to be an accurate assessment of in vivo platelet function, the patient should avoid the use of aspirin or aspirin-like drugs for seven days prior to the bleeding time test since the ingestion of aspirin and many aspirinlike drugs will result in a prolonged BT (∞ Chapter 36). Likewise, a

TABLE 39-1

Conditions Associated with a Prolonged Bleeding Time (∞ Chapter 36)

von Willebrand disease
Bernard-Soulier syndrome
Glanzmann's thrombasthenia
Congenital storage pool disease
Afibrinogenemia
Severe hypofibrinogenemia
Certain vascular bleeding disorders like Ehlers-Danlos syndrome
Uremia

platelet count should be performed prior to the BT test since a platelet count of $<100 \times 10^9/L$ will result in a prolongation of the bleeding time. If the above conditions are met, a prolonged bleeding time usually indicates platelet dysfunction (Table 39-1 ⚙).

PLATELET AGGREGOMETRY

Platelet aggregation studies are the foundation of platelet function testing in the laboratory. The addition of an **aggregating reagent** (platelet agonist) to a stirred suspension of platelet-rich plasma results in platelet shape change and aggregation.[7,8] These changes can be monitored as an increase in light transmission through the PRP suspension as aggregation occurs. An aggregometer records the changes in percent transmittance in the form of a graph (curve). A battery of aggregating reagents is used in the performance of platelet aggregation studies. Commonly used aggregating reagents include ADP, epinephrine, collagen, ristocetin, and arachidonic acid. Platelet aggregation studies should not be performed on any patient who has ingested aspirin seven days prior to the test. Aspirin inhibits platelet aggregation and may mask the presence of a qualitative platelet abnormality (∞ Chapter 34).

Depending upon the aggregating reagent used, aggregation occurs in one or two waves. The primary wave represents the direct response of the platelets to the aggregating reagent. It represents platelet shape change and the formation of small aggregates. The secondary wave represents complete aggregation, which occurs as a result of endogenous ADP release from the platelet dense bodies.

An aggregating reagent that results in both a primary and secondary wave is said to produce a biphasic curve, whereas an aggregating reagent that results in only one wave is said to produce a monophasic curve. Aggregating reagents produce typical aggregation patterns (Figure 39-1 ■). **Ristocetin** is unique among the aggregating reagents in that its action is dependent upon the interaction

of von Willebrand factor and the platelet membrane receptor glycoprotein Ib (GPIb/IX) and technically represents platelet agglutination rather than aggregation (∞ Chapter 34). Changes in platelet aggregation curves are interpreted to identify qualitative platelet disorders (Table 39-2 ⚙). Careful attention to detail is required to obtain reproducible platelet function studies. Results are influenced by choice of anticoagulant, pH, time of storage, rate of stirring, and platelet count.[9]

Although ristocetin induced platelet agglutination may be abnormal in both von Willebrand disease (VWD) and Bernard-Soulier syndrome (BSS), plasma ristocetin cofactor activity (discussed later) is usually decreased in the former but is normal in the latter disorder. Additionally, the defect in ristocetin-induced platelet agglutination observed in VWD can be corrected by the addition of normal plasma to the patient's PRP because the defect is a deficiency of a plasma protein and not a defect in platelets. The agglutination defect in BSS is not corrected because the defect is due to a deficiency of the GPIb/IX complex on the patient's platelet membrane and is not corrected by the addition of normal plasma.

ADDITIONAL TESTS EVALUATING PLATELET FUNCTION

Platelet Secretion Studies   Although not available in most clinical laboratories, studies of platelet secretion are usually available in coagulation reference laboratories. The secretion of granule contents is monitored by following the agonist-induced release of ^{14}C-serotonin from platelet dense bodies or of ADP release by a chemiluminescence procedure.[9]

Flow Cytometry   The development of monoclonal antibodies reactive with platelet surface receptors now offers new approaches for laboratory diagnosis of platelet disorders. Bernard-Soulier syndrome (GPIb/IX deficiency) and Glanzmann's thrombasthenia (GPIIb/IIIa complex deficiency) can be evaluated by flow cytometry using antibodies directed against GPIb/IX and IIb/IIIa, respectively. A panel of antibodies has been developed that recognize the resting, activated, and ligand-occupied forms of the GPIIb/IIIa complex.[9] These antibodies can be used in flow cytometry to assess the presence as well as functional activity of the complex. These assays will likely play an increasing role in the evaluation of platelet function in the near future.

✓ **Checkpoint! #2**

What effect will aspirin have on the bleeding time of a patient who takes aspirin daily for a heart condition? Explain.

Normal Platelet Aggregation Curves

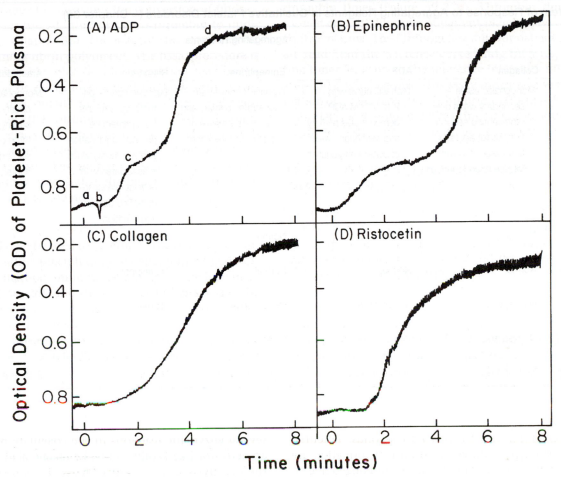

■ **FIGURE 39-1** Normal platelet aggregation curves. Normal responses to the commonly used aggregating reagents: ADP, epinephrine, collagen, ristocetin. Point *a* represents the baseline before addition of the reagent; point *b* is the initial increase in absorbance that occurs immediately following the addition of reagent and represents a change in platelet shape; point *c* represents the primary wave of aggregation; point *d* represents the secondary wave of aggregation.

▶ **LABORATORY INVESTIGATION OF SECONDARY HEMOSTASIS**

Laboratory tests of secondary hemostasis evaluate coagulation factors and also can detect inhibitors of coagulation.

SCREENING TESTS

Screening tests include the prothrombin time, activated partial thromboplastin time, thrombin time, and fibrinogen. Abnormalities in these tests will help in selection of more specific tests to assist diagnosis.

Prothrombin Time

The prothrombin time (PT) is an important screening test for the laboratory evaluation of patients with inherited or acquired deficiencies in the extrinsic or common pathway of the coagulation cascade and for monitoring the effectiveness of **oral anticoagulant therapy** (∞ Chapters 35, 38). This test utilizes a crude preparation of tissue factor (a thromboplastin-calcium reagent) to activate the coagulation cascade via formation of the TF/factor VII complex.[10] The time required for clot formation is recorded. This procedure is provided on the text's companion Web site. Clot formation may be detected by optical or electromechanical methods using manual, semiautomated, or automated devices. The general

other inhibitors.[21,23,24] Freeze–thawed (ruptured) platelets serve as a source of phospholipid. The patient's PPP is mixed with a suspension of ruptured platelets and APTT reagent. The addition of 0.025M calcium chloride activates the coagulation system. The clotting time is determined and compared with the APTT clotting times of the patient PPP and the saline control (1:2 dilution of saline and patient PPP). If lupus anticoagulants are present, the clotting time with added phospholipids will be significantly shorter than the original APTT and the saline control APTT. False positive results may be seen with patients receiving heparin or those with extremely high titer inhibitors to other clotting factors.

Hexagonal Phospholipids.   Molecules of purified **phosphatidyl ethanolamine** undergo structural rearrangement into hexagonal H_{II} phase structures at 37°C in aqueous solution. Hexagonal phase phosphatidyl ethanolamine consists of hexagonally packed cylinders of lipid surrounding central aqueous channels toward which the polar head groups are orientated. LLAC antibodies specifically recognize these structures.[25] The addition of H_{II} phase phosphatidyl ethanolamine to a plasma containing LLAC will correct the prolonged APTT. An advantage of this procedure over the PNP is the elimination of false positive results for patients receiving heparin as seen with the PNP.

Dilute Russell's Viper Venom Test   Unlike the platelet neutralization procedure where LLAC activity is inactivated in the presence of increased phospholipids, the dilute **Russell's viper venom** test (dRVVT) is based on the premise that lupus-like anticoagulant activity will be increased in the presence of reduced phospholipids.[24,26] The reagent used in this procedure contains dilute Russell's viper venom, calcium chloride, and phospholipids. In this procedure, the reagent is added to patient PPP and RVV activates factor X, resulting in clot formation. Clot formation may be detected by optical or electromechanical methods using manual, semiautomated, or automated devices. If lupus-like anticoagulant is present, the patient's dRVVT will be greater than the normal control plasma's dRVVT. The ratio of patient's clotting time to the clotting time of normal control plasma is determined. The normal ratio is less than 1.2. (A deficiency in factor X, II, or V will have been ruled out by the previously performed mixing studies since factor deficiencies are associated with corrected mixing study results and lupus-like anticoagulant with uncorrected results.)

Factor VIII Inhibitor Assay

A factor VIII inhibitor is quantitated by preparing various dilutions of the patient plasma with a normal pooled plasma containing a known amount of factor VIII activity. If factor VIII inhibitor is present it inactivates factor VIII. After incubation, the residual factor VIII activity is measured by a factor VIII assay.[14] The residual factor VIII activity is calculated from the comparison of factor VIII activity in the patient plasma dilution with the activity in normal pooled plasma

(Web Figure 39-2 ■). Multiple dilutions of patient plasma help confirm the presence of an inhibitor. In the case of a true factor deficiency, the result is independent of the plasma dilution, whereas the effect of an inhibitor is dilution-dependent. A weak factor VIII inhibitor may not be detected by this procedure. To detect weaker inhibitors, the incubation temperature and time should be altered. The dilutions should be incubated at 37°C for an increased period of time. The inhibitor titer does not correlate with or predict bleeding. The characteristics of an inhibitor vary from patient to patient.

The results of a factor VIII inhibitor assay are reported in Bethesda units. The residual factor VIII activity is converted to a Bethesda unit using Web Table 39-5 ✪ and the calculation formula (Web Figure 39-3 ■). One Bethesda unit of inhibitor is defined as the amount of inhibitor that will inactivate 50% of the factor VIII activity present. Although the Bethesda titer assay was originally developed to measure factor VIII inhibitors, the assay can be modified to assay factor V and factor IX inhibitors as well.

✔ Checkpoint! #6

Why are ruptured platelets able to neutralize lupus-like anticoagulants?

▶ LABORATORY INVESTIGATION OF THE FIBRINOLYTIC SYSTEM

Abnormalities in the fibrinolytic system are not usually detected using the PT and APTT screening tests. The patient's primary disease and the physician's clinical findings (bleeding or thrombosis) may suggest a fibrinolytic system problem and indicate diagnostic laboratory testing.

FIBRIN DEGRADATION PRODUCTS

The detection of fibrin and/or fibrinogen degradation products (FDP) in patient plasma indicates increased fibrinolytic activity (∞ Chapter 35). Conditions associated with increased FDPs include disseminated intravascular coagulation (DIC), liver disease, alcoholic cirrhosis, kidney disease, cardiac disease, postsurgical complications, carcinoma, myocardial infarction, pulmonary embolism, deep vein thrombosis, and eclampsia. The FDP assay represents one of the screening tests used in the diagnosis of DIC and other thrombotic disorders.

Fibrin and/or fibrinogen degradation products (FDPs) are identified through a specific antigen–antibody reaction.[27] For this procedure, patient sample is collected in a collection tube containing thrombin to assure all fibrinogen is removed (clotted) and a fibrinolytic inhibitor to prevent in vitro fibrino(geno)lysis. The patient's serum is mixed with latex particles coated with monoclonal antihuman FDP antibodies on a glass slide for a specific time period (e.g., 2 minutes). At the end of this time period, the reaction mixture is observed macroscopically for the presence of agglutination. The sensitivity of the test system and the choice of specimen will vary dependent on the manufacturer. Most procedures require the preparation of two dilutions for each sample (i.e., 1:2 and 1:8), which allows a semiquantitation of FDP. Macroscopic agglutination in both dilutions corresponds to an FDP level greater than 20 μg/mL. If macroscopic agglutination is observed in the 1:2 dilution but not in the 1:8 dilution, the results correspond to an FDP level greater than 5 μg/mL but less than 20 μg/mL. No macroscopic agglutination in either dilution indicates an FDP level less than 5 μg/mL. Normally, individuals have FDP levels less than 5 μg/mL. The standard FDP assay does not distinguish between fibrin degradation products and fibrinogen degradation products because the antigenic epitopes recognized by the antibodies are expressed on both types of degradation products. Samples that clot poorly (e.g., due to the presence of a high concentration of heparin) may result in artifactually elevated levels of FDP.

D-DIMER

The D-dimer is a marker specific for plasmin degradation (lysis) of fibrin.[28] The D-dimer is a fibrin degradation product generated from factor XIIIa crosslinked fibrin (∞ Chapter 35), and is an excellent marker for disseminated intravascular coagulation with secondary fibrinolysis. However, D-dimers are also elevated in pulmonary embolism, deep vein thrombosis, arterial thromboembolism, recent trauma or surgery, cirrhotic liver disease, and renal failure (∞ Chapter 38). Patients with hyperfibrinogenolysis without thrombin generation will have elevated FDPs but normal (negative) D-dimer levels.

The D-dimer assay can be performed on plasma (citrated, EDTA, or heparinized) as well as serum. The extra step of preparing serum (as in the standard FDP test) is avoided, as fibrinogen and fibrin do not cross-react with the D-dimer monoclonal antibodies used in this test. In this procedure, the patient specimen is mixed with latex particles coated with monoclonal antibodies (directed against D-dimer) on a glass slide for a specific time (e.g., 2 minutes). At the end of this time the reaction mixture is observed macroscopically for the presence of agglutination. Most procedures test undiluted and a 1:2 diluted plasma sample, which allows a semiquantitation of results. Macroscopic agglutination in neither sample corresponds to a D-dimer level of less than 0.5 μg/mL. If macroscopic agglutination is observed in the undiluted plasma but not in the 1:2 dilution, the results correspond to a D-dimer level of 0.5–1.0 μg/mL. The observation of macroscopic agglutination in both samples corresponds to a D-dimer level of greater than 1.0 μg/mL. Normal individuals will have less than 0.5 μg/mL.

EUGLOBULIN CLOT LYSIS

The euglobulin clot lysis is useful in the detection of increased fibrinolytic activity.[14,15] Conditions associated with increased fibrinolytic activity include DIC, liver disease, surgery, certain malignancies, and women receiving oral contraceptives or during menstruation. The euglobulin fraction of plasma consists of fibrinogen, plasminogen, and the activators of plasminogen (but no fibrinolytic inhibitors). This fraction is isolated from plasma by precipitation with 1% acetic acid. The precipitated euglobulin fraction is dissolved in buffered saline, and thrombin is added to clot the euglobulins. The resulting clot serves as substrate for plasmin, which is generated within the clot from plasminogen activation by the plasminogen activators. The resulting clot is incubated at 37°C for two hours. At 30-minute intervals, the clot is observed for evidence of lysis. The euglobulin lysis of the clot is the time required for complete degradation of the clot. In normal individuals, the time required for complete euglobulin clot lysis is greater than 2 hours. Increased fibrinolytic activity is indicated by clot lysis in less than 2 hours. A fibrinogen level of <100 mg/dL can produce a false positive euglobulin clot lysis test.[29]

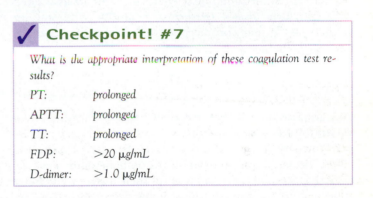

> ✓ **Checkpoint! #7**
>
> *What is the appropriate interpretation of these coagulation test results?*
>
> | | |
> |---|---|
> | PT: | *prolonged* |
> | APTT: | *prolonged* |
> | TT: | *prolonged* |
> | FDP: | *>20 μg/mL* |
> | D-dimer: | *>1.0 μg/mL* |

▶ LABORATORY INVESTIGATION OF HYPERCOAGULABLE STATES

If individuals have repeated thrombotic episodes, they have a hypercoagulable state. Laboratory tests can assist in determining if the thrombosis is due to hereditary or acquired abnormalities in the hemostatic system.

ANTITHROMBIN III

Antithrombin III (AT III) activity can be measured by a variety of assays. Immunologic methods measure the concentration of the protein using enzyme immunoassays (EIA) or enzyme-linked immunoassays (ELISA), radial immunodiffusion (RID), or microlatex particle immunologic assay.

Functional assays may assess inhibitor activity in the presence or absence of heparin. Functional assays use either thrombin or factor Xa as targets for inhibition by AT and may utilize either clotting of fibrinogen (natural substrate) or cleavage of a synthetic chromogenic substrate as the end-point of enzymatic activity. The AT III activity in the presence of heparin is determined using a two-part assay. In the first part, plasma is incubated with a known excess of thrombin in the presence of heparin. The second part of the assay determines the residual thrombin activity by its enzymatic activity on an appropriate substrate (fibrinogen or a chromogenic substrate).

In the **chromogenic assay,**[30] thrombin activity results in the release of p-nitroaniline (pNA) from the chromogenic substrate, which is measured spectrophotometrically at 405 nm. The residual thrombin activity in the second part of the assay is inversely proportional to the AT III level in the plasma. A reference (standard) curve is prepared by plotting the AT III activity (%) for each reference plasma dilution against its corresponding absorbance. The results for patients and controls are read from this curve using their respective absorbance readings. The general reference interval for AT-III is 85–122%.

Inherited deficiencies of AT III may involve a decrease in the protein level or the presence of a dysfunctional protein (∞ Chapter 38). Acquired deficiencies of AT III are associated with DIC, liver disease (cirrhosis), nephrotic syndrome, in women taking oral contraceptives or on estrogen therapy, and malignancy.

PROTEIN C

Like antithrombin III, protein C (PC) can be measured by a variety of methods. Quantitative (antigen) analyses can be performed by EIA or ELISA procedures. Functional assays use either thrombin or the thrombin/thrombomodulin complex to activate PC. Enzyme activity is then assessed either by using a chromogenic (synthetic) substrate or by measuring its anticoagulant activity in a clot-based assay. Chromogenic functional assays may be less informative than clot-based assays when screening for PC defects. Several individuals have been described with normal PC antigen (immunologic) measurements, who have reduced PC anticoagulant activity in clot-based assays but normal amidolytic activity in chromogenic assays.[31] These individuals may have defects in the ability of activated PC (APC) to interact with platelet membranes or the factor Va or VIIIa substrates and would be missed by routine chromogenic assays.

In spite of this limitation, the chromogenic assay for protein C is widely used. In the chromogenic assay, protein C is incubated with a specific activator derived from the venom of *Agkistrodon c. contotrix* (Protac, American Diagnostica, Inc.).[32] The quantity of APC is measured by its enzymatic activity on a chromogenic substrate. The enzymatic activity results in the release of p-nitroaniline (pNA) from the chromogenic substrate, which is measured spectrophotometrically at 405 nm. The absorbance of pNA is directly propor-

tional to the quantity of activated protein C. A reference (standard) curve is prepared by plotting the protein C activity (%) for each reference plasma dilution against its corresponding absorbance. The results for patients and controls are read from this curve using their respective absorbance readings. The general reference interval for protein C is 60–150%.

The clotting assay is based on the ability of APC to prolong the APTT via inactivation of factor Va and factor VIIIa. Patient's plasma is incubated with PC deficient plasma (to compensate for any factor deficiency other than PC), PC activator, and APTT reagent. Calcium chloride is added and the time for clot formation is measured. In PC deficient patients the clotting time is about 30 seconds, while with normal PC levels the time is about 150 seconds. This assay is affected by heparin.

Inherited deficiencies of protein C include quantitative deficiencies characterized by decreased antigenic and functional levels of PC, and qualitative deficiencies characterized by dysfunctional protein C (∞ Chapter 38). Clot-based or chromogenic assays will detect most quantitative and qualitative deficiencies, while immunologic assays fail to detect qualitative deficiencies. Acquired deficiencies of protein C are associated with DIC, vitamin K deficiency, liver disease, oral anticoagulant therapy, and postsurgery.

PROTEIN S

Circulating protein S (PS) exists in two forms: free (40%) and bound to C4b binding protein (60%). Only free protein S serves as a cofactor for APC, enhancing its anticoagulant activity. Laboratory evaluation of PS includes assays of total PS antigen (ELISA assays) and free PS (immunoassays using a monoclonal antibody specific for the free form).[33] Functional PS assay methods are based on the ability of PS to serve as a cofactor for the anticoagulant effect of APC. Activated protein C resistance (see later section) may cause false positive PS test results if clotting (functional) assays are used to diagnose PS deficiency.

In a typical clot-based procedure for measuring the cofactor activity of PS,[34] four reagents are used including: (1) PS deficient plasma, to assure optimal levels of all coagulation factors except PS; (2) activated protein C; (3) activated factor V, to serve as substrate for activated protein C; and (4) calcium chloride. Patient PPP is mixed with PS deficient plasma. To this mixture, activated protein C and activated factor V reagents are added and incubated at 37°C. Following incubation, calcium chloride is added to initiate clot formation. The clotting time is proportional to the PS activity (i.e., the higher the level of PS, the longer the clotting time).

A reference (standard) curve is prepared using dilutions of pooled normal plasma representing 100%, 75%, 50%, and 25% PS activity. The PS activity for each plasma and control is read from this curve. The general reference interval for protein S is 66–122%.

Inherited deficiencies of protein S may involve a decrease in the protein or a dysfunctional protein (∞ Chapter 38). The clot-based procedure will detect both quantitative and qualitative deficiencies of PS. Immunologic methods will not detect qualitative deficiencies of PS. Acquired deficiencies of PS are associated with liver disease, pregnancy, oral contraceptives, DIC, type I diabetes mellitus, and oral anticoagulant therapy.

PLASMINOGEN/PLASMINOGEN ACTIVATION

Functional assays of plasminogen are based on its conversion to plasmin by an excess of activator and are determined by a coupled enzymatic procedure.[35] The first reaction involves the incubation of plasma with a known excess of streptokinase. A plasminogen–streptokinase complex is formed that possesses plasmin-like activity. The second reaction determines the quantity of plasminogen–streptokinase complex by its enzymatic activity on a chromogenic substrate. The enzymatic activity results in the release of p-nitroaniline (pNA) from the chromogenic substrate, which is measured spectrophotometrically at 405 nm. The absorbance of pNA is directly proportional to the quantity of plasminogen. A reference (standard) curve is prepared by plotting the plasminogen activity (%) for each reference plasma dilution against its corresponding absorbance. The results for patients and controls are read from this curve using their respective absorbance readings. The general reference interval for plasminogen level is 74–124%.

Plasminogen activators and plasminogen activator inhibitors (PAI) can be measured similarly. Plasminogen activator may be quantitated by cleavage of specific chromogenic substrates or in a coupled system in which the plasminogen activator content is measured indirectly by the amount of plasminogen converted to plasmin through the use of the plasmin chromogenic substrate. PAI-1 activity is measured by assessment of its activation–neutralization capacity.

Measurement of circulating plasminogen levels is useful in monitoring hepatic regeneration of plasminogen during discontinuous treatment with streptokinase and to control and adjust the rate of infusion if plasminogen is being given to the patient. Tissue plasminogen activator (t-PA), PAI-1, α_2-antiplasmin, and plasmin–α_2-antiplasmin (PAP) complex measurements are useful in assessing the functional status of the fibrinolytic system in patients with excessive primary or secondary fibrinolysis (∞ Chapter 37).

Inherited deficiencies of plasminogen include quantitative deficiencies characterized by decreased antigenic and functional levels, and qualitative deficiencies characterized by dysfunctional protein (∞ Chapter 38). Acquired deficiencies of plasminogen are associated with DIC, liver disease, and leukemias. Deficiency of t-PA or excess of PAI-1 have been reported in inflammatory states and linked with a hypercoagulable tendency (∞ Chapter 38).

Antigenic levels of plasminogen, plasminogen activators (e.g., t-PA), plasminogen activator inhibitors (PAI-1) and PAP complex are determined by immunologic techniques such as enzyme-linked immunoassays (ELISA) or radial immunodiffusion (RID).

ANTIPLASMIN

The primary biochemical inhibitor of plasmin is α_2-antiplasmin (α_2AP). The concentration of functional inhibitor can be analyzed by a coupled reaction using the plasmin chromogenic substrate.[36] The first reaction involves the incubation of plasma with a known excess of plasmin. The second reaction determines the residual plasmin activity by its enzymatic activity on a chromogenic substrate. Plasmin activity results in the release of pNA from the chromogenic substrate, which is measured spectrophotometrically at 405 nm. The residual plasmin activity is inversely proportional to the α_2AP level in the plasma. A reference (standard) curve is prepared by plotting the α_2AP activity (%) for each reference plasma dilution against its corresponding absorbance. The results for patients and controls are read from this curve using their respective absorbance readings. Each laboratory should establish its own reference interval. The normal antiplasmin level for this procedure is 80–120%.

Measurement of circulating α_2AP levels is useful in monitoring fibrinolytic therapy. A decrease in α_2AP reflects the efficacy of the therapy. Acquired deficiencies of α_2AP are associated with severe liver disease, DIC (excessive secondary fibrinolysis), primary fibrinolysis, and septicemia.

ACTIVATED PROTEIN C RESISTANCE

Detection of factor V Leiden mutation (FVL) is important since it represents the most common inherited thrombophilic disorder (∞ Chapter 38). The presence of the FVL mutation results in the resistance of activated factor V to degradation by activated protein C, commonly referred to as activated protein C resistance (APCR).[37] Laboratory tests for APCR are either clot-based functional tests or molecular techniques. A modified APTT, comparing results in the presence or absence of activated protein C, is often used as a screening test. In this test, patient PPP is first mixed with an equal volume of factor V deficient substrate to enhance the sensitivity of the test. A standard APTT is performed on this mixture, and the clotting time is determined. A modified APTT is then performed on the mixture following the addition of a specific amount of purified activated protein C. The modified APTT should be prolonged, due to the APC-mediated destruction of factors Va and VIIIa. The APCR ratio is calculated using the clotting times of the modified APTT and standard APTT (Web Figure 39-4 ■). APCR is indicated by an APCR ratio less than 2.2. For the screening test to be reliable, the initial APTT should be within normal limits; no coumadin, heparin, factor deficiencies, or lupus-like anticoagulant can be present. The sensitivity and specificity of

KEY TERMS

Biphasic antibody
Column chromatography
Densitometer
Hereditary erythroblastic multinuclearity with positive acidified serum test (HEMPAS)
Isopropanol precipitation
Radial immunodiffusion
Supernatant

BACKGROUND BASICS

The information in this chapter will build on concepts learned in the previous chapters. To maximize your learning experience you should review these concepts before starting this unit of study.

Level I

▶ Erythropoiesis: Describe normal erythropoiesis. (Chapter 4)
▶ Hemoglobin synthesis: Summarize the basics of hemoglobin synthesis and name the components that are required. (Chapter 5)
▶ Classification of anemias: Outline the classification systems for the anemias. (Chapter 10)

Level II:

▶ Hemoglobinopathies: Describe the hemoglobinopathies including hemoglobin S and hemoglobin C. (Chapter 12)
▶ Thalassemias: Compare and contrast alpha thalassemia, beta thalassemia, and hereditary persistance of fetal hemoglobin. (Chapter 13)
▶ Anemias characterized by membrane defects: Describe these anemias including the pathophysiology of hereditary spherocytosis. (Chapter 17)
▶ Anemias characterized by metabolic defects: Describe these anemias including the pathophysiology of glucose-6-phosphate dehydrogenase deficiency. (Chapter 18)
▶ Immune hemolytic anemias: Describe these anemias including hemolytic disease of the newborn, transfusion-induced hemolytic anemia, cold hemagglutinin disease, and paroxysmal nocturnal hemoglobinuria. (Chapter 19)

▶ OVERVIEW

Routine hematology tests such as the CBC, differential, and reticulocyte count are used as screening tests to determine the presence of a primary disease in the hematopoietic system or to identify hematologic changes that provide clues to the presence of nonhematologic diseases. Analysis of the results of these screening tests together with clinical signs and symptoms of the patient will help to determine if further

testing is necessary. Algorithms or critical pathways assist in the choice of follow-up testing (reflex testing) to abnormal screening test results. These reflex tests are used in the definitive diagnosis of a variety of anemias. With a definitive diagnosis, the appropriate treatment plan may be implemented and monitored with additional laboratory procedures such as the reticulocyte count. This chapter describes laboratory procedures used in reflex testing. The principles, procedures, and results of the tests for specific anemias are summarized.

▶ HEMOGLOBIN ELECTROPHORESIS USING CELLULOSE ACETATE

Electrophoresis is the movement of charged molecules in an electric field. The detection and preliminary identification of hemoglobinopathies and thalassemias may be obtained using this procedure (∞ Chapters 12, 13). In hemoglobin electrophoresis, hemoglobin A (adult hemoglobin) takes on a net negative charge at an alkaline pH and moves the farthest toward the anode (positive electrode). Many abnormal hemoglobin variants will have altered charges due to single amino acid substitutions within their globin chains (∞ Chapter 12). This change in the degree of the negative charge allows for the separation of the majority of abnormal hemoglobin variants from hemoglobin A at an alkaline pH.[1, 2] The electrophoretic patterns and hemoglobin percentages of the unknown specimens are compared to those of the control sample containing HbA, -F, -S, and -C and a known adult sample.

In this procedure, EDTA-anticoagulated whole blood is centrifuged to obtain packed erythrocytes. The erythrocytes are washed, and a hemolysate is obtained by lysing the erythrocytes with a hemolysate reagent (e.g., 0.005 M EDTA). The hemolysate (i.e., patient, control, or known adult sample) is applied to a cellulose acetate plate. The plate is then placed in the electrophoresis chamber. An alkaline buffer, pH 8.6, permits the flow of electrons from the cathode to the anode within the chamber, alters the charge of the hemoglobin molecules based on their amino acid composition, and allows for the migration and separation of the hemoglobin molecules based on the strength of their negative charge. The hemoglobin molecules are allowed to electrophorese (migrate) for 25 minutes. Following the electrophoresis, the cellulose acetate plate is stained with Ponceau S, a protein dye-binding stain. The stained plate is cleared to remove the cellulose acetate and create a transparent plate with the stained hemoglobin bands representing the hemoglobin electrophoretic pattern for each sample. This plate can then be evaluated visually or with a **densitometer** to determine the percentage of hemoglobin present in each band or region.

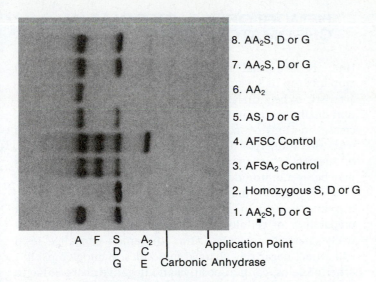

8. AA$_2$S, D or G

7. AA$_2$S, D or G

6. AA$_2$

5. AS, D or G

4. AFSC Control

3. AFSA$_2$ Control

2. Homozygous S, D or G

1. AA$_2$S, D or G

| A | F | S D G | A$_2$ C E | Application Point |

Carbonic Anhydrase

■ **FIGURE 40-1** Electrophoretic mobilities of hemoglobins on cellulose acetate at pH 8.6. (Key: A, A$_2$, D, G, S, F, C, E = hemoglobin variants) (Courtesy of Helena Laboratories, Beaumont, TX)

Cellulose acetate electrophoresis allows for the separation of HbA, -F, -S, and -C into distinct bands (Figure 40-1 ■). However, other abnormal hemoglobin variants have the same electrophoretic mobility as HbS and HbC. HbD and HbG have the same mobility as HbS whereas, HbE and HbO$_{Arab}$ have the same mobility as HbC. Thus, additional tests must be used to confirm the presence of these abnormal hemoglobin variants. The solubility test may be used to

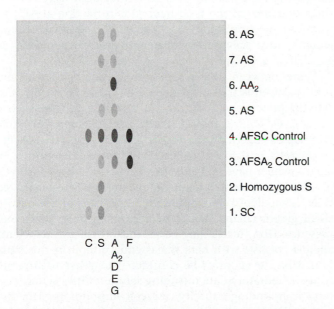

8. AS

7. AS

6. AA$_2$

5. AS

4. AFSC Control

3. AFSA$_2$ Control

2. Homozygous S

1. SC

| C | S A$_2$ D E G | A | F |

■ **FIGURE 40-2** Electrophoretic mobilities of hemoglobins on citrate agar at pH 6.2, showing separation of hemoglobins S and C from other hemoglobins. (Key: A, A$_2$, S, F, C, D, E, G = hemoglobin variants)

confirm HbS, and citrate agar electrophoresis may be used to confirm the presence of HbS and HbC.

Citrate agar electrophoresis at pH 6.2 also separates HbA, -F, -S, -C into distinct bands (Figure 40-2 ■). Since no other hemoglobin variants travel with HbS and HbC on citrate agar, it is used to confirm their presence.[3] It is also useful in differentiating other hemoglobin variants that travel together with HbS and HbC on cellulose acetate electrophoresis; these hemoglobin variants (HbD, HbG, HbE, and HbO$_{Arab}$) have the same mobility as HbA on citrate agar. Rare abnormal hemoglobin variants may be positively identified with DNA analysis of the globin genes (∞ Chapter 25).

Due to the small amount of sample used, the presence of low concentrations of hemoglobin variants or increases in HbA$_2$ concentration may not be detected. A more accurate method to detect increases in HbA$_2$ is anion exchange **column chromatography.**

✓ **Checkpoint! #1**

What is the basis for hemoglobin separation in the hemoglobin electrophoresis procedures?

▶ **ACID ELUTION FOR HEMOGLOBIN F**

The acid elution test for fetal hemoglobin (HbF) may be used in the differentiation of hereditary persistence of fetal hemoglobin (HPFH) from other conditions associated with high levels of HbF (∞ Chapters 12, 13). HPFH is characterized by an even or uniform distribution of HbF within the erythrocytes, whereas other conditions with high levels of HbF are characterized by an uneven or nonuniform distribution of HbF within the erythrocytes. Conditions such as beta thalassemia minor, beta thalassemia major, sickle cell anemia, hereditary spherocytosis, and aplastic anemia are associated with high levels of HbF but nonuniform distribution. This stain may also be used to detect the presence of fetal cells in the maternal circulation (fetal-maternal bleed) during problem pregnancies.

In an acid solution, all hemoglobins are eluted from the erythrocytes except hemoglobin F (fetal hemoglobin).[4] Blood smears are fixed in 80% ethanol and then incubated in the elution buffer, citrate-phosphate (pH 3.3). The slide is stained with acid hematoxylin and counterstained with eosin. The slide is observed microscopically using the oil immersion lens to determine the distribution of HbF within the erythrocytes and the percentage of HbF-containing erythrocytes. Erythrocytes containing fetal hemoglobin stain bright pink or red with the eosin B stain (Figure 40-3 ■). The rest of the erythrocytes appear as pale ghosts. Intermediate erythrocytes (pink colored, but not intense) are sometimes seen. The acid hematoxylin stains the leukocyte's nuclei a faint gray purple.

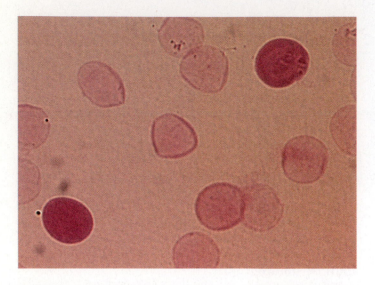

■ **FIGURE 40-3** Acid elution test for determination of hemoglobin F. Erythrocytes containing hemoglobin F appear as bright pink staining cells. The light staining cells are erythrocytes that contain adult hemoglobins.

▶ QUANTITATION OF HEMOGLOBIN F BY ALKALI DENATURATION

Fetal hemoglobin (HbF) is resistant to denaturation by strong alkali solutions, while other hemoglobins are not resistant. The addition of a strong alkali solution (1.27 M NaOH) to a hemolysate containing a known concentration of hemoglobin results in hemoglobin denaturation.[5,6] The denaturation process is stopped by adding a saturated solution of ammonium sulfate. Ammonium sulfate lowers the pH of the reaction mixture and precipitates all denatured hemoglobins. After filtration, the concentration of the remaining alkali-resistant hemoglobin is determined. The alkali-resistant hemoglobin is expressed as a percentage of the total hemoglobin concentration. The hemoglobin concentrations (alkali-resistant and total) are determined by the cyanmethemoglobin method (∞ Chapter 7). The general reference interval for an adult is less than 2%.

HbF levels may also be determined by column chromatography or **radial immunodiffusion** techniques. Column chromatography is more accurate at HbF levels greater than 40%, and radial immunodiffusion is more accurate at HbF levels less than 2%.

✓ Checkpoint! #2

Alkali denaturation revealed a HbF level of 70%, and the acid elution for HbF demonstrated an uneven distribution of HbF within the erythrocytes. Why are both alkali denaturation and acid elution performed to evaluate HbF?

▶ HEMOGLOBIN A₂ BY COLUMN CHROMATOGRAPHY

HbA_2 is a normal adult hemoglobin present in small amounts (up to 3.5%). Increased amounts of HbA_2 are characteristic of beta thalassemia minor. Therefore, the quantitation of HbA_2 is useful in its presumptive diagnosis. Slight increases in HbA_2 concentration have been noted in persons with HbS trait, HbS disease, unstable hemoglobin variants, or megaloblastic anemia. Decreased HbA_2 concentrations may be seen in iron deficiency anemia or alpha thalassemia.

Hemoglobin A_2 may be quantitated with anion exchange column chromatography. The anion exchange resin is a preparation of cellulose covalently coupled to small positively charged molecules. Thus, the anion exchange resin will attract negatively charged molecules. Hemoglobins, like other proteins, contain positive and negative charges due to the ionizing properties of their component amino acids. In the anion exchange chromatography of hemoglobin A_2, the ionic strength of the buffer, and pH levels are controlled to cause different hemoglobins to possess different net negative charges.[7,8] These negatively charged proteins are attracted to the positively charged cellulose and bind accordingly. Following binding, the hemoglobins are removed selectively from the resin by altering the pH or ionic strength of the elution buffer. Due to the solubility of hemoglobin A_2 in the elution buffer, hemoglobin A_2 is eluted from the resin as the elution buffer moves through the column. The other normal, and most abnormal, hemoglobins are retained by the resin. The percentage of hemoglobin A_2 is determined by comparing the absorbance of the hemoglobin A_2 fraction to the absorbance of the total hemoglobin fraction at 415 nm using a spectrophotometer. The CDC National Hemoglobinopathy Laboratory reference interval for HbA_2 is 1.8–3.5%.

Values between 3.5% and 8% are considered indicative of beta thalassemia trait (∞ Chapter 13). Values above 8% indicate the presence of additional hemoglobin variants such as S, C, E, O, D, S-G hybrid, and F, which elute with HbA_2 (∞ Chapter 12). HbA_2 cannot be differentiated from several abnormal hemoglobin variants such as hemoglobins C, E, and O, which have a net electrical charge similar to HbA_2 at pH 8.6. If abnormal hemoglobin variants are suspected, other hemoglobin electrophoretic techniques or DNA analysis of globin chains should be performed to confirm their presence. HbA_2 levels may be normal when iron deficiency anemia coexists with beta thalassemia minor. In this situation, HbA_2 levels must be considered together with family history, laboratory data including serum ferritin, serum iron, total iron-binding capacity, red cell morphology, Hb, Hct, and MCV. HbA_2 may also be quantitated using cellulose acetate electrophoresis followed by elution or densitometry. However, these methods are less accurate than HbA_2 measurement by anion exchange column chromatography.

▶ HEAT DENATURATION TEST FOR UNSTABLE HEMOGLOBIN

Unstable hemoglobins are hemoglobin variants that result from a variety of amino acid substitutions or deletions that affect the intramolecular interactions of the hemoglobin molecule (∞ Chapter 12). These hemoglobin variants are susceptible to spontaneous denaturation resulting in Heinz body formation and erythrocyte hemolysis. In the laboratory, blood samples can be manipulated so that unstable hemoglobins become insoluble and form flocculent precipitate at higher temperatures (50°C), whereas normal hemoglobin remains soluble.[9] The hemoglobin concentrations for heated and unheated fractions are determined by the cyanmethemoglobin method. The concentration of unstable hemoglobin is expressed as a percentage of the total hemoglobin concentration (unheated fraction).

Unstable hemoglobins are a cause of congenital nonspherocytic hemolytic anemias (∞ Chapter 12). Examples of unstable hemoglobins are: hemoglobin Koln, hemoglobin Hammersmith, hemoglobin Zurich, hemoglobin Seattle, and hemoglobin Bristol. A positive heat denaturation test should be confirmed by other test methods that identify unstable hemoglobins, such as tests for erythrocyte inclusions and the **isopropanol precipitation** test. Low concentrations of unstable hemoglobin result in false negative results.

▶ HEINZ BODY STAIN

Heinz bodies represent denatured hemoglobin inclusions. These inclusions are usually round or oval and appear refractile. They tend to locate adjacent to the erythrocyte membrane. Heinz bodies are visible only on supravital stained smears and are not visible on Wright-stained smears. Heinz bodies may be present in glucose-6-phosphate dehydrogenase deficiency and related enzyme disorders when the individual is exposed to oxidizing agents such as primaquine or sulfanilamide (∞ Chapter 18). In addition, they may be found in individuals with unstable hemoglobins or thalassemias. They are occasionally found in senescent erythrocytes of normal individuals.

A specific dye for Heinz bodies is brilliant green.[10] Using this method, EDTA-anticoagulated whole blood is first mixed with 0.5% neutral red. The mixture is counterstained with 0.5% brilliant green. Several thick smears are prepared from the final mixture. The smears are observed microscopically for the presence of Heinz bodies. Heinz bodies stain green, while reticulocytes and Howell-Jolly bodies stain a deep red. The erythrocytes will stain light red. The percentage of erythrocytes containing Heinz bodies may be determined by counting the number of erythrocytes containing Heinz bodies within 500 erythrocytes.

The specificity of the brilliant green dye for eliminates problems that arise with the use of other supravital stains such as methyl violet or crystal violet. With these other supravital stains, Howell-Jolly bodies, basophilic stippling, and reticulum stain the same as Heinz bodies. This often leads to difficulties in the interpretation of the stain.

▶ FLUORESCENT SPOT TEST FOR GLUCOSE-6-PHOSPHATE DEHYDROGENASE

The fluorescent spot test for glucose-6-phosphate dehydrogenase (G6PD) is a screening test to detect G6PD deficiency (∞ Chapter 18). In this procedure, EDTA- or heparin-anticoagulated whole blood is added to a mixture of glucose-6-phosphate, NADP, and saponin.[11] Saponin hemolyzes the erythrocytes releasing their contents into solution. If the erythrocytes contain G6PD, NADP will be converted to NADPH. Using ultraviolet light, the presence of NADPH is detected by its fluorescence. Lack of G6PD is identified by the absence of fluorescence, since NADP will not fluoresce under ultraviolet light. The fluorescent spot test should not be used to assess the degree of G6PD deficiency. A quantitative measurement of G6PD activity should be performed for this purpose.

▶ OSMOTIC FRAGILITY TEST

In this procedure, heparin-anticoagulated whole blood is added to increasingly hypotonic solutions of buffered sodium chloride (0.85% to 0.00%) and the solutions are incubated 20 minutes at room temperature.[12] The amount of hemolysis at each concentration is determined by measuring the absorbance of the **supernatants** spectrophotometrically. An osmotic fragility graph is prepared by plotting the percentage hemolysis of each solution against its concentration, and the results are compared to a normal control. In normal individuals, an almost symmetrical sigmoid shaped curve is obtained (Figure 40-4 ■). Normal erythrocytes will begin to hemolyze around 0.50% sodium chloride (NaCl) concentration, and hemolysis will be complete at 0.30% NaCl. The normal values for osmotic fragility with each sodium concentration are given in Table J ✪ in the inside book cover.

In the osmotic fragility test, spherocytes with a decreased surface-area-to-volume ratio have a limited ability to expand in hypotonic solutions. They will lyse at higher concentrations of sodium chloride than normal biconcave erythrocytes and are said to have an increased osmotic fragility. Target cells or sickle cells have a large surface-area-to-volume ratio. This increased surface-area-to-volume ratio translates into a greater ability to expand in hypotonic solutions. These cells will lyse at lower concentrations of sodium

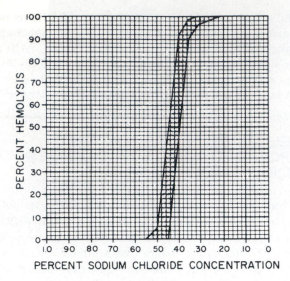

FIGURE 40-4 Normal osmotic fragility curve. The osmotic fragility curve of a normal individual would fall within the area defined by the two sigmoid curves. A curve to the left of normal indicates increased fragility, and a curve to the right decreased fragility.

chloride than normal cells and are said to have a decreased osmotic fragility.

An increased osmotic fragility is associated with hemolytic anemias in which spherocytes are present, in particular, hereditary spherocytosis (∞ Chapter 17). Conditions associated with a decreased osmotic fragility include thalas-

semia, sickle cell anemia, and those conditions in which target cells are observed. Figure 40-5 ■ depicts the increased osmotic lysis of spherocytes in a hypotonic medium.

An incubated osmotic fragility test is performed to identify patients with mild hereditary spherocytosis in which the standard osmotic fragility test is normal. In the incubated osmotic fragility test, patient's blood and control blood are incubated for 24 hours at 37°C under sterile conditions. A significantly increased osmotic fragility after incubation is characteristic of hereditary spherocytosis.

✓ **Checkpoint! #3**

A patient's osmotic fragility test shows beginning hemolysis at 0.60% NaCl and complete hemolysis at 0.50% NaCl. How should these results be interpreted?

▶ **SUGAR-WATER SCREENING TEST**

A sugar-water solution (10%) provides a low-ionic-strength solution that promotes the attachment of complement to susceptible paroxysmal nocturnal hemoglobinuria erythrocytes.[13] Upon attachment of complement, the erythrocytes hemolyze. Normal erythrocytes do not hemolyze under these conditions. A positive sugar-water test (sucrose hemolysis test) is presumptive evidence for paroxysmal nocturnal hemoglobinuria (PNH) (∞ Chapter 17). The acidified serum

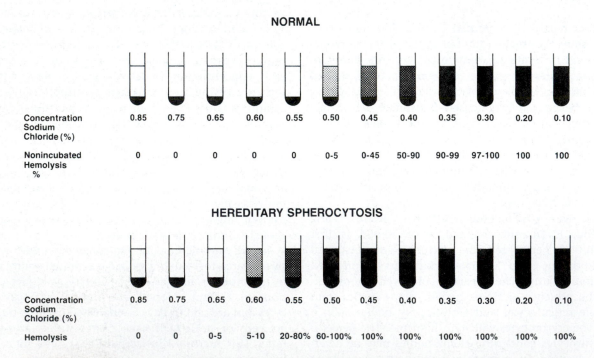

NORMAL

Concentration Sodium Chloride (%)	0.85	0.75	0.65	0.60	0.55	0.50	0.45	0.40	0.35	0.30	0.20	0.10
Nonincubated Hemolysis %	0	0	0	0	0	0-5	0-45	50-90	90-99	97-100	100	100

HEREDITARY SPHEROCYTOSIS

Concentration Sodium Chloride (%)	0.85	0.75	0.65	0.60	0.55	0.50	0.45	0.40	0.35	0.30	0.20	0.10
Hemolysis	0	0	0-5	5-10	20-80%	60-100%	100%	100%	100%	100%	100%	100%

FIGURE 40-5 The osmotic fragility test demonstrates the increased osmotic lysis of spherocytes in a hypotonic medium compared with normal erythrocytes. (Key: clear supernatant = no hemolysis; patterned supernatant = partial hemolysis; black supernatant = complete hemolysis)

test should be used to confirm PNH, since the sugar-water test is not specific. If the sugar-water test is negative, no further testing is required because the test is sensitive for PNH.

▶ ACIDIFIED SERUM TEST

The erythrocytes of paroxysmal nocturnal hemoglobinuria (PNH) are unusually sensitive to hemolysis by complement. In the acidified serum test (Ham test), complement attaches to the erythrocytes at a slightly acidic pH (6.5–7.0) and is activated by an alternate pathway not involving the presence of antibodies.[14] The activation of complement results in the hemolysis of the erythrocytes. Table 40-1 ✪ outlines the procedural setup for the acidified serum test and the expected results in PNH. A diagnosis of paroxysmal nocturnal hemoglobinuria is suggested if hemolysis occurs in tubes #2 and #5. No hemolysis should be seen in tube #3 since PNH erythrocytes require complement for hemolysis.

A false positive test may be seen in hereditary spherocytosis. Spherocytes may undergo hemolysis in test tubes #2, #3, and #5. If hemolysis occurs in test tubes #2 and #7 but not in test tube #5, a warm hemolysin antibody may be present in the patient's serum. The acidified serum test may also be positive in the **hereditary erythroblastic multinuclearity with positive acidified serum test (HEMPAS)**. Two differentiating features of this disorder are: (1) the patient's (HEMPAS) erythrocytes are not lysed by the patient's own acidified serum, and (2) the sucrose hemolysis test is negative.

▶ DONATH-LANDSTEINER TEST FOR PCH

The Donath-Landsteiner test is a screening test for paroxysmal cold hemoglobinuria (PCH).[15] PCH is characterized by the presence of the Donath-Landsteiner antibody, a **biphasic antibody** with anti-P specificity (∞ Chapter 19). This IgG antibody is capable of activating complement resulting in hemolysis. The Donath-Landsteiner test should be performed when an individual presents with hemoglobinuria and a positive direct antiglobulin test due to C3 only, with no evidence of autoantibody activity in the serum. In this procedure, a series of test tubes is set up to detect the biphasic nature of complement activation (Table 40-2 ✪). Normal serum serves as a source of complement since individuals with PCH may express low levels of complement. The 50% suspension of group O erythrocytes with P antigen serves as the antibody receptors. Following the appropriate incubation schedule, the tubes are centrifuged and observed for hemolysis. If anti-P is present in the patient's serum, it will bind to the erythrocyte's P antigen during the incubation time in the melting ice bath. During the second incubation time at 37°C the antibody dissociates from the erythrocytes, and complement is activated leading to hemolysis. Therefore, the test is considered positive for PCH if tubes A1 and/or A2 demonstrate hemolysis and the remaining tubes have no hemolysis. Proper specimen collection and processing are essential to the outcome of this test. Patient's blood should be allowed to clot at 37°C and the serum separated at this temperature to avoid cold autoabsorption and loss of antibody prior to testing.

▶ ERYTHROPOIETIN

Erythropoietin (EPO) levels are determined by enzyme-linked immunosorbent assay (ELISA). In this procedure, microtiter plate wells are coated with a monoclonal mouse antihuman antibody directed against EPO.[16] This antibody represents the capture antibody since it will bind EPO from the serum, either patient, control, or standard. Following a washing step, the wells are incubated with a polyclonal rabbit anti-EPO that is enzyme-labeled with horseradish peroxidase. This second antibody will bind to the initial antigen–antibody complex. Hence, EPO is sandwiched between two specific antibodies (Figure 39-4 ■). A substrate specific for the enzyme label (i.e., tetramethylbenzidine) is added to the microtiter plate wells, and a colorimetric reaction occurs. The absorbance of each microtiter well is determined using a microtiter plate reader, an adaptation of a spectrophotometer. The amount of absorbance measured in a given microtiter well is directly proportional to the concentration of EPO in the sample. The control and patient results are determined from a reference (standard) curve that is prepared using known concentrations of EPO. The general reference interval for serum EPO is 3.0–16.6 mIU/mL.

Measurement of EPO levels is useful in the diagnosis of certain anemias and polycythemia. For example, secondary polycythemias like chronic obstructive pulmonary disease or cyanotic heart disease are associated with elevated levels of EPO, while the myeloproliferative disorder polycythemia

✪ TABLE 40-1							
Schematic Outline of Acidified Serum Test Procedure and Expected Results in PNH							
Tube	1	2	3	4	5	6	7
Patient serum (mL)	0.5	0.5				0.5	0.5
Control serum (mL)			0.5*	0.5	0.5		
0.2 N HCl (mL)		0.05	0.05		0.05		0.05
Patient RBC (mL)	0.05	0.05	0.05	0.05	0.05		
Control RBC (mL)						0.05	0.05
Results observed in PNH	0	+	0	0	+	0	0

PNH is suggested if hemolysis occurs in tubes #2 and #5. No hemolysis should be seen in tube #3. Key: * = Serum is heat inactivated; 0 = no hemolysis; + = hemolysis.

✪ TABLE 40-2

Schematic Outline of Donath-Landsteiner Test Procedure for Detecting PCH

Incubation Set	Tube 1	Tube 2	Tube 3	Incubation Protocol
A	Patient's serum	Patient's serum	_____	1. 30 minutes in melting ice bath
	_____	Normal serum	Normal serum	⟶ 2. 60 minutes @ 37°C
	50% Group O cells	50% Group O cells	50% Group O cells	
B	Patient's serum	Patient's serum	_____	1. 90 minutes in melting ice bath
	_____	Normal serum	Normal serum	⟶
	50% Group O cells	50% Group O cells	50% Group O cells	
C	Patient's serum	Patient's serum	_____	1. 90 minutes @ 37°C
	_____	Normal serum	Normal serum	⟶
	50% Group O cells	50% Group O cells	50% Group O cells	

PCH is indicated if hemolysis occurs in tubes A1 and/or A2 and remaining tubes have no hemolysis. Tubes A3, B3, and C3 represent controls for complement activity and should not demonstrate hemolysis. Tubes B1 and B2 represent controls for the presence of cold-reacting antibodies, and tubes C1 and C2 represent controls for the presence of warm-reacting antibodies. It is important to include these controls to eliminate possible false positive interpretations.

vera is associated with normal to low EPO levels (∞ Chapter 27). Decreased levels of EPO are observed in anemia of renal failure, anemia of chronic disease, and anemia of hypothyroidism (∞ Chapters 11, 15).

► SOLUBLE TRANSFERRIN RECEPTOR

Soluble transferrin receptor (sTfR) represents a truncated form of the membrane transferrin receptor that is normally found on the surface of cells that require iron. sTfR levels are determined by enzyme-linked immunosorbent assay (ELISA). In this procedure, microtiter plate wells are coated with a monoclonal antihuman antibody directed against sTfR.[17] This antibody represents the capture antibody since it will bind sTfR from the serum, either patient, control, or standard. Following a washing step, the wells are incubated with a second monoclonal anti-sTfR that is enzyme-labeled with horseradish peroxidase. This second antibody will bind to the initial antigen–antibody complex. Hence, sTfR is sandwiched between two specific antibodies (Figure 39-4 ■).

A substrate specific for the enzyme label is added to the microtiter plate wells, and a colorimetric reaction occurs. The absorbance of each microtiter well is determined using a microtiter plate reader. The amount of absorbance measured in a given microtiter well is directly proportional to the concentration of sTfR in the sample. The control and patient results are determined from a reference (standard) curve that is prepared using known concentrations of sTfR. The general reference interval for serum sTfR is 8.7–26.1 nmol/L.

Measurement of sTfR levels is useful in the differential diagnosis of iron deficiency anemia from anemia of chronic disease since sTfR levels are elevated in iron deficiency anemia but normal in anemia of chronic disease (∞ Chapter 11).

✓ Checkpoint! #4

A patient was recently diagnosed with a hypochromic, microcytic anemia. Additional laboratory testing revealed: EPO 1.5 mIU/mL and sTfR 15.8 nmol/L. Which anemia is consistent with these results?

SUMMARY

This chapter reviewed reflex tests used in the definitive diagnosis of anemias including sickle cell anemia, beta thalassemias, glucose-6-phosphate dehydrogenase deficiency, hereditary spherocytosis, paroxysmal nocturnal hemoglobinuria, paroxysmal cold hemoglobinuria, iron deficiency, and anemia of chronic disease. It is important for clinical laboratory professionals to have a thorough understanding of each procedure in order to understand appropri-

ate use, troubleshoot potential sources of error, identify other problems in the performance of the test, and to understand the meaning of test results. With a definitive diagnosis of the patient's anemia, the appropriate choice of treatment can be made, followed by the determination of relevant laboratory tests to be used to monitor treatment.

REVIEW QUESTIONS

LEVEL I

1. Which hemoglobin travels the slowest in hemoglobin electrophoresis using cellulose acetate? (Checklist #1)
   a. hemoglobin A
   b. hemoglobin F
   c. hemoglobin A_2
   d. hemoglobin S

2. In the acid elution test for hemoglobin F, the purpose of the citrate phosphate buffer is: (Checklist #2)
   a. to fix the erythrocytes and other blood cells
   b. to elute all hemoglobins except hemoglobin F from erythrocytes
   c. to stain the leukocytes
   d. to counterstain the erythrocytes containing HgF

3. Which abnormal erythrocyte morphology is associated with decreased osmotic fragility? (Checklist #2)
   a. microcytes
   b. spherocytes
   c. target cells
   d. dacrycytes

4. Hemoglobin electrophoresis using cellulose acetate reveals the major percentage of hemoglobin traveling in the S region, and the solubility test was negative. Which of the following is the most likely abnormal hemoglobin? (Checklist #2)
   a. hemoglobin C
   b. hemoglobin S
   c. hemoglobin E
   d. hemoglobin D

5. When examining an acid elution test for hemoglobin F, the clinical laboratory professional observed uniformly stained erythrocytes on the control slide (mixture of adult erythrocytes and cord cells) and the patient's slide. What is the source of this error? (Checklist #2)
   a. fixative
   b. stain
   c. elution buffer
   d. counterstain

6. A patient's Wright-stained peripheral blood smear reveals the presence of numerous disc-shaped erythrocytes that appear slightly smaller than normal and have a decreased to absent area of central pallor. Which is the most appropriate reflex test? (Checklist #2)
   a. osmotic fragility test
   b. hemoglobin electrophoresis
   c. acidified serum test
   d. solubility test

LEVEL II

1. A patient with a hypochromic, microcytic anemia has a hemoglobin A_2 level of 4.8%. Which of the following is the most likely diagnosis? (Checklist #2)
   a. beta thalassemia minor
   b. iron deficiency anemia
   c. aplastic anemia
   d. heterozygous hemoglobin C

2. Which supravital stain best distinguishes Heinz bodies from other erythrocyte inclusions? (Checklist #1)
   a. crystal violet
   b. brilliant green stain
   c. Wright's stain
   d. methyl violet

3. A diagnosis of PNH is suspected. What screening test is appropriate? (Checklist #2)
   a. hemoglobin electrophoresis
   b. sugar-water test
   c. HAM test
   d. acid elution test

4. In the Ham test, what is the purpose of the 0.2N HCl reagent? (Checklist #1)
   a. stabilize the erythrocyte membrane
   b. hemolyze the normal erythrocytes
   c. denature erythrocyte membrane proteins
   d. promote complement binding to erythrocyte membrane

5. Which laboratory test is used to distinguish iron deficiency anemia from anemia of chronic disease? (Checklist #2)
   a. sTfR
   b. HbA_2
   c. HbF
   d. serum iron

6. In performing a reticulocyte count, the clinical laboratory professional observes erythrocyte inclusions suggestive of denatured hemoglobin. What is the best stain to confirm the identity of these inclusions? (Checklist #2)
   a. crystal violet stain
   b. brilliant green stain
   c. Wright's stain
   d. methyl violet stain

7. The following results were observed on a Donath-Landsteiner test: only tube A1 shows hemolysis. What is the appropriate interpretation for these results? (Checklist #2)
   a. warm autoimmune hemolytic anemia
   b. normal erythrocytes
   c. paroxysmal cold hemoglobinuria
   d. spherocytosis

REVIEW QUESTIONS (continued)

LEVEL I

7. Which test is best to quantitate HbF? (Checklist #1)
   a. hemoglobin electrophoresis
   b. acid elution test
   c. alkali denaturation test
   d. column chromatography

8. A patient with a suspected diagnosis of hereditary sphero-cytosis has a normal osmotic fragility test. What further test should be done? (Checklist #2)
   a. no further test required
   b. incubated osmotic fragility
   c. hemoglobin electrophoresis
   d. acid elution for HbF

9. The anticoagulant of choice for the osmotic fragility test is: (Checklist #1)
   a. oxalate
   b. EDTA
   c. citrate
   d. heparin

10. Electrophoresis using cellulose acetate reveals a band of hemoglobin with HbC mobility. Citrate agar electrophoresis does *not* show a HbC band. The most likely explanation is: (Checklist #2)
    a. the abnormal hemoglobin may be HbE or HbO$_{Arab}$
    b. the citrate agar electrophoresis result is erroneous
    c. the abnormal hemoglobin may be HbG or HbD
    d. the cellulose acetate electrophoresis is not reliable

LEVEL II

8. A patient had the following results:

RBC	2.90×10^{12}/L	MCV	76 fL
Hb	6.2 g/dL	MCH	21 pg
Hct	22.0%	MCHC	28 g/dL
Serum iron	55 µg/dL		
sTfR	28.5 nmol/L		

What is the most appropriate diagnosis? (Checklist #2)
   a. iron deficiency anemia
   b. beta thalassemia minor
   c. anemia of chronic disease
   d. sideroblastic anemia

9. Which laboratory test would be useful in the differential diagnosis of polycythemia? (Checklist #2)
   a. HbA$_2$
   b. sTfR
   c. Ham test
   d. EPO

10. A patient has a positive acidified serum test with hemolysis in tube #5 but *not* tube #2. The sugar-water test is negative. This may indicate: (Checklist #2)
    a. PNH
    b. PCH
    c. HEMPAS
    d. G6PD deficiency

www.prenhall.com/mckenzie

Use the above address to access the free, interactive Companion Web site created for this textbook. Get hints, instant feedback, and textbook references to chapter-related multiple choice questions.

REFERENCES

1. NCCLS. *Detection of Abnormal Hemoglobin Using Cellulose Acetate Electrophoresis,* 2nd ed. Wayne, PA: NCCLS; 1994.

2. *Hemoglobin Electrophoresis Procedure.* Beaumont, TX: Helena Laboratories; 1985.

3. NCCLS. *Citrate Agar Electrophoresis for Confirming the Identification of Variant Hemoglobins.* Vol. 8, no. 6. Wayne, PA: NCCLS; 1988.

4. *Fetal Hemoglobin-Acid Elution: Semi-Quantitative Procedure for Blood Smears.* St. Louis: Sigma Diagnostics; 1990.

5. NCCLS. *Quantitative Measurement of Fetal Hemoglobin Using the Alkali Denaturation Method.* Vol. 9, no. 18. Wayne, PA: NCCLS; 1989.

6. International Committee for Standardization in Haematology. Recommendations for fetal hemoglobin reference preparations and fetal hemoglobin determination by the alkali denaturation method. *Br J Haematol.* 1979; 42:133.

7. NCCLS. *Chromatographic (Microcolumn) Determination of Hemoglobin A$_2$.* Vol. 9, no. 17. Wayne, PA: NCCLS; 1989.

8. *Sickle-Thal Quik Column Procedure.* Beaumont, TX: Helena Laboratories; 1988.

9. Huisman THJ, Jonxis JHP. *The Hemoglobinopathies: Techniques of Identification.* New York: Marcel Decker; 1977.

10. Schwab ML, Lewis AE. An improved stain for Heinz bodies. *Am J Clin Pathol.* 1969; 39:673.

11. *Glucose-6-Phosphate Dehydrogenase Deficiency: Qualitative, Visual Fluorescence Screening Procedure.* St. Louis: Sigma Diagnostics; 1989.

12. *UNOPETTE RBC Osmotic Fragility Determination for Manual Methods Procedure.* Rutherford, NJ: Becton, Dickinson and Company; 1996.

13. Hartmann RC, Jenkins DE. The "sugar-water" test for paroxysmal nocturnal hemoglobinuria. *New Engl J Med.* 1966; 275:155.

14. Ham TH. Studies on destruction of erythrocytes. *Arch Int Med* 1939; 66:1271.

15. *American Association of Blood Banks: Technical Manual,* 13th ed. Bethesda, MD: AABB; 1999.

16. *Quantikine IVD Human Epo Immunoassay Procedure.* Minneapolis, MN: R&D Systems; 1999.

17. *Quantikine IVD Human sTfR Immunoassay Procedure.* Minneapolis, MN: R&D Systems; 1999.

41

Automation in Hematology

Cheryl Burns, M.S.

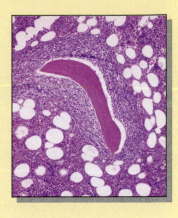

■ CHECKLIST - LEVEL I

At the end of this unit of study the student should be able to:

1. Cite the electrical impedance principle of cell counting and identify the instruments that use this technology.

2. Describe the use of radio frequency in cell counting and identify the instruments that use this technology.

3. State the principles of light scatter used in cell counting and identify the instruments that use this technology.

4. List the reported parameters for each blood cell counting instrument.

5. Categorize cell parameters as directly measured, derived from a histogram, scattergram or cytogram, or calculated.

6. Describe the principle of reticulocyte count enumeration by automated blood cell counting instruments.

7. State the electromechanical principle of clot detection and identify instruments that use this technology.

8. State the photo-optical principle of clot detection and identify instruments that use this technology.

■ CHECKLIST - LEVEL II

At the end of this unit of study the student should be able to:

1. Compare/contrast the methods of analysis for the described histograms, scatterplots, scattergrams, and cytograms and interpret results.

2. Describe and interpret the automated reticulocyte parameters.

KEY TERMS

Aperture
Backlighting
Cellular hemoglobin concentration mean (CHCM)
Cluster analysis
Coincidence
Continuous flow analysis
Contour gating
Hemoglobin distribution width (HDW)
Histogram
Hydrodynamic focusing
Isovolumetric sphering
Mean platelet volume (MPV)
Platelet distribution width (PDW)
Radar chart
Random access
Reagent blank
Scatterplot
Threshold limit
Viscosity

BACKGROUND BASICS

The information in this chapter will build on the concepts learned in previous chapters. To maximize your learning experience you should review these concepts prior to beginning this unit of study.

Level I

▶ State the principles of cell enumeration by hemacytometer. (Chapter 7)

▶ State the principle of the cyanmethemoglobin method for hemoglobin determination. (Chapter 7)

▶ Calculate the erythrocyte indices. (Chapter 7)

▶ Describe the peripheral blood smear examination process and correlate peripheral blood smear findings with complete blood counts (CBC). (Chapter 8)

▶ Describe and state the principle of the manual reticulocyte count procedure. (Chapter 7)

▶ Describe the basic procedures for evaluation of secondary hemostasis (i.e., prothrombin time and activated partial thromboplastin time). (Chapter 39)

Level II

▶ Summarize the diagnostic use of the reticulocyte count in the evaluation of hematologic disorders and in monitoring various therapies such as iron replacement and bone marrow transplant. (Chapters 10, 11, 32)

▶ OVERVIEW

Automation is firmly established within the hematology/coagulation laboratory. This chapter reviews examples of instrumentation that are currently utilized. The basic principles of operation are discussed, and samples of normal test results are displayed for each instrument.

▶ AUTOMATED BLOOD CELL COUNTING INSTRUMENTS

The evolution of instrumentation in hematology began in the mid-1950s. Until that time, clinical laboratory professionals were performing manual hemacytometer blood cell counts, spun hematocrits, spectrophotometrically determined hemoglobins, and microscopic blood smear evaluations. With the advent of the first single automated blood cell counter, manual hemacytometer blood cell counts for erythrocyte enumeration and leukocyte enumeration were replaced. In general, automated blood cell counters provide data with increased reliability, precision, and accuracy.

With the many advances in hematology instrumentation, automation currently encompasses the primary testing in the hematology laboratory. A complete blood cell count including the platelet count, a five-part leukocyte differential, and absolute reticulocyte count can be done by automated instruments. A number of principles for cell counting and differential analysis have been utilized in the past. The two principles of blood cell counting currently used by the hematology instruments are impedance and optical light scattering.

The impedance principle of blood cell counting is based on the increased resistance that occurs when a blood cell with poor conductivity passes through an electrical field. The number of pulses indicate the blood cell count, and the amplitude of each pulse is proportional to the volume of the cell.[1] Examples of instruments using this principle are the Beckman-Coulter instruments, the Sysmex Corporation instruments, and the Abbott CELL-DYN instruments.

The optical light scattering principle of blood cell counting is based on light scattering measurements obtained as a single blood cell passes through a beam of light (optical or laser). Blood cells create forward scatter and side scatter that are detected by photodetectors. The degree of forward scatter is a measurement of cell size, while the degree of side scatter is a measurement of cell complexity or granularity.[2] The Technicon H Systems and Bayer ADVIA instruments utilize this principle.

This section will review the basic operating principles of several hematology instruments that may be seen in the field. Other instruments use a combination of these principles.

 Checkpoint! #1

What is the basis of the impedance principle for cell counting?

IMPEDANCE INSTRUMENTS

Described here are six instruments that use the impedance principle in cell counting. Three are Coulter instruments, two are Sysmex instruments and one is the CELL-DYN.

Coulter S-Plus Series

In 1983, Coulter Corporation introduced the Coulter Counter S-Plus IV, a multiparameter, automated analyzer.[3–5] Blood cell counting was based on the Coulter principle of impedance. Blood cells were diluted in an electrically conductive diluent and two electrodes separated by an **aperture** were suspended in this dilution (Figure 41-1 ■). As individual blood cells pass through the aperture, there is an increase in resistance between the two electrodes proportional to the volume of the cell. **Threshold limits** were established for the enumeration of each cell population based on cell volume. Like previous Coulter instruments, the Coulter S-Plus series has two counting chambers that operate simultaneously (one counting chamber for erythrocyte and platelet enumeration and another for leukocyte enumeration). Each counting chamber has three separate apertures for triplicate analysis and internal checking for error.

Histograms (size distribution curves) are created for erythrocyte (RBC), leukocyte (WBC), and platelet (PLT) populations based on cell volume and relative cell number (Figure 41-2 ■). These histograms allow the visualization of subpopulations of cells, their average size in relation to the rest of the population, and their relative number.

The data obtained from the erythrocyte/platelet dilution includes the RBC count by direct measurement (particles greater than 36 fL), mean cell volume (MCV), and red cell distribution width (RDW), which are derived from the RBC

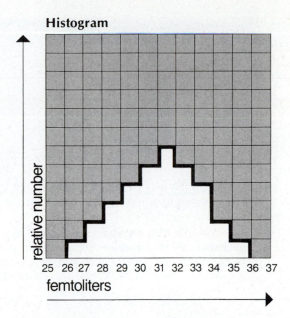

Histogram

■ **FIGURE 41-2** Histogram, or size distribution curve, allows the visualization of the blood cell population based on the relative cell number and its volume (in fL). (Reprinted, with permission, from *Significant Advances in Hematology*. Hialeah, FL: Coulter Electronics, Inc.; 1983.)

histogram (Figure 41-3 ■). The hematocrit is calculated from the MCV and the RBC count. The mean cell hemoglobin (MCH) is calculated from the RBC count and the hemoglobin concentration, and the mean cell hemoglobin concentration (MCHC) is calculated from the hemoglobin concentration and hematocrit. The hemoglobin concentration is obtained from the WBC counting chamber.

The platelet count is also obtained from the RBC dilution. Particles between 2 and 20 fL are counted as platelets, and a raw platelet histogram is obtained (Figure 41-4 ■). The raw platelet histogram is evaluated to determine if it is a log normal curve. The raw platelet histogram is electronically smoothed and extrapolated over 0–70 fL. The platelet count is derived from the extrapolated histogram. Two additional parameters are obtained from the platelet histogram: **mean platelet volume (MPV)**, which is analogous to the MCV, and **platelet distribution width (PDW)**, which is analogous to the RDW.

The leukocyte count is directly measured from the leukocyte dilution after a lytic agent has been added. The lytic agent serves to lyse the erythrocytes, convert free hemoglobin to cyanmethemoglobin, and shrink the leukocyte cell membrane and cytoplasm. Therefore, the leukocyte count represents a measure of the cell volume rather than native cell size as it passes through the aperture. Particles greater than 35 fL are counted as leukocytes. A WBC histogram is created from the data obtained as the cells pass through the aperture. A three-part differential is obtained based on the relative sizes of the leukocytes evaluated. Lymphocytes are

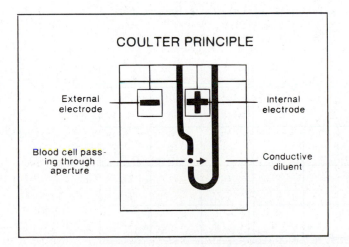

■ **FIGURE 41-1** Coulter principle. Increased electrical resistance, or impedance, occurs when the poorly conductive blood cell passes through the aperture. (Reprinted, with permission, from Pierre R. *Seminar and Case Studies: The Automated Differential*. Hialeah, FL: Coulter Electronics, Inc.; 1985.)

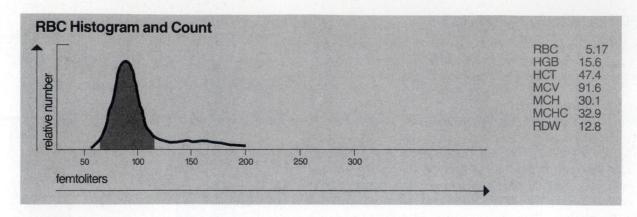

RBC	5.17
HGB	15.6
HCT	47.4
MCV	91.6
MCH	30.1
MCHC	32.9
RDW	12.8

■ FIGURE 41-3 RBC histogram and count. The shaded area represents those cells used in the RDW calculation. The excluded cells may represent large platelets, platelet clumps, or electrical interference on the left and RBC doublets, RBC triplets, RBC agglutinates, or aperture artifacts on the right. (Reprinted, with permission, from *Significant Advances in Hematology.* Hialeah, FL.: Coulter Electronics, Inc.; 1983.)

found between 35 and 90 fL; mononuclear cells are found between 90 and 160 fL; granulocytes are found between 160 and 450 fL (Figure 41-5 ■).

The concentration of cyanmethemoglobin is determined by photometry at 525 nm. Through the application of Beer's law, the concentration of cyanmethemoglobin is proportional to the concentration of free hemoglobin. Additionally, this instrument utilizes a **reagent blank** at the beginning of each operating cycle.

The analyzer's computer analyzes the data obtained from the erythrocyte/platelet dilution and the leukocyte dilution. The analyzer's computer corrects the counts for **coincidence** (two or more cells passing through the aperture at the same time) and evaluates the triplicate results from each dilution for replication. If two or three results do not agree, the result is not reported but recorded as "vote-out." If the

results are accepted they are averaged and displayed on a computer screen or printed to a hard copy for the clinical laboratory professional's review. If abnormalities are detected by the analyzer, the abnormal results are either backlighted or flagged. **Backlighting**, or highlighting, is primarily utilized for out-of-range results or vote-out situations. Region flags are utilized for the WBC histogram and differential (Table 41-1 ✪). These flags alert the clinical laboratory professional to the presence of interferences within one or more of the WBC histogram regions. For example, the presence of nucleated erythrocytes or clumped platelets is indicated if the Region 1 flag is reported.

✔ **Checkpoint! #2**

Why is lytic agent added to the leukocyte dilution?

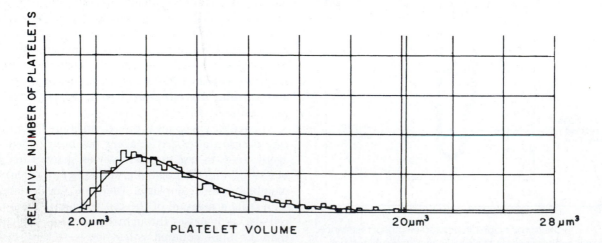
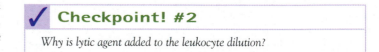

■ FIGURE 41-4 Normal platelet histogram, Coulter Counter S Plus. The jagged line represents the raw data collected from 2–20 fL. The smooth line represents the extrapolated histogram from 0–70 fL. (Reprinted, with permission, from *Significant Advances in Hematology.* Hialeah, FL: Coulter Electronics, Inc.; 1983.)

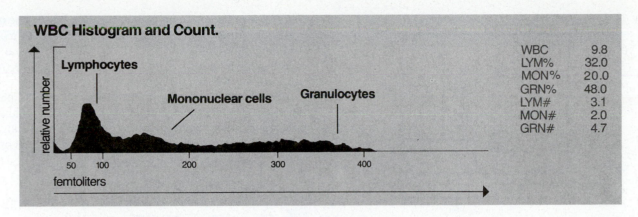

WBC Histogram and Count.

WBC	9.8
LYM%	32.0
MON%	20.0
GRN%	48.0
LYM#	3.1
MON#	2.0
GRN#	4.7

■ **FIGURE 41-5** WBC histogram and count. In a normal patient, the lymphocyte region represents lymphocytes, the mononuclear region represents monocytes, and the granulocyte region represents neutrophils, eosinophils, and basophils. (Reprinted with permission, from *Significant Advances in Hematology.* Hialeah, FL: Coulter Electronics, Inc.; 1983.)

Coulter STKS

The Coulter STKS utilizes a combination of technologies to enumerate erythrocytes, platelets, and leukocytes and to determine a five-part differential.[6–11] The basic counting principle of impedance is utilized to enumerate the cell counts and derive the erythrocyte and platelet histograms. The five-part differential is determined by VCS (volume · conductivity · scatter) technology.

The instrument aspirates a sample of EDTA anticoagulated blood and divides this sample three ways. As with previous Coulter instruments, erythrocyte and platelet counts are determined within one aperture bath, and leukocyte counts and hemoglobin determinations are obtained from a second aperture bath. The data from each bath are accumulated and reviewed by the analyzer. The cell counts, histograms, and other erythrocyte and platelet parameters are sent to the data management system. (See Web Table 41-1 ✪ for the reported parameters.)

The third portion of the blood sample is sent to a mixing chamber where a dilution is prepared utilizing a lytic agent that removes erythrocytes but maintains leukocytes in their near-native state. A stabilizer is also added to preserve the integrity of the leukocytes. This dilution is analyzed within the flow cell of the triple transducer to obtain the five-part differential. The cells pass through the flow cell singly by **hydrodynamic focusing.** As each cell passes through the flow cell, three separate measurements are taken simultaneously. These measurements include cell volume, cell conductivity, and the cell's light scatter characteristics. Cell volume is determined by impedance; cell conductivity that evaluates internal physical and chemical constituents is determined by a high-frequency electromagnetic probe; and light scatter characteristics are determined by helium–neon laser. The analyzer system analyzes these measurements and classifies the cell into one of five normal populations. From these measurements, the percentage value of each cell type is obtained and the absolute number is calculated. The two-dimensional **scatterplots** are created and displayed by the data management system. The DF1 (discriminant function 1) scatterplot is the two-dimensional scatterplot most commonly included in the STKS report form and shows data derived from volume and light scatter (Figure 41-6 ■). The DF2 scatterplot shows data derived from volume and conductivity analysis (Web Figure 41-1 ■). The basophil population, which is hidden by the neutrophil and eosinophil populations on other scatterplots, is observed on the DF3 scatterplot (Web Figure 41-2 ■). Scatter-

✪ TABLE 41-1

Coulter S-Plus WBC Histogram Region Flags

Region Flag	Affected Position	Possible Abnormalities
R1	Lymphocyte population does not begin at baseline (~35 fL)	Nucleated erythrocytes, large platelets, clumped platelets, or intracellular parasites (e.g., malaria)
R2	No valley between lymphocyte and mononuclear populations (~90 fL)	Reactive lymphocytes, blast cells
R3	No valley between mononuclear and granulocyte populations (~160 fL)	Eosinophilia, basophilia, immature neutrophils
R4	Granulocyte population does not return to baseline (~450 fL)	Granulocytosis
RM	Interference detected in multiple positions	

Other impedance-based instruments providing three-part leukocyte differentials use a flagging system similar to the Coulter S-Plus instrument.

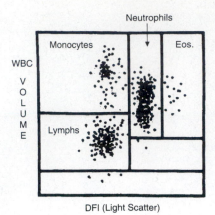

■ **FIGURE 41-6** Discriminant function 1 (DF1) scatterplot, Coulter STKS. DF1 scatterplot graphs volume vs light scatter and reveals the locations of four leukocyte populations. The basophil population is located behind the lymphocytes. (Courtesy of Coulter Electronics, Inc., Hialeah, FL)

plots and histograms may also be utilized to detect abnormalities or subpopulations of cells (Figure 41-7 ■).

The microcomputer system analyzes and compiles all data obtained from the instrument. The results are displayed on a computer screen or printed to a hard copy for the clinical laboratory professional's review (Figure 41-8 ■). Abnormalities in the results are identified by a cell classification system. This system consists of software-generated flags (sus-

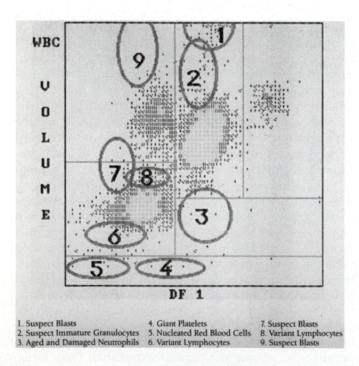

1. Suspect Blasts
2. Suspect Immature Granulocytes
3. Aged and Damaged Neutrophils
4. Giant Platelets
5. Nucleated Red Blood Cells
6. Variant Lymphocytes
7. Suspect Blasts
8. Variant Lymphocytes
9. Suspect Blasts

■ **FIGURE 41-7** Location of abnormal cell types on the scatterplot, Coulter STKS. (Courtesy of Coulter Electronics, Inc., Hialeah, FL)

pect flags) or user-defined flags (definitive flags). The clinical laboratory professional uses this information to correlate complete blood count (CBC) data with peripheral blood morphology to improve the identification and confirmation of abnormalities.

The Coulter STKS instrument is also capable of performing a separate reticulocyte analysis. Reticulocyte analysis utilizes the supravital stain, new methylene blue, to stain residual RNA. The stained sample is analyzed by VCS technology to determine the reticulocyte count.

✔ ## Checkpoint! #3

Explain how the additional methodologies used by the Coulter STKS improved the leukocyte differential.

Coulter Gen·S

The Gen · S is Beckman-Coulter's top-of-the-line multiparameter blood cell counting instrument.[12,13] From a single blood sample aspiration, the Gen·S is capable of determining a CBC, five-part differential, and reticulocyte count. The basic principles of analysis are similar to the Coulter STKS; however, several improvements have been made. Like other instruments, the blood sample is aspirated by a closed tube system. The aspirated blood sample is divided into four aliquots. The first aliquot is sent to the RBC/platelet dilution chamber, where analyses of erythrocytes and platelets are carried out in the same manner as previously discussed for the Coulter S-Plus instrument. The second aliquot is sent to the WBC dilution chamber, where the leukocyte count and hemoglobin determination are made as discussed for the Coulter S-Plus instrument.

A third aliquot is sent to the orbital mixing chamber. Within this chamber, blood is mixed by gentle agitation with heated lysing reagent to remove the erythrocytes while leaving the leukocytes in their near native state. A second stabilizing reagent is added to stop the lytic reaction. This dilution is sent to the VCS flow cell for analysis. The same characteristics are evaluated as described in the Coulter STKS section. The difference between the STKS and Gen·S is in the internal system used to monitor and adjust reaction characteristics and the data analysis of the VCS-derived characteristics to differentiate the leukocyte cell types. The Intellikinetics application monitors and reacts to changes in the external environment (e.g., changes in ambient room temperature). With this application, the Gen·S system is able to maintain consistent reaction conditions and eliminate cellular analysis problems due to inconsistent location of cells within three-dimensional space. Data analysis is improved through the use of the AccuGate computer program. With this data analysis program, **contour gating** is used to identify and classify the different leukocytes. The advantage of

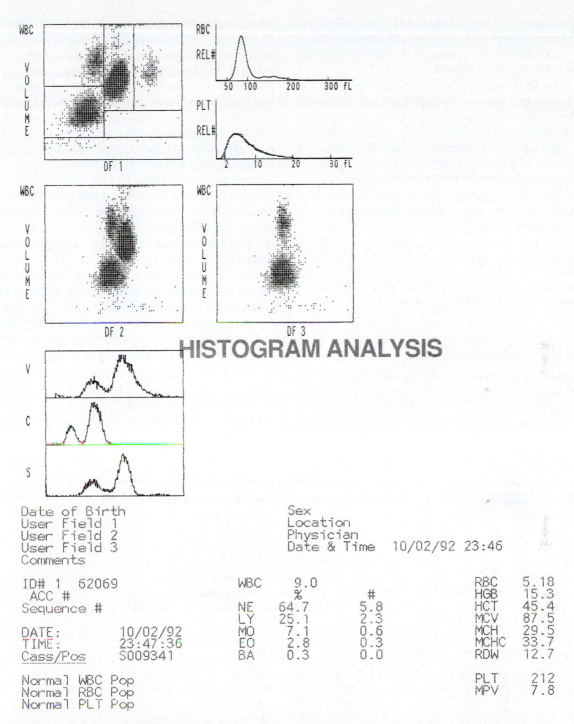

HISTOGRAM ANALYSIS

■ **FIGURE 41-8** Coulter STKS report from a normal individual. (Courtesy of Linda Nash, MT(ASCP), Southwest Texas Methodist Hospital, San Antonio, TX)

contour gating over linear gating is the ability to differentiate overlapping cell populations (e.g., monocytes from reactive lymphocytes).

In the heated reticulocyte dilution chamber, the fourth aliquot is mixed with new methylene blue reagent. The residual RNA is precipitated within the reticulocytes. The stained sample is then mixed with a hypotonic solution that (1) elutes hemoglobin from the erythrocytes, but permits precipitated RNA to remain, and (2) spheres the erythrocytes. This dilution is sent to the VCS flow cell for analysis. Contour gating of the VCS-derived characteristics is used to classify reticulocytes vs mature erythrocytes and identify the immature reticulocyte fraction (Web Figure 41-3 ■; ∞ Chapter 10). The reticulocyte parameters obtained by this analysis include absolute reticulocyte count, reticulocyte percentage, immature reticulocyte fraction, and mean reticulocyte volume.

The computer system compiles all data obtained from the instrument's analysis, evaluates the data to detect abnormalities, and determines the reported parameters (Web Table 41-1 ✪). The reported results and selected histograms/scatterplots are displayed on the computer screen or printed to a hard copy (Figure 41-9 ■). If abnormalities are detected, the clinical laboratory professional is alerted by suspect flags or user-defined flags. This information can then be used in a more thorough evaluation of the patient's data and examination of a peripheral blood smear.

 Checkpoint! #4

How does the method of analysis for the five-part leukocyte differential differ between the Coulter STKS and Coulter Gen·S?

Sysmex NE-8000

The Sysmex NE-8000 is a fully automated hematology instrument manufactured by Sysmex Corporation, Ltd.[14] This instrument is capable of performing blood cell counts, hemoglobin determinations, and five-part differentials. Blood cell counting is based on the impedance principle with both cell counts and histograms obtained through the analysis of a blood cell dilution. The five-part differential is obtained through a combination of technologies: impedance, radio frequency, and differential cell lysis.

Erythrocytes and platelets are counted from one dilution, and the leukocyte count and hemoglobin determination are obtained from a second dilution, which contains a mild lytic agent. The lytic agent lyses the erythrocytes and converts the free hemoglobin to cyanmethemoglobin but maintains leukocytes in their native state. The use of hydrodynamic focusing in the cell counting process minimizes the problems due to coincidence, erythrocyte deformability, and the recirculation of counted cells. Instead of utilizing established

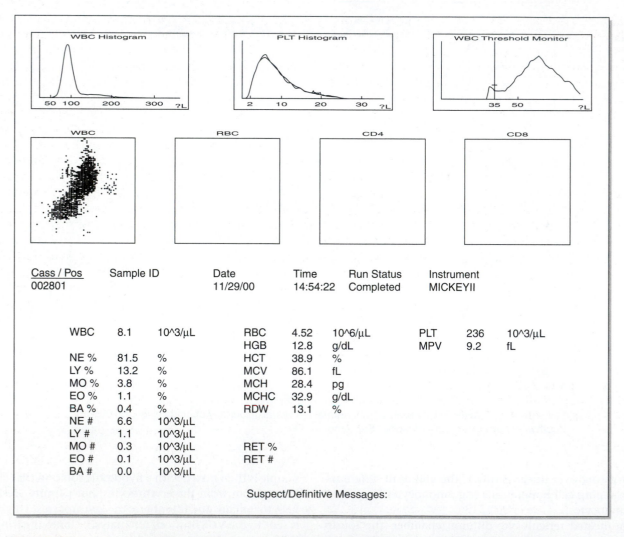

■ **FIGURE 41-9** Coulter GEN·S report from a normal individual. (Courtesy of Celia Jimeniz, MT(ASCP), San Antonio, TX)

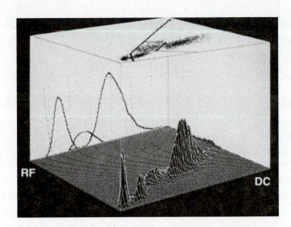

■ **FIGURE 41-10** Isometric histogram from normal individual, Sysmex NE-8000. RF refers to radio frequency and reflects the complexity of the cell. DC refers to direct current (impedance) and reflects the volume of the cell. (Courtesy of Sysmex Corporation, Kobe, Japan)

threshold limits for the differentiation of cell populations, the NE-8000 utilizes automatic discrimination. Automatic discriminators (floating threshold limits) allow for patient-to-patient variation by adjusting with each sample, therefore more clearly defining each cell population. In addition to the cell counts, histograms are also generated for the erythrocyte and platelet counts. Like other impedance counters, the analyzer's computer reviews the data obtained from each dilution and derives or calculates additional erythrocyte and platelet parameters (Web Table 41-1 ✪).

Information obtained from three separate detection blocks is compiled to give the five-part differential. The first detection block utilizes a combination of impedance and radio frequency to generate a trimodal histogram and two-dimensional scattergram representing the lymphocyte, monocyte, and granulocyte populations (Web Figures 41-4 and 41-5 ■). Radio frequency provides information on nuclear size and cellular density, and impedance reflects the cell size. Automatic discriminators allow clearer delineation of the three cell populations. By combining this information with particle numbers, a three-dimensional histogram is created (Figure 41-10 ■). Eosinophils and basophils are enumerated in separate detection blocks utilizing specific cell lytic agents and impedance. Histograms are generated for these two cell populations. The neutrophil count is obtained by subtracting the eosinophil and basophil counts from the granulocyte population.

All data, including cell counts, histograms, and scattergrams are analyzed by the computer system. The results are displayed on the computer screen or printed to a hard copy (Figure 41-11 ■). An extensive flagging program with interpretive comments alerts the clinical laboratory professional to abnormal results. Use of the flagging system and observation of the scattergrams and histograms allows the clinical laboratory professional to focus on specific abnormalities when performing a peripheral blood smear evaluation.

Sysmex SE-9500

The SE-9500 is a **random access,** discrete hematology analyzer that is capable of performing selected testing of the CBC components (i.e., Hb, Hct, PLT only) through user-defined menus or preset menus.[15,16] The basis of cell counting is similar to that of the NE-8000. The differences are in the measurement of hemoglobin, determination of the five-part differential, and performance of reticulocyte analysis. The hemoglobin measurement is a cyanide-free determination. Surfactants lyse the erythrocytes and release the hemoglobin. Sodium lauryl sulfate (SLS) converts ferrous iron to ferric iron, forming methemoglobin. Methemoglobin combines with SLS to form an SLS-hemichrome molecule. The absorbance of this molecule is measured to determine the hemoglobin concentration.

Five separate channels evaluate the leukocyte population: the "diff" channel, the immature cell channel (IMI), the leukocyte enumeration channel, and two channels specific for eosinophils and basophils. For the diff channel, the blood sample is diluted, erythrocytes are lysed, and leukocytes are maintained in their native state. Direct current and radio frequency characteristics of each cell are determined, and three leukocyte subpopulations are identified: the granulocytes, monocytes, and lymphocytes (Figure 41-12 ■).

In the IMI channel, reagents act selectively on the lipid membranes of the leukocytes. Mature leukocytes with phospholipid-rich membranes are completely lysed, leaving only bare nuclei. The immature myeloid cells remain intact. In the IMI channel, the cells are analyzed by direct current and radio frequency to determine the degree of immaturity (Figure 41-13 ■). This channel allows a clear delineation of immature neutrophils and blasts. In addition, this channel provides a new parameter, the hematopoietic progenitor cell (HPC) count. Studies have shown that the hematopoietic progenitor cell count correlates well with the CD34+ cell count by flow cytometry. Thus, HPC counts, like CD34+ cell counts, can be used for determination of peripheral blood, stem cell counts to assess optimal harvesting time following peripheral blood stem cell mobilization[17,18] (∞ Chapter 32).

The third leukocyte channel is used for leukocyte enumeration and comparison to the previously discussed leukocyte channels to identify potential discrepancies. The eosinophils and basophils are enumerated in dedicated channels with specific lysing reagents as discussed for the NE-8000 instrument.

From the leukocyte channels, scattergrams or histograms are created from the information gathered by direct current and radio frequency, and **cluster analysis** is used to separate the individual leukocyte populations. Together, the five-part differential and the data from the immature cell channel may be used by the clinical laboratory professional for the interpretation of specific abnormalities.

An additional feature is the **radar chart** that is created by the data analysis component from the patient's results for eight CBC parameters (Figure 41-14 ■). The comparison of

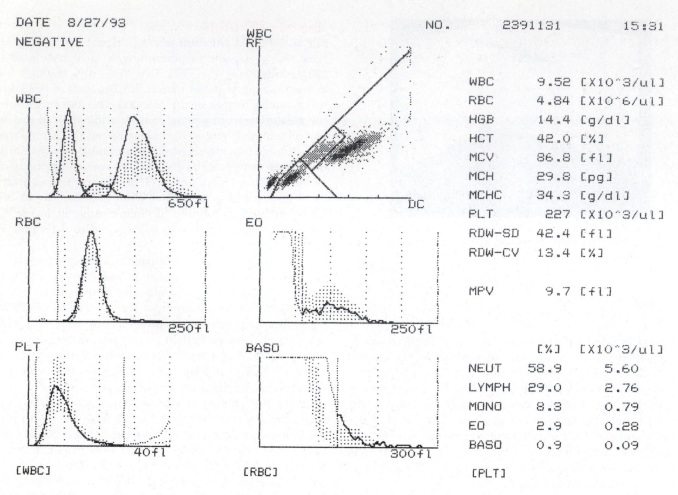

DATE 8/27/93
NEGATIVE

WBC

RBC

PLT

[WBC]

WBC
RF

EO

BASO

[RBC]

NO.   2391131   15:31

WBC	9.52	[X10^3/ul]
RBC	4.84	[X10^6/ul]
HGB	14.4	[g/dl]
HCT	42.0	[%]
MCV	86.8	[fl]
MCH	29.8	[pg]
MCHC	34.3	[g/dl]
PLT	227	[X10^3/ul]
RDW-SD	42.4	[fl]
RDW-CV	13.4	[%]
MPV	9.7	[fl]

	[%]	[X10^3/ul]
NEUT	58.9	5.60
LYMPH	29.0	2.76
MONO	8.3	0.79
EO	2.9	0.28
BASO	0.9	0.09

[PLT]

■ **FIGURE 41-11** Sysmex NE-8000 report from a normal individual. (Courtesy of Dora Mae Parker, MS, MT(ASCP), Baylor University Medical Center, Dallas, TX)

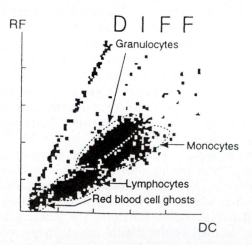

■ **FIGURE 41-12** SE-9500 leukocyte differential scatterplot, "diff" channel. Three populations of leukocytes are identified based on their direct current and radio frequency characteristics. (Courtesy of Sysmex Corporation, Kobe, Japan)

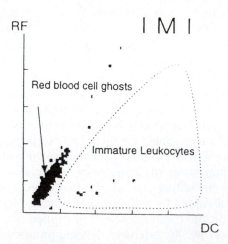

■ **FIGURE 41-13** SE-9500 leukocyte differential scatterplot, IMI channel. Immature neutrophils and blasts are identified by differential cell membrane lysis. Mature leukocytes are completely lysed, while immature leukocytes are not lysed. (Courtesy of Sysmex Corporation, Kobe, Japan)

the patient's radar chart to a normal radar chart may be used by the clinical laboratory professional as another tool in the investigation of hematologic abnormalities such as iron deficiency anemia (Figure 41-14).

The reticulocyte analysis module (RAM-1) uses flow cytometry and supravital staining to determine the absolute reticulocyte count, reticulocyte percentage, low fluorescence ratio, middle fluorescence ratio, and high fluorescence ratio. This methodology is discussed in detail in the section on the Sysmex R-3500 reticulocyte analyzer.

The SE-Alpha R is an integrated system consisting of the SP-100 slide preparation unit and the SE-9500 hematology analyzer. This integrated system performs a complete CBC and reticulocyte analysis and prepares a Wright-stained peripheral blood smear in a closed-tube, walk-away environment.

> ✓ ### Checkpoint! #5
>
> *In the Sysmex instruments, how are eosinophils and basophils isolated for enumeration?*

Abbott CELL-DYN 4000

Like other automated cell analyzers, the CELL-DYN 4000 utilizes a combination of technologies to enumerate erythrocytes, leukocytes, platelets, and reticulocytes and determine

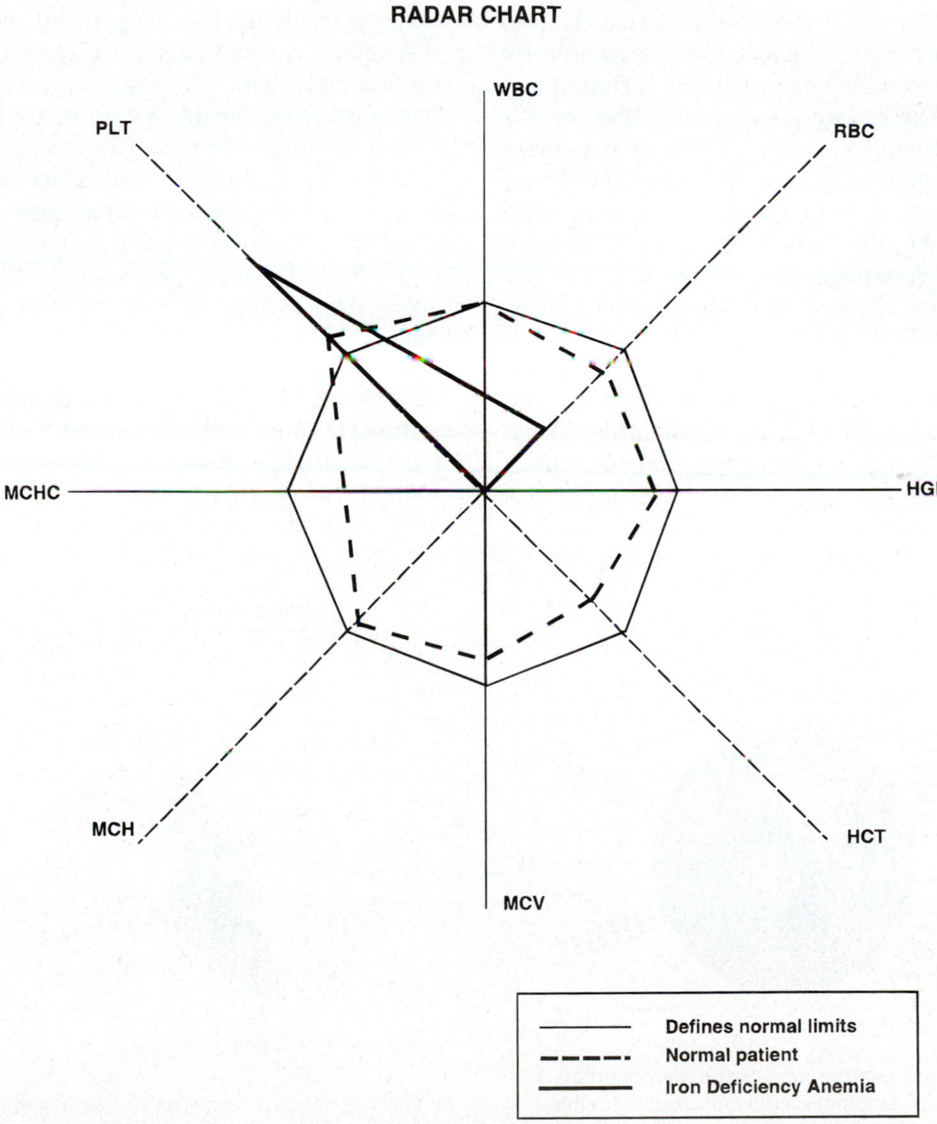

RADAR CHART

	Defines normal limits
	Normal patient
	Iron Deficiency Anemia

■ FIGURE 41-14 A radar chart from the Sysmex SE-9500 showing a comparison of the pattern seen in iron deficiency (bold line) to the pattern of a normal patient (dotted line). The solid octagonal line defines normal reference points.

a five-part leukocyte differential.[19,20] Flow cytometry, fluorescence staining, and impedance are used to make these determinations.

The instrument aspirates a sample of EDTA anticoagulated blood and sends a portion of this sample to one of three dilution cup assemblies. The hemoglobin dilution is prepared in the front dilution cup assembly. Hemoglobin reagent serves to dilute the blood sample, lyse erythrocytes, and convert free hemoglobin to a single chromagen by a reaction with imidazole. The hemoglobin concentration is determined spectrophotometrically at 540 nm. A reagent blank is used to minimize optical interferences, whereas leukocyte interference is minimal since the reagent destroys leukocytes and their nuclei. This cyanide-free reaction shows good correlation with the cyanmethemoglobin reference method.

In the middle dilution cup assembly, the sample is diluted for the determination of leukocytes and nucleated erythrocytes. The WBC reagent dilutes the leukocytes, lyses erythrocytes, strips the cytoplasmic membrane from nucleated erythrocytes and fragile leukocytes, and stains DNA of the exposed nuclei with a fluorescence dye. This dilution is sent to the optical flow cell. Hydrodynamic focusing directs cells single file through the flow cell. An argon-ion laser interacts with each cell to create light scatter and fluorescence. The following characteristics are determined: (1) 0° light scatter or forward scatter that reflects cell size; (2) 7° light scatter that reflects cell complexity; (3) 90° light scatter or side scatter that reflects nuclear lobularity; and (4) 90° depolarized light scatter that reflects cytoplasmic granularity (Figure 41-15 ■). Discriminant line analysis is used to isolate and identify various cell populations. A histogram is created based on one-dimensional data (e.g., size) or two-dimensional data (e.g., size vs DNA). The data management system identifies the valley between the cell populations and sets a discriminant line (Web Figure 41-6 ■). Scatterplots and contour plots are used to further classify subpopulations of leukocytes. The 0° (size) vs 7° (complexity) scatterplot allows differentiation of neutrophils, monocytes, and lymphocytes (Figure 41-16 ■). Eosinophils are differentiated from neutrophils in the 90°D (granularity) vs 90° (lobularity) scatterplot (Web Figure 41-7 ■). Finally, lymphocytes are separated from basophils based on size and complexity. Additional information obtained from evaluation of this dilution includes the enumeration of nucleated erythrocytes and identification of nonviable or fragile leukocytes, which are based on fluorescence intensity (DNA content) and light-scatter characteristics. The data management system analyzes these characteristics to determine the total leukocyte count and the five-part leukocyte differential.

Two different dilutions are prepared in the rear dilution cup assembly. One dilution represents the erythrocyte/platelet dilution. The diluent serves to dilute the blood sample and sphere the erythrocytes. Using the principles of hydrodynamic focusing and impedance, the erythrocytes and platelets are evaluated as they pass singly through the impedance transducer. From the impedance transducer, the erythrocyte count, erythrocyte size distribution curve (histogram), platelet size distribution curve, and platelet count are obtained. A second portion of the erythrocyte/platelet dilution is sent to the optical flow cell for enumeration of these cells based on light-scatter characteristics. The erythrocyte count from the optical flow cell and the platelet count from the impedance transducer are used as internal quality control checks against the reported erythrocyte count from the impedance transducer and the reported

■ FIGURE 41-15 Four light scatter measurements from the CELL-DYN 4000. The 0° scatter reflects cell size; 7° scatter reflects cell complexity; 90° scatter reflects nuclear lobularity; and 90° depolarized scatter reflects cytoplasmic granularity. (Courtesy of Abbott Laboratories, Diagnostic Division, Abbott Park, IL)

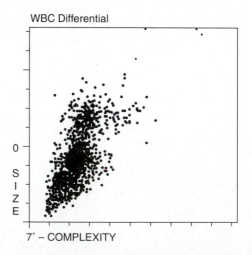

■ FIGURE 41-16 0° (size) vs 7° (complexity) scatterplot, CELL-DYN 4000. Neutrophils, monocytes, and lymphocytes are identified. Lymphocytes are located lower left in the scatterplot; the middle cell population is monocytes; and neutrophils are located upper center in the scatterplot.

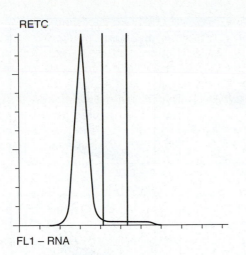

RETC

FL1 – RNA

■ FIGURE 41-17 Reticulocyte histogram, CELL-DYN 4000. Reticulocytes are found between the two gates. The peak to the left represents mature erythrocytes.

platelet count from the optical flow cell. The second dilution represents the reticulocyte dilution. The sample is diluted by the isotonic diluent, and nucleic acids are stained with a fluorescence dye. This dilution is sent to the optical flow cell, where the number of reticulocytes is determined based on fluorescence intensity and light-scatter characteristics. From this information, a reticulocyte histogram is created that allows the determination of the reticulocyte count and the immature reticulocyte fraction (Figure 41-17 ■).

The data management system analyzes and compiles all data obtained from the instrument and determines the reported parameters (Web Table 41-1 ✪). The results are displayed on a computer screen or printed to a hard copy for the clinical laboratory professional's review (Figure 41-18 ■). System-initiated messages and data flags alert the clinical laboratory professional to potential abnormalities or errors in the results. This information is used to correlate complete blood count (CBC) data with peripheral blood morphology to improve the identification and confirmation of abnormalities.

 Checkpoint! #6

Which CELL-DYN scatterplot allows differentiation of eosinophils from neutrophils?

LIGHT-SCATTERING INSTRUMENTS

Two instruments will be described here, the Technicon H*1 and the Bayer Advia 120.

Technicon H*1

Technicon Instruments Corporation (now Bayer Corporation) has been involved in hematology instrumentation since the early 1970s. The first instruments were based on continuous flow analysis similar to their chemistry instruments. The Hemolog D performed leukocyte differentials based on continuous flow analysis and peroxidase cytochemical staining. The Technicon H-6000 was capable of performing a complete blood cell count and five-part differential utilizing continuous flow analysis and an improved cytochemical staining method. The Technicon H*1 was the first of a series of instruments that combined these principles of cell detection and identification with flow cytometry.[21–28]

The Technicon H*1 aspirates a sample of EDTA anticoagulated blood and processes portions of that sample through four separate channels. The erythrocyte/platelet channel determines erythrocyte and platelet counts by the analysis of light-scattering measurements obtained as the diluted cells pass singly through a helium–neon laser beam. The diluent utilized for erythrocyte and platelet counts causes **isovolumetric sphering** of the erythrocytes. Isovolumetric sphering of erythrocytes eliminates cell volume errors due to variations in erythrocyte shape. The erythrocytes are counted and sized by both high-angle and low-angle light-scattering measurements. Individual erythrocyte hemoglobin concentration and cell volume can be determined from these measurements; thus, the mean cell volume (MCV) and **cellular hemoglobin concentration mean (CHCM)** are obtained. The red cell distribution width (RDW) and the **hemoglobin distribution width (HDW)** are derived from these measurements. Platelet enumeration and sizing are accomplished using one detector that is set at an increased gain. Together, these measurements allow for the generation of an erythrocyte cytogram and of erythrocyte, hemoglobin concentration, and platelet histograms (Figure 41-19 ■).

Within the hemoglobin channel, a portion of EDTA-anticoagulated blood is mixed with the hemoglobin diluent. The erythrocytes are lysed and free hemoglobin is converted to cyanmethemoglobin. The concentration of cyanmethemoglobin is determined photometrically at 546 nm.

The leukocyte count and five-part differential are obtained utilizing two different methods and two separate channels, the peroxidase channel and the basophil/lobularity channel. In the peroxidase channel, neutrophils, monocytes, and eosinophils are identified by the degree of peroxidase positivity and the amount of forward light scatter. Lymphocytes and large unstained cells (LUCs) are identified by the amount of forward light scatter and the fact that they remain unstained by this peroxidase cytochemical staining method. Erythrocytes are removed prior to peroxidase staining by lytic action. The amount of forward scatter and degree of peroxidase positivity are detected as the cells pass through a tungsten halogen-based flow cell. As a result, neutrophils are located in the upper right quadrant, eosinophils in the lower right quadrant, and monocytes in the center triangular region, while lymphocytes are located adjacent to the y-axis in the center left quadrant and LUCs are located in the upper left quadrant of the peroxidase cytogram

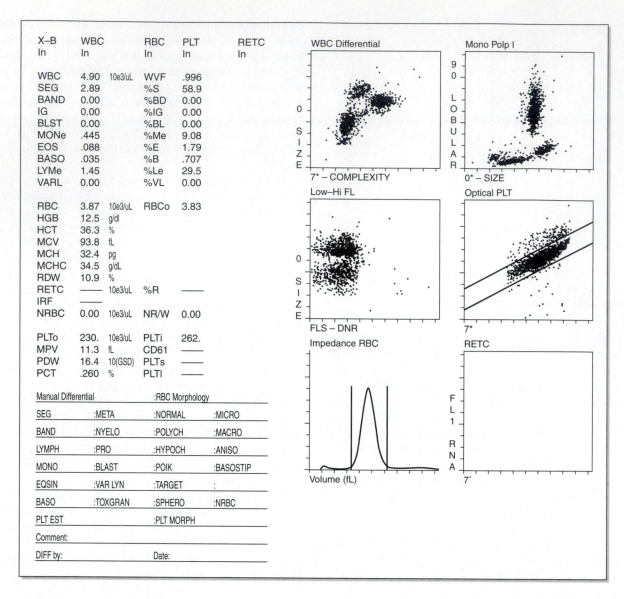

X–B In	WBC In		RBC In	PLT In	RETC In
WBC	4.90	10e3/uL	WVF	.996	
SEG	2.89		%S	58.9	
BAND	0.00		%BD	0.00	
IG	0.00		%IG	0.00	
BLST	0.00		%BL	0.00	
MONe	.445		%Me	9.08	
EOS	.088		%E	1.79	
BASO	.035		%B	.707	
LYMe	1.45		%Le	29.5	
VARL	0.00		%VL	0.00	
RBC	3.87	10e3/uL	RBCo	3.83	
HGB	12.5	g/dl			
HCT	36.3	%			
MCV	93.8	fL			
MCH	32.4	pg			
MCHC	34.5	g/dL			
RDW	10.9	%			
RETC	——	10e3/uL	%R	——	
IRF	——				
NRBC	0.00	10e3/uL	NR/W	0.00	
PLTo	230.	10e3/uL	PLTi	262.	
MPV	11.3	fL	CD61	——	
PDW	16.4	10(GSD)	PLTs	——	
PCT	.260	%	PLTI	——	

Manual Differential		:RBC Morphology	
SEG	:META	:NORMAL	:MICRO
BAND	:NYELO	:POLYCH	:MACRO
LYMPH	:PRO	:HYPOCH	:ANISO
MONO	:BLAST	:POIK	:BASOSTIP
EQSIN	:VAR LYN	:TARGET	:
BASO	:TOXGRAN	:SPHERO	:NRBC
PLT EST		:PLT MORPH	
Comment:			
DIFF by:		Date:	

WBC Differential   7* – COMPLEXITY

Mono Polp I   0* – SIZE

Low–Hi FL   FLS – DNR

Optical PLT   7*

Impedance RBC   Volume (fL)

RETC   7°

FIGURE 41-18 CELL-DYN 4000 report from a normal individual. (Courtesy of Faye Summerfield, MT(ASCP), University Hospital, San Antonio, TX)

(Figure 41-19 ■). Within the basophil/lobularity channel, a fourth portion of EDTA-anticoagulated blood is mixed with basophil diluent. The basophil diluent lyses erythrocytes and platelets and strips all leukocytes except basophils of their cytoplasm. The helium–neon laser flow cell measures this dilution. Basophils will have large, low-angle scattered signatures, and the remaining cell nuclei will be classified as mononuclear or polymorphonuclear based on their high-angle scatter signatures. The normal cell pattern as depicted on the basophil/lobularity cytogram is referred to as the worm, with the head region representing the mononuclear cells and the body region representing the polymorphonu-

clear cells. The basophils are located in the region above the worm (Figure 41-19 ■).

The absolute count for each leukocyte population is obtained from both channels. The computer compares the corresponding cell counts and generates flags if the results do not compare. The percentage values are calculated from the absolute cell counts. In the peroxidase channel, basophils and lymphocytes fall in the same region; therefore, the total lymphocyte count is determined by subtracting the basophil count obtained from the basophil/lobularity channel. An advantage of this method of determining cell counts is the capability of performing WBC counts and differen-

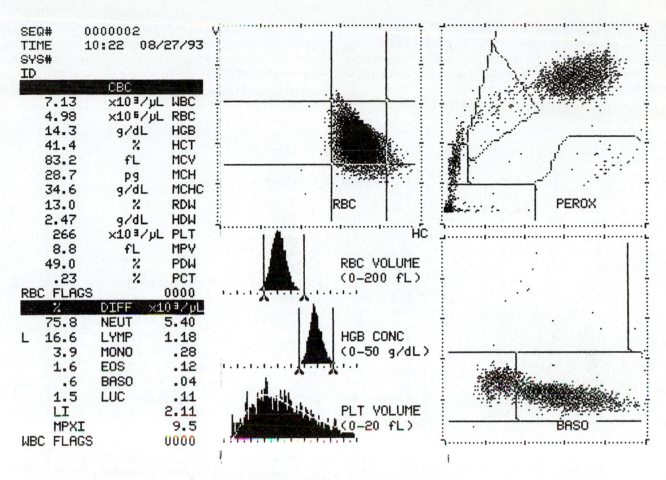

■ **FIGURE 41-19** Technicon H*1 report from a normal individual depicting the erythrocyte cytogram, erythrocyte and platelet histogram, a hemoglobin concentration histogram, a WBC peroxidase cytogram, and basophil/lobularity cytogram.

tials on specimens with very low counts (WBC<0.1 × 10⁹/L).

The Technicon H*1 evaluates the information from the two flow cells and displays the information on the computer screen. The results can be printed to hard copy for the records (Figure 41-19 ■). If abnormalites are detected in cell counts, histograms, or cytograms, the instrument flags the appropriate result or results. The flagging criteria assist the clinical laboratory professional in defining the abnormalities to be reviewed by peripheral blood smear examination.

Bayer ADVIA 120

Like the newest models from other manufacturers, the Bayer ADVIA 120 is capable of performing a CBC, five-part leukocyte differential, and reticulocyte count.[29] The ADVIA 120 has five measurement channels. The hemoglobin channel utilizes the same methodology and provides the same data as the Technicon H*1 instrument. The erythrocyte/platelet channel is similar to the Technicon H*1. The difference is in the measurement of platelets. Platelets are evaluated simulta-

neously with the erythrocytes using both high-angle light scatter and low-angle light scatter. From this information a platelet cytogram is determined. The actual platelet count is obtained from the integrated analysis of the erythrocyte cytogram and platelet cytogram in order to include large platelets while excluding erythrocytes, erythrocyte fragments, and erythrocyte ghosts. Other data obtained from this channel are the same as from the Technicon H*1. The peroxidase and basophil/lobularity channels utilize the same methodologies and provide the same data as the Technicon H*1. The data management system uses cluster analysis to identify individual cell populations within a cytogram. Each population is identified by its position, area, and density. Thresholds are set, and the number of cells in each population is determined.

The fifth channel is the reticulocyte channel, where cellular RNA of the reticulocytes is stained with oxazine 750, a nucleic acid dye. The helium–neon laser flow cell is used to evaluate the erythroid cells for light-scattering and absorbance characteristics. Reticulocytes are differentiated from mature erythrocytes based on their RNA content. In addition to the absolute reticulocye count and relative reticulocyte percentage, reticulocyte analysis includes a measure of the reticulocyte mean cell volume and the reticulocyte cellular hemoglobin concentration mean.

Like the Technicon H*1, the ADVIA's data management system evaluates the information from the two flow cells, determines the reported parameters, and displays the information on the computer screen (Web Table 41-1 ✪). The results can be printed to hard copy for the records (Figure 41-20 ■). If

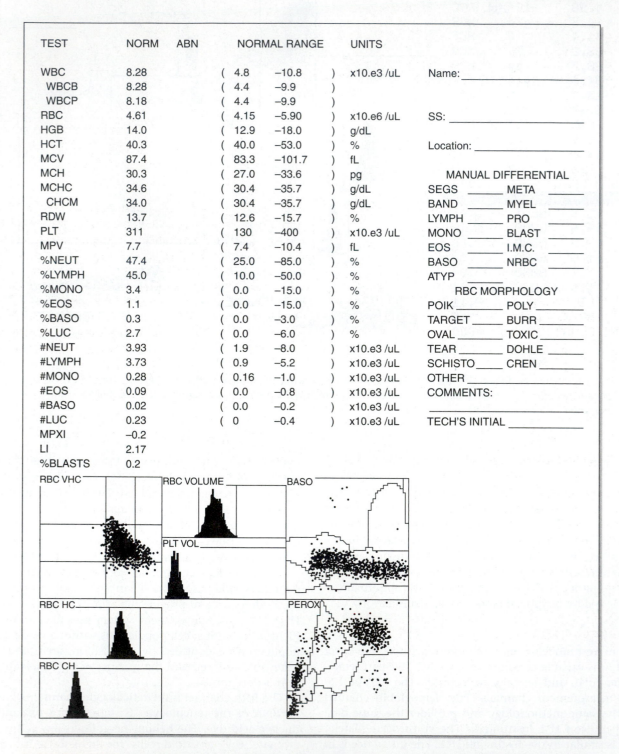

TEST	NORM	ABN	NORMAL RANGE			UNITS
WBC	8.28		(4.8	−10.8	)	x10.e3 /uL
WBCB	8.28		(4.4	−9.9	)	
WBCP	8.18		(4.4	−9.9	)	
RBC	4.61		(4.15	−5.90	)	x10.e6 /uL
HGB	14.0		(12.9	−18.0	)	g/dL
HCT	40.3		(40.0	−53.0	)	%
MCV	87.4		(83.3	−101.7	)	fL
MCH	30.3		(27.0	−33.6	)	pg
MCHC	34.6		(30.4	−35.7	)	g/dL
CHCM	34.0		(30.4	−35.7	)	g/dL
RDW	13.7		(12.6	−15.7	)	%
PLT	311		(130	−400	)	x10.e3 /uL
MPV	7.7		(7.4	−10.4	)	fL
%NEUT	47.4		(25.0	−85.0	)	%
%LYMPH	45.0		(10.0	−50.0	)	%
%MONO	3.4		(0.0	−15.0	)	%
%EOS	1.1		(0.0	−15.0	)	%
%BASO	0.3		(0.0	−3.0	)	%
%LUC	2.7		(0.0	−6.0	)	%
#NEUT	3.93		(1.9	−8.0	)	x10.e3 /uL
#LYMPH	3.73		(0.9	−5.2	)	x10.e3 /uL
#MONO	0.28		(0.16	−1.0	)	x10.e3 /uL
#EOS	0.09		(0.0	−0.8	)	x10.e3 /uL
#BASO	0.02		(0.0	−0.2	)	x10.e3 /uL
#LUC	0.23		(0	−0.4	)	x10.e3 /uL
MPXI	−0.2					
LI	2.17					
%BLASTS	0.2					

Name: _____

SS: _____

Location: _____

MANUAL DIFFERENTIAL

SEGS _____   META _____
BAND _____   MYEL _____
LYMPH _____   PRO _____
MONO _____   BLAST _____
EOS _____   I.M.C. _____
BASO _____   NRBC _____
ATYP _____

RBC MORPHOLOGY

POIK _____   POLY _____
TARGET _____   BURR _____
OVAL _____   TOXIC _____
TEAR _____   DOHLE _____
SCHISTO _____   CREN _____
OTHER _____
COMMENTS:
_____

TECH'S INITIAL _____

RBC VHC   RBC VOLUME   BASO
PLT VOL
RBC HC   PEROX
RBC CH

■ **FIGURE 41-20** Advia 120 report from a normal individual. (Courtesy of David Teplicek, MT(ASCP), Audie Murphy Memorial Veterans Administration Hospital, San Antonio, TX)

abnormalites are detected in cell counts, histograms, or cytograms, the instrument flags the appropriate result or results. The flagging criteria assist the clinical laboratory professional in defining the abnormalities to be reviewed by peripheral blood smear examination.

 Checkpoint! #7

For instruments using optical light scatter to determine blood cell counts, which cellular characteristic is determined by the degree of forward scatter?

► AUTOMATED RETICULOCYTE ANALYZERS

Reticulocyte enumeration is utilized to evaluate the bone marrow's erythropoietic activity. Evaluation of the erythropoietic activity is useful in the differentiation of anemias, the monitoring of a patient's response to therapy, and the assessment of erythropoietic activity following a bone marrow or stem cell transplant. Traditionally, the reticulocyte count has been performed manually using a supravital stain (e.g., new methylene blue) and microscopic enumeration. However, the newer automated blood cell counting instruments and dedicated automated reticulocyte analyzers are replacing the manual method. With automation, more cells are analyzed, improving the precision, accuracy, and reliability of these counts.

Automated instruments provide additional reticulocyte parameters such as reticulocyte hemoglobin concentration (CHr), reticulocyte mean volume (MCVr), and immature reticulocyte fraction (IRF). The reticulocyte hemoglobin concentration is determined from the direct measurement of reticulocyte volume and hemoglobin concentration by light-scattering and absorbance characteristics. The reticulocyte mean cell volume is derived from the reticulocyte cytogram and reflects the average size of the reticulocyte population. The immature reticulocyte fraction, or high-intensity ratio, reflects those reticulocytes with an increased amount of RNA or the early immature reticulocytes. An increased number of immature reticulocytes may be an indication of an erythropoietic response. For this reason, these parameters have proven useful in measuring bone marrow engraftment following transplant and determining bone marrow response to iron or erythropoietin therapy.[30–32]

SYSMEX R-3500

The Sysmex R-3500 is a fully automated instrument for reticulocyte analysis.[33,34] A blood sample is reacted with fluorescence dye auramine-O and sent to an argon laser flow cell for analysis. Two different detectors determine forward scat-

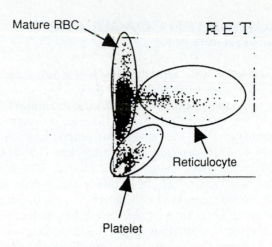

■ **FIGURE 41-21** Sysmex R-3500 reticulocyte scattergram. (Courtesy of Sysmex Corporation Kobe, Japan)

ter, reflecting cell size, and fluorescence, reflecting RNA content. The data analysis system integrates these two characteristics to create the reticulocyte scattergram (Figure 41-21 ■). From the scattergram, cells are classified as mature erythrocytes, reticulocytes, and platelets. The reticulocytes are further classified based on fluorescent activity to determine reticulocyte maturity (Figure 41-22 ■). Reported parameters include absolute reticulocyte count, reticulocyte percentage, erythrocyte count, low fluorescence ratio (LFR), middle fluorescence ratio (MFR), high fluorescence ratio (HFR), immature reticulocyte fraction (IRF), and platelet count. The IRF represents the MFR and HFR combined and is reported as a percentage of the total reticulocyte count.

 Checkpoint! #8

When performing a reticulocyte analysis, what cellular component is stained?

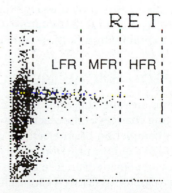

■ **FIGURE 41-22** Sysmex R-3500 reticulocyte scattergram depicting the three subpopulations of reticulocytes: low fluorescence ratio (LFR), middle fluorescence ratio (MFR), and high fluorescence ratio (HFR). (Courtesy of Sysmex Corporation Kobe, Japan)

► AUTOMATED COAGULATION INSTRUMENTS

Instrumentation was actually introduced into coagulation testing in the early twentieth century. These first instruments, like the majority of instruments utilized today, analyzed the coagulation system through the detection of clot formation.[35,36] The coaguloviscometer developed by Kottman in 1910 determined clotting times by measuring the change in blood **viscosity** as it clotted. The change in viscosity was determined by plotting the voltage against time. A second method of clot detection was introduced by Kugelmass in 1922. He adapted the nephelometer to coagulation testing. In nephelometry, the clotting time was determined by measuring variations in transillumination as registered by a galvenometer. The photoelectric technique for the determination of clotting times was introduced by Baldes and Nygaard in 1936. With their instrument, clotting times were determined by the measurement of increasing optical density as the plasma clotted. Coagulation instrumentation continued to improve, and by the 1960s semiautomated coagulation instruments began to replace manual coagulation techniques in the clinical laboratory. These first instruments were based on electromechanical methods or optical density methods of clot detection. The 1970s saw an evolvement in coagulation testing with the introduction of fully automated instruments capable of performing multiple coagulation assays.

With the new directions in coagulation testing including chromogenic and immunologic methods, coagulation instruments are now capable of performing these test methods, as well as the clot-based tests. The introduction of instrumentation into coagulation testing has led to increased precision and accuracy and, therefore, improved diagnostic testing and monitoring of therapeutic interventions.

The two principles of clot-based detection currently used by coagulation instruments are electromechanical and optical density. This section will review these principles and how they have been adapted to several coagulation instruments that may be seen in the clinical laboratory. Other available instruments use a combination of these principles.

ELECTROMECHANICAL INSTRUMENTS

These instruments measure the time for a clot to form in plasma by detecting changes in the reaction mixture. One instrument detects completion of an electrical circuit between two electrodes when a clot forms (Fibrometer). The other detects a decrease in movement of an iron ball in an electromagnetic field when a clot forms (STArt 4 Clot Detection).

BBL FibroSystem

The FibroSystem, a semiautomated coagulation instrument, was introduced in the 1960s. This system is composed of a Fibrometer coagulation timer, a thermal prep block to pre-warm reagents and samples to 37°C, and an automatic pipet to deliver the appropriate amount of sample or reagent to the test cuvette.[37] The Fibrometer probe, which is an integral part of the Fibrometer coagulation timer, serves as the clot detector. The probe consists of two sensory electrodes (stationary and moving) and a probe foot, which is an extension of the moving electrode extending beyond the base of the probe assembly. In the timing sequence, the moving electrode cycles through the reaction mixture in an elliptical pattern created by the raising and lowering of the probe foot. The stationary electrode remains in the reaction mixture and is responsible for establishing the electric potential between the two electrodes. The moving electrode becomes electrically active when it is above the reaction mixture. As the fibrin clot is formed, it is picked up by the small hook on the tip of the moving electrode. The electric circuit is completed when the moving electrode becomes activated as it moves out of the reaction mixture; current flows from the stationary electrode through the reaction mixture and fibrin clot to the moving electrode. The creation of this electric circuit causes the timing device to stop, and the clotting time in seconds is recorded. Thus, the principle of clot detection is the electromechanical principle. An advantage of the FibroSystem is that it can be adapted to any coagulation assay that is clot based.

American Bioproducts STArt 4 Clot Detection Instrument

The STArt 4 Clot Detection instrument is a semiautomated instrument for coagulation testing that is based on the electromechanical clot detection principle.[38,39] This is a stand-alone instrument consisting of four independently timed incubation stations with 16 wells, a dispensing pipet, room temperature and 37°-thermostated reagent storage wells, four measurement channels, and a microprocessor system. This variation of the electromechanical clot detection principle is based on the increasing viscosity of plasma as clot formation occurs. The increasing viscosity is detected by the movement of an iron ball located at the bottom of the reaction cuvette. A constant pendular swing of the ball is created by alternating an electromagnetic field on opposite sides of the cuvette utilizing two independent driving coils. As clot formation begins, the plasma viscosity increases and there is a corresponding decrease in ball movement. The clotting time is determined from an algorithm of the variations in oscillation amplitude. Clotting time results are displayed on the liquid crystal display (LCD) screen, and printed results are obtained from the thermal printer. This instrument can be adapted to any coagulation assay that is clot based.

 Checkpoint! #9

Compare the clot detection methods for the Fibrometer system and the STArt 4 system.

OPTICAL DENSITY INSTRUMENTS

Organon Teknika Coag-A-Mate XM

The Coag-A-Mate XM is a semiautomated instrument utilizing the change in optical density that occurs with clot formation as its principle of clot detection.[40] The instrument consists of a reagent storage compartment, incubation test plate, photodetection system, and microprocessing system. The test procedures are programmed using the touch entry keypad. Reagents and patient specimens are manually pipeted into the test cuvettes. The reaction mixture is warmed to 37°C in the incubation test plate. For determination of the clotting time, the test cuvette is placed in one of two measuring stations. The addition of the final reagent to the test cuvette initiates the timer. The photoelectric cell detects the sudden increase in optical density occurring with fibrin formation, and the timer is stopped. The results are displayed on the LCD panel below each measuring station. This instrument is capable of performing two tests simultaneously. All clot-based coagulation assays may be performed by this instrument.

CHROMOGENIC/CLOT DETECTION INSTRUMENTS

Several coagulation instrument manufacturers currently market coagulation instruments that combine the traditional clot-based detection principle with chromogenic analysis.

Since the coagulation cascade is a series of enzymatic reactions catalyzed by serine proteases, the activity of these enzymes can be measured by conventional clinical chemistry methods. Chromogenic analysis is an example of a clinical chemistry methodology that has been adapted to coagulation testing. In a chromogenic analysis, the enzyme of interest (activated coagulation factor) cleaves the chromogenic substrate at a specific site, releasing the chromophore tag. The color intensity is measured spectrophotometrically and is proportional to the concentration of the enzyme. Through the choice of substrates used in a specific assay, chromogenic assays can be used for the testing of individual coagulation proteins, biochemical inhibitors, and fibrinolytic proteins. In addition to coagulation instruments, chromogenic assays have been adapted for use on a number of spectrophotometric chemistry analyzers.

MLA Electra 1800C

The MLA Electra 1800C is a fully automated coagulation instrument consisting of two components, an analyzer and an automated closed tube sampler. The instrument is capable of performing clot-based assays and chromogenic assays in random access.[41] The operator chooses the appropriate tests from user-defined test panels or individual test options. Reagents are stored on board in six refrigerated positions and preheated to 37°C immediately before addition to the sample. Both clot-based and chromogenic assays are based on a change in optical density. In the clot-based assays, the amount of light detected by the photodetector decreases as the fibrin clot forms, causing a change in the electrical signal output from the detector. The electrical signal is analyzed by the computer to determine the clotting time. For chromogenic assays the photodetector monitors the rate of change in optical density as the colored product is formed. The reaction between reagent substrate and the analyte releases the chromophore paranitroaniline, which is measured at 405 nm. The instrument takes a series of optical density readings and determines the linearity of the data and the change in absorbance per minute. This absorbance change is compared to the reference calibration curve programmed into the instrument by the laboratory. The final result is determined from this curve and is reported in the appropriate units. A hard-copy printout of the results, temperature status, error messages, and standard curve is obtained from the thermal printer, and results can be interfaced with a laboratory information system (LIS).

Sigma AMAX CS-190

The AMAX CS-190 is a random access, fully automated coagulation analyzer that is capable of performing three different methodologies: electromechanical, optical density, and chromogenic.[42] The instrument can perform all three methodologies simulatenously. Both samples and reagents are stored at 15°C. A temperature-controlled probe (37°C) is used to transfer the appropriate amount of sample or reagent to the reaction cuvette for measurement.

Electromechanical measurement of clot formation is based on the Amelung ball method. The test cuvette contains a stainless steel ball. After sample and reagent (e.g., activated partial thromboplastin) are added to the cuvette, it is placed in a mechanical measurement well. The addition of the starting reagent (e.g., calcium chloride) initiates the rotation of the ball. The rotating ball is held in a predetermined position within the cuvette by a magnet. As the fibrin clot forms, fibrin strands draw the ball away from its steady state position. A sensor detects the change in ball position, and the timer is stopped. The clotting time represents the elapsed time between addition of starting reagent and detection of ball movement. The advantage of this measurement is the small volumes of sample and reagent that may be used.

The second method of clot detection available on the AMAX CS-190 is optical density. After sample and reagent (e.g., activated partial thromboplastin) are added to the cuvette, it is placed in a photo-optical measurement well. When the starting reagent (e.g., calcium chloride) is added to the cuvette, the instrument measures the initial absorbance of the reaction mixture and monitors the change in absorbance over time. The rate of change in absorbance between the initial reading and the final reading is used to calculate the clotting time. The use of both the initial absorbance reading and final absorbance reading in th' calculation minimizes the effect of lipemia or icterus on the final clotting time result.

The chromogenic assays are performed in the photo-optical measurement well. The temperature-controlled probe delivers the appropriate amount of sample and reagent to the test cuvette. The final enzymatic reaction in the chromogenic assays yields paranitroaniline. The photodetector cell monitors the change in optical density over the reaction period at 405 nm. A clotting curve created by plotting the change in optical density against time is compared to the appropriate calibration curve. The patient results are calculated from this comparison and are reported in the appropriate units.

The data management system analyzes all data for potential problems or errors and alerts the clinical laboratory professional. Results may be printed to a hard copy, or the system can be interfaced with an LIS system.

 Checkpoint! #10

For the optical density instruments, what is the basis of clot detection?

SUMMARY

This chapter briefly reviewed the ever-increasing technology within the automated hematology laboratory. The blood cell counting instruments include those using impedence and light scattering priniciples. Some can also measure reticulocytes. Automated coagulation instruments include those that use electromechanical, optical density, and chromogenic methods to detect clot formation in a plasma mixture. To operate these instruments to their fullest potential, it is important that qualified clinical laboratory profession-als evaluate the data created by the instrument's analysis of individual cell's characteristics or clotting characteristics. Through careful review of that data, new applications of these instruments may arise that will aid in the early detection of abnormalities. Automation has increased precision and accuracy within the hematology laboratory and shortened the amount of time needed for analysis, but it has also increased the need for the individual's interpretive skills.

REVIEW QUESTIONS

LEVEL I

1. Blood cell counting by this instrument is based on optical light scattering: (Checklist #3)
   a. Coulter GEN·S instrument
   b. Sysmex NE-8000 instrument
   c. CELL-DYN 4000 instrument
   d. Bayer ADVIA 120

2. In automated blood cell counting instruments, hydrodynamic focusing is used to: (Checklist #3)
   a. assure that only a single cell enters the detection area at any given time
   b. direct the beam of light onto the center of the photodetector
   c. select the appropriate wavelength of light for analysis
   d. focus the beam of light on the detection area

3. For the Coulter GEN·S instrument, which parameter is calculated? (Checklist #5)
   a. erythrocyte count
   b. MCV
   c. reticulocyte percentage
   d. absolute neutrophil count

4. Which dye is used to stain cellular RNA for reticulocyte counting on the Bayer ADVIA 120? (Checklist #6)
   a. thiazole orange
   b. oxazine 750
   c. new methylene blue
   d. auramine-O

LEVEL II

1. What information is needed to create an erythrocyte histogram? (Checklist #1)
   a. cell volume and relative cell number
   b. cell size and cell complexity
   c. nuclear size and cellular density
   d. cell forward scatter and cell side scatter

2. For the Sysmex SE-9500, which of the following technologies is *not* used in the categorization of leukocyte cell types? (Checklist #1)
   a. impedance
   b. radio frequency
   c. optical light scatter
   d. differential cell lysis

3. Using the Bayer ADVIA 120 instrument, which leukocyte cell type is located in the body of the worm of the basophil/lobularity cytogram? (Checklist #1)
   a. basophils
   b. mononuclear leukocytes
   c. polymorphonuclear leukocytes
   d. eosinophils

REVIEW QUESTIONS *(continued)*

LEVEL I

5. For this coagulation instrument, clot formation is detected by the flow of current between two sensory electrodes: (Checklist #7)
   a. Sigma AMAX CS-190 instrument
   b. BBL Fibrometer instrument
   c. MLA Electra 1800C instrument
   d. American Bioproducts STArt 4 instrument

6. Both electromechanical and photo-optical principles of clot detection are available on the: (Checklist #7)
   a. BBL Fibrometer instrument
   b. MLA Electra 1800C instrument
   c. American Bioproducts STArt 4 instrument
   d. Sigma AMAX CS-190 instrument

7. The photo-optical principle of clot detection is based on the: (Checklist #8)
   a. observation of increased light transmission as a fibrin clot forms
   b. optical detection of ball movement as a fibrin clot forms
   c. observation of increased absorbance as a fibrin clot forms
   d. photometric detection of an oscillating magnetic force as a fibrin clot forms

8. For the Abbott CELL-DYN 4000, which parameter is directly measured? (Checklist #5)
   a. hematocrit
   b. platelet count
   c. relative neutrophil percentage
   d. absolute reticulocyte count

9. Which automated blood cell counting instrument uses the analysis of fluorescence intensity and light scatter to determine the reticulocyte count? (Checklist #6)
   a. Coulter STKS
   b. Technicon H*1
   c. Abbott CELL-DYN 4000
   d. Coulter GEN·S

10. For the Sysmex NE-8000 instrument, which parameter is derived from a histogram or scattergram? (Checklist #5)
    a. absolute monocyte count
    b. erythrocyte count
    c. mean cell volume
    d. hematocrit

LEVEL II

4. The Coulter GEN·S five-part differential is determined by the analysis of cellular characteristics as defined by: (Checklist #1)
   a. light scatter, cytochemical staining, and radio frequency
   b. light scatter and radio frequency
   c. impedance and cytochemical staining
   d. impedance, conductivity, and light scatter

5. The reticulocyte hemoglobin concentration (CHr) is determined by the measurement of the cell's: (Checklist #2)
   a. absorbance and light scatter characteristics
   b. absorbance and radio frequency characteristics
   c. fluorescence intensity and impedance characteristics
   d. fluorescence intensity and conductivity characteristics

www.prenhall.com/mckenzie

Use the above address to access the free, interactive Companion Web site created for this textbook. Get hints, instant feedback, and textbook references to chapter-related multiple choice questions.

REFERENCES

1. Mattern CFT, Brackett FS, Olson B. Determination of number and size of particles by electrical gating: Blood cells. *J Appl Physiol*. 1957; 10:56.

2. Jovin TM, et al. Automatic sizing and separation of particles by ratios of light scattering intensities. *J Histochem Cytochem*. 1976 24:269.

3. Cox CJ, et al. Evaluation of the Coulter Counter Model S-Plus IV. *Am J Clin Path.* 1985; 84:297.

4. Griswold DJ, Champagne VD. Evaluation of the Coulter S-Plus IV three-part differential in an acute care hospital. *Am J Clin Path.* 1985; 82:49.

5. Allen JK, Batjer JD. Evaluation of an automated method for leukocyte differential counts based on electronic volume analysis. *Arch Path Lab Med.* 1985; 109:534.

6. Barnard DF, et al. Detection of important abnormalities of the differential count using the Coulter STKR blood counter. *J Clin Path.* 1989; 42:772.

7. Krause JR. Automated differentials in the hematology laboratory. *Am J Clin Path.* 1990; 93:S11.

8. Warner BA, Reardon DM. A field evaluation of the Coulter STKS. *Am J Clin Path.* 1991; 95:207.

9. Corberand JX. Discovery of unsuspected pathological states using a new hematology analyser. *Med Lab Sci.* 1991; 48:80.

10. Poulsen KB, Bell CA. Automated hematology: Comparing and contrasting three systems. *Clin Lab Sci.* 1991; 4:16.

11. *Coulter STKS Operator's Guide.* Hialeah, FL: Coulter Corporation; 1991.

12. *Coulter GEN·S System Reference.* Miami, FL: Coulter Corporation; 1996.

13. *Clinical Case Studies: Coulter GEN·S System Enhanced VCS Technology.* Bulletin 9165. Brea, CA: Beckman Coulter; Inc., 2000.

14. *NE-8000 Operator's Manual;* McGaw, IL: Baxter Scientific Products Division; 1988.

15. Peng L, Gao X, Jiang H, Peng Z, Su J. Laboratory evaluation of the Sysmex SE-9500 automated haematology analyser. *Clin Lab Haem.* 2001; 23:237–42.

16. *Sysmex SE-9500 Operator's Manual.* Kobe, Japan: TOA Medical Electronics Co., Ltd.; January 1997.

17. Pollard Y, Watts MJ, Grant D, Chavda N, Linch DC, Machin SJ. Use of the haemopoietic progenitor cell count of the Sysmex SE-9500 to refine apheresis timing of peripheral blood stem cells. *Br J Haem.* 1999; 106(2):538–44.

18. Peng L, Yang J, Yang H, Peng Z, Xu C, Liu T. Determination of peripheral blood stem cells by the Sysmex SE-9500. *Clin Lab Haem.* 2001; 23:231–36.

19. *CELL-DYN 4000 System Operator's Manual.* Abbott Park, IL: Abbott Laboratories, Diagnostic Division; March 1999.

20. Grimaldi E, Scopacasa F. Evaluation of the Abbott CELL-DYN 4000 hematology analyzer. *Am J Clin Pathol.* 2000; 113(4):497–505.

21. Watson JS, Davis RA: Evaluation of the Technicon H*1 Hematology System. *Lab Med.* 1987; 18:316.

22. Bollinger PB, et al. The Technicon H*1: An automated hematology analyzer for today and tomorrow. *Am J Clin Pathol.* 1987; 87:71.

23. Nelson L, Charache S, Wingfield S, Keyser, E. Laboratory evaluation of differential white blood cell count information from the Coulter S-Plus IV and Technicon H*1 in patient populations requiring rapid "turnaround" time. *Am J Clin Pathol.* 1989; 91:563.

24. Kim YR, Ornstein L. Isovolumetric sphering of erythrocytes for more accurate and precise cell volume measurement by flow cytometry. *Cytometry.* 1983; 3:419.

25. Ross DW, Bardwell A. Automated cytochemistry and the white cell differential in leukemia. *Blood Cells.* 1980; 6:455.

26. Mohandas N, et al. Accurate and independent measurement of volume and hemoglobin concentration of individual red cells by laser light scattering. *Blood.* 1986; 68:506.

27. Swaim WR. Laboratory and clinical evaluation of white blood cell differential counts: Comparison of the Coulter VCS, Technicon H*1, and 800-cell manual method. *Am J Clin Pathol.* 1991; 95:381.

28. *Technicon H*1 System Operator's Guide.* Tarrytown, NY: Technicon Instruments Corp.; 1985.

29. *Bayer ADVIA 120 System Operator's Guide.* Tarrytown, NY: Bayer Corporation; 1999.

30. Brugnara C. Reticulocyte cellular indices: A new approach in the diagnosis of anemias and monitoring of erythropoietic function. *Critical Rev in Clin Lab Sciences.* 2000; 37(2):93–130.

31. Grotto HZ, Vigoritto AC, Noronha JF, Lima GA. Immature reticulocyte fraction as a criterion for marrow engraftment: Evaluation of a semi-automated reticulocyte method. *Clin & Lab Haematol.* 1999; 21(4):285–87.

32. Brugnara C. Use of reticulocyte cellular indices in the diagnosis and treatment of hematological disorders. *Int J Clin Lab Res.* 1998; 28(1):1–11.

33. *Sysmex R-3500 Operator's Manual.* Kobe, Japan: Sysmex Corporation, Ltd.; October 2000.

34. Takarada K. Overview of the Sysmex R-3500, an automated reticulocyte analyzer. *Sysmex J International.* 1998; 8(1):43–47.

35. Ens GE, Jensen R. Coagulation instrumentation review. *Clin Hemostasis Rev.* 1993; 7(5):1.

36. Sabo MG. Coagulation instrumentation and reagent systems. In: *Laboratory Evaluation of Coagulation.* D. A. Triplett, ed. Chicago: ASCP Press; 1982.

37. *The FibroSystem Manual.* Cockeysville, MD: Division of Becton Dickinson and Company; June 1976.

38. *STArt-4 Operator's Manual.* Parsipanny, NJ: American Bioproducts Company; 1990.

39. Ledford MR, Kaczor DA. Evaluation of the ST4 Clot Detection instrument. *Lab Med.* 1992; 23:172.

40. *Coag-A-Mate XM Operations Manual.* Durham, NC: Organon Teknika Corp; 1990.

41. *Electra 1800C Operator's Manual.* Pleasantville, NY: Medical Laboratory Automation, Inc.; 1998.

42. *Amelung AMAX CS-190 Operator's Manual.* St. Louis: Sigma Diagnostics, Inc.; 1997.

42

Quality Assurance in the Hematology Laboratory

Cheryl Burns, M.S., Lucia More, M.S.

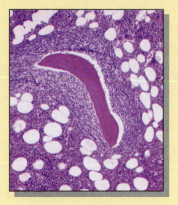

■ CHECKLIST - LEVEL I

At the end of this unit of study the student should be able to:

1. Identify the components of a quality assurance program and match sources of error with component.
2. State the importance of a quality assurance program.
3. State the importance of documentation in a quality assurance program.
4. Describe the use of proficiency testing in the clinical laboratory including required frequency.
5. Given data, employ an appropriate method to determine the reference range for an analyte.
6. Define *universal precautions* and identify the source.
7. Demonstrate knowledge of OSHA standards and their application in the clinical laboratory.
8. Given a material safety data sheet (MSDS), identify critical information.
9. Define: *accuracy, precision, control material, mean,* and *standard deviation*.
10. Given the appropriate data, calculate the mean and standard deviation and create the quality control chart.
11. Interpret quality control results utilizing established control charts.
12. Given test results, recognize CBC data and/or histogram variations that indicate the presence of WBC, RBC, and platelet abnormalities.
13. Recognize CBC data that indicate the presence of interfering substances, such as lipemia, hemolysis, and icteria.
14. Identify coagulation test results that indicate a problem with specimen integrity.

■ CHECKLIST - LEVEL II

At the end of this unit of study the student should be able to:

1. Design methods of competency testing.
2. Apply and interpret statistics used in method evaluation.
3. Determine the components and interpret the results of a method evaluation study.
4. Determine and appraise a method's reportable range.
5. Interpret the Westgard rules and use in evaluating quality control results.

■ CHECKLIST - LEVEL II (continued)

6. Describe the use of moving averages to monitor RBC data.

7. Assess the use of patient specimens to monitor daily quality control in hematology.

8. Select the appropriate actions to be taken when abnormalities are detected in hematology or coagulation results.

9. Recommend procedures to correct for the presence of lipemia, hemolysis, and icteria.

10. Demonstrate the ability to use Delta checks in a quality control program.

KEY TERMS

Analytical time
Blinded preanalyzed samples
Clinical Laboratory Improvement Amendments
Competency assessment
Correlation coefficient (r)
Delta check
Internal quality control program
Linearity
Material safety data sheet (MSDS)
Medical decision levels
NCCLS
Outlier
Proficiency testing
Quality control (QC) limit
Random variation
Reference interval
Reportable range
Sensitivity
Slope (b)
Specificity
Split sample
Standard deviation (SD)
Systematic variation
Transcription errors
Turnaround-time (TAT)
Universal precautions
y-intercept (a)

BACKGROUND BASICS

Levels I and II

▶ Specimen collection: Describe the specimen collection protocol for hematology and hemostasis procedures. (Chapters 7, 39)

▶ Routine hematology procedures: Summarize each of the routine hematology procedures and give potential sources of error. (Chapter 7)

▶ Peripheral blood smear: Summarize the characteristics of an optimally stained peripheral blood smear and give potential sources of error. (Chapter 8)

▶ Laboratory testing in coagulation: Summarize each of the screening coagulation procedures and give potential sources of error. (Chapter 39)

▶ Automation in hematology: Describe the principles of cell counting used by the automated hematology analyzers and principles of clot detection for the automated coagulation analyzers. (Chapter 41)

▶ OVERVIEW

One of a clinical laboratory professional's most important responsibilities is to ensure the quality of test results. To accomplish this, laboratories must have in place quality assurance and quality control programs. These programs consist of guidelines designed to assure accurate testing and reporting of results. This includes a protocol for reviewing patient results in order to determine if results can be reported. This chapter will address the components of these programs.

▶ QUALITY ASSURANCE

Laboratories must have an established quality assurance program as mandated by subpart P of the **Clinical Laboratory Improvement Amendments** of 1988 (CLIA '88).[1] A laboratory's quality assurance program should be designed to monitor all aspects related to testing of patient specimens.[2] The goal of the program is to assure accurate testing and reporting of results from all specimens submitted to the laboratory. Accrediting agencies such as the College of American Pathologists (CAP) or the Joint Commission on Accreditation of Healthcare Organizations (JCAHO) monitor the comprehensiveness and quality of the program. This chapter will review the various aspects to consider in the design of a comprehensive quality assurance program.

BASIC COMPONENTS

A common approach to the development of a quality assurance program is to divide it into three components: (1) preanalytical, which deals with all aspects affecting the test outcome occurring prior to the testing procedure; (2) analytical, which incorporates all aspects affecting the testing procedure itself; and (3) postanalytical, which deals with aspects affecting the test outcome occurring after the testing procedure (Table 42-1 ◐).

TABLE 42-1

Comprehensive Quality Assurance Program*

Preanalytical Components
1. Patient requisitions
2. Patient preparation
3. Specimen collection protocol
4. Specimen transport protocol
5. Specimen processing protocol
6. Specimen storage
7. Phlebotomy training

Analytical Components
1. Test method/procedure
2. Reagents
3. Internal quality control
4. External quality control
5. Maintenance of instrumentation
6. Linearity/reportable range determination
7. Method evaluation (instrument comparison)
8. Reference range determination
9. Personnel requirements
10. Competency testing
11. Continuing education

Postanalytical Components
1. Review of patient results
2. Posting of patient results
3. Maintenance of patient records
4. Monitoring of turnaround time
5. Surveying of customer satisfaction
6. Maintaining of all documentation

*Factors to be considered in each component part, preanalytical, analytical, and postanalytical are given.

TABLE 42-2

Potential Sources of Error in Specimen Collection and Their Effect on Test Outcome

Source of Error	Effect on Test Outcome
Patient misidentification	Inaccurate test results
Hemolyzed specimen	Dilutional effect on analytes and decreased erythrocyte counts
Failure to invert collection tubes properly	Clotted specimen and falsely decreased cell counts or prolonged coagulation test results
Failure to fill collection tube properly	Under- or over-anticoagulated specimen for coagulation testing with citrate tube
Failure to follow the order of the draw*	Cross-contamination with collection tube additives
Length of tourniquet application greater than 1 minute	Hemoconcentration of specimen
Collection from an IV site	Dilutional effect on analytes
Time of draw	Analyte dependent; e.g., hemoglobin is highest in the morning
Patient anxiety or crying	Analyte dependent; e.g., increases leukocyte count

*Order of the draw refers to the suggested order in which different anticoagulant and nonanticoagulant collection tubes are filled from a single venipuncture. For example, a collection tube with no additive should be filled prior to an EDTA collection tube to avoid contamination of the nonanticoagulant tube with EDTA (∞ Chapter 7).

Preanalytical Component

The testing process begins with the test order. Patient requisitions should be designed to be user friendly and provide adequate patient information. This information should include at a minimum the patient's name, identification number (e.g., social security number), age, sex, diagnosis, and tests to be performed. The patient should receive appropriate information to prepare for the tests. For example, the patient should be informed on the fasting requirements for a cholesterol test. This information should be provided in the laboratory's specimen collection procedure manual and in a format easily distributed to and understood by the patient.

One of the most important factors affecting a test's outcome is specimen collection (∞ Chapters 7, 39).[3–5] As we often hear, "The test result is only as good as the quality of the specimen." Many variables enter into the specimen collection process that may effect the outcome (Table 42-2). Each potential source of error should be addressed in the specimen collection procedure manual and by a thorough educational program for the phlebotomist or the individual designated to perform the phlebotomy (i.e., nursing person-nel). Periodic continuing education should be provided to address specimen collection problems or introduce new protocols.

Once the specimen is collected, it must be properly labeled and transported to the laboratory for processing and testing. If testing cannot be done immediately, the specimen should be properly stored. For example, a specimen for routine coagulation testing requires separation of plasma from cells and storage at room temperature if testing will be performed within 4 hours (∞ Chapter 39). All this information should be found within the specimen collection procedure manual and will vary dependent on the test to be performed.

Analytical Component

The analytical component addresses all issues involving the testing procedure itself. A test method procedure manual should be available in all laboratories. Within this manual, each test should be addressed as to its purpose, principle, specimen requirements, reagents, quality control, step-by-step procedure, interpretation of results, and potential sources of error.[6,7]

An **internal quality control program** should be established to monitor the testing process and assure accurate patient test results. Quality control will be addressed in more detail later in this chapter. In addition, overall quality control should be assessed through an external quality control program also known as **proficiency testing.** Proficiency testing monitors the testing process by comparison to peer laboratories.[8] This is addressed in a subsequent section of this chapter.

Maintenance of analytical instruments (e.g., automated blood cell counting instrument) must be followed as directed by the manufacturer and documentation of all maintenance activities must be easily accessible for troubleshooting quality control problems.

Individuals performing the testing procedures must meet the personnel requirements established by CLIA '88 and will vary depending on the test procedure. Continuing education is also required to keep testing personnel abreast of changes within the testing procedures and the practice of the profession.

Post Analytical Component

Factors that may affect the test outcome and its use after the testing process are addressed by the postanalytical component.[9] Procedures should be established for the review of patient results and identification of those results that require further attention. For example, a specimen should be repeated if the hemoglobin and hematocrit do not match (e.g., $Hb \times 3 = Hct$).

Automated instruments can be interfaced with the laboratory information system (LIS) for electronic transfer of patient results. The LIS may also be interfaced with the hospital's or outpatient facility's computer system for reporting of patient results directly to the patient's chart. Electronic transfer of results minimizes **transcription errors.** The records of patient test results should be maintained within the laboratory. Procedures should be established for the archiving and retrieval of patient test results.

The laboratory is a business enterprise. Therefore, customer satisfaction (e.g., physician or patient) and communication are important issues to be addressed in the quality assurance program. An important factor affecting satisfaction level is **turnaround-time (TAT)** for test results. Critical patient care decisions are often dependent on a laboratory test result. Computerization has made monitoring of TAT more manageable. If a TAT problem is identified, laboratory management or the quality assurance committee should investigate the problem and recommend appropriate action.

In addition, protocols should be established to address customer complaints and other communication issues to minimize customer dissatisfaction. Surveys may be used to assess customer satisfaction and identify areas that need to be addressed. A quality assurance committee should be established to oversee the quality assurance program and determine changes that need to be made and how they should be implemented.

Finally, documented records of all aspects of the quality assurance program should be maintained and retrievable upon request. These documents provide important information regarding the recognition of a problem, the process used to resolve it, and the change that occurred as a result of that process.

 Checkpoint! #1

Explain the importance of each component of the quality assurance program to its ultimate goal.

PROFICIENCY TESTING

Proficiency testing is an external quality control program that monitors long-term accuracy of the different test systems (e.g., prothrombin time by the Sigma AMAX CS-190 instrument) through comparison to peer laboratories. Clinical laboratories have participated in proficiency testing surveys such as the College of American Pathologists (CAP) survey program since the 1960s. CLIA '88, however, mandated that clinical laboratories participate in a proficiency testing survey at least three times a year.[10] Failure to achieve an acceptable rating for any given analyte (e.g., prothrombin time) in two out of three surveys results in suspension of the certification to perform that test procedure. Reinstatement of a test procedure involves taking the appropriate action to correct the problem and successful performance in two consecutive proficiency testing surveys.

Clinical laboratories contract with organizations like CAP or the American Association of Bioanalysts to provide the proficiency testing service. A proficiency testing survey consists of proficiency samples, whole blood, or lypholized serum/plasma representing the full range of values that would be expected in patient specimens. These samples are sent to the laboratory at specified time intervals, usually three times per year. Proficiency samples should be tested as part of a typical patient specimen run. Results are returned to the survey provider for statistical analysis. The survey provider determines the target value for each test result and establishes the limits for acceptable *vs* unacceptable results through comparison studies with peer laboratories. For example, in a proficiency survey for hemoglobin determinations the acceptable limit may be within $\pm 2s$ (**standard deviation**) of the target value. The survey provider notifies the clinical laboratory of its findings.

Each laboratory should have a comprehensive program to respond to an unsatisfactory result. The source of the problem may be identified by checking for changes in the test procedure or reagents, reviewing the instrument's maintenance log and previous quality control results, and identifying changes in testing personnel. With the problem identified, corrective action can be taken to solve it. Proficiency testing survey results and documentation of corrective action should be maintained within the laboratory.

Checkpoint! #2

If a clinical laboratory loses its certification to perform protein C assays, what is involved in regaining that certification?

COMPETENCY TESTING

An additional requirement under CLIA '88 is **competency assessment** of all testing personnel. CLIA '88 requires that this assessment take place twice during the first year of employment and annually thereafter.[11–13] The exact mechanisms to evaluate testing personnel's competency were not clearly outlined in the *Federal Register,* and laboratory directors, managers, and supervisors have struggled to determine the appropriate methods to evaluate competency within their laboratories. Clearly, this assessment must be more than a simple evaluation of one's knowledge of the material. The ability to score high on a multiple-choice test regarding laboratory test procedures within one's job description does not evaluate the individual's ability to perform and troubleshoot the test procedures. Direct observation checklists, random assignment of proficiency testing materials, or **"blinded" preanalyzed samples** may be used to evaluate these competencies (see Web Table 42-1 ✪ for an example of a direct observation checklist). For each assessment tool, criteria must be established to judge acceptable performance. In the case of a 100-cell leukocyte differential, acceptable criteria might be based on the 95% confidence limits of the expert results (e.g., hematology supervisor or pathologist).

No single method of assessing competency will be appropriate for all test procedures. It remains the responsibility of the laboratory supervisor, manager, or director to make that choice for the particular laboratory setting. Additionally, educational materials (i.e., textbooks, selected journal articles, slide study sets, videotapes, or computer-based instruction) should be available to assist clinical laboratory professionals in improving their competency.

 Checkpoint! #3

What is an appropriate method of assessing a clinical laboratory professional's competency in performing PT and APTT using an automated coagulation instrument?

METHOD EVALUATION/ INSTRUMENT COMPARISON

Selection, evaluation, and implementation of a new methodology or instrument in the hematology/hemostasis laboratory should follow an established protocol. Each laboratory should design its own protocol. This section will discuss several important components to be included in the protocol.

Selection

Selection of a new methodology or instrument is a daunting task. In the ideal setting, a committee should be formed to make this selection. For the selection of a new instrument, committee membership may include the hematology/hemostasis supervisor, several clinical laboratory professionals, laboratory information system (LIS) personnel, quality assurance supervisor, biomedical engineer, and laboratory manager.

The first task of this committee is to determine the desirable characteristics of the new instrument.[14,15] A needs assessment survey could be used for this purpose. The needs assessment survey should be completed by those individuals who will be using the instrument, as well as by those individuals who may be affected by the use of that instrument (Web Table 42-2 ✪). Desirable characteristics identified by this survey can then be used to solicit proposals from vendors (e.g., sales personnel for Beckman-Coulter, Roche-Sysmex, or Abbott Laboratories) (see Web Table 42-3 ✪ for these characteristics).

The careful evaluation of the vendor's proposal packet by the selection committee will begin to narrow the selection process to several possible instruments. Members of the selection committee should also seek input from colleagues and the literature with regards to new instrumentation available and other laboratories' experiences with that instrumentation. The in-house evaluation of each instrument is a crucial step in the selection process. At this time, all interested parties would have a hands-on opportunity to assess the actual performance of the instrument in a real-time laboratory. Thus, a more meaningful evaluation can be obtained with regard to whether the instrument meets the laboratory's needs. The more information the committee has to base its selection on, the better the selection will be. Ultimately, the selection of the instrument comes down to a particular laboratory's needs and the cost of meeting those needs.

With regard to the selection of a new methodology or test system, the selection process will be similar. The selection committee must take into account the cost per test, reagents, reagents' shelf-life and storage requirements, quality control program, test's **sensitivity** (the ability to detect small quantities of the analyte), **specificity** (ability to determine only the analyte in question), and **linearity** (range of concentration over which the test method can be used), required instrumentation and equipment, **analytical time,** and specimen types that can be analyzed (i.e., whole blood, serum, CSF, etc.). Both testing personnel and potential clients should be consulted for their input during the selection process.

Analytical Reliability

With the purchase of a new instrument or the introduction of a new methodology, the laboratory must verify the instrument's and/or method's performance through a series of performance studies. To verify analytical reliability of an instrument, the clinical laboratory professional must evaluate the instrument with regard to **random variation** (variation due to chance) and **systematic variation** (variation within the instrument that alters results, but is predictable). Precision studies are used to assess random variation and evaluate the reproducibility of the test method.[16,17] To check within run precision, the clinical laboratory professional should run 10–20 aliquots of a patient sample in the same run. This should be done using patient samples of different concentration levels that correspond to **medical decision levels** of the analyte. For example, to check within run precision for hemoglobin, three patient samples may be chosen: sample #1 Hgb = 8.0 g/dL; sample #2 Hgb = 12.0 g/dL; sample #3 Hgb = 19.0 g/dL. Each sample is separated into 10 aliquots, and each aliquot is analyzed. For each set of data, the mean, standard deviation, and coefficient of variation are calculated (Table 42-3 ✪). Precision can be determined by applying a statistical test called the F-test or by comparing the calculated CV to the manufacturer's CV. Within run precision is acceptable if the CV is less than or equal to the manufacturer's CV. If the CV is greater than the manufacturer's CV, the clinical laboratory professional should check the data for **outliers.** Any outlier should be discarded and the data reevaluated. If the CV is still unacceptable, signifi-

cant random variation exists within this method, or reagent and/or testing personnel errors have affected the study.

Systematic variation is assessed through the methods comparison procedure, which allows comparison of patient results between the new method and a method that is known to be accurate. **Split samples** (division of a single sample into two or more aliquots) are used. The **NCCLS** recommends the use of at least 40 samples and preferably 100.[16–19] The samples should be random so they are representative of the clinical range of samples. Ideally, they should represent different pathologic conditions as well. With the samples identified, each sample is split for analysis by each method. The samples are run in duplicate for each method, but the duplicate run should be done at a different time period. All analysis should be completed on the same day, preferably within 4 hours.[19] Several statistical tools are used to analyze the results. The paired-t test compares the mean of the differences of test results between the two methods and determines if a statistically significant difference exists between the current method and the new method (see Web Table 42-4 ✪ for an example of paired-t test). The calculated t value for the two sets of results is compared to the critical t value from a statistical table. If the calculated t value is less than the critical t value, no significant difference exists between the two methods.

Linear regression analysis allows determination of the **y-intercept (a), slope (b),** standard error of the estimate ($s_{y/x}$), **correlation coefficient (r),** and coefficient of determination (r^2) (Figure 42-1 ■). The general formula for the linear regression line is $y = a + bx$, where y is the predicted mean value of y for a given x value. The coefficient of determination evaluates the strength of the relationship between the two methods. For example, an r^2 value of .90 for a comparison between current and new methods would mean that 90% of the variability in the new method is directly predictable from the variability in the current method. Therefore, a strong relationship would exist between the two methods.

Linear regression analysis is also used to detect systematic (constant or proportional) errors and random errors. Constant systematic errors are identified by a change in the y-intercept. If the y-intercept is a value other than 0 (y > 0 or y < 0), this indicates that a constant difference exists between the new method and the current method regardless of the analyte's concentration. The observation of a constant systematic error usually indicates a calibration problem. Proportional systematic errors are identified by changes in the slope. If there is no difference between the current method and the new method, the slope will be 1.00 ± 5%. A change in the slope represents a difference between the new method and the current method that is proportional to the analyte's concentration. That is, the higher the concentration, the greater the difference is between the two methods. A proportional systematic error is most frequently associated with erroneous calibration. Random error can be detected by an in-

---

✪ TABLE 42-3

Within Run Precision Study for Hemoglobin Determination by Daman EXCELL-16

	Sample #1	Sample #2	Sample #3
1	7.9	12.0	19.2
2	8.1	12.3	19.4
3	8.0	12.2	19.4
4	8.1	12.2	19.4
5	8.1	12.2	19.3
6	8.0	12.3	19.4
7	8.0	12.3	19.4
8	8.1	12.4	19.5
9	8.1	12.4	19.3
10	8.1	12.3	19.6
Mean	8.1	12.3	19.4
s	0.07	0.11	0.11
CV	0.86%	0.89%	0.57%
Manufacturer's CV	<1.0%	<1.0%	<1.0%

Three patient samples were chosen, and 10 aliquots of each sample were tested. The mean, standard deviation (s), and coefficient of variation (CV) were determined for each patient sample. Comparison of each calculated CV to the manufacturer's CV reveals acceptable precision for the hemoglobin procedure since the calculated CV is less than the manufacturer's CV. This procedure demonstrates the reproducibility of this hemoglobin determination.

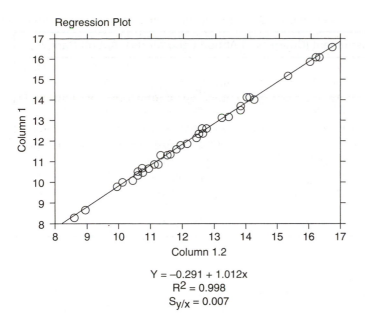

Regression Plot

$$Y = -0.291 + 1.012x$$
$$R^2 = 0.998$$
$$S_{y/x} = 0.007$$

■ **FIGURE 42-1** Linear regression analysis for comparison of hemoglobin by automated cell analyzer (column 1.2) and point-of-care analyzer (column 1). Data sets are those given in Web Table 42-4 ✪. Interpretation of the linear regression analysis reveals a strong relationship $R^2 = 0.998$ between the automated cell analyzer's hemoglobin method and the point-of-care analyzer's hemoglobin method. No proportional systematic error exists since the slope (1.012) is between 0.95 and 1.05. The y-intercept (−0.291) is slightly less than 0, which indicates a small degree of negative bias or constant systematic error. This may be considered negligible by most laboratories. Random error also is not indicated since the standard error of the estimate (0.007) is nearly 0. Overall, this analysis demonstrates excellent comparison of methods.

crease in the standard error of the estimate. Increased dispersion of results about the regression line results in an increased standard error of the estimate.

✓ Checkpoint! #4

Linear regression analysis was performed on results from a method comparison of an automated prothrombin time method (current) and a point-of-care prothrombin time method. The following results were obtained:

$$y\text{-}intercept = 1.014$$

$$slope = 0.978$$

What conclusions can be drawn from these results?

Linearity and Reportable Range Determinations

The manufacturer typically determines an instrument's linearity. For hematology instruments, the linearity is determined for each directly measured parameter (e.g., leukocyte count, hemoglobin, and MCV). This is accomplished by analyzing serial dilutions of a linearity check material multiple times to minimize effects of imprecision.[20] Regression analysis is used to establish the linear range and the tolerance limits (Table 42-4 ✪). The tolerance limits represent the maximum allowable difference between the measured result and the reference value for a given dilution. A similar procedure is used to determine linearity for coagulation instruments.

Verification of the instrument's **reportable range** should be included within the method evaluation for a new hematology or coagulation instrument or as one of the installation procedures for that new instrument.[21] To verify the reportable range, the clinical laboratory professional should analyze in duplicate at least three different levels of calibrators or linearity check materials that fall within the reportable range.[16] If these results fall within the instrument's defined tolerance limits, the reportable range is verified. In addition, these data may be plotted to visualize the linearity. If the data do not fall within tolerance limits or are nonlinear, the process should be repeated using more calibrators in the affected part of the range. If the data do not verify the instrument's reportable range, the laboratory should modify the reportable range to reflect the instrument's performance characteristics in its current setting.

With the verification of the reportable range, each laboratory should establish its protocol for handling results that exceed the reportable range, either above or below. For example, results above the reportable range may be diluted, reanalyzed, and the result multiplied by the dilution factor to determine the accurate result. Hematology results below the reportable range may require reanalysis of the sample and review of the peripheral blood smear before the result is reported as less than the lower limit of the reportable range.

REFERENCE INTERVAL DETERMINATION

Hematology and coagulation **reference intervals** are available from various recognized hematology textbooks or hematology/coagulation instrument and reagent manufacturers. However, it is ideal for each laboratory to determine its own reference intervals. Reference intervals are influenced by the diversity of instrumentation, choice of reagents, and patient population served by the laboratory. The laboratory may choose to establish its own reference intervals or validate the manufacturer's reference intervals. The process of validating a reference interval is less time-consuming and more cost effective. The recommended procedure for validation of a reference interval is described in Web Table 42-5 ✪.[22] Once validated, the reference intervals can be used as representative for the laboratory and its patient population. If the reference intervals are not validated, the more rigorous process of establishing a reference interval should be performed.

Establishing a reference interval is an arduous task. It involves careful planning to define the criteria for subject

REVIEW QUESTIONS (continued)

LEVEL I

8. How should the clinical laboratory professional interpret the prothrombin time control results for the current control run if the ±2s control limits are 11.8–14.2 seconds for Level I and 25.0–28.0 seconds for Level II? (Checklist #11)

   Current Run Level I   11.6 seconds
   Level II   24.6 seconds

   a. acceptable
   b. unacceptable

9. Which of the following parameters will be effected by the presence of lipemia? (Checklist #13)
   a. RBC, Hb, Hct, MCV, MCH, MCHC
   b. RBC, Hct, MCV, MCHC
   c. Hb, MCH, MCHC
   d. Hct, MCV, MCHC

10. In interpretation of a patient's CBC results, the clinical laboratory professional notes the platelet count is 25×10^9/L. Which of the following may be associated with this finding? (Checklist #12)
    a. observation of erythrocyte fragments on the blood smear
    b. presence of cryoglobulins
    c. observation of platelet clumps at the feather edge of the blood smear
    d. presence of intracellular parasites like malaria

LEVEL II

7. For the automated hematology analyzers, moving averages can be used to monitor the instrument's performance in determining: (Checklist #6)
   a. leukocyte parameters
   b. erythrocyte parameters
   c. platelet parameters
   d. reticulocyte parameters

8. Initial interpretation of a patient's CBC results showed an MCHC of 38 g/dL. The clinical laboratory professional warmed the specimen to 37°C and reanalyzed it. No change was observed. What is the appropriate course of action? (Checklist #8)
   a. observe the blood smear for the presence of spherocytes
   b. replace patient's plasma with equal volume of saline and reanalyze.
   c. recollect patient specimen using sodium citrate and analyze
   d. examine the blood smear for the presence of nucleated erythrocytes

9. The following coagulation test results were obtained: PT = 7.5 seconds and APTT = 20 seconds. How should the clinical laboratory professional approach these findings? (Checklist #8)
   a. report results to patient's chart
   b. observe specimen for the presence of hemolysis
   c. check sample for small clots
   d. examine collection tube to determine if it was underfilled

10. Which source of error would be detected by a delta check? (Checklist #10)
    a. depleted reagent supply
    b. improper calibration of the instrument
    c. deteriorating light source
    d. failure to correctly label the patient's specimen

www.prenhall.com/mckenzie
Use the above address to access the free, interactive Companion Web site created for this textbook. Get hints, instant feedback, and textbook references to chapter-related multiple choice questions.

REFERENCES

1. Clinical Laboratory Improvement Amendments of 1988; Final Rule, 42 CFR Part 405, Subpart P (493.1701), *Federal Register* 57(40):7183–84, 1992.

2. Carver CJ. Establishing a thorough quality assurance program. *Advance for Medical Laboratory Professionals*. 2000; 12(9):6.

3. Tarapchak P. Identify, eliminate the "error" of your ways. *Advance for Medical Laboratory Professionals*. 2000; 10(3):64–71.

4. King D. A variety of variables. *Advance for Medical Laboratory Professionals*. 2000; 12(24):14–17.

5. Drew N. Monitoring specimen collection errors. *Advance for Medical Laboratory Professionals*. 2000; 12(15):12–15.

6. NCCLS. *Clinical Laboratory Technical Procedure Manuals*, 3rd ed. GP2-A3. Wayne, PA: NCCLS; 1996.

7. Clinical Laboratory Improvement Amendments of 1988; Final Rule, 42 CFR Part 405, Subpart K (493.1211), *Federal Register* 57(40):7164, 1992.

8. Shahangian S, Holmes EH, Taylor RN. Toward optimal PT use. *MLO.* 2000; 32(4):32–43.

9. Carver C. A closer look at post-analytical policies and procedures. *Advance for Medical Laboratory Professionals.* 2000; 12(7):6.

10. Clinical Laboratory Improvement Amendments of 1988; Final Rule, 42 CFR Part 405, Subpart I (493.901), *Federal Register* 57(40): 7151–62, 1992.

11. Clinical Laboratory Improvement Amendments of 1988; Final Rule, 42 CFR Part 405, Subpart P (493.1713), *Federal Register* 57(40):7184, 1992.

12. Gerbasi S. Competency assessment in a team-based laboratory. *MLO.* 2000; 32(9): 46–54.

13. Leach AP, Haun DE. Assessing competence in finding and reporting abnormal morphologic features while scanning peripheral blood smears. *Clin Lab Science.* 2000; 13(3):160–65.

14. Barglowski M. The instrument selection process: Beyond the sales pitch. *MLO.* 2001; 33(2):45–51.

15. O'Brien JA. The acquisition and maintenance of laboratory instrumentation. *MLO.* 2001; 33(2):36–44.

16. Polancic J, Roncancio G. *Method Verification and Instrument Selection Procedures.* The Laboratory Consultants, Inc. of Illinois; October 1994.

17. Plaut D. Analytical accuracy: Verifying performance. *MT Today.* 1994; 14–16.

18. NCCLS. *Approved Guideline for Method Comparison and Bias Estimation Using Patient Samples.* Document EP9-A. Wayne, PA: NCCLS; 1995.

19. Cembrowski GS, Sullivan AM, Hofer TL. Quality control and statistics. In: *Clinical Chemistry: Principles, Procedures, Correlations,* 4th ed. Bishop ML, Duben-Engelkirk JL, and Fody EP, Eds. Philadelphia: Lippincott Williams & Wilkins; 2000.

20. *CELL-DYN 4000 System Operator's Manual.* Abbott Park, IL: Abbott; March 1999:4–12.

21. Clinical Laboratory Improvement Amendments of 1988; Final Rule, 42 CFR Part 405, Subpart K (493.1213), *Federal Register* 57(40): 7164, 1992.

22. NCCLS. *Approved Guideline for How to Define and Determine Reference Intervals in the Clinical Laboratory.* Document C28-A. Wayne, PA: NCCLS; 1995.

23. Winsten S. The ecology of normal values in clinical chemistry. *Crit Rev Clin Lab Sci.* 1976; 6:319.

24. Centers for Disease Control. Acquired immunodeficiency syndrome (AIDS): Precautions for clinical and laboratory staffs. *MMWR.* 1982; 31:577–80.

25. Centers for Disease Control. Public health service guidelines for the management of health-care worker exposures to HIV and recommendations for postexposure prophylaxis. *MMWR.* 1998; 47:1–28.

26. West KH, Cohen ML. Standard precautions: A new approach to reducing infection transmission in the hospital setting. *J IV Nursing.* 1997; 20(6):S7–S10.

27. Occupational Safety and Health Administration Ergonomics Program Standard, Proposed Standard, 29 CFR Part 1910 Subpart Y, 2000.

28. Occupational Safety and Health Administration Hazard Communication; Final Rule, 29 CFR, *Federal Register* 59:6126–84, 1994.

29. Westgard JO. QC: The calculations. Westgard JO, ed. In: *Basic QC Practices: Training in Statistical Quality Control for Healthcare Laboratories.* Madison, WI: Westgard Quality Corporation; 1998.

30. Westgard JO, Barry PL, Hunt MR, Groth T. A multi-rule Shewhart chart for quality control in clinical chemistry. *Clin Chem.* 1981; 27:493–501.

31. Westgard JO. QC: The multirule procedure. Westgard JO. ed. In: *Basic QC Practices: Training in Statistical Quality Control for Healthcare Laboratories.* Madison, WI: Westgard Quality Corporation; Madison, WI.

32. Bull BS, Elashoff RM, Heilbron DC, et al. A study of various estimators for the derivation of quality control procedures from patient erythrocyte indices. *Am J Clin Pathol.* 1974; 61:473–81.

33. Dotson MA. Methods to monitor and control systematic error. Stiene-Martin EA, Lotspeich-Steininger CA, Koepke JA, eds. In: *Clinical Hematology: Principles, Procedures, Correlations,* 2nd ed. Philadelphia: J. B. Lippincott; 1998.

34. Cornblcet J. Spurious results from automated hematology cell counters. *Lab Med.* 1983; 14(8):509–14.

35. Brigden ML, Dalal BI. Spurious and artifactual test results I: Cell counter-related abnormalities. *Lab Med.* 1999; 30(5):325–334.

36. Houwen B, Duffin D. Delta checks for random error detection in hematology tests. *Lab Med.* 1989; 20(6):378–81.

APPENDIX A

Answers to Case Study Questions

CHAPTER 1

Case Summary: Aaron had clinical signs of infection and a past history of ear infections. The CBC results revealed a high WBC count, consistent with an infectious process. The diagnosis of otitis media usually can be made by history and physical examination. Laboratory tests are not required.

Question:

1. If Aaron was diagnosed with otitis media, what cellular component(s) in his blood would be playing a central role in fighting this infection?

Explanation:

The leukocytes, or white blood cells, are the cells that are central in fighting infection.

Question:

2. Aaron's physician ordered a CBC. The results are Hb 115 g/L; Hct 0.34L/L; RBC 4.0 × 10^{12}/L; WBC 18 × 10^9/L. What parameters, if any, are outside the reference range? Why do you have to take Aaron's age into account when evaluating these results?

Explanation:

The WBC count is increased. The upper reference range for WBC in a 2-year-old is 17 × 10^9/L. It is important to take Aaron's age into account because the reference ranges for blood cell concentrations are different in children of various ages and are different from those in adults.

CHAPTER 3

Case Summary: Francine had an acute lymphocytic leukemia. This is a type of leukemia that is characterized by a malignant proliferation of immature lymphocytic cells.

Question:

1. Refer to the tables on the inside cover of the book and determine which blood cell parameters are abnormal, if any.

Explanation:

The hemoglobin is decreased. The WBC is normal but the platelets are markedly decreased.

Question:

2. Describe Francine's bone marrow as normal, hyperplastic, or hypoplastic.

Explanation:

The bone marrow is hyperplastic. Normal bone marrow cellularity is <50%.

Question:

3. What conditions can cause this bone marrow finding?

Explanation:

Conditions associated with an increased celluarity of bone marrow may include anemia and leukemia.

Question:

4. What do you think is the cause of the splenomegaly?

Explanation:

The splenomegaly could be due to extramedullary hematopoiesis. Malignant cells may be proliferating in the spleen.

Question:

5. Why might the peripheral blood reveal changes associated with hyposplenism when the spleen is enlarged?

Explanation:

Tumor cells can incapacitate the spleen, causing functional hyposplenism.

Question:

6. What might explain the lymphadenopathy?

Explanation:

The malignant lymphocytic cells may be proliferating in the lymph nodes causing enlargement.

CHAPTER 4

Case Summary: This is a case of a 28-year-old Caucasian male of Italian descent with an acute hemolytic anemia. An initial diagnosis of malaria was presumptively made. The patient, however, was negative for malaria. He was eventually diagnosed as having G6PD deficiency and a hemolytic anemia induced by the antimalarial drug primaquine.

Question:

1. Predict Stephen's reticulocyte count: low, normal, or increased.

Explanation:

From the erythrocyte count, HGB, and HCT, we know the patient is moderately anemic. The increase of polychromatic erythrocytes on a blood smear suggests an increased number of reticulocytes.

Question:

2. What is the cellular mechanism that results in hemolysis due to a deficiency in G6PD?

Explanation:

In the hexose monophosphate shunt, the reduction of NADPH and glutathione depends on the enzyme glucose-6-phosphate dehydrogenase (G6PD). When this enzyme is deficient, hemoglobin denatures under oxidant stress, and intracellular hemoglobin precipitates form.

Question:

3. Explain how Heinz body inclusions cause damage to the erythrocyte membrane.

Explanation:

Hemoglobin precipitates known as Heinz bodies form along the inner surface of the erythrocyte membrane. This results in a loss of membrane flexibility, cell lysis, and splenic trapping.

Question:

4. Would you predict Stephen's serum erythropoietin levels to be low, normal, or increased? Why?

Explanation:

Hemolytic anemias result from factors outside the marrow. Erythroid production and maturation is normal. The loss of erythrocytes results in a systemic decrease in cellular oxygen tension. This stimulates EPO production from the kidneys, which in turn stimulates erythropoiesis in the marrow.

Question:

5. Explain why Stephen has a low haptoglobin value.

Explanation:

The oxidant stress caused by the malarial drug primaquine was out of balance due to the patient's erythrocyte deficiency of G6PD. This resulted in hemoglobin precipitation (Heinz bodies) and cell destruction. Some of the hemoglobin is released into the peripheral blood and is bound by haptoglobin. The haptoglobin reserves become depleted quickly.

CHAPTER 5

Case Summary: Jerry lost a substantial amount of blood from the fractures and surgery. If his hemoglobin was normal before the accident

(14–16 g/dL), he lost about one-half the volume of his blood. With the loss of this much blood, he also lost a substantial amount of iron. Although he was given iron supplements, it will take time for his hemoglobin to reach normal again. He had symptoms of anemia with lethargy and pallor. This results from a loss of hemoglobin and hence a decrease in the amount of oxygen delivered to the tissue. The blood transfusions will bring his hemoglobin concentration up more rapidly and give his body the energy it needs to repair itself.

Question:

1. If Jerry is iron deficient, what is the effect on synthesis of ALAS, transferrin receptor, and ferritin?

Explanation:

Lack of iron promotes the binding of IRE-BP to the IRE of the mRNA of ALAS, transferrin receptor, and ferritin. This causes a decreased synthesis of ALAS, increased synthesis of transferrin receptor, and decreased synthesis of ferritin.

Question:

2. What was the rationale for giving Jerry the iron?

Explanation:

Since Jerry had lost the blood through bleeding, he also lost a substantial amount of iron. Even if body storage iron is normal, iron supplements are often given, in this case to provide the iron needed for rapid and increased hemoglobin synthesis.

Question:

3. Explain why Jerry may have these symptoms.

Explanation:

Jerry's hemoglobin was very low, which means that his tissues were not getting the oxygen they needed. This leads to a decrease in metabolic activity and consequently a decrease in energy. Pallor is a classic sign of anemia because blood is preferentially circulated to critical areas of the body including the brain, heart, etc. The skin's blood supply decreases, causing a loss of the pinkish color of the skin, especially apparent in Caucasians.

Question:

4. Explain why Jerry may have had more energy after the transfusions.

Explanation:

The transfusions boosted Jerry's hemoglobin level and, thus, increased the amount of oxygen that could be transported to the tissues for critical metabolic processes.

CHAPTER 6

Case Summary: Mr. Mertzig had a physical as a prerequisite to buying a life insurance policy. His results were within the reference range for his sex and age except for the WBC count, which was above the reference range.

Question:

1. Are any of these results outside the reference range? If yes, which one(s)?

Explanation:

The WBC count is above the reference range.

Question:

2. If this were a newborn, would you change your evaluation? Why?

Explanation:

Newborns have a higher reference range for WBC; therefore, if this were a newborn, the WBC bount would fall within the reference range.

Question:

3. Are any of the WBC concentrations outside the reference range (relative or absolute)?

Explanation:

All the results, both percents and absolute values, are within the reference range.

Question:

4. Is there a need for reflex testing on Mr. Mertzig? Explain your answer.

Explanation:

Although Mr. Mertzig's WBC count is slightly above the reference range, his absolute individual white cell numbers are within reference range. Given the fact that he has no symptoms, the physical examination was normal, and no abnormal cells were noted on the blood smear, there is probably no need to do further testing. The reference range is usually set by calculating the mean and adding and subtracting two standard deviations. This range will include 95% of normal individuals. About 5% of individuals will have a result outside this range and still be normal. This may be the case with Mr. Mertzig.

CHAPTER 9

Case Summary: Mr. Jones was pancytopenic. Clinical history and further laboratory tests revealed no cause for the pancytopenia. A bone marrow aspirate and biopsy was obtained. Evaluation revealed the presence of many blasts. The diagnosis based on bone marrow testing was acute myelocytic leukemia.

Question:

1. Is a bone marrow evaluation indicated for this patient?

Explanation:

CBC data indicate that the patient is pancytopenic. Presence of pancytopenia in a young patient is worrisome. The common causes of pancytopenia in a young patient include HIV infection, alcoholism, medications, and B_{12} and folic acid deficiency. Presence of teardrop cells with pancytopenia indicates marrow fibrosis or marrow infiltration by leukemia, lymphoma, or granulomas. Bone marrow is definitely indicated in this patient. Patient does not have lymphadenopathy, hepatomegaly, or splenomegaly, so the chance of lymphoma involving the marrow is very unlikely.

Question:

2. How should you proceed with the marrow evaluation?

Explanation:

Fortunately, the laboratorian made several touch imprints from the biopsy. There is no reason for doing cytochemical stains on the aspirate smear if one has a good quality and good number of touch imprint slides. These touch imprints were of good quality and showed many blasts. The touch imprints were stained with cytochemical stains. No differentiation was present among these blasts. The cells stained consistent with myeloblasts. The hemodiluted marrow was sent for flow cytometry and cytogenetics. The aspirate can be sent for flow cytometry, as flow is more sensitive in detecting the lineage of blasts. Flow cytometry was positive for myeloid markers and negative for lymphoid markers. The remainder of the aspirate was sent for cytogenetics with a hope that some cells might be able to grow and show any specific cytogenetic abnormality.

Question:

3. Can a diagnosis be made from tests on the aspirate rather than waiting for the biopsy slides?

Explanation:

Yes. The presence of many blasts in the bone marrow aspirate smears and on the touch imprints indicates acute leukemia. The lineage of blasts can be determined based on cytochemical stains and/or flow cytometry. Bone marrow biopsy in this case would not provide any added information.

CHAPTER 10

Case Summary: This patient had a severe macrocytic, hyperchromic anemia as revealed by the red cell indices. The anemia developed slowly over time, which gave his body the opportunity to adapt to a low hemoglobin level. If a patient had lost this much blood quickly, the probability of shock and death would have been high. The yellowness of his eyes suggests a high bilirubin concentration, which is typical of a hemolytic anemia. This patient had a test that revealed antibodies and complement on his red blood cells. This supports the diagnosis of an immune hemolytic anemia. The presence of spherocytes supports this diagnosis as they are a sign that the spleen has removed antibody/antigen complexes from the cell membrane. Note that the MCHC is increased, which is typical of spherocytes. The high reticulocyte count and presence of polychromatophilic erythrocytes indicates the bone marrow is responding appropriately by increasing output of erythrocytes. The high reticulocyte count is probably responsible for the increased MCV.

Question:

1. Calculate the erythrocyte indices. Does the information given suggest acute or chronic blood loss? What is the significance of the RDW?

Explanation:

MCV 113 fL; MCH 43.7 pg; MCHC 38.8 g/dL. The case history suggests chronic blood loss. The hemoglobin is very low, and the patient probably would be in shock if he lost this much blood suddenly. The RDW suggests significant anisocytosis.

Question:

2. Calculate the absolute reticulocyte count. His RBC count is 0.71 $\times 10^{12}$/L and the reticulocyte count is 22%. Is this increased, decreased, or normal?

Explanation:

The absolute reticulocyte count is:
$22\% \times 0.71 \times 10^{12}$/L $= 0.156 \times 10^{12}$/L $= 156 \times 10^{9}$/L
This is at the high end of the reference range.

Question:

3. George's blood smear revealed marked spherocytosis. Explain the importance of this finding.

Explanation:

Spherocytes are cells that have lost membrane. They are significant in this case because they indicate a hemolytic anemia.

Question:

4. Explain George's abnormal indices.

Explanation:

The indices are all elevated: MCV 113 fL; MCH 43.6 pg; MCHC 38.8 g/dL. The increased MCV may be due to the high reticulocyte count. The MCH is elevated due to the presence of these large cells that are able to hold more hemoglobin than a smaller cell. The MCHC is elevated due to the marked spherocytosis.

Question:

5. Classify George's anemia morphologically and functionally.

Explanation:

George's anemia is morphologically classified as macrocytic, hyperchromic. Functionally, it is classified as a survival defect. It appears that the cells are being destroyed by an immune hemolytic process. The bone marrow has increased production of cells as indicated by the increased reticulocyte count.

CHAPTER 11

Case Summary: This patient is suffering from IDA due to chronic blood loss from the GU tract. He has the typical blood picture of microcytic, hypochromic erythrocytes. His iron studies reveal a lack of total body iron. The serum iron and % transferrin saturation are low.

Question:

1. How would you describe his anemia morphologically?

Explanation:

MCV = 63 fL; MCH = 19.5 pg. The anemia is microcytic, hypochromic.

Question:

2. Calculate % saturation.

Explanation:

Serum iron/TIBC = 4%. The serum iron is low and TIBC increased resulting in a low % saturation.

Question:

3. Is this value normal, decreased, or increased?

Explanation:

Decreased. Less than 15% saturation is decreased.

Question:

4. What disease, if any, is suggested by this value?

Explanation:

Iron deficiency (ID). The percent saturation of transferrin is decreased in ID, usually to less than 10%.

Question:

5. Do the iron studies in our patient suggest sideroblastic anemia?

Explanation:

No. Iron studies in this patient reveal a lack of total body iron. In sideroblastic anemia there is a defect in the incorporation of iron into the porphyrin ring. Iron accumulates in the red cell and macrophage. Thus the total body iron is increased in sideroblastic anemia.

Question:

6. Do the laboratory test results and clinical history of our patient indicate that a bone marrow examination is necessary?

Explanation:

No, adequate information is present from other laboratory tests. In ID anemia, the CBC and iron studies give important clues to diagnosis. A bone marrow may be performed in difficult cases but is usually not necessary.

Question:

7. How do the iron study results of our patient help in differentiating the diagnosis of iron deficiency from ACD and sideroblastic anemia?

Explanation:

In ACD, the serum iron is low and TIBC and % saturation are normal or decreased. In sideroblastic anemia the TIBC is decreased but serum iron and % saturation are increased. In both ACD and sideroblastic anemia, the total body iron is normal to increased. In ID, total body iron is decreased.

Question:

8. What additional iron test that was not done would be most helpful in this case?

Explanation:

Serum ferritin is a good indicator of iron stores and is less invasive than a bone marrow.

CHAPTER 12

Case Summary: This patient, previously diagnosed with a hemoglobinopathy, was admitted to the hospital with symptoms of vaso-occlusive crisis. Testing revealed he had pneumonia and sickle cell disease. The infection was probably responsible for precipitating the crisis.

Question:

1. Identify a laboratory test needed to determine Shane's hemoglobinopathy.

Explanation:

Hemoglobin electrophoresis is needed to identify a hemoglobinopathy.

Question:

2. What is the abnormal hemoglobin causing this patient's disease?

Explanation:

HbS.

Question:

3. Is the patient heterozygous or homozygous for the disorder?

Explanation:

We can assume that the patient is homozygous because of the very high concentration of HbS present and lack of HbA.

Question:

4. What is this disorder called?

Explanation:

This disorder is referred to as sickle cell disease or sickle cell anemia.

Question:

5. What physiological condition does this patient have that may lead to sickling of his erythrocytes?

Explanation:

This patient has fever, suggesting infection or inflammation. The chest radiograph indicated pneumonia. It is possible that the infection is causing hypoxia and other physiological alterations that promote sickling.

Question:

6. What is the cause of this patient's pain and acute distress?

Explanation:

The patient is experiencing a vaso-occlusive crisis as a result of sickling of erythrocytes in the microvasculature. (Physicians refer to this as a "pain" crisis.) It is possible he is also experiencing acute chest syndrome.

Question:

7. Why might Shane be more susceptible to pneumonia than an individual without sickle cell disease?

Explanation:

It is likely that he has functional asplenia as a result of repeated sickling episodes in the spleen. Without a functioning spleen, he is more susceptible to certain bacterial infections. Often sickle cell patients are treated with prophylactic antibiotics to prevent infections.

Question:

8. Which of the patient's hematologic test results are consistent with a diagnosis of sickle cell anemia?

Explanation:

His hemoglobin is markedly reduced and in the range typically seen in sickle cell disease. There are also increased leukocytes and platelets, which are common findings. The presence of sickle cells and other findings on the blood smear are all consistent with a diagnosis of sickle cell disease.

Question:

9. What does the presence of polychromatophilic erythrocytes signify?

Explanation:

Polychromatophilic erythrocytes are actually reticulocytes. This indicates that the bone marrow is attempting to compensate for the deficit of erythrocytes in the peripheral blood by releasing these slightly immature cells.

Question:

10. Why is the absolute neutrophil count elevated?

Explanation:

Neutrophilia is associated with bacterial infection.

Question:

11. What is the significance of ovalocytes on the blood smear?

Explanation:

These cells are probably irreversibly sickled cells.

Question:

12. What is the significance of Howell–Jolly bodies on the smear?

Explanation:

The patient's spleen is not functional and is incapable of removing these inclusions from the erythrocytes.

Question:

13. What is the significance of the patient's elevated LD?

Explanation:

Lactic dehydrogenase is an enzyme found in high concentration in erythrocytes. Elevated LD levels are associated with increased hemolysis of erythrocytes, a typical finding in sickle cell disease.

CHAPTER 13

Case Summary: John had the typical symptoms of anemia. His CBC revealed a microcytic, hypochromic anemia. Tests for iron deficiency were negative. Hemoglobin electrophoresis was abnormal with the presence of hemoglobins H and Bart's. These hemoglobins indicate a deficiency of α-chains. The presence of some HbA, HbA$_2$, and HbF indicate that some α-chains are being produced. This suggests the presence of α-thalassemia. The parents also exhibit symptoms of anemia and should be tested to determine if they have a form of α-thalassemia. This will help confirm the diagnosis in the child.

Question:

1. Based on the indices, classify the anemia morphologically.

Explanation:

Microcytic, hypochromic

MCV = 69 fL

MCH = 21 pg

MCHC = 29.2 g/dL

The MCV is below the lower limit of normal (80 fL) indicating microcytic erythrocytes. The MCHC is the best indicator of hemoglobin content and is also below the lower limit of normal (32 g/dL) suggesting hypochromasia. The below normal MCH (<27 pg) corroborates the decreased hemoglobin content.

Question:

2. Name the dominant poikilocyte observed in this peripheral blood smear.

Explanation:

Target cells are the dominant poikilocytes.

Question:

3. Name three disorders that frequently present with the same poikilocyte that dominates in this peripheral blood smear.

Explanation:

Thalassemia

Hemoglobinopathy

Iron deficiency anemia

Question:

4. List two additional lab tests that would help confirm the diagnosis and predict the results of each.

Explanation:

Disorder	Hb Electrophoresis	Hb Solubility Test	Iron Panel
Thalassemia (α)	HbH Hb Bart's $\downarrow$ HbA, A$_2$, and F	Negative	Normal
Thalassemia (β)	Hb Bart's $\downarrow$ HbA $\uparrow$ HbA$_2$ and HbF	Negative	Normal
Hemoglobinopathy	HbS or HbC or HbE, etc. $\downarrow$ HbA	Positive with some (HbS, etc.)	Normal
Iron deficiency anemia	Normal	Negative	$\downarrow$ Serum iron $\downarrow$ Ferritin $\downarrow$ % Saturation $\downarrow$ BM iron $\uparrow$ TIBC

Question:

5. Is the hemoglobin electrophoresis normal or abnormal?

Explanation:

Abnormal.

Question:

6. If abnormal, list hemoglobins that are elevated, decreased, or abnormally present.

Explanation:

Elevated	Decreased	Abnormal
None	HbA	Hb Bart's
	HbF	HbH
	HbA_2	

Question:

7. If abnormal, which globin chains are decreased?

Explanation:

α-chains and all α-chain containing hemoglobins (HbA, F, and A_2) are decreased.

Question:

8. If abnormal, which globin chains are produced in excess?

Explanation:

β-chain containing HbH and γ-chain containing Hb Bart's are elevated, ruling out a β-, γ-, $\delta\beta$-, and $\gamma\delta\beta$-thalassemia.

Question:

9. Is the iron panel normal or abnormal?

Explanation:

Normal.

Question:

10. If the iron tests are abnormal, list those tests outside the normal range and indicate if they are elevated or decreased.

Explanation:

Normal, so nonapplicable.

Question:

11. If abnormal, state the disorder(s) consistent with the abnormal iron panel.

Explanation:

An abnormal iron panel usually presents with a pattern consistent with one of the iron metabolism disorders (i.e., iron deficiency, lead poisoning, anemia of chronic disease, sideroblastic anemia, etc.). A normal iron panel, as is the case here, rules out iron deficiency anemia.

Question:

12. Given all the data supplied, what is the definitive diagnosis of John's anemia?

Explanation:

A microcytic, hypochromic anemia with target cells suggests a thalassemia, hemoglobinopathy, or iron deficiency anemia. The other microcytic, hypochromic anemias involving abnormal iron metabolism are also possibilities but usually do not present with significant numbers of target cells. The normal iron panel rules out iron deficiency anemia and the other disorders of iron metabolism. The negative hemoglobin solubility rules out some hemoglobinopathies. The abnormal hemoglobin electrophoresis confirms the diagnosis by further ruling out iron deficiency (which shows a normal Hb electrophoresis) and hemoglobinopathies by absence of structural hemoglobin variants that have an amino acid substitution (i.e., HbS, HbC, HbE, etc.). The decreased concentration of all three α-containing hemoglobins, HbA, HbA_2, and HbF, suggest an α-thalassemia. The presence of the abnormal hemoglobins, HbH and Hb Bart's, rule out a β- and γ-thalassemia, respectively. The severity of the symptoms, the inherited nature of the disease, the early age of onset, the microcytic, hypochromic peripheral blood picture with target cells, and the presence of HbH and Hb Bart's on Hb electrophoresis indicate a severe form of α-thalassemia called HbH disease.

CHAPTER 14

Case Summary: This is a case of a 36-year-old female with a megaloblastic anemia. An initial diagnosis of moderate anemia, jaundice, and neurological complications was made. Based on the patient's laboratory test results, she was diagnosed as having a vitamin B_{12} deficiency. The Schilling test demonstrated that the deficiency was due to the absence of intrinsic factor. This patient can be diagnosed with a megaloblastic anemia due to a lack of intrinsic factor. The patient is suffering from the adult form of pernicious anemia with demonstrated anti-intrinsic factor antibodies.

Question:

1. What is the morphologic classification of the patient's anemia?

Explanation:

Macrocytic. The morphologic classification of anemia includes normocytic, microcytic, and macrocytic. Macrocytic is the classification when the MCV >100 fL.

Question:

2. Based on the information obtained so far, what is the most likely diagnosis?

Explanation:

There is a vitamin B_{12} deficiency. The patient was admitted with signs of a moderate hemolytic anemia and neurological symptoms. Her CBC shows she has a macrocytic anemia. Her leukocyte and platelet counts are at the lower end of the normal range, indicating a developing pancytopenia. The blood smear revealed hypersegmented neutrophils, ovalocytes, and Howell-Jolly bodies. Her bilirubin values support a diagnosis of hemolysis due to an increased indirect bilirubin. On a differential diagnosis, neurological symptoms typically accompany vitamin B_{12} deficiency rather than a folate deficiency. Based on her serum vitamin B_{12} and folate results, she can be definitively diagnosed as having a megaloblastic anemia due to a vitamin B_{12} deficiency.

Question:

3. What is the significance of the AST/ALT results?

Explanation:

There is no liver disease. These are both liver enzymes. Since they are normal, liver disease is ruled out as a source of jaundice or the macrocytic anemia.

Question:

4. What further testing can be done to obtain a definitive diagnosis?

Explanation:

Testing for intrinsic factor antibodies, Schilling test, gastric analysis. A common cause of vitamin B_{12} deficiency in a patient with no previous gastrointestinal history is pernicious anemia. The Schilling test can determine if the deficiency is due to absence of intrinsic factor or some malabsorption disorder.

Question:

5. What is this patient's definitive diagnosis?

Explanation:

Pernicious anemia. The Schilling test result in Part I showed less than 7% of the initial radioactively tagged dose of oral vitamin B_{12} in the urine 24 hours later. When the test was repeated with intrinsic factor, a greater amount of the B_{12} dose was found in the urine after 24 hours. Gastric analysis provides stomach pH levels. The diagnosis of pernicious anemia is supported by the finding of intrinsic factor blocking antibodies in her blood.

Question:

6. How would the diagnosis change if the special testing results were as follows?
Schilling Test:
Part I, before intrinsic factor: 1%
Part II, After intrinsic factor: 3%
Instrinsic factor-blocking antibodies: Negative

Explanation:

The diagnosis is not pernicious anemia. The vitamin B_{12} deficiency is due to some other malabsorption disorder. An abnormal Schilling test result following Part II with oral intrinsic factor and the absence of

autoantibodies suggest that her vitamin B_{12} deficiency was due to some sort of malabsorption disorder such as Crohn's disease or bowel blindloop syndrome.

Question:

7. What would you predict this patient's reticulocyte count to be?

Explanation:

Normal to low. The patient's reticulocyte count would probably be normal to decreased. Megaloblastic anemia results from ineffective erythropoiesis with intramedullary hemolysis, which blunts the number of reticulocytes in the marrow storage pool. In addition, polychromasia was *not* found on the patient's blood smear, which is a sign of reticulocytosis.

CHAPTER 15

Case Summary: Rachael had symptoms of anemia and a bleeding disorder when she was first seen by her physician. Her past medical history was significant in that she had recently recovered from a viral infection. Her laboratory results revealed pancytopenia and a low reticulocyte count. Bone marrow examination showed hypoplasia. These findings suggest acquired aplastic anemia associated with past viral infection.

Question:

1. Select laboratory tests appropriate for screening for aplastic anemia.

Explanation:

The CBC is an important screening test for all anemias.

Question:

2. Justify the selection of laboratory screening tests based on Rachael's clinical signs and symptoms.

Explanation:

It is important to know the patient's hemoglobin and hematocrit, as anemia may be one cause of weakness and shortness of breath. A low platelet count may explain the presence of petechiae and bruises.

Question:

3. Evaluate the relationship between Rachael's age and the likelihood of having aplastic anemia.

Explanation:

Because approximately 25% of cases occur in persons less than age 20, it is possible she may have aplastic anemia. Overall, however, the incidence of aplastic anemia is quite low.

Question:

4. If aplastic anemia is present, would you expect her to have an idiopathic or secondary form? Explain your answer.

Explanation:

It is difficult to estimate whether she has an idiopathic or secondary form without a more complete history. Idiopathic forms are more common in this age group, however. Approximately 50–70% of all cases of aplastic anemia cannot be linked to a specific cause.

Question:

5. What aspect of this patient's history may be associated with the occurrence of aplastic anemia?

Explanation:

The fact that we now know about the previous infection with hepatitis is helpful. There are some data to suggest an association between aplasia and infections with viruses.

Question:

6. Is it likely that Rachael has a constitutional form of aplastic anemia? Explain your answer.

Explanation:

It is unlikely that a constitutional form of aplastic anemia would be detected at such an advanced age. Fanconi's anemia is first observed in much younger children who typically have other congenital abnormalities.

Question:

7. Correlate these clinical findings with her laboratory screening test results.

Explanation:

The patient's weakness and shortness of breath are related to the degree of anemia indicated by her decreased hemoglobin and hematocrit. Petechiae and bruising are caused by her severe thrombocytopenia. Recurrent fevers are suggestive of infection. She is severely neutropenic and, therefore, at high risk for infection.

Question:

8. Evaluate each of the patient's laboratory results by comparing them to reference ranges.

Explanation:

All CBC parameters are below reference range for a person of this age.

Question:

9. Which of the patient's routine laboratory results are consistent with those expected for aplastic anemia?

Explanation:

All are consistent with expected results for patients with aplastic anemia.

Question:

10. Classify the morphologic type of anemia.

Explanation:

The patient's MCV is 100 fL and MCHC is 29. The anemia is macrocytic, normochromic. This finding is consistent with aplastic anemia.

Question:

11. Calculate the absolute lymphocyte count. Are her lymphocytes truly elevated as suggested by the relative lymphocyte count?

Explanation:

The absolute lymphocyte count is 1.1×10^9/L, which is slightly decreased. The relative lymphocyte count (94%) is very high due to the patient being severely neutropenic. Thus, examining the relative count without considering the total leukocyte count can be very misleading.

Question:

12. Correct the reticulocyte count. Why is this step important?

Explanation:

The patient's corrected reticulocyte count is 0.4%, which is below reference range. All reticulocyte counts need to be corrected when anemia is present in order to assess the bone marrow's degree of compensation for the anemia.

Question:

13. Calculate the absolute reticulocyte count.

Explanation:

The patient's absolute reticulocyte count is 0.1%, which is consistent with a diagnosis of aplastic anemia.

Question:

14. Compare these results with those expected for a person with aplastic anemia.

Explanation:

A markedly hypocellular marrow is consistent with a diagnosis of aplastic anemia. There was insufficient hematopoietic material to aspirate an adequate sample.

Question:

15. Interpret the significance of the lack of malignant cells and hematopoietic blasts.

Explanation:

If malignant cells were present in the marrow, a diagnosis of metastatic disease or lymphoma rather than aplastic anemia would have been likely. Bone marrows of patients with leukemias and myelodysplastic syndromes typically are hyperplastic with increased numbers of hematopoietic blasts present.

Question:

16. Suggest a means of improving the validity of bone marrow examination results for this patient.

Explanation:

When aplastic anemia is suspected, it may be advisable to sample multiple areas of the bone marrow.

Question:

17. Appraise the prognosis for Rachael.

Explanation:

Prognosis is rather poor for patients with aplastic anemia unless a compatible donor can be found for bone marrow transplant.

Question:

18. Predict a treatment regimen.

Explanation:

Treatment would consist of supportive therapy using blood components. A platelet transfusion would probably be ordered immediately. If the aplasia did not resolve, a bone marrow transplant would be considered.

Question:

19. What other hematologic conditions must be ruled out for this patient?

Explanation:

Other causes of pancytopenia of the peripheral blood include myelodysplastic syndromes (MDS) and megaloblastic anemia.

Question:

20. What laboratory test is most beneficial in differentiating aplastic anemia from these other disorders? Compare the expected results for aplastic anemia with those of the other disorders.

Explanation:

Serum B_{12} and folic acid levels could be used to rule out anemia due to a deficiency of one of these nutrients. However, a bone marrow examination is essential to make a diagnosis in this case. If the patient had megaloblastic anemia, megaloblastic changes would be evident in the hematopoietic cells. Myelodysplastic changes and increased numbers of myeloblasts would support a diagnosis of MDS.

CHAPTER 16

Case Summary: Ms. Nummi had a severe drop in her hemoglobin after pancreatic surgery. Thinking that she was bleeding internally, the physician was ready to take her back to surgery. Laboratory tests revealed a high reticulocyte count indicating her bone marrow was producing erythrocytes at an accelerated rate. Her bilirubin was increased indicating accelerated hemolysis. The blood smear revealed the presence of spherocytes, which suggests cell membrane damage and grooming by the spleen. Patient history revealed that the patient had received multiple transfusions for previous illness as well as several units on this hospitalization. Workup for a delayed transfusion reaction revealed the presence of alloantibodies and suggested that the spherocytes were due to antigen/antibody complexes on the cell membrane. Based on laboratory results, the decision was made that the patient was not bleeding internally but that her low hemoglobin was due to extravascular hemolysis of red cells.

Question:

1. What type of anemia is suggested by the laboratory results and clinical history?

Explanation:

Decreased survival is suggested by the laboratory results. This is most probably an immune hemolytic anemia because spherocytes are present. The bone marrow's production of cells is increased as indicated by reticulocytosis (285 $\times$ 10^9/L, RPI >2).

Question:

2. Do the laboratory test results indicate intravascular or extravascular hemolysis? Explain.

Explanation:

Extravascular, as suggested by laboratory results and presence of spherocytes on the blood smear. The haptoglobin is probably decreased because of severity of hemolysis.

Question:

3. Is this anemia due to an intrinsic or extrinsic erythrocyte defect?

Explanation:

Extrinsic. Patient history suggests an acquired defect. Presence of spherocytes, a positive AHG, and presence of antibodies suggest immune hemolytic anemia, probably as a result of the transfusions given.

CHAPTER 17

Case Summary: Jack is a 12-year-old with a life-long history of hemolytic crises suggesting a hereditary condition. Laboratory results reveal a microcytic, hyperchromic anemia. The blood smear shows a variety of poikilocytes suggestive of hemolysis. The osmotic fragility test is increased. The test that is most helpful in this case is the thermal sensitivity test. The cells are heat sensitive, which together with the other laboratory results and clinical history, suggests hereditary pyropoikilocytosis.

Question:

1. Calculate the erythrocyte indices.

Explanation:

$$MCV = \frac{29.2 \times 10}{4.0} = 73\ fL \qquad MCH = \frac{10.8 \times 10}{4.0} = 27\ pg$$

$$MCHC = \frac{10.8 \times 100}{29.2} = 37 g/dL$$

Question:

2. Based upon the calculated indices, describe the patient's red blood cells.

Explanation:

The patient's erythrocytes are microcytic, hyperchromic. The term *hyperchromic* is technically correct, but most laboratorians use this term sparingly. This term signifies that the erythrocytes have too much hemoglobin, when in essence that is not true. Instead, these erythrocytes have lost part of their membrane, which causes a decrease in the surface-area-to-volume ratio. This changes the erythrocyte from a discocyte to a spherocyte. The only erythrocyte that will reflect an MCHC of >36g/dL is the spherocyte.

Question:

3. What additional lab tests should be ordered?

Explanation:

This patient has a hemolytic type of anemia with erythrocytes that are microcytic. Erythrocyte morphology on the peripheral smear revealed elliptocytes, spherocytes, and fragmented erythrocytes. It is important to know whether or not this problem is the result of a stimulated immune system (antibodies present). An AHG test should be ordered to determine if this is true. If the AHG is negative, the patient may have an inherited erythrocyte membrane defect. Lab tests that could be used to differentiate the erythrocyte membrane disorders include the osmotic fragility test and the thermal sensitivity test.

Question:

4. Interpret the results of the osmotic fragility test.

Explanation:

The patient's erythrocytes lysed at a higher NaCl concentration than the control cells. This signifies that the patient's erythrocytes cannot take on as much water as a normal cell and, thus, they are said to have increased osmotic fragility.

Question:

5. What do the results of the thermal sensitivity test reveal about the patient's erythrocytes?

Explanation:

The results of the thermal sensitivity test reveal that the patient's erythrocytes are abnormally heat sensitive. Normal erythrocytes will not fragment until heated to 49°–50°C.

Question:

6. What disorder is suggested by the patient's lab findings?

Explanation:

The patient has a hemolytic anemia that is not a result of a stimulated immune system. The erythrocyte morphology reveals microcytosis, spherocytes, elliptocytes, teardrop cells, and micropoikilocytes. The osmotic fragility is increased and the thermal sensitivity test shows that the erythrocytes are heat sensitive. These findings suggest that the patient has hereditary pyropoikilocytosis.

CHAPTER 18

Case Summary: A 25-year-old black male experienced fever, chills, and general malaise 3 days after receiving prophylactic primaquine. Laboratory testing revealed that he was anemic and the bilirubin was increased. In addition, haptoglobin was decreased. Review of the blood smear revealed bite cells and spherocytes. A Heinz body stain was positive. Based on these results, a hemolytic anemia was suspected. He received two units of packed red blood cells. A test for G6PD was performed and results were borderline low. Follow-up testing revealed a low G6PD.

Question:

1. What test should be considered after finding bite cells on a blood smear?

Explanation:

The appearance of bite cells on a blood smear suggests physical damage to the RBCs as the spleen attempts removal of Heinz bodies. Therefore, a Heinz body stain can be employed to reveal their presence as a cause of the anemia.

Question:

2. Why were the initial G6PD test result normal and the repeat test abnormal?

Explanation:

The initial test for G6PD was normal for two reasons. First, the older, more deficient erythrocytes were selectively destroyed during the hemolytic crisis, leaving younger cells with more normally functioning enzyme. Second, the patient had been transfused, and therefore any blood sample would not be representative of the patient's own cells but would contain G6PD contributed by the donor erythrocytes.

Question:

3. What was the precipitating cause of the patient's anemia?

Explanation:

The patient developed anemia because of treatment with the oxidant drug primaquine. Oxidant damage to hemoglobin due to lack of reducing power supply by G6PD in the hexose-monophosphate shunt leads to erythrocyte destruction.

CHAPTER 19

Case Summary: This patient's data demonstrate reactions seen in warm autoimmune hemolytic anemia secondary to systemic lupus erythematosus. Spherocytes indicate extravascular hemolysis, and reticulocytosis suggests compensation by increased bone marrow production of erythrocytes. The positive DAT (anti-IgG) is a clue that the cell destruction is immune-mediated. Her serum reacts with all antibody screening cells and panel cells after addition of antihuman globulin. The diagnosis of systemic lupus erythematosus (SLE)—an autoimmune disease characteristically diagnosed in women between the ages of 24 and 40—provides additional support for the secondary nature of the immune mediated hemolysis. Patients with SLE often develop not only antibodies against nuclear components of all cells in the body but also to erythrocytes, as demonstrated in this patient. Treatment would begin initially with steroids, and if the patient were nonresponsive, then other modalities would be considered. Transfusion is discouraged unless the hemoglobin value drops to a very low level.

Question:

1. What are some reasons that this person may have a low hemoglobin value?

Explanation:

Low hemoglobin may be due to iron deficiency, occult bleeding, extravascular hemolysis.

Question:

2. What is the significance of the spherocytes?

Explanation:

They indicate damage to the cell membrane and extravascular hemolysis.

Question:

3. Based on these results what do you suspect is going on with this patient? Explain.

Explanation:

Some type of immune-mediated hemolysis is occurring due to the presence of IgG on the erythrocyte.

Question:

4. What type of antibody appears to be present in this patient? Explain.

Explanation:

Autoantibody. The patient's serum is reacting with her own cells, which indicates that the antigen is present on her own cells.

Question:

5. What is the relationship of the patient's primary disease, systemic lupus erythematosus, and her anemia?

Explanation:

SLE is an autoimmune disease in which the patient often develops a WAIHA secondary to the disease.

Question:

6. How would knowing that the patient had not been transfused in the last several months help you make a decision on the underlying cause of the antibody?

Explanation:

If the patient had been transfused, then the foreign antigens on the transfused cells could have stimulated an alloantibody. However, the alloantibody would not be reacting with the patient's own cells.

Question:

7. What would you tell the clinician about giving a transfusion?

Explanation:

Transfusions are not indicated in WAIHA because the transfused cells contain an antigen that will react with the antibody and be destroyed just as the patient's own cells are.

Question:

8. What kind of therapy might be used?

Explanation:

The most common therapy is use of corticosteroids, which depress the immune reaction. If the patient does not respond to this drug then other cytotoxic drugs or splenectomy may be indicated.

CHAPTER 20

Case Summary: This case demonstrates the sequence of testing that might be used to determine the cause of microangiopathic hemolytic anemia. The presence of schistocytes may be seen in a number of conditions, but additional laboratory tests such as platelet count and coagulation studies will help in identifying the underlying cause. In addition, medical history such as age, diarrheal episodes, pregnancy status, or other physical conditions (acquired or inherited) will help in differential diagnosis and in deciding a sequence of additional testing. In this case age and lack of diarrheal prodrome rule out HUS. The low platelet count but normal coagulation tests help rule out DIC. The most likely condition is TTP. The lack of an identifiable precipitating condition and the adult age onset indicate it is most likely of the single episode, nonrecurring type.

Question:

1. What are some conditions that result in the presence of schistocytes?

Explanation:

Some conditions that result in the presence of schistocytes include disseminated intravascular coagulation, hemolytic uremic syndrome, thrombotic thrombocytopenic purpura, mechanical trauma due to artificial heart valves, malignant hypertension, and burns (thermal injury).

Question:

2. What is the significance of these results?

Explanation:

The platelet count indicates a thrombocytopenia, which correlates with the patient's increased tendency to bruising. Her reticulocyte count was elevated and indicates a response by the bone marrow.

Question:

3. Why might the clinician order coagulation tests?

Explanation:

The presence of unexplained bruises may indicate an abnormality in the hemostatic mechansim. This can be screened for by coagulation tests.

Question:

4. What do these findings indicate about the underlying problem?

Explanation:

The PT and APTT showed slightly prolonged levels, and the fibrinogen was only slightly decreased. This rules out DIC because in DIC you would expect greatly prolonged PT and APTT values, decreased fibrinogen, and increased FDP.

Question:

5. Based on these results, what is the most likely condition associated with these clinical and laboratory results? Explain.

Explanation:

TTP. The patient's age, normal urinary volume, and lack of diarrheal prodrome help rule out HUS. The neurological symptoms in concert with the other laboratory values point to TTP.

Question:

6. What therapy might be used?

Explanation:

Plasma exchange with either fresh frozen plasma (FFP) or with cryo-poor FFP can be used.

CHAPTER 21

Case Summary: This trauma patient had surgery to repair bone fractures. After surgery the WBC count was elevated with a predominance of bands. The platelet count and hemoglobin were also below the reference range for his age and sex. Although a bacterial infection was suspected based on the CBC, cultures were negative. Despite the high WBC count and shift-to-the-left there were no toxic changes of the

leukocytes. After further review it was determined that the patient had Pelger-Huët anomaly. The bands were actually mature neutrophils whose nucleus failed to segment.

Question:

1. What results, if any, are abnormal?

Explanation:

The white blood count and number of bands are elevated.

Question:

2. What is the most likely reason for these results?

Explanation:

The most likely reason for an elevated white count and left shift on a trauma patient who has had emergency surgery is a bacterial infection acquired either from the original trauma or during surgery. Leukocytosis without toxic changes present or a shift-to-the-left may occur in postsurgical patients.

Question:

3. Given the leukocyte morphology and cultures, what additional condition must now be considered?

Explanation:

Since the cultures are all negative and there are no other indications of a reactive process, such as toxic granulation, Döhle bodies, or vacuoles, it is unlikely the patient has an infection. Pelger-Huët anomaly is a benign inherited condition where the neutrophils have hyposegmentation. The nuclei are shaped like dumbbells or wire-rimmed eyeglasses and have very condensed chromatin.

Question:

4. Explain the clinical significance of the nuclear anomaly described in this patient.

Explanation:

Pelger-Huët anomaly is benign and the neutrophils appear to function normally. The greatest significance of this disorder is that it be recognized and cells not mistakenly identified as bands leading to an incorrect diagnosis of infection. In this case, the patient had additional tests (the cultures) performed that probably were not necessary if the condition had been diagnosed previously.

Question:

5. Why is the white count elevated?

Explanation:

Pelger-Huët does not typically present with leukocytosis unless accompanied by another condition. The white count is probably increased due to tissue damage from the accident trauma and/or the surgery. Also, although the patient's hemoglobin is only low normal, it is likely that a young previously healthy man had a higher value before the accident. He could have lost blood from the accident and/or during the surgery. Acute blood loss and surgery are associated with leukocytosis.

CHAPTER 22

Case Summary: This young infant had recurrent infections since birth. Her WBC was normal but there was an absolute lymphocytopenia. Further investigation suggested an immune deficiency disorder and led to additional laboratory tests. These tests revealed high levels of erythrocyte adenosine and deoxyadenosine indicating a deficiency in adenosine deaminase. This deficiency occurs from a gene deletion resulting in an autosomal inherited severe combined immunodeficiency. Normal immune function is restored when (1) toxic metabolites are cleared, (2) a normal adenosine deaminase gene is inserted into the patient's lymphocytes, or (3) the patient has a bone marrow transplant.

Question:

1. Does this patient have a leukocytosis or leukopenia? Explain.

Explanation:

No, there is not a leukocytosis or leukopenia. The WBC count is within normal range.

Question:

2. Does this patient have an abnormal lymphocyte count? Explain.

Explanation:

The absolute lymphocyte count = $7.6 \times 10^9/L \times 0.04 = 0.304 \times 10^9/L$. This is abnormally low as the reference range at this age is $2.5–16.5 \times 10^9/L$.

Question:

3. What is the absolute lymphocyte count?

Explanation:

At 54 days, the absolute lymphocyte count is only $12.3 \times 10^9/L \times 0.01 = 0.123$ lymphocytes $\times 10^9/L$, a condition of lymphocytopenia.

Question:

4. What possible causes exist for these opportunistic infections?

Explanation:

Two causes of immunodeficiency are suspected with opportunistic infection and severe lymphocytopenia: (1) AIDS, and (2) severe combined immunodeficiency syndrome.

Question:

5. Is this child more likely to have a congenital or acquired immune deficiency?

Explanation:

A congenital immune deficiency is more probable as the child has had recurrent infections and lymphocytopenia since birth.

Question:

6. If she has a congenital immune deficiency, is it more likely she has X-linked or autosomal SCIDS?

Explanation:

Autosomal SCIDS. Females who carry the abnormal X-linked SCIDS gene have normal immunity. Only normal X chromosomes are found in the lymphocytes of females who carry the abnormal X-linked SCIDS gene.

Question:

7. Are the lymphocytes more likely to be morphologically heterogeneous or homogeneous? Why?

Explanation:

Homogeneous. The congenital immune deficiency disorders are characterized by normal appearing lymphocytes but the lymphocytes are either defective or decreased in concentration or both. Heterogeneous lymphocytes are normally reactive lymphocytes. They are stimulated by infectious agents.

Question:

8. What confirmatory test is indicated?

Explanation:

A test to determine a decreased adenosine deaminase level or increased purine metabolites of deoxyadenosine triphosphate and deoxyguanosine triphosphate confirm an enzyme deficiency.

CHAPTER 23

Case Summary: The case is an example of chronic lymphocytic leukemia involving the peripheral blood. It demonstrates the technique of gating the cells of interest, how to determine a phenotype, and the use of a characteristic phenotype in establishing a diagnosis of a subtype of lymphoid malignancy.

Question:

1. What is the optimal specimen?

Explanation:

The CBC revealed peripheral blood lymphocytosis. Therefore, flow cytometry of the peripheral blood would be appropriate. An EDTA anticoagulated specimen is ideal. The CBC sample could be used if it was processed within 24 hours of being drawn. Other anticoagulants are adequate (e.g., heparin and ACD).

Question:

2. Which cells are of interest and should be included in the gate?

Explanation:

The cells of interest are the lymphocytes.

Question:

3. What are the typical forward and side scatter properties of the cells of interest?

Explanation:

Lymphocytes have low side scatter (granularity) and variable forward scatter (size).

Question:

4. What is the phenotype?

Explanation:

The majority of the lymphocytes have the following abnormal phenotype: CD45+, CD19+, CD20+, CD23+, CD5+, lambda+, kappa−.

Question:

5. Which features indicate clonality?

Explanation:

Expression of only one immunoglobulin light chain (lambda, but not kappa) and the aberrant expression of CD5 indicate a clonal population of B cells.

Question:

6. What is the diagnosis?

Explanation:

The diagnosis is chronic lymphocytic leukemia, B cell (CLL), or small lymphocytic lymphoma (SLL). CD5-positive B cells are characteristic of CLL, SLL, or mantle cell lymphoma (MCL). CD23 expression is found in CLL and SLL but not MCL. Although lymphoma primarily involves the lymph nodes and other lymphoid organs, there may be secondary involvement of the peripheral blood and bone marrow.

Question:

7. Which of the flow cytometry results presented in this case indicate that this is a malignancy of mature lymphocytes (chronic lymphocytic leukemia) and not acute lymphoblastic leukemia?

Explanation:

The strong expression of CD45, presence of surface immunoglobulin, and absence of CD34 and CD10 expression all indicate a mature B lymphocyte phenotype.

CHAPTER 24

Case Summary: Gregory had leukocytosis and a shift to the left when initially seen. The differential diagnosis was important in order to determine if this abnormal blood picture was due to a benign or neoplastic process. Cytogenetic studies revealed an acquired clonal aberration (t9;22) diagnostic of CML. Gregory had a bone marrow transplant with his sister's donated cells. Five years later, cytogenetic studies revealed a relapse and impending blast crisis.

Question:

1. What is the most appropriate specimen to submit for cytogenetic analysis and how should it be processed?

Explanation:

The most appropriate specimen to submit for chromosome analysis of CML is a bone marrow sample. If the bone marrow is not aspirable, peripheral blood can be used but sometimes will not yield mitosis. The processing must be performed by direct harvest and/or unstimulated cultures.

Question:

2. Is this a congenital or acquired aberration?

Explanation:

This is an acquired aberration that is only present in the hematopoietic cells—RBC precursors, WBC precursors, megakaryocytes, and some lymphocytes.

Question:

3. Is it a clonal aberration?

Explanation:

This is a clonal aberration, as it is present in more than one cell (in this case, it was present in 100% of cells analyzed, which is typical for CML).

Question:

4. What is the significance of this finding for the diagnosis?

Explanation:

The finding of the t(9;22) confirms the diagnosis of CML.

Question:

5. What is the significance of this finding?

Explanation:

This finding confirms the engraftment of female donor cells in the recipient bone marrow. While no cells with the t(9;22) are found by cytogenetic methods, molecular studies may show the presence of the BCR gene rearrangement, as these techniques are more sensitive than routine cytogenetics.

Question:

6. What other studies could be performed that would be informative as to the status of the donor and recipient cells?

Explanation:

FISH analysis can be performed on the interphase nuclei using probes for the X and Y chromosome to demonstrate the sex of the cells present. In addition, probes for the t(9;22) can be used if male cells are present to determine if they are leukemic cells. Molecular studies can also be obtained for the BCR gene rearrangement.

Question:

7. What is the significance of these findings?

Explanation:

The cytogenetic results performed at 5 years posttransplant show not only a relapse of the CML, but also a cytogenetic transformation indicative of pending blast crisis, as evidenced by the +8 and i(17q) that were not seen in the original leukemic cells.

CHAPTER 25

Case Summary: This patient had a high blast percentage in the peripheral blood and bone marrow that is typical of acute leukemia. However, she also had the Philadelphia chromosome, which is associated with chronic myelogenous leukemia (CML). This mutation involves the BCR/ABL translocation with p210 breakpoints. Thus, this patient could be suffering from a blast crisis of CML. There are times when the chronic phase of CML may not be diagnosed before blast crisis. The other possibility here is that the patient has de novo acute leukemia. These leukemias also may harbor a Philadelphia chromosome, but the breakpoints in the BCR gene at the molecular level are different from the breakpoints in CML. This patient had the de novo form of acute lymphocytic leukemia (ALL) as the molecular analysis revealed the BCR/ABL p190.

Question:

1. What is the classification of this neoplastic hematologic disorder based on the peripheral blood and bone marrow results?

Explanation:

This patient has an acute leukemia as the blast count is >30% in both the peripheral blood and bone marrow.

Question:

2. What molecular defect is consistent with the presence of the Philadelphia chromosome?

Explanation:

The BCR/ABL translocation is the molecular equivalent of the Philadelphia chromosome. There is a reciprocal translocation between the ABL gene on chromosome 9 and the BCR gene on chromosome 22. The Philadelphia chromosome represents the shortened chromosome

22. This fusion gene produces a new protein having increased tyrosine kinase activity.

Question:

3. Would molecular analysis assist in diagnosis? Explain.

Explanation:

Molecular analysis would assist in diagnosis. This patient has the Philadelphia chromosome associated with CML but has a peripheral blood and bone marrow picture of acute leukemia. Thus, she may be in the blast crisis of CML or have a de novo acute leukemia. In de novo acute leukemia, the breakpoint in the BCR gene is often different, producing a fusion gene encoding a p190 protein.

Question:

4. If molecular analysis should be done, which laboratory procedure should be used and what specimen should be obtained?

Explanation:

The rt-PCR analysis of BCR/ABL should be done. Alternatively, the Southern blot procedure can be performed to detect a rearranged BCR gene. A bone marrow specimen or peripheral blood may be used.

Question:

5. The molecular analysis revealed BCR/ABL translocation consistent with a p190 breakpoint. What is the diagnosis?

Explanation:

This defect is found in some cases of de novo ALL.

Question:

6. Why is this molecular finding helpful in therapy decisions?

Explanation:

It identifies a set of patients who are less responsive to standard chemotherapy, and the prognosis is poor compared to Philadelphia-negative ALL.

CHAPTER 26

Case Summary: This patient has chronic lymphocytic leukemia. The patient is elderly and had been in good health, and the symptoms of the leukemia had progressed slowly. The predominant cell present on the peripheral blood smear is a mature lymphocyte. The patient's prognosis should be good, with a life span of 5 years or more with supportive therapy.

Question:

1. Given the patient's laboratory results, would this most likely be considered an acute or chronic leukemia?

Explanation:

Chronic leukemia. The peripheral blood shows an accumulation of mature lymphocytic cells with an increased white blood cell count.

Question:

2. What group of leukemia (cell lineage) is suggested by the patient's blood cell differential results?

Explanation:

Lymphocytic leukemia. The patient exhibits an increased percentage of mature lymphocytes with an increased white blood cell count and a lack of myelocytic cells.

Question:

3. What would you expect the blast count on the bone marrow to be according to the FAB classification system? The WHO classification system?

Explanation:

<30%, FAB definition; <20%, WHO definition. In acute leukemias, blasts constitute more than 30% of the nonerythroid marrow nucleated cells; in MDS, MPD, and chronic leukemia, blasts compose less than 30% (WHO <20%) of the marrow cells.

Question:

4. Would you expect Agnes to survive more than 3 years or succumb fairly quickly after treatment?

Explanation:

Survive more than 3 years. Chronic leukemias progress slowly, and the course of the disease is measured in years rather than months, as is typical for the acute leukemias.

Question:

5. Is Agnes a suitable candidate for a bone marrow transplant? Why or why not?

Explanation:

No. The highest rate of success with bone marrow transplants has occurred in those younger than 40 years of age in a first remission with a closely matched donor. Because this patient is 72 years old and CLL patients usually do well with supportive therapy, it would be unlikely that she would be a candidate for a bone marrow transplant.

Question:

6. What types of treatment are available for our patient Agnes?

Explanation:

Chemotherapy, radiation, bone marrow transplant, immunotherapy. Permanent remission in CLL is rare. Treatment is conservative and usually reserved for patients with more aggressive forms of the disease.

CHAPTER 27

Case Summary: The clinical findings of abdominal discomfort, increasing splenomegaly, weakness, and bone pain are consistent with chronic myeloproliferative disorders. The laboratory findings of increased uric acid, left shift, increased platelet count, difficult bone marrow aspiration, dacryocytes on peripheral blood smear, and cytogenetic abnormalities are all characteristic of MMM. Malignant stem cells give rise to abnormal leukocytes, erythrocytes, and megakaryocytes. The megakaryocytes secrete excessive PDGFs that stimulate fibroblasts to lay down excessive fibrin in the bone marrow cavity. This fibrosis leads to the extramedullary hematopoiesis causing splenomegaly and hepatomegaly.

In this case, the peripheral blood film with a leukoerythroblastic picture of immature myeloid cells, nucleated red blood cells, and dacryocytes should rule out causes of marrow infiltration by nonhematopoietic tumor cells, granulomas, or fungus.

The diagnosis of this case is myeloid metaplasia with myelofibrosis. Myelofibrosis can evolve into any of the chronic myeloproliferative disorders or acute leukemia. A moderate leukocytosis (WBC <30.0 $\times 10^9$/L), leukoerythroblastosis, dry tap, and lack of the Philadelphia chromosome distinguish MMM from the other myeloproliferative disorders.

Question:

1. What are the patient's MCV and MCHC?

Explanation:

MCV = 35/3.6 × 10 = 97 fL and MCHC = 11.6/35 × 100 = 33%.

Question:

2. How would you morphologically classify the patient's anemia?

Explanation:

The patient has a normochromic, normocytic anemia.

Question:

3. Based on the patient history and current laboratory data, what other tests should be performed?

Explanation:

Because of the hepatosplenomegaly and laboratory results, a bone marrow and Philadelphia chromosome analysis should be considered.

Question:

4. What diagnoses are suggested?

Explanation:

All MPD (CML, essential thrombocytosis, polycythemia vera, or myelofibrosis with myeloid metaplasia) can produce a leukocytosis and fibrotic bone marrow.

Question:

5. Give a reason for the unsuccessful, dry-tap, bone marrow aspiration.

Explanation:

Increased fibrosis in the bone marrow makes aspiration difficult. Excess PDGF and TGF-β stimulate collagen proliferation and fibrosis in the bone marrow. Dry taps may also result from improper placement of the needle into the marrow cavity, a marrow that is hypocellular, or one that is packed tightly with neoplastic cells.

Question:

6. What characteristic peripheral blood morphologies correlate with the bone marrow picture and physical exam?

Explanation:

You would expect to see dacryocytes and should look for micromegakaryocytes in the peripheral blood.

Question:

7. What is the most likely explanation for the increased splenomegaly?

Explanation:

The progressive bone marrow fibrosis causes anemia, resulting in extramedullary hematopoiesis in the spleen and liver. This increases splenic blood flow, red cell pooling, and enlargement of the spleen.

Question:

8. What are possible outcomes of this disorder?

Explanation:

Myelofibrosis with myeloid metaplasia can show progressive fibrosis or evolve into polycythemia vera, essential thrombocythemia, CML, or acute leukemia.

CHAPTER 28

Case Summary: Mr. Hancock had bicytopenia (anemia and thrombocytopenia) with a shift to the left and dysplastic erythrocyte and granulocyte features. The bone marrow was hypercellular with an increased M:E ratio. There was trilineage dysplasia. Based on the FAB criteria for subgrouping the MDS, he most probably has RAEB.
The results of the CBC on Mr. Hancock were:
RBC: 1.60×10^{12}/L
Hb: 58 g/L
Hct: 0.17 L/L
WBC: 10.5×10^9/L
Platelets: 39×10^9/L
Reticulocyte count: 0.8%
Differential: 44% segmented neutrophils
        7% band neutrophils
        6% lymphocytes

            28% eosinophils
            1% metamyelocytes
            1% myelocytes
            9% promyelocytes
            4% blasts
The neutrophilic cells show marked hyposegmentation and hypogranulation. RBC morphology included anisocytosis and poikilocytosis, teardrop cells, ovalocytes, and schistocytes.

Question:

1. Cytopenia is present in what cell lines?

Explanation:

Cytopenia is present in the erythrocytic and megakaryocytic cell lines (RBCs and platelets are decreased).

Question:

2. What abnormalities are present in the differential?

Explanation:

The abnormalities present in the differential are: shift to the left including metamyelocytes, myelocytes, promyelocytes, and a few blasts; also a marked increase in eosinophils.

Question:

3. What evidence of dyspoiesis is seen in the leukocyte morphology?

Explanation:

Hyposegmentation and hypogranulation in the leukocyte morphology are evidence of dyspoiesis.

Question:

4. Calculate the MCV. What peripheral blood findings are helpful to rule out megaloblastic anemia?

Explanation:

The MCV is calculated as 106 fL (170/1.6). The following peripheral blood findings help to rule out megaloblastic anemia: hyposegmentation of neutrophils rather than hypersegmentation, WBC count slightly elevated rather than decreased as is typical in megaloblastic anemia, and shift to the left with blasts is not characteristic of megaloblastic anemia.

Question:

5. What features of the differential resemble CML? What helps to distinguish this case from CML?

Explanation:

Increased eosinophils and all stages of granulocytes in the peripheral blood are found in both MDS and CML. The characteristics that differentiate these two groups are that the WBC count is too low for typical CML and RBC, and platelet counts are not usually decreased to this extent in CML.

Question:

6. Which of the hematopoietic cell lines exhibit dyshematopoiesis in the bone marrow?

Explanation:

All three cell lines (myeloid, erythroid, and megakaryocytic) exhibit dyshematopoiesis in the bone marrow.

Question:

7. How would you classify the bone marrow cellularity?

Explanation:

The bone marrow shows increased cellularity for a 65 year old; normal cellularity is 50% and decreases with age.

Question:

8. What does the M:E ratio indicate?

Explanation:

The M:E ratio indicates myeloid hyperplasia; a normal M:E ratio is 3:1 or 4:1.

Question:

9. Identify at least two features of the bone marrow that are compatible with a diagnosis of MDS.

Explanation:

Features in the bone marrow compatible with a diagnosis of MDS are increased blasts in the bone marrow (<30%), dyserythropoiesis, dysleukopoiesis, dysmegakaryopoiesis, and hypercellularity.

Question:

10. What chemistry tests would be helpful to rule out megaloblastic anemia?

Explanation:

Vitamin B_{12} and folate levels would be helpful to rule out megaloblastic anemia; values should be normal to increased, not decreased as would be seen in megaloblastic anemia.

Question:

11. What is the most likely MDS subgroup? Based upon what criteria?

Explanation:

The most likely MDS subgroup is RAEB based upon the following criteria: <5% blasts in the peripheral blood, 5–20% blasts in the bone marrow, cytopenia in at least two cell lines, and qualitative abnormalities in all cell lines.

Question:

12. Using the International Prognostic Scoring System (IPSS), what is the prognosis for this patient?

Explanation:

Use of the International Prognostic Scoring System (IPSS) on this patient is: 2 cytopenias = 0.5; 12% blasts in bone marrow = 1.5; complex karyotype with multiple abnormalities = 1.0. Total = 3.0 (high risk—median survival 0.4 yr).

CHAPTER 29

Case Summary: Mr. Guerro had bleeding symptoms when he was seen in the emergency room. A CBC was performed and revealed leukocytosis, anemia, and thrombocytopenia. The differential was abnormal with blasts and promyelocytes present. A bone marrow was performed. The M:E ratio was elevated at 7.8:1. The predominant cell was an abnormal promyelocyte. These cells had very heavy granulation and multiple Auer rods. The diagnosis is AML-M3 of the hypergranular type.

Question:

1. What clues do you have that this patient may have an acute leukemia?

Explanation:

There is anemia, increased WBC, decreased platelets, and most significantly blasts and promyelocytes on the peripheral blood smear.

Question:

2. Based on the presenting data, what additional testing might be of value?

Explanation:

A bone marrow should be performed. Other tests could include cytogenetics, molecular testing for the RAR-α/PML translocation.

Question:

3. Based on the peripheral blood examination, what cytochemical stain results would you expect to find on Mr. Guerro's neoplastic cells?

Explanation:

Myeloperoxidase, Sudan black B, and specific esterase should be positive as these cells are myeloid in origin.

Question:

4. If the cells from Mr. Guerro's bone marrow were immunophenotyped, which of the following would be positive? CD13, CD33, CD34, CD19, CD10, CD7, CD2.

Explanation:

When the APTT is abnormal and the PT is normal, the possible factor deficiencies are VIII, IX, XI, XII, prekallikrein, and high molecular weight kininogen.

Question:

7. What is the most likely factor deficiency? Why?

Explanation:

The most likely factor deficiency is factor VIII because it is the most common.

Question:

8. What do the results of the APTT on the mixture of Scott's plasma with normal plasma indicate?

Explanation:

The results of the mixing studies indicate that normal plasma corrected the patient's result. This indicates a factor deficiency rather than an inhibitor.

Question:

9. What test should be performed next?

Explanation:

A factor VIII assay should be performed next.

Question:

10. If a factor VIII assay was done with results of <1 U/dL, what molecular studies should be done?

Explanation:

Molecular studies for the inversion mutation in intron 22 should be done for all patients with severe factor VIII deficiency.

Question:

11. What therapy is indicated for this patient?

Explanation:

Therapy for factor VIII deficiency includes heat inactivated factor VIII concentrates and recombinant factor VIII.

Question:

12. What complications from the therapy are possible?

Explanation:

A complication of therapy that occurs in patients with hemophilia A, particularly those with the inversion mutation in intron 22, is the development of an inhibitor.

CHAPTER 38

Case Summary: The patient is a 37-year-old female who was diagnosed with deep vein thrombosis of the leg. She is dehydrated. She is on oral contraceptives and coumadin. Her family history revealed that paternal uncles and maternal cousins had thrombotic episodes. Testing for AT, PC, PS, fibrinogen, D-dimer, and plasminogen was done during the DVT episode and again 6 months later after she was off coumadin. All tests were within the reference range. Several years later she was tested and found to be heterozygous for Factor V_{Leiden} and prothrombin G20210.

Question:

1. What risk factors, if any, are revealed in the patient's history?

Explanation:

This patient had several risk factors for thrombosis, including dehydration and oral contraceptives. There is also a strong family history of thrombosis, suggesting a hereditary component in the etiology of her acute thrombotic event.

Question:

2. What other possibilities could explain the thrombotic event in this patient?

Explanation:

She was initially tested twice, since testing during an acute thrombotic episode or while on coumadin is not as informative as testing after the episode has resolved or when off anticoagulants. Unfortunately, neither set of tests helped establish a diagnosis, based on the available tests. Additional causes of hereditary thrombophilia could include activated protein C resistance; prothrombin mutation 20210; hyperhomocysteine; deficiencies of heparin cofactor II, TFPI, t-PA or factor XII; elevated fibrinogen, factor VIII, or PAI-1.

Question:

3. Why is the patient at greater risk for a thrombotic event than her mother or her two sisters?

Explanation:

Specific molecular assays were subsequently done of the family, and they revealed two mutations: both the V_{Leiden} and prothrombin 20210 mutations. The fact that both these mutations were found in the same family probably accounts for the strong family history. The patient had inherited two different genetic mutations, both of which carry an increased risk of thrombosis. In addition she had several other clinical risk factors, probably contributing to her thrombotic event. Since the mother and sisters had a single genetic mutation, their risk of thrombosis was probably less than that of A.C. The patient was taken off oral contraceptives and put back on coumadin.

APPENDIX B

Answers to Checkpoints

Chapter 1

Checkpoint! #1

What cellular component of blood may be involved in disorders of hemostasis?

Answer:

The platelets are involved in hemostasis.

Checkpoint! #2

Is reflex testing suggested by these results?

Answer:

The girl has a decreased hemoglobin and increased WBC count. Reflex testing is suggested to help identify the cause of these abnormal results. A differential will identify the types of leukocytes that are present in increased concentrations and give clues to the diagnosis. Further laboratory testing can also help identify the cause of the anemia.

Chapter 2

Checkpoint! #1

A cell undergoing mitosis fails to attach one of its duplicated chromosomes to the microtubules of the spindle apparatus during metaphase. The cell's metaphase checkpoint malfunctions and does not detect the error. What is the effect (if any) on the daughter cells produced?

Answer:

If one of the paired (duplicated) sister chromatids fails to attach to the mitotic spindle during metaphase, the duplicated chromosomes will not separate during anaphase and telophase. If the cell does not catch this mistake, and cytokinesis completes anyway, one daughter cell will have two copies of that chromosome and the other daughter cell will have none. Both cells are said to be aneuploid (i.e., have an abnormal number of chromosomes).

Checkpoint! #2

What would be the effect on the hematopoietic system homeostasis if the expanded clone of antigen-activated B lymphocytes failed to undergo apoptosis after the antigenic challenge was removed?

Answer:

The result would be an accumulation of excess lymphocytes and a progressive lymphocytosis.

Checkpoint! #3

Hematopoietic stem cells that have initiated a differentiation program are sometimes described as undergoing death by differentiation. Explain.

Answer:

When a hematopoietic stem cell makes the commitment to differentiate, it begins a maturation process that will culminate in what we call terminally differentiated cells—i.e., cells that have lost the capacity to divide and have a finite (limited) life span. Thus the process of differentiation "dooms" the cell to eventual death.

Checkpoint! #4

Cytokine control of hematopoiesis is said to be characterized by redundancy and pleiotrophy. What does this mean?

Answer:

Redundancy refers to the fact that many different cytokines do the same thing—i.e., GM-CSF and IL-3 have overlapping (nearly identical) activities. IL-11 and TPO both stimulate platelet production (although TPO is the more important cytokine, physiologically). Redundancy is a good thing, as it assures the organism that if a mutation knocks out a regulatory gene, there are additional cytokines that can take over and substitute for the lost activity. At least part of the explanation for redundancy may be the "shared receptor chains" that have been identified for certain groups of cytokines.

Pleiotrophy refers to the fact that a single cytokine often has multiple activities, often on multiple target cells.

Checkpoint! #5

Individuals with congenital defects of the γ-chain of the IL-2 receptor suffer from profound defects of lymphopoiesis, far greater than individuals with congenital defects of the α-chain of the IL-2 receptor. Why?

Answer:

The γ-chain of the IL-2 receptor is shared with five other cytokines, all important in regulating lymphopoiesis—IL-4, IL-7, IL-9, IL-11, and IL-15. Thus a disabling mutation of the γ-chain results in loss of physiologic activity of all six cytokines, whereas mutations affecting the α-chain only compromise the physiologic activity of a single cytokine, IL-2.

Checkpoint! #6

Mutations of proto-oncogenes predisposing to malignancy are said to be dominant mutations, while mutations of antioncogenes are said to behave as recessive mutations, requiring loss of both alleles. Explain this difference in behavior of the gene products.

Answer:

Immunophenotyping is necessary to differentiate T cell ALL from B cell ALL, and mature B cell ALL from precurser B cell ALL. Treatment and prognosis in these different subtypes differ.

Checkpoint! #6

What is the absolute CD4 count? Is this count compatible with a diagnosis of AIDS in an HIV infected individual?

Answer:

$5 \times 10^9/L \times 0.30 = 1.5 \times 10^9/L \times 10\% = 0.15 \times 10^9/L$ (150/μL)
A CD4 count less than 200/μL is diagnostic of AIDS in an HIV infected individual.

Checkpoint! #7

What are the advantages of automated reticulocyte counting over manual counts?

Answer:

Many more cells are counted in automated counts than in manual counts. Automated counts by flow cytometry can determine the maturity of the cells.

Chapter 24

Checkpoint! #1

A newborn baby boy has multiple congenital malformations, and a chromosome abnormality is suspected as the cause. What is the most appropriate specimen to submit for chromosome analysis? How should the laboratory professional process the specimen?

Answer:

The most appropriate specimen to determine the presence of a congenital aberration is peripheral blood. The specimen should be processed by culture stimulated with phytohemagglutinin to stimulate mitosis of the circulating lymphocytes.

Checkpoint! #2

Cytogenetic studies were performed on a bone marrow specimen from a female patient with a myelodysplastic state with the following results:

> *one cell—47,XX,+8*
> *one cell—45,XX,–20*
> *five cells—46,XX,del(5)(q13q34),–7,+21*

Which of these aberrations are clonal? What term would apply to the five cells?

Answer:

The clonal aberrations are the del(5), –7, and +21. The +8 and –20 are seen in only one cell each and are therefore nonclonal. The five abnormal cells would be referred to as pseudodiploid.

Checkpoint! #3

A 35-year-old man has acute leukemia. Cytogenetic studies of the bone marrow reveal the following: 46,XY,t(15;17)(q22;q11.2). What type of leukemia does this patient have, and what will cytogenetic studies show after treatment if he achieves complete remission?

Answer:

The t(15;17) is diagnostic for acute promyelocytic leukemia, AML-M3. If the patient achieved complete remission, cytogenetic analysis of bone marrow cells would show a normal male karyotype.

Checkpoint! #4

Five years ago a 46-year-old woman received chemotherapy and radiation treatment for breast cancer. She now has pancytopenia. Cytogenetic analysis of the bone marrow is performed and shows 10 of 20 cells with the following: 45,XX,del(5)(q13q34),–7. What is the significance of this finding?

Answer:

These results show clonal acquired aberrations indicative of a malignant cell line. The del(5) and –7 are consistent with a secondary myelodysplastic state/acute leukemia.

Checkpoint! #5

A 5-year-old girl has fatigue and easy bruising. A CBC shows a leukocyte count of 40 × 10⁹/L with 85% blasts. Bone marrow cytogenetic studies are performed and show all cells with the following karyotype: 53,XX,+X,+4,+6,+10,+18,+20,+21. What is the prognostic significance of this finding?

Answer:

This karyotype in a pediatric aged patient with acute lymphocytic leukemia would correlate with a good prognosis.

Chapter 25

Checkpoint! #1

A 40-year-old male is diagnosed with an inherited disease for which a specific point mutation is responsible. His mother died of a similar disease 10 years ago. For purposes of family counseling, the physician wants to know if she had the same mutation. The histology laboratory has archival paraffin-embedded tissue from the mother. What laboratory method(s) are best for detecting the gene mutation?

Answer:

PCR and DNA sequencing are often used to detect point mutations in paraffin-embedded tissue. In most cases, paraffin-embedded tissue is not amenable to Southern blot analysis. In situ hybridization and FISH are not good choices for detecting point mutations.

Checkpoint! #2

A patient with CML was treated with chemotherapy. On subsequent marrow samples the physician ordered molecular testing for residual disease after treatment. The BCR/ABL mutation was not detected 4 months after treatment but was detected at the 8th and 9th months after treatment. Interpret this result.

Answer:

The BCR/ABL translocation may be detected for several months after successful therapy, presumably because some of the tumor cells have been damaged but have not yet died. However, the longer after therapy it is found, and if it is persistent over several tests or if it reappears after previous negative testing, the greater the likelihood of relapse.

Checkpoint! #3

An enlarged lymph node was biopsied and sent to the laboratory for molecular analysis. Lymphoma was suspected. What molecular test(s) could be done on the specimen to determine if the node is malignant and to determine if the cells are of T or B cell origin?

Answer:

Detection of clonal immunoglobulin or TCR gene rearrangement by PCR or Southern blot can be used to differentiate clonal from polyclonal proliferation. Clonal gene rearrangement is characteristic of malignant tumors. B cell tumors usually have clonal rearrangements of Ig heavy chain and kappa light chains. T cell tumors usually have clonal rearrangement of TCRβ and TCRγ genes. Further classification of a lymphoma is aided by molecular tests for translocations such as BCL1/IgH in mantle cell lymphoma, BCL2/IgH in folicular lymphoma, or MYC translocation in Burkitt's lymphoma.

Chapter 26

Checkpoint! #1

A 62-year-old male presents with an elevated leukocyte count, mild anemia, and a slightly decreased platelet count. His physician suspects leukemia. Explain why the erythrocytes and platelets would be affected.

Answer:

Leukemia is a stem cell disorder in which all cell progeny are involved. If the patient has the suspected leukemia, he would experience an unregulated production of neoplastic cells. As the neoplastic cell population increases, the concentration of normal cells, like the platelets and erythrocytes, decreases.

Checkpoint! #2

Does a 3-year-old child with Down syndrome have an increased likelihood of developing leukemia? Why or why not?

Answer:

Yes, some individuals with congenital abnormalities associated with karyotypic abnormalities have a markedly increased risk of developing acute leukemias.

Checkpoint! #3

A patient has 50% monoblasts in the bone marrow. Which of the four major types of leukemia does he have, AML, CML, ALL, or CLL?

Answer:

A patient with 50% monoblasts in the bone marrow has AML. ALL and CLL can be eliminated due to their lymphoid lineage, and CML <30% (WHO <20%) blasts in the bone marrow.

Checkpoint! #4

Why is the finding of Auer rods an important factor in the diagnosis of leukemia?

Answer:

Auer rods can be found in the blast cells and promyelocytes of some acute myeloid leukemias. The finding of Auer rods can help establish the diagnosis because these unique, pink-staining inclusions are not found in ALL.

Checkpoint! #5

A pathology resident is evaluating the peripheral blood smear of a 40-year-old male. He suspects a diagnosis of CML. In order to confirm his suspicion, he ordered a LAP score. Do you think that ordering a LAP score will help him in making the right diagnosis?

Answer:

The LAP score is usually decreased in patients with CML. It can be used to differentiate a leukemoid reaction from CML. However, patients with CML in blast crisis, who have a high number of circulating blasts, can have an increased score. Although a leukemoid reaction has a shift to the left, it is not characterized by the presence of blasts.

Checkpoint! #6

A 30-year-old male presented to the emergency room complaining of fatigue, weakness, and gum bleeding. The CBC showed anemia, thrombocytopenia, and a WBC of 30 × 10⁹/L. Evaluation of the peripheral blood smear showed numerous intermediate to large blasts with fine nuclear chromatin and abundant cytoplasm. The bone marrow biopsy contained 60% blasts. No Auer rods were seen after careful evaluation. Several cytochemical stains were then performed. The blasts failed to stain with myeloperoxidase, Sudan black B, and specific esterase; however, the majority of blasts reacted intensely with α-naphthyl esterase. Incubation with sodium fluoride inhibited the staining seen with α-naphthyl esterase. What type of leukemia do you think this patient has?

Answer:

Alpha-naphthyl esterase stains primarily monocytes and its precursors; therefore, it is useful in the diagnosis of acute leukemias with a monocytic component such as acute monocytic and myelomonocytic leukemias. However, other bone marrow elements can also show staining with α-naphthyl esterase. That is why the fluoride inhibition test is recommended. In this test, sodium fluoride is added to the α-naphthyl esterase incubation mix. Sodium fluoride inhibits the monocytic enzyme. In our patient the blasts failed to stain in the mix containing the fluoride, confirming the monocytic differentiation. The predominance of staining with α-naphthyl esterase and the absence of staining with myeloperoxidase, Sudan black B, and specific esterase indicate that this patient most likely has acute monocytic leukemia (AML-M5).

Checkpoint! #7

A pathologist is reviewing the slides from the pleural fluid of a 50-year-old male who has hepatosplenomegaly and minimal lymphadenopathy. It is not clear if the mononuclear cells are mature lymphoma cells or leukemic blasts. There is not enough material for flow cytometry to do immunophenotyping, but there is enough to make a few extra cytospin smears. Which stain do you think can be useful in this case?

Answer:

A TdT stain will be very useful. TdT is a DNA polymerase found in the nuclei of immature lymphocytes and is present in the majority of ALL cases. TdT is a primitive cell marker and is of value in distinguishing ALL from malignant lymphoma. It is also helpful in defining leukemic cells in body fluids.

Checkpoint! #8

A patient has 35% blasts in the bone marrow. They do not show any specific characteristics that will allow them to be classified according to cell lineage. What are the next steps that the CLS should take with this specimen?

Answer:

Cytochemistry will help establish cell lineage as myeloid or lymphoid. An immunologic analysis would provide information on what specific membrane antigens are on the blast cells. By using a panel of monoclonal antibodies, the cells' lineage can usually be determined because specific surface markers are characteristically found on each particular cell line. Genetic analysis can also be performed as some cytogenetic chromosome karyotypes are commonly found in certain types of leukemia.

Chapter 27

Checkpoint! #1

In essential thrombocythemia, all hematopoietic lines have increased cell proliferation. Which lineage has the greatest increase?

Answer:

The megakaryocytic cell line is increased in essential thrombocythemia.

Checkpoint! #2

A patient has the CML phenotype but the genetic karyotype does not show the Philadelphia chromosome. If this is truly a CML, what should molecular analysis show?

Answer:

Molecular analysis would show a BCR/ABL gene rearrangement in a new fused hybrid gene.

Checkpoint! #3

Describe the peripheral blood differential of a CML patient.

Answer:

There is a shift to the left in granulocytes with high numbers of myelocytes and promyelocytes. If blasts are present, they compose less than 30% of cells (<20% with WHO classification).

Checkpoint! #4

What clinical, peripheral blood, and genetic features differentiate CML from an infectious process?

Answer:

An extreme peripheral blood leukocytosis—segmented neutrophils with a left shift showing many myelocytes, some promyelocytes, and blasts are found in CML. Age of the patient and absence of infection, low LAP score, and presence of the Philadelphia chromosome or BCR/ABL translocation all are hallmarks for CML.

Checkpoint! #5

What one feature separates other forms of MPD from CML?

Answer:

The Philadelphia chromosome occurs in CML.

Checkpoint! #6

What growth factors are primarily responsible for stimulating fibrogenesis in the bone marrow?

Answer:

Platelet derived growth factor (PDGF) and transforming growth factor-beta (TGF-ß) are increased and associated with marrow fibrosis.

Checkpoint! #7

What erythrocyte morphologic feature is a hallmark for myelofibrosis?

Answer:

The finding of dacryocytes (teardrop erythrocytes) is a hallmark for myelofibrosis with myeloid metaplasia.

Checkpoint! #8

Which of the following conditions are associated with an absolute increase in red cell mass? Iron deficiency, smoking, emphysema, pregnancy, or dehydration.

Answer:

Smoking, emphysema, and pregnancy are conditions in which additional red cells are needed to prevent a physiologic anemia. Iron deficiency prevents the formation of additional red cells. Dehydration causes a relative red cell mass increase due to decreased plasma volume.

Checkpoint! #9

Renal tumors may produce an inappropriate amount of EPO, resulting in what type of polycythemia?

Answer:

Secondary polycythemia, or increase of red cell mass due to an identifiable cause.

Checkpoint! #10

Is a patient who has a platelet count of 846 × 10⁹/L, splenomegaly, and abnormal platelet function tests of hyperaggregation likely to have reactive or essential thrombocytosis?

Answer:

This patient is likely to have essential thromobocytosis. Patients with reactive thrombocytosis rarely have platelet counts greater than 1,000 × 10⁹/L, but neither would they have splenomegaly or thrombotic complications.

Chapter 28

Checkpoint! #1

How does the typical peripheral blood picture in MDS differ from aplastic anemia?

Answer:

The typical blood picture in aplastic anemia is pancytopenia, a significant decrease in all three cell populations (∞ Chapter 15). In MDS, cytopenia is present in the peripheral blood in one cell line or more. Pancytopenia has been estimated to occur in only 19% of cases of MDS. Both MDS and aplastic anemia can be macrocytic. MDS exhibits more frequent qualitative abnormalities indicating dyspoiesis, such as anisocytosis, poikilocytosis, basophilic stippling, Howell-Jolly bodies, and nucleated RBCs. The neutrophils often show abnormal granulation and pseudo–Pelger-Huët cells. Giant and hypogranular platelets may be seen. The bone marrow would be the best way to differentiate the two syndromes. A hypoplastic bone marrow is typical in aplastic anemia. MDS usually shows a hypercellular marrow but if it is hypocellular, it may be difficult to differentiate from aplastic anemia.

Checkpoint! #2

Why is serum vitamin B$_{12}$, serum folate level, or bone marrow iron stain important in the diagnosis of MDS?

Answer:

Some features of the blood picture in MDS resemble the megaloblastic anemias (macrocytosis, megaloblastoid changes in erythrocytic precursor cells). A normal serum vitamin B$_{12}$ and/or folate level would rule out megaloblastic anemia. An iron stain on the bone marrow will allow assessment of the presence of ringed sideroblasts, which would be necessary for a diagnosis of RA or RARS.

Checkpoint! #3

Why is it important to correctly identify the number of blasts when evaluating the peripheral blood or bone marrow smear of a patient suspected of having MDS?

Answer:

The number of blasts is used to classify the MDS into different subtypes and to predict prognosis and treatment. It is also used to differentiate MDS from acute leukemia.

Chapter 29

Checkpoint! #1

What results would you expect to find on the CBC and differential in a suspected case of acute leukemia?

Answer:

You would expect a normocytic, normochromic anemia, decrease in platelets with some large forms present, neutropenia, monocytosis, and on the differential blast cells, an increase in eosinophils and basophils.

Checkpoint! #2

What is the major difference between the FAB and WHO classification systems in differentiating acute leukemia from the other neoplastic hematologic disorders?

Answer:

In the WHO classification the minimum blast count compatible with AL is 20%, while in the FAB classification the minimum is 30%.

Checkpoint! #3

Explain why molecular analysis is not performed on all suspected cases of AL.

Answer:

The molecular aberrations are not known for all AL and, thus, probes are not available. Those in which an aberration is commonly present and can be probed for are AML-M3 and the ALL.

Checkpoint! #4

What hematologic feature helps differentiate M0 from M1?

Answer:

Cytochemical stains in M0 are negative, but some of the blasts in M1 have a positive reaction with myeloperoxidase and/or Sudan black B. Both have myeloid antigens, CD13 and CD33.

Checkpoint! #5

A patient with AML has a peripheral blood differential that includes 91% myeloblasts, 3% promyelocytes, 3% granulocytes, and 3% monocytes. Is this an M1 or M2 AML? Explain.

Answer:

This is an M1. There are >90% myeloblasts. In M2 there are <90% myeloblasts.

Checkpoint! #6

Why is it important to do molecular studies on patients with AML-M3?

Answer:

The RAR-α/PML abnormality is diagnostic of M3. Those with this translocation respond to therapy with all trans-retinoic acid. If the translocation disappears after therapy and then reappears, relapse can be predicted.

Checkpoint! #7

How are M5A and M5B differentiated, and what is the significance of making the distinction?

Answer:

In M5A, >80% of the monocytic cells are monoblasts. In M5B, there are <80% monoblasts. Classification, as in all the AL, is important as it may provide information on the aggressiveness of disease and the response to therapeutic regimens.

Checkpoint! #8

What is the differentiating hematologic feature of M6 that allows it to be subgrouped?

Answer:

More than 50% of the bone marrow cells are erythroid and 30% or more of the remaining cells are blasts.

Checkpoint! #9

Predict the peripheral blood picture of a patient on antifolate chemotherapy.

Answer:

There would be a megaloblastic blood picture including pancytopenia with a macrocytic anemia.

Chapter 30

Checkpoint! #1

Compare the typical age groups in which AML and ALL are found.

Answer:

The AMLs are characteristically found in adults, while the ALLs are typically found in children. The ALL-L2 subgroup is the most common ALL found in adults. The AML-MI is most common in adults and in infants less than one year of age.

Checkpoint! #2

Contrast the malignant neoplastic cells in ALL with those found in AML.

Answer:

Myeloblasts are generally larger than lymphoblasts. They have more abundant grayish cytoplasm. The nucleus has fine chromatin and prominent nucleoli. Lymphoblasts have scant, blue cytoplasm. The nucleus has coarser chromatin, and the nucleoli are inconspicuous. The ALL and AML blasts cannot be definitively identified by morphology alone as there is considerable heterogeneity from that described above. Cytochemistry is helpful in determining cell lineage. The myeloperoxidase and Sudan black B are positive in myeloblasts and negative in lymphoblasts. Immunophenotyping is helpful also. The myeloblasts are positive for CD13 and CD33, while lymphoblasts are negative for these antigens.

Checkpoint! #3

Contrast the morphology of blasts found in L1, L2, and L3.

Answer:

The L1 blasts are small and homogeneous. The nucleus is regular in shape with occasional clefts or indentations, and the chromatin is fine. Nucleoli are not prominent and may not be visible. The cytoplasm is scant. The L2 blasts are heterogenous and larger than in L1. The nucleus is irregular in shape with prominent nucleoli. There is a moderate to abundant amount of cytoplasm. The L3 blasts are large cells with abundant, intensely blue cytoplasm. There are prominent vacuoles in the cytoplasm. Nucleoli are visible.

Checkpoint! #4

Why is it necessary to immunophenotype the lymphoblasts in ALL if they have been identified as lymphoblasts morphologically?

Answer:

The lymphoblasts should be immunophenotyped to determine if they are of T or B cell origin. This information has treatment and prognostic implications.

Checkpoint! #5

A patient has 50% blasts in his bone marrow. Cytochemical stains are negative with peroxidase and Sudan black B. Immunophenotyping is CD19-positive, but CD20-, CD2-, CD10-, and CD7-negative. What additional testing may be helpful to distinguish the immunologic subgroup of this leukemia?

Answer:

These appear to be lymphoblasts by cytochemistry results. The cells have the B cell antigen CD19, but are negative for other B cell markers, CD10 and CD20. Cells are negative for the T cell markers CD2 and CD7. This may be a very early progenitor B ALL. It would be helpful to test for the CD34 marker and the presence of TdT. These are markers of very early cells. Molecular testing for the rearrangement of the immunoglobulin genes may also help determine if these are B cells.

Checkpoint! #6

A 3-year-old patient has 45% lymphoblasts in the bone marrow. The blasts are slightly larger than lymphocytes and appear to be a homogeneous population. The nuclear membrane is regular, and nucleoli are not prominent. There is a small amount of moderately basophilic cytoplasm. What is the most likely FAB group of this leukemia? If the cells tested positive for CD19, CD10, and CD34, what is the most likely immunologic subgroup? Why should cytogenetics be done on this patient?

Answer:

The description of the blasts best fits the L1 FAB subgroup. These markers suggest the early pre-B immunologic subgroup. Cytogenetics is important in ALL to provide prognostic information.

Checkpoint! #7

A patient with acute leukemia has two morphologically different types of blasts. One population is positive for CD7 and CD2. The other is positive for CD33 and CD13. What is the most appropriate classification of this leukemia?

Answer:

This is most likely an acute leukemia with lineage heterogeneity. Since the lineage associated markers are found on two different sets of blasts, it is most likely a bilineage acute leukemia. The blasts appear by immunophenotype to be myeloblasts and T lymphoblasts.

Checkpoint! #8

How can the neoplastic cells in myeloid/NK cell AL be differentiated from the neoplastic cells of AML-M3 if they appear morphologically similar?

Answer:

There are no faggot cells in myeloid/NK AL but they are typically found in AML-M3 cells. The diagnostic translocation, t(15;17), of AML-M3 is not found in myeloid/NK AL. The cells in myeloid/NK AL have cell-mediated cytotoxicity, while the AML-M3 cells do not.

Chapter 31

Checkpoint! #1

How does the BCL-2 gene rearrangement differ from most other oncogenes?

Answer:

The BCL-2 gene rearrangement leads to persistence of cells due to an inhibition of apoptosis rather than uncontrolled cell proliferation.

Checkpoint! #2

How does staging differ from grading in defining and classifying the lymphoid malignancies?

Answer:

Stage is the extent and distribution of disease, while classification is the separation of grades of lymphoma and often uses a combination of morphology, phenotype, and genotype.

Checkpoint! #3

The chronic lymphoid leukemic malignancies are a heterogeneous group. What characteristics allow them to be grouped together?

Answer:

The chronic lymphoid leukemic malignancies are grouped together because the malignant cell is a mature lymphocyte, and these cells are found in the blood and bone marrow (leukemic distribution).

Checkpoint! #4

What cell characteristically distinguishes Hodgkin lymphoma from non-Hodgkin lymphoma? Describe this cell.

Answer:

The Reed-Sternberg cell characteristically distinguishes Hodgkin lymphoma from non-Hodgkin lymphoma. It has two or more nuclear lobes containing inclusion-like nucleoli and an area of perinucleolar clearing (owl's eye appearance).

Checkpoint! #5

What clinical finding differentiates multiple myeloma from other plasma cell neoplasms?

Answer:

The presence of multiple lytic bone lesions differentiates multiple myeloma from other plasma cell neoplasms.

Chapter 32

Checkpoint! #1

A physician is evaluating a 28-year-old patient with a history of acute lymphoblastic leukemia for PBSC transplantation. The laboratory professional found circulating leukemic blasts in the peripheral blood. Is this patient a candidate for an autologous PBSC transplant?

Answer:

Presence of circulating blasts in a patient who is being evaluated for the autologous PBSC is not a good sign. Since PBSCs are collected from the person's peripheral blood by apheresis technology, the stem cell product in this patient would definitely contain leukemic blasts. It would be almost impossible to separate these leukemic blasts from the normal stem cells even by purging. Therefore autologous PBSC transplant is not an option for this patient at least at this point. The search for the matched allogeneic stem cell donor should be made.

Checkpoint! #2

A patient with CML needs a stem cell transplant. What would be the best form of transplant for him, and what antigen type needs to be matched?

Answer:

CML is a stem cell disorder, which means the patient's own stem cells are affected by the disease. Therefore the best form of transplant for this patient is an allogeneic stem cell transplant. For this allogeneic transplant, the patient and donor should be matched for HLA-A, -B and -DR antigens. ABO antigens are tested for both donor and patient; however, the matching is not required for the allogeneic stem cell transplant.

Checkpoint! #3

You receive a peripheral blood specimen in the hematology laboratory with a request for a mononuclear cell count and analysis of CD34+ cells. Without any further information, why should you consider this a STAT request?

Answer:

The volume of cells necessary to achieve a successful engraftment may be determined indirectly by the MNC count or the CD34+ count. A clinical decision can be made to collect more cells depending on these counts. The timing of the collection of the stem cells also may be determined based on these counts.

Checkpoint! #4

A physician wants to evaluate the engraftment on a male patient who received SCT from his brother four months ago. What laboratory tests should be performed to make this assessment?

Answer:

To evaluate the long-term engraftment of HSCs, various laboratory methods have evolved. Currently, the most widely used tests are in situ hybridization (ISH) with sex chromosome and typing of variable number tandem repeat (VNTR) polymorphism by DNA amplification. The ISH is applicable in cases when the donor and recipient are of different sex. In this case, the VNTR polymorphism by DNA amplification to distinguish donor and recipient cells must be performed.

Checkpoint! #5

A CMV-seronegative patient requires SCT. Two HLA-matched donors are available. Is it important to know the CMV status of the stem cell donor? If the stem cell donor is CMV-seronegative and the patient requires red cell transfusion during the peritransplant period, what blood components (in terms of CMV status) would you select for this patient?

Answer:

The CMV-seropositive person (i.e., a subject who shows serologic evidence of prior CMV exposure) can be an SCT donor to a CMV-seronegative recipient. However, if two HLA-compatible donors are available for a CMV-seronegative patient, the preference is given to the donor who is seronegative for CMV. The rationale is that CMV infection can be fatal in the peritransplant setting. However, if the CMV-seronegative donor is not available but a matched CMV-seropositive donor is available, transplant can still be performed. Most transplant physicians believe that a CMV-seronegative recipient should receive CMV-seronegative cellular blood components if the stem cells' donor is also CMV-seronegative. If the CMV-negative blood component is not available, transfusing a leukocyte reduced filtered component may effectively prevent the transmission of CMV disease.

Chapter 33

Checkpoint! #1

To obtain a sample of cerebrospinal fluid for anlaysis, the needle must be inserted into what area of the central nervous system?

Answer:

Subarachnoid space.

Checkpoint! #2

A 32-year-old woman has right-sided chest pain and shortness of breath that has worsened over a two-week period. Chest radiologic studies reveal a right pleural effusion, and a thoracentesis is performed. The pleural fluid specimen on cytocentrifuged, Wright-stained slide reveals cells similar to that seen in Figure 33-7. What is the best interpretation of this finding? If there is a strong concern that this may represent a low-grade lymphoma, what would be the best way to determine whether these are benign or malignant lymphocytes?

Answer:

These cells are benign lymphocytes with the artifact of a pale staining area resembling nucleoli. These are not blasts because of the mature chromatin. Immunophenotyping by flow cytometry of the pleural fluid would be the best way to determine whether this is a benign or malignant population of lymphocytes.

Checkpoint! #3

When examining a cytocentrifuged, Wright-stained slide of a body fluid specimen, what are the best features to use in determining if tissue cells are benign or malignant?

Answer:

Nuclear features are the best features to use to distinguish benign and malignant cells. These include: nuclear membrane (smooth or irregular), chromatin pattern (regular or irregular distribution), and nucleoli (present or absent, nucleolar membrane smooth or irregular).

Checkpoint! #4

A 47-year-old man is found comatose at home by his wife. During examination in the emergency room a spinal tap is performed and grossly bloody spinal fluid is obtained. The total red blood cell count in the first tube is the same as that in the third tube. A cytocentrifuged, Wright-stained slide shows findings similar to that seen in Figure 33-54. What is the most appropriate interpretation?

Answer:

There has been a true subarachnoid hemorrhage.

Checkpoint! #5

A 57-year-old man has an acutely swollen, painful, reddened joint in his left great toe. Joint fluid is aspirated, and a photomicrograph is taken (Figure 33-69). This picture is taken with polarized light using a quartz compensator. What is the most appropriate interpretation of this finding?

Answer:

There are both monosodium urate and calcium pyrophosphate crystals present.

Chapter 34

Checkpoint! #1

Think about the last time that you injured your finger with a paper cut. Did your finger bleed immediately? If not, what might have prevented immediate bleeding?

Answer:

No. Vasoconstriction of the blood vessels.

Checkpoint! #2

What actions of the endothelial cells prevent clotting from occurring within the blood vessels?

Answer:

They have a negatively charged surface that repels clotting factors and platelets in the normal peripheral blood circulation. They synthesize heparan sulfate and thrombomodulin, which inhibit fibrin formation. They synthesize PGI_2, which inhibits platelet activation. They synthesize tPA and PAI-1, which control fibrinolysis.

Checkpoint! #3

What would be the effect on the platelet count if a patient had a mutation in the gene for thrombopoietin that resulted in inability of the gene to code for functional mRNA?

Answer:

The platelet count would be decreased.

Checkpoint! #4

If a patient has a mutation in the gene for thrombopoietin that resulted in inability of the gene to code for mRNA, how would you expect the number of megakaryocytes seen on bone marrow smears to be affected?

Answer:

The number of megakaryocytes in the bone marrow would be decreased.

Checkpoint! #5

If a patient inherited a mutation of the gene for glycoprotein IIIa that resulted in its absence, what two platelet antigens would be decreased or absent?

Answer:

HPA-1 and HPA-3.

Checkpoint! #6

If a patient with Bernard-Soulier disease or von Willebrand disease cut a finger, would you expect bleeding to stop as fast as the bleeding stops when you cut your own finger? Why?

Answer:

No. Because their platelets would be unable to adhere to collagen and the primary hemostatic plug would take longer to form to halt the bleeding.

Checkpoint! #7

Your finger is still bleeding at this point, but the platelets are aggregating to form the primary hemostatic plug. Let's review the key events:
a. To what do platelets first adhere?

b. *What bridge and what platelet membrane receptor are needed for platelet adhesion?*

c. *What bridge and what platelet membrane receptor are needed for platelets to attach to one another?*

d. *What is the attachment of platelets to one another called?*

Answer:

a. Collagen

b. Von Willebrand factor and glycoprotein Ib/IX

c. Fibrinogen and glycoprotein IIb/IIIA

d. Platelet aggregation

Checkpoint! #8

Your finger has now stopped bleeding. Outline the steps of primary hemostasis that have occurred.

Answer:

The blood vessels have undergone vasoconstriction and are by now possibly beginning to dilate. Platelet adhesion, platelet aggregation, platelet secretion, and formation of the primary hemostatic plug have occurred.

Chapter 35

Checkpoint! #1

What is the major distinction between the so-called extrinsic and intrinsic pathways?

Answer:

Both pathways require enzymes and protein cofactors originally present in plasma; however, the extrinsic pathway also requires an activator (tissue factor) that is not found in the blood under normal circumstances.

Checkpoint! #2

Will a patient who is vitamin K-deficient produce any of the vitamin K-dependent factors? Why is vitamin K so vital to the formation of coagulation complexes?

Answer:

A patient who is vitamin K-deficient will still synthesize the proteins but will fail to attach the extra carboxyl group to the γ-carbon of glutamic acid residues in the GLA domains of the protein, which is required for full functional activity of the proteins. The γ-carboxy-form of the proteins is required for Ca^{2+}-mediated interaction with phospholipid surfaces, which is required for formation of the coagulation activation complexes.

Checkpoint! #3

Why are the domains of the serine proteases involved in blood clotting so important in the hemostatic mechanism?

Answer:

The catalytic domain of the protease converts a zymogen to its active form. The various noncatalytic domains of the serine proteases contain the regulatory elements of the proteins, and are responsible for conferring the specificity of activation and activity of each enzyme. They bind calcium, promote interaction with phospholipids, cofactors, receptors, and substrates.

Checkpoint! #4

Which components of the intrinsic pathway are believed to be essential for in vivo hemostasis?

Answer:

Factors IX, VIII, and possibly factor XI. Factor XII, prekallikrein, and HMW kininogen are not essential for normal in vivo hemostasis.

Checkpoint! #5

Historically, the major importance for initiating coagulation was assigned to either the intrinsic or the extrinsic pathway. What are some observations that suggest that the classic concepts were not accurate?

Answer:

Thrombin can activate factor XI, bypassing the need for contact activation by factor XII/kallikrein/HK. Factor IX can be activated by factor VIIa, as well as factor XIa (again, bypassing the need for contact activation). Thus, initiation of coagulation by tissue factor/factor VII is sufficient to initiate activation of both pathways. However, full escalation of the coagulation system requires proteins of both pathways.

Checkpoint! #6

What are the three steps in the formation of an insoluble fibrin clot?

Answer:

(1) Hydrolytic **cleavage** of fibrinopeptides A and B by thrombin, forming a fibrin monomer. (2) Spontaneous **polymerization** of fibrin monomers to form fibrin polymers. (3) **Stabilization** of the fibrin polymers by factor XIIIa.

Checkpoint! #7

Why is the process of fibrinolysis a vital part of the hemostatic mechanism? Why must it be closely regulated and controlled?

Answer:

Fibrinolysis is needed to restore the blood vessel structure and function to normal when the fibrin clot is no longer needed. It is essential to balance the activity of the procoagulant proteins. If activity of fibrinolysis is deficient, the result is thrombosis; if fibrinolysis is excessive, the result is hemorrhage.

Checkpoint! #8

Why are the plasmin degradation products of fibrinogen and fibrin different?

Answer:

Plasmin cleaves at the same place on molecules of either fibrin or fibrinogen (at the coiled regions, midway between the terminal D domains and the C-central domain). In fibrinogen, this produces separate D and E fragments. However, because fibrin monomers have been covalently crosslinked by factor XIIIa, complexes of various combinations (particularly the so-called D-dimer) are formed. The presence of D-dimer confirms that both the procoagulant system (thrombin) and the fibrinolytic system (plasmin) have been activated.

Checkpoint! #9

Why are naturally occurring inhibitors important in the hemostatic mechanism?

Answer:

Naturally occurring inhibitors help control the activity of the coagulation and fibrinolytic proteases, so that they are inactive when distant from a site of vessel damage, which helps to limit clot formation to areas of vessel injury. They are essential in preventing unwarranted initiation or excessive amplification of the coagulation cascade.

Chapter 36

Checkpoint! #1

Assume that you are the clinical laboratory scientist collecting a blood specimen from a patient with a suspected bleeding disorder. You noticed petechiae and several bruises on the patient's arm. What screening tests would the physician likely have ordered? What results of these tests would your expect (normal or abnormal) in this patient?

Answer:

The physician would likely have ordered a platelet count, prothrombin time, and activated partial thromboplastin time as screening tests. The presence of petechiae indicates a platelet abnormality. The most common platelet abnormality is thrombocytopenia. Therefore, you would expect the platelet count to be decreased. The prothrombin and activated partial thromboplastin times are normal in platelet abnormalities that are not complicated or accompanied by abnormalities of fibrin formation.

Checkpoint! #2

If you observed an average of 14 platelets on a peripheral blood smear prepared from the needle tip and your laboratory allowed correlation between the direct instrument count and the blood smear estimate of 20%, what range would you expect the instrument count to be? Is this platelet estimate within an acceptable reference range?

Answer:

Average of 14 platelets $\times$ 15 $\times$ 10^9/L = 210 $\times$ 10^9/L. An acceptable range of the instrument count would be 168–252 $\times$ 10^9/L. Yes, this is within the acceptable reference range.

Checkpoint! #3

How many platelets per 1000$\times$ field would you expect to observe on the peripheral smear of a patient with acute ITP?

Answer:

You would expect to see an average of fewer than six platelets per field. It can be difficult to find platelets on the blood smear of some ITP patients.

Checkpoint! #4

A 6-year-old boy was brought to his pediatrician because the mother noticed small pinkish spots on the boy's legs. Upon examination he also had several bruises on his arms and legs. Laboratory tests were ordered. His platelet count was 20 $\times$ 10^9/L and PT and APTT were within normal limits. The CBC was normal except for the low platelet count. There was no previous history of bleeding. The mother said she noted the spots after he was given the hepatitis vaccine. What is the most probable type of thrombocytopenia? Should other coagulation tests be performed at this time?

Answer:

The most probable type of thrombocytopenia experienced by this patient is an immune type of increased destruction, which is reportedly associated with viral infections in some children. Other coagulation tests are not necessary.

Checkpoint! #5

What is the pathophysiology of the thrombocytopenia in megaloblastic anemia?

Answer:

Thrombocytopenia occurs in megaloblastic anemia because of ineffective production of all myeloid cell lines in the bone marrow.

Checkpoint! #6

Explain why primary thrombocytosis is often associated with abnormal platelet function while secondary thrombocytosis is not.

Answer:

Primary thrombocytosis is associated with the myeloproliferative disorders, which are clonal disorders of the pluripotential stem cell. The abnormal clone grows autonomously and not in response to normal regulatory factors. It is likely that abnormalities in platelet function are acquired along with the ability to grow autonomously. In secondary thrombocytosis the platelets are increased because of the normal regulatory routes in response to a need for more platelets.

Checkpoint! #7

Compare the results of platelet aggregation studies in platelet adhesion, aggregation, and secretion disorders.

Answer:

Platelet adhesion to collagen requires that von Willebrand factor attached to platelet GPIb/IX receptors bridge the platelet to the collagen fiber. Platelet aggregation studies are abnormal with ristocetin in these disorders because ristocetin takes the place of collagen in the test. Other routine agonists require the platelet GPIIb/IIIa receptor and fibrinogen as the bridge to attach one platelet to another platelet. Platelet aggregation disorders involve abnormalities in the GPIIb/IIIa receptor or in fibrinogen. Therefore, platelet aggregation studies will be abnormal with all agonists except ristocetin. In platelet secretion disorders platelets are able to respond to agonists in the primary wave of aggregation but are unable to release their own ADP and manufacture their own thromboxane A$_2$, so that the secondary wave of aggregation seen with ADP and epinephrine and the wave of aggregation with collagen are abnormal.

Checkpoint! #8

Why are the bleeding time test and the closure time abnormal for up to 7 days following ingestion of aspirin?

Answer:

Aspirin inhibits the platelet enzyme, cyclooxygenase, which is necessary for production of thromboxane A$_2$. TXA$_2$ is necessary in the activated platelet for secretion of granule contents and, therefore, the function of the platelets is impaired. The defective platelets continue to circulate for their normal life span, which is about 10 days. Since they are circulating, the bone marrow is not stimulated to produce new platelets to replace the defective ones.

Chapter 37

Checkpoint! #1

A. Why do patients with type 1 VWD have 25–50% of vWf in their plasma? B. Why do they have a corresponding decrease in factor VIII in their plasma?

Answer:

A. Type 1 VWD is inherited as an autosomal dominant characteristic. Patients have symptoms with abnormalities of only one gene. The second gene is still functional. Theoretically, 50% of vWf would be present but other variations such as the blood type O may result in less than 50% in some patients.

B. Patients with type 1 VWD have a corresponding decrease in factor VIII in their plasma because factor VIII requires the presence of vWf to be functional.

Checkpoint! #2

A. If a patient with VWD has an equal decrease in factor VIII assay, vWf:RCo, and vWf:Ag assay, does this more likely indicate that there is a true decrease in the amount of vWf or does it indicate that the patient has a type of VWD that is characterized by abnormal function of vWf. Support your answer.
B. What type of VWD is most likely in a patient with these laboratory test results?

Answer:

A. There is a true decrease in the amount of vWf because the tests for function and immunologic activity are both decreased.
B. These results are characteristic of VWD, type 1.

Checkpoint! #3

What abbreviation is acceptable for:
A. the antigenic properties of vWf?
B. the function of factor VIII?
C. the complex of factor VIII and vWf?

Answer:

A. vWf:Ag
B. VIII:C
C. Factor VIII/vWf complex

Checkpoint! #4

Referring to Table 37-3, explain the reason why the platelet function tests are abnormal in VWD and not in factor VIII or IX deficiencies.

Answer:

Platelet function tests are abnormal in VWD because vWf is necessary for platelets to adhere to collagen. This affects the closure time, the bleeding time, and platelet aggregation studies with ristocetin. Ristocetin takes the place of collagen in the platelet aggregation test system. In the absence of vWf, platelets do not adhere and do not aggregate. vWf is not needed for platelets to aggregate with other agonists. In factor VIII and IX deficiencies there is a decrease in these coagulation proteins that affects fibrin formation, but platelets are normal and vWf is present.

Checkpoint! #5

Explain why the thrombin time will be abnormal in patients with afibrinogenemia and dysfibrinogenemia.

Answer:

The thrombin time is dependent on the adequate conversion of soluble fibrinogen to fibrin. Patients with afibrinogenemia have no fibrinogen to convert to fibrin, and patients with dysfibrinogenemia have fibrinogens with abnormal ability to convert to fibrin.

Checkpoint! #6

Explain why the prothrombin time but not the APTT is prolonged in factor VII deficiency.

Answer:

Factor VII is activated by tissue thromboplastin, which is the first step in fibrin formation. The reagent for the prothrombin time is tissue thromboplastin; therefore, when the factor VII is deficient, fibrin formation will be delayed. In the APTT tissue thromboplastin is not present in the test system. Instead, fibrin is formed by activating the contact factor system and factor VII is bypassed.

Checkpoint! #7

Explain why the laboratory screening tests are normal in patients with factor XIII deficiency.

Answer:

The laboratory screening tests all depend on fibrin formation in the test container. Factor XIII functions after fibrin formation to stabilize the fibrin in vivo. It is not necessary for fibrin to form.

Checkpoint! #8

A. Why is thrombocytopenia usually present in a patient with DIC?
B. Which hemostasis laboratory screening tests (PT and APTT), if any, will the following affect?
  Decreased factor V?
  Decreased factor VIII?
  Decreased fibrinogen?
  Decreased antithrombin?
C. Which laboratory test results would distinguish DIC from hemophilia A?

Answer:

A. Thrombocytopenia is present because platelets are consumed in DIC. They are activated by thrombin and are incorporated into the fibrin clots within the circulation.
B. Decreased factor V: PT and APTT
  Decreased factor VIII: APTT
  Decreased fibrinogen: PT and APTT
  Decreased antithrombin: neither
C. The APTT is abnormally increased and the factor VIII assay decreased in hemophilia A. All other tests are normal. In DIC all factors and inhibitors that are consumed as blood clots are abnormal, and fibrinolytic products are increased because blood is clotting and

lysing in DIC. This affects all of the hemostasis tests that are routinely performed, as well as the platelet count.

Chapter 38

Checkpoint! #1

Why would defects of fibrinolysis result in hypercoagulability?

Answer:

Under normal conditions, hemostasis depends on a delicate balance between clot-promoting factors (procoagulant influences) and clot-inhibiting factors (anticoagulants and fibrinolysis). Defects in fibrinolysis result in hypercoagulability because the delicate balance has now been disturbed, and the clot-promoting factors dominate the clinical picture.

Checkpoint! #2

Why is thrombotic disease associated with hereditary thrombophilia considered a multigene (or multirisk factor) disease?

Answer:

Individuals who have inherited a thrombophilia gene generally do not experience thrombotic episodes unless they have a second either genetic or acquired predisposing factor. Thus, many individuals who carry thrombophilia genes do not have acute thrombotic events and may be diagnosed only when family screening is done for another family member who has had a thrombosis.

Checkpoint! #3

Why are both immunologic and functional assays recommended when screening a patient suspected of having a familial thrombophilic defect?

Answer:

Inherited defects of the hemostatic proteins involved in familial thrombophilia can be either quantitative or qualitative defects. Immunologic assays for total protein will fail to diagnose qualitative defects (dysfunctional proteins) which typically give normal antigen levels but reduced functional levels. Functional assays are generally considered the better screening assay if a familial thrombophilia is suspected.

Checkpoint! #4

Why should heparin therapy overlap initiation of oral anticoagulant therapy when treating a patient with an acute thrombosis?

Answer:

Oral anticoagulants (vitamin-K antagonists) decrease functional levels of procoagulant protein factors II, VII, IX, and X, as well as the anticoagulant proteins PC and PS. However, this action is not immediate (as is the anticoagulant effect of heparin), and the decrease in activity of each of the above proteins varies, depending on the half-life of each in the circulation. Because PC has a relatively short half-life, clearance of biologically active molecules (presynthesized before oral anticoagulants were begun) occurs more quickly for PC than for the procoagulant protein factors II, IX, and X. Thus for the first few days after initiating coumadin therapy, there is an imbalance between clot-inhibiting influences (PC) and clot-promoting influences (factors II, VII, and X). The net effect is a period of hypercoagulability before the full anticoagulant effect of

coumadin is realized. For a patient who already has a hemostatic system that is presumably not in balance, this could further aggravate it. Thus, heparin anticoagulant therapy should be continued through the first 4–5 days of oral anticoagulant therapy, until the full effect of coumadin is achieved.

Chapter 39

Checkpoint! #1

Why have most clinical laboratories switched from 3.8% to 3.2% sodium citrate for specimen collection in coagulation studies?

Answer:

The use of 3.2% sodium citrate minimizes the chances of over-anticoagulating a specimen due to a high hematocrit or an inadequately filled collection tube.

Checkpoint! #2

What effect will aspirin have on the bleeding time of a patient who takes aspirin daily for a heart condition? Explain.

Answer:

Aspirin irreversibly inhibits cyclooxygenase, which is responsible for thromboxane A_2 synthesis. Thromboxane A_2 is required for platelet aggregation; therefore the bleeding time will be prolonged. Since aspirin's action is irreversible, the platelet is effected for its life span (~7–10 days).

Checkpoint! #3

Routine coagulation testing was performed on a properly collected and processed specimen. The PT was prolonged, but APTT was normal. What is the best interpretation of these results?

Answer:

These results indicate a factor VII deficiency. The PT evaluates factors in the extrinsic and common pathways, while the APTT evaluates factors in the intrinsic and common pathways. Since only the PT is prolonged, the factor deficiency must be in the extrinsic pathway.

Checkpoint! #4

Given the following coagulation test results, what is the appropriate follow-up or reflex test?

PT: normal
APTT: prolonged
Mixing studies: no correction

Answer:

The appropriate follow-up or reflex test would be the platelet neutralization procedure or dilute Russell's viper venom time. Either test would identify the presence of lupus-like anticoagulant.

Checkpoint! #5

What is the function of the factor deficient substrate reagent and the reference plasma in a factor assay?

Answer:

The factor deficient substrate reagent assures that all coagulation factors except the coagulation factor to be assayed are at optimal activity levels. In this way, only the activity level of a single coagulation factor will be evaluated. Reference plasma contains a known activity level for each coagulation factor and is used to establish the factor activity curve from which the patient's factor activity can be determined (similar to a standard curve).

Checkpoint! #6

Why are ruptured platelets able to neutralize lupus-like anticoagulants?

Answer:

Platelet membrane phospholipids are exposed when platelets rupture. Since lupus-like anticoagulants are antiphospholipid antibodies, they will bind to the exposed phospholipids and will no longer interfere with the test reagent phospholipids.

Checkpoint! #7

What is the appropriate interpretation of these coagulation test results?

PT:	prolonged
APTT:	prolonged
TT:	prolonged
FDP:	>20 µg/mL
D-dimer:	>1.0 µg/mL

Answer:

These coagulation test results are indicative of disseminated intravascular coagulation (DIC). D-dimer is a specific indicator of fibrin clot degradation that is observed in DIC.

Checkpoint! #8

In diagnostic laboratory evaluation of a hypercoagulable state such as antithrombin III deficiency, why is it important to determine the functional activity of the coagulation protein as well as its antigenic level?

Answer:

Several hypercoagulable states are characterized by a normal antigenic level of protein but have decreased functional activity. In other words, the hypercoagulable state is the result of a dysfunctional coagulation protein. The diagnosis would be missed if only the antigenic level was assessed.

Checkpoint! #9

A patient has been diagnosed with a deep vein thrombosis and placed on heparin therapy. The patient's current APTT level is 92 seconds. If the patient's weight is 75 kg, should the heparin dose be changed, and if so, how should the dose be altered?

Answer:

With an APTT of 92 seconds, this patient is at the supratherapeutic range. Using the weight-based nomogram, the patient's heparin dose should be decreased by 150 units/h (2 units/kg/h · 75 kg = 150 units/h).

Chapter 40

Checkpoint! #1

What is the basis for hemoglobin separation in the hemoglobin electrophoresis procedures?

Answer:

The net charge of hemoglobin molecules can be altered by the pH of the buffer. When placed in an electric field, the hemoglobin molecules will be separated based on their net charge. For example, at pH 8.6 hemoglobin molecules will have a net negative charge with hemoglobin A possessing the strongest net negative charge and traveling the fastest.

Checkpoint! #2

Alkali denaturation revealed HbF level of 70%, and the acid elution for HbF demonstrated an uneven distribution of HbF within the erythrocytes. Why are both alkali denaturation and acid elution performed to evaluate HbF?

Answer:

The alkali denaturation test quantitates HbF, while the acid elution test helps determine the distribution of HbF within the erythrocyte population. Together, these two tests help differentiate diagnosis of disorders characterized by an increase in HbF.

Checkpoint! #3

A patient's osmotic fragility test shows beginning hemolysis at 0.60% NaCl and complete hemolysis at 0.50% NaCl. How should these results be interpreted?

Answer:

These results indicate increased osmotic fragility that is associated with hereditary spherocytosis.

Checkpoint! #4

A patient was recently diagnosed with a hypochromic, microcytic anemia. Additional laboratory testing revealed: EPO 1.5 mIU/mL and sTfR 15.8 nmol/L. Which anemia is consistent with these results?

Answer:

These results are consistent with anemia of chronic disease. A normal sTfR level but decreased EPO are characteristic findings in this disorder.

Chapter 41

Checkpoint! #1

What is the basis of the impedance principle for cell counting?

Answer:

The impedance principle is based on the fact that blood cells are poorly conductive particles. Increased resistance is observed when a poorly conductive particle passes through an electrical field.

Checkpoint! #2

Why is lytic agent added to the leukocyte dilution?

Answer:

Lytic agent is added to the leukocyte dilution to lyse the erythrocytes and convert the released hemoglobin to cyanmethemoglobin. Cyanmethemoglobin is used to measure hemoglobin concentration. If erythrocytes were not lysed, they would cause falsely increased leukocyte counts.

Checkpoint! #3

Explain how the additional methodologies used by the Coulter STKS improved the leukocyte differential.

Answer:

The Coulter STKS utilizes conductivity and light scatter, in addition to cell volume, to determine the leukocyte differential. The additional characteristics of each cell revealed by conductivity and light scatter enhance the ability to differentiate leukocytes from the traditional three-part differential (granulocytes, mononuclear cells, and lymphocytes) to a five-part differential (neutrophils, monocytes, lymphocytes, eosinophils, and basophils).

Checkpoint! #4

How does the method of analysis for the five-part leukocyte differential differ between the Coulter STKS and Coulter Gen·S?

Answer:

The Coulter Gen·S uses contour gating, compared to linear gating used by the Coulter STKS. Contour gating allows the differentiation of overlapping cell populations like monocytes and reactive lymphocytes.

Checkpoint! #5

In the Sysmex instruments, how are eosinophils and basophils isolated for enumeration?

Answer:

Eosinophils and basophils are isolated by specific lytic agents that destroy all leukocytes except the cell, eosinophil, or basophil to be counted. Isolated cells are counted by impedance.

Checkpoint! #6

Which CELL-DYN scatterplot allows differentiation of eosinophils from neutrophils?

Answer:

The 90°D vs 90° scatterplot allows differentiation of eosinophils from neutrophils based on their different granularity and lobularity characteristics.

Checkpoint! #7

For instruments using optical light scatter to determine blood cell counts, which cellular characteristic is determined by the degree of forward scatter?

Answer:

Forward scatter reflects cell size.

Checkpoint! #8

When performing a reticulocyte analysis, what cellular component is stained?

Answer:

In reticulocyte analysis, cellular RNA is stained.

Checkpoint! #9

Compare the clot detection methods for the Fibrometer system and the STArt 4 system.

Answer:

For the Fibrometer system, the completion of an electric circuit between two electrodes by the fibrin strand indicates clot formation. The STArt 4 system detects clot formation by a decrease in the iron ball's movement as plasma viscosity increases.

Checkpoint! #10

For the optical density instruments, what is the basis of clot detection?

Answer:

Detection of clot formation is based on an increase in absorbance (optical density) or decreased transmittance as measured by a photodetector.

Chapter 42

Checkpoint! #1

Explain the importance of each component of the quality assurance program to its ultimate goal.

Answer:

The preanalytical component is critical to the quality assurance program because the test outcome is only as good as the specimen from which it is determined. The QA program must assure proper collection and handling of specimens prior to testing. The analytical component represents all factors that impact the testing system. The test outcome will be affected if there is a breakdown in the testing system due to lack of a proper QA program. A breakdown in the QA program within the postanalytical component will affect the recording/reporting of the test outcome. This may delay appropriate treatment for the patient.

Checkpoint! #2

If a clinical laboratory loses its certification to perform protein C assays, what is involved in regaining that certification?

Answer:

The clinical laboratory should determine the reason for the failure, correct the problem, and document the process. Following the corrective action, successful participation in two consecutive proficiency testing surveys for protein C would result in the laboratory's recertification to perform protein C assays.

Checkpoint! #3

What is an appropriate method of assessing a clinical laboratory professional's competency in performing PT and APTT using an automated coagulation instrument?

Answer:

To assess competency in performing PT and APTT, a combination of direct observation checklist and blinded preanalyzed samples would provide an appropriate method of assessment.

Checkpoint! #4

Linear regression analysis was performed on results from a method comparison of an automated prothrombin time method (current) and a point-of-care prothrombin time method. The following results were obtained: y-intercept = 1.014 and slope = 0.978. What conclusions can be drawn from these results?

Answer:

Based on the linear regression results, there is a constant difference between the automated prothrombin time procedure and the point-of-care prothrombin time procedure since the y-intercept is greater than zero. That is, the automated prothrombin time method gives consistently higher results than the point-of-care method. Therefore, a constant systematic error exists. The slope indicates there is not a proportional systematic error between the two methods as the slope is between 0.95 and 1.05.

Checkpoint! #5

Define the term reference interval.

Answer:

For a given analyte, the reference interval represents the usual results for a healthy population. For example, the reference interval for hemoglobin in the adult male population is 13.3–17.7 g/dL.

Checkpoint! #6

If a spill occurred when handling the EXCELL differential diluent, what would be the appropriate procedure to clean it up? Refer to Figure 42-2.

Answer:

Absorbent material should be used to wipe up the diluent, and the area should be washed with water.

Checkpoint! #7

To establish the control limits for a new lot number of level 1 prothrombin time coagulation control, the following data points were collected: 11.8, 11.6, 12.1, 12.0, 12.3, 12.6, 11.9, 12.2, 12.0, 11.5, 12.7, 12.1, 11.2, 12.3, 12.9, 13.0, 12.3, 11.9, 12.4, 12.5 (results are in seconds). What are the ±2s control limits?

Answer:

The ±2s control limits are 11.2–13.2 seconds with a mean of 12.2 seconds.

Checkpoint! #8

After performing daily quality control on the automated hematology analyzer, the clinical laboratory professional observes a 4_{1s} violation for the hemoglobin parameter. What type of error is indicated?

Answer:

The 4_{1s} violation indicates a systematic error that may be due to expired reagent or a deteriorating hemoglobin lamp.

Checkpoint! #9

In reviewing a patient's CBC results, the clinical laboratory professional notes an MCHC of 37 fL. What corrective action should be taken?

Answer:

The clinical laboratory professional should check the patient's specimen for lipemia, cold agglutinins, or icteria since these interfering substances are associated with an elevated MCHC. The clinical laboratory professional should also perform a manual hematocrit to determine if the automated hematocrit is falsely decreased.

Checkpoint! #10

The clinical laboratory professional observes that the 3.2% sodium citrate tube for a prothrombin time and activated partial thromboplastin time is only two-thirds full. Explain the effect this will have on the patient's coagulation results.

Answer:

If the specimen collection tube is only two-thirds full, there will be excess anticoagulant present, and the plasma will be overanticoagulated. Therefore, the coagulation results will be falsely prolonged.

APPENDIX C

Answers to Review Questions

CHAPTER 1
1. a
2. d
3. a
4. c
5. b
6. a
7. c
8. b
9. d
10. d

CHAPTER 2
Level I
1. b
2. c
3. d
4. c
5. a
6. a
7. b
8. a
9. d
10. b

Level II
1. c
2. b
3. c
4. a
5. d
6. b
7. c
8. c
9. a
10. b

CHAPTER 3
Level I
1. a
2. b
3. a
4. d
5. a

Level II
1. a
2. d
3. d

4. a
5. b

CHAPTER 4
Level I
1. a
2. b
3. b
4. c
5. a
6. c
7. d
8. d
9. c
10. b

Level II
1. a
2. d
3. c
4. d
5. d
6. b
7. c
8. a
9. a
10. c

CHAPTER 5
Level I
1. a
2. b
3. b
4. c
5. d
6. c
7. b
8. d
9. c
10. a

Level II
1. d
2. b
3. a
4. c
5. b
6. d
7. c

8. b
9. a
10. b

CHAPTER 6
Level I
1. c
2. b
3. b
4. d
5. c
6. b
7. a
8. a
9. b
10. c

Level II
1. a
2. d
3. a
4. b
5. b
6. d
7. d
8. d
9. c
10. c

CHAPTER 7
Level I
1. c
2. d
3. b
4. c
5. c
6. d
7. c
8. d
9. c
10. b
11. b
12. a
13. d
14. a
15. c

Level II
1. b
2. b

3. b
4. d
5. a

CHAPTER 8
Level I
1. b
2. a
3. c
4. b
5. c
6. b

Level II
1. c
2. b
3. a
4. b

CHAPTER 9
Level I
1. c
2. a
3. b
4. d
5. a
6. a
7. c
8. b
9. a
10. a

Level II
1. b
2. c
3. c
4. a
5. a
6. c
7. b
8. c
9. c
10. b

CHAPTER 10
Level I
1. d
2. a
3. b
4. b
5. b
6. d
7. a
8. d
9. c
10. b

Level II
1. c
2. d

3. c
4. d
5. a
6. c
7. d
8. b
9. a
10. d

CHAPTER 11
Level I
1. b
2. a
3. c
4. c
5. d
6. d
7. d
8. b
9. d
10. c

Level II
1. a
2. d
3. b
4. c
5. b
6. c
7. b
8. a
9. b
10. a

CHAPTER 12
Level I
1. b
2. a
3. c
4. c
5. b
6. d
7. d
8. b
9. a
10. c

Level II
1. a
2. d
3. b
4. c
5. d
6. d
7. a
8. b
9. a
10. c

CHAPTER 13
Level I
1. c
2. a
3. d
4. a
5. d
6. c
7. b
8. a
9. c
10. b

Level II
1. a
2. c
3. a
4. a
5. d
6. b
7. b
8. d
9. a
10. a

CHAPTER 14
Level I
1. b
2. a
3. c
4. c
5. d
6. a
7. b
8. c
9. a
10. c

Level II
1. b
2. c
3. c
4. b
5. a
6. a
7. b
8. d
9. c
10. b

CHAPTER 15
Level I
1. b
2. a
3. d
4. a
5. c
6. c
7. d
8. a

9. d
10. b

Level II
1. c
2. b
3. c
4. d
5. a
6. c
7. a
8. d
9. b
10. c

CHAPTER 16
Level I
1. d
2. b
3. b
4. a
5. c

Level II
1. c
2. a
3. d
4. a
5. b

CHAPTER 17
Level I
1. a
2. c
3. d
4. b
5. b
6. d
7. c
8. c
9. d
10. b

Level II
1. c
2. b
3. c
4. a
5. b
6. c
7. a
8. d
9. c
10. b

CHAPTER 18
Level I
1. d
2. b
3. c

4. d
5. a
6. a
7. d
8. c
9. a
10. d

Level II
1. c
2. b
3. a
4. b
5. a
6. c
7. b
8. d
9. d
10. a

CHAPTER 19
Level I
1. b
2. c
3. a
4. a
5. d
6. c
7. c
8. b
9. c
10. d

Level II
1. b
2. b
3. a
4. a
5. a
6. d
7. c
8. a
9. c
10. d

CHAPTER 20
Level I
1. b
2. d
3. a
4. d
5. c
6. d
7. a
8. a
9. c
10. a

Level II
1. a
2. c

3. d
4. b
5. a
6. c
7. d
8. b
9. c
10. d

CHAPTER 21
Level I
1. b
2. d
3. a
4. b
5. a
6. b
7. a
8. d
9. c
10. c

Level II
1. d
2. c
3. d
4. b
5. c
6. a, b, d, e
7. a, b, c, d, e
8. a, d, e
9. a, b, d, e
10. a, c, d
11. a, d

CHAPTER 22
Level I
1. c
2. b
3. c
4. c
5. a
6. c
7. c
8. d
9. d
10. c

Level II
1. d
2. b
3. a
4. a
5. a
6. a
7. c
8. d
9. a
10. c

CHAPTER 23
Level I
1. d
2. c
3. d
4. d
5. d
6. c
7. d
8. b
9. a
10. b

Level II
1. b
2. a
3. b
4. d
5. c
6. b
7. d
8. a
9. c
10. b

CHAPTER 24
Level I
1. a
2. c
3. c
4. a
5. a
6. a
7. a
8. b
9. c
10. d

Level II
1. b
2. d
3. c
4. a
5. b
6. a
7. b
8. a
9. d
10. d

CHAPTER 25
Level II
1. c
2. b
3. a
4. b
5. a
6. c
7. b
8. d

9. d
10. d

CHAPTER 26
Level I
1. a
2. a
3. b
4. b
5. b
6. d
7. b
8. a
9. d
10. b
11. a

Level II
1. a
2. c
3. d
4. c
5. a
6. b
7. c
8. b
9. d
10. b
11. a
12. c

CHAPTER 27
Level I
1. b
2. a
3. b
4. c
5. b
6. b
7. d
8. a
9. c
10. b

Level II
1. b
2. a
3. c
4. b
5. c
6. d
7. d
8. d
9. d
10. a

CHAPTER 28
Level I
1. a
2. b

3. c
4. a
5. c
6. c
7. d
8. a
9. d
10. c

Level II
1. d
2. d
3. a
4. b
5. a
6. d
7. d
8. a
9. b
10. c

CHAPTER 29
Level I
1. c
2. a
3. c
4. b
5. a
6. c
7. c
8. c
9. d
10. d

Level II
1. d
2. b
3. d
4. b
5. d
6. c
7. c
8. a
9. d
10. c

CHAPTER 30
Level I
1. b
2. d
3. b
4. a
5. c
6. a
7. d
8. d
9. b
10. b

Level II
1. d
2. a
3. a
4. b
5. d
6. a
7. b
8. a
9. c
10. c

CHAPTER 31
Level I
1. d
2. b
3. d
4. c
5. c
6. b
7. d
8. b
9. d
10. a

Level II
1. a
2. c
3. a
4. c
5. a
6. b
7. a
8. a
9. a
10. a

CHAPTER 32
Level I
1. d
2. d
3. b
4. c
5. b
6. a
7. a
8. d
9. c
10. b

Level II
1. c
2. c
3. a
4. d
5. d
6. d
7. c
8. b
9. c

10. a

CHAPTER 33
Level I
1. d
2. c
3. d
4. d
5. a
6. d
7. d
8. d
9. d
10. a

Level II
1. d
2. a
3. b
4. a
5. b
6. a
7. c
8. a
9. c
10. c

CHAPTER 34
Level I
1. b
2. c
3. d
4. c
5. c
6. b
7. d
8. d
9. b
10. d

Level II
1. b
2. c
3. a
4. d
5. a
6. c
7. b
8. d
9. a
10. b

CHAPTER 35
Level I
1. b
2. a
3. d
4. c
5. b
6. b

7. b
8. c
9. c
10. a

Level II
1. a
2. d
3. d
4. c
5. b
6. b
7. d
8. a
9. b
10. a

CHAPTER 36
Level I
1. d
2. d
3. a
4. b
5. a
6. c
7. d
8. d
9. d
10. b

Level II
1. c
2. a
3. c
4. a
5. b
6. d
7. c
8. d
9. c
10. a

CHAPTER 37
Level I
1. d
2. a
3. b
4. b
5. c
6. d
7. a
8. d
9. b
10. b

Level II
1. b
2. a
3. c
4. c
5. b

6. a
7. c
8. b
9. d
10. b

CHAPTER 38
Level I
1. a
2. a
3. c
4. d
5. b
6. d
7. d
8. c
9. a
10. a

Level II
1. a
2. c
3. b
4. d
5. a
6. a
7. c
8. d
9. a
10. b

CHAPTER 39
Level I
1. b
2. c
3. b
4. a
5. a
6. b
7. b
8. a

9. c
10. a

Level II
1. d
2. a
3. d
4. c
5. a
6. d
7. c
8. b
9. b
10. a

CHAPTER 40
Level I
1. c
2. b
3. b
4. d
5. c
6. a
7. c
8. b
9. d
10. a

Level II
1. a
2. b
3. b
4. d
5. a
6. b
7. c
8. a
9. d
10. c

CHAPTER 41
Level I
1. d
2. a
3. d
4. b
5. b
6. d
7. c
8. b
9. c
10. c

Level II
1. a
2. c
3. c
4. d
5. a

CHAPTER 42
Level I
1. c
2. c
3. b
4. b
5. b
6. c
7. c
8. b
9. c
10. c

Level II
1. a
2. a
3. d
4. c
5. b
6. c
7. b
8. a
9. b
10. d

► **A**

Abetalipoproteinemia (hereditary acanthocytosis) – rare, autosomal recessive disorder characterized by the absence of serum β-lipoprotein, low serum cholesterol, low triglyceride, and low phospholipid and an increase in the ratio of cholesterol to phospholipid.

Acanthocyte – an abnormally shaped erythrocyte with spicules of varying length irregularly distributed over the cell membrane's outer surface; also known as a spur cell. There is no central area of pallor.

Achlorhydria – the absence of hydrochloric acid in stomach gastric secretions.

Acquired aberration – chromosome aberration (either numerical or structural) that occurs at some time after birth and involves only one cell line.

Acquired immune deficiency syndrome (AIDS) – a disease caused by infection with human immunodeficiency virus type I (HIV-1). The virus selectively infects helper T lymphocytes (CD4+) causing rapid depletion of these cells. This causes a deficiency in cell-mediated immunity. The patients have repeated infections with multiple opportunistic organisms and an increase in malignancies.

Acrocentric – refers to a chromosome that has the centromere close to the terminal end so that the short arm is much shorter than the long arm. The short arm consists only of a stalk and a small amount of DNA called a satellite.

Acrocyanosis – *see* Raynaud's phenomenon.

Activated lymphocyte – *see* reactive lymphocyte.

Activated protein C resistance (APCR) – a condition in which activated protein C is not able to inactivate factor V, which may cause or contribute to thrombosis. In most cases it is due to a mutation in factor V in which Arg 506 is replaced with Gln (factor V Leiden).

Acute leukemia – a malignant hematopoietic stem cell disorder characterized by proliferation and accumulation of immature and nonfunctional hematopoietic cells in the bone marrow and other organs.

Acute lymphocytic leukemia (ALL) – a malignant lymphoproliferative disorder characterized by proliferation and accumulation of lymphoid cells in the bone marrow. Peripheral blood smear reveals the presence of many undifferentiated or minimally differentiated cells.

Acute myelocytic leukemia (AML) – a malignant myeloproliferative disorder characterized by proliferation and accumulation of primarily undifferentiated or minimally differentiated myeloid cells in the bone marrow.

Acute phase reactant – plasma protein that rises rapidly in response to inflammation, infection, or tissue injury.

Acute undifferentiated leukemia (AUL) – a malignant proliferation and accumulation of immature cells in the bone marrow that do not have characteristics of either myeloid or lymphoid cells.

Adipocyte – cell whose cytoplasm is largely replaced with a single fat vacuole; fat cell.

Adsorbed plasma – platelet-poor plasma that is adsorbed with either barium sulfate or aluminum hydroxide to remove the coagulation factors II, VII, IX, X (the prothrombin group). Factors V, VIII, XI, XII, and fibrinogen (I) are present in adsorbed plasma. This plasma is one of the reagents used in the substitution studies to determine a specific factor deficiency.

Afibrinogenemia – a condition in which there is absence of fibrinogen in the peripheral blood. It may be caused by a mutation in the gene controlling the production of fibrinogen or by an acquired condition in which fibrinogen is pathologically converted to fibrin.

Aged serum – serum that lacks coagulation factors fibrinogen (I), prothrombin (II), V, VIII. Aged serum is prepared by incubating normal serum for 24 hours at 37°C. Factors VII, IX, X, XI, and XII are present in aged serum. This serum is one of the reagents used in the substitution studies to determine a specific factor deficiency.

Agglutinate – clumping together of erythrocytes as a result of interactions between membrane antigens and specific antibodies.

Aggregating reagent – chemical substance (agonist) that promotes platelet activation and aggregation by attaching to a receptor on the platelet's surface.

Agonist – a term used to describe substances that can attach to a platelet membrane receptor and activate platelets causing them to aggregate (e.g., collagen, ADP). These agonists are used in the laboratory to test platelet function using a platelet aggregometer.

Agranulocytosis – absence of granulocytes in the peripheral blood.

AIDS related complex (ARC) – the second recognized clinical stage of a person infected with the HIV virus. Immune compromised patients with mild symptoms of weight loss, fever, lymphadenopathy, thrush, chronic rash, or intermittent diarrhea are included in this category.

Alder-Reilly anomaly – a benign condition characterized by the presence of leukocytes with large purplish granules in their cytoplasm when stained with a Romanowsky stain. These cells are functionally normal.

Aleukemic leukemia – leukemia in which the abnormal malignant cells are found only in the bone marrow.

Allele – one of two or more genes that correspond to the same trait and occupy the same position on paired chromosomes.

Alloantibodies – antibodies produced in one individual in response to the antigens of another individual of the same species.

Allogeneic – pertaining to an allograft in which donor and host belong to the same species but are not genetically identical.

Allogeneic stem cell transplantation – transplantation of stem cells between genetically dissimilar animals of the same species.

Alloimmune hemolytic anemia – a hemolytic anemia generated when blood cells from one person are infused into a genetically unrelated person. Antigens on the infused donor cells are recognized as foreign by the recipient's lymphocytes, stimulating the production of antibodies. The antibodies react with donor cells and cause hemolysis.

Alpha granules – platelet storage granules containing a variety of proteins that are released into an area after an injury.

Analytical time – the time between specimen entry into the test system and the reporting of the result by the instrument.

Anemia – a decrease in the normal concentration of hemoglobin or erythrocytes. This may be caused by increased erythrocyte loss or decreased erythrocyte production. Anemia may result in hypoxia.

Aneuploid – number of chromosomes per cell that does not equal a multiple of the haploid number, n. For example, in human cells a chromosome count of 45, 47, 48, etc.

Anisocytosis – a term used to describe a general variation in erythrocyte size.

Antibody – an immunoglobulin produced in response to an antigenic substance.

Anticardiolipin antibody (ACA) – an autoantibody directed against negatively charged phospholipids. *See* antiphospholipid antibody.

Anticoagulant – chemical substance added to whole blood to prevent blood from coagulating. Depending on the type of anticoagulant, in vitro coagulation is prevented by the removal of calcium (EDTA) or the inhibition of the serine proteases such as thrombin (heparin).

Antigen – any foreign substance that evokes antibody production (an immune response) and reacts specifically with that antibody.

Antigen-dependent lymphopoiesis – development of immunocompetent lymphocytes into effector T and B lymphocytes that mediate the immune response through production of lymphokines and antibodies. The process is initiated when mature lymphocytes come into contact with an antigen. This process occurs in secondary lymphoid tissue.

Antigen-independent lymphopoiesis – development of lymphoid stem cells into immunocompetent T and B lymphocytes (virgin lymphocytes). This process occurs in the primary lymphoid tissue under the regulation of hematopoietic growth factors.

Antihuman globulin (AHG) – a globulin used in a laboratory procedure that is designed to detect the presence of antibodies directed against erythrocyte antigens on the erythrocyte membrane.

Antioncogene – a gene that codes for a normal substance that suppresses tumor formation. Maturation and/or absence of both alleles allows tumor growth. Also called a tumor-suppressor gene.

Antiphospholipid antibody – an autoantibody directed against antigens that consist of a negatively charged phospholipid. Clinically important antiphospholipid antibodies include anticardiolipin antibody (ACA) and lupus anticoagulant (LA). In some individuals, these antibodies are associated with thrombosis and other hemostatic defects.

Antiphospholipid antibody syndrome – a clinical condition characterized by the presence of high titers of antiphospholipid antibodies, thrombocytopenia, recurrent arterial and venous thromboses. Often affects young males.

Aperture – a small opening through which blood cells are drawn into an electronic cell counter. Electrodes are located on either side of the aperture, and electrical resistance is detected as the cell passes through the aperture.

Apheresis – to separate or remove. Whole blood is withdrawn from the donor or patient and separated into its components. One of the components is retained, and the remaining constituents are recombined and returned to the individual.

Aplasia – the failure of hematopoietic cells to generate and develop in the bone marrow.

Aplastic anemia – an anemia characterized by peripheral blood pancytopenia and hypoplastic marrow. It is considered a pluripotential stem cell disorder.

Apoferritin – cellular protein that combines with iron to form ferritin. It is only found attached to iron, not in the free form.

Apoptosis – programmed cell death resulting from activation of a predetermined sequence of intracellular events; "cell suicide."

APSAC – acylated plasminogen streptokinase activator complex; a modification of the enzyme, streptokinase, that is a chemically altered complex of streptokinase and plasminogen and is used as a thrombolytic agent in the treatment of thrombosis.

APTT – a laboratory test that measures fibrin forming ability of coagulation factors in the intrinisic coagulation cascade.

Arachidonic acid (AA) – an unsaturated essential fatty acid, usually attached to the second carbon of the glycerol backbone of phospholipids, released by phospholipase A_2 and a precursor of prostaglandins and thromboxanes.

Arachnoid mater – delicate membrane that covers the central nervous system; middle layer of the meninges.

Ascites – effusion and accumulation of fluid in the peritoneal cavity.

Ascitic fluid – fluid that has abnormally collected in the peritoneal cavity of the abdomen.

Atypical lymphocyte – *see* reactive lymphocyte.

Auer rods – reddish blue staining needle-like inclusions within the cytoplasm of leukemic myeloblasts that occur as a result of abnormal cytoplasmic granule formation. Their presence on a Romanowsky stained smear is helpful in differentiating acute myeloid leukemia from acute lymphoblastic leukemia.

Autoantibodies – antibodies in the blood that are capable of reacting with the subject's own antigens.

Autohemolysis – lysis of the subject's own erythrocytes by hemolytic agents in the subject's serum.

Autoimmune hemolytic anemia (AIHA) – anemia that results when individuals produce antibodies against their own erythrocytes. The antibodies are usually against high incidence antigens.

Autologous stem cell transplantation – transplantation or infusion of a person's own stem cells.

Autosome – chromosomes that do not contain genes for sex differentiation; in humans, chromosome pairs 1–22.

Autosplenectomy – extensive splenic damage secondary to infarction. This is often seen in older children and adults with sickle cell anemia.

Azurophilic granules – the predilection of some granules (primary granules) within myelocytic leukocytes for the aniline component of a Romanowsky type stain. These granules appear bluish purple or bluish black when observed microscopically on a stained blood smear. They first appear in the promyelocyte.

 B

Backlighting – highlighting a parameter that falls outside its reference interval or a user-defined action limit. Backlighting alerts the clinical laboratory professional of a potential problem or error that requires further investigation.

Band neutrophil – the immediate precursor of the mature granulocyte. These cells can be found in either the bone marrow or peripheral blood. The nucleus is elongated and nuclear chromatin condensed. The cytoplasm stains pink, and there are many specific granules. The cell is 9–15 μm in diameter. Also called a stab or unsegmented neutrophil.

Basophil – a mature granulocytic cell characterized by the presence of large basophilic granules. These granules are purple blue or purple black with Romanowsky stain. The cell is 10–14 μm in diameter, and the nucleus is segmented. Granules are cytochemically positive with periodic acid-schiff (PAS) and peroxidase. The granules contain histamine and heparin peroxidase. Basophils constitute <0.2 × 10^9/L or 0–1% of peripheral blood leukocytes. The basophil functions as a mediator of inflammatory responses. The cell has receptors for IgE.

Basophilia – an increase in the concentration of circulating basophils.

Basophilic normoblast – a nucleated precursor of the erythrocyte that is derived from a pronormoblast. The cell is 10–16 μm in diameter. The nuclear chromatin is coarser than the pronormoblast, and nucleoli are usually absent. Cytoplasm is more abundant and it stains deeply basophilic. The cell matures to a polychromatophilic normoblast. Also called a prorubricyte.

Basophilic stippling – erythrocyte inclusions composed of precipitated ribonucleoprotein and mitochondrial remnant. Observed on Romanowsky stained blood smears as diffuse or punctate bluish black granules in toxic states such as drug (lead) exposure. Diffuse, fine basophilic stippling may occur as an artifact.

B cell ALL – an immunologic type of ALL in which the neoplastic cell is a B lymphoid cell. There are subtypes.

BCL-2 gene – gene on chromosome 18 producing bcl-2 protein. The translocation t(14;18) found in follicular lymphoma leads to bcl-2 overexpression and inhibition of lymphocyte cell death.

Bence-Jones protein – excessive immunoglobulin light chains in the urine.

Benign – nonmalignant. Formed from highly organized, differentiated cells that do not spread or invade surrounding tissue.

Bernard-Soulier disease – a rare hereditary platelet disorder characterized by a genetic mutation in the gene coding for platelet glycoprotein Ib resulting in inability of the platelets to adhere to collagen.

Bilineage leukemia – a leukemia that has two separate populations of leukemic cells, one of which phenotypes as lymphoid and the other as myeloid.

Bilirubin – a breakdown product of the heme portion of the hemoglobin molecule. Initial steps in the degradation of hemoglobin result in a water insoluble form (unconjugated or direct bilirubin) that travels in the blood stream to the liver, where it is converted to a water soluble form (conjugated or indirect bilirubin) that can be excreted into the bile.

Bioavailability – the amount of free drug available to produce its effect.

Biphasic antibody – antibody that binds to erythrocytes at room temperature or below and causes hemolysis when the blood warms to 37°C.

Biphenotypic leukemia – an acute leukemia that has myeloid and lymphoid markers on the same population of neoplastic cells.

Birefringent – characteristic of a substance to change the direction of light rays that are directed at the substance; can be used to identify crystals.

Bleeding time and PFA 100 – a screening test that measures platelet function.

Blinded preanalyzed samples – previously analyzed samples that are integrated randomly into a specimen run and possess no identifying feature (e.g., number or designation) to indicate that they are different from the current patient specimens. These samples can only be identified by the individual who selected and relabeled them. Used as a part of a quality control program.

Blood coagulation – formation of a blood clot, usually considered a normal process.

Bohr effect – the effects of pH on hemoglobin-oxygen affinity. This is one of the most important buffer systems in the body. As the H$^+$ concentration in tissues increases, the affinity of hemoglobin for oxygen is decreased, permitting unloading of oxygen.

Bone marrow aspirate – fluid withdrawn from the bone marrow by aspiration using a special needle (e.g., Jamshidi needle) and syringe. It represents the specialized soft tissue that fills the medullary cavities between the bone trabeculae. Examination of the bone marrow aspirate is useful in evaluating hematopoietic cellular morphology, distribution, and development; observing for presence of abnormal cells; and estimating cellularity.

Bone marrow trephine biopsy – removal of a small piece of the bone marrow core that contains marrow, fat, and trabeula. Examination of the trephine biopsy is useful in observing the bone marrow architecture and cellularity and allows interpretation of the spatial relationships of bone, fat, and marrow cellularity.

Bordatella pertussis – a gram-negative aerobic coccobacilli that is the cause of whooping cough. The hematologic picture in whooping cough is leukocytosis with lymphocytosis. The lymphocytes are small cells with folded nuclei.

Buffy coat – the layer of white blood cells and platelets that lies between the plasma and erythrocytes in centrifuged blood sample.

Burkitt's cell – lymphoblast that is found in Burkitt's lymphoma.

Butt cell – circulating neoplastic lymphocyte with a deep indentation (cleft) of the nuclear membrane. Butt cells may be seen when follicular lymphoma involves the peripheral blood.

 C

Cabot ring – reddish-violet erythrocyte inclusion resembling the figure 8 on Romanowsky stained blood smears that can be found in some cases of severe anemia.

Capitated payment – a reimbursement method for health care by third-party payers in which the insurer contracts with certain health care providers who agree to provide services for a defined population on a per member fee schedule. The insurer determines who the providers will be.

Carboxyhemoglobin – compound formed when hemoglobin is exposed to carbon monoxide; it is incapable of oxygen transport.

Carboxylation – in coagulation it refers to the addition of a carboxyl group to a coagulation factor (II, VII, IX, X). This occurs in the liver. The factor is not functional until it is carboxylated. Vitamin K is required for this reaction.

Cardiac tamponade – critical clinical situation in which the pericardial sac fills with fluid and restricts the heartbeat and venous return to the heart.

Caspase – cysteine proteases responsible for cell alterations in apoptosis.

Catalytic domain – a molecular area of a molecule that is common to all serine proteases involved in blood clotting. Cleavage of a peptide bond occurs here and converts the proenzyme to its active form.

CD designation – cluster of differentiation; refers to a group of monoclonal antibodies recognizing the same protein marker antigen on a cell. They are used to classify cell types and stages of maturation.

Cell cycle – the biochemical and morphological stages a cell passes through leading up to cell division; includes G1, S, G2, and M phases.

Cell cycle checkpoint – point in the cell cycle where progress through the cycle can be halted until conditions are suitable for the cell to proceed to the next stage.

Cell mediated immunity – an event in the immune response mediated by T lymphocytes. The event requires interaction between histocompatible T lymphocytes and macrophages with antigen. At least three important T lymphocyte subsets are involved: helper, suppressor, and cytotoxic.

Cellular hemoglobin concentration mean (CHCM) – an erythrocyte index that represents the average hemoglobin concentration of the individual cells analyzed. CHCM is derived from the hemoglobin histogram. Interference with the hemoglobin determination due to turbidity or lipemia can be identified by comparing the CHCM to the MCHC.

Central nervous system (CNS) – part of the nervous sytem that consists of the brain and spinal cord.

Centriole – cytoplasmic organelle that is the point of origin for the contractile protein known as the spindle fiber.

Centromere – primary constriction that attaches sister chromatids in a chromosome, dividing the chromatids into long and short arms.

Cerebrospinal fluid (CSF) – fluid that is normally produced to protect the brain and spinal cord. It is produced by the choroid plexus cells, absorbed by the arachnoid pia and circulates in the subarachnoid space.

Cheidak-Higashi anomaly – a multisystem disorder inherited in an autosomal recessive fashion and characterized by recurrent infections, hepatospleomegaly, partial albinism, CNS abnormalities; neutrophil chemotaxis and killing of organisms is impaired. There are giant cytoplasmic granular inclusions in leukocytes and platelets.

Chemotaxins – chemical messengers that cause migration of cells in one direction.

Chimerism – cells from two different zygotes expressed in one individual.

Cholecystitis – inflammation of the gallbladder.

Cholelithiasis – formation of calculi or bilestones in the gallbladder or bile duct.

Chromatid – structure of DNA during G_0 and G_1 of the cell cycle. After S-phase, DNA has replicated and the chromosome consists of two parallel, identical chromatids held together at the centromere.

Chromogenic assay – spectrophotometric measurement of an enzyme's activity based on the release of a colored pigment following enzymatic cleavage of the pigment-producing substrate (chromogen).

Chromosome – nuclear structure seen during mitosis and meiosis consisting of supercoiled DNA with histone and nonhistone proteins. Consists of two identical (sister) chromatids attached at the centromere.

Chronic idiopathic thrombocytopenic purpura (ITP) – an immune form of thromboyctopenia that occurs most often in young adults and lasts longer than six months.

Chronic lymphocytic leukemia (CLL) – a lymphoproliferative disorder characterized by a neoplastic growth of lymphoid cells in the bone marrow and an extreme elevation of these cells in the peripheral blood. It is characterized by leukocytosis, <30% blasts, and a predominance of mature lymphoid cells.

Chronic myelocytic leukemia (CML) – a myeloproliferative disorder characterized by a neoplastic growth of primarily myeloid cells in the bone marrow and an extreme elevation of these cells in the peripheral blood. There are two phases to the disease: chronic and blast crisis. In the chronic phase, there are less than 30% blasts in the bone marrow or peripheral blood, whereas in the blast crisis phase there are more than 30% blasts. Individuals with this disease have the BCR/ABL translocation, which codes for a unique P210 protein. Also referred to as chronic granulocytic leukemia (CGL).

Chronic myelomonocytic leukemia (CMML) – a subgroup of the myelodysplastic syndromes. There is anemia and a variable total leukocyte count. An absolute monocytosis ($>1 \times 10^9/L$) is present and immature erythrocytes and granulocytes may also be present. There are less than 5% blasts in the peripheral blood. The bone marrow is hypercellular with proliferation of abnormal myelocytes, promonocytes, and monoblasts, and there are <20% blasts.

Chronic nonspherocytic hemolytic anemia – a group of chronic anemias characterized by premature erythrocyte destruction. Spherocytes are not readily found, differentiating these anemias from hereditary spherocytosis.

Chylous – a body effusion that has a milky, opaque appearance due to the presence of lymph fluid and chylomicrons.

Circulating inhibitor (anticoagulant) – acquired pathologic protein, primarily immunoglobulins (IgG or IgM), with antibody specificity toward a factor involved in fibrin formation. Circulating inhibitors interfere with the activity of the factor. The inhibitors are associated with a number of conditions, such as hemophilia, autoimmune diseases, malignancies, certain drugs, and viral infections.

Circulating leukocyte pool – the population of neutrophils actively circulating within the peripheral blood stream.

Clinical Laboratory Improvement Amendments (CLIA) – regulations that mandate standards in clinical laboratory operations and testing signed into federal law in 1988.

Clonality – the presence of identical cells derived from a single progenitor. Can be detected by the identification of only one of the immunoglobulin light chains (kappa or lambda) on B cells or the presence of a population of cells with a common phenotype.

Clonogenic – giving rise to a clone of cells.

Clot – extravascular coagulation, whether occurring in vitro or in blood shed into the tissues or body cavities.

Clot retraction – the cohesion of a fibrin clot that requires adequate, functionally normal platelets. Retraction of the clot occurs over a period of time and results in the expression of serum and a firm mass of cells and fibrin.

Cluster analysis – a type of analysis in which floating thresholds cluster specific cell populations together based on size and staining or absorption characteristics. With cluster analysis, an instrument is able to accommodate for shifts in abnormal cell populations from one sample to another sample.

Coagulation factors – soluble inert plasma proteins that interact to form fibrin after an injury.

Cobalamin – a cobalt-containing complex that is common to all subgroups of the vitamin B_{12} group.

Codocytes – *see* target cell.

Codon – a sequence of three nucleotides that encodes a particular amino acid.

Coefficient of determination (r^2) – represents the square of the correlation coefficient. Coefficient of determination is a measure of the strength of the relationship between two data sets.

Coefficient of variation – the relative standard deviation or standard deviation expressed as a percentage of the mean for a set of data.

Cofactor – coagulation factors V and VII function as cofactors. Required for the conversion of specific zymogens to the active enzyme form.

Coincidence – in an electronic cell counter, a phenomenon of two or more cells crossing the sensing zone at the same time and evaluated as only one cell.

Cold agglutinin disease – condition associated with the presence of cold-reacting autoantibodies (IgM) directed against erythrocyte surface antigens. This causes clumping of the red cells at room or lower temperatures.

Colony forming unit – a visible aggregation (seen in vitro) of cells that developed from a single stem cell.

Colony stimulating factor – cytokine that stimulates the growth of immature leukocytes in the bone marrow.

Column chromatography – a laboratory separation method based on the differential distribution of a liquid or gaseous sample (mobile phase) that flows through a column of specific substance (stationary phase). Depending on the chemical characteristics of the stationary phase, the substance of interest may bind to the stationary phase and remain in the column or directly pass through the column and remain in the mobile phase. If the substance remains in the column, a second mobile phase (elution buffer) is used to release the substance from the stationary phase and allow it to pass through the column.

Committed/progenitor cells – parent or ancestor cells that differentiate into one cell line.

Common coagulation pathway – one of the three interacting pathways in the coagulation cascade. The common pathway includes three rate-limiting steps: (1) activation of factor X by the intrinsic and extrinsic pathways, (2) conversion of prothrombin to thrombin by activated factor X, and (3) cleavage of fibrinogen to fibrin.

Compensated hemolytic disease – a disorder in which the erythrocyte life span is decreased but the bone marrow is able to increase erythropoiesis enough to compensate for the decreased erythrocyte life span; anemia does not develop.

Competency assessment – mechanism of assessing the requisite ability of testing personnel to perform a given laboratory procedure. This includes recognition of specimen collection errors, interpretation of test results to detect possible instrument or specimen problems, interpretation of quality control results, troubleshooting instrument or specimen problems, proper reporting of results.

Complement – any of the eleven serum proteins that when sequentially activated causes lysis of the cell membrane.

Complementary DNA – synthetic DNA transcribed from an RNA template by the enzyme reverse transcriptase. Also known as cDNA.

Complete blood count (CBC) – a hematology screening test that includes the white blood cell (WBC) count, red blood cell (RBC) count, hemoglobin, hematocrit, and often, platelet count. It may also include red cell indices.

Compression syndrome – an altered physiological function of an organ or tissue due to impingement by an abnormal mass.

Conditioning regimen – high-dose chemotherapy and/or irradiation given to the patient before stem cell transplantation.

Congenital – present at birth.

Congenital aberration – chromosome aberration (either numerical or structural) that is present at the time of birth in all cell lines, or in several cell lines in the case of mosaicism.

Congenital Heinz body hemolytic anemia – inherited disorder characterized by anemia due to decreased erythrocyte lifespan. Erythrocyte hemolysis results from the precipitation of hemoglobin in the form of Heinz bodies, which damages the cell membrane and causes cell rigidity.

Consolidation – the second phase of cancer chemotherapy; its function is to damage or kill those malignant cells that were not destroyed during the induction phase.

Contact group – a group of coagulation factors in the intrinsic pathway that is involved with the initial activation of the coagulation system and requires contact with a negatively charged surface for activity. These factors include factors XII, XI, prekallikrein, and high molecular weight kininogen.

Continuous flow analysis – an automated method of analyzing blood cells that allows measurement of cellular characteristics as the individual cells flow singly through a laser beam.

Contour gating – subclassification of cell populations based on two characteristics such as size (x-axis) and nuclear density (y-axis) and the frequency (z-axis) of that characterized cell type. This information is used to create a three-dimensional plot. A line is drawn along the valley between two peaks to separate two cell populations.

Correlation coefficient (r) – determines the distribution of data about the estimated linear regression line.

Coverglass smear – blood smear prepared by placing a drop of blood in the center of one coverglass, then placing a second coverglass on top of the blood at a 45° angle to the first coverglass. The two coverglasses are pulled apart, creating two coverglass smears.

CRM– – cross-reacting material negative; a clotting factor that is defective and can be identified by abnormal functional and immunologic tests.

CRM+ – cross-reacting material positive; a functionally defective clotting factor that is identified by immunologic means.

Crossover – reciprocal exchange of genetic material between chromatids that normally occurs in meiosis to increase the diversity of the species.

Cryoprecipitate – a preparation of proteins containing fibrinogen, von Willebrand factor, and factor VIII and used for replacement therapy in patients with hemophilia A and von Willebrand disease. It is prepared by freezing and thawing plasma.

Cryopreservation – the maintaining of the viability of cells by storing at very low temperatures.

Cryosupernatant – product that lacks large vWf multimers that are present in fresh frozen plasma, yet still contains the vWf cleaving protease missing in thrombotic thrombocytopenic purpura (TTP) patients.

Culling – filtering and destruction of senescent/damaged red cells by the spleen.

Cyanosis – develops as a result of excess deoxygenated hemoglobin in the blood, resulting in a bluish color of the skin and mucous membranes.

Cyclins/Cdks – kinase proteins that regulate the transition between the various phases of the cell cycle.

Cytochemistry – chemical staining procedures used to identify various constituents (enzymes and proteins) within white blood cells. Useful in differentiating blasts in acute leukemia, especially when morphologic differentiation on Romanowsky stained smears is impossible.

Cytokine – protein produced by many cell types that modulates the function of other cell types; cytokines include interleukins, colony stimulating factors, and interferons.

Cytomegalovirus (CMV) – a herpes virus that replicates only in human cells. The virus has a widespread distribution and is spread by close contact with an infected person.

Cytoplasm – the protoplasm of a cell outside the nucleus.

 D

D-dimer – a cross-linked fibrin degradation product that is the result of plasmin's proteolytic activity on a fibrin clot. The presence of D-dimers is specific for fibrinolysis.

Decay accelerating factor – a regulating complement protein found on cell membranes that accelerates decay (dissociation) of membrane bound complement (C3bBb). An absence of this factor leads to excessive sensitivity of these cells to complement lysis.

Deep vein thrombosis (DVT) – formation of a thrombus, or blood clot, in the deep veins (usually a leg vein).

Delayed bleeding – a symptom of severe coagulation factor disorders in which a wound bleeds a second time after initial stoppage of bleeding. This occurs because the primary hemostatic plug is not adequately stabilized by the formation of fibrin.

Delta (δ) storage pool disease – an autosomal dominant disease characterized by a decrease in dense granules in the platelets.

Demarcation membrane system – a cytoplasmic membrane system in the megakaryocyte that separates small areas of the cell's cytoplasm. These areas will eventually become the platelets.

Dense bodies – platelet storage granules containing nonmetabolic ADP, calcium, and serotonin along with other compounds that are released into an injured area.

Dense tubular system (DTS) – a membrane in the platelet that originates from the smooth endoplasmic reticulum of the megakaryocyte. It is one of the storage sites for calcium ions within platelets. The channels of the DTS do not connect with the surface of the platelet.

Densitometry – a laboratory testing method that determines the pattern and concentration of protein fractions separated by electrophoresis. It measures the amount of light absorbed by each dye-bound protein fraction as the fraction passes a slit through which light is transmitted. The amount of light absorbed (optical density) is directly proportional to the protein's concentration.

Deoxyhemoglobin – hemoglobin without oxygen.

Diamond-Blackfan anemia – congenital, progressive erythrocyte hypoplasia that occurs in very young children. There is no leukopenia or thrombocytopenia.

Diapedese – passage of blood cells through the unruptured capillary wall. For leukocytes, this involves active locomotion.

Differentiation – appearance of different properties in cells that were initially equivalent.

Diploid – number of chromosomes in somatic cells that is 2n. For human cells 2n = 46.

Direct antiglobulin test (DAT) – a laboratory test used to detect the presence of antibody and/or complement that is attached to the erythrocyte. The test uses antibody directed against human immunoglobulin and/or complement.

Disseminated intravascular coagulation (DIC) – a complex condition in which the normal coagulation process is altered by an underlying condition resulting in complications such as thrombotic occlusion of vessels, bleeding, and ultimately organ failure. DIC is initiated by damage to the endothelial lining of vessels.

DNA (deoxyribonucleic acid) – the blueprint that cells use to catalog, express, and propagate information. DNA is the fundamental substance of heredity that is carried from one generation to the next. It is a double-stranded molecule composed of complementary nucleotide sequences. The two strands of DNA are held together by hydrogen bonds formed according to the following rules of complementary nucleotide pairing: G bonds with C; A bonds with T; other combinations cannot bond.

Döhle bodies – an oval aggregate of rough endoplasmic reticulum that stains light gray blue (with Romanowsky stain) found within the cytoplasm of neutophils and eosinophils. It is associated with severe bacterial infection, pregnancy, burns, cancer, aplastic anemia, and toxic states.

Donath-Landsteiner antibody – a biphasic IgG antibody associated with paroxysmal cold hemoglobinuria. The antibody reacts with erythrocytes in capillaries at temperatures below 15°C and fixes complement to the cell membrane. Upon warming, the terminal complement components on erythrocytes are activated, causing cell hemolysis.

Downey cell – an outdated term used to describe morphologic variations of the reactive lymphocyte.

Drug-induced hemolytic anemia – hemolytic anemia precipitated by ingestion of certain drugs. The process may be immune mediated or nonimmune mediated.

Dura mater – dense membrane covering the central nervous system. Outermost layer of the meninges.

Dutcher bodies – intranuclear membrane bound inclusion bodies found in plasma cells. The body stains with periodic acid-Schiff (PAS) indicating it contains glycogen or glycoprotein. Appearance is finely distributed chromatin, nucleoli, or intranuclear inclusions.

Dysfibrinogenemia – a hereditary condition in which there is a structural alteration in the fibrinogen molecule.

Dyshematopoiesis – abnormal formation and/or development of blood cells within the bone marrow.

Dysplasia – abnormal cell development.

Dyspoiesis – abnormal development of blood cells frequently characterized by asynchrony in nuclear to cytoplasmic maturation and/or abnormal granule development.

▶ **E**

Ecchymosis – bruise (bluish black discoloration of the skin) that is greater than 3mm in diameter caused by bleeding from arterioles into subcutaneous tissues without disruption of intact skin.

Echinocyte – a spiculated erythrocyte with short, equally spaced projections over the entire outer surface of the cell.

Edematous – refers to the swelling of body tissues due to the accumulation of tissue fluid.

Effector lymphocytes – antigen stimulated lymphocytes that mediate the efferent arm of the immune response.

Efficacy – ability to produce the desired effect (e.g., anticoagulation).

Effusion – abnormal accumulation of fluid.

Elliptocyte – an abnormally shaped erythrocyte. The cell is an oval to elongated ellipsoid with a central area of pallor and hemoglobin at both ends; also known as ovalocyte, pencil cell, or cigar cell.

Embolism – the blockage of an artery by embolus, usually by a portion of blood clot but can be other foreign matter, resulting in obstruction of blood flow to the tissues.

Embolus – a piece of blood clot or other foreign matter that circulates in the blood stream and usually becomes lodged in a small vessel obstructing blood flow.

Endomitosis – nuclear DNA synthesis without cytoplasmic division.

Endoplasmic reticulum (ER) – a cytoplasmic organelle in eukaryocytic cells that consists of a network of interconnected tubes and flattened membranous sacs. If the ER has ribosomes attached, it is known as granular or rough endoplasmic reticulum (RER), and if ribosomes are not attached, it is known as smooth endoplasmic reticulum (SER).

Endothelial cells – flat cells that line the cavities of the blood and lymphatic vessels, heart, and other related body cavities.

Engraftment – homing of infused stem cells into the bone marrow microenvironment resulting in hematopoietic recovery.

Enzyme – a protein that catalyzes a specific biochemical reaction but is not itself altered in the process.

Eosinophil – a mature granulocyte cell characterized by the presence of large acidophilic granules. These granules are pink to orange pink with Romanowsky stains. The cell is 12–17 μm in diameter, and the nucleus has 2–3 lobes. Granules contain acid phosphatase, glycuronidase cathepsins, ribonuclease, arylsulfatase, peroxidase, phospholipids, and basic proteins. Eosinophils have a concentration of less than 0.45×10^9/L in the peripheral blood. The cell membrane has receptors for IgE and histamine.

Eosinophilia – an increase in the concentration of eosinophils in the peripheral blood ($>0.5 \times 10^9$/L). Associated with parasitic infection, allergic conditions, hypersensitivity reactions, cancer, and chronic inflammatory states.

Epistaxis – hemorrhage from the nose.

Epitope – a structural portion of an antigen that reacts with a specific antibody. Also called the antigenic determinant.

Epstein-Barr virus (EBV) – a virus that attaches to B lymphocytes by a specific receptor designated CD21 on the B lymphocyte membrane surface.

Error detection – the ability of a laboratory's multirule quality control procedure to detect a true error in the testing system and reject the control run.

Erythroblastic island – a composite of erythroid cells in the bone marrow that surrounds a central macrophage. These groups of cells are usually disrupted when the bone marrow smears are made but may be found in erythroid hyperplasia. The central macrophage is thought to transfer iron to the developing cells. The least mature cells are closest to the center of the island and the more mature cells on the periphery.

Erythroblastosis fetalis – hemolytic anemia occurring in newborns as a result of fetal-maternal blood group incompatibility involving the Rh factor of ABO blood groups. It is caused by an antigen-antibody reaction in the newborn when maternal antibodies traverse the placenta and attach to antigens on the fetal cells.

Erythrocyte – red blood cell (RBC) that has matured to the nonnucleated stage. The cell is about 7 μm in diameter. It contains the respiratory pigment hemoglobin, which readily combines with oxygen to form oxyhemoglobin. The cell develops from the pluripotential stem cell in the bone marrow under the influence of the hematopoietic growth factor, erythropoietin, and is released to the peripheral blood as a reticulocyte. The average life span is about 120 days, after which the cell is removed by cells in the mononuclear-phagocyte system. The average concentration is about 5×10^{12}/L for males and 4.5×10^{12}/L for females.

Erythrocytosis – an abnormal increase in the number of circulating erythrocytes as measured by the erythrocyte count, hemoglobin, or hematocrit.

Erythrophagocytosis – phagocytosis of an erythrocyte by a histiocyte; the erythrocyte can be seen within the cytoplasm of the histiocyte as a pink globule or, if digested, as a clear vacuole on stained bone marrow or peripheral blood smears.

Erythropoiesis – formation and maturation of erythrocytes in the bone marrow; it is under the influence of the hematopoietic growth factor, erythropoietin.

Erythropoietin – a hormone secreted by the kidney that regulates erythrocyte production by stimulating the stem cells of the bone marrow to mature into erythrocytes. Its primary effect is on the committed stem cell, CFU-E.

Essential thrombocythemia – a myeloproliferative disorder affecting primarily the megakaryocytic element in the bone marrow.

There is extreme thrombocytosis in the blood (usually >1,000 × 10^9/L). Also called primary thrombocythemia, hemorrhagic thrombocythemia, and megakaryocytic leukemia.

Euchromatin – region of the chromosome that contains genetically active DNA, is lighter staining and replicates early in S phase of the cell cycle. (*See* heterochromatin.)

Evan's syndrome – a condition characterized by a warm autoimmune hemolytic anemia and concurrent severe thrombocytopenia.

Exchange transfusion – simultaneous withdrawal of blood and infusion with compatible blood.

Extracellular matrix – noncellular components of the hematopoietic microenvironment in the bone marrow.

Extramedullary erythropoiesis – red blood cell production occurring outside the bone marrow.

Extramedullary hematopoiesis – the formation and development of blood cells at a site other than the bone marrow.

Extravascular – occurring outside of the blood vessels.

Extrinsic pathway – one of the three interacting pathways in the coagulation cascade. The extrinsic pathway is initiated when tissue factor comes into contact with blood and forms a complex with factor VII. The complex activates factor X. The term *extrinsic* is used because the pathway requires a factor extrinsic to blood, tissue factor.

Extrinsic Xase – a complex of tissue factor and factor VIIa that forms when a vessel is injured.

Exudate – effusion that is formed by increased vascular permeability and/or decreased lymphatic resorption. This indicates a true pathologic state in the anatomic region, usually either infection or tumor.

▶ F

FAB classification – the current internationally accepted scheme for the classification of the acute leukemias. It is based on a combination of bright-light microscopy and cytochemical testing. (FAB = French-American-British)

Factor V Leiden – a mutant form of factor V in which Arg 506 is replaced with Gln. This makes the molecule resistant to activated protein C.

Factor VIII:C assay – a method that determines the amount of factor VIII.

Factor VIII concentrate – a lyophilized preparation of concentrated factor VIII used for replacement therapy of factor VIII in patients with hemophilia A.

Factor VIII inhibitor – an IgG immunoglobulin with antibody specificity to factor VIII. The inhibitor inactivates the factor. The antibodies are time and temperature dependent. Factor VIII inhibitors are associated with hemophilia.

Factor VIII/vWf complex – the plasma form of vWf associated with factor VIII.

Faggot cell – a cell in which there is a large collection of Auer rods and/or phi bodies.

False rejection – rejection of a control run that is not truly out of control. The result falling outside the control limits or violating a Westgard rule is due to the inherent imprecision of the test method.

Fanconi's anemia (FA) – an autosomal recessive disorder characterized by chromosomal instability. Patients have a complex assortment of congenital anomalies in addition to a progressive bone marrow hypoplasia.

Favism – sensitivity to a species of bean, *Vicia faba*. It is commonly found in Sicily and Sardinia in individuals who have inherited glucose-6-phosphate dehydrogenase deficiency. It is characterized by fever, acute hemolytic anemia, vomiting, and diarrhea after ingestion of the bean or inhalation of the plant pollen.

Fee-for-service – a payment method for health care in which consumers choose their own health care providers and the provider determines the fees for the services. The fees may be paid by the patient or a third-party payer.

Ferritin – an iron-phosphorus-protein compound formed when iron complexes with the protein apoferritin; it is a storage form of iron found primarily in the bone marrow, spleen, and liver. Small amounts can be found in the peripheral blood proportional to that found in the bone marrow.

Fibrin degradation products (FDP) – the breakdown products of fibrin or fibrinogen that are produced when plasmin's proteolytic action cleaves these molecules. The four main products are fragments X, Y, D, and E. The presence of fibrin degradation products is indicative of either fibrinolysis or fibrinogenolysis.

Fibrin monomer – the structure resulting when thrombin cleaves the A and B fibrinopeptides from the α and β chains of fibrinogen.

Fibrinogen group – a group of coagulation factors that are consumed during the formation of fibrin and therefore absent from serum. Includes factors I, V, VIII, and XIII. Also called the consumable group.

Fibrinolysis – breakdown of fibrin.

Fibrin polymer – a complex of covalently bonded fibrin monomers. The bonds between glutamine and lysine residues are formed between terminal domains of γ chains and polar appendages of α chains of neighboring residues.

Fibronectin – extracellular-matrix glycoprotein capable of binding heparin.

Fibrosis – abnormal formation of fibrous tissue.

Flame cell – a plasma cell with reddish purple cytoplasm. The red tinge is caused by the presence of a glycoprotein and the purple by ribosomes.

Flow chamber – the specimen handling area of a flow cytometer where cells are forced into single file and directed in front of the laser beam.

Fluorochrome – molecules that are excited by light of one wavelength and emit light of a different wavelength.

Forward light scatter – laser light scattered in a forward direction in a flow cytometer. Forward light scatter is related to particle size (e.g., large cells produce more forward scatter).

Free erythrocyte protoporphyrin (FEP) – protoporphyrin within the erythrocyte that is not complexed with iron. The concentration of FEP increases in iron-deficient states. It is now known that in the absence of iron, erythrocyte protoporphyrin combines with zinc to form zinc protoporphyrin (ZPP).

F-test – statistical tool used to compare features of two or more sets of data.

Functional hyposplenism – reduced splenic function due not to the loss of splenic tissue but to the accumulation of cells sequestered in the spleen.

 G

Gammopathy – an abnormal condition in which there is an increase in serum immunoglobulins.

Gating – in flow cytometry, isolating cells with the same light scattering or fluorescence properties by placing a gate around them electronically.

Gene – a functional segment of DNA that serves as a template for RNA transcription and protein translation. Regulatory sequences control gene expression, so that only a small fraction of the estimated 100,000 genes are ever transcribed by a given cell.

Gene cluster – a group of closely linked genes that can be affected as a group.

Gene promoter – a DNA sequence that RNA polymerase binds to, to begin transcription of a gene.

Gene rearrangement – a process in which segments of DNA are cut and spliced to produce new DNA sequences. During normal lymphocyte development, rearrangement of the immunoglobulin genes and the T cell receptor genes results in new gene sequences that encode the antibody and surface antigen receptor proteins necessary for immune function.

Gene therapy – introduction of a normally functioning gene into the appropriate target cell of an affected individual.

Genome – the total aggregate of inherited genetic material. In humans, the genome consists of 3 billion base pairs of DNA divided among 46 chromosomes, including 22 pairs of autosomes numbered 1–22 and the two sex chromosomes.

Genotype – the genetic constitution of an individual, often referring to a particular gene locus.

Germinal center – lightly staining center of a lymphoid follicle where B cell activation occurs.

Germline – cell lineage that consists of germ cells.

Glanzmann's thrombasthenia – a rare hereditary platelet disorder characterized by a genetic mutation in one of the genes coding for the glycoproteins IIb or IIIa and resulting in the inability of platelets to aggregate.

Globin – the protein portion of the hemoglobin molecule.

Glossitis – an inflammation of the tongue.

Glucose-6-phosphate-dehydrogenase (G6PD) – an enzyme within erythrocytes that is important in carbohydrate metabolism. It dehydrogenates glucose-6-phosphate to form 6-phosphogluconate in the hexose monophosphate shunt. This reaction produces NADPH from NADP. This provides the erythrocyte with reducing power, protecting the cell from oxidant injury.

Glutathione – a tripeptide that takes up and gives off hydrogen and prevents oxidant damage to the hemoglobin molecule. Deficiency of this enzyme is associated with hemolytic anemia.

Glycocalin – a portion of glycoprotein Ib of the platelet membrane that is external to the platelet surface and contains binding sites for von Willebrand factor and thrombin.

Glycocalyx – an amorphous coat of glycoproteins and mucopolysaccharides covering the surface of cells, particularly the platelets and endothelial cells.

Glycolysis – the anaerobic conversion of glucose to lactate and pyruvic acid resulting in the production of energy (ATP).

Glycoprotein Ib – a glycoprotein of the platelet surface that contains the receptor for von Willebrand factor and is critical for initial adhesion of platelets to collagen after an injury.

Glycoprotein IIb/IIIa complex – a complex of membrane proteins on the platelet surface that is functional only after activation by agonists and then becomes a receptor for fibrinogen and von Willebrand factor. It is essential for platelet aggregation.

Glycosylated hemoglobin – hemoglobin that has glucose irreversibly attached to the terminal amino acid of the beta chains. Also called HbA$_{1c}$.

Golgi apparatus – a cytoplasmic organelle composed of flattened sacs or cisternae arranged in stacks. In secretory cells it functions in concentrating and packaging secretory products. It does not stain with Romanowsky stains and appears as a clear area usually adjacent to the nucleus.

Gower hemoglobin – an embryonic hemoglobin detectable in the yolk sac for up to eight weeks gestation. It is composed of two zeta (ζ) chains and two epsilon (ε) chains.

Graft-versus-host disease (GVHD) – tissue injury secondary to HLA-mismatch grafts resulting from immunocompetent donor T lymphocytes that recognize HLA antigens on the host cells and initiate a secondary inflammatory response.

Graft versus leukemia – favorable effect seen when immunocompetent donor T cells present in the allograft destroy the recipient's leukemic cells.

Granulocytopenia – a decrease in granulocytes below 2×10^9/L.

Granulocytosis – an increase in granulocytes above 6.8×10^9/L. Usually seen in bacterial infections, inflammation, metabolic intoxication, drug intoxication, and tissue necrosis.

Granulomatous – a distinctive pattern of chronic reaction in which the predominant cell type is an activated macrophage with epithelial-like (epithelioid) appearance.

Gray platelet syndrome – a rare hereditary platelet disorder characterized by the lack of alpha granules.

 H

Hairy cell – the neoplastic cell of hairy cell leukemia characterized by circumferential, cytoplasmic, hairlike projections.

Ham test – a specific laboratory test for paroxysmal nocturnal hemoglobinuria (PHN). When erythrocytes from a patient with PNH are incubated in acidified serum, the cells lyse due to complement activation. Also called the acid-serum lysis test.

Haploid – number of chromosomes in a gamete that is n; consists of one of each of the autosomes and one of the sex chromosomes. For human cells n = 23.

Haplotypes – Referring to one of the two alleles at a genetic locus.

Haptoglobin – serum α_2-globulin glycoprotein that transports free plasma hemoglobin to the liver.

Heinz bodies – an inclusion in the erythrocyte composed of denatured or precipitated hemoglobin. Appears as purple staining body on supravitally (crystal violet) stained smears.

HELLP syndrome – an obstetric complication characterized by hemolysis (H), elevated liver enzymes (EL), and a low platelet count (LP). The etiology and pathogenesis are not well understood.

Helmet cell – abnormally shaped erythrocyte with one or several notches and projections on either end that look like horns. Also called keratocyte and horn-shaped cells. The shape is caused by trauma to the erythrocyte.

Hematocrit – the packed cell volume of erythrocytes in a given volume of blood following centrifugation of the blood. Expressed as a percentage of total blood volume or as liter of erythrocytes per liter of blood (L/L). Also, referred to as packed cell volume (PCV).

Hematogones – precursor B lymphocytes present normally in the bone marrow.

Hematology – the study of formed cellular blood elements.

Hematoma – a localized collection of blood under the skin or in other organs caused by a break in the wall of a blood vessel.

Hematopoiesis – the production and development of blood cells normally occurring in the bone marrow under the influence of hematopoietic growth factors.

Hematopoietic microenvironment – specialized, localized environment in hematopoietic organs that supports the development of hematopoietic cells.

Hematopoietic progenitor cell – hematopoietic precursor cell developmentally located between stem cells and the morphologically recognizable blood precursor cells; includes multilineage and unilineage cell types.

Hematopoietic stem cell – hematopoietic precursor cell capable of giving rise to all lineages of blood cells.

Heme – the nonprotein portion of hemoglobin and myoglobin that contains iron nestled in a hydrophobic pocket of a porphyrin ring (ferroprotoporphyrin). It is responsible for the characteristic color of hemoglobin.

Hemochromatosis – a clinical condition resulting from abnormal iron metabolism. Characterized by accumulation of iron deposits in body tissues.

Hemoconcentration – refers to the increased concentration of blood components due to loss of plasma from the blood.

Hemoglobin – an intracellular erythrocyte protein that is responsible for the transport of oxygen and carbon dioxide between the lungs and body tissues.

Hemoglobin distribution width – a measure of the distribution of hemoglobin within an erythrocyte population. It is derived from the hemoglobin histogram generated by the Bayer/Technicon instruments.

Hemoglobin electrophoresis – method of identifying hemoglobins based on differences in their electrical charges.

Hemoglobinemia – presence of excessive hemoglobin in the plasma.

Hemoglobinopathy – disease that results from an inherited abnormality of the structure or synthesis of the globin portion of the hemoglobin molecule.

Hemoglobinuria – the presence of hemoglobin in the urine.

Hemolysis – a destruction of erythrocytes resulting in the release of hemoglobin. In hemolytic anemia this term refers to the premature destruction of erythrocytes.

Hemolytic anemia – a disorder characterized by a decreased erythrocyte concentration due to premature destruction of the erythrocyte.

Hemolytic disease of the newborn (HDN) – an alloimmunne disease characterized by fetal red blood cell destruction as a result of incompatibility between maternal and fetal blood groups.

Hemolytic transfusion reaction – interaction of foreign (nonself) erythrocyte antigens and plasma antibodies due to the transfusion of blood. There are two types of transfusion reactions: immediate (within 24 hours) or delayed (occurring 2 to 14 days after transfusion).

Hemolytic uremic syndrome (HUS) – a disorder characterized by a combination of microangiopathic hemolytic anemia, acute renal failure, and thrombocytopenia.

Hemopexin – a plasma glycoprotein (β-globulin) that binds the heme molecule in plasma in the absence of haptoglobin.

Hemophilia A – a sex-linked (X-linked) hereditary hemorrhagic disorder caused by a genetic mutation of the gene coding for coagulation factor VIII.

Hemophilia B – a sex-linked (X-linked) hereditary hemorrhagic disorder caused by a genetic mutation of the gene coding for coagulation factor IX.

Hemorrhage – loss of a large amount of blood, either internally or externally.

Hemorrhagic disease of the newborn – a severe bleeding disorder in the first week of life caused by deficiencies of the vitamin K-dependent clotting factors due to vitamin K deficiency.

Hemosiderin – a water insoluble, heterogeneous iron–protein complex found primarily in the cytoplasm of cells (normoblasts and histocytes in the bone marrow, liver, and spleen); the major long-term storage form of iron. Readily visible microscopically in unstained tissue specimens as irregular aggregates of golden yellow to brown granules. It may be visualized with Prussian-blue stain as blue granules. The granules are normally distributed randomly or diffuse.

Hemosiderinuria – presence of iron (hemosiderin) in the urine; result of intravascular hemolysis and disintegration of renal tubular cells.

Hemostasis – the localized, controlled process that results in arrest of bleeding after an injury.

Heparin – a polysaccharide that inhibits coagulation of blood by preventing thrombin from cleaving fibrinogen to form fibrin. Commercially available in the form of a sodium salt for therapeutic use as an anticoagulant.

Heparin induced thrombocytopenia (HIT) – thrombocytopenia associated with heparin therapy in some patients.

Hereditary elliptocytosis – an autosomal dominant condition characterized by the presence of increased numbers of elongated and oval erythrocytes. The abnormal shape is due to a horizontal interaction defect with abnormal spectrin, deficiency or defect in band 4.1, or deficiency of glycophorin C and abnormal band 3.

Hereditary erythroblastic multinuclearity with positive acidified serum test (HEMPAS) – type II congenital dyserythropoietic anemia

(CDA). CDA is characterized by both abnormal and ineffective erythropoiesis. Type II is distinguished by a positive acidified serum test but a negative sucrose hemolysis test.

Hereditary pyropoikilocytosis (HPP) – a rare but severe hemolytic anemia inherited as an autosomal recessive disorder. Characterized by marked erythrocyte fragmentation. The defect is most likely a spectrin abnormality in the erythrocyte cytoskeleton.

Hereditary spherocytosis – a chronic hemolytic anemia caused by an inherited erythrocyte membrane disorder. The vertical interaction defect is most commonly due to a combined spectrin and ankyrin deficiency. The defect causes membrane instability and progressive membrane loss. Secondary to membrane loss, the cells become spherocytes and are prematurely destroyed in the spleen. The condition is usually inherited as an autosomal dominant trait.

Hereditary stomatocytosis – a rare hemolytic anemia inherited in an autosomal dominant fashion. The erythrocyte membrane is abnormally permeable to sodium and potassium. The cell becomes overhydrated, resulting in the appearance of stomatocytes. The specific membrane abnormality has not been identified.

Hereditary xerocytosis – a hereditary disorder in which the erythrocyte is abnormally permeable to sodium and potassium, with an increased potassium efflux. The erythrocyte becomes dehydrated and appears as either target or spiculated cells. The cells are rigid and become trapped in the spleen.

Heterochromatin – region of the chromosome that contains genetically inactive DNA, is dark staining, and replicates late in S phase of the cell cycle.

Heterologous – refers to morphologically nonidentical chromosomes that have different gene loci.

Heterophil antibodies – antibodies that can react against a heterologous antigen that did not stimulate the antibody's production. In infectious mononucleosis, heterophil antibodies are produced in response to infection with Epstein-Barr virus, and react with sheep, horse, and beef erythrocytes.

Heterozygous – different genes at a gene locus.

Hexose-monophosphate shunt – a metabolic pathway that converts glucose-6-phosphate to pentose phosphate. This pathway couples oxidative metabolism with the reduction of nicotinamide adenine dinucleotide-phosphate (NADPH) and glutathione. This provides the cell with reducing power and prevents injury by oxidants.

Histogram – a graphical representation of the number of cells within a defined parameter such as size.

HIV-I (human immunodeficiency virus type-I) – a virus that causes acquired immunodeficiency syndrome (AIDS).

Hodgkin lymphoma (disease) – malignancy that most often arises in lymph nodes and is characterized by the presence of Reed-Sternberg cells and variants with a background of varying numbers of benign lymphocytes, plasma cells, histiocytes, and eosinophils. The origin of the malignant cell is still controversial.

Homologous – consists of two morphologically identical chromosomes that have identical gene loci, but may have different gene alleles as one member of a homologous pair is of maternal origin and the other is of paternal origin.

Homozygous – identical genes at a gene locus.

Horizontal interactions – side-by-side interactions involving the proteins of the erythrocyte membrane.

Howell-Jolly bodies – erythrocyte inclusion composed of nuclear remnants (DNA). On Romanowsky stained blood smears, it appears as a dark purple spherical granule usually near the periphery of the cell. Commonly associated with megoblastic anemia and splenectomy.

Humoral immunity – immunity imparted as a result of B lymphocyte activation. The B lymphocyte differentiates to a plasma cell that produces antibodies specific to the antigen that stimulated the response.

Hybridization – the process in which one nucleotide strand binds to another strand by formation of hydrogen bonds between complementary nucleotides.

Hydrodynamic focusing – a phenomenon that allows cells/particles to flow in a single column due to differences in the pressures of two columns of fluid in a flow chamber of a flow cytometer. The particles are contained in an inner column of sample fluid that is surrounded by a column of stream sheath fluid. The gradient between the sample and sheath fluid keeps the fluids separate (laminar flow) and is used to control the diameter of the column of sample fluid. The central column of sample fluid is narrowed to isolate single cells that pass through a laser beam like a string of beads.

Hydrops fetalis – a genetically determined hemolytic disease (thalassemia) resulting in production of an abnormal hemoglobin (hemoglobin Bart's, γ_4) that is unable to carry oxygen. No alpha(α)-globin chains are synthesized.

Hypercoagulable state – a condition associated with an imbalance between clot promoting and clot inhibiting factors. This leads to an increased risk of developing thrombosis.

Hyperdiploid – number of chromosomes per cell that is more than 2n. For human cells, this would be >46.

Hypereosinophilic syndrome – a term used to describe a persistent blood eosinophilia over 1.5×10^9/L with tissue infiltration and no apparent cause.

Hyperhomocysteinemia – elevated levels of homocysteine in the blood as a result of impaired homocysteine metabolism. It can be due to acquired or congenital causes. It is associated with premature atherosclerosis and arterial thrombosis.

Hyperplasia – an increase in the number of cells per unit volume of tissue. This can be brought about by an increase in the number of cells replicating, by an increase in the rate of replication, or by prolonged survival of cells. The cells usually maintain normal size, shape, and function. The stimulus for the proliferation may be acute injury, chronic irritation, or prolonged, increased hormonal stimulation; in hematology, a hyperplastic bone marrow is one in which the proportion of hematopoietic cells to fat cells is increased.

Hypersplenism – a disorder characterized by enlargement of the spleen and pancytopenia in the presence of a hyperactive bone marrow.

Hypocellularity – decreased cellularity of hematopoietic precursors in the bone marrow.

Hypochromic – a lack of color; used to describe erythrocytes with an enlarged area of pallor due to a decrease in the cell's hemoglobin content. The mean corpuscular hemoglobin concentration (MCHC) and mean corpuscular hemoglobin (MCH) are decreased.

Hypodiploid – number of chromosomes per cell that is less than 2n. For human cells, this would be <46.

Hypofibrinogenemia – a condition in which there is an abnormally low fibrinogen level in the peripheral blood. It may be caused by a mutation in the gene controlling the production of fibrinogen or by an acquired condition in which fibrinogen is pathologically converted to fibrin.

Hypogammaglobulinemia – a condition associated with a decrease in resistance to infection as a result of decreased γ-globulins (immunoglobulins) in the blood.

Hypoplasia – a condition of underdeveloped tissue or organ usually caused by a decrease in the number of cells. A hypoplastic bone marrow is one in which the proportion of hematopoietic cells to fat cells is decreased.

Hypoproliferative – decreased production of any cell type.

Hypoxia – a deficiency of oxygen to the cells.

 I

Idiopathic – pertains to disorders or diseases in which the pathogenesis is unknown.

Idiopathic (or immune) thrombocytopenic purpura (ITP) – an acquired condition in which the platelets are destroyed by immune mechanisms faster than the bone marrow is able to compensate. Platelets are decreased.

Immature reticulocyte fraction (IRF) – an index of reticulocyte maturity provided by flow cytometry. The IRF may be helpful in evaluating bone marrow erythropoietic response to anemia, monitoring anemia, and evaluating response to therapy.

Immune hemolytic anemia – an anemia that is caused by premature, immune mediated, destruction of erythrocytes. Diagnosis is confirmed by the demonstration of immunoglobulin (antibodies) and/or complement on the erythrocytes.

Immune response – body's defense mechanism, which includes producing antibodies to foreign antigens.

Immunoblast – a T or B lymphocyte that is mitotically active as a result of stimulation by an antigen. The cell is morphologically characterized by a large nucleus with prominent nucleoli, a fine chromatin pattern, and abundant, deeply basophilic cytoplasm.

Immunocompetent – the ability to respond to stimulation by an antigen.

Immunoglobulin – molecule produced by B lymphocytes and plasma cells that reacts with antigen. Consists of two pairs of polypeptide chains: two heavy and two light chains linked together by disulfide bonds. Also called an antibody.

Immunohistochemical stains – application of stains using immunologic principles and techniques to study cells and tissues; usually a labeled antibody is used to detect antigens (markers) on a cell.

Immunophenotyping – identification of antigens using detection antibodies.

Immunosuppressed – the inability to produce antibodies to antigens.

Immunotherapy – a form of therapy in which different immune cells are manipulated in vivo or in vitro and later infused to alter the immune function of other cells.

Indirect antiglobulin test (IAT) – laboratory test used to detect the presence of serum antibodies against specific erythrocyte antigens.

Induction therapy – the initial phase of cancer chemotherapy; its function is to rapidly drop the tumor burden and induce a remission back to a normal state.

Ineffective erythropoiesis – premature death of erythrocytes in the bone marrow preventing release into circulation.

Infectious lymphocytosis – an infectious, contagious disease of young children that may occur in epidemic form. The most striking hematologic finding is a leukocytosis of $40–50 \times 10^9$/L with 60–97% small, normal-appearing lymphocytes.

Infectious mononucleosis – a self-limiting lymphoproliferative disease caused by infection with Epstein-Barr virus (EBV). The leukocyte count is usually increased, which is related to an absolute lymphocytosis. Various forms of reactive lymphocytes are present. Serologic tests to detect the presence of heterophil antibodies are helpful in differentiating this disease from more serious diseases. Also known as the kissing disease.

In situ hybridization – detection of specific DNA or RNA sequences in tissue sections or cell preparations using a labeled complementary nucleic acid sequence or probe.

Integral proteins – proteins embedded between phospholipids within a cell membrane.

Internal quality control program – program designed to verify the validity of laboratory test results that is followed as part of the daily laboratory operations. Typically, monitored using Levey-Jennings plots and Westgard rules.

International Normalized Ratio (INR) – method of reporting prothrombin time results when monitoring long-term oral anticoagulant therapy. Results are independent of the reagents and methods used.

International Sensitivity Index (ISI) – value provided by the manufacturer of thromboplastin reagents. It indicates the responsiveness of the particular lot of reagent compared to the international reference thromboplastin.

Intrinsic coagulation pathway – one of the three interacting pathways in the coagulation cascade. The intrinsic pathway is initiated by exposure of the contact coagulation factors (factors XII, XI, prekallikrein, and high molecular weight kininogen) with vessel subendothelial tissue. The intrinsic pathway activates factor X. The term *intrinsic* is used because all intrinsic factors are contained within the blood.

Intrinsic factor – a glycoprotein secreted by the parietal cells of the stomach that is necessary for binding and absorption of dietary vitamin B_{12}.

Intrinsic Xase – a complex of factors IXa, VIIIa, phospholipid, and calcium that assembles on membrane surfaces.

IRE-BP (iron responsive element-binding protein) – a protein that binds to a stem-loop structure of ferritin and transferrin receptor mRNA. The stem-loop structure of mRNA is known as the iron responsive element (IRE). The binding affinity of IRE-BP for the IRE is determined by the amount of cellular iron. The IRE-BP is involved in the regulation of transferrin receptors and ferritin.

Irreversibly sickled cells (ISC) – rigid cells that have been exposed to repeated sickling events and cannot revert to a normal discoid shape. They are ovoid or boat-shaped and have a high MCHC and low MCV.

Ischemia – deficiency of blood supply to a tissue, caused by constriction of the vessel or blockage of the blood flow through the vessel.

Isoelectric focusing – movement of charged particles through a support medium with a continuous pH gradient. Individual proteins will move until they reach the pH that is equal to their isoelectric point.

Isopropanol precipitation – precipitation technique that identifies the presence of unstable hemoglobins due to their insolubility in isopropanol as compared to normal hemoglobins.

Isovolumetric sphering – a method employed by the Bayer/Technicon instruments in which a specific buffered diluent is used to sphere and fix the blood cells without altering their volume.

▶ **J**

Jaundice – yellowing of the skin, mucous membranes, and the whites of the eye caused by accumulation of bilirubin.

▶ **K**

Karyolysis – destruction of the nucleus.

Karyorrhexis – disintegration of the nucleus resulting in the irregular distribution of chromatin fragments within the cytoplasm.

Karyotype – a systematic display of a cell's chromosomes that determines the number of chromosomes present and their morphology.

Keratocytes – abnormally shaped erythrocytes with one or several notches and projections on either end that look like horns. Also called helmet cells and horn-shaped cells. The shape is caused by trauma to the erythrocyte.

Killer cell – population of cytolytic lymphocytes identified by monoclonal antibodies. Involved in several activities such as resistance to viral infections, regulation of hematopoiesis, and activities against tumor cells.

Knizocytes – an abnormally shaped erythrocyte that appears on stained smears as a cell with a dark stick-shaped portion of hemoglobin in the center and a pale area on either end. The cell has more than two concavities.

▶ **L**

L&H/popcorn cell – the neoplastic cell variant found in LP Hodgkin lymphoma characterized by a delicate multilobated nucleus and multiple, small nucleoli. The L&H cell has a B cell phenotype: LCA+ (leukocyte common antigen), CD20+, CD 15–.

Lacunar cell – the neoplastic cell variant found in NS Hodgkin lymphoma characterized by abundant pale staining cytoplasm. Characterized by cytoplasmic clearing and delicate, multilobated nuclei.

Lambert-Beer's law – law forming the mathematical basis for colorimetry; the absorbance (A) of a colored solution is equal to the product of the concentration of the substance being measured (C), times the depth of solution through which the light travels (L), times a constant (K). $A = C \times L \times K$.

Large granular lymphocyte – null cells with a low nuclear-to-cytoplasmic ratio, pale blue cytoplasm, and azurophilic granules. They do not adhere to surfaces or phagocytose.

Lecithin:cholesterol acyl transferasse (LCAT) deficiency – rare autosomal disorder that affects metabolism of high density lipoproteins. It is characterized by a deficiency of an enzyme that catalyzes the formation of cholesterol esters from cholesterol. Onset is usually during young adulthood.

Leptocyte – an abnormally shaped erythrocyte that is thin and flat with hemoglobin at the periphery. It is usually cup-shaped.

Leukemia – a progressive, malignant disease of the hematopoietic system characterized by unregulated, clonal proliferation of the hematopoietic stem cells. The malignant cells eventually replace normal cells. It is generally classified into chronic or acute, and lymphocytic or myelocytic.

Leukemic hiatus – a gap in the normal maturation pyramid of cells, with many blasts and some mature forms but very few intermediate maturational stages. Eventually, the immature neoplastic cells fill the bone marrow and spill over into the peripheral blood, producing leukocytosis (e.g., acute leukemia).

Leukemoid reaction – a transient, reactive condition resulting from certain types of infections or tumors characterized by an increase in the total leukocyte count to greater than 25×10^9/L and a shift to the left in leukocytes (usually granulocytes).

Leukocyte – white blood cell (WBC). There are five types of leukocytes: neutrophils, eosinophils, basophils, lymphocytes, and monocytes. The function of these cells is defense against infection and tissue damage. The normal reference range for total leukocytes in peripheral blood is $3.5–11.0 \times 10^9$/L.

Leukocyte alkaline phosphatase (LAP) – an enzyme present within the specific (secondary) granules of granulocytes (from the myelocyte stage onward). Useful in distinguishing leukemoid reaction/reactive neutrophilia (high LAP) from chronic myelogenous leukemia (low LAP).

Leukocytosis – an increase in WBCs in the peripheral blood; WBC count over 11×10^9/L.

Leukoerythroblastic reaction – a condition characterized by the presence of nucleated erythrocytes and a shift-to-the-left in neutrophils in the peripheral blood. Often associated with myelophthisis.

Leukopenia – decrease in leukocytes below 4×10^9/L.

Leukopoiesis – the production of leukocytes.

Linearity – the range of concentration over which the test method can be used without modifying the sample (i.e., diluting the sample).

Linearity check material – commercially available material with known concentrations of the analytes and no interfering substances or conditions. Linearity check material is used to determine an instrument's or method's linearity.

Linear regression analysis – statistical tool used to determine a single line through a data set that describes the relationship between two methods, X and Y. General equation is $Y = a + bx$, where a denotes the y-intercept; b is the slope; and Y is the predicted mean value of Y for a given x value.

Linkage analysis – the process of following the inheritance pattern of a particular gene in a family based on its tendency to be inherited together with another locus on the same chromosome.

Locus – a specific position on the chromosome.

Low molecular weight heparin (LMWH) – heparin molecules of M.W. 2,000–12,000 Daltons.

Lupus-like anticoagulant – a circulating anticoagulant that arises spontaneously in patients with a variety of conditions (originally found in patients with lupus erythematosus) and directed against phospholipid components of the reagents used in laboratory tests for clotting factors. *See* antiphospholipid antibody.

Lymphadenopathy – abnormal enlargement of lymph nodes.

Lymphoblast – a lymphocytic precursor cell found in the bone marrow. The cell is 10–20 μm in diameter and has a high nuclear/cytoplasmic ratio. The nucleus has a fine (lacy) chromatin pattern with one or two nucleoli. The cytoplasm is agranular and scant. It stains deep blue with Romanowsky stain. The cell contains terminal deoxynucleotidyltransferase (TdT) but no peroxidase, lipid, or esterase.

Lymphocyte – a mature leukoctye with variable size depending on the state of cellular activity and amount of cytoplasm. The nucleus is usually round with condensed chromatin and stains deep, dark purple with Romanowsky stains. The cytoplasm stains a light blue. Nucleoli are usually not visible. A few azurophilic granules may be present. These cells interact in a series of events that allow the body to attack and eliminate foreign antigen. Lymphocytes have a peripheral blood concentration in adults from 1.5 to 4.0×10^9/L (20–40% of leukocytes). The concentration in children less than 10 years old is higher.

Lymphocytic leukemoid reaction – characterized by an increased lymphocyte count with the presence of reactive or immature-appearing lymphocytes. Reactions are associated with whooping cough, chickenpox, infectious mononucleosis, infectious lymphocytosis, and tuberculosis.

Lymphocytopenia – a decrease in the concentration of lymphocytes in the peripheral blood ($<1.0 \times 10^9$/L). Also called lymphopenia.

Lymphocytosis – an increase in peripheral blood lymphocyte concentration ($>4 \times 10^9$/L in adults or $>9 \times 10^9$/L in children).

Lympho-epithelial lesion – infiltration of epithelium by groups of lymphocytes. Infiltration of mucosal epithelium by neoplastic lymphocytes is characteristic of MALT lymphoma.

Lymphoid follicle – sphere of B cells within lymphatic tissue.

Lymphokines – substances released by sensitized lymphocytes and responsible for activation of macrophages and other lymphocytes.

Lymphoma – malignant proliferation of lymphocytes. Most cases arise in lymph nodes, but it can begin at many extranodal sites. The lymphomas are classified as to B or T cell and low, intermediate, or high grade.

Lymphoma classification – division (grading) of lymphomas into groups, each with a similar clinical course and response to treatment. Current schemes use a combination of morphologic appearance, phenotype, and genotype.

Lypholized – serum or plasma sample that has been freeze-dried. Sample is reconstituted with a diluent, typically distilled or deionized water.

Lysosmal granules – granules containing lysosomal enzymes.

Lysosome – membrane bound sacs in the cytoplasm that contain various hydrolytic enzymes.

▶ **M**

Macrocyte – an abnormally large erythrocyte. The MCV is >100 fL. Oval macrocytes are characteristically seen in megaloblastic anemia.

Macro-ovalocyte – an abnormally large erythrocyte with an oval shape. This cell is characteristically seen in megaloblastic anemia.

Macrophage – a large tissue cell (10–20 μm) derived from monocytes. The cell secretes a variety of products that influence the function of other cells. It plays a major role in both nonspecific and specific immune responses.

Maintenance therapy – the third and final phase of cancer chemotherapy, its function is to prevent the repair and/or return of the malignant clone, thus allowing the normal immune system to clear away all remaining disease.

Malignant neoplasm – a clone of identical, anaplastic (dedifferentiated), proliferating cells. Malignant cells can metastasize.

Marginating pool – the population of neutrophils that are attached to or marginated along the vessel walls and not actively circulating. This is about one-half the total pool of neutrophils in the vessels.

Maturation – a process of attaining complete development of the cell.

Maturation index – a mathematical expression that attempts to separate AML-M5 and AML-M1 with and without maturation.

Mean cell hemoglobin (MCH) – an indicator of the average weight of hemoglobin in individual erythrocytes reported in picograms. The reference interval for MCH is 26–34 pg. This parameter is calculated from the hemoglobin and erythrocyte count: MCH (pg) = Hemoglobin (g/dL) ÷ Erythrocyte count ($\times 10^{12}$/L) × 10.

Mean cell hemoglobin concentration (MCHC) – a measure of the average concentration of hemoglobin in grams per deciliter of erythrocytes. The reference interval is 32–36 g/dL. The MCHC is useful when evaluating erythrocyte hemoglobin content on a stained smear. This parameter will correlate with the extent of chromasia exhibited by the stained cells and is calculated from the hemoglobin and hematocrit. MCHC (g/dL) = hemoglobin (g/dL) ÷ hematocrit (L/L).

Mean cell volume (MCV) – an indicator of the average volume of individual erythrocytes reported in femtoliters. The reference interval for MCV is 80–100 fL. This parameter is useful when evaluating erythrocyte morphology on a stained blood smear. The MCV usually will correlate with the diameter of the erythrocytes observed microscopically. The MCV can be calculated from the hematocrit and erythrocyte count: MCV (fL) = hematocrit (L/L) ÷ Erythrocyte count ($\times 10^{12}$/L) × 1000.

Mean platelet volume – mean volume of a platelet population; analogous to the MCV of erythrocytes.

Medical decision level – concentration of an analyte where medical intervention is required for proper patient care.

Medullary hematopoiesis – blood cell production and development in the bone marrow.

Megakaryocyte – a large cell found within the bone marrow characterized by the presence of large or multiple nuclei and abundant cytoplasm. Gives rise to the blood platelets.

Megaloblastic – asynchronous maturation of any nucleated cell type characterized by delayed nuclear development in comparison to the cytoplasmic development. The abnormal cells are large and are characteristically found in pernicious anemia or other megaloblastic anemia.

Metacentric – chromosome that has the centromere near center so that the short arm and long arms are equal in length.

Meninges – the three membranes covering the brain and spinal cord.

Metamyelocyte – a granulocytic precursor cell normally found in the bone marrow. The cell is 10–15 µm in diameter. The cytoplasm stains pink and there is a predominance of specific granules. The nucleus is indented with a kidney-bean shape. The nuclear chromatin is condensed and stains dark purple.

Methemoglobin – hemoglobin with iron that has been oxidized to the ferric state (Fe^{+++}); it is incapable of combining with oxygen.

Methemoglobin reductase pathway – a metabolic pathway that uses methemoglobin reductase and NADH to maintain heme iron in the reduced state (Fe^{++}).

Microangiopathic hemolytic anemia (MAHA) – any hemolytic process that is caused by prosthetic devices or lesions of the small blood vessels.

Microcyte – an abnormally small erythrocyte. The MCV is typically less than 80 fL and its diameter less than 7.0 µm on a stained smear.

Microenvironment – a unique environment in the bone marrow where orderly proliferation and differentiation of precursor cells take place.

Micromegakaryocyte – small, abnormal megakaryocyte sometimes found in the peripheral blood in MDS and the myeloproliferative syndromes.

Microtubule – a cylindric structure (20–27 µm in diameter) composed of protein subunits. It is a part of the cytoskeleton, helping some cells maintain shape. The microtubules increase during mitosis and form the mitotic spindle fibers. They also assist in transporting substances in different directions. In the platelet, a band of tubules located on the circumference is thought to be essential for maintaining the disc shape in the resting state.

Minimum residual disease – the presence of malignant cells detected by molecular tests when all other tests are negative.

Mitotic pool – the population of cells within the bone marrow that is capable of DNA synthesis. Also called the proliferating pool.

Mixed lineage acute leukemia – an acute leukemia that has both myeloid and lymphoid populations present or blasts that possess myeloid and lymphoid markers on the same cell.

Monoblast – the monocytic precursor cells found in bone marrow. It is about 14–18 µm in diameter with abundant agranular, blue gray cytoplasm. The nucleus may be folded or indented. The chromatin is finely dispersed and several nucleoli are visible. The monoblast has nonspecific esterase activity that is inhibited by sodium fluoride.

Monoclonal gammopathies – an alteration in immunoglobulin production that is characterized by an increase in one specific class of immunoglobulin.

Monocyte – a mature leukocyte found in bone marrow or peripheral blood. Its morphology depends upon its activity. The cell ranges in size from 12–30 µm with an average of 18 µm. The blue-gray cytoplasm is evenly dispersed with fine dust-like granules. There are two types of granules. One contains peroxidase, acid phosphatase, and arylsulfatase. Less is known about the content of the other granule. The nuclear chromatin is loose and linear forming a lacy pattern. The nucleus is often irregular in shape.

Monocyte-macrophage system – a collection of monocytes and macrophages, found both intravascularly and extravascularly. Plays a major role in initiating and regulating the immune response.

Monocytopenia – a decrease in the concentration of ciruculating monocytes ($<0.2 \times 10^9$/L).

Monocytosis – an increase in the concentration of circulating monocytes ($>1.0 \times 10^9$/L).

Monosomy – one daughter cell with a missing chromosome (one copy instead of two).

Morulae – basophilic, irregularly shaped granular, cytoplasmic inclusions found in leukocytes in an infectious disease called ehrlichiosis.

Mosaic – occurs in the embryo shortly after fertilization, resulting in congenital aberrations in some cells and some normal cells.

Mott cell – pathologic plasma cell whose cytoplasm is filled with colorless globules. These globules most often contain immunoglobulin (Russell bodies). The globules form as a result of accumulation of material in the RER, SER, or Golgi complex due to an obstruction of secretion. The cell is associated with chronic plasmocyte hyperplasia, parasitic infection, and malignant tumors. Also called grape cells.

Multimer analysis – an analysis that determines the structure of vWf multimers.

Multiple myeloma – plasma cell malignancy characterized by increased plasma proteins.

Mutation – any change in the nucleotide sequence of DNA. In instances where large sequences of nucleotides are missing, the alteration is referred to as a deletion.

Myeloblast – the first microscopically identifiable granulocyte precursor. It is normally found in the bone marrow. The cell is large (15–20 µm) with a high nuclear/cytoplasmic ratio. The nucleus has a fine chromatin pattern with a nucleoli. There is moderate amount of blue, agranular cytoplasm.

Myelocyte – a granulocytic precursor cell normally found in the bone marrow. The cell is 12–18 µm in diameter with a pinkish granular cytoplasm. There are both primary and secondary granules present.

Myelodysplastic syndromes (MDS) – a group of primary neoplastic pluripotential stem cell disorders characterized by one or more cytopenias in the peripheral blood together with prominent maturation abnormalities (dysplasia) in the bone marrow.

Myelofibrosis with myeloid metaplasia – a myeloproliferative disorder characterized by excessive proliferation of all cell lines as well as progressive bone marrow fibrosis and blood cell production at sites other than the bone marrow, such as the liver and spleen. Also called agnogenic myeloid metaplasia and primary myelofibrosis.

Myeloid-to-erythroid ratio (M:E ratio) – the ratio of granulocytes and their precursors to nucleated erythroid precursors derived from performing a differential count on bone marrow nucleated hematopoietic cells. Monocytes and lymphocytes are not included. The normal ratio is usually between 1.5:1 and 3.5:1, reflecting a predominance of myeloid elements.

Myeloid/NK cell acute leukemia – an acute leukemia in which the neoplastic cells coexpress myeloid antigens (CD33, CD13, and/or CD15) and NK cell-associated antigens (CD56, CD11b), while they lack HLADR and T lymphocyte associated antigens CD3 and CD8.

Myeloperoxidase – an enzyme present in the primary granules of myeloid cells including neutrophils, eosinophils, and monocytes.

Myelophthisis – replacement of normal hematopoietic tissue in bone marrow by fibrosis, leukemia, or metastatic cancer cells.

Myeloproliferative disorders (MPD) – a group of neoplastic clonal disorders characterized by excess proliferation of one or more cell types in the bone marrow.

▶ N

National Committee for Clinical Laboratory Standards (NCCLS) – national agency that establishes laboratory standards.

Necrosis – pathologic cell death resulting from irreversible damage; "cell murder."

Neonatal idiopathic thrombocytopenic purpura (neonatal ITP) – a form of ITP that occurs in newborns due to the transfer of maternal alloantibodies.

Neoplasm – abnormal formation of new tissue (such as a tumor) that serves no useful purpose. May be benign or malignant.

Neutropenia – a decrease in neutrophils below 2×10^9/L.

Neutrophil – a mature white blood cell with a segmented nucleus and granular cytoplasm. These cells constitute the majority of circulating leukocytes. The absolute number varies between 2.0 and 6.8 $\times 10^9$/L. They are also called granulocytes or segs.

Neutrophilia – an increase in neutrophils over 6.8×10^9/L. Seen in bacterial infections, inflammation, metabolic intoxication, drug intoxication, and tissue necrosis.

Nondisjunction – an error in segregation that occurs in mitosis or meiosis so that sister chromatids do not disjoin. A spindle fiber malfunction results in one daughter cell with an extra chromosome (trisomy) and one daughter cell with a missing chromosome (monosomy).

Nonspecific granules – large, blue-black granules found in promyelocytes. The granules have a phospholipid membrane and stain positive for peroxidase.

Nonthrombocytopenic purpura – a condition in which platelets are normal in number but purpura are present; purpura is considered to be caused by damage to the blood vessels.

Normal pooled plasma – platelet-poor plasma collected from at least 20 individuals for coagulation testing. Plasmas should give PT and APTT results within the laboratory's reference interval. The plasma is pooled and used in mixing studies to differentiate a circulating inhibitor from a factor deficiency.

Normoblast – nucleated erythrocyte precursor in the bone marrow. Also known as erythroblast.

Normogram – a chart that displays the relationship between numerical variables.

Nuclear-cytoplasmic asynchrony – a condition in which the cellular nucleus matures slower than the cytoplasm, suggesting a disturbance in coordination. As a result, the nucleus takes on the appearance of a nucleus associated with a younger cell than its cytoplasmic development indicates. This is a characteristic of megaloblastic anemias.

Nuclear-to-cytoplasmic ratio (N:C ratio) – the ratio of the volume of the cell nucleus to the volume of the cell's cytoplasm. This is usually estimated as the ratio of the diameter of the nucleus to the diameter of the cytoplasm. In immature hematopoietic cells the N:C ratio is usually greater than in more mature cells. As the cell matures, the nucleus condenses and the cytoplasm expands.

Nucleolus (pl: nucleoli) – a spherical body within the nucleus in which ribosomes are produced. It is not present in cells that are not synthesizing proteins or that are not in mitosis or meiosis. It stains a lighter blue than the nucleus with Romanowsky stains.

Nucleotide – the basic building block of DNA, composed of nitrogen base (A = adenine, T = thymine, G = guanine, or C = cytosine) attached to a sugar (deoxyribose) and a phosphate molecule.

Nucleus (pl: nuclei) – the characteristic structure in the eukaryocytic cell that contains chromosomes and nucleoli. It is separated from the cytoplasm by a nuclear envelope. The structure stains deep bluish-purple with Romanowsky stain. In young, immature hematopoietic cells, the nuclear material is open and dispersed in a lacy pattern. As the cell becomes mature, the nuclear material condenses and appears structureless.

Null cell – *see* large granular lymphocytes.

▶ O

Oncogene – an altered gene that contributes to the development of cancer. Most oncogenes are altered forms of normal genes that function to regulate cell growth and differentiation. The normal gene counterpart is known as a proto-oncogene.

Open canalicular system (OCS) – a membrane system in the platelet that surrounds twisted channels that lead from the platelet surface to the interior of the platelet. It is a remnant of the demarcation membrane system of the megakaryocyte.

Opportunistic organisms – organisms that are usually part of the normal flora but can cause disease if there is a significant change in host resistance or within the organism itself.

Opsonin – an antibody or complement that coats microorganisms or other particulate matter found within the blood stream so that the foreign material may be more readily recognized and phagocytized by leukocytes.

Optimal counting area – area of the blood smear where erythrocytes are just touching but not overlapping; used for morphologic evaluation and identification of cells.

Oral anticoagulant – a group of drugs (e.g., coumadin, warfarin) that prevent coagulation by inhibiting the activity of vitamin K. Vitamin K is required for the synthesis of functional prothrombin group coagulation factors.

Orthochromatic normoblast – a nucleated precursor of the erythrocyte that develops from the polychromatophilic normoblast. It is the last nucleated stage of erythrocyte development. The cell normally is found in the bone marrow.

Osmotic fragility – a laboratory procedure employed to evaluate the ability of erythrocytes to withstand different salt concentrations; this is dependent upon the erythrocyte's membrane, volume, surface area, and functional state.

Osteoblast – cell involved in formation of calcified bone.

Osteoclast – cell involved in resorption and remodeling of calcified bone.

Outlier – data point that falls outside the expected range for all data. An outlier is not considered to be part of the population that was sampled.

Oxygen affinity – the ability for hemoglobin to bind and release oxygen. An increase in CO_2, acid, and heat decrease oxygen affinity, while an increase in pO_2 increases oxygen affinity.

Oxyhemoglobin – the compound formed when hemoglobin combines with oxygen.

 P

P_{50} value – partial pressure of oxygen at which 50% of hemoglobin is saturated with oxygen.

P53 gene – normally functions as an antioncogene by preventing proliferation of DNA-damaged cells, promoting apoptosis of these damaged cells, and preventing unwanted DNA amplification. When mutated, this gene may lose its tumor suppressive effect.

Paired t test – statistical tool used to compare the difference between two paired data sets. Paired t test determines if a statistically significant difference exists between the two paired data sets.

Pancytopenia – marked decrease of all blood cells in the peripheral blood.

Panhypercellular – increase in all blood cells in the peripheral blood.

Pappenheimer bodies – iron-containing particles in mature erythrocyte. On Romanowsky stain, visible near the periphery of the cell and often occur in clusters.

Paroxysmal cold hemoglobinuria (PCH) – an autoimmune hemolytic anemia characterized by hemolysis and hematuria upon exposure to cold.

Paroxysmal nocturnal hemoglobinuria (PNH) – a stem cell disease in which the erythrocyte membrane is abnormal, making the cell more susceptible to hemolysis by complement. There is a lack of decay accelerating factor (DAF) and C8 binding protein (C8bp) on the membrane, which is normally responsible for preventing amplification of complement activation. The deficiency of DAF and C8bp is due to the lack of glycosyl phosphatidyl inositol (GPI), a membrane glycolipid that serves to attach (anchor) proteins to the cell membrane. Intravascular hemolysis is intermittent.

Pelger-Huët anomaly – an inherited benign condition characterized by the presence of functionally normal neutrophils with a bilobed or round nucleus. Cells with the bilobed appearance are called pince-nez cells.

Percent saturation – the portion of transferrin that is complexed with iron.

Pericardial cavity – body cavity that contains the heart.

Pericardium – membrane that lines the pericardial cavity.

Peripheral membrane protein – protein that is attached to the cell membrane by ionic or hydrogen bonds but is outside the lipid framework of the membrane.

Peritoneal cavity – space between the inside abdominal wall and outside of the stomach, small and large intestines, liver, superior aspect of the bladder, and uterus.

Peritoneum – lining of the peritoneal cavity.

Pernicious anemia – megaloblastic anemia resulting from a lack of intrinsic factor. The intrinsic factor is needed to absorb cobalamin (vitamin B_{12}) from the gut.

Petechiae – small, pinhead-sized purple spots caused by blood escaping from capillaries into intact skin. These are associated with platelet and vascular disorders.

Phagocytosis – cellular process of cells engulfing and destroying a foreign particle through active cell membrane invagination.

Phagolysosome – a digestive vacuole (secondary lysosome) formed by the fusion of lysosomes and a phagosome. The hydrolytic enzymes of the lysosome digest the phagocytosed material.

Phagosome – the formation of an isolated vacuole within the process of opsonization.

Pharmacokinetics – quantitative study of a drug's disposition in the body over time.

Phase microscopy – a type of light microscopy in which an annular diaphragm is placed below or in the substage condenser, and a phase shifting element is placed in the rear focal plane of the objective. This causes alterations in the phases of light rays and increases the contrast between the cell and its surroundings. This methodology is used to count platelets.

Phenotype – the physical manifestation of an individual's genotype, often referring to a particular genetic locus.

Phi body – a smaller version of the Auer rod.

Pia mater – thin membrane directly covering the central nervous system; middle layer of the meninges.

Pica – a perversion of appetite that leads to bizarre eating practices; a clinical finding in some individuals with iron deficiency anemia.

Pitting – removal of abnormal inclusions from erythrocytes by the spleen.

PIVKA (protein-induced by vitamin-K absence or antagonist) – these factors are the nonfunctional forms of the prothrombin group coagulation factors. They are synthesized in the liver in the absence of vitamin K and lack the carboxyl (COOH) group necessary for binding the factor to a phospholipid surface.

Plasma cell – a transformed, fully differentiated B lymphocyte normally found in the bone marrow and medullary cords of lymph nodes. May be seen in the circulation in certain infections and disorders associated with increased serum γ-globulins. The cell is characterized by the presence of an eccentric nucleus containing condensed, deeply staining chromatin and deep basophilic cytoplasm. The large Golgi apparatus next to the nucleus does not stain, leaving an obvious clear paranuclear area. The cell has the PC-1 membrane antigen and cytoplasmic immunoglobulin.

Plasma cell neoplasm – a monoclonal neoplasm of immunoglobulin secreting cells.

Plasmacytosis – the presence of plasma cells in the peripheral blood or an excess of plasma cells in the bone marrow.

Plasmin – a proteolytic enzyme with trypsin-like specificity that digests fibrin or fibrinogen as well as other coagulation factors. Plasmin is formed from plasminogen.

Plasminogen – a β-globulin, single-chain glycoprotein that circulates in the blood as a zymogen. Large amounts of plasminogen are absorbed with the fibrin mass during clot formation. Plasminogen is activated by intrinsic and extrinsic activators to form plasmin.

Plasminogen activator inhibitor-1 (PAI-1) – the primary inhibitor of tissue plasminogen activator (t-PA) and urokinase-like plasminogen activator (tcu-PA) released from platelet α granules during platelet activation.

Plasminogen activator inhibitor-2 (PAI-2) – an inhibitor of tissue plasminogen activator and urokinase-like plasminogen activator. Secretion of PAI-2 is stimulated by endotoxin and phorbol esters. Increased levels impair fibrinolysis and are associated with thrombosis.

Platelet – a round or oval structure in the peripheral blood formed from the cytoplasm of megakaryocytes in the bone marrow. Platelets play an important role in primary hemostasis adhering to the ruptured blood vessel wall and aggregating to form a platelet plug over the injured area. Platelets are also important in secondary hemostasis by providing platelet factor 3 (PF3) important for the activation of coagulation proteins. The normal reference range for platelets is $150–440 \times 10^9$/L.

Platelet activation – stimulation of a platelet that occurs when agonists bind to the platelet's surface and transmit signals to the cell's interior. Activated platelets form aggregates known as the primary platelet plug.

Platelet adhesion – platelet attachment to collagen fibers.

Platelet aggregation – platelet-to-platelet interaction that results in a clumped mass; may occur in vitro or in vivo.

Platelet clump – aggregation of platelets; may occur when blood is collected by capillary puncture (due to platelet activation) and when blood is collected in EDTA anticoagulant (due to unmasking of platelet antigens that can react with antibodies in the serum).

Platelet distribution width (PDW) – coefficient of variation of platelet volume distribution; analogous to RDW.

Platelet factor 4 – protein present in platelet's alpha granules that is capable of neutralizing heparin.

Plateletpheresis – a procedure in which platelets are removed from the circulation.

Platelet-poor plasma (PPP) – citrated plasma containing less than 15×10^9/L platelets. It is prepared by centrifugation of citrated whole blood at a minimum RCF of $1000 \times g$ for 15 minutes. PPP is used for the majority of coagulation tests.

Platelet procoagulant activity – the property of platelets that enables activated coagulation factors and cofactors to adhere to the platelet surface during the formation of fibrin.

Platelet-rich plasma (PRP) – citrated plasma containing approximately $200–300 \times 10^9$/L platelets. It is prepared by centrifugation of citrated whole blood at an RCF of $150 \times g$ for 10 minutes. PRP is used in platelet aggregation studies.

Platelet satellistism – adherence of platelets to neutrophil membranes in vitro; this can occur when blood is collected in EDTA anticoagulant.

Pleura – lining of the pleural cavities.

Pleural cavity – space between the chest wall and the lungs.

Plethora – excess of blood.

Plumbism – lead poisoning.

Pluripotential cell – cell that differentiates into many different cell lines. Has the potential to self-renew, proliferate, and differentiate into erythrocytic, myelocytic, monocytic, lymphocytic, and megakaryocytic blood cell lineages.

Poikilocytosis – a term used to describe the presence of variations in the shape of erythrocytes.

Point of care (POC) instrument – instrument that allows for analytical testing of patient specimens outside the laboratory setting (e.g., home testing or physician's office testing).

Polychromatophilia – the quality of being stainable with more than one stain; the term is commonly used to describe erythrocytes that stain with a grayish or bluish tinge with Romanowsky stains due to residual RNA, which takes up the blue portion of the dye.

Polychromatophilic erythrocyte – an erythrocyte with a bluish tinge when stained with Romanowsky stain; contains residual RNA. If stained with new methylene blue, these cells would show reticulum and would be identified as reticulocytes.

Polyclonal – arising from different cell clones.

Polyclonal gammopathy – an alteration in immunoglobulin production that is characterized by an increase in immunoglobulins of more than one class.

Polycythemia – condition associated with increased erythrocyte count.

Polymerase chain reaction – a procedure for copying a specific DNA sequence manyfold.

Polymorphic variants – variant morphology of a portion of a chromosome that has no clinical consequence.

Polymorphonuclear neutrophil (PMN) – a mature granulocyte found in bone marrow and peripheral blood. The nucleus is segmented into 2 or more lobes. The cytoplasm stains pinkish and there is abundant specific granules. This is the most numerous leukocyte in the peripheral blood ($2–6.8 \times 10^9$/L). Its primary function is defense against foreign antigens. It is active in phagocytosis and killing of microorganisms. Also called a segmented neutrophil or seg.

Polyploid – number of chromososmes per cell that is a multiple of n (23) other than one or two (e.g., 3n(69), 4n(92), etc.).

Porphyrins – a highly unsaturated tetrapyrrole ring bonded by four methane (–CH=) bridges. Substituents occupy each of the eight peripheral positions on the four pyrrole rings. The kind and order of these substituents determine the type of porphyrin. Porphyrins are only metabolically active when they are chelated.

Portland hemoglobin – an embryonic hemoglobin found in the yolk sac and detectable up to eight weeks gestation. It is composed of two zeta (ζ) and two gamma (γ) chains.

Postmitotic pool – also called the maturation-storage pool; the neutrophils in the bone marrow that are not capable of mitosis. These cells include metamyelocytes, bands, and segmented neutrophils. Cells spend about 5–7 days in this compartment before being released to the peripheral blood.

Primary aggregation – the earliest association of platelets in an aggregate that is reversible.

Primary fibrinolysis – a clinical situation that occurs when there is a release of excessive quantities of plasminogen activators into the blood in the absence of fibrin clot formation. Excess plasmin degrades fibrinogen and the clotting factors, leading to a potentially dangerous hemorrhagic condition.

Primary hemostasis – the initial arrest of bleeding that occurs with blood vessel/platelet interaction.

Primary hemostatic plug – an aggregate of platelets that initially halts blood flow from an injured vessel.

Primary thrombocytosis – an increase in platelets that is not secondary to another condition. Usually refers to the thrombocytosis that occurs in neoplastic disorders.

Probe – a tool for identifying a particular nucleotide sequence of interest. A probe is composed of a nucleotide sequence that is complementary to the sequence of interest and is therefore capable of hybridizing to that sequence. Probes are labeled in a way that is detectable, such as by radioactivity.

Procoagulant – an inert precursor of a natural substance that is necessary for blood clotting or a property of anything that favors formation of a blood clot.

Proficiency testing – utilizes unknown samples from an external source (e.g., College of American Pathologists) to monitor the quality of a given laboratory's test results.

Progenitor cell – parent or anscestor cells that differentiate into mature, functional cells.

Prolymphocyte – the immediate precursor cell of the lymphocyte; normally found in bone marrow. It is slightly smaller than the lymphoblast and has a lower nuclear to cytoplasmic ratio. The nuclear chromatin is somewhat clumped, and nucleoli are usually present. The cytoplasm stains light blue and is agranular.

Promonocyte – a monocytic precursor cell found in the bone marrow. The cell is 14–18 μm in diameter with abundant blue-gray cytoplasm. Fine azurophilic granules may be present. The nucleus is often irregular and deeply indented. The chromatin is finely dispersed and stains a light purple-blue. Nucleoli may be present. Cytochemically, the cells stain positive for nonspecific esterase, peroxidase, acid phosphatase, and arylsulfatase. The cell matures to a monocyte.

Promyelocyte – a granulocytic precursor cell normally found in the bone marrow. The cell is 15–21 μm in diameter. The cytoplasm is basophilic and the nucleus is quite large. The nuclear chromatin is lacy, staining a light purple-blue. Several nucleoli are visible. The distinguishing feature is the presence of large blue-black primary (azurophilic) granules. The granules have a phospholipid membrane that stains with Sudan black B. The granules contain acid phosphatase, myeloperoxidase, acid hydrolases, lysozyme, sulfated mucopolysaccharides, and other basic proteins. The promyelocyte matures to a myelocyte. Also called a progranulocyte.

Pronormoblast – a precursor cell of the erythrocyte. The cell is derived from the pluripotential stem cell and is found in the bone marrow. The cell is 12–20 μm in diameter and has a high nuclear-cytoplasmic ratio. The cytoplasm is deeply basophilic with Romanowsky stains. The nuclear chromatin is fine, and there is one or more nucleoli. Also called a rubriblast. The cell matures to a basophilic normoblast.

Prothrombinase complex – a complex formed by coagulation factors Xa and V, calcium, and phospholipid. This complex activates prothrombin to thrombin.

Prothrombin group – the group of coagulation factors that are vitamin K-dependent for synthesis of their functional forms and that require calcium for binding to a phospholipid surface. Includes factors II, VII, IX, and X. Also known as vitamin K-dependent factors.

Prothrombin time (PT) – a screening test used to detect deficiencies in the extrinsic or common pathway of the coagulation cascade and for monitoring the effectiveness of oral anticoagulant therapy.

Prothrombin time ratio – a calculation derived by dividing the patient's prothrombin time result by midpoint of the laboratory's normal range and used to calculate the International Normalized Ratio (INR).

Prourokinase – an immature, single-chain form of urokinase that is prepared from urine and by recombinant DNA techniques and can be activated to a two-chain form by plasmin.

Pseudochylous – fluid that appears chylous due to the presence of many inflammatory cells; does not contain lymph fluid or chylomicrons.

Pseudodiploid – a cell that has a chromosome count of *2n* (46), however, with a combination of numerical and/or structural aberrations, e.g., 46, XY, −5, −7, 2D8, 2D21.

Pseudoneutrophilia – an increase in the concentration of neutrophils in the peripheral blood ($>6.8 \times 10^9$/L) occurring as a result of cells from the marginating pool entering the circulating pool. The response is immediate but transient. This redistribution of cells accompanies vigorous exercise, epinephrine administration, anesthesia, convulsion, and anxiety states; also called immediate or shift neutrophilia.

Pseudo–Pelger-Huët cells – an acquired condition in which neutrophils display a hyposegmented nucleus. Unlike the real Pelger-Huët anomaly, the nucleus of this cell contains a significant amount of euchromatin and stains more lightly. A critical differentiation point is that all neutrophils are equally affected in the genetic form of Pelger-Huët anomaly, but only a fraction of neutrophils will be hyposegmented cells in the acquired state. Associated with MDS and MPD; may also be found after treatment for leukemias.

Pulmonary embolism – obstruction of the pulmonary artery or one of its branches by a clot or foreign material that has been dislodged from another area by the blood current.

Pure red cell aplasia (PRCA) – anemia with selective decrease in erythrocyte precursors in the marrow.

Purging – a technique by which undesirable cells that are present in the blood or bone marrow products are removed.

Purpura – (1) purple discoloration of the skin caused by petechiae and/or ecchymoses; (2) a diverse group of disorders that are characterized by the presence of petechiae and ecchymoses.

Pyknotic – pertaining to degeneration of the nucleus of the cell in which the chromatin condenses to a solid, structureless mass and shrinks.

 Q

Quality control limit – expected range of results. These limits are used to determine if a test method is in control, and to minimize the chance of inaccurate patient results. If the test method is out of control, an intervention is required to reconcile the problem.

Quiescence (G_0) – a phase in a cell that has exited the cell cycle and is in a nonproliferative state.

► **R**

R (relaxed) structure – conformational change in hemoglobin that occurs as the molecule takes up oxygen.

Radar chart – graphical representation of eight CBC parameters: WBC, RBC, Hb, Hct, MCV, MCH, MCHC, and PLT. Lines are drawn to connect the parameters; resembles a radar oscilloscope. Changes in the shape of the radar chart are indicative of different hematologic disorders.

Radial immunodiffusion – diffusion technique in which antibody is incorporated into agarose gel and antigen is placed into wells in the gel. The antigen is quantitated by the size of a precipitin ring that forms as antigen diffuses from a sample well into the gel.

Random access – capability of an automated hematology instrument to process specimens independently of one another; may be programmed to run individual tests (e.g., Hb or platelet counts) or a panel of tests (e.g., CBC with reticulocyte count) without operator intervention.

Random variation – variation within an instrument or test method that is due to chance. This type of variation can be either positive or negative in direction and affects precision.

Rapoport-Leubering shunt – a metabolic pathway in which 2,3-diphosphoglycerate (2,3-DPG) is synthesized from 1,3-diphosphoglycerate. 2,3-DPG facilitates the release of oxygen from hemoglobin in the erythrocyte. 2,3-DPG is also referred to as 2,3-BPG (bisphosphoglycerate).

Raynaud's phenomenon – secondary disorder resulting from vaso-arterial spasms in the extremities of the body when exposed to the cold. Characterized by blanching of the skin, followed by cyanosis, and finally redness when the affected area is warmed; also referred to as acrocyanosis.

RBC indices – the RBC indices help classify the erythrocytes as to their size and hemoglobin content. Hemoglobin, hematocrit, and erythrocyte are used to calculate the three indices: mean corpuscular volume (MCV), mean corpuscular hemoglobin concentration (MCHC), and mean corpuscular hemoglobin (MCH). The indices give a clue as to what the erythrocytes should look like on a stained blood film.

Reactive lymphocyte – an antigen stimulated lymphocyte that exhibits a variety of morphologic features. The cell is usually larger than the resting lymphocyte and has an irregular shape. The cytoplasm is more basophilic. The nucleus is often elongated and irregular with a finer chromatin pattern than that of the resting lymphocyte. Often this cell is increased in viral infections; also called a virocyte, or stimulated, transformed, atypical, activated, or leukocytoid lymphocyte.

Reactive neutrophilia – an increase in the concentration of peripheral blood neutrophils ($>6.8 \times 10^9$/L) as a result of reaction to a physiologic or pathologic process.

Reagent blank – measurement of absorbance due to reagent alone; eliminates false increase in sample absorbance due to reagent color.

Red thrombus – thrombus composed mostly of red blood cells; so named because of its red coloration.

Reed-Sternberg cell – cell found in the classic form of Hodgkin lymphoma. It is characterized by a multilobated nucleus and large inclusion-like nucleoli.

Reference interval – test value range that is considered normal. Generally the range is determined to include 95% of the normal population.

Reflex testing – follow-up testing that is performed based on results of screening tests.

Refractive Index – the degree to which a transparent object will deflect a light ray from a straight path.

Refractory – pertains to disorders or diseases that do not respond readily to therapy.

Refractory anemia – a subgroup of the FAB classification of the myelodysplastic syndromes. Anemia refractory to all conventional therapy is the primary clinical finding. Blasts constitute <1% of nucleated peripheral blood cells. The bone marrow shows signs of dyserythropoiesis.

Refractory anemia with excess blasts (RAEB) – a subgroup of the FAB classification of the myelodysplastic syndromes. There are usually cytopenias and signs of dyspoiesis in the peripheral blood with <5% blasts. The bone marrow is usually hypercellular with dyspoiesis in all hematopoietic cell lineages. Bone marrow blasts vary from 5% to 20%.

Refractory anemia with excess blasts in transformation (RAEB-T) – a subgroup of the FAB classification of the myelodysplastic syndromes. There is/are cytopenia(s) in the peripheral blood with more than 5% blasts. The bone marrow is usually hyperceullular with dyspoiesis and 20–30% blasts. In the WHO classification this would be considered acute leukemia (>20% blasts).

Refractory anemia with ringed sideroblasts (RARS) – a subgroup of the FAB classification of the myelodysplastic syndromes characterized by <1% blasts in the peripheral blood, anemia, and/or thrombocytopenia and/or leukopenia. There are more than 15% ringed sideroblasts and <5% blasts in the bone marrow.

Remission – a diminution of the symptoms of a disease.

Replication – the process by which DNA is copied during cell division. Replication is carried out by the enzyme DNA polymerase, which recognizes single-stranded DNA and fills in the appropriate complementary nucleotides to produce double-stranded DNA. Synthesis is initated at a free 5' end where double-stranded DNA lies adjacent to single-stranded DNA, and replication proceeds in the 5' direction. In the laboratory, DNA replication can be induced as a means of copying DNA sequences, as exploited in the polymerase chain reaction.

Reportable range – range that is defined by a minimum value and a maximum value of calibration material.

Restriction endonuclease – an enzyme that cleaves double-stranded DNA at specific nucleotide sequences. For example, HindIII cleaves DNA only where the sequence 5'-AAGCTT-3' is present. A variety of other enzymes are known to cut various specific target sequences. Examples of common restriction endonucleases are BamH1, EcoR1, Mnl1, MstII, Pst1, and Xba1.

Restriction point – occurs in late G1; point when cell cycle progression becomes autonomous.

Reticulocyte – first nonnucleated stage of erythrocyte development in the bone marrow. Contains RNA that is visualized as granules or filaments within the cell when stained supravitally with new methylene blue. Normally reticulocytes constitute approximately 1% of the circulating erythrocyte population.

Reticulocyte production index (RPI) – an indicator of the bone marrow response in anemia. The calculation corrects the reticulocyte count for the presence of marrow reticulocytes in the peripheral blood. Calculated as follows:

(Patient hematocrit [L/L] ÷ 0.45 [L/L]) × reticulocyte count (%) × (1 ÷ maturation time of shift reticulocytes) = RPI

Reticulocytosis – the presence of excess reticulocytes in the peripheral blood.

Rh null disease – disorder associated with the lack of the Rh antigen on erythrocytes.

Rhopheocytosis – an energy and temperature dependent process by which iron enters cells.

Ribosomes – a cellular particle composed of ribonucleic acid (RNA) and protein whose function is to synthesize polypeptide chains from amino acids. The sequence of amino acids in the chains is specified by the genetic code of messenger RNA. Ribosomes appear singly or in reversibly dissociable units and may be free in the cytoplasm or attached to endoplasmic reticulum. The cytoplasm of blood cells that contain a high concentration of ribosomes stains bluish purple with Romanowsky stains.

Richter's transformation – transformation from CLL to another disease, usually large B cell lymphoma.

Ringed sideroblasts – erythroblasts with abnormal deposition of excess iron within mitochondria resulting in a ring formation around the nucleus.

Ristocetin – aggregating reagent that specifically evaluates vWF interaction with glycoprotein Ib on platelets.

Ristocetin induced platelet aggregation (RIPA) – measures function of patient's vWf to bind platelets to collagen.

RNA (ribonucleic acid) – a single-stranded molecule composed of ribonucleotides (A, C, G, and U). RNA is produced by transcription of genes from a DNA template; RNA in turn serves as a template for protein translation.

Romanowsky-type stain – any stain consisting of methylene blue and its oxidation products and eosin Y or eosin B.

Rouleaux – erythrocyte distribution characterized by stacking of erythrocytes like a roll of coins. This is due to abnormal coating of the cell's surface with increased plasma proteins, which decreases the zeta potential between cells.

Russell bodies – a globule filled with immunoglobulin found in pathologic plasma cells called Mott cells (see Mott cell).

Russell's viper venom – venom that possesses thromboplastin-like activity and activates factor X.

▶ **S**

Satellite DNA – DNA containing many tandem repeats. Morphologically, it appears as a small ball-like structure making up the short arm of acrocentric chromosomes. This is the locus of the nucleolar organizing region.

Scatterplot – a dot-plot histogram of two cellular characteristics. Together, the two characteristics allow definition of the leukocyte subpopulations.

Schistocyte – fragment of an erythrocyte; a schistocyte may have a variety of shapes including triangle, helmet, and comma.

Secondary aggregation – irreversible aggregation of platelets that occurs over time.

Secondary fibrinolysis – a clinical condition characterized by excessive fibrinolytic activity in response to disseminated intravascular clotting.

Secondary hemostasis – the formation of fibrin that stabilizes a primary platelet plug.

Secondary hemostatic plug – a primary platelet aggregate that has been stabilized by fibrin formation during secondary hemostasis.

Secondary thrombocytosis – an increase in platelet concentration in the blood. The increase is in response to stimulation by another condition.

Secretion – energy dependent discharge or release of products usually from glands in the body but also pertaining to the contents of platelet granules that are released after stimulation of the platelets by agonists; also, the product that is discharged or released.

Self-renewal – the property of regenerating the same cells.

Sensitivity – refers to the ability of a test method to detect small quantities of the analyte.

Serine protease – the family of serine proteases includes thrombin, factors VIIa, IXa, Xa, XIa, XIIa, and the digestive enzymes chymotrypsin and trypsin. They selectively hydrolyze arginine- or lysine-containing peptide bonds of other zymogens converting them to serine proteases. Each serine protease involved in the coagulation cascade is highly specific for its substrate.

Serpin – a family of serine protease inhibitors that inhibit target molecules by formation of a 1:1 stoichiometric complex.

Severe combined immunodeficiency syndrome (SCIDS) – a heterogeneous group of disorders based on diverse genetic origins, different inheritance patterns, and severity of clinical manifestations. The disease may be inherited either as a sex-linked trait or as an autosomal-recessive trait. This is the most severe immune deficiency disease.

Sézary's cell – circulating neoplastic cell found in Sézary's syndrome characterized by a very convoluted (cerebriform) nuclear outline.

Shelf life – the time period for which a reagent or control is stable given appropriate storage conditions. Shelf life will change once the reagent or control is reconstituted if lypholyzed or opened if liquid.

Shift neutrophilia – *see* pseudoneutrophilia.

Shift-to-the-left – the appearance of increased numbers of immature leukocytes in the peripheral blood.

Sickle cell (drepanocyte) – elongated crescent shaped erythrocyte with pointed ends. Sickle cell formation may be observed in wet preparations or in stained blood smears from patients with sickle-cell anemia.

Sickle-cell anemia – a genetically determined disorder in which hemoglobin S is inherited in the homozygous state. No hemoglobin A is present. Hemoglobins S, F, A_2 are present.

Sickle-cell trait – a genetically determined disorder in which hemoglobin S is inherited in the heterozygous state. The patient has one normal β-globin gene and one $β^S$-globin gene. Both hemoglobin A and hemoglobin S are present.

Side light scatter – laser light scattered at a 90° angle due to internal complexity and granularity of the particle (e.g., neutrophils produce a lot of side scatter because of their numerous cytoplasmic granules).

Sideroacrestic – a defect in iron utilization.

Siderocyte – an erythrocyte that contains stainable iron granules.

Sideropenic – lack of iron.

Slope – the angle or direction of the regression line with respect to the x and y axes. The slope is used to identify the presence of proportional systematic error.

Small lymphocytic lymphoma (SLL) – identical to CLL, but primarily involves the lymph nodes. The two disorders appear to belong to one disease entity with differing clinical manifestations.

Smooth endoplasmic reticulum (SER) – *see* endoplasmic reticulum.

Smudge cell – cell whose cytoplasmic membrane has ruptured, leaving a bare nucleus. Increased numbers of smudge cells are observed in lymphoproliferative disorders like chronic lymphocytic leukemia. Can also be seen in reactive lymphocytosis and in other neoplasms.

Southern blot – a procedure first described by Ed Southern for determining DNA structure. In this procedure, DNA is cleaved with restriction endonucleases that cut DNA at specific nucleotide sequences. The resulting DNA fragments are electrophoresed in an agarose gel to separate them by size and then treated with a solution of high pH that separates double-stranded DNA into two single-stranded parts. The single-stranded fragments are then transferred to a membrane where they can be hybridized to a complementary labeled probe. Probe hybridization permits identification of the DNA fragments containing the sequence of interest. The size and number of those fragments reflects the structure of the DNA.

Specificity – the ability of a test method to determine only the analyte meant to be detected or measured.

Specimen run – an interval, period of time, or number of specimens for which the accuracy and precision of the laboratory procedure is expected to remain stable.

Spherocyte – an abnormally round erythrocyte with dense hemoglobin content (increased MCHC). The cell has no central area of pallor as it has lost its biconcave shape.

Splenectomy – removal of the spleen.

Splenomegaly – abnormal enlargement of the spleen.

Split sample – division of a single sample into two or more aliquots for the purpose of testing on two or more instruments within the same time period or retesting the sample at another time.

Spur cell anemia – an acquired hemolytic condition associated with severe hepatocellular disease such as cirrhosis, in which there is an increase in serum lipoproteins, leading to excess of erythrocyte membrane cholesterol. The total phospholipid content of the membrane, however, is normal.

Stab – *see* band.

Stage – the stage of a neoplasm is the extent and distribution of disease. Determining the stage of disease usually involves radiologic studies, peripheral blood examination, and bone marrow aspiration and biopsy.

Standard deviation – distribution of a set of data about the mean.

Standard error of the estimate ($s_{y/x}$) – a measure of the variation in the regression line. The $s_{y/x}$ is used to identify random error.

Starry sky – morphologic appearance characteristic of high-grade lymphoma produced by numerous tingible body macrophages (stars) and a diffuse sheet of neoplastic cells (sky).

Stomatocyte – an abnormal erythrocyte shape characterized by a slit-like area of central pallor. This cell has a uniconcave, cup shape.

Streptokinase – a bacterial enzyme derived from group C-beta hemolytic steptococci that activates plasminogen to plasmin and is used as a thrombolytic agent in the treatment of thrombosis.

Stroma – extracellular matrix or microenvironment that supports hematopoietic cell proliferation in the bone marrow.

Stromal cells – cellular elements of the hematopoietic microenvironment in the red portion of bone marrow.

Submetacentric – chromosome that has the centromere positioned off-center so that the short arm is shorter than the long arm.

Sucrose hemolysis test – a screening test to identify erythrocytes that are abnormally sensitive to complement lysis. In this test, erythrocytes, serum, and sucrose are incubated together. Cells abnormally sensitive to complement will lyse. The test is used to screen for paroxysmal nocturnal hemoglobinuria. Also called the sugar-water test.

Sulfhemoglobin – stable compound formed when a sulfur atom combines with each of the four heme groups of hemoglobin; it is incapable of carrying oxygen.

Supernatant – clear liquid remaining on top of a solution after centrifugation of the particulate matter.

Supravital stain – a stain used to stain cells or tissues while they are still living.

Syngeneic stem cell transplantation – transplantation of stem cells between genetically identical twins.

Synovium – continuous membrane that lines the bony, cartilaginous, and connective tissue surfaces of a joint.

Systematic variation – variation within an instrument or test method that occurs in one direction and can be predicted. This type of variation affects accuracy.

► T

Target cell – an abnormally shaped erythrocyte. The cell appears as a target with a bull's-eye center mass of hemoglobin surrounded by an achromic ring and an outer ring of hemoglobin. The osmotic fragility of this cell is decreased; also called Mexican hat cell.

Tartrate resistant acid phosphatase (TRAP) – acid phosphatase staining following tartrate incubation.

T cell ALL – an immunologic subgroup of ALL. There are two types of T-ALL: early T precursor ALL and T-ALL. T-ALL are differentiated using only two CD markers, CD7 (gp40 protein) and CD2 (E-receptor), and TdT.

Teardrop (dacryocytes) – erythrocyte that is elongated at one end to form a teardrop or pear-shaped cell. Teardrop may form after erythrocytes with cellular inclusions have transversed the spleen. A teardrop cell cannot return to its original shape because it has either been stretched beyond the limits of deformability of the membrane or has been in the abnormal shape for too long a time.

Telangiectasia – persistent dilation of superficially located veins.

Thalassemia – a group of genetically determined microcytic, hypochromic anemias resulting from a decrease in synthesis of one or more globin chains in the hemoglobin molecule. The disorder may occur in the homozygous or heterozygous state. Heterozygotes may be asymptomatic but homozygotes typically have a severe, often fatal, disease. Thalassemia occurs most frequently in populations from the Mediterranean area and Southeast Asia.

Therapeutic range – level of a drug that is beneficial but not toxic to the individual.

Threshold limit – the level above which voltage pulses of particles will be counted. Adjusting the threshold limit allows different types of cells to be counted.

Thrombocyte – *see* platelet.

Thrombocytopenia – a decrease in the number of platelets in the peripheral blood below the reference range for an individual laboratory (usually below 150×10^9/L).

Thrombocytosis – an increase in the number of platelets in the peripheral blood above the reference range for an individual laboratory (usually over 440×10^9/L).

Thromboembolism – blockage of a small blood vessel by a blood clot that was formed in the heart, arteries, or veins, dislodged and moved through blood vessels until reaching a smaller vessel and blocking further blood flow.

Thrombogenic – tendency to thrombose.

Thrombolytic therapy – therapy designed to dissolve or break down a thrombus.

Thrombomodulin – an intrinsic membrane glycoprotein present on endothelial cells that serves as a cofactor with thrombin to activate protein C. It forms a 1:1 complex with thrombin inhibiting thrombin's ability to cleave fibrinogen to fibrin but enhances thrombin's ability to activate protein C.

Thrombophilia – a tendency to form blood clots abnormally. Also referred to as hypercoagulability.

Thrombophlebitis – thrombosis within a vein that is accompanied by an inflammatory response, pain and redness of the area.

Thrombopoietin – a humoral factor that regulates the maturation of megakaryocytes and the production of platelets.

Thrombosis – formation of a blood clot or thrombus, usually considered to be under abnormal conditions within a blood vessel.

Thrombotic thrombocytopenia purpura (TTP) – acute disorder of unknown etiology that affects young adults. Characterized by microangiopathic anemia, decreased number of platelets, and renal failure as well as neurological symptoms.

Thrombus – a blood clot within the vascular system.

TIBC – total iron binding capacity; this refers to the total amount of iron that transferrin can carry, about 253–435 μg/dL.

Tingible body macrophage – macrophages phagocytosing fragments of dying cells. They are found in areas of extensive apoptosis (reactive germinal centers and high-grade lymphoma).

Tissue factor – a coagulation factor present on subvascular cells that forms a complex with factor VII when the vessel is ruptured. This complex activates factor X. Tissue factor is an integral protein of the cell membrane.

Tissue homeostasis – maintenance of an adequate number of cells to carry out the functions of the organism. Homeostasis is controlled by cell proliferation, cell differentiation, and cell death (apotosis).

Tissue plasminogen activator (t-PA) – a serine protease that activates plasminogen to plasmin. It forms a bimolecular complex with fibrin increasing the catalytic efficiency of t-PA for plasminogen activation.

Toxic granules – large, dark blue-black primary granules in the cytoplasm of neutrophils that are present in certain infectious states. Usually seen in conjunction with Döhle bodies.

Toxoplasmosis – a condition that results from infection with *Toxoplasma gondii*. Acquired infection may be asymptomatic, or symptoms may resemble infectious mononucleosis. There is a leukocytosis with relative lymphocytosis or rarely an absolute lymphocytosis and the presence of reactive lymphocytes.

Trabecula – projection of calcified bone extending from cortical bone into the marrow space; provides support for marrow cells.

Transcription – synthesis of RNA from a DNA template.

Transferrin – a plasma β_1-globulin responsible for the binding of iron and its transport in the bloodstream. Each gram of transferrin can bind 1.25 mg of iron. The capacity of transferrin to bind iron is functionally measured as the total iron binding capacity (TIBC).

Transglutaminase – factor XIIIa is the only coagulation protein with transglutaminase activity. It catalyzes the formation of isopeptide bonds between glutamine and lysine residues on fibrin, forming stable covalent cross-links.

Transient erythroblastemia of childhood (TEC) – a temporary suppression of erythropoiesis that frequently occurs after a viral infection in infants and children. Therapy is supportive, and patients usually recover within two months.

Translation – synthesis of protein from an RNA template.

Translocation – an abnormal chromosomal rearrangement whereby part of one chromosome breaks off and becomes attached to another chromosome. The site of juxtaposition between the two chromosomes is referred to as the breakpoint.

Transplancental idiopathic thrombocytopenic purpura – a form of ITP that is present in newborns because of maternal transfer of platelet-destroying antibodies.

Transudate – effusion that is formed due to increased hydrostatic pressure or decreased osmotic pressure; does not indicate a true pathologic state in the anatomic region.

Trisomy – one daughter cell with an extra chromosome (three copies instead of two).

T-structure (tense) – the conformational change in a hemoglobin molecule that occurs when oxygen is released from hemoglobin.

Turnaround time – time between specimen collection and reporting of a test result.

2,3-diphosphoglycerate (2,3-DPG) – a product of the glycolytic pathway that affects the oxygen affinity of hemoglobin. It serves in the biochemical feedback system that regulates the amount of oxygen released to the tissues. As the concentration of 2,3-DPG increases, hemoglobin's affinity for oxygen decreases and more oxygen is released to the tissue. Also referred to as 2,3-biphosphoglycerate (2,3-BPG).

Type 1 VWD (classic VWD) – quantitative decrease of structurally normal vWf.

Type 2 VWD – qualitative disorder of vWf, four subtypes are possible: 2A, 2B, 2M, 2N.

Type 3 VWD – severe, rare quantitative deficiency of vWf.

Type I myeloblasts – the classic description of myeloblasts. These cells contain no granules and have a highly immature nucleus.

Type II myeloblasts – more mature than the type I myeloblasts, these cells can contain Auer rods, phi bodies, and/or primary granules.

Tyrosine kinase protein – protein that regulates metabolic pathways and serves as receptor for growth factors.

▶ U

UIBC (unsaturated iron binding capacity)– the portion of transferrin that is not complexed with iron. (TIBC − serum iron = UIBC).

Universal precautions – preventative guidelines to minimize the potential exposure of health care workers to blood-borne pathogens. These guidelines include the use of gloves whenever handling any body fluid.

Urokinase – an enzyme found in urine that activates plasminogen to plasmin and is used as a thrombolytic agent in the treatment of thrombosis.

▶ V

Variable number tandem repeats – DNA sequences that are tandemly repeated in a genome and that can vary among different individuals.

Vascular permeability – the property of endothelial cells of blood vessels that selectively allows for exchange of gases, nutrients, and waste products.

Vasculitis – inflammation of a blood vessel.

Vasoconstriction – narrowing of the lumen of blood vessels that occurs immediately following an injury.

Vaso-occlusive crisis – an acute event caused by spontaneous blockage of microvasculature by rigid sickle cells. The crisis may be triggered by infection, dehydration, decreased oxygen pressure, or slow blood flow. Often the crisis occurs without a known cause.

Vertical interactions – up-and-down interactions involving the skeletal lattice and proteins of the erythrocyte membrane. These interactions stabilize the lipid bilayer membrane.

Viral load – measuring the number of copies of HIV-1 RNA indicates a patient's viral load.

Viscosity – resistance to flow; physical property is dependent on the friction of component molecules in a substance as they pass one another.

Vitamin K-dependent factors – *see* prothrombin group.

Vitronectin – serum or extracellular-matrix glycoprotein capable of binding heparin.

von Willebrand disease – an autosomal dominant hereditary bleeding disorder in which there is a lack of von Willebrand factor (vWf). This factor is needed for platelets to adhere to collagen. Platelet aggregation is abnormal with ristocetin. The bleeding time is also abnormal. The APTT may be prolonged due to a decrease in the factor VIII molecule secondary to a decrease in vWf.

von Willebrand factor (vWf) – a plasma factor needed for platelets to adhere to collagen. It binds to the platelet glycoprotein Ib. It is synthesized in megakaryocytes and endothelial cells. The vWf is a molecule of multimers. It is noncovalently linked to factor VIII in plasma.

von Willebrand factor (vWf):Ag assay – a test that determines the amount of vWf.

von Willebrand factor (vWf) multimer – a vWf molecule consisting of identical subunits.

▶ W

Warm autoimmune hemolytic anemia – anemia resulting from the presence of IgG autoantibodies that are reactive at 37°C with antigens on subject's erythrocytes. The antibody/antigen complex on the cell membrane sensitizes the erythrocyte, which is removed in the spleen or liver.

Wedge smear – blood smear prepared on a glass microscope slide by placing a drop of blood at one end and with a second slide pulling the blood the length of the slide.

White thrombus – thrombus composed mostly of platelets and fibrin that appears light gray.

▶ Y

y-intercept – the point where the regression line intersects the y-axis. The y-intercept is used to identify the presence of constant systematic error.

▶ Z

Zymogen – an inactive precursor that can be converted to the active form by an enzyme, alkali, or acid. The inert coagulation factors are zymogens. Also called a proenzyme.

INDEX

TABLE D

Differential Counts of Bone Marrow Aspirates from 12 Healthy Men

	Mean (%)	Observed Range (%)	95% Confidence Limits (%)
Neutrophilic series (total)	53.6	49.2–65.0	33.6–73.6
Myeloblasts	0.9	0.2–1.5	0.1–1.7
Promyelocytes	3.3	2.1–4.1	1.9–4.7
Myelocytes	12.7	8.2–15.7	8.5–16.9
Metamyelocytes	15.9	9.6–24.6	7.1–24.7
Band	12.4	9.5–15.3	9.4–15.4
Segmented	7.4	6.0–12.0	3.8–11.0
Eosinophilic series (total)	3.1	1.2–5.3	1.1–5.2
Myelocytes	0.8	0.2–1.3	0.2–1.4
Metamyelocytes	1.2	0.4–2.2	0.2–2.2
Band	0.9	0.2–2.4	0–2.7
Segmented	0.5	0–1.3	0–1.1
Basophilic and mast cells	0.1	0–0.2	—
Erythrocytic series (total)	25.6	18.4–33.8	15.0–36.2
Pronormoblasts	0.6	0.2–1.3	0.1–1.1
Basophilic	1.4	0.5–2.4	0.4–2.4
Polychromatophilic	21.6	17.9–29.2	13.1–30.1
Orthochromatic	2.0	0.4–4.6	0.3–3.7
Lymphocytes	16.2	11.1–23.2	8.6–23.8
Plasma cells	1.3	0.4–3.9	0–3.5
Monocytes	0.3	0–0.8	0–0.6
Megakaryocytes	0.1	0–0.4	—
Reticulum cells	0.3	0–0.9	0–0.8
M:E ratio	2.3	1.5–3.3	1.1–3.5

Reprinted, with permission, from Lee GR, Bithell TC, Foerster J, Athens JW, Lukens JN. *Wintrobe's Clinical Hematology*, 10th ed. Philadelphia: Lippincott, Williams & Wilkins; 1999.

TABLE F

Reference Values for Tests to Monitor Erythrocyte Destruction

Analyte	Age	Conventional Unit
Bilirubin	<1day	1–6 mg/dL
	1–2 days	6–7.5 mg/dL
	2–<5 days	4–8 mg/dL
	>5 days to adult	0.2–1.0 mg/dL (total; high critical limit 15 mg/dL with SD 5)
		0–0.2 mg/dL (conjugated)
Haptoglobin	—	19–204 mg/dL

TABLE E

Reference Values for Common Coagulation Test Reference Values (compiled from multiple sources)

Analyte	Reference Value
Activated partial thromboplastin time (APTT)	36–40 seconds (birth to 1 week)
	23–35 seconds (1 week to adult)
Prothrombin time	11–14 seconds
	1.0–1.6 INR (birth to 6 months)
	0.8–1.2 INR (6 months to adult)
	2.0–3.0 INR range for anticoagulant therapy for venous thrombosis
	2.5–3.5 INR range for anticoagulant therapy for mechanical heart valve
Bleeding Time	2.5–9.5 minutes
Thrombin time	10–22 seconds
Fibrinogen	190–465 mg/dL
Reptilase time	18–22 seconds
Protein S functional	55–174%
Protein S free	70–160%
Protein S total	70–160%
Protein C functional	70–140%
Protein C antigen	65–150%
Factor IX	50–200%
Factor V	60–130%
Factor VII	40–200%
Factor VIII	55–180%
Factor X	45–170%
Factor II	70–130%
Factor II, V, VII, VIII, IX, X, XI inhibitors	<0.5 BU/mL
D-dimer	25–95 ng/mL
Fibrin degradation products (FDP)	<5 µg/mL
Dilute Russell's viper venom time (DRVVT)	<40 seconds
Lupus anticoagulant	negative
Antithrombin (AT)	80–125%
AT antigen	22–40 mg/dL
Activated protein C resistance (APCR)	>2.1
Plasminogen	75–142%
Plasminogen activator inhibitor-1 (PAI-1)	78–142% activity; 4–43 µg/mL antigen
von Willebrand factor activity	42–139%
von Willebrand factor antigen	60–150%